Mental Health and Collaborative Community Practice

An Australian Perspective

Fourth Edition

Edited by

Graham Meadows
John Farhall
Ellie Fossey
Brenda Happell
Fiona McDermott
Sebastian Rosenberg

with

Vrinda Edan
Merinda Epstein
Hamilton Kennedy
Cath Roper

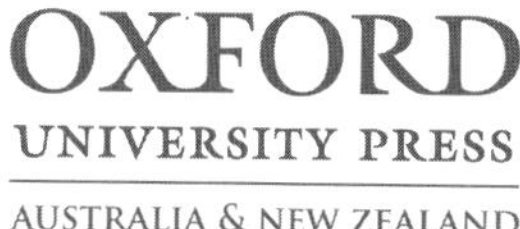

OXFORD
UNIVERSITY PRESS

Oxford University Press is a department of the University of Oxford. It furthers the University's objective of excellence in research, scholarship, and education by publishing worldwide. Oxford is a registered trademark of Oxford University Press in the UK and in certain other countries.

Published in Australia by
Oxford University Press
Level 8, 737 Bourke Street, Docklands, Victoria 3008, Australia

First published 2001
Second edition 2007
Third edition 2012
Fourth Edition
Reprinted 2022

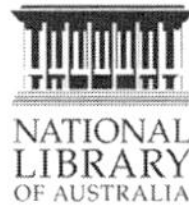

A catalogue record for this book is available from the National Library of Australia

ISBN 9780190309916

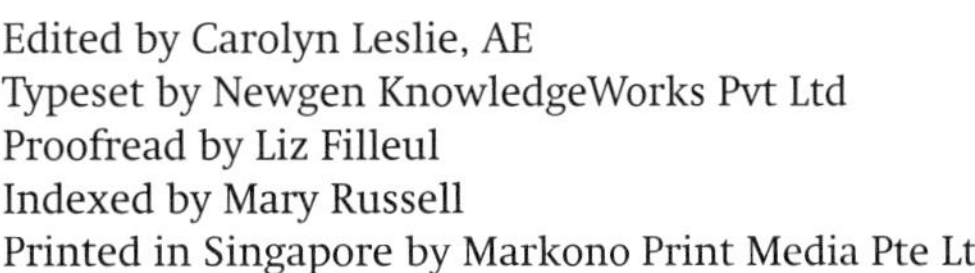
Edited by Carolyn Leslie, AE
Typeset by Newgen KnowledgeWorks Pvt Ltd
Proofread by Liz Filleul
Indexed by Mary Russell
Printed in Singapore by Markono Print Media Pte Ltd

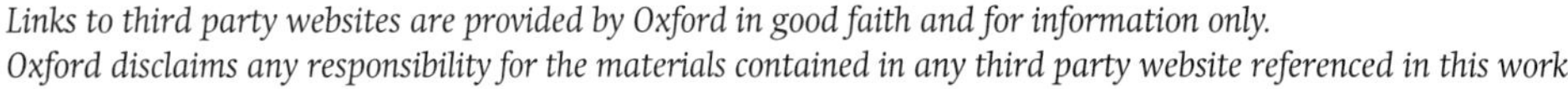

CONTENTS

ACRONYMS

5HT-TLPR	Serotonin (5HT) transporter linked promoter polymorphism
AASP	Adult/Adolescent Sensory Profile
ABF	Activity Based Funding
ABS	Australian Bureau of Statistics
ACAS	aged care assessment service
ACBS	Association for Contextual Behavioural Science
ACCHS	Aboriginal Community Controlled Health Services
ACE-R	Addenbrooke's Cognitive Examination-Revised
ACLS	Allen's Cognitive Levels Screen
ACMHN	Australian College of Mental Health Nurses
ACT	Australian Capital Territory
ACT	Acute Care Teams
ACT	Acceptance and Commitment Therapy
ACT	assertive community treatment
ADD	Attention-deficit disorder
ADHD	attention deficit hyperactivity disorder
ADL	activities of daily living
ADM	Antidepressant Medication
AHMAC	Australian Health Ministers' Advisory Council
AHPRA	Australian Health Practitioner Regulation Agency
AICA-S	Assessment of Internet and Computer game Addiction Scale
AIDA	Australian Indigenous Doctors Association
AIFS	Australian Institute of Family Studies
AIHW	Australian Institute for Health and Welfare
AIPA	Australian Indigenous Psychologists Association
ALP	Australian Labour Party
AMHOCN	Australian Mental Health Outcomes and Classification Network
AMHRU	Adult Mental Health Rehabilitation Unit
AMHS	Aged Persons Mental Health Services
AMHU	Adult Mental Health Unit
AMPD	Alternative Model of Personality Disorders
AMPS	Assessment of Motor and Process Skills
AMSANT	Aboriginal Medical Services Alliance Northern
AMYOS	Acute Mobile Youth Outreach Service
AN	Anorexia Nervosa
AOD	Alcohol and Other Drugs
APA	American Psychiatric Association
APS	Australian Psychological Society
ARAFMI	Association of Relatives and Friends of the Mentally Ill
ARFID	Avoidant/Restrictive Food Intake Disorder
ASD	Autism Spectrum Disorder
ASGS	Australian Statistical Geography Standard

ASPD	Antisocial personality disorder
ATAPS	Access to Allied Psychological Services
ATISISPEP	Aboriginal and Torres Strait Islander Suicide Prevention Project
AUDIT	Alcohol Use Disorders Identification Test
BA	Behavioural activation
BASIS 32	Behaviour and Symptom Identification Scale
BCA	Brief Cognitive assessment
B-CATS	Brief Cognitive Assessment Tool for Schizophrenia
BDD	Body Dysmorphic Disorder
BDD	Bodily Distress Disorder
BDHP	Brisbane Diamantina Health Partners
BED	binge eating disorder
BEST	Borderline Evaluation of Severity over Time
BID	Body Integrity Dysphoria
BMI	Body Mass Index
BNLA	Building a New Life in Australia
BPD	Borderline Personality Disorder
BPDD	Behavioural or psychological disturbances in dementia
BPQ	Borderline Personality Questionnaire
BPSD	behavioural and psychological symptoms of dementia
BPSL	Biopsychosocial and Lifestyle Model
BRIDGES	Building Recovery of Individual Dreams & Goals through Education & Support
CALD	Culturally and Linguistically Diverse
CAM	Confusion Assessment Method
CAM	Complementary and Alternative Medicines
CAMHS	Child and Adolescent Mental Health Service
CAMHS	Central Australia Mental Health Services
CAN	Consumer Activity Network
CANSAS	Camberwell Assessment of Need Short Appraisal Schedule
CAPS-5	Clinician-Administered PTSD Scale for DSM-5
CASP	Critical Appraisal Skills Program
CAT	Cognitive Analytic Therapy
CATIE	Clinical Antipsychotic Trials of Intervention Effectiveness
CATSINaM	Congress of Aboriginal and Torres Strait Islander Nurses and Midwives
CATT	Crisis and Assessment Treatment Team
CBCL	Child Behaviour Checklist
CBPATSISP	Centre of Best Practice in Aboriginal and Torres Strait Islander Suicide Prevention
CBS	Charles Bonnet syndrome
CBT	Cognitive Behaviour Therapy
CBT-AN	Cognitive-behaviour therapy specific for anorexia nervosa
CBT-BN	CBT for bulimia nervosa
CBT-E	CBT-Enhanced
CCAA	Christian Counsellors Association of Australia
CD	conduct disorder
CDM	clinical decision-making
CE	Chief Executive

CES-D	Center for Epidemiologic Studies Depression Scale
CET	Cognitive Enhancement Therapy
CFOS	Community Forensic Outreach Service
CFS	Chronic fatigue syndrome
CFT	compassion focused therapy
CGAS	Children's Global Assessment Scale
CGI-S	Clinical Global Impression - Severity scale
CHCCAG	Cairns and Hinterland Consumer and Carer Advisory Group
CHIME	Connectedness, Hope, Identity, Meaning and purpose & Empowerment
CI	Concentration Index
CIDI	Composite International Diagnostic Interview
CIMHA	Consumer Integrated Mental Health Application
CISD	Critical Incident Stress Debriefing
CL	Consultation Liaison
CLIPP	Consultation and Liaison in Primary-Care Psychiatry
CLS	community living supports
CMA	chromosomal microarray
CMHSS	community mental health support service
CMO	community managed organisation
CMT	compassionate mind training
CMV	cytomegalovirus
CNS	Central nervous system
COAG	Council of Australian Governments
COMT	Catechol-O-methyltransferase
CONSORT	Consolidated Standards of Reporting Trials
COO	Chief Operating Officer
COPD	Chronic Obstructive Pulmonary Disease
COPM	Canadian Occupational Performance Measure
COPMI/KOPING	children whose parents have a severe mental illness
COVID	Coronavirus disease
CPD	Continuing Professional Development
CPIP	Clinical Practice Improvement Program
CPR	Cardio pulmonary resuscitation
CPT	Cognitive processing therapy
CRM	Collaborative Recovery Model
CRPD	Convention on the Rights of Persons with Disabilities
CRPS	Complex Regional Pain Syndrome
CRT	Cognitive remediation therapy
CT	Computerised tomography
CT	computed tomography
CTO	Community Treatment Order
CYMHS	Child and Youth Mental Health Services
D/FV	Domestic and Family Violence
DALYs	Disability-Adjusted Life-Years
DBT	Dialectical Behaviour Therapy

DD	depression disorders
DES	Disability Employment Services
DID	Dissociative identity disorder
DIP-DM	Diagnostic Interview for Psychosis
DOCS	Dimensional Obsessive-Compulsive Scale
DoH	Department of Health
DSM	Diagnostic and Statistical Manual
DSS	Department of Social Security
DTI	Diffusion tensor imaging
DTT	difficult to treat
DUP	Duration of Untreated Psychosis
DVA	Department of Veterans Affairs
DVA	Department of Veterans Affairs
EBCD	Experience-Based Co-Design
EBP	evidence-based practice
ECATT	Emergency Crisis and Assessment Treatment Team
ECT	Electroconvulsive Therapy
ED	Eating Disorder
EE	Expressed Emotion
EEA	Emergency Examination Authorities
EEG	Electro-Encephalogram
EEG	Electroencephalography
EEO	Emergency Examination Order
EMDR	eye movement desensitisation and reprocessing
EPPIC	Early Psychosis Prevention and Intervention Centre
EPS	extrapyramidal side-effects
FAB	Frontal Assessment Battery
FACT	Function ACT
FAS	foetal alcohol syndrome
FDG-PET	Fluorodeoxyglucose (FDG)-positron emission tomography
FEDU	Feeding or eating disorders, unspecified
FEP	First Episode Psychosis
FFT	Family-focused therapy
FIHS	Factors Influencing Health Status
fMRI	functional magnetic resonance imaging
FSS	functional somatic syndromes
FT	Family Therapy
FTAC	Fixated Threat and Assessment Centre
FTE	full-time equivalent
GA	Generalised Anxiety
GABA	gamma amino butyric acid
GAD	generalised anxiety disorder
GAF	Global Assessment of Functioning
GDP	Gross Domestic Product
GDS	Geriatric Depression Scale

GP	General Practitioner
GPM	General psychiatric management
G-SAS	Gambling Symptom Assessment Scale
GWAS	Genome Wide Association Studies
HASI	Housing and Accommodation Support Initiative
HASP	Housing and Support Program
HCC	Health Complaints Commissioner
HCR	Historical, Clinical and Risk-management
HD	Hoarding disorder
HELP	Hospital Elder Life Program
HHOT	Homeless Health Outreach Teams
HHS	Hospital and Health Services
HIRF	Herston Imaging Research Facility
HIV	Human immunodeficiency virus
HoNOS	Health of the Nation Outcome Scales
HoNOS 65+	Health of the Nation Outcome Scales 65+
HoNOSCA	Health of the Nation Outcome Scales for Children and Adolescents
HOPE	Hospital Outreach Post-suicide Engagement
HPA	hypothalamic-pituitary-adrenal
HYPE	Helping Young People Early
IAHA	Indigenous Allied Health Association
IAHP	Indigenous Australian's Health Programme
IBS	irritable bowel syndrome
ICD	International Classification of Diseases
ICLS	Individualised Community Living Strategy
ICM	intensive case management
ICMJE	International Committee of Medical Journal Editors
ICOT	intensive community (rehabilitation) outreach teams
ID	Intellectual disability
IGD	Internet Gaming Disorder
IGDT-10	Internet Gaming Disorder Test-10
IHPA	Independent Hospital Pricing Authority
IMR	Illness Management and Recovery
INT	Integrated Neurocognitive Therapy
IPC	Interpersonal Counselling
IPD	individual patient data
IPDE	International Personality Disorder Examination
IPS	Intentional Peer Support
IPS	Individual Placement and Support
IPSRT	Interpersonal and Social Rhythm Therapy
IPT	Integrated Psychological Therapy
IQ	intelligence quotient
IRSD	Index of Relative Socio-Economic Disadvantage
ITP	Interpersonal Psychotherapy
K-10	Kessler-10

KPIs Key performance indicators
LAI Long Acting Injectable
LBD Lewy body disease
LEC-5 Life Events Checklist for DSM-5
LGBTIQ Lesbian Gay Bisexual Transgender, Intersex & Queer
LGBTIQ+SB Lesbian Bisexual Transgender, Intersex & Queer (denoting sister girl and brother boy)
LHD Local Health District
LHDs Local Health Districts
LHNs Local Health Networks
LSD lysergic acid diethylamide
LSP Life Skills Profile
MANTRA Maudsley Anorexia Nervosa Treatment for Adults
MAO-A Monoamine Oxidase A
MAOI MonoAmine Uptake Inhibitor
MBCT mindfulness based cognitive therapy
MB-EAT mindfulness-based eating awareness treatment
MBS Medicare Benefits Schedule
MBSR mindfulness based stress reduction
MBT Mentalization-based therapy
MCD Mild Neurocognitive
MCI Mild Cognitive Impairment
MCT meta-cognitive therapy
MCV mean corpuscular volume
MD Major Depression
MDD Major Depressive Disorder
MH ECO Mental Health Experience Co-Design
MHA Mental Health Australia
MHAODB Mental Health Alcohol and Other Drugs Branch
MHC Mental Health Commission
MHCSS mental health community support services
MHI Mental Health Inventory
MHIT Mental Health Intervention Team
MHPC Mental Health Principal Committee
MHRT Mental Health Review Tribunal
MHS Mental Health Services
MHSSU Mental Health Short Say Unit
MHTP Mental Health Treatment Plan
MiCBT mindfulness-integrated cognitive behaviour therapy
MIET Mindfulness-based Interoceptive Exposure Task
MIR Magnetic resonance imaging
MIRF Mental Illness Research Fund
MIRT Mobile Intensive Rehabilitation Teams
MMPI Minnesota Multiphasic Personality Inventory
MMSE Mini Mental State Examination
MOCA Montréal Cognitive Assessment

MOHO	Model of Human Occupation
MOICD	Medical Outreach Indigenous Chronic Disease
MRI	Magnetic Resonance Imaging
MSAC	Medical Services Advisory Committee
MSAD	McLean Study of Adult Development
MSC	mindful self-compassion
MSE	Mental State Examination
MSE	mental status examination
MT	Marital Therapy
NACCHO	National Aboriginal Community Controlled Health Organisation
NAMI	National Alliance of Mental Illness
NAP	National Action Plan
NATSIHWA	National Aboriginal and Torres Strait Islander Health Workers Association
NATSILMH	National Aboriginal & Torres Strait Islander Leadership in Mental Health
NDIA	National Disability Insurance Agency
NDIS	National Disability Insurance Scheme
NDSHS	National Drug Strategy Household Survey
NGO	non-government organisation
NHMRC	National Health and Medical Research Council
NHS	National Health Service
NHS	National Health Survey
NIH	National Institutes of Health
NMBA	Nursing and Midwifery Board of Australia
NMDA	N-methyl-D-aspartate
NMDA-R	N-methyl-D-aspartate Receptor
NMH	National Mental Health
NMHC	National Mental Health Commission
NNH	Number Needed to Harm
NNT	Number Needed to Treat
NOCC	National Outcomes and Casemix Collection
NODS	NORC DSM-IV Screen for Gambling Problems
NPD	Narcissistic Personality Disorder
NPV	Negative predictive value
NRT	nicotine replacement treatments
NSMHW	National Surveys of Mental Health and Wellbeing
NSMHWB	National Survey of Mental Health and Well-being
NUCOG	Neuropsychiatry Unit Cognitive Assessment Tool
OCCWG	Obsessive-Compulsive Cognitions Working Group
OCD	obsessive-compulsive disorder
OCPD	Obsessive-compulsive personality disorder
ODD	oppositional defiant disorder
OECD	Organisation for Economic Co-operation and Development
OED	Oxford English Dictionary
OPCRIT	Operational Criteria Checklist for Psychotic Illness and Affective Illness
OPHI-II	Occupational Performance History Interview II

OQ	Outcome Questionnaire
OS/UFED	Other Specified/Unspecified Eating Disorder
OSA	Occupational Self Assessment
OSA	Obstructive sleep apnoea
OSFED	Other specified feeding or eating disorders
OTC	Over the counter
OTI	Opiate Treatment Index
OYH	Orygen Youth Health
PACE	Personal Assessment and Crisis Evaluation
PACER	Police Ambulance Crisis Emergency Response
PAI	Personality Assessment Inventory
PANSS	Positive and Negative Syndrome Scale
PARCS	Prevention and Recovery Centres
PASS	Performance Assessment of Self-Care Skills
PBA	Psychology Board of Australia
PBS	Pharmaceutical Benefits Scheme
PCL-5	PTSD Checklist for DSM-5
PCLI	Pathways to Community Living Initiative
PCOS	Polycystic Ovarian Syndrome
P-CRT	parallel cluster randomised trial
PD	Personality Disorders
PDCA	plan-do-check-act
PDD NOS	pervasive developmental disorder not otherwise specified
PD-NOS	personality disorder not otherwise specified
PECC	Psychiatric Emergency Care Centres
PEDro	Physiotherapy Evidence Database
PET	positron emission tomography
PGSI	Problem Gambling Severity Index
PG-YBOCS	Pathological Gambling – Yale Brown Obsessive Compulsive Scale
PHaMS	Personal Helpers and Mentors Program
PHN	Primary Health Network
PHNC	Physical Health Nurse Consultant
PHNs	Primary Health Networks
PHQ-9	Patient Health Questionnaire
PICO	P – population or patient or consumer; I – intervention; C – control or comparison intervention; O – outcome(s).
PIR	Partners in Recovery
PNCQ	Perceived Need for Care Questionnaire
PoC	Phase of Care
POES	Profiles of Occupational Engagement
PP	psychodynamic psychotherapy
PPV	Positive Predictive Value
pROMs	Patient-reported outcome measures
PRPP	Perceive Recall Plan Perform
PST	Planning Support Tool

PST	Problem Solving Therapy
PTSD	Post Traumatic Stress Disorder
PULSAR	Principles Unite Local Services Assisting Recovery
QA	Quality Assurance
QALYs	Quality-Adjusted Life-Years
QFTAC	Queensland Fixed Threat Assessment Centre
QI	Quality Improvement
QMHC	Queensland Mental Health Commission
RANZCP	The Royal Australian & New Zealand College of Psychiatrists
RCA	Root Cause Analysis
RCT	randomised controlled trial
RDF	Resource Distribution Formula
REM	Rapid Eye Movement
RFT	Relational frame theory
ROGS	Report on Government Services
ROM	routine outcome measurement
RTW	Return-to-work
RUDAS	Rowland Universal Dementia Assessment Scale
RUG-ADL	Resource Utilisation Groups-Activities of Daily Living Scale
SAD	Seasonal Affective Disorders
SADQ-C	Severity of Alcohol Dependence Questionnaire Form C
SARS-COV-2	Severe acute respiratory syndrome coronavirus 2
SCARP	Substantial Comparability Assessment Review Panel
SCHN	Sydney Children's Hospitals' Network
SCID	Structured Clinical Interview for DSM-5
SCID-II	Structured Clinical Interview for DSM-IV Axis II Disorders
SCOFF	Sick, control, one-stone, fat, food (selected words from the question set)
SDA	Sex Discrimination Amendment
SDQ	Strengths and Difficulties Questionnaire
SEIFA	Socio-Economic Indices for Areas
SEWB	Social & Emotional Well Being
SFT	Schema Focussed Therapy
SGA	Second generation antipsychotics
SHIP	Study of High Impact Psychosis
SHIP	Survey of High Impact Psychosis
SI-R	Savings Inventory-Revised
SMART	Self-Management And Recovery Technology
SMHRU	Secure Mental Health Rehabilitation Units
SNRI	serotonin and noradrenaline reuptake inhibitor
SODQ	Severity of Opiate Dependence Questionnaire
SOFAS	Social and Occupational Functioning Assessment Scale
SOGS	South Oaks Gambling Screen
SPECT	Single Photon Emission Tomography
SPT	Supportive Psychotherapy
SRT	Social rank theory

SSAMHS	State-wide Specialist Aboriginal Mental Health Service
SSCM	specialist supportive clinical management
SSFC	Single Session Family Consultation
SSRIs	Serotonin Specific Reuprake Inhibitors
SSU	short stay units
STPP	Short-term Psychodynamic Psychotherapy
SW-CRT	stepped wedge cluster randomised trial
TAFE	Technical And Further Education
TAU	treatment as usual
TCAs	tricyclic antidepressants
TEMHS	Top End Mental Health Services
TF CBT	trauma focussed cognitive behavioural therapy
TFP	Transference-focused psychotherapy
TGA	Therapeutic Goods Administration
TICP	Trauma-informed Care and Practice
TMS	Transcranial Magnetic Stimulation
TPS	Triple P-Positive parenting program
UNCRPD	United Nations Convention on the Rights of Persons with Disabilities
UNHCR	United Nations High Commissioner for Refugees
UPSA	University of California San Diego Performance-based Skills Assessment
VMIAC	Victorian Mental Illness Awareness Council
VNS	Vagus Nerve Stimulation
WAIS	Wechsler Adult Intelligence Scale
wDST	Web Decision Support Tool
WEIS	Work Environment Impact Scale
WHO	World Health Organization
WMRLC	Western Massachusetts Recovery Learning Community
WRAP	Wellness Recovery Action Plan
WRI	Worker Role Interview
YBOCS	Yale-Brown Obsessive-compulsive Scale
YES	Your Experience of Service
ZAN-BPD	Questionnaire and clinician-scored ZAN-BPD

ABOUT THE AUTHORS

EDITORIAL GROUP

Graham Meadows (lead editor) is a Professor in the School of Clinical Sciences at Monash Health and in the School of Primary and Allied Health Care at Monash University, a Consultant Psychiatrist with Monash Health and an Honorary Professorial Fellow with The University of Melbourne School of Global and Population Health. He is the Director of Southern Synergy, the Monash Health Adult Psychiatry Research, Training and Evaluation Centre, a Research Centre in the Faculty of Medicine, Nursing and Health Sciences at Monash University. He has been an investigator on over 30 research grants for over 8 million $AUD and authored well over 150 journal papers or book chapters. A prominent figure in innovation in mental health care in Australia, he has national and international research profiles in areas of epidemiology, mental health of disadvantaged and marginalised groups, equity in resource distribution and mindfulness in mental health practice.

John Farhall is jointly appointed as Associate Professor in the Department of Psychology and Counselling at La Trobe University and as Consultant Clinical Psychologist at NorthWestern Mental Health in Melbourne - a role designed to enhance research, clinical practice and post-graduate training by bringing together expertise from public mental health services and academia. John has worked as a clinical psychologist in community mental health centres and psychiatric hospital settings, led a state-wide staff training unit for Psychiatric Services, served as a Director of Mind Australia and as a professional member of the Victorian Civil and Administrative Tribunal. His research has centred on understanding and responding to the needs of people with psychotic disorders, including evaluating and disseminating new community mental health service types, trialling evidence-based innovative psychotherapies and digital interventions promoting recovery-oriented practice. His teaching includes psychopathology, psychological therapies, and mental health services, and his practice has focussed on CBT and ACT for psychosis. John has over 130 research and professional publications.

Ellie Fossey is Professor and Head of the Department of Occupational Therapy in the School of Primary and Allied Health Care at Monash University, an Adjunct Professor in the Living with Disability Research Centre at La Trobe University, and a registered Occupational Therapist. Her academic and professional career spans undergraduate and postgraduate teaching, curriculum development and research in occupational therapy and in mental health at universities in England and Australia, and professional practice principally in community mental health settings. Ellie's previous research has predominantly focused on participation and disability, experiences of everyday living with mental health issues, and the impacts of ongoing health conditions on people's occupations, and primarily used qualitative and participatory research approaches. Recent projects focus on tertiary education experiences of students with mental health issues, disability supports in tertiary education, employment barriers and workplace supports for employees experiencing ongoing mental health issues, and recovery-oriented practice in mental health services; and typically involve research teams that draw on lived expertise and interdisciplinary perspectives.

Brenda Happell is Professor of Nursing and Executive Director, Synergy, Nursing and Midwifery Research Centre, University of Canberra and ACT Health. With 28 years' experience in teaching, curriculum development, supervision of higher degrees, assessment and educational research, Brenda has directed Research Centres at the University of Melbourne and at Central Queensland University. Brenda has approximately 400 publications in refereed journals and approximately 12 million $AUD in competitive research funding, including lead investigator on an NHMRC grant. She was Editor in Chief of the International Journal of Mental Health Nursing from 2004 to 2014, Brenda is currently the Associate Editor of Issues in Mental Health Nursing and a member of Editorial Boards of five international health and nursing journals. Brenda is a current Director of the Board of the Australian College of Mental Health Nurses. Her research interests include: Consumer/service user participation in mental health services, physical health of people experiencing mental illness and mental health nursing education and practice roles.

Fiona McDermott is adjunct Associate Professor in the Department of Social Work, Faculty of Medicine, Nursing & Health Sciences, Monash University. She is Editor of *Australian Social Work*. Fiona has published four books, many journal articles and book chapters. These publications reflect her interest in the ways in which knowledge is advanced in social work and health and mental health care and how such knowledge is used in practice. She has a particular interest in teaching and supervising higher degree research, undertaking research in health and mental health including in the areas of multiple and complex needs.

Dr Sebastian Rosenberg is the Head of the Mental Health Policy Unit at the Centre for Mental Health Research at the Australian National University and Senior Lecturer in Mental Health Policy at the Brain & Mind Centre, University of Sydney. Prior, he was Deputy CEO of the Mental Health Council of Australia from 2005–2009, assisting in publication of the seminal Not for Service report (2005) among others, and before this he worked as a public servant in both federal and state health departments. Sebastian has also worked as a consultant on many significant mental health projects, including in relation to the establishment of mental health commissions. Sebastian's research interests are in health policy, particularly in relation to mental health and accountability, working towards understanding the extent to which Australia's mental health system is helping people get better.

Vrinda Edan is an experienced consumer worker with 20 years' work in the consumer field. She has a background as a health professional, and her work is shaped by both her personal experiences and her work in strategic leadership positions in health services, on Ministerial committees and in large research projects bringing a consumer voice. Vrinda uses a Human Rights framework, supporting consumers to regain choice and control in their lives. This approach is sustained by her role as Chair of the Board of the Victorian Mental Illness Awareness council (VMIAC), member of the Speaking from experience group (Victorian Legal Aid), and member of Ministerial and departmental committees. Vrinda has completed a Graduate Certificate in Organisational Dynamics, Intentional Peer Support training, Level 2 of MBCT, and has recently graduated from Monash University with a M Nursing. Vrinda is currently undertaking a PhD at the University of Melbourne.

Merinda Epstein has for three decades been a leading thinker and writer in the consumer movement. Working in the 1990s on the Understanding & Involvement project pioneering fourth-generation evaluation methodology in mental health, other roles have included: Victorian Representative on the National Mental Health Consumer Network; Independent Consumer Member of the National Community Advisory Group on mental health, and member of the Australian Health Ministers Advisory Committee Evaluation Sub Committee for the First National Mental Health Strategy. The citation for her 2004 Australian Human Rights Award, praising her bravery, moral integrity and insight, identified Merinda as '... one of Australia's leading mental health consumer advocates and internationally recognised for her contribution to mental health service development'. Her pioneering work in the area of Complex Post Traumatic Stress, driven by deeply held ethical values and a keen intellectual interest, is her greatest challenge and most valued accomplishment.

Hamilton Kennedy is a 26 year old Melbourne resident who has been a consumer of mental health services for the past decade. They have grown critical of traditional mental health services and believes that consumer input is vital to correcting them. They are currently a peer worker as part of the Victorian Expanding Post Discharge Support initiative. Hamilton also works in consumer research and consultancy and has a strong interest in ensuring that research, policy and literature accurately caters to the needs of consumers. Hamilton has also completed their Bachelors of Social Work degree and is currently undertaking a Masters in Narrative Therapy and Community Practice. However, Hamilton firmly believes that their lived experience of mental illness is their number one qualification and what drives their passion and contribution.

Cath Roper held one of four pioneering staff-consumer consultant positions in mental health services in Victoria between 1995 and 1999 and later became the first consumer academic in Australia, at the Centre for Psychiatric Nursing, University of Melbourne. She has a teaching background and holds a Masters in Social Health from the University of Melbourne. Cath had annual involuntary admissions to mental health services over a thirteen-year period and these experiences continue to drive her research, teaching, training and policy work particularly around exposing the human rights breaches caused by mental health laws. Cath believes that madnesss and distress are meaningful experiences and she has a particular interest in all forms of consumer scholarship especially 'mad studies'.

EDITORIAL BOARD MEMBERS

Dr Fiona Best is a Consultant Psychiatrist, having been a Fellow of the Royal Australian and New Zealand College of Psychiatrists since 2009. Completing her medical degree at the University of Melbourne in 2000, a Masters of Psychiatry (Melbourne) in 2006, and a Masters of Mental Health Science – Forensic (Monash) in 2016, Dr. Best has also completed RANZCP advanced training in forensic psychiatry (2015) and RANZCP advanced training in the psychotherapies (2016). An accredited member of the RANZCP Forensic Faculty, she has been employed by Forensicare as a Consultant Forensic Psychiatrist since 2009 and worked previously as a registrar. She has been the RANZCP Director of Advanced Training, Forensic, (Vic) since 2015, sits on the RANZCP Victorian Psychiatry Training Committee and is the Deputy Chair of the RANZCP Sub Committee for Advanced Training Forensic Psychiatry. Dr. Best is also employed as a teaching associate with the Department of Psychiatry, Monash University and is the Chief Examiner for two units of a Masters of Psychiatry at Monash University. A sessional member of the Mental Health Tribunal since 2013, she is active in supervision and training of registrars; Dr. Best also has a BA(Hons), Fine Arts from the UK.

Pat Dudgeon is from Bardi people of the Kimberley. She is a psychologist and is known for her role in Indigenous higher education and as Head of the Centre for Aboriginal Studies at Curtin University, having worked there from 1990 and led the organization through significant growth and change. Amongst many projects, grants and awards achieved during her time as Head, of significance was the Curtin Indigenous Research Centre (CIRC), established in 1997. Her doctorate was entitled Mothers of Sin: Indigenous Women's Perceptions of their Identity and Sexuality. As well as leadership in Indigenous higher education, Pat Dudgeon has also had significant involvement in psychology and Indigenous issues for many years. She was the first convener of the Australian Psychological Society Interest Group: Aboriginal Issues, Aboriginal People and Psychology and has been instrumental in convening many conferences and discussion groups at national levels to ensure that Indigenous issues are part of the agenda in the discipline. She has many publications in this area and is considered one of the 'founding' people in Indigenous people and psychology. Currently she is the Chair of the Indigenous Australian Psychologists Association and in 2008, was the first Aboriginal psychologist to be awarded the grade of Fellow in the Australian Psychological Society. Pat is actively involved with the Aboriginal community and has a commitment to social justice for Indigenous people. Currently, she is a research fellow and an associate professor at the University of Western Australia.

Jonathan Harms has worked as a plaintiff lawyer, a public servant, policy advisor and stakeholder manager for a variety of State and Federal Ministers, government departments, private corporations, and non-government organisations. In the course of this career he has gained significant experience in the development of policy including regulatory schemes. From 2012 forwards, as CEO of Mental Health Carers New South Wales ('MHCN'), the peak body for carers of people with lived experience of mental illness in NSW, Jonathan has worked to enhance stakeholder participation in MHCN policy development; and, to enhance external networks for carer support workers and mental health carers across NSW for consultation and advocacy purposes.

Dr Caroline Johnson is a general practitioner in Melbourne with a special interest in primary mental health care. Alongside her long-standing clinical practice, she has extensive experience from undergraduate through to postgraduate training of doctors in mental health skills and is currently a Senior Medical Educator at EV GP Training and a Senior Lecturer in the Department of General Practice, University of Melbourne. She has published on recovery from depression, mental health treatment plans and the important role of general practice in providing care for common mental disorders. Her PhD was an exploration of the way people experiencing depression are monitored in the primary care setting. She has held numerous mental health advocacy positions including as Clinical lead in mental health on the RACGP Expert Committee in Quality Care and a board member of Mental Health Australia.

Harry Minas is the Head of the Global and Cultural Mental Health Unit in the Centre for Mental Health at the School of Population and Global Health in the University of Melbourne. Harry is a psychiatrist whose work is in three broad areas: mental health system development, particularly in low-resource and post-conflict settings; culture and mental health, with a focus on mental health of immigrant and refugee communities and the development of services for culturally diverse societies; and the human rights of people with mental illness. He is a distinguished fellow of the Pacific Rim College of Psychiatrists and is the Founder and Editor-in-Chief of the International Journal of Mental Health Systems.

Sally Morris holds extensive knowledge and expertise in mental health and suicide prevention within the context of LGBTIQ people and communities. Sally has worked in mental health and suicide prevention over the last 20 years and her work has had a primary focus on improving the mental health of LGBTIQ people and communities by identifying, challenging, and addressing practices of structural stigma that has a detrimental impact on health and wellbeing. Sally's work within the community sector has included case management, group facilitation, project management, writing policy and procedures, service coordination, community capacity building, sector development, development and delivery of professional development training, and network building and facilitation. Sally is an advocate for building the capacity of peers at a community level to play an active role in suicide prevention and has a particular interest in the role of social inclusion and belonging in mental health. In 2014 Sally co-founded Wendybird in 2014 with her partner Chantel Keegan, named in honour of her younger sister who died of suicide in 2007. Wendybird brings together a passionate and skilled group of LGBTIQ people that build and facilitate community spaces that foster belonging for those who are often excluded. Sally has published a number of articles in the areas of LGBTIQ people, suicide prevention, and disaster recovery, and regularly presents at conferences on LGBTIQ mental health, suicide prevention and inclusive practice.

CONTRIBUTORS

Tareq Abuelroos is a Consultant Psychiatrist at the Victorian Dual Disability Service.
June Alexander is a Lecturer at Flinders University, specialising in disability support.
Marlies Alvarenga is a Consultant Clinical Psychologist with the Monash Cardiovascular Research Centre, also with an appointment in the Department of Psychiatry, School of Clinical Sciences at Monash Health, Monash University.

Andrew Baillie is a Clinical Psychologist and Professor of Allied Health (conjoint) with Sydney Local Health District and co-Research leader of eHealth at the School of Health Sciences, University of Sydney.

Richard Baldwin is a Senior Policy Officer at Mental Health Carers NSW, specialising in the health and aged care sectors.

Michelle Banfield is a mental health consumer and Head of Lived Experience Research at the Centre for Mental Health Research, Australian National University.

Mike Barry is a Clinical Psychologist in private practice specialising in trauma and mood disorders and working with military, veterans and emergency service personnel.

Eddie Bartnik was inaugural Commissioner at the Western Australian Mental Health Commission. He is an Independent Consultant and International Lead for the International Initiative for Disability Leadership.

Bridget Bassilios is a Senior Research Fellow at the Centre for Mental Health at the University of Melbourne and an independently practising clinical and health psychologist.

Tarun Bastiampillai is a Professor in the College of Medicine and Public Health at Flinders University.

Malcolm Battersby is Professor and Head of Psychiatry at the College of Medicine and Public Health, Flinders University, and Senior Consultant Psychiatrist at Southern Adelaide Local Health Network, Mental Health Division.

Richard Benjamin is a public sector psychiatrist and psychotherapist. He is particularly interested in the long-term effects of child abuse, their manifestations in adults presenting with mental illness, and the benefits of incorporating an understanding of both trauma and relationship in therapeutic responses.

Chad Bennet is Clinical Director and Consultant Psychiatrist with the Victorian Dual Disability Service based at St Vincent's Hospital, Melbourne.

Grant Blashki is an Associate Professor at the Nossal Institute and the Melbourne Sustainable Society Institute at the University of Melbourne, and Lead Clinical Advisor for Beyond Blue.

Kylie Boucher is Senior Project Lead at the Centre for Mental Health Learning and has a passion for supported decision-making and human rights focussed practice.

Jacques Boulet is an interdependent researcher, General Editor at *New Community Quarterly*, and Director, Borderlands Cooperative, Melbourne.

Jillian Broadbear is an Adjunct Clinical Associate Professor at Monash University and Senior Research Fellow at Spectrum Personality Disorder Service for Victoria.

Lisa Brophy is a Professor and Discipline Lead in Social Work and Social Policy at La Trobe University. She is also an honorary principal research fellow in the Centre for Mental Health at the University of Melbourne.

Rita Brown is President of the Australian Borderline Personality Disorder Foundation and Carer Consultant at Spectrum, Personality Disorder Service.

Sally Buchanan-Hagen is a Lecturer in the School of Nursing and Midwifery, Faculty of Health at Deakin University.

Susie Burke is a psychologist at the Australian Psychological Society, looking at ways of using psychological knowledge to enhance community wellbeing and promote social justice.

Louise Byrne is currently a Vice Chancellor's Postdoctoral Fellow in the School of Management at RMIT University.

David Castle is a Professor of Psychiatry at St Vincent's Health, Melbourne and the University of Melbourne.

Jaz Chisholm is a PhD candidate in the Department of Social Work at Monash University.

David Clarke is Medical Program Director of the Mental Health Program at Monash Health and a Professor in the Department of Psychiatry at Monash University.

Laura Collister is Chief Executive at Wellways Australia, a mental health and disability support organisation.

Rose Cuff is the state-wide FaPMI Coordinator, The Bouverie Centre, within the School of Psychology and Public Health at La Trobe University.

Marilyn Cugnetto is a Research Assistant at North Western Mental Health (Melbourne Health), and an Honorary Research Fellow in the School of Psychology and Public Health at La Trobe University.

Indigo Daya is a Consumer Academic at the Centre for Psychiatric Nursing, Faculty of Health Sciences, the University of Melbourne.

Sagarika De Fonseka is a Consultant Psychiatrist. She is specialized in Psychogeriatrics (old-age psychiatry) and provides specialist psychiatry care to adults of all ages and the elderly.

Nikki Dowling is an associate professor within the School of Psychology at Deakin university.

Lorna Downes has held roles in the mental health sector including individual carer, support and advocacy. She is currently at the Centre for Mental Health Learning Victoria.

Brett Emmerson is an Associate Professor of Psychiatry at the University of Queensland and Executive Director, Metro North Mental Health.

Priscilla Ennals is Senior Manager - Research & Evaluations at Neami National.

Joanne Enticott is a Senior Research Fellow and Biostatistician, at Monash Centre for Health Research and Implementation and Southern Synergy, Department of Psychiatry, Monash University.

Daniel Fassnacht is a Lecturer in Psychology at Flinders University in the College of Education, Psychology and Social Work, and an Honorary Research Fellow at the Australian National University.

Sabin Fernbacher is a consultant with experience in mental health services and State Government.

Sarah Francis is a clinical psychologist in private practice working towards a PhD in the area of mindfulness-based interventions.

Cherrie Galletly is Professor of Psychiatry and Department Head, Medical Specialities, at the University of Adelaide.

Flick Grey is a researcher and mental health consultant and recipient of the 2015 Hocking Fellowship to investigate the 'Open Dialogue' model.

Margaret Grigg is Chief Executive Officer at Forensicare, Victoria's forensic mental health service.

Aaron Groves is Chief Civil Psychiatrist and Chief Forensic Psychiatrist at Department of Health Tasmania.

Bridget Hamilton is Associate Professor and Director of the Centre for Psychiatric Nursing at University of Melbourne.

Sabine Hammond is Professor, School of Behavioural & Health Sciences at the Australian Catholic University.

Meredith Harris is Associate Professor, and Principal Research Fellow in the School of Public Health, University of Queensland, specialising in the field of mental health services research and evaluation.

Carol Harvey is a Professor at the Department of Psychiatry, University of Melbourne, and a consultant psychiatrist with NorthWestern Mental Health.

Cassandra Hastie has worked as a policy officer at Mental Health Carers NSW.

Phillipa Hay is Chair of Mental Health at the School of Medicine, University of Sydney, and a past president of the Australian Academy for Eating Disorders.

Tara Hickey is a clinical psychologist whose PhD work with Monash University was in the area of mindfulness and compassion practices.

Judy Hope is Associate Professor, psychiatrist and researcher in mental health services, suicide prevention and psychopharmacology, with appointments at Monash Unviersity and Eastern Health.

David Huppert is Consultant Psychiatrist at Alfred Health, Melbourne and Deputy Chief Psychiatrist, Department of Health and Human Services, Victoria.

Akshay Ilango is a consultation liaison psychiatrist with Monash Health where he is deputy director of the mental health program, and an adjunct academic with Monash University.

Brett Inder is a Professor and Deputy Head of the Department of Econometrics and Business Statistics, Monash University.

Anton Isaacs is a public health physician and Senior Lecturer at the Department of Rural & Indigenous Health, Monash University.

Danielle Jaeger is a consumer who is passionate about sharing her lived experience of Borderline Personality Disorder.

Darren Jiggins is a leader in the peer workforce in Australia, contributing to mental health services policy development as a consumer consultant on national committees.

Nikolaos Kazantzis is a Professor of Clinical Psychology at the Institute for Social Neuroscience (Psychology), training, practicing and researching in Cognitive Behaviour Therapy.

Barbara Keeble-Devlin, now retired, worked and lectured in mental health care for over forty years.

Nicholas Keks is a Professor of Psychiatry at Monash University and a consultant psychiatrist with Delmont Hospital.

Daniel King is a Senior Research Fellow and clinical psychologist in the School of Psychology at the University of Adelaide.

Robert King is an Adjunct Professor in the School of Psychology and Counselling, Queensland University of Technology and a board member for Richmond Fellowship Queensland.

Marlena Klaic is an OT and leader of translational research in Allied Health at Melbourne Health, and has a PhD focused in Evidence Based Practice from Monash University.

Michael Kyrios is Vice President and Executive Dean at Flinders University in the College of Education, Psychology and Social Work.

Rhoda Lai is a research assistant specialising in Aged Mental Health. She has held research positions at Monash University Aged Psychiatric Unit, Monash Health, and the University of Melbourne, Aged Mental Health Psychiatry.

Catherine Lourey is the NSW Mental Health Commissioner and an experienced mental health leader working in public policy and human services.

Roxxanne MacDonald is a Youth Advisory Council Member at Orygen.

Lyn Mahboub is a Lecturer and Lived Experience Academic at Curtin University and a Strategic Recovery Advisor and Hearing Voices Network Liaison for Richmond Wellbeing, Western Australia.

Bernie McCormick has worked in the mental health system as a consumer consultant, telephone advocate, university lecturer, board director and a consumer adviser to the Melbourne Magistrates Court.

Patrick McGorry is Executive Director of Orygen and Professor of Youth Mental Health at the University of Melbourne.

Peter McKenzie is a lecturer at The Bouverie Centre, School of Psychology and Public Health, La Trobe University.

Cristina Mei is a research fellow at Orygen, and Academic Research and Publications Officer at the Centre for Youth Mental Health, University of Melbourne.

Annette Mercuri is Carer Consultant at Inner West Area Mental Health Service, Melbourne.

Stephanie Merkouris is a Research Fellow within the School of Psychology at Deakin University with experience in problem gambling and treatment.

Louise Mewton is Scientia Senior Lecturer at the Centre for Healthy Brain and Ageing, University of NSW, and researches in the epidemiology, assessment and prevention of problematic alcohol use.

Helen Milroy is a Consultant Child and Adolescent Psychiatrist and Winthrop Professor at the University of Western Australia. Her work and research interests include holistic medicine, child mental health, recovery from trauma and grief, application of Indigenous knowledge, cultural models of care, Aboriginal health and mental health, and developing and supporting the Aboriginal medical workforce.

Mark Morel is Peer Support Worker with the STEP program at Neami National, and a Peer Advisor with Way2Home in Darlinghurst, Sydney.

Vera Morgan is Head of the Neuropsychiatric Epidemiology Research Unit in the University of Western Australia (UWA) School of Population and Global Health, Director of the Centre for Clinical Research in Neuropsychiatry in the UWA Division of Psychiatry, and Operational Epidemiologist at the North Metropolitan Health Service Mental Health.

Gerry Naughtin is Strategic Adviser, Mental Health, in the Strategic Advisers and Research Division of the NDIA. Gerry has an extensive career in human services in the disability and aged care sectors and has a strong history of engagement on consumer and carer participation.

Daniel O'Connor is an Emeritus Professor in the Faculty of Medicine, Nursing and Health Sciences, Monash University and was Deputy Chief Psychiatrist for Aged Persons Mental Health in the State of Victoria.

Brendan O'Hanlon is a researcher in mental health and families at The Bouverie Centre, La Trobe University. He has a strong interest in how family-based approaches can be best implemented in service settings.

Erin Parker is a sessional academic in the Research School of Psychology at the Australian National University and an allied health private practitioner at headspace Canberra.

Melissa Petrakis is Senior Lecturer in Social Work at Monash University and Chair of the Board of Tandem, the Victorian mental health family and friends peak body.

Allan Pinches, a former journalist, has worked in the consumer movement for more than 28 years as a consultant, researcher, and writer.

Chris Plakiotis is Unit Head at the Aged Persons Mental Health Service, Monash Health, and Adjunct Senior Lecturer at the Department of Psychiatry, Monash University. As a consultant psychiatrist he works primarily in acute inpatient and consultation-liaison psychiatry settings to provide comprehensive, multidisciplinary treatment for a wide range of mental health conditions affecting adults of all ages.

Abner Poon is a Senior Lecturer in Social Work at the School of Social Sciences, Faculty of Arts and Social Sciences, University of NSW. His research focuses on the impact of mental illness on families and caregivers within the context of social work practice.

Rory Randall is a Consumer Academic in the Melbourne School of Health Sciences, University of Melbourne.

Sathya Rao is Executive Clinical Director of Spectrum, Personality Disorder Service for Victoria, Vice President of Australian BPD Foundation and Adjunct Clinical Associate Professor at Monash University.

Helena Roennfeldt is a lived experience researcher, academic and social worker specialising in community mental health.

Carmela Salomon is a 3DN Project Officer at the University of NSW, specialising in a range of initiatives to support responsible psychotropic prescribing and cardiometabolic health in people with an intellectual disability.

Neeraj Sareen is Head of Adult Community Mental Health at Alfred Health, Melbourne. He is a fellow of the Royal Australian and New Zealand College of Psychiatrists and a member of the Royal College of Psychiatrists UK.

Jaydip Sarkar is a Consultant of the Women's Unit and the Personality Disorder Initiative in Forensicare, Victoria's forensic services.

Faye Scanlan is a research fellow at Orygen and a psychologist at headspace.

Justin Scanlan is Senior Lecturer and Course Director for the Bachelor of Applied Science (Occupational Therapy) at the Faculty of Health Sciences, University of Sydney.

Brett Scholz is a Research Fellow in the Medical School, ANU College of Health and Medicine, specialising in ways in which barriers to consumer leadership can be challenged, the role of allies to the consumer movement, and co-production between consumers and other mental health professionals.

James Scott leads the Child and Youth Research Group at the QIMR Berghofer Medical Research Institute, specialising in developing preventative strategies and cost-effective real-world interventions for mental illness in children and youth.

Frances Shawyer is a clinical psychologist and researcher in mindfulness and mental health services research, as well as Deputy Director and a Research Fellow at Southern Synergy, the Southern Adult Mental Health Research, Training and Evaluation Centre, Monash University.

Fiona Smith is a Lecturer and Director of Field Education, Social Work and Social Policy at the School of Allied Health, Human Services and Sport, La Trobe University.

Kate Sommerville is an anti-pokies advocate based in Melbourne.

Bob Stanton is a Senior Lecturer in the School of Health, Medical and Applied Sciences, Central Queensland University, with 25 years' experience working with the sport, health, fitness and rehabilitation sectors.

Louise Stone, a General Practitioner, is an Associate Professor in the College of Health and Medicine at ANU. She has a clinical, teaching, research and policy interest in mental health.

Suresh Sundram is a Professor of Psychiatry at Monash University and Head of the Department of Psychiatry in the School of Clinical Sciences at Monash Health, also a Consultant Psychiatrist with Monash Health.

Maree Teesson AC is Director of the Matilda Centre; Director of the NHMRC Centre of Research Excellence in Prevention and Early Intervention in Mental Illness and Substance Use; and an NHMRC Leadership Fellow at the University of Sydney.

Neil Thomas is an Associate Professor in the Department of Psychological Sciences, Swinburne University; Deputy Director at the Centre for Mental Health; Director of the National eTherapy Centre; and Honorary Consultant Clinical Psychologist with Alfred Health.

Yoland Wadsworth is Adjunct Professor at the Social & Global Studies Centre at RMIT University and is one of Australia's pioneers in transformative social research and evaluation.

Timothy Wand is Associate Professor at the Sydney Nursing School and a nurse practitioner in mental health liaison at Royal Prince Alfred Hospital.

Kay Wilhelm is Consultation Liaison Psychiatrist and Clinical Lead at St Vincent's Hospital, Sydney; Professor and Head of Psychiatry at the University of Notre Dame, Sydney Campus; and Conjoint Professor at the School of Psychiatry, University of NSW.

Anne Williams is a Lecturer in Occupational Therapy at Swinburne University, specialising in factors that support people experiencing severe mental illnesses to participate in meaningful occupations.

Alan Woodward is currently serving on the National Mental Health Commission. He has worked in the fields of mental health, crisis support and suicide prevention for 20 years as an executive leader, a service and program developer, an evaluator and researcher and as an expert advisor to governments and peak bodies.

Jeff Young is the Director of The Bouverie Centre, La Trobe University. He is a clinical psychologist and family therapist and has worked, published and presented in the area of Mental Health for over 25 years.

PREFACE

This book is a resource for anyone working or interested in mental health care systems and services in Australia. Much material here should be of value to case managers and others in clinical mental health services, including those engaged in post-graduate study and aiming to take on senior clinical or supervisory roles. Many staff working in the community managed mental health sector also will find information of relevance to their roles here. In addition, we have considered undergraduates in nursing and allied health disciplines, for whom this might serve as a useful reference text. Further, it may be useful for medical students and doctors in exploring the mental health service system, which can seem very different from other settings in the health care system. For psychiatrists, including those in training, there will be useful material on systemic approaches to mental health care, while chapters on clinical matters may provide some alternative perspectives to more traditional texts, as well as including material useful for revision. In addition, the content may be useful for people receiving mental health services, and to families or carers who may be interested in the way that the services are organised and how things are thought about and done. Likewise it may be helpful for people in managerial positions within mental health care, perhaps without having worked in this specific branch of health care previously. In alignment with this broad range of possible audiences, the scope of the book is broad. In this substantially revised edition, the content is divided into four parts:

Part One - *The Context for Contemporary Mental Health Care*. Content here addresses societal and cultural issues in mental health care; influences on policy and strategy from global, national, state and local levels; the interface between research and practice; how services are evaluated; and what we understand about the frequency with which mental health problems occur in the community and what the determinants of this may be. It features the perspectives of different participants in the service system and consideration of how they might work together.

Part Two - *Principles for Collaborative Community Practice* moves into a consideration of the skills, knowledge and understandings that underpin community mental health practice and how to support and assist people with mental health problems. Coordination, working collaboratively and relationship-building skills are included here. Treatments with medications, psychological treatments and the complex suite of ideas surrounding supporting people in their recovery are also addressed in this Part.

Part Three - *Mental Health Problems Considered in the Context of the Lifespan* concentrates on disorders that are typically identified and treated in the lifespan periods of childhood and adolescence, youth, and older age. Both the developmental context and the relevant service system are highlighted.

Part Four - *Mental health problems considered in terms of disorders*. Here the chapter order for the most part reflects the order of presentation in the ICD-11 classification system and the focus is primarily on adults. Both high and low prevalence disorders have profound significance for individuals, families and society; these chapters aim to bring to life the nature of the disorders and their most important treatments.

Each part has a brief introductory section and the reader who is planning to use this book extensively may find it useful to review these sections for further orientation.

There is a logical progression to the work and for some readers working through this sequence may be useful. We expect that many readers will wish to explore specific sections or issues and we have worked to ensure that cross-referencing within assists movement through the text.

A firm intent in the preparation of this text has been to present the range of opinions and perspectives that contribute to the rich and challenging task of working in the interest of those with mental health issues. This is intended to facilitate the challenge which presents itself to all working in the field: integrating the fullest possible range of conceptual, informational and human contributions in the pursuit of quality in community mental health practice. Accordingly, the contributions to this book come from a wide range of authors whose perspectives reflect the varying viewpoints in the field of mental health care. We have not set out to reconcile the possibly conflicting viewpoints that this inclusion generates since to do so would present an unrealistic picture. Rather, the reality of mental health practice involves making effort towards tolerance and understanding of those with perspectives other than one's own, and respect for the diversity of views within and outside the professional team. Many different voices and opinions are contained within the book, and we believe this is a particular strength of the work. Authors contributing to a chapter may not share all the views expressed in the chapter, so that authorship within each chapter is identified in relation to each specific contribution within the text. Where chapters feature a large number of authors contributing different sections, the author attribution may be listed alphabetically rather than reflecting priority or size of individual contributions.

Graham Meadows, John Farhall, Ellie Fossey, Brenda Happell, Fiona McDermott and Sebastian Rosenberg

Note: The authors, editors and publisher have taken care to ensure that the information presented in this work is accurate and current at the time of publication. However, we acknowledge that a work of this size and scope may contain errors, and information that has been superseded or soon will be. Guidelines and directives that govern clinical practice in various settings might differ from content presented here. In the matters of drug prescription and administration particularly, readers should consult manufacturers' information and other reputable sources. The authors, editors and publisher accept no responsibility for the outcomes of clinical or other decisions that may be made drawing on the content of the book.

INTRODUCTION

Mental health practice has complexity manifest in a multiplicity of related theories, concepts, policies, organisations, and services; this has profound repercussions for mental health consumers and carers who often experience confusion along with multiple disadvantages personally and structurally. They encounter head-on the impacts of this complexity, frequently seeking help across organisations, exposed to competing discourses, paradigms, interventions and practitioners. There is a tendency to accept the complex nature of the field and of practice as the status quo. This is just 'how things are'. This book aims to challenge this unhelpful position and explore the different elements, characteristics and implications of this complexity.

This book is primarily addressed to service providers. It may also be of interest to a broader group of people, including researchers, policy-makers, funders and the general community. In this book we bring together the range of actors and systems, programs and interventions through which mental health services in Australia are constructed and delivered. Throughout, we rely on hearing and learning from consumers and carers. We need their critique and analysis of this complex system. What is it that consumers and carers want people working in the mental health sector to know in order to provide the most helpful services? How can their unique knowledge derived from lived experience be recognised, respected and effectively utilised to improve mental health service delivery? Their contributions to theory development, conceptual understanding, policy and practice are the sine qua non of good mental health services.

The mental health system cannot be understood by reducing it to its parts or by looking at the whole as an inextricable combination of interrelated parts. This is where Complexity Theory can be of assistance. It argues that systems are affected by the entangled relationships between those parts and that the relations among the parts are contingent, employing four key concepts of non-linearity; feedback; emergence; and adaptiveness. Contexts then in which mental health service providers and consumers find themselves are characterized by unpredictability and uncertainty. A complexity theory-informed approach helps us to recognize that we and those we work with have agency, we can act unpredictably and we can adapt to and influence our environment. This brings us to collaborative practice.

Collaborative community practice frames the content of this book. It underlines the importance of collaboration as a pre-requisite for the delivery of the best possible mental health services. As we have noted above, the mental health field comprises and crosses many social structures and organisational boundaries. The differences in approaches and understanding of what is meant by the experience of mental illness and of the policies and services designed to address the needs of consumers, carers and communities may be varied and sometimes contradictory. Collaboration requires recognition of these differences, the identification of areas of shared ground as well as identification of what is not known. It is often from the foundation of what is not known by all actors that effective policies or programs might emerge.

Our aim in this book is to bring together the perspectives, knowledge, and experiences of those engaged in the mental health field. These chapters comprise what is known and by whom. By default, they also tell us what is not yet known or where gaps in knowledge and understanding exist. Further, they also provide insight into research and evaluation, offering guidelines for how we might go about knowing more and enhancing the evidence base for interventions. However, bearing in mind the perspective derived from Complexity Theory, this is unlikely to be a seamless process and will at times create tensions. Such an approach may on occasions challenge the value of predictive instruments or assessments that influence practice. However, it can simultaneously encourage greater focus on the informal or spontaneously occurring events and processes that can provide critical insights into the development of policies, organisations, programs and interventions. In the preparation of this fourth edition the following has guided our thinking and guidance to authors:

1. While use of terms shifts and changes, we have sought to integrate a 'Recovery Oriented Practice' focus into the general structure and composition of the book.
2. We have aimed to continue the established inclusive and pluralistic nature of the book particularly inclusion of lived experience or consumer perspectives; we have strengthened the wider editorial team to that end.
3. We have taken a stance that sharing of information with consumers about the diagnostic and clinical reasoning process is necessary to make these first two points a reality. For that reason, among others, the primary diagnostic system in the book is ICD-11. DSM remains copyright to the American Psychiatric Association, while ICD-11 is readily available on the internet. Where necessary, DSM categories are described by contrast with ICD.
4. We have sought more than in previous editions throughout to ensure that the book is engaged with the realities of practice in the complex, varied, rapidly changing, and multicultural setting that this country represents with all its inequities of opportunity and disadvantage including those that profoundly affect the Indigenous peoples of this country.
5. We have sought to bring some greater uniformity into this edition - so bringing greater consistency to the structure of chapters and sections where various contributions seek to treat of similar material. While continuing to accommodate a plurality of perspectives we also wish to strive for somewhat greater consistency in use of language.
6. In aiming to bring the fourth edition text in at under 400,000 words of text, there has been a striving for abridgement and concise treatment throughout.

A central tenet of determining content in the successive editions of this book has been the aim of providing readers from differing perspectives with an understanding of the ways in which others encountered in the mental health service system may see things. It is also a critically important purpose of the book to give readers some sense of how and why the mental health care system may have been formed, and to understand that service systems are in constant evolution. We hope that by describing some frameworks for understanding how systems change and may be changed this content may empower people to engage and work effectively in systems development. Also, to be able when necessary better to tolerate and accept the frustrations and unavoidable uncertainties as services go through stages of transition.

Mental Health care is a political issue at many levels. In party political terms, periods of consensus politics around governmental responses are the exception rather than the rule; mental health services can be an arena in which political games are fought out between sides of politics and levels of government. Politics can be seen as including any assignment of power between groups and persons so inter-personal, inter-disciplinary and inter-sectoral relationships in the area also are in many respects political. Issues surrounding: Indigenous peoples; migrants and refugees; influences of wealth inequities and of access to quality service provision for instance through radically reorganised disability-support services - all need some political analysis to create a coherent picture of developments through time. The book seeks not to shy away from broadly political considerations, rather to acknowledge and accommodate a range of perspectives, on occasions locating these within relevant socio- political frameworks.

There have been recent shifts in the political environment that have very practical implications. At the time of writing the first edition of this book many changes in mental health care delivery were being driven by the National Mental Health Strategy. The accomplishments of the strategy have been enormous: in many parts of Australia the driving force of the strategy has led to services that are much better organised and much more coherently structured than previously. However, the role of the strategy has changed now compared with when the journey that this book represents began. The strategy effectively lapsed between 2014 and 2017, with no National Mental Health Plan in place. Though reactivated with a fifth plan released in 2017, this strategy is not the driving force at this point that it was in the 1990s. Australian health reform processes are changing the relationship between governments in the federal system and the Commonwealth's proportional share of funding is growing compared with that of the States and Territories. The advent of the National Disability Insurance Scheme and the changing role of the Primary Health Networks represent dynamic areas of change. Traditional roles such as psychiatrist and psychiatric nurse are changing as funding models change and there are new or growing roles. The COVID-19 pandemic has shifted many long-standing assumptions regarding how services need to be delivered.

The perspective and contribution of the people we typically have referred to as consumers in the writing of this text has remained a distinguishing feature in the fourth edition. A new editorial board structure includes four new Associate Editors with a role in improving this aspect of the fourth edition. The use of terms here - such as consumer - is a sensitive issue. There are problems from some perspectives with any of the available terminology - people may variously be described - or choose to be - as having lived experience of mental health problems, having used mental health services, to be consumers, clients or patients of the services, or simply people. Some may prefer to describe themselves as survivors of their passage through such services or having made progress with recovery in spite of them - or in the absence of service experience at all. In much of the book the term consumer will be used, as well as all of the others above when they seem best suited to the specific context - but the limitations of the term will be discussed and alternatives will be used when indicated by context.

Research and advocacy from within the consumer field has advanced understanding of issues relevant to consumers and the services they receive, including the manner in which services are developed and resourced. The ideas around personal recovery originated in this context. A challenge for writing about recovery in such a book is that while personal recovery as contrasted with clinical recovery was first given voice from consumers it has become incorporated into policy and strategy in ways that can serve to expropriate a set of ideas that originated in the context of something sharing features with those of a resistance movement. We are hoping that the involvement of our additional Associate Editors will have helped us strike a reasonable balance in this area.

In another departure from previous editions, six members of an editorial board have joined with the editors and associate editors in the task, either helping with alignment of content in regards to issues presenting in the context of particular groups in the population or in alignment with some specific professional interests.

We also have made further efforts to give due recognition and consideration of the roles and contributions of families and carers and the implications these have for responses to people with mental health problems as well as to their own needs and the social and political implications of these.

Our sincere hope then as the editors is that, extending as it does the content and contributions of the first three editions, the fourth edition of this book will contribute further to better mental health in the Australian community.

ACKNOWLEDGMENTS

The developmental process for this edition took around five years, and the edition has substantial changes reflected in the new title. The work towards this has involved editors from earlier editions John Farhall, Ellie Fossey, Fiona McDermott and Graham Meadows, also with a much-extended editorial group into which came Brenda Happell and Seb Rosenberg, while Margaret Grigg left that group during the early part of the edition development (though she re-joined as an author later). Margaret's editorial contribution to two of the earlier editions and that of Professor Bruce Singh in initiation of the project and as an editor in all three earlier editions is warmly acknowledged. Also joining in editorial roles have been Associate Editors with lived experience including Merinda Epstein, Cath Roper, Hamilton Kennedy and Vrinda Edan. An advisory group (including Caroline Johnson, Fiona Best, Harry Minas, Sally Morris, Jonathan Harms and Pat Dudgeon) allowed input from the perspectives of general practice, psychiatry, cultural and linguistic diverse communities, LGBTIQ communities, carers and Indigenous people. Administration support has involved Debbie Lang and Kellie Youngs. Debra James has stayed with the book as OUP editor for another edition and has been a key helper in negotiating the many stages and challenges involved in such a substantial and complex work, assisted through time and in different aspects of the work by Melpo Christofi, Erin O'Loughlin, Amy Shields, Sanam Goodman; while as copy editor, Carolyn Leslie was meticulous and supportive. Over the length of time involved participation of individuals has changed, some have left and others joined but to all involved there is thanks and appreciation of commitment, goodwill and active engagement with the visioning and realisation of this work.

Some authors involved in earlier editions have not contributed to this one but their content has been retained as part of the base for the writing and this is signified by listing them as 'with' on the author lists. As noted for the third edition, we have sought to identify and request permissions as indicated for copyright material and again would be keen to hear of any omissions in this which we could correct.

A special note of thanks goes to Debbie Lang who has provided administrative support throughout to the writing coordination, referencing, project management and meeting support through the different editorial stages.

The publishers would like to express our sincere thanks to the lead editors, and to all the authors, for contributing their knowledge, experience and wisdom to this comprehensive new edition.

PART 01

THE CONTEXT FOR CONTEMPORARY MENTAL HEALTH CARE

Mental health care can be considered as located in various contexts, so important material explored here comes from conceptual, historical, ecological, environmental, cultural, scientific, ethical, strategic and informational sources—to name but a few. These involve different basic assumptions and approaches to the development of knowledge—reflecting and constructing different paradigms and epistemologies. The chapters in this part then purposively scan a series of bodies of knowledge and understanding.

A useful potentially integrative process introduced early on involves: considerations of critical and reflective thinking; working with and in complexity; and addressing tensions between ideas and perspectives through a dialectical approach. These concepts are returned to at multiple points in this part and in the text as a way to encourage integration of this broadly framed material.

Chapter 1.1 starts the text with information from several perspectives that may be helpful in approaching thinking about mental health problems. We introduce early on some ideas from complexity science as well as historical material. Perspectives from consumers and carers are introduced.

Chapter 1.2 brings into focus environmental and social issues that form important contemporary contexts to mental health issues. Climate change and societal determinants, including the influences of inequities in wealth and income distribution, are considered here.

Chapter 1.3 investigates two important identifiable groupings in the Australian population where these backgrounds may be relevant to understanding how problems arise and how they may be better addressed. The Indigenous population and the LGBTIQ communities are considered here.

Chapter 1.4 considers how knowledge is advanced in the field through research or evaluation. A wide range of paradigms and epistemological approaches are described or illustrated here including how different approaches may engage with different values and conceptual systems and how they may influence policy making and practice.

Chapter 1.5 brings into focus some issues in development and planning of mental health services and some contemporary challenges in enabling those services to make differences to public mental health.

Chapter 1.6 considers a wide range of sources of information on mental health care in Australia, including population needs and service provision seeking to address those needs.

Chapter 1.7 takes a policy and strategy focus at national and state/territory levels, and through this describes some of the shaping of services across the breadth of Australia.

1.1

MENTAL HEALTH CARE AS A COMPLEX SYSTEM

GRAHAM MEADOWS, FIONA MCDERMOTT, SEBASTIAN ROSENBERG, MERINDA EPSTEIN, ALLAN PINCHES, JACQUES BOULET, JONATHAN HARMS, RICHARD BALDWIN & CASSANDRA HASTIE

1.1.1 MENTAL HEALTH SYSTEMS AND COMPLEXITY SCIENCE

FIONA MCDERMOTT, SEBASTIAN ROSENBERG, GRAHAM MEADOWS, MERINDA EPSTEIN & JACQUES BOULET

COMPLEXITY THINKING IN CLINICAL DECISION MAKING

In considering development of a proficient, expert or even masterful practitioner, four strands of thinking can be identified: reflective, critical, complexity and dialectical (Higgs, Jensen, Loftus, & Christensen, 2018; see Sections 1.1.5 and 1.5.10). An appraisal of complexity and a typical feature of mental health care can be seen as permeating these four kinds of thinking and so we will begin with some consideration of how complexity can be understood and used. Practitioners and others have different places in what is often referred to as a mental health care system so we will begin with consideration of application of complexity to the mental health care system, through which we will explore some key concepts in complexity science which we will then return to at various points in the text (see, for instance, Chapters 1.2, 1.5 and 2.3).

COMPLEXITY AND THE MENTAL HEALTH CARE SYSTEM

> Anyone who isn't confused really doesn't understand the situation.
>
> *Ed Murrow*

The idea of a mental health system is important in considering delivery of mental health service but also may be misleading. Using the term 'system' suggests that policies, programs and actors provide mental health services through a consistently organised and interconnected set of actions and elements. These may operate on different levels and in different ways. But if considered as a *system* they might be expected to be structured and patterned to rationally and logically meet particular ends and needs, with identified inputs supporting specified processes leading to desired outputs in a stable and predictable way. However, this description would rarely reflect the experience of mental health service providers, consumers, or other key stakeholders for whom engagement with the mental health system is often disorganised, messy, complicated and unreliable, lacking the consistent causal connection associated with the *system* concept.

Conceptualisation of what a mental health service system might be involves, at least, environmental, political, economic, organisational, social, interpersonal, biological, physical, psychological and cultural considerations, all modified according to context. Typically, a system observed as such will have interactions outside the scope of observation, so may be considered 'open' rather than 'closed' and this is one source of uncertainty. But here also, Complexity Science can be of assistance and particularly ideas around complex adaptive systems (CAS). CAS are affected by the relationships between their parts but these relationship effects may not be consistent—understanding the workings of the parts of the system may not lead to a correct understanding or prediction

Table 1.1 Key concepts in considering properties of complex adaptive systems

Concept	Definition	Example
Emergence	Properties of the system as a whole which are emergent and cannot be predicted from individual parts or the sum of parts.	The behaviour of consumer groups: many agents can be much smarter than the few, or a large number of people tip into a forceful movement for change that gives rise to unexpected structures and events (see Section 1.1.6).
Feedback	The way systems or organisms create their environment and are in turn moulded by that environment i.e. how they coevolve. One element affects others which in turn can affect the original element. Feedback can be positive or negative and can occur between levels (micro, meso, macro) so that micro-level interactions between the subunits generate some pattern in the macro-level that then back-reacts onto the subunits, causing them to generate a new pattern.	If mental health attendances at emergency departments (EDs) increase, those responsible for system design may increase resources to provide care there or in other acute services, potentially diverting resources away from, for instance, services supporting primary mental health care. But if an important contributor factor to the increased ED presentation is compromised, primary care capacity then may become a positive feedback loop (see Section 1.5.11).
Adaptation	System behaviour changes in response to an intervention; the system spontaneously orders itself, and never settles in to a steady state of behaviour. Systems are in a state of transformation, incorporating resources from outside themselves.	A multidisciplinary team making a decision about how best to work with a patient brings together agents who have interactions across boundaries of different systems; the decision and the process involved in reaching it reflects this and simultaneously sets up another system (the intervention; see Section 2.2.6).
Self-organisation	Overall organisation and order is achieved as the outcome of spontaneous local interaction rather than as a result of a plan.	Private mental health care providers in Australia are generally free to practice where they prefer. This self-organisation leads to an emergent property of inequity (see Chapters 1.2, 1.5 and 1.7).

of how the system behaves. Sometimes there may be little consistency in correspondence between input into such systems and the outputs that follow. Nevertheless, there are concepts that can help us better predict how such systems may work—or understand better why our intuitive or otherwise informed predictions may prove incorrect. Four relevant concepts in complexity theory are non-linearity; feedback; emergence; and adaptiveness (see Table 1.1). In this context, these four concepts—along with acknowledgement that these systems typically are open—recognise and affirm the deeply relational way in which humans live and survive, their interrelationship with their environment and their sensitivity to the influence of outside factors, which in turn are changeable in ways that often are unpredictable and uncertain. Minas provides a helpful analysis of Australia's mental health from within a complexity science perspective, noting the impact of these four factors in creating what he terms a 'zone of complexity' (Minas, 2005, p. 36), characterised by the simultaneous press of forces for stability and for chaos.

1.1.2 UNDERSTANDING MENTAL DISORDER

FIONA MCDERMOTT & GRAHAM MEADOWS

What follows in this chapter is an account of the key elements—perspectives, decisions, innovations and experiments—which characterise important historical developments in understanding (or failing to understand) and responding to (or failing to respond to) mental disorder. The partiality and contested nature of knowledge and understanding, the creativity and successes of various responses and innovations, and the failures, are all part of this story

We believe it is helpful to examine this history in terms of continuing and unresolved debates about:

1. how to make sense of mental illness, its causes and effects
2. how to respond to mental illness
3. who it is who should do something about or for or with people with mental illness.

These questions arise from a sociological perspective, which views history as evolving and emerging from the debates and events that make up social life and are expressed in social practices. In this chapter, we will discuss each of them. The considerations raised by point 3 in the above list then lead us into discussions reflecting the perspectives of consumers and carers, contributions which in turn are central to influential forces such as the recovery movement (see Sections 1.1.6, 1.5.2 and 2.6.2).

1.1.3 MAKING SENSE OF THE HISTORY OF MENTAL DISORDER

FIONA MCDERMOTT & GRAHAM MEADOWS

INTRODUCTION

There are numerous choices about how to convey this history, each of which would provide us with different, perhaps rival, interpretations of the past and the present. As Eghigian, in his introduction to *The Routledge History Of Madness And Mental Health* comments, '(m)adness...has a history—or perhaps better put, it has histories. As societies and their institutions and values have changed, so too have the ways in which madness has been experienced, understood, and treated' (Eghigian, 2017, p. 2). While much of the history of mental disorder discussed in this chapter refers to the history of mental disorder in UK, Europe, US, Canada and Australia, Eghigian's recent edited book includes chapters discussing the history and development in Asia, Africa, Japan and South Asia. The history of madness, as Eghigian points out, references that array of experiences which are part of what is integral to being human. Thus, this history is not a story about 'others' but rather a set of stories about ourselves.

BEGINNINGS

We can cite streams of thought in ancient Greece that held that mental disturbance could be seen as an outcome of brain disease and hence to be treated by physicians. However, these beliefs subsequently lost influence through much of Western Europe, where the legacy of thinking from the Middle Ages was that bizarre thoughts and behaviour were likely to be construed as evidence of demonic possession or witchcraft. Although relatives might care for individuals or local communities might tolerate people with mental illness, in many settings they were at risk of being subject to harsh treatment. With increased population and urbanisation came a trend towards institutional confinement of the mentally ill, along with others seen as deviant, with little or no notion of rights to humane treatment. Large institutions, variously labelled as hospitals, jails, madhouses or asylums, contained many people who would now be seen as suffering from mental illness.

THE AGE OF REASON

The intellectual movement of the seventeenth and eighteenth centuries, referred to as the Enlightenment, gave privilege to reason as a way of approaching understanding the world, and in time this change of view affected the way in which those seen as mad were treated. During the Enlightenment, when rationality was privileged, the position of the mad and the irrational provided a particular challenge (Jones, 1996). There was considerable debate over whether or not, with the right kind of 'moral treatment', the mad could become rational once more. Moral treatment here consisted of placing the patient in an environment that encouraged behaviour in line with accepted social standards, and was pervaded by religious teachings. The Enlightenment belief that progress would proceed on the basis of scientific study gave increasing influence to medicine as a scientific practice, and held hope that psychiatry, as a branch of medicine, could devise specialist medical treatment for the insane. Scull argues that the outcome of these debates over the virtues and benefits of moral versus medical treatment of the insane was a finding in favour of science: mental illness was thereby 'captured' in the late eighteenth century by the medical profession (Scull, 1989). Mental disorder achieved the status of an illness, to be conceptualised, diagnosed and treated as other somatic ailments. The asylums were thought of not only as places for confinement but also as places with programs aimed at treating and rehabilitating sufferers.

As we have noted, a key aspect of Enlightenment thinking had been the attainment of rationality, a desire to gather and order knowledge. This ordering of knowledge took the form of sorting, grouping, dividing and classifying phenomena, to generate categories and make distinctions on the basis of those characteristics identified as descriptive of a group. In medicine, this expressed itself in work from Linnaeus and Sydenham on medical classification systems (nosologies). In the nineteenth century, in the mental health field the nosological work of the German psychiatrist Kraepelin is particularly significant; many of the conceptual structures established by Kraepelin and other psychiatrists and philosophers of this time persist, largely unchanged, to the present.

POSITIVISM AND ITS CHALLENGERS

The positivist tradition, arising in the twentieth century, is exemplified in the belief that reality is driven by immutable natural laws and mechanisms, and is knowable, provided that the knower or inquirer remains distant, noninteractive and value free. This intellectual posture had its origins in the Enlightenment, and emphasised the separation of mind and body. The power of expert knowledge, knowledge that is objective and value free, assured the influence of the medical profession in understanding and treating mental illness.

In the late twentieth century, we saw the emergence of nonpositivist epistemologies (theories of knowledge). These are characterised by an increased valuing of personal knowledge and experience, and a recognition of the person as fundamentally self-interpreting. Here the notion of a positivist view of the progressive pursuit of a single valid truth through systematic method is largely discarded. This posture of presenting a model of multiple viewpoints, each with their own 'validity', is one of the characteristics of 'postmodern' philosophies.

Within the mental health field, this broadening of perspectives has added to our recognition of the complexity of the field, and has led to attempts to respond adequately and with a variety of approaches to mental distress

MODERN PSYCHIATRY

Following Kraepelin, the development of a system of diagnostic categories describing psychopathology has become indispensable, both in general psychiatry and the field of psychiatric epidemiology. Epidemiological studies, with their dependence on classification systems, have enabled the undertaking of large-scale research studies into the prevalence, causes, consequences, and amount and effectiveness of care of the mentally ill (Robbins, 1990; Tsuang, Tohen, & Jones, 2011; Prince, Stewaart, Ford, & Hotopf, 2003). Undoubtedly this trend towards classification has had great benefits. However, it has also led, at times, to a reduction of the person to a description of his or her disorder, as in the practice of referring to 'schizophrenics'.

Throughout the twentieth century, other significant strands of thought have contributed to the underpinning of mental health practice. Sigmund Freud founded psychoanalysis as we understand it today, though it has undergone many changes since his pioneering work. Freud worked closely with people with mental disorders, accessing their inner lives through talk. The forces proceeding to mental disturbance were seen as being within the unaware, unconscious mind, and conflicts at this level produced disturbance in the aware self. By the beginning of the twentieth century, Freud was advancing a model of mental disturbance that no longer placed it as something alien, or the result of demonic possession. Instead, psychopathology could be seen as a part of everyday life, as the outcome of repressed trauma was present in everyone to some degree.

Through the early part of the twentieth century, the experimental science of psychology made great advances. Conditioned reflexes, as described by Pavlov, and operant conditioning, as first set out by Skinner, provided the core framework of behaviourism, which then developed through work on motivation and other aspects of psychology towards the complementing of behavioural approaches with the cognitive approach. The sophistication of linkage between these approaches has progressively increased—also with benefits from integration with concepts from other aspects of psychological treatment and with source ideas from other philosophical and spiritual traditions (see Section 2.6.7).

PHILOSOPHY AND NEUROSCIENCE

In struggling to make sense of the phenomenon of mental disorder, various attempts have been made to conceptualise it. These include philosophical considerations of the nature of mind, the interconnections between mind and body, the characteristics distinguishing human beings, the impact of social structure on individual life and making sense of the experience of mental disorder from within one's own mind. Developments in neuroscience have increasingly made observable events in the brain accompanying conscious experiences that hitherto were objects only of introspective analysis. For at least the last 25 years, the field of consciousness studies has been in active ferment (Dennett, 1991; Blackmore & Troscianko, 2018); and there is increasing recognition of the physicality of emotion, with arguments arising against separating mind from body (see, for instance, Damasio, 2000).

SOCIOLOGY OF MENTAL HEALTH AND ILLNESS

During the early twentieth century, theoretical developments in sociology gave a different kind of access to the lived experience of people previously segregated: those experiencing mental illness, criminals and people of different ethnic backgrounds. Mental disturbance came to be understood in terms of being an outcome of social processes as well as being described as illness.

ETHNOGRAPHY IN THE MENTAL HOSPITAL

In the 1960s and 1970s, the focus of research by Goffman (1961) and others, including Rosenhan (1973), was on the institutional treatment of mental patients in hospitals. It included striking studies on simulated patients. These volunteers expressed fairly limited psychiatric symptomatology, but often successfully secured hospital admission. Thereafter they found that, by virtue of their position as patients, their subsequent relatively normal behaviour was often described as pathological by the observing staff. This work has contributed significantly to our understanding of the relationship between social structures and roles, and the power of labelling to circumscribe the interpretation of behaviour. However, much work from this period might not meet contemporary methodological standards and/or have been influenced by personal experiences. So the emergent narrative from some of these projects is receiving some questioning as the twenty-first century unfolds (Cahalan, 2020; Shalin, 2014).

STRUCTURALIST PERSPECTIVES

The structuralists are associated with critical and feminist theorists, who recognise that such factors as social regulation, an unequal distribution of resources and power relations influence social practices and life chances. In the mental health field, the most notable workers were the 'anti-psychiatrists' Laing, Cooper and Esterson, who analysed the power relationships they saw as influential in both the emergence of patients' symptoms and in psychiatrists' diagnostic and treatment practices. The power relationships within capitalist societies were held responsible for the disintegration of personality and for psychiatry itself becoming an actor in the perpetuation of oppression. Such analyses provided arguments for challenges to the authority of the medical model in understanding deviance and mental illness. The meeting of this challenge was in part the force behind the emergence of broader synthetic models, such as the conceptualisation of the biopsychosocial model of mental illness, which will be discussed later in the text (see Sections 2.2.3 and 2.3.4).

The work of Michel Foucault in the late 1960s and 1970s, in particular his text, *The History of Madness*, has been a significant (and continuing) influence on structuralist and post-structuralist thought in relation to understanding and analysis of mental disorder. Foucault's book is both an historical and philosophical critique of the ways in which society excluded unreason, physically demonstrated by the incarceration of the mad, in great numbers, in asylums. However, historians such as Andrew Scull (in Eghigian, 2017) and others (Porter, 1985) contest the basis of his argument by presenting a contrasting account of the actual numbers of people and their health, mental health and socioeconomic status who were institutionalised during the nineteenth century.

Nevertheless, it is apparent that since the mid-1970s there has been a radical change in ways in which mental health problems have been thought about. These changes have created challenges to earlier epistemologies of practice and research.

A recent issue of *Medical History* (Bacopoulos-Viau & Fauvel, 2015) presents several papers carrying forward the work of Porter (1985) and his call for a 'patient-centred' account of the history of psychiatry, the construction of a history 'from below'. This call occurs amid many changes (discussed in Sections 1.1.5, 1.1.6, 1.1.7, 1.7.2, 1.1.8, 2.3, 2.3.2 and Chapter 2.5)—deinstitutionalisation, advances in pharmacology, the continuing use of standardised diagnostic tools and the consistently emerging and more-audible voices of patients, service users, activists, advocates and carers. Recognition is increasingly being given to the understanding that individuals are embedded within cultural networks which shape sense of self, illness and identity. A perspective further exploring and analysing the history of psychiatry and mental health services informed by complexity theory (see Sections 1.1.1, 1.5.10 and 1.5.11) might enable us to better see how psychiatric patients and consumers are in fact integral to the construction and coevolution of the psychiatric, mental health and allied health professions.

FEMINIST PERSPECTIVES ON MENTAL ILLNESS

Feminist researchers and writers began to challenge dominant perspectives in the mental health field in the 1970s, proposing a different reading of the incidence, prevalence and meaning of women's mental illness. Emphasis began to be placed on understanding the conditions of women's lives as implicated in the causation of mental or emotional distress. Previous research and understanding of women's mental illness had focused on the belief that women were innately inferior to men, and had a biologically based tendency to mental pathology because of their reproductive and hormonal processes. Menstruation, childbirth and menopause were heavily implicated in creating a vulnerability to mental illness.

Against this explanation and viewpoint, feminist researchers have been critical of the adequacy of the evidence linking the impact of reproductive biology and specific mental states. In place of this link, arguments have been put that women's mental distress refers to the effect of the material, social and political constraints of their lives under the oppressive conditions of patriarchy. Their discontent is expressed through symptoms that have been interpreted as illness or disorder. The devaluing and disempowerment of women, which has been reflected throughout history, was understood to be present in tendencies to diagnose women as mentally ill more frequently than men, and in the apparently higher rates of depression prevalent among women. Feminist perspectives proposed that women's madness might be better understood as a manifestation of the emotional frustration, narrowness and confinement of their lives (Al-Issa, 1982; Astbury, 1996; Busfield, 1996; Chesler, 1989; Chesler, 1972; Jimenez, 1997; Penfold & Walker, 1983; Russell, 1995; Saltman, 1991; Stoppard, 1999; Stoppard & McMullen, 2003; Ussher, 1992; Willie, 1995).

In 2019, Women's Health Victoria's Submission to the Productivity Commission highlighted that the WHV considered gender '...a critical, overlaying social determinant of mental health and mental illness: Gender determines the differential power and control men and women have over the socioeconomic determinants of their mental health and lives, their social position, status and treatment in society and their susceptibility and exposure to specific mental health risks (Women's Health Victoria, 2019, p. 1).

There has also been increasing recognition of the impact of exposure to violence, in particular domestic and family violence (D/FV), on the health and mental health of women (Western, 2018). Disturbing statistics indicate the high incidence of reported exposure to violence in Australia: two in every five women (41%) have experienced violence since the age of 15 years. Around one in three (34%) has experienced physical violence and almost one in five (19%) has experienced sexual violence. The negative impacts of violence on women's health include poor mental health, in particular anxiety and depression, as well as alcohol and illicit drug use and suicide (Western, 2018).

The mental health consumer movement and the women's movement have tended to develop their agendas separately although sharing some political views, particularly with regard to issues of power and prejudice. Lewis discussed the reasons for this in the United Kingdom, noting that the women's movement has been particularly successful in applying pressure for change in service provision in other sectors by advancing models of 'good' women-sensitive practice (Lewis, 2009). In Victoria, policy concerning women's mental health services was raised in 1997 in *Tailoring Services to Meet the Needs of Women* (Victorian Department of Human Services, 1997). Eighteen years later, in 2016, the Australian Health Policy Collaboration published *Investing in Women's Mental Health: Strengthening the Foundations for Women, Families and the Australian Economy* (Duggan, 2016), noting the lack of attention to gender-sensitive mental health services in the National Mental Health Plans and arguing that there is a need for a gendered mental health policy. This report notes that there remains an absence of '... comprehensive recognition that gender influences the risks, impacts and consequences of mental illness. Overall, the service landscape remains extremely fragmented and gender-blind at best and in certain situations, particularly in inpatient units and prisons, lack of gender-sensitivity and specialist provision can amplify and perpetuate the risks of abuse and violence which may have already had adverse impacts on mental health. Moreover, there is clear evidence that women often do not receive appropriate mental health services whether they are in hospitals, prisons, nursing homes, addiction programs or community settings' (Duggan, 2016). The Fifth National Mental Health and Suicide Prevention Plan, while placing priority on Aboriginal and Torres Strait Islander people and safety issues for service users, consumers and carers, does not directly address the issue of gender-sensitive service provision. However, the Victorian Women and Mental Health Network (Women's Mental Health Network Victoria, 2020), active since 1988, continues to advocate for, among a number of issues and as a priority, inpatient safety for women in public and private psychiatric wards.

INCREASING RECOGNITION OF THE ROLE OF SOCIAL DETERMINANTS AND INEQUITY

Along with gender, many other demographic and social determinants influence occurrence, onset and severity of mental health problems. This has received increasing attention in the literature including in policy documents from the WHO (World Health Organization and the Calouste Gulbenkian Foundation, 2014). Beyond individual effects there also is considerable evidence that levels of inequity in societies are related to the rates of mental health problems in those societies (Wilkinson & Pickett, 2018). This is an issue of importance for both mental health practice and also social policy—it will be given extensive attention later in the text (see Chapter 1.2, and Sections 1.2.4, 1.2.5 and 1.6.3).

1.1.4 RESPONDING TO MENTAL DISORDER

FIONA MCDERMOTT & GRAHAM MEADOWS

INTRODUCTION

The struggle to understand mental illness proceeded simultaneously with attempts to intervene and treat those experiencing it. Tensions and contradictions evident in these attempts highlight the mix of motives and beliefs as to the nature of mental illness and the rights and responsibilities incumbent on those who intervened.

TREATMENT AS AN EMERGENT IDEA

The belief characterising Enlightenment thinking that the social and natural worlds could be transformed by human intervention and need not be taken as 'givens' was reflected during the late eighteenth and nineteenth centuries in the sequestering of those identified as poor, insane or criminal. Indeed, as Giddens points out (1991, pp. 155–60), the notion of deviance was constructed out of the desire to achieve regulation in social life. Those who could not be regulated (the poor, the insane and the criminal) were constructed as deviants. However, this deviant status required that special settings (poorhouses, prisons and asylums) be established for them, whereby remedial treatment and regularised control could be asserted over them. An outcome of this was their increasing invisibility as they were excluded from social and community life. The threat that their disturbing modes of behaviour may have posed to the maintenance of social order had been, it was hoped, screened out.

Contemporary debates in the eighteenth century over the virtues of both medical and moral treatments (Scull, 1989) suggest that the Enlightenment philosophy of attaining cures and remedies for the insane was firmly in evidence. The mental hospital, as Giddens points out (1991, p. 159), had as its purpose the creation of a humane environment that would methodically correct for deficiencies and reform the afflicted personality.

INNOVATION AND EXNOVATION

Following the increasingly systematic and experimental approach taken to medicine after the Enlightenment, a body of demonstratively effective treatments accumulated. This process gathered momentum during the twentieth century, because of developments of technologies and strategies for the empirical testing of treatments. As will be introduced elsewhere in this text (see Chapter 2.5), advances can be considered in terms of efficacy advances or practice improvements (better tolerated or easier to prescribe treatments)—both forms of innovation. The term 'exnovation' (Frank & Glied, 2006b) has been coined to describe abandonment of practice no longer seen as beneficial.

TREATMENTS FOR NEUROLOGICAL DISEASES

Before 1900, the asylums had contained large numbers of people suffering not with what would now be seen as psychiatric disorders but with consequences of syphilis and uncontrolled epilepsy. This changed through the early part of the twentieth century, with increasingly effective treatments for these conditions.

For syphilis, salvarsan treatment was introduced in Germany in 1909, and from the 1940s and 1950s, penicillin treatment further improved the outcomes for people with this disorder.

For treatment of seizure disorders, barbital in 1903, phenobarbital in 1912 and a host of other anticonvulsants since, have transformed these problems into predominantly manageable conditions.

PHYSICAL TREATMENTS

Better drug treatments for mental illness

Research utilising randomised controlled clinical trial methodology has, since the 1940s, proved highly suitable for conducting trials of various psychotropic drugs (see Chapter 1.4). Significant outcomes were achieved in the development of medication for people suffering from schizophrenia, depression and bipolar mood disorders. Before these improvements in psychotropic drugs, the majority of people with serious mental illnesses were in many countries receiving institution-based treatment, spending the greater part of their lives in hospitals and asylums.

There was a burst of activity in the production of new psychotropic drugs in the years after World War II, and in the 1950s many drugs still in wide use today were introduced. An early contribution to this was Australian: the introduction of lithium by John Cade for the treatment of mania in 1949. The drug was adopted widely in the 1960s after being shown to be effective in maintenance treatment of bipolar disorder. The first generation of effective antipsychotic medications was ushered in by chlorpromazine, initially reported as effective in treating psychosis in 1952 in France, and coming into use more widely through the 1950s. The antidepressant effect of imipramine was reported in 1957, introducing the tricyclic antidepressants, and in the same year the first of the benzodiazepine tranquillisers (chlordiazepoxide or librium) was synthesised.

Sometimes new drugs offer increased effectiveness; for example, clozapine, an early second-generation antipsychotic drug (see Chapter 2.5), may often treat schizophrenia effectively where the condition has not responded to other interventions. More commonly, the new drugs constitute *practice advances*—having similar effectiveness to the older drugs, but fewer side effects, or being less dangerous in overdose. Hence, there are changed terms of exchange surrounding the drug: the amount of side-effect that has to be undergone to attain the therapeutic effect, making the drugs much more attractive to many consumers. In this category we can put fluoxetine, sertraline and other drugs in this class of the serotonin specific reuptake inhibitors for depression, and also risperidone, olanzapine, quietiapine and others (see Chapter 2.5) as novel antipsychotics. What we are describing here is by way of a pattern where a period of dramatic efficacy advances has been followed by developments more typically in the way of practice advances (Frank & Glied, 2006a).

Electroconvulsive therapy

Electroconvulsive therapy (ECT), an Italian invention dating from 1938, was first used in schizophrenia, but has proved most effective in severe depression. In ECT, passage of an electrical current through the brain causes a seizure, and it is this seizure that has therapeutic effect. When initially used on patients who were conscious before application of the shock, this technique was a desperate measure, horrifying in application and with high risks of broken bones from the unmodified seizures. Memory disturbance following the seizures could be severe. Understandably, ECT gained a reputation as a barbaric practice. The technique has been progressively refined and, with the use of anaesthetic and paralytic agents, brought into line with appropriately humane modern standards. Measurement of the brain seizure response through monitoring of brain electrical activity with the EEG has added to the sophistication of the technique. It now ranks among the safest of medical interventions for depression (see Chapters 2.5 and 4.2). Understandably, though, in the minds of many, the practice still carries a fearful set of associations.

Other physical treatments

Some previously widely used treatments have become understood to be ineffective or even potentially harmful and so have been subject to exnovation as termed here (see Section 1.1). Insulin coma therapy, deep sleep therapy and earlier crude forms of psychosurgery would fall in this category. Newer and innovative approaches, including deep brain stimulation and transcutaneous magnetic stimulation, are coming into wider use as demonstrably efficacious once hurdles to their dissemination are overcome.

PSYCHOLOGICAL TREATMENTS

Psychological interventions have progressed dramatically in efficacy through the later part of the twentieth century as the behavioural and cognitive revolutions brought new and often highly efficacious treatments into play and further waves of treatments are now finding their places (see Section 2.6.7). Psychodynamic therapy, though still having its place in treatments for some problems and being of value for personal development for many choosing to spend time in therapy, has been generally abandoned in regards to some of its earlier uses, such as in primary treatments of schizophrenia, this being another example of exnovation.

RECOVERY

Recovery as a term permeating the rhetoric of contemporary mental health care burst onto the Australian scene in the first decade of this century. Although coined in its modern professional usage nearly 30 years ago (Anthony, 1993), the term does not appear in either of the first two national Mental Health Plans (1993–98, 1998–2003), but by the third (2003–08) and later plans (see Sections 1.7.1, 1.7.2, 1.4.11 and 1.5.4), it is present on almost every page. This has been followed by articulation of a national framework for recovery oriented mental health services that includes policy and practice guidance (Commonwealth of Australia, 2013), and in direction setting in all states and territories (see Section 1.7.2). The intent is clear in recent government policy making that services should seek to transform service delivery towards the adoption of effective models that will serve to enhance recovery.

'Applications of recovery' as a term will be explored at multiple sites in this text (see Sections 1.1.6, 1.5.2, 1.7.2 and 2.6.2) and further understanding of how it may usefully be understood will typically develop through exposure to the term in a range of different contexts. At one level, the concept of recovery is a reflection of the episodic nature of much of mental illness. Periods of recovery are common. Recovery has also been associated with relapse prevention, or the steps to be taken to prolong periods of wellness between episodes of illness (Rickwood, 2005). However, and beyond this, we can observe that over time 'recovery' has taken on the qualities of a movement, initially with aspects of a protest movement led by consumers against psychiatric practices that were often seen as oppressive, and not giving due recognition or value to consumers' first-hand experiences. Over time it has come to have positive attributes strongly connected with values of agency, empowerment and choice for consumers. It also has been adopted, or it could be critically argued co-opted (Russo & Sweeney, 2016), into approaches described as 'recovery oriented practice' (see Section 2.6.2). The task of aligning working practices with recovery for most services at time of writing is something of a work in progress. It is something that may involve critical and reflective consideration of values through interpersonal and intrapersonal dialectical discussion as well as acknowledgement of complexity. In practice terms, to borrow from concepts above, it will challenge us to both innovation and exnovation in working practices.

1.1.5 WHO SHOULD DO SOMETHING TO/FOR/ WITH PEOPLE WITH MENTAL ILLNESS?

FIONA MCDERMOTT & GRAHAM MEADOWS

Questions concerning the best ways to respond to the problems posed by mental illness demonstrate the linkages between knowledge and interests of stakeholder groups. The history of developments in the mental health field over the last 250 years reflects a gradual opening up of a field of interests. These interests represent a broader base of involvement, demonstrated by the active participation of allied health service providers, service users and consumers, and carers. The move towards deinstitutionalisation has undoubtedly been driven by a number of historical forces, including, as set out above, treatments for neurosyphilis and epilepsy in the early part of the twentieth century, and better psychotropics, beginning in the 1950s.

Movements in the 1960s and 1970s aimed at ensuring civil rights of all citizens also played their part in the move towards community treatment, as did the empirical testing of models for delivery of care in the community in the 1970s and 1980s. Today, in many service settings, we can truly be seen as being in a post-institutional stage of mental health practice, with many clinicians and clients never having had experience of working or being cared for in the large institutional asylum settings.

The achievements of psychotropic drug research and development have, as we have noted, contributed to helping people experiencing mental disorders spend less time in hospital, and typically for brief rather than long-term admissions. However, these advances have certainly not allowed psychiatry to bask in the glory of its therapeutic triumphs. The civil rights movements of the mid and late twentieth century have been critical of institutions, and the role of medicine in practices associated with them, which have been seen as oppressive and even abusive. In the United States, in particular, this played a part in provoking a neo-Kraepelinian revival in the 1970s (Klerman, 1990). The neo-Kraepelinian paradigm emphasised the role of the psychiatrist as expert diagnostician, and held that 'psychiatry was the specialty of medicine, concerned with mental disorders and their scientific understanding, as well as with the diagnosis and treatment of individuals suffering from these disorders' (Klerman, 1990, p. 29). Thus, in the United States, psychiatry in many ways sought to 'remedicalise' and thereby regain some lost aspects of its reputation and credibility. This movement was much less pronounced in the United Kingdom, and the Australian position could be seen as lying somewhere between these strands.

The movement towards deinstitutionalisation and community care has meant that people experiencing mental illness are now more visible and audible. The responsibility for their care (and control) has shifted to community-based clinical and rehabilitation services. Where previously services were provided almost solely by psychiatrists and hospital-based workers, the shift to community-based programs was intended to open up treatment and intervention provision to a range of service providers: social workers, occupational therapists, psychologists, nurses, general practitioners and psychiatrists. Each of these professions shows differing epistemologies of practice and research. Deinstitutionalisation and community care initiatives have also meant that families are more frequently involved in the care and accommodation of mentally ill members. Where community services are weak, this can lead to difficulties, both for familial caregivers and the people themselves.

The rapid changes wrought by deinstitutionalisation and community care have presented a challenge for delivery of care. While there are many community agencies, resources are scarce and these agencies are fragmented in ways in which the asylums, as total institutions, were not (see Chapter 1.7). There are three principal provider groups: professionals from a range of disciplines (including medical, allied health, legal, psychosocial rehabilitation, criminal justice and religious groups); family members and carers; and service user and/or consumer-survivor groups. Each interest group varies in the particular issues and concerns that motivate it. Professional groups differ in their perspectives on the place and the various merits of clinical treatment and psychosocial rehabilitation practices. Family and carer groups have been concerned to advocate improved services. Consumer-survivor groups have lobbied for a range of empowering services and the opportunity to establish and maintain self-help initiatives. Indeed, the involvement of consumers, service users and survivors in their own treatment and as a critical voice in evaluating intervention treatment responses, as will be discussed below, has been one of the most significant developments in the mental health field, and in contemporary times, offering increasingly sophisticated theoretical understanding, most notably the concept of 'consumer perspective', which will be a feature of many other contributions to the text (see, for example, Sections 1.1.6 and 1.1.7). Throughout this text, and starting in this first chapter, we are seeking to accommodate these perspectives. Here we are in alignment with the idea that the development of higher-level decision making and practice capacities are supported by relatively conventional critical thinking, but also importantly by the capacity to see things from multiple viewpoints, tolerating complexity and with an ability to constructively contain internal dialogue and dialectical process. Section 1.1.6 provides two consumer perspectives that may serve a function of opening the reader up to such processes, one on service and policy development and another on the role of consumers in professional and other training activities.

1.1.6 CONSUMER PERSPECTIVES AND CONTRIBUTIONS

ALLAN PINCHES

STRATEGIC THINKING AND PRACTICAL PROGRAMS FOR CHANGE: KEY OUTPUTS OF AUSTRALIA'S MENTAL HEALTH CONSUMER MOVEMENT

Over recent decades, the mental health consumer movement in Australia has made a significant contribution to a wave of innovation and change in the mental health field, with the widespread deinstitutionalisation of mental health services.

INTRODUCTION

In a historically transformative period, like developments overseas, there was a gradual build-up toward deinstitutionalisation, followed by a time of 'lift-off', in the mid-1990s in Victoria and soon after in other states. The consumer movement was to play a crucial role in the changes but was still a relatively modest operation.

The mental health field underwent sweeping reforms, with new thinking and continuing on-the-ground restructure of services, helping to form something of a two-way street with the consumer movement experiencing an enormous period of growth and development, emerging as a major catalyst and strategic partner for change.

Major trends included:

- A massive shift away from large, long stay, institutional psychiatric hospitals and relocation of most services 'in the community' including small psychiatric inpatient units co-located with general hospitals. Mental health patients were intended to live and re-integrate into the community, with policies stating adequate backup services would be in place.

- Mental health consumers, on the strength of research and development projects, notably including the landmark 'U & I' (Understanding and Involvement) project (see Section 1.4.8) auspiced by the Victorian Mental Illness Awareness Council, prepared the ground for governments and services for their adoption of a policy of consumer participation in the planning and development of mental health services. This aligns with UN Covenants on mental health and disability maintaining the right of consumers to have their say in services, as well as full social participation.
- A range of non-government psychosocial rehabilitation and support services were also set up—often amid much community debate, the advocacy of concerned family carers and expressed needs of consumers themselves. These services provided varied levels of supports in local areas—such as group housing with support, community linkages, and social activities and groups via day programs, but in recent years day programs have largely been taken out of the service mix, with stated intentions of enhancing individual support.
- These organisations proved an important seeding ground for consumer participation, and consumers gave back enormously.
- Building upon extensive developmental work of consumers and key allies here and abroad, mental health psychosocial support services and later, clinical services, began to include recovery-based approaches in mental health service provision.
- The foundational and multifaceted work of consumer consultants led to a progression of lived experience roles, including peer support workers, consumer advocates, consumer academics, educators, researcher, and other roles still evolving.
- Consumer workers have contributed to public inquiries and legislative reform over the years, and have a growing role in mental health governance, public information, service accreditation standards, staff selection panels, advocacy and appeals, and other functions.
- There has been a rapidly increasing range of consumer-designed research projects, services, programs, consumer-led conferences and training courses, many publications, including a proliferation of sites and stories on consumer issues on social media.
- Consumers are becoming more widely involved as Educators and Trainers for service providers and with their own consumer colleagues, a focus on recovery-based methods, peer support, and trauma-informed approaches.
- High profile organisations, which employ some consumers, have been running awareness campaigns aimed at reducing stigma and discrimination around mental health, which seems to have increased recognition of these issues and the need for wider discussion.

A PRACTICAL SLICE OF A MOVEMENT'S LARGER, MORE INSPIRATIONAL HISTORY

Influences are clearly discernible today of the consumer movement's proud history and origins, including continuing links to human rights and social justice causes. These influences included: the black Civil Rights Movement of the 1960s in the United States; the Peace Movement and counter-culture; feminism and emerging critical social theories; the LGBTIQ struggles; the disability movement's campaigns under the banner 'Nothing about us without us' and the independent living movement; the Indigenous *First People's* movement; and the work of US consumer rights campaigner, Ralph Nader.

The local context was also important: how mental health services were developing; how the thinking of many about society or government was changing; and what possibilities were opening for more professionalised and instrumental movement.

THE GROWING AND EVOLVING MENTAL HEALTH CONSUMER MOVEMENT

The mental health consumer movement in Australia has, in recent years, undergone a major growth in numbers, influence, sophistication of its operations, and range and capacity in relation to issues it can deal with. The movement continues to provide a vital consumer advocacy voice about problems and possible solutions in mental health systems. Its advocacy work has evolved and diversified into many different streams, which seem likely to become distinct sub-disciplines.

In part this has been about responding to a broad panoply of social and economic issues, many of which are prominent in public debate about groups of people suffering disadvantage, and growing perceptions among some in the community that these issues had intersected with 'mental health issues' all along. Inexorably, many ways are emerging of applying a growing body of consumer knowledge to questions raised in services and in the wider community.

LEADERSHIP STYLES, MEMBERSHIP ENGAGEMENT AND MORE JOINED-UP APPROACHES

The consumer movement has experienced a major replenishment of leadership in recent years, and many of these key people seem to take pride in their own lived experience and their attempts to help deploy the collective consumer movement knowledge, philosophies and methods into the work of organisations.

There is a trend towards setting up working teams and trying harder to be inclusive of the voices of consumers, including providing opportunities for people to gather together, work together, and enjoy some collegial satisfaction of being active in such a movement. Consumer leaders come from varied backgrounds but tend to affirm concepts like human rights and social justice, empowerment, participatory democracy, education and information sharing, community development, participatory action research (see Sections 1.4.1 and 1.4.8), and above all, respecting the lived experience of consumers.

There are still many areas where the consumer movement will probably always need to monitor and explore its balances around leadership and grassroots participation, with tensions inherent to advocacy messaging and free expression: especially with a growing critique of the notion of 'Representation' (Happell & Roper, 2006).

Constructive partnerships and collaboration with other organisations, including with mental health services and government, are often viewed as desirable for progress, and when critique of the systemic problems is required, diplomacy and balance, with evidence-based advocacy backed by consumer research, can make a big difference. In 2018, NSW, Victoria, WA and other consumers renewed proposals to the Federal Government for a dedicated National Mental Health Consumer Peak Organisation, along similar lines to a 1996–2008 organisation which had been defunded, and had been a national advocacy voice, a coordination body and a research and policy engine. The consumer movement also became further activated by the Victorian Government's announcement of a Royal Commission into Mental Health, which sparked widespread and varied interest.

There has also been an influx of young people into the movement, with fresh hopes and dreams, tech savvy, broad educational and working backgrounds, with energy and enthusiasm, and a belief in equality of opportunity. Some older consumers say it is hard to get over the institutional past, and cope with social and economic difficulties when support services in the community and welfare benefits are becoming increasingly tenuous. An example is the difficulties mental health consumers encounter in the funding and eligibility rules of the National Disability Insurance Scheme (NDIS).

LIVED EXPERIENCE CONSUMER WORK GROWING AND DIVERSIFYING

Lived experience consumer workers are now employed in mental health in a growing range of roles, with many in the foundational and multi-faceted role of Consumer Consultant where they facilitate a relationship between services and consumers, conduct surveys, hold forums, and disseminate newsletters, design and maintain complaints/feedback systems, facilitate consumer advisory groups, and lead many innovative research and development projects, and many activities broadly under the heading of service improvement. The value of consumer consultants has been noted in several consumer-based participatory action research reports, and while there have been significant improvements in the take-up of the CCs' work in organisations, many still encounter problems and constraints. These include issues around employment pay and conditions; heavy and sometimes too open-ended workloads; lack of tailored training, lack of peer-based supervision or definition of career paths; a continuing shortage of funding; and service culture and degree of acceptance of consumer roles by other staff are still cited as problematic among consumers (Bennetts, 2009; Pinches, 2004; Byrne, Roper, Happell, & Reid-Searl, 2019).

CONSUMERS AS PIONEERS IN DEVELOPING RECOVERY-BASED APPROACHES

Consumers are noted to have played a major part in the introduction of recovery approaches in mental health since the late 1990s (see Sections 1.1.6, 1.5.2 and 2.6.2), in the United States and elsewhere, and recovery topics occupied many articles and conference sessions for many years, beginning as early as the 1980s.

Consumer-oriented notions of recovery tend to be less concerned with questions of *diagnosis, symptoms, or cure,* but rather, maintain that the consumer's lived experience is an area where change can happen, with or without symptoms. The consumer movement tends to refer to this as *personal recovery.* Based on the explorations of consumers who have sought to understand life lessons accompanying mental health challenges, including myself and friends and my own research, recovery approaches often aim to support and encourage the person to seek an enhanced sense of hope, empowerment, and introduce a range of knowledge and resources, to help gain a greater degree of control over one's life and possibilities (Pinches, 2011, p. 7).

Major elements may include: personal empowerment based on learning new skills; getting a better compass on the world; good referrals to genuinely worthwhile community resources; building confidence and social connection; linking to education, employment and other options genuinely aligned to one's interest.

A leading ally to the consumer movement on recovery approaches, Professor Larry Davidson, a US psychologist, with colleagues, wrote:

> In addition to hope, recovery from mental illness, broadly defined, involves a process of overcoming some of the consequences of the illness; gaining an enhanced sense of identity; empowerment, and meaning, and purpose in life; and developing valued social roles, citizenship, and community connections despite a person's symptoms profile or continued disability. In recent years there has been a growing emphasis on mental health care that supports rather than hinders people's opportunities to participate in such processes of healing (Davidson, O'Connell, Tondora, Staeheli, & Evans, 2005; Slade, Leese, Cahill, Thornicroft, & Kuipers, 2005).

The influential recovery approach writings of a 'lived experience' consumer–psychologist, Dr Patricia Deegan—have also been enormously influential to the consumer movement and particularly with concepts around recovery and social justice.

Deegan wrote:

> For many of us who are [psychosocially] disabled, recovery is a process, a way of life, an attitude, and a way of approaching the day's challenges. It is not a perfectly linear process. At times our course is erratic, and we falter, slide back, regroup and start again...
>
> The need is to meet the challenge of the disability and to re-establish a new and valued sense of integrity and purpose within and beyond the limits of the disability. The aspiration is to live, work, and love in a community in which one makes significant contribution (Deegan, 1988, p. 11-19).

CONSUMERS WORKING IN PEER SUPPORT: A BIG BREAKTHROUGH

For a long time, both consumers and carers have aspired to augment the mental health workforce with peer support workers (see Sections 1.1.7, 1.6.6, 2.2, and 2.3.10). This growth has begun, with these workers now a more common feature, employed within both clinical and psychosocial rehabilitation and support services across Australia. Out of a total mental health workforce of 28 600, in 2017-18, there were 184 consumer full-time equivalent (FTE) workers employed in public mental health services and 68 carer FTE.

Peer workers are supporting consumers on inpatient units as they move towards discharge, and providing short-term follow-up support for consumers being discharged back into the community. Many other clinical and community rehabilitation and support services now include an element of peer support, including some of the larger, more regulated facilities such as Region-based Peer Hubs, Community Care Units, Secure Extended Care Units, and forensic services. Considerable work is going into improving the quality and consistency of training opportunities and peer supervision arrangements for peer support workers.

Shery Mead, a consumer-based psychologist in the United States, along with several consumer colleagues, developed an approach called Intentional Peer Support (IPS), upon which several Peer Crisis Centres were developed, and the model exported to other countries including Australia.

Mead wrote in an essay explaining some theoretical underpinnings of IPS:

> Traditional research methodologies and hypotheses are founded on the belief that we won't get over having a mental illness; we are only capable of 'functional' healing as we attain certain socially prescribed goals—housing, job security, social integration, and so forth. There is no dialogue about wellness or about how we might exist, even thrive, within a culture that values and evaluates based on our own personal goals. If researchers would let go of methodology and epistemology that defines mental illness as a permanent disability we could, through dialectical evaluation of how people have recovered, explore the relationship of peer support and self-help to recovery (Mead, Hilton, & Curtis, 2001).

IPS has emerged as a leading consumer-based trauma-informed approach to peer support, originating from peer support centre models aiming for a person-centred, recovery-based approach. A rich tradition of peer support service models from here and abroad, which have been consumer developed, has much to offer and can often be licensed for Australian use. Examples are: Intentional Peer Support, (US) PeerZone, Flourish, and WRAP (from Wellness Recovery Action Plan operating in UK and US and Australia) and TePou (NZ).

An example of innovative large-scale service based largely on peer support is CAN (Consumer Activity Network), in Sydney, which includes mental health aftercare *Hospital in the Home* support, 'warm lines' involving conversations rather than counselling, encouragement of self-advocacy, educative discussions, 'drop-in' times, and meaningful roles for volunteers. Another notable Sydney organisation is the Richmond Psychiatric Rehabilitation Association, which has a large range of activities, with about 30% of staff coming from lived experience.

OTHER CONSUMER DEVELOPED AND RUN SUPPORT INITIATIVES

These include:

- New methods like Recovery Colleges, Recovery Camps, Hearing Voices Network, which aim to be *non-judgemental* of the experiences of consumers and affirm their search for what is meaningful to them.
- Trauma-informed services which have had consumers involved in all stages of development and delivery, including the Open Dialogue approach and Intentional Peer Support.
- Consumer-run services now exist to support, inform, and help advocate for consumers applying for NDIS coverage (e.g., VMIAC.)
- Mental Health First Aid and alternative methods of suicide prevention, such as Alt2Su (Alternatives to Suicide).
- Consumer-run internet, social media, video, community radio, arts, music, drama, community education projects, 'Mad Pride' comedy events, alternative cultural spaces. The movement has increasing links with alternative community venues such as creative writing, storytelling for social change, performance poetry events, pop-up community learning venues, including numerous 'Meetup' groups (Byrne et al., 2019).

CONSUMERS' GROWING ROLE AS RESEARCHERS AND EDUCATORS

The Centre for Mental Health Research at the Australian National University hosts ACACIA—the Australian Capital Territory's Consumer and Carer Mental Health Research Unit. It was established in 2013 with funding from ACT Health and aims to undertake research which is relevant to and benefits the lives of mental health consumers and carers in the ACT. All the research is conducted in partnership with consumers and carers. ACACIA staff members and students are mental health consumers or carers with academic expertise and qualifications. ACACIA also has an Advisory Group comprising local consumers and carers as well as the heads of the key ACT consumer and carer organisations. This kind of formal consumer and carer mental health academic unit remains rare.

There are increasing numbers of consumer-generated research and development reports, articles, and social media materials, building up daily, within the realms of consumer organisations, academic organisations and service provider sites. There are growing numbers of consumer academics carrying out specialised work at universities in Australia, reflecting trends here, and including the United States, UK, New Zealand, and parts of Europe.

A project called Learning Together: Education and Training Partnerships in Mental Health, in 1999 (Department of Health and Aged Care, 1999) as part of the National Mental Health Strategy has become known as 'The Deakin Papers', and made an enduring case for consumers as educators and researchers. Merinda Epstein and Daniel Rechter, as reference for group delegates, wrote:

> If we can guarantee the valuing of consumer perspectives, then we can begin to differentiate various roles users might have as representatives of our body of expert knowledge: as consultants, educators and trainers...As consultants to services our role is one of change agent. Where individual users are unable to articulate what they want, because such services cannot be imagined in the present, or more commonly they are not being listened to, consumer consultants can function as a kind of 'litmus test' for change (Epstein & Rechter, p. 24).

While there has been considerable progress towards the aspiration of consumers working in highly integrated ways as lived experience educators and researchers in services and academia, a great deal of potential lies ahead.

CONSUMER RESEARCH 'MANIFESTOS' IN UK AND AUSTRALIA

Comprehensively designed prospective research agendas—or 'manifestos'—have been formulated by the Australia-based Consumer Led Research Network (NSW Consumer Led Research Network, 2016), and the UK's National Survivor Research Network, with many project ideas (Survivor Researcher Network, 2018).

Australian network convenor Dr Katherine H Gill wrote about the growing role of consumer researchers in mental health, and growing official recognition.

> Consumer researchers are not just researchers with a lived experience of mental illness/mental distress, but researchers who are skilled at harnessing their lived experience purposefully, alongside their professional training, experience and qualifications, to contribute to the research at all stages throughout the research processes... (Gill, 2017, p. 51).

According to Gill, there was no shortage of qualified consumer researchers but there was a shortage of opportunities to participate.

In 2000 Cath Roper was appointed as Australia's first consumer academic at the Centre for Mental Health Nursing Research and Practice, Melbourne University. She wrote about what consumer perspectives could contribute to co-production research.

> Over time consumers have developed unique ways of knowing, theorising and thinking about those experiences that constitute a unique discipline in the field of mental health, known in Australia

as 'consumer perspective'. When using consumer perspective, consumers 'offer their own *analyses* of their experience and the services and systems they encountered'.

An explicit goal of co-production is to reposition people who have traditionally been thought of as passive 'consumers' of services to being regarded as people with necessary expertise who can lead thinking and innovation (Byrne et al., 2019; Roper, 2016a, pp. 18, 19).

The consumer movement over time has contributed to the development of various 'new' or 'alternative' qualitative research methods, including participatory action research, facilitated workshops and focus groups, co-production research, Experience Based Co-Design, adaptable satisfaction or exit surveys, agile ways of utilising online tools like Survey Monkey, and myriad forms of consumer participation.

Such methods can support consumer perspective approaches (see Sections 1.4.1, 1.4.9 and 1.4.10), with an enhanced focus on consumers' experiences, responses, and suggestions for change; they can encourage a sense of inclusion and collaboration for participants; and foster a reflective, holistic approach to solution seeking, including a focus on factors which can contribute towards consumer recovery and enhanced awareness of broader social determinants of health.

1.1.7 THE CONTRIBUTION OF CONSUMERS TO PROFESSIONAL TRAINING OF THE MENTAL HEALTH WORKFORCE

MERINDA EPSTEIN

INTRODUCTION

Students and clinicians working in mental health need to know that the contribution of consumers is not an extra add on to the professional training. It is an essential part of it.

CLINICAL PERSPECTIVE

Every clinician brings to their practice a clinical perspective. This is gained through professional education, an apprenticeship model of learning and often an influential hidden curriculum. This perspective feeds the professional views and skills clinicians profess and act upon. Within these are the various specific world views of the different clinical groups. Thus interpretations of medical knowledge and practice are always filtered through a specific perspective (or lens); that of being a clinician.

VIEWS OF CLINICIANS

Every clinician also holds and sometimes promulgates both personal and professional views. These views might have been developed through experience as a student and clinician but their roots will be influenced by personal life experiences of influential social institutions: a child of migrants, a survivor of family violence, a secret of mental illness, a father of a child with a disability or an experience of a good school.

Complicating any analysis is the way that some professional groups use the term 'clinical view' to mean 'clinical opinion'. This needs clarification. Important to this discussion is the idea of 'view' which means that we all, including all clinicians and all consumers, bring with us a worldview based on our knowledge of life in all its vagaries, uncertainties and complexities. Views are very different from a perspective and different from a 'clinical opinion'.

Views as experiences of life are not just about the psycho-disposition of the individual or the characteristics of the group such as the 'competitive urge' in doctors or the 'caring urge' in nurses or, perhaps, the political urge in active consumers. It is also about the large social forces that create the society in which we live; one that often re-creates our social world in the image of only some of us. If perspective is the lens through which we view mental distress then views are the many salient meanings we 'see' when we move through this prism to our own understandings.

CONSUMER PERSPECTIVE

Clinicians involved in the provision of mental health services have a perspective born of destiny. This is not debatable. Theirs is a perspective that holds authority and power–divided unevenly admittedly. Consumers also have a fundamental perspective. It is situated in powerlessness not power. There are considerable ethical considerations to be made about the subjective position of the consumer voice. The lens through which we undertake to make a commentary on service provision is one of being done 'on' and 'to' (Wadsworth, 2011) by systems of care. This is the consumer perspective. Our venture is to challenge such powerlessness but it is the lack of power that references us. It is very tempting for better educated consumers, consumers who are also clinicians, consumers who are also family carers, for example, to step outside their consumer perspective. Although the content of the views they put forward may be garnered, soundly, by gathering information and ideas from others, the consequence of skewing consumer perspective is to earn points towards sameness with clinicians, use power–even on behalf of others–feel less ashamed or market themselves in the burgeoning consumer worker market place. The problem is that only some consumers, in some situations, are able to speak directly and this is not 'a consumer perspective'. The extent to which this is ethical given the perspective we claim to bring to the table is questionable. This is not a matter of differing views. It is a matter of fundamental perspective, power and discourse.

THE CLINICAL-CONSUMER PERSPECTIVE: A PROBLEM FOR HEALTH EDUCATORS

Too often clinical educators (and others) get caught up in an idea that clinicians provide the technical knowledge, professional perspective and expertise, and consumers, if included at all, simply provide the story. This is empowering for many consumers who want their experience of health systems heard. Consumer perspective is egalitarian and non-competitive. However, health educators often want consumer views (especially as stories) without adequately understanding the need for and respect of consumer perspective. Powerless people are easily picked off and it is in the interest of the powerful to pit story against story, experience against experience and diagnosis against diagnosis. Society takes our power away and university students may, at least, give us back some recognition and admiration. This can be attractive. Some clinical educators seem to be searching for the 'real consumer' and some clinicians search for people 'just like my patients' or 'just like my clients'. The refusal to share power in these instances is obvious. To argue for the purity of the non-political consumer is to be political. To search for consumers who will only tell the stories you want and are willing to hear simply amplifies the forces that work against truly collaborative mental health practice.

CONSUMER VIEWS

If consumer perspective, like nursing perspective, is a way of looking at the world, then what consumers see or remember or don't want to remember, like what individual nurses see and remember and don't want to remember, can be just about anything. Whereas perspective is singular, views are infinite–for all groups in the sector. They are based on training but they are also based on society, our place in society and individual life circumstances. The political reality is that the views of people who align themselves with professional groups are always privileged in relation to consumer views. This reality is denied mainly because those with privilege rarely recognise they have privilege, which is very different from many consumers who are acutely aware their views are too often seen as an adornment. Clinical perspectives are not uniform. Professional groups interact hierarchically. Nurses, for example, don't feel that their views are always privileged. They are but they don't feel it. Individual consumer knowing is often tokenistic or patronised in complex realities of ideology and power. Views are important but they will have little traction if ways cannot be found to bring them together and analyse memories and events in a coherent way guided by a perspective of what it means to be diagnosed with a mental illness. There

Table 1.2 Lemon Tree Learning perspectives

Acquisition	• Consumer perspective is acquired as a result of receiving, or being unable to receive when you wish to, services in the mental health system.
The 'lens'	• Consumer perspective is about looking at madness and mental health institutions through the eyes of someone who has experienced it first-hand as a 'patient'. Closely tied to this... is the experience of having viewed the world... through eyes that have been categorised as in some way 'mad' or perhaps... [distressed] enough to require intervention from a mental health professional.
Basic assumptions	• That individual consumers are 'the experts' about their own life and being, carrying the wisdom to best articulate their own needs if they are accorded the time, space and means to do so.
Consumer perspective is:	• Developed out of a collective consciousness and political solidarity that grew from the consumer/user/survivor movement. • Like feminist perspective, wog perspective, and from the women's movement etc. • About 'belonging' to a group of people who are marginalised and discriminated against.
It is often, at an individual level, where politics is located—the politics of powerlessness	• Not just a political arm or a dedicated movement. • Camaraderie on acute units described by many. • Valiant personal attempts to protect other consumers sometimes in dangerous spaces. • Training sessions run by consumers which resonate. • Black humour shared by many. • Learning the ropes from old hands more useful than systems information. • Holding back personal information on others when it is required by staff. • Lying for sound reasons. • Not dobbing. • Unusual places for bonding.
Non-consumer perspective	• To interpret someone else's behaviour using the tools supplied by the medical establishment as this is not consumer perspective language for all. • Being aware that 'stories', experiences and views are not always shared even when perspective is. It is not consumer perspective to speak on others' behalf without permission.
Themes representing consumer perspective culture	• Questioning the medical model. • Defining what has happened to you in your own way. • Choosing what you want to happen next. • Staff behaviour which is health promoting rather than health assaulting. • Questioning taken-for-granted definitions of professionalism.
Consumer-including practice	• ...minimise observing through professional perspective eyes or assuming righteous authority simply because of an affiliation with an established professional base.
Consumer intelligence	• We know more than you think. • Consumer-common sense. • Not all that is seen from outside as powerlessness actually is. Sometimes disempowerment is mined by consumers to actually deal with powerlessness. This is not 'manipulation' and what is described as manipulation in services is sometimes a very healthy component of consumer perspective communication.
	Consumer perspective is an historically wary one.

Source: Epstein, 1997

is nothing wrong with personal stories in principle, indeed they can be powerful. They are seductive for many consumers and they might be good for the mental health of all, but there's a question mark around whether they actually lead to changes in practice. The challenge for the consumer movement is whether story without consumer-driven analysis is actually useful.

THE LEMON TREE LEARNING PROJECT

In Australia the idea of a consumer perspective was first articulated by Shaw and Epstein in 1997. Their argument was that there are certain characteristics of being a consumer that could be brought together as shared. They called these shared attributes 'perspective'. Although they described some attributes of a consumer perspective their emphasis was on the consumer way of looking at things—the lens. Table 1.2 summarises the main points about perspective from the Lemon Tree Learning work.

1.1.8 THE CARER PERSPECTIVE

RICHARD BALDWIN, JONATHAN HARMS & CASSANDRA HASTIE

INTRODUCTION

Informal carers play an important role in the lives of people with a mental illness. In most cases they provide care for a much longer period than formal mental health services. Mental health services provide a complementary role to that of the informal carer and for this reason it is important to understand the role that carers provide and how they must be involved in the planning and delivery of mental health services.

WHO IS A CARER?

A 'carer' is a person who cares for an individual requiring assistance. While the term can refer to either paid or unpaid carers, and the reason for the need for care covers a wide range of disabilities, the focus of this discussion is on unpaid carers of people with a mental disability and/or illness. Some publications refer to family members and carers, which can be confusing as not all family members are carers. For simplicity here, the term 'carers' should be read as including family members who provide care.

Unpaid carers are bearing the burden of care for people who identify as having a psychosocial disability. According to the Australian Bureau of Statistics (ABS) (2015a), there were 823 000 people in Australia with a psychosocial disability in 2015. Of these over 600 000 people reported receiving care of some form from an informal carer. By comparison only about 180 000 people with a psychosocial disability relied solely on formal care providers. As these data emerge from the routine ABS survey of people who identify as having a disability, they underestimate the number of people with a mental illness who are assisted by carers, but don't identify as having a psychosocial disability.

The relationship between a carer and the person with a mental illness in need of care can vary between close and extended family members, friends, neighbours, volunteers and people with ethnic or kinship relationships. The ABS report that in Australia more than 50% of the assistance provided to people with psychosocial disability was provided by the partner or parent of person with a disability (Australian Bureau of Statistics (ABS), 2015). The remaining assistance was provided, in approximately equal distribution, by the children, other relatives, or a friend of the person with a psychological disability.

The range of activities provided by informal carers for people with a psychosocial disability is broad and is illustrated in Figure 1.2. Cognitive and emotional tasks and assistance with mobility are the activities most frequently provided for this group, however the other activities provided are significant and together define the caring role. However, it is also important to recognise that carers are not defined by the activities they provide, the number of hours per week spent giving support and whether the carer lives with the person to whom care is provided. Some people providing care may not identify themselves as a carer.

Figure 1.1 Australia, informal carers for people with a disability in 2015

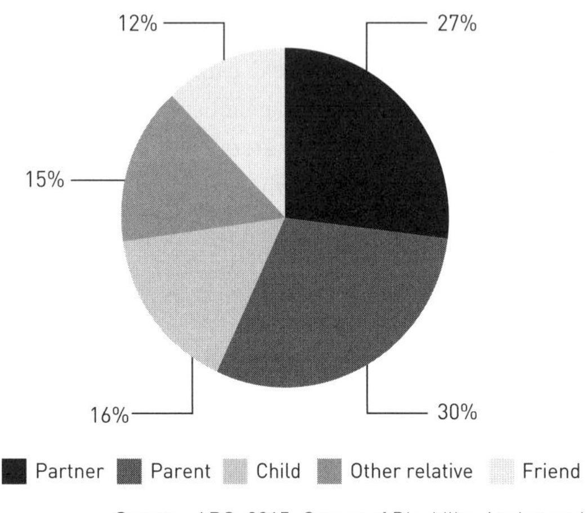

Source: ABS, 2015, *Survey of Disability, Ageing and Carers: Psychosocial Disability*, table 8.1, 44300DO088

Because carers vary in age, gender, cultural identity and sexuality, issues may emerge in the caring role over time and impact the carer's capacity to continue in the caring role. Carers may not be able or willing to continue to provide the range of services needed and may experience fatigue, particularly if they perceive that the recognition and support they need for their caring role is inadequate or absent. For example, children as carers, as they mature, may face the dilemmas of balancing the caring role with the competing demands of study, career and their own family. Older carers, caring for their adult children, may find the assistance required difficult to provide as they age. In addition, the informal nature of the relationship, for example with a carer who is an unmarried partner (including same sex partner), a friend or neighbour, can sometimes generate challenges when these carers interact with a health care or other service provider.

Figure 1.2 Australia, distribution of the broad area of activity for which assistance is provided by an informal carer for a person with a psychosocial disability, ABS 2017

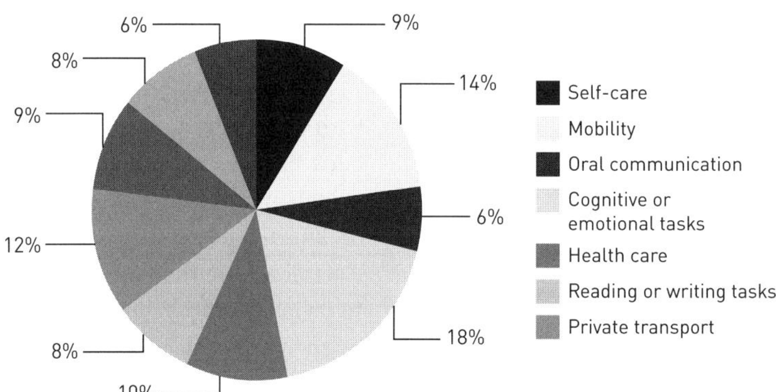

Source: ABS, 2015, *Survey of Disability, Ageing and Carers: Psychosocial Disability*, table 8.1, 44300DO088

The Australian Government (2010a) and most states have adopted legislation that recognise the role and rights of carers. These Acts recognise the broad range of carers and generally place no restriction on who is a carer for the purpose of the rights and responsibilities provided by the Act. This carer role is also defined in other legislation. Later in this chapter, we explore the similarities and differences of the recognition of the rights of carers in Mental Health Acts across the states and territories in Australia.

EVOLUTION OF THE CARER PERSPECTIVE IN AUSTRALIA

The recognition of the challenges faced by carers of people with a mental illness commenced in 1974. That year Margaret Lukes (a social worker with the NSW Association for Mental Health) convened a small group of relatives of people with experience of mental illness to discuss carer issues. Inspired by this meeting a seminar in early 1975 confirmed the need for better support for carers and family members and the Association of Relatives and Friends of the Mentally Ill (ARAFMI) was established. By comparison the Carers Association of NSW, which advocated on behalf of carers more generally, would not be established until 1980 (Mental Health Carers Australia, 2019). Mental health carer associations are now established in most states and territories as well as nationally.

Advocacy activity and local support groups are now conducted in most states and territories in Australia by local and national organisations. These organisations are active in agitating for the health funding of psychosocial support and education for mental health carers. They also provide information and assistance to carers about navigating the health care system and preserving the carers' own mental wellbeing.

The establishment of carer organisations has improved the recognition of the rights and benefits of carers and subsequent legal and policy reforms have improved the capacity of carers to advocate. However, the recognition of carers' rights of access to the treating team can generate tension between the carer's desire to help achieve recovery for that person, and the desire of the individual for autonomy and rights to self-determination. This tension is often fuelled by the limitations of contemporary treatments for mental illness. As some treatments can have serious side effects, the carer is often placed in a position between the individual and the treating professionals, especially when treatment is administered against the will of the person concerned. Recognition by the treating team of these tensions and dilemmas can go some way to assist the carer to find the right balance in their relationships with both the mental health service providers and the individual with the mental illness.

Box 1.1: Carers and restrictive practices

Policy and guidelines issued by health authorities can specify that carers should be informed when a consumer's freedom to move is restricted in a mental health facility. Restrictive practice includes manual, physical or mechanical restraint, and/or placing the person in a room alone and preventing them from leaving. While circumstances often prevent the carer being notified in advance of this restriction, where this policy applies, the clinical team should ensure that the nominated/designated carer is notified as soon as possible of any decision to restrict a consumer's free movement.

CULTURAL NORMS AND CARER RIGHTS

The recognition of carers' rights and responsibilities is influenced by cultural norms reflected in the Australian legal and health care systems. These cultural norms, which, like in other English-speaking countries, place a strong emphasis on the rights of the individual and the concept of 'negative liberty'. Negative liberty is the right of the individual for freedom from interference so long as that individual is doing no harm to anyone else (The Stanford Encyclopedia of Philosophy, 2016). This right has its basis in the concept of individualism. Individualism is contrasted with collectivism, or the social pattern in which individuals construe themselves as parts of collectives and are primarily motivated by duties to those collectives (The Stanford Encyclopedia of Philosophy, 2011). Cultures vary in their preference for individualist or collectivist approaches. Societies immersed in Anglo-Saxon cultures tend to favour individualist approaches which are likely to foster policies and practices which are more risk tolerant of individualistic behaviours than collectivist ones. Societies based in Asia and the Middle East tend to favour a more collectivist approach, which has less tolerance for individual freedoms. Based on their cultural background this variation in approach may influence an individual and their family in the context of carer advocacy and decisions in relation to care and treatment.

The way we conceptualise individual liberty influences the supportive systems our society creates. Some argue that in our current system we have a 'deal or no deal' approach, that is, a person is either deprived

Box 1.2: Carers and smoking policy

Administration of the policy banning smoking in inpatient mental health facilities is a continuing challenge for clinicians, carers and consumers. This policy is often thought to be a trigger for aggression although the evidence for this association is equivocal. The recent review of Seclusion and Restraint in Mental Health units in NSW recognised the tensions in implementation of this policy as leading to incidents related to aggression resulting in restraint and seclusion. This can be a challenging issue for carers, who often want to provide cigarettes to inpatients. Proactive efforts by mental health workers and professionals can reduce or help avoid confrontation and aggression if they seek early to establish a productive relationship with carers of smokers, inform them of the smoking policy and educate them on the facility's nicotine replacement therapy that is available to inpatients.

of their rights to make decisions or completely free to make any they choose. Such an approach can create systems of care that do not deal well with situations where people need to be supported (but not excluded) from decision making. Many aspects of decision making in mental health treatment and support occupy this middle ground. This occurs where people need to be encouraged and assisted to make better decisions for themselves but due to their illness may be inclined to make destructive decisions. Clinicians also vary in their approach to decision making and risk taking. A recovery approach to mental health care is based on the concept of providing the most possible freedom for the individual with a mental illness but this freedom needs to also recognise the rights of family and carers.

Box 1.3: Carers and mental health tribunals

In most jurisdictions in Australia, carers have the specific right to be involved in the hearings of the judicial tribunal established under the relevant legislation to determine whether a consumer should be involuntarily detained in a mental health facility. These tribunals also hear appeals and other matters, such as application to administer ECT to involuntarily consumers. In some jurisdictions, carers have the right to request a hearing of the tribunal.

In most jurisdictions the Mental Health Act makes specific provision for carers to be notified of the planned hearing so they can exercise their right to be involved. 'All reasonable steps' must be made to notify carers of the time, date and location of the hearing. The mental health facility and clinicians may be responsible for this timely notification of carers (and consumers). The consumer's health record should record that carers have been notified in a timely manner to exercise their right to participate.

In these hearings, consumers can often be linked in via video or telephone if it is not possible to appear in person.

RECOGNITION OF CARER RIGHTS IN LEGISLATION

The rights of the carers of people with a mental illness, who are being treated in a health care facility or service, are recognised in all the Mental Health Acts of the Australian states and territories (ACT Government, 2015; Northern Territory Government, 2002; NSW Government, 2007; Queensland Government, 2016; Government of South Australia, 2009; Tasmanian Government, 2013; Victoria State Government, 2014; Government of Western Australia, 2014). While there are variations in the provision of these Acts, they generally recognise the following rights of carers:

- to be involved in decisions related to care and discharge

- to have contact, to be able to visit and support the person with a mental illness
- to receive reports, be advised, informed or notified
- to be consulted or be able to express their views or have their views considered
- to request or seek review, appeal or revocation of an assessment or treatment order
- to raise issues with, request to see or have a visit by an official/community visitor
- to make a complaint.

While the Acts vary in the specific clauses that deal with the rights of carers they largely all provide some coverage of each of these rights. Some Acts (such as South Australia and the ACT) deal in some detail with the rights of carers to be informed and to have the right to express their view about care and treatment. All the Acts (except for those of the Northern Territory and Tasmania) have specific provisions allowing the consumer to nominate or designate their preferred carer.

Two jurisdictions (Northern Territory and Western Australia) also specifically include the right of consumers to make a complaint, and two (the ACT and South Australia) specifically include carers on advisory tribunals and other panels.

INVOLVING CARERS

Involving carers and family members in the care and treatment of people with a mental illness is consistent with relational recovery principles (Price-Robertson, Obradovic, & Morgan, 2017). Recovery principles emphasise that individuals exist within a community of relationships, and recovery practice needs to recognise these relationships. These principles (Australian Government, 2010a) particularly emphasise 'listening to, learning from and acting upon communications from carers' and 'working in partnership with them ... in a way that makes sense' to them. Mental health services must involve carers if they are to comply with National Standards and some state and territory legislation.

Box 1.4: National Standards

The National Standards for Mental Health Services (Australian Government, 2010b) includes a standard on carers. This standard (number 16) requires that the mental health service 'recognises, respects, values and supports the importance of carers to the wellbeing, treatment, and recovery of people with a mental illness' (p. 16). To meet this standard, services must:

- have documented policies and practices to identify carers as soon as possible in the episode of care and record their details in the health record and these policies will also detail how they will involve carers in planning care
- implement and maintain continuing engagement with carers as partners in the delivery of care as soon as possible and in all episodes of care
- involve carers in care and discharge planning
- consider the special needs of carers from particular segments of the population and inform carers of their rights and responsibilities
- provide information about and access to services that maximise the wellbeing of carers
- involve carers in policy development and evaluation, and provide training and support to these carers.

The responsibility for complying with these principles, standards and legislation rests with frontline line staff, both health professionals and other health workers regardless of whether they work in emergency departments, inpatient mental health services, community health services, primary care settings and non-government services.

These principles and standards mean that health professionals and employees must engage with, and include, carers. Moreover, that involvement and inclusion should commence with the first encounter of an individual with the health service, despite the challenges this initial involvement may create. The exceptions to early involvement of carer can occur when the individual has specifically determined that their carers not be informed and has the right to do so under the relevant Act, or where there are reasons known to the treating team that involvement of the carers would not be in the best interests of the individual at that time.

'Involving' and 'including' means much more than simply collecting and recording information. In some jurisdictions the relevant Mental Health Act includes provision which requires the treating medical officer or accredited person to consider the views of family members and carers when assessing whether the person is mentally ill or mental disorder (see, for example, the *Mental Health Act 2007* (NSW), s 72B or the *Mental Health Act 2009* (SA), s 41 (2)).

Box 1.5: When carers should not be involved

While carer involvement is encouraged and now enshrined in legislation, there are exceptions where family, friends, or carers should not be involved. This may be decided by the consumer or, in some circumstances, an authorised medical officer. Mental health consumers can have the right to nominate people who are to be excluded from communication and involvement. Reasons for this vary. It is important to remember that experiences of mental illness may not be the only experience affecting the consumer. Family, friend, and carer relationships are not exempt from domestic and family violence, child abuse, and elder abuse among other things. In NSW specifically, nominated persons may not be notified if an authorised medical officer or director of community treatment believes that doing so would put the patient at risk of serious harm. Despite the rights of carers to be involved and informed in some circumstances, involvement of carers can have a negative impact on a consumer's safety or their progress towards recovery.

Carers provide a different insight into the individual's mental health condition than can be gained from discussions and examination of him or her alone. The views and preferences of carers and family members are also often crucial to decisions about treatment and care and about planning for the future for a variety of reasons, particularly if they are to be the continuing care provider. Carers may have knowledge of the individual's past encounters with health services and past treatments and care. They are likely to know what the individual's preferences are and how he or she is likely to comply with or tolerate treatments. Carers are often likely to know what a consumer will agree to, or not agree to, and what his or her living situation and relationships are likely to be in the future.

Often the initial engagement with a health service or a specialist mental health service can occur during a crisis for the individual. In these circumstances, which can involve conflict between an individual and his or her carer, determining the nature and importance of these relationships can be challenging for the assessing health professionals. Although encounters between the health professional, carer and consumer may be 'challenging', due to the underlying conflict, this is not enough reason for excluding carers in early decisions concerning treatment and care. In some cases, it may be a necessary to interview carers separately from the individual with mental health issues, or to interview them at a different location or time. These interviews need to be balanced with the need to gain and maintain the consumer's trust and build a therapeutic relationship.

Despite the standards and legislation, carers often report dissatisfaction with their involvement by health professionals around care decision and care planning. Cree and colleagues found that 'many carers perceive a lack of recognition and appreciation of their role from health professionals' (Cree et al., 2015). In addition to structural barriers to their involvement (such as the timing and location of meetings that are not convenient to the carer), they identified barriers related to power imbalances within the system and issues related to confidentiality and privacy. Carers should normally be informed when specific events occur involving the individual, such as the application of restraint, the use of seclusion, major changes of treatment, if a patient leaves without medical advice or an involuntary patient goes absent without leave.

PRIVACY AND THE ROLE OF CARERS

Often there is a balance to be achieved between the consumer's rights to privacy and the carer's need for information. Guidelines for Australian providers suggest that health professionals are sometimes not clear as to boundaries of legal and ethical practice regarding confidentiality and information sharing and, to be on the safe side, will tend to exclude carers (National Mental Health Consumer and Carer Forum, 2011; Carers Trust, 2013). While each situation needs to be assessed individually, it may be useful for health professionals to engage in an explicit discussion with both consumers and carers on what information can be shared and the agreements reached should be documented. There may also be circumstances where the treating team determine that sharing information with carers is necessary even though this is against the explicit wishes of the consumer, and where it may result in a loss of trust and cause further trauma.

The balance of an individual's rights to privacy and confidentiality and the carer's need for information, support and continuing involvement, supported by policy and legislation, is not always easy to achieve. While the general weight of advice and policy is in favour of the involvement of carers, legislation, in some states (such as the *Mental Health Act 2007* (NSW), s 72(3)), allows for the individual to nominate persons 'who are excluded from being given notice or information about the person'. However, the right of the individual to exclude the carer from having information on them is not absolute.

SUMMARY

The role of carers has evolved, become better recognised and formalised over recent decades. This is most welcome and begins to put in place a more holistic and recovery-focused response to mental illness for many people. It provides due respect to a role many played despite minimal support previously. Families have long borne the major responsibility for caring.

However, being a carer often comes at a cost. Carers face mental ill health as a direct consequence of their caring role and experience higher rates of mental ill health than the general population (Aadil, Shah, Wadoo, & Latoo, 2010). As the role of carer continues to evolve, it is important to be mindful of strategies that can minimise the stress associated with this role.

1.1.9 COMMENTARY AND REFLECTION

FIONA MCDERMOTT & GRAHAM MEADOWS

Our purpose so far in this beginning chapter has been to sketch the evolving history of mental health conceptualisations, practices and developments. Framed within a complexity science perspective, the challenges posed by competing understandings, multiple stake holders and a context of service and treatment innovation and exnovation demonstrates the constant flux in emergent systemic responses and adaptations to mental illness. In contemporary times the contributions of consumers as critical actors in progressing both understanding and action for changes is highlighted.

Having sketched out some concepts of complexity science, as this text is being finalised, we note that individually, in our communities, at different levels of government and globally, humanity is confronting the highly complex challenges presented by the COVID-19 pandemic. In Chapter 1.2, we will briefly consider pandemics and mental health, while the spread and full range of effects and implications of SARS-CoV-2 will continue to be researched and analysed—hopefully with increasing understanding—in coming years. If viewed through a complexity science lens, the COVID-19 pandemic provides a currently evolving exemplar of how such a perspective might enable the development of knowledge about the intersections, systemic adaptations and impact of a phenomenon which impacts on biological, personal, organisational, environmental, political, and economic levels, exposing the inequalities characterising the pandemic's impact on vulnerable populations, in particular those experiencing mental ill health.

1.2

CRITICAL ENVIRONMENTAL AND SOCIAL DETERMINANTS OF MENTAL HEALTH PROBLEMS AND THEIR CARE

SUSIE BURKE, JOANNE ENTICOTT, ANTON ISAACS, GRAHAM MEADOWS & SEBASTIAN ROSENBERG

1.2.1 INTRODUCTION

ANTON ISAACS, GRAHAM MEADOWS & SEBASTIAN ROSENBERG

There are things to celebrate as the twenty-first century unfolds. Prior to the COVID-19 pandemic, the size of all global economies combined had increased roughly ninefold in the last 50 years and doubled in the last 20 years (World Bank, 2019a). The proportion of the world that lives in extreme poverty has been progressively going down. Most of the world's population now lives in middle rather than low income countries, with the greater resource access this implies. Nationally, in the two decades that form the span of the four editions of this text, Australian GDP in current per capita US dollars has increased from $22 000 per capita to $54 000 per capita, and mental health expenditure has more than doubled in that time. In health broadly, smallpox is an increasingly distant memory and the eradication of polio may be in sight. The great majority of children receive at least some immunisation protection and many more of them survive through to their first, fifth or later birthdays than used to be the case (Rosling, Rosling, & Rönnlund, 2018).

But the start of the twenty-first century is also a time of inexorable accumulation of evidence, with wider and wider recognition, that the Earth as a whole has not simply buffered the changes that expansions of human activity have brought about. Human societies over time have on many occasions compromised their local or regional environments with sometimes severe consequences for particular societies (Diamond, 2011) but this task of facing up to the current challenge of ecological disruption on a planetary scale is newer. Presenting as it does a source of existential threat to humanity as well as a source of specific impacts on individuals and communities. In this chapter, we will provide consideration of climate change, its implications for mental health and mental health care.

Of course, climate change is not the whole story as regards societal or service delivery considerations for mental health care. Beyond the impact of the pandemic, a wide range of environmental and social determinants need to be considered in social policy and in understanding the influences on individual or family presentations. Over time the UN has provided influential direction as to how to consider understanding and address such issues and our next section summarises some key UN statements.

A critical influence here is that the material advances and health gains or improvements in service provisions have not been shared equally around either between or within countries–in ways that particularly have changed since the 1980s. In recent years the recognition of this has involved economist writers such as Thomas Piketty (Piketty & Goldhammer, 2017) demonstrating how things have turned around. A period in which many inequalities reduced up until the 1980s has been followed by several decades of increasing disparities. The ascendant monetarism or neo-liberalism of the 1980s and forward led to the taking away of many safeguards against inequities within societies and the relative gap between rich and poor has widened since in many nations (Piketty & Goldhammer, 2017; Milanovic, 2016). So as we move on through the chapter to consider the role of social determinants in mental health, illness and disorder (see Chapter 1.2), and responses to these problems, we also will consider the role that increasing inequality and inequity, things that in turn may be exacerbated by climate change, play as influences on mental health, wellbeing and illness, and to what extent policy and other interventions either work to balance inequality and inequity, or not.

1.2.2 CLIMATE CHANGE AND MENTAL HEALTH

SUSIE BURKE

> The eyes of all future generations are upon you. And if you choose to fail us, I say–we will never forgive you.
>
> *Greta Thunberg, UN Climate Summit, New York, 23 September 2019*

INTRODUCTION

Climate change is regarded as one of the most serious global health threats of the twenty-first century (Costello et al., 2009), overall the greatest threat to humanity, and an existential risk to our world–a threat that could annihilate most people on Earth.

As well as physical health impacts, climate change also affects people's mental health and psychosocial wellbeing via the direct effects of increasingly frequent and severe extreme weather events (EWEs), like fires, floods, cyclones and heatwaves, but also via the flow-on effects of its gradual and insidious changes, like sea level rises, prolonged droughts, changed growing seasons, land degradation, food and water shortages. Then there are the psychological effects of seeing climate change as an existential threat to civilisation as we know it, and the impact that this has on people's mental health and wellbeing.

Understanding the mental health and psychosocial impacts of the climate crisis is critically important. The risks and impacts of the climate crisis on mental health are already rapidly accelerating, and disproportionally affect people who are most marginalised around the world. Interventions must be urgently implemented at all levels of society, both to reduce the threat by swift and effective action to halt global warming, as well as adaptive measures to anticipate the threats and build resilience around the world as we learn to cope with escalating and accelerating changes to our world.

THE CLIMATE EMERGENCY

Excessive production of greenhouse gas emissions over the last few hundred years trapping additional heat in the lower atmosphere has resulted in a pattern of increasing average global temperatures and subsequent instability in global weather patterns. As this text is being finalised in 2020, the ten warmest years in history have occurred since 1998, and the Earth has not been so warm for 115 000 years (NOAA 2017). The Earth has already reached 1.1 degree of warming relative to pre-industrial temperatures, with dire consequences all around the planet: increasingly frequent and intense extreme weather event disasters, loss of species, loss of summer sea ice, melting ice caps, and coral reefs in a death spiral.

Emissions are still rising. Even if the Paris Accord target of a 1.5 to 2.0 rise in temperature is met, scientists 'cannot exclude the risk that a cascade of feedbacks could push the Earth System irreversibly onto a 'Hothouse Earth' pathway' (Steffen et al., 2018). These extreme conditions would be outside those that have occurred over the past few hundred thousand years, which have been cycles of ice ages with milder periods in between. This level of temperature increase would be catastrophic (IPCC, 2014). This would be a world of unprecedented heatwaves, severe drought, bushfires, flooding and major storms in many regions, with serious impacts on all human systems and ecosystems.

To return to below 1.5 degree of warming is essential to stabilise the Earth's climate, but will require urgent and strong action all over the globe (IPCC 2018). However, despite knowing about dangerous climate change, this awareness has not yet led to actions around the world that are commensurate with the threat.

PSYCHOLOGICAL EFFECTS OF CLIMATE CHANGE

Even just knowing about climate change and the existential threat it poses to our very survival can have a significant psychological impact. The reality is truly frightening. However the impact of climate change on our psychological health and wellbeing is far more varied and complex than this.

When we talk about the mental health consequences of climate change it is useful to separate out the different types of climate hazards that impact us. Berry and colleagues (2010) organise climate change related hazards into three categories: acute hazards, like fires, floods and other extreme weather events; sub-acute hazards, like pervasive drought; and chronic hazards like rising sea level and increasing temperatures. Australia is ranked as highly sensitive to the physical risks of climate change, with predictions of more storms, floods, rain and bushfires (HSBC, 2018).

These climate hazards lead to a variety of direct and indirect or vicarious psychological impacts (Berry et al., 2010; Clayton et al., 2017; Hayes et al., 2018; Doherty & Clayton, 2011). The composite term 'mental health and psychosocial wellbeing' is often used to capture the full spectrum of psychological impacts from mild stress responses to chronic stress and significant mental health problems. In addition, it's also important to consider the negative impacts of climate change on community health.

Specific groups of people in society are at higher risk of distress and other adverse mental health consequences from exposure to climate change. According to a recent major report on climate change and health (Dodgen, Donato, Kelly, La Greca, & Morganstein, 2016) groups especially at risk are poor people, people living in areas most susceptible to specific climate change events, people from marginalised groups, as well as those living in communities that rely on the natural environment for sustenance and livelihood. In Australia, Indigenous people are at high risk, as well as people living in rural and remote parts of the country.

DIRECT EFFECTS

There is a well-established literature documenting the mental health impacts of the direct effects of climate change in the form of extreme weather event disasters like bushfires, cyclones, floods, severe storms and heatwaves.

Natural disasters can have devastating consequences for individuals and communities. People can die, they can lose family members, friends, or neighbours, be injured, lose pets, livestock, livelihoods, homes, properties, and all their possessions. They can lose their schools, workplaces, and familiar places. They may be displaced from their communities and have to move away to find new homes, new jobs, and start over.

The trauma related to extreme weather events brings a significant risk of mental health problems, most commonly post-traumatic stress disorder (PTSD), depression, complicated grief, followed by substance use, other anxiety disorders (e.g., Norris et al., 2002; Simpson et al., 2011). There have also been increasing reports of suicide and suicidal ideation following extreme weather events (Dudgeon et al., 2016).

Extreme heat and humidity can initiate or exacerbate mental health problems in populations already suffering from mental illness and stress-related disorders. In addition, some psychiatric medications can interfere with the body's ability to regulate temperature, meaning that people who are being treated with these drugs could be at risk of overheating during extreme heat events (Martin-Latry, et al., 2007).

It should be noted, also, that mental health problems are not the only psychological consequence of disasters, and there is a growing understanding of a range of complex psychosocial consequences which can also include more positive experiences like post-traumatic growth and resilience (Weissbecker, 2011).

INDIRECT EFFECTS

There is also a range of psychological impacts that flow on from social, economic and environmental disruptions caused by all manner of climate related hazards. For example, extreme weather events or the more gradual effects of rising temperatures and sea levels can cause damages to physical infrastructure, physical health effects, food and water shortages, land degradation, financial losses, rising prices of food, water, services, forced migration, violent conflict and so on. All of these disruptions can have flow-on effects on people's wellbeing, increasing stress, grief, anxiety, depression, trauma (Clayton et al., 2017).

Environmental psychologists Susan Clayton and colleagues also talk about climate change impacts on community health. These types of impacts are understudied, but may include things like a diminishment in community cohesion, loss of community identity, threats to a sense of continuity and sense of belonging as people are forced to move in and out of communities because of environmental stressors; an undermining of cultural integrity if people have to leave their homelands. Threats to community health also include an increased likelihood of criminal behaviour, violence and aggression as community members experience various stressors related to climate change (Clayton et al., 2017).

VICARIOUS, OVERARCHING EFFECTS

There is a growing understanding of the ways in which climate change as a global environmental threat may create emotional distress and anxiety about the future or vicarious distress for the plight of people in other places who are being directly affected by climate hazards.

Qualitative research finds evidence of some people being deeply affected by feelings of loss, helplessness and frustration as they engage with the problems of global climate change (Moser, 2013). Many people may also feel seriously concerned, frightened, angry, pessimistic, or guilty in response to climate change. New terms such as 'eco-anxiety', 'climate change anxiety', are being coined to describe the growing angst around knowing that humans are contributing to global warming, species extinction, dwindling natural resources, and increased pollution. People's distress can be greatly compounded by their awareness of society's current failure to act swiftly enough to mitigate the growing threat of the climate crisis.

ADDRESSING CLIMATE CHANGE AND MENTAL HEALTH

Understanding what to do to reduce these threats (climate change mitigation) and adapt to these threats (adaptation, disaster preparedness), as well as how to care for people who are adversely affected by climate change impacts, are an essential part of mental health practitioners' work.

Addressing the mental health implications of climate change requires changes at all levels, from global to local. It requires policy changes and frameworks, but also concrete action by mental health practitioners in their workplaces and professional bodies, in the community and in their consulting rooms.

Understanding the psychological impacts of climate change is important so that we can help people come to terms with and psychologically adapt to a climate-changed world and reality. The more we know about how people are feeling, thinking and doing in relation to climate change, then the more we are able to help them respond in useful ways—in ways that both reduce the threats of climate change as well as prepare people to adapt to the changes that cannot be avoided.

MITIGATION

Climate change mitigation refers to the things that we do to minimise the threat of climate change, which in turn reduces the negative psychological impacts. These are priority actions because, above all else, we need a liveable planet. Mitigation actions include activities to reduce greenhouse gas emissions as well as to draw down excess carbon which is already in the atmosphere.

There are several levels of influence that mental health practitioners can use within their organisations, and as advocates in the health care sector, to reduce emissions, encourage others to do the same, and take a leadership role on the importance of effective action to curb climate change. Arguably, mental health professionals have a moral and ethical responsibility to take leadership on climate change mitigation to address an issue which is caused by human behaviour, and which threatens human health and wellbeing.

Important mitigation activities range from mental health professionals advocating for strong climate policies with governments, decision makers and opinion leaders, and also within their own professional organisations. There are several climate and health advocacy bodies that have been established globally (e.g. Health Care without Harm) and within countries (e.g., the Climate and Health Alliance (CAHA) in Australia), who advocate collectively for swift climate action and are calling for the climate crisis to be treated as an emergency.

ADAPTATION

Even with dramatic mitigation efforts, there are still going to be severe effects of climate change which will be felt all over the globe. Climate change threatens people in ways that their previous experience will not have prepared them for. Climate change adaptation refers to the things that we do to lower the risks, and prepare for unavoidable threats.

In the following section, we will look at what adaptation means from the perspective of the health care sector, and then for mental health practitioners within their workplaces. Adaptation also includes a range of coping actions that individuals and communities may take in response to climate change (Reser, Bradley & Ellul, 2012). So, from a psychological perspective, adaptation to climate change is also about 'coming to terms with' climate change, and includes how people perceive and understand the problems, how they cope with the feelings that are elicited in response to climate change, and how they decide what to do in response to the problems.

ADAPTATION IN THE HEALTH CARE SECTOR

There is a range of adaptation measures that ought to be considered to support population level mental health in a changing climate. Hayes et al (2018) include things like policy responses, such as building public health systems that fully take into account the profound implications and consequences of the connections between climate change and human health (McMichael et al., 2009), and planning (e.g., identifying at-risk populations, developing action plans for responding to climate hazards to meet the psychosocial needs of the population). The health sector needs to develop alternative, more effective, practices to manage the complex issues related to climate change while continuing to implement their traditional primary, secondary and tertiary preventive models (Walter et al., 2014). Experts recognise that the current ways in which the health care sector operates is not fully able to take into account the profound implications and consequences of the connections between climate change and human health (McMichael et al., 2009; Walter et al., 2014), nor deliver progress on the scale and with the speed required (Hanlon et al., 2012; Morris, 2010).

Adaptation tasks within a mental health practitioner's workplace or organisation are also extremely important as a way of preparing for future shocks. They first need to develop a clear understanding of climate change as an important issue; then they have to become aware of their organisations' own climate change vulnerability, and take on a sense of responsibility for developing a solution or response (Gardener et al. 2010). Then, organisations are likely to perform a range of tasks to prepare for possible future shocks, including developing organisational disaster plans to incorporate increased scale and intensity of extreme weather events, retrofitting buildings for better protection against increased intensity of extreme weather events (e.g., heat waves, severe storms), mobilising resources for assistance in the event of extreme weather events, like generators for backup power. (For specific examples of organisations performing tasks to prepare for climate change impacts, see Walker & Mason, 2015.)

Beyond the workplace, mental health practitioners also have roles they can play to help prepare their communities for climate change impacts. This could include communicating about climate change threat in a way that helps people to see that the climate threat is relevant and important to them, and one that they therefore need to do something about. Letting people know that we already have concrete, plausible solutions to drastically reduce carbon emissions, and showing them that they can contribute to these solutions, and also that many of these solutions can simultaneously create a healthier environment and more resilient communities, can help to counter feelings of helplessness about the problem (CRED, 2014). Moreover, when people believe there are solutions available, they are more likely to perceive climate change as a problem worth addressing.

There is a large literature of social science research on effective communication around climate change and risk, and several institutions have a strong focus on this. One of the lessons learned is the value of 'trusted communicators' to help engage people with the problems. Most people value and highly respect the views of scientists and academics (see for example the Yale climate surveys (Yale Program on Climate Change Communication, 2020), the Stanford surveys (Political Psychology Research Group, 2020) and the Griffith University NCAARF (Griffith University NCCARF, 2020) surveys which report this). Health practitioners fall within the 'trusted' category of scientists and academics, and thus have a powerful voice for communicating about climate change, and particularly for raising the importance of climate change as a health threat.

Finally, there is also the role of helping people to 'psychologically' adapt to climate change. This psychological adaptation to the threat of climate change requires a similar set of responses. It requires an acknowledgement of this grave and global threat. It requires using coping strategies to manage the feelings and thoughts that arise so that people can face up to and come to terms with the threat and not try to avoid it by distraction etc. Then it also requires behavioural and psychological engagement, in which people change and adjust their behaviour and lifestyle in order to reduce the threat and protect themselves.

People can, of course, react in all sorts of unhelpful ways to the threat of climate change—minimise the threat, distract themselves, put hope in god, or silver bullet solutions, become helpless, hopeless. This is why psychological adaptation involves managing the thoughts and feelings so that people can stay engaged with the problem and also the solutions.

Knowing how climate change affects us psychologically is profoundly important for increasing mitigation and adaptation. 'Coming to terms' with it requires psychological preparedness, adaptation, and adjustment as well as behavioural and lifestyle adaptation and change.

CONCLUSION

The climate crisis affects people's mental health and psychosocial wellbeing in a variety of ways, from increasing the risk of significant mental health problems, through to a range of complex psychosocial impacts including increased anxiety, stress and profound grief.

Distilling the precise impact of climate change on mental health can be difficult to separate from other social determinants, but articulating climate change as a determinant of mental health is an increasingly important part of a contemporary response to mental health needs in the twenty-first century.

1.2.3 SOME INTERNATIONAL POLICY BACKGROUND

GRAHAM MEADOWS

UNIVERSAL DECLARATION OF HUMAN RIGHTS, ARTICLE 25(1)

Dating back to 1948, the Universal Declaration of Human Rights, Article 25(1) states:

> Everyone has the right to a standard of living adequate for the health and well-being of himself and of his family, including food, clothing, housing and medical care and necessary social services, and the right to security in the event of unemployment, sickness, disability, widowhood, old age or other lack of livelihood in circumstances beyond his control (United Nations, 2019).

THE UN SUSTAINABLE DEVELOPMENT GOALS

In 1992 the United Nations Conference on Environment and Development, held in Rio de Janeiro, set out Agenda 21, looking forward to the imperatives for global development in the twenty-first century. This agenda has been developed through time and notably given specific goals through the Millennium Goals, then from 2015, with the UN Sustainable Development Goals (SDGs), intended to run until 2030. These are reproduced here to promote consideration of how these bear on mental health, and the extent to which even in a high income nation such as Australia, our society, institutions, fiscal and financial policy may be seen as falling short of what might be hoped for in pursuit of the goals.

1. End poverty in all its forms everywhere
2. End hunger, achieve food security and improved nutrition and promote sustainable agriculture
3. Ensure healthy lives and promote wellbeing for all at all ages
4. Ensure inclusive and equitable quality education and promote lifelong learning opportunities for all
5. Achieve gender equality and empower all women and girls
6. Ensure availability and sustainable management of water and sanitation for all
7. Ensure access to affordable, reliable, sustainable and modern energy for all
8. Promote sustained, inclusive and sustainable economic growth, full and productive employment and decent work for all
9. Build resilient infrastructure, promote inclusive and sustainable industrialisation and foster innovation
10. Reduce inequality within and among countries
11. Make cities and human settlements inclusive, safe, resilient and sustainable
12. Ensure sustainable consumption and production patterns
13. Take urgent action to combat climate change and its impacts
14. Conserve and sustainably use the oceans, seas and marine resources for sustainable development
15. Protect, restore and promote sustainable use of terrestrial ecosystems, sustainably manage forests, combat desertification, and halt and reverse land degradation and halt biodiversity loss
16. Promote peaceful and inclusive societies for sustainable development, provide access to justice for all and build effective, accountable and inclusive institutions at all levels
17. Strengthen the means of implementation and revitalise the global partnership for sustainable development (Agenda 21, 1992).

The relationship between the SDGs and mental health has been considered in *The Lancet* Commission on Global Mental Health, from which Figure 1.3 is reproduced.

Figure 1.3 The relationship between the SDGs and mental health

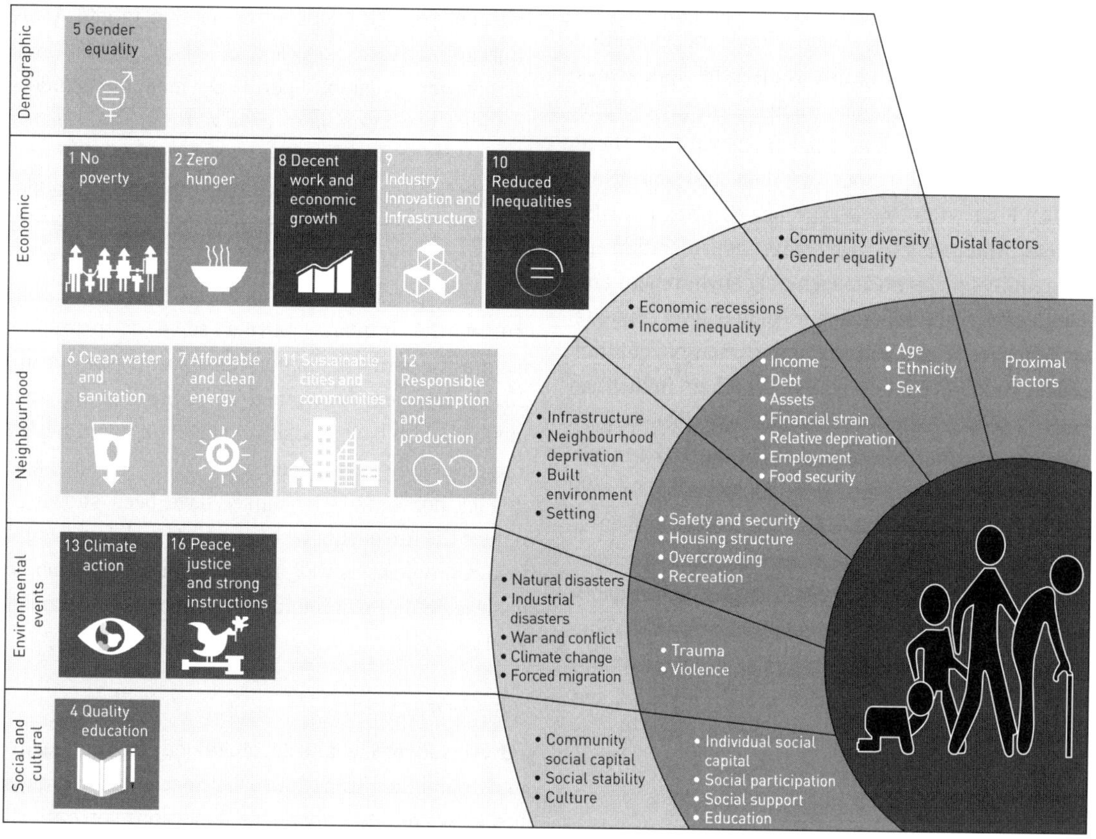

Source: Patel et al., 2018, figure 6

1.2.4 SOCIAL DETERMINANTS OF MENTAL HEALTH AND ILLNESS

ANTON ISAACS & GRAHAM MEADOWS

INTRODUCTION AND KEY CONCEPTS

Social determinants refers to the factors in the social environment that have a significant influence on an individual's health (Wilkinson & Marmot, 2003). The fact that people who are less well-off have more illnesses and live shorter lives than those who are rich, is a well-recognised social injustice (Wilkinson & Marmot, 2003). Social determinants also impact the mental health of populations. Those who are poor and disadvantaged are at greater risk of mental disorders (Allen, Balfour, Bell, & Marmot, 2014; Fisher & Baum, 2010). Operating in parallel with social determinants, and sometimes causally interconnected, are biological determinants including genetic, epigenetic, infective, toxic and other environmental factors which can influence mental health outcomes at different stages of life (Patel et al., 2018).

Critical in consideration of this are two definitions from the *Oxford English Dictionary*:

> *Inequality*, The state or condition of being unequal; want of equality.
>
> Compare this with 'inequity':
>
> *Inequity*, Want of equity or justice; the fact or quality of being unfair.

A MULTILEVEL FRAMEWORK

In order to consider how inequalities and inequities may influence mental health we need to work across the range of factors that may influence these two. Here we make use of an influential framework for these considerations, as set out by Allen and colleagues (2014). First, a life course approach covering prenatal periods through old age, next consideration of community-level contexts including environment and health care systems; and finally country level contexts including political and economic factors, cultural norms, and specific policies. Another influential body of work is that of Wilkinson and Pickett who have advanced and developed (2011, 2018a) a thesis around how more unequal societies may fare less well on multiple indicators including indicators of mental health, with an underlying proposition that wherever problems have a social gradient, then greater inequality makes the overall rate of the problem worse. This proposition may usefully be borne in mind as we work through the range of identified social indicators and their possible influences on mental health and illness.

LIFE COURSE

Introduction

A life course approach recognises that disadvantage can influence mental health outcomes by impacting upon all stages of life starting before birth and accumulating over one's lifetime (World Health Organization and Calouste Gulbenkian Foundation, 2014). This approach has been shown to be useful in understanding and addressing mental health inequalities and proposes action to be taken at different stages of life (World Health Organization, 2013a).

Prenatal experience

The health and development of a foetus is strongly influenced by the health and welfare of his or her mother. Maternal risk factors such as poor health and nutrition, smoking, alcohol and drug misuse, stress, and highly demanding physical labour can all adversely affect prenatal development (World Health Organization, 2013). For instance, children of depressed mothers are at greater risk of being underweight and low birthweight is an independent risk factor for depression in later years (Surkan, Kennedy, Hurley, & Black, 2011). Risk factors for common perinatal mental disorders include: socioeconomic disadvantage; unintended pregnancy; being younger; experiencing intimate partner violence and having insufficient emotional and practical support (Fisher et al., 2012). On the other hand, factors such as being more educated, having a permanent job, and having a kind and trustworthy intimate partner serve as protective factors for perinatal mental disorders (Fisher et al., 2012). Interventions aimed at improving maternal mental health have a positive impact on infant health and development (Rahman et al., 2013). Prenatal and infancy home visits by nurses have been shown to reduce the use of substances and internalising mental health problems as well as improvement in academic achievement of children until the age of 12 (Kitzman et al., 2010).

The early years

Poverty adversely affects childhood mental health and children from lower socioeconomic groups are less likely to experience conditions for optimal development (Schady, 2011). These factors can affect children as young as three years of age (Kelly, Sacker, Del, M., & Marmot, 2011). Socioeconomic status, which includes family income, maternal education and neighbourhood disadvantage, is an independent contributor to the mental health of a child aged 4 and these effects mostly persist over time (Christensen, Fahey, Giallo, & Hancock, 2017). Racial discrimination has been shown to adversely affect the physical and mental health of Aboriginal children aged 5–10 (Shepherd, Li, Cooper, Hopkins, & Farrant, 2017).

Adverse family conditions and poor quality of parenting that results in a 'lack of secure attachment, neglect, lack of quality stimulation, and conflict' in early life are also associated with higher risk of mental disorders in later years (Bell, Donkin, & Marmot, 2013). Exposure to direct physical and psychological abuse and growing up in families with domestic violence is particularly harmful for children (Fryers & Brugha, 2013). Childhood abuse leading to trauma is associated with psychotic experiences in adulthood (Janssen et al., 2004). Parental mental health also influences children's mental health outcomes. For instance, children whose mothers have a mental illness are much more likely to develop a mental disorder (Leijdesdorff, van Doesum, Popma, Klaassen, & van Amelsvoort, 2017; Melzer, Fryers, Jenkins, Brugha, & McWilliams, 2003; O'Donnell et al., 2015).

However, the adverse effects of poverty and socioeconomic disadvantage can be offset by good social and emotional interactions with parents (Kelly, Sacker, et al., 2011). Moreover, family support including support in maternal and child care, and maternal education can buffer the impacts of early-year inequalities (World Health Organization, 2013a). Strengthening family and community links is also important in improving the mental health and wellbeing of Aboriginal children (Williamson et al., 2010). The Triple P-Positive parenting program (TPS) developed in Queensland is an excellent example of improving the mental health of parents and young children (Bodenmann, Cina, Ledermann, & Sanders, 2008; Sanders et al., 2008). The Incredible Years (IY) Teacher Classroom Management and Child Social and Emotion curriculum (Dinosaur School) is another example of an early childhood program for the prevention of mental disorders in early childhood (Webster-Stratton, Jamila Reid, & Stoolmiller, 2008).

Later childhood

Mental disorders are very common in adolescents—the most common of which are anxiety disorders, behaviour disorders, mood disorders and substance use disorders (Merikangas et al., 2010; Sawyer et al., 2001). Financial difficulties are an important social determinant for this age group particularly when they are students (Richardson, Elliott, Roberts, & Jansen, 2017). Children from low socioeconomic backgrounds are also more likely to be expelled from school causing high levels of psychological distress (Ford et al., 2018). Depressive symptoms in adolescents are due to both adverse childhood and current experiences (Bell et al., 2013; Wickrama, Conger, Lorenz, & Jung, 2008). Aboriginal young people in the age group 10–24 have been found to have high levels of psychological distress, mental disorders and substance use as well as intentional and unintentional injuries (Azzopardi et al., 2018).

Adolescents need to be supported socially and emotionally in order to enable positive interactions with peers, family, and the wider community. Schools can play an important role in improving mental health of older children and adolescents in different ways. Schools can work directly with students and with services to ensure they get the care they need as well as help parents with parenting skills and financial support (World Health Organization and Calouste Gulbenkian Foundation, 2014).

Working age

Studies have clearly demonstrated strong associations between undesirable employment or financial situations and higher levels of psychological distress which are associated with common mental disorders such as depression and anxiety (Catalano et al., 2011). In Australia, people who reside in areas of socioeconomic disadvantage and whose income levels are in the lowest decile are at higher risk of mental disorders (Enticott, Meadows, Shawyer, Inder, & Patten, 2016; Isaacs, Enticott, Meadows, & Inder, 2018). Job loss is associated with symptoms of depression and anxiety and this relationship is more pronounced with long-term unemployment (Catalano et al., 2011). Those on disability support and other forms of welfare have a higher risk of mental disorders (Kiely & Butterworth, 2013; Milner et al., 2017).

Strategies to reduce risks of mental health problems among the working age group include lessening long-term unemployment, improving quality of work across the social gradient, and developing greater flexibility and security of employment (Marmot Review Team, 2010). Policies aimed at social protection and minimum wages as well as employment practices that promote higher rewards, more control and balance at work have been shown to reduce stress, depression and anxiety at work as well as increase productivity (Bambra, Egan, Thomas, Petticrew, & Whitehead, 2007; Egan et al., 2007). Policies to reduce alcohol consumption in this group are also being considered as a method of reducing mental health problems (Stockwell, Auld, Zhao, & Martin, 2012; Wahlbeck & McDaid, 2012).

Family building

The family is the fundamental unit in social hierarchy that provides the physical and psychological milieu within which children grow and develop (World Health Organization, 2013a). A healthy society is made up of healthy families. There are several groups of people in Australia where circumstances in the family such as parental separation, unemployment, domestic violence, migration and alcohol and drug addiction can cause enduring mental health problems among children. Families at risk of these issues include refugees, Indigenous and low socioeconomic status families or where parents are from different cultures. Some ways of building families where natural bonds are broken include helping parents who played previously harmful roles to get a second chance at developing new healthy parenting skills and helping young people who are challenging to identify and build good relationships with more than one significant adult (Jesuit Social Services, 2009). A strengths-based perspective is considered to be a good approach when working with at-risk families (Early & GlenMaye, 2000).

Older people

Risk factors for mental disorders among the elderly include social isolation, particularly in women (World Health Organization and Calouste Gulbenkian Foundation, 2014). The mental health of older people can be affected when they lose the ability to live independently, become bereaved due to the loss of a life partner or experience a sudden loss of income due to retirement from the labour force. These factors lead to social isolation and psychological distress (World Health Organization, 2013a).

Education, being married and volunteering appear to be protective factors for mental disorders among the elderly (Ploubidis & Grundy, 2009; Lum & Lightfoot, 2005). Those who are physically independent, but isolated by the loss of a partner or relocation, would benefit from community housing where they can develop new relationships and be close to social support facilities (Mead, Lester, Chew-Graham, Gask, & Bower, 2010). Those who have physical disabilities can be supported with better access to medical facilities, and assistance with daily activities (Australian Institute of Health and Welfare, 2015a).

COMMUNITY LEVEL CONTEXTS

Building community connectedness and combating social isolation is necessary for improving mental health (Kelly, Lewin, et al., 2011). Studies from the United Kingdom have shown increased psychiatric correlates among adolescents who were unhappy with their neighbourhoods (Shiue, 2014).

Engaged communities

Community engagement refers to actions 'involving communities in decision making and in the planning, design, governance and delivery of services' (Swainston & Summerbell, 2008). Community engagement interventions have been shown to be effective in reducing health inequalities as well as improving health behaviours and health consequences (O'Mara-Eves et al., 2013). This is particularly so with disadvantaged communities (O'Mara-Eves et al., 2015). Lower socioeconomic status communities including migrants, refugees and Aboriginal communities are known to benefit much more when they are meaningfully engaged (Ellis, Miller, Baldwin, & Abdi, 2011; Isaacs & Sutton, 2016; O'Mara-Eves et al., 2015).

There are different models of community engagement (Brunton et al., 2017) such as peer or lay delivered interventions delivered by community health workers who are from the community itself (Cyril, Smith, Possamai-Inesedy, & Renzaho, 2015). Other models include those of empowerment where decisions are taken by the community with help from outsiders (Brunton et al., 2017). Examples of community engagement in Australia include the Latrobe Health Innovation Zone in Victoria where there is concerted involvement of community groups and agencies in the planning and delivery of better health and wellbeing outcomes following the Hazelwood Mine Fire Inquiry (Victorian Government, 2018) and the place-based suicide prevention program in Victoria and Tasmania where communities are engaged as active partners in developing solutions (Victorian and Tasmanian PHN Alliance, 2018).

Actions in primary care

It is acknowledged that if people with mental health problems and their families are to access mental health care, the latter needs to be integrated into primary care services (World Health Organization, 2018a) because general practitioners (GPs) are considered to be the gateway to mental health services. While much has been achieved in improving skills of GPs in Australia, there is still considerable variability in competence and interest in this section of the health workforce. Despite the desirability of establishment of 'stepped care' models and an injunction to Primary Health Networks to attend to this going back several years (see Section 1.5.6), implementation is inconsistent across the country so there may not be clear structured escalation pathways from GPs to mental health services (General Practice New South Wales, 2014). In addition, current funding mechanisms are a disincentive for GPs to provide care for individuals with mental health problems (General Practice New South Wales, 2014). Actions in primary care therefore require redesigned models of care, investment in implementation research, financial and human resources and supportive government policy (World Health Organization, 2018a).

Actions in humanitarian settings

Asylum seekers and refugees are often among the most vulnerable people in Australia, having experienced torture and trauma prior to displacement and flight. Detained asylum seekers are particularly at risk of PTSD, depression and anxiety (Filges, Montgomery, Kastrup, & Jørgensen, 2015). Even while in the community, refugees facing difficulties with social integration experience a higher prevalence of mental disorders due to isolation, discrimination and unemployment (WHO Regional Office for Europe, 2018).

Actions targeted at improving the mental health and wellbeing of such communities should start with providing basic needs such as food security, accommodation and general subsistence (WHO Regional Office for Europe, 2018). Once basic needs are provided, actions that focus on providing a safe and healthy school environment for children and adolescents as well as employment for adults are recommended (WHO Regional Office for Europe, 2018).

Targeted interventions to improve mental health and access to mental health services include providing information on entitlement to both users and providers of mental health care, establishing outreach services that provide a bridge to mainstream mental health care, coordinating mental and physical health care with social services, providing cultural mediators and interpretation services to enable better patient-clinician interactions and cultural competence training for clinicians and other health care providers (WHO Regional Office for Europe, 2018).

Actions targeting the natural and built environment

It is widely acknowledged that health is created and lived by people in the settings of their everyday lives and it depends on all of society's combined action on the physical and social environment (Tsouros, 1991). Actions that aim to support mental health can directly influence mental and physical health outcomes. In addition to the built environment, the natural environment and outdoor spaces are also important for good mental health. Engaging in outdoor activities such as walking, cycling and gardening have been shown to reduce stress, anxiety and depression (Barton, Hine, & Pretty, 2009; Pretty et al., 2007).

Towards this end, the WHO launched the European Healthy Cities Network in 1987-88 (Tsouros, 2015) which has since expanded across the globe (de Leeuw & Simos, 2017). A healthy city is 'one that is conscious of health and health equity and strives to improve it' (Tsouros, 2015). There are 11 parameters recommended for a healthy city such as a clean and safe physical environment with a sustainable ecosystem and the establishment of a mutually supportive community who have control over the decisions affecting their lives and wellbeing (de Leeuw, 2011). Goal 11 of the Sustainable Development Goals also promises to make cities and other human settlements 'safe, inclusive, resilient and sustainable by 2030' (United Nations, 2020).

Onkaparinga near Adelaide and Kiama on the South Coast of NSW are Australian attempts at replicating the Healthy Cities approach (de Leeuw & Simos, 2017). However, it has been argued that the continuation of the monetarist market-driven order sustains inequities and poses a challenge to this approach (Shepherd et al., 2017).

COUNTRY LEVEL CONTEXTS

Country level studies on social determinants have shown that increase in unemployment such as that which occurred due to the financial crisis of 2008 was associated with an increased number of suicides, particularly in men (Barr, Taylor-Robinson, Scott-Samuel, McKee, & Stuckler, 2012; Chang, Stuckler, Yip, & Gunnell, 2013; Stuckler, Basu, Suhrcke, Coutts, & McKee, 2009). Times of economic hardship tend to exacerbate social exclusion of people with mental illness, particularly males and those with lower education status (Evans-Lacko, Knapp, McCrone, Thornicroft, & Mojtabai, 2013) and job insecurity is associated with poorer mental health (Virtanen et al., 2011). Strong social welfare schemes appear to protect against unemployment risks for poor mental health (Stuckler et al., 2009). Australia's National Mental Health Policy 2008 expanded its framework to include housing, education and employment as well as getting different sectors to come together to work collaboratively in the promotion, prevention and early intervention services (Commonwealth of Australia, 2009).

PRINCIPLES FOR ACTION TO ADDRESS SOCIAL DETERMINANTS

Rawls veil of ignorance

We briefly account here an example of a reasoning approach to morality in social and other policy decision making (see Chapters 1.1 and 1.5) which has been an important contribution of John Rawls, an influential twentieth century American egalitarian moral and political philosopher. With reference to earlier philosophical traditions, this was an idea grounded in a frequently used philosophical method, the thought experiment. Thought experiments may not necessarily be practical in reality but imagining them can help us work through philosophical problems and challenges. Rawls proposed that political decision making can helpfully be considered as ideally operating from behind a *veil of ignorance* (Rawls, 1999). That is to say, if the decision maker is unaware of where they may be placed in society, considered in terms of level of resources or power for instance, then they may make decisions that are more purely based on morals than personal vested interest. In this context then, we may consider that purely morally based decisions about policy as it bears on mental health care, might be made from a position of ignorance about where the individual might be placed on a range of levels of influence of social determinants of mental health and illness. The sections that follow will consider specific principles and actions advocated for within key headings as set out by the WHO and implicitly represent considerations largely made as if from behind a Rawlesian Veil of Ignorance.

Proportionate universalism

Services and health programs that are targeted to the poor and disadvantaged often become poorly funded and implemented and are ultimately withdrawn because they do not enjoy the support of the entire population. Furthermore, those for whom the service is meant for, usually do not have the power to complain about its poor quality or withdrawal. As a result, most services and programs targeted at disenfranchised groups do not succeed in reducing the health inequalities that they are designed to achieve.

Inequalities in mental health (and physical health) exist along a social class gradient where every member of the population experiences some degree of health inequity. Targeted services are likely to miss most of these inequities by creating 'unfair cut offs' of certain groups. The concept of proportionate universalism aims to overcome the limitations of targeted programs by providing services according to the level of need of people across the entire social gradient.

Action across sectors

Risk and protective factors of mental health problems occur at different levels such as the family, community, structural and population level. A social determinants approach includes health, education, employment, transport, accommodation, etc which requires strong collaboration between health and non-health sectors. A reduction in health inequalities can be achieved when health equity is a central theme in all policies across all sectors. Implementing intersectoral collaboration requires innovation and a joint sense of purpose. An Australian example of successful intersectoral collaboration was showcased in the Partners in Recovery initiative (Isaacs, Sutton, Dalziel, & Maybery, 2017).

Life course approach

When a life course perspective is adopted, it implies that there is a recognition that mental health at each stage of life is influenced by both unique and common factors and that mental health and illness accumulates throughout life. Accordingly, strategies aimed at prevention and treatment should be appropriately designed to the different stages of life and in so doing, appropriate organisations such as early learning centres, schools and employers must be involved. Special attention will also need to be paid to the promotion of positive mental health and the prevention of mental disorders in old age, given the expected upsurge in the proportion of older people

Early intervention

The life course approach specifies that it is vital that every child gets the best possible start in life. In order to achieve this, it is imperative that parents are supported to increase both their chances and that of their children, of having better mental health. Interventions for persons with a mental illness who have children can not only improve mental illness outcomes for the parent but also promote positive determinants of the child's wellbeing and reduce the risk of the child developing a mental illness later on (Siegenthaler, Munder, & Egger, 2012).

Healthy mind and healthy body

Social determinants of health impact both physical and mental health. In addition, physical illness can impact on the mental health of a person and vice versa. Therefore reducing mental health inequalities will require actions to reduce physical health inequalities as well. A social determinants approach will therefore need to consider both physical and mental health implications.

Prioritising mental health

Mental health needs to be prioritised across all policy areas in the entire population—not just in health (McQueen, Wismar, Lin, Jones, & Davies, 2012)—by highlighting its strong links to productivity (Jenkins & Minoletti, 2013). Increased awareness and understanding of mental health needs to coincide with more financial, medical and human resource allocations towards addressing mental health inequalities.

Avoiding short-termism

A common criticism of policy making is that it is often short-sighted or is obstructed by short-term thinking. A social determinants approach to mental health cannot afford to be so because it includes a life course perspective requiring long-term and sustainable policies. It is therefore vital that policy makers consider durable strategies with long-term implications such as building of communities, capacities, partnerships and local institutions across the life course.

Mental health equity in all policies

Just as mental health needs to be prioritised by all policy areas, it is also necessary for all sectors to ensure that policies do not in any way harm or potentially worsen mental health inequities. There are a number of tools that can be used for the assessment of the impact of policy on physical health equity. These can be modified or redeveloped to include mental health equity.

Knowledge for action at the local level

Different types of information is necessary in order to implement action to prevent and improve mental health at the local level. National level strategies should provide the framework and support for local level action

Types of information necessary for action at the local level:

- burden of mental disorders such as distribution of mental disorders and unmet need for services and programs
- public knowledge and understanding of mental illness
- socioeconomic stressors and mechanisms
- help-seeking behaviours, pathways to treatment
- evaluation of services and programs for mental health problems
- local views on potential solutions and interventions
- availability of local assets and resources

- knowledge about synergies between interventions in education, housing, transport, income generation schemes and community development
- knowledge about evidence-based interventions in other settings.

Country-wide strategies

Country-wide strategies have the greatest potential to reach large populations and are most likely to have a significant impact on reducing mental health inequalities. Strategies aimed at alleviation of poverty, effective social protection across the life course, reduction of discrimination, promoting access to employment, health care, housing, and education, can have positive benefits for mental health.

Areas such as treatment of maternal depression, early childhood development, disadvantaged families where there is mental illness and alcohol dependence which have particularly strong associations with mental disorders and a clear social class gradient must be specifically targeted by policy initiatives.

INEQUALITY AND MENTAL HEALTH PROBLEMS

> Everybody knows the fight was fixed; The poor stay poor, the rich get rich; That's how; it goes; Everybody knows
>
> *Leonard Cohen*

Wilkinson and Pickett (2011; 2018b) have shown that a host of social and health problems are more frequent in societies where there is a large difference in income levels between the rich and poor. The more the inequality the worse the problems. Combining internationally comparable data, they demonstrate that the highest rates of mental illness are in the United States, followed by Australia, UK, New Zealand and Canada, the most unequal of the rich developed countries (2018b, p. 35). Their book, *The Inner Level* (2018b), describes psychological effects of inequality. They suggest that people who live in more unequal societies have higher psychological distress which in turn results in higher rates of depression, anxiety and suicide. Schizophrenia and psychotic disorders are also higher in more unequal societies. People respond differently to this distress. For instance, they can become depressed or anxious or develop self enhancement and narcissistic behaviour–which also seem to increase in more unequal societies. Inequality affects not just health and mental health, but also the quality of social relations and behavioural outcomes. In more unequal countries diminished levels of trust and increasing rates of isolation and loneliness prevail, taking their toll on emotional and mental wellbeing. Income differences can be reduced by progressive taxation and increasing economic democracy. However changes such as this may not be readily influenced by mental health policy frameworks. The SDGs introduced earlier include as goal 10 reducing inequities, but there is evidence that income and wealth trends in Australia as in many other nations, in fact are going in the opposite direction (see Chapters 1.5 and 1.6).

1.2.5 PANDEMICS AND MENTAL HEALTH

ANTON ISAACS & GRAHAM MEADOWS

Epidemics are significant increases in disease prevalence in one community or country, while pandemics involve simultaneous worldwide disease spread. Recorded examples of pandemics go back for millennia and a list of the most damaging ones, some of which have killed tens of millions of people, would include several of each of influenza and cholera, bubonic plague, HIV/AIDS and–at time of writing–COVID-19. The mental and psychological effects of the latest pandemic appear to be immense due to increased global interconnectedness (Ventriglio, Watson, & Bhugra, 2020). It can be that the most important public impact of a pandemic is the lockdown of societal activities resulting in job losses, economic downturns and social isolation. This in turn can cause individuals and households to experience financial stress (Australian Bureau of Statistics, 2020), loneliness (Banerjee & Rai, 2020) and decreased access to community and religious support (Reger, Stanley, & Joiner, 2020). Given the causal contribution these and other affected social determinants (see Section 1.2.4) make to mental health problems and to extended episodes, we can expect that the incidence and prevalence of depression, anxiety, post-traumatic stress disorders and insomnia in the population will increase during such times (Torales, O'Higgins, Castaldelli-Maia, & Ventriglio, 2020).

For people with disorders such as schizophrenia, effects may be considered in terms of interference with a recovery journey—social isolation and job loss or insecurity for instance may interfere with this journey across domains of connectedness, hope, identity, meaning and purpose, and empowerment (CHIME; see Section 2.6.2). Mental health effects of pandemics are therefore widespread. As well as presenting heavy, even overwhelming impacts on general health systems, they also can over-tax mental health services (Li et al., 2020; Percudani, Corradin, Moreno, Indelicato, & Vita, 2020). Health care workers in particular—who may be at increased disease risk through patient-exposure—may also experience fatigue and lower levels of performance (Torales et al., 2020) and the occupational stress may increase their risk of mental illness. So in that context, health care workers also have needs to be heard, supported, protected, and cared for (Shanafelt, Ripp, & Trockel, 2020) as well as potentially having needs for specific mental health care.

Considering trends in the ever-changing world order that increase the risk and severity of mental health impacts during pandemics (see Sections 1.2.2 and 1.2.4), it becomes imperative to identify, prepare for and manage these situations. The COVID-19 pandemic has thrust epidemiological modelling of different kinds—including simulation modelling (see Section 1.5.11) into at times front-page news and it is to be anticipated that modelling of mental health impacts will feature in future planning for such events. We have proposed (see Section 1.1.8) that this is a compelling example of complexity as a challenge. The balancing of attention to addressing social determinants, suppression or possible eradication of disease spread, and provision of accessible health care may be informed by well-constructed and validated simulation models. Telehealth has great potential as a way of reaching people in this context with psychological interventions. But unless this mode delivers more equitable services than the existing Australian system (see Section 1.2.5), it may not have the hoped-for population health effects.

1.2.6 APPLYING THESE CONCEPTS AROUND SOCIAL DETERMINANTS TO AUSTRALIA

GRAHAM MEADOWS, JOANNE ENTICOTT & SEBASTIAN ROSENBERG

FINDINGS ON SOCIAL DETERMINANTS

As noted in the previous chapter on epidemiology, our best most recent data on levels of mental health problems in Australian communities comes from studies using the Kessler 10 scale. As Jorm noted (2018), 'Studies on Australian samples have shown that psychological distress is associated with unemployment (Reavley, Jorm, Cvetkovski, & Mackinnon, 2011), low income (Enticott et al., 2018); low social capital (Phongsavan, Chey, Bauman, Brooks, & Silove, 2006), low social connectedness and social support (Atkins, Naismith, Luscombe, & Hickie, 2013; Levula, Harr, & Wilson, 2018); workplace characteristics (Considine et al., 2017); poor quality diet (Hodge, Almeida, English, Giles, & Flicker, 2013; Nguyen, Ding, & Mihrshahi, 2017), limitations on physical functioning (Atkins et al., 2013); and physical diseases (Byles et al., 2014)'.

INCREASING INEQUALITY

Inequity in service responses

Introduction

As Jorm noted in assessing population health impacts of the Better Access Scheme, 'There may be limits on how much change treatment can produce where such risk factors (unemployment, low income, low social capital, connectedness and support, poor diet, physical diseases and limitations on physical functioning) are present and persisting. Dealing with these risk factors may require a greater emphasis on prevention (Jorm, 2014) and on social factors that lie outside the domain of mental health services (Mulder, Rucklidge, &

Wilkinson, 2017).' However, if we take as a standpoint that services should be reasonably evenly accessible to all in need, as might be guided by consideration of decision making from behind a Rawlesian Veil of Ignorance position (see Chapter 1.2), then we should find that services work to some measure to balance the inequalities that result from the impact of factors such as socioeconomic disadvantage. Authors (including some working on this text) examined this in an article in *The Conversation (Three Charts On...)* which is reproduced here under terms of the Creative Commons licence. *The Conversation* is a useful source for academically well-informed accounts of contemporary issues and has a good amount of material relevant to mental health care.

The National Mental Health Services Planning Framework

Some information on this, with its key component of a planning support tool (PST) can be found in Section 1.2.5. One key point in relation to the issue of social determinants as under consideration here is that the PST estimates service need and response for communities generally typical of Australia–apart from consideration of the very general demographic features of age and sex of the population. It does not yet feature adjustments of planning estimates for any of the social determinants identified in this chapter.

BOX 1.6: THREE CHARTS ON—WHY RATES OF MENTAL ILLNESS AREN'T GOING DOWN DESPITE HIGHER SPENDING

Successive Australian governments have increased their spending on mental health over the last few decades, which is a good thing. But when the rate of mental illness isn't going down, we need to step back and ask why.

Our research shows there is unfairness in how Australia's mental health care is delivered. Improving mental health will depend at least in part on fairer distribution. While this means increasing spending in regional and remote Australia, it also means getting more resources to poorer urban areas.

Higher spending, but no effects

Major funding streams into mental health care come from state and territory governments (60%), the Australian Government (35%) and private health insurance funds (5%). The rising blue line in the below graph represents this total dollar spend, which has been increasing. Today it is around AU$150 more per person than in 1999–2000.

Figure 1.4 Annual mental health expenditure per capita versus % of population with a very high Kessler 10 (K10) mental health score

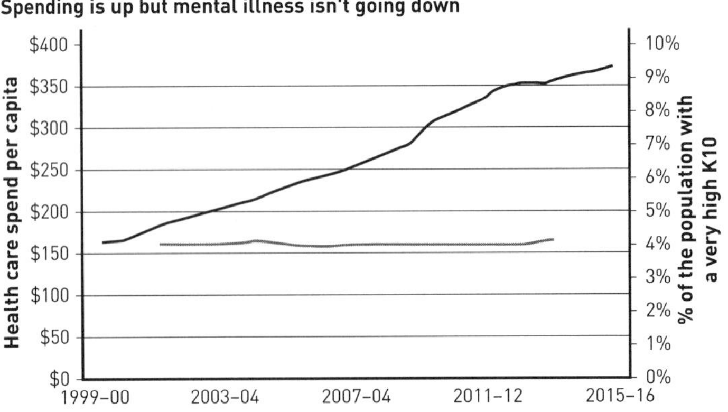

We might hope the proportion of the population with active mental health problems would be going down with the increase in spending. But the bottom red line shows this isn't the case. This line represents the rate of the population with higher levels of psychological distress, as quantified by the Kessler 10.

The Kessler 10 (K10) is a questionnaire answered by around 20 000 Australians in national surveys every three years. It asks about depressive and anxiety symptoms in the last 30 days. Your GP might have asked you to fill out this questionnaire if mental health has been discussed.

People with increased scores are likely to have clinical anxiety or depressive problems, so the rate of very high K10 (30 or more) is a useful measure of mental illness in the population.

The slug-like creep of an essentially flat (red) line shows that the percentage of Australians with very high K10 scores has stayed steady at a bit over 4% since 1999–2000.

Funding isn't getting to the right people

So why is increased spending not affecting the very high K10 rate? Perhaps it needs to reach some higher dollar threshold to make a difference. Maybe other cultural changes are pushing up the underlying rate, or money needs to be spent differently—perhaps more on, say, effective prevention.

However, we suggest a major reason is that the increased spending is not getting care to people in the areas that need it most.

Figure 1.5 Mental health service use versus % of population with a very high K10 score, by area

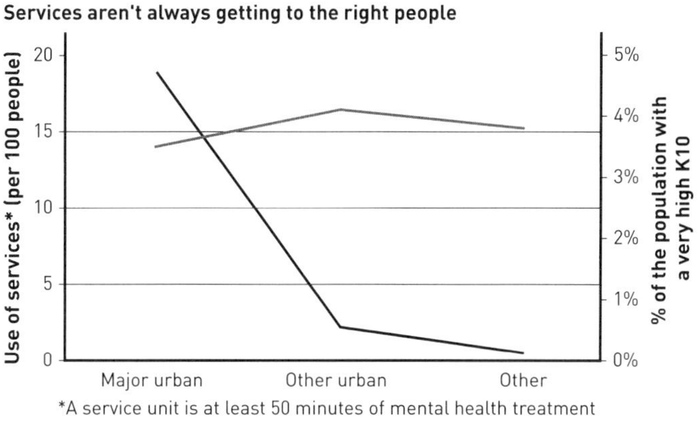

Medicare data reveal something of how this is happening. The left axis of the second graph has a blue line showing the annual use for each 100 people of Medicare item 80010—a session of about an hour with a clinical psychologist—over four years, across various regions. Once you leave the major urban areas, this rate just about falls off a cliff.

It's important to note the rate of very high K10 (represented by the red line) isn't appreciably higher outside the big cities. While there will be specific remote areas with higher rates, overall living in regional and remote Australia doesn't seem to mean you're more likely to have clinical anxiety or depression.

But, as the graph shows, you are much less likely to get to consult with a clinical psychologist to help you with the condition if you live in a regional or remote area.

Socioeconomic disadvantage

Another big problem is socioeconomic disadvantage. This is measured with the Index of Relative Socioeconomic Disadvantage (IRSD), which the next graph groups into five bands: from most deprived (poorest, left) to least (richest, right).

Figure 1.6 Mental health service use versus % of population with a very high K10 score, by area of socioeconomic disadvantage (IRSD scale)

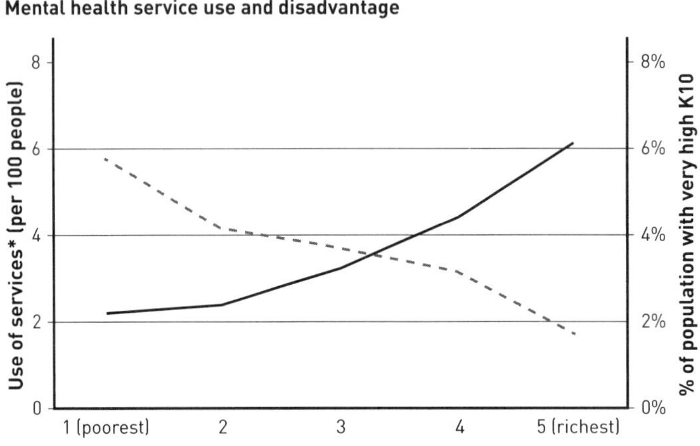

*A service unit is at least 50 minutes of mental health treatment

The left axis and bold line show how people living in deprived areas—and there's a lot of them, mostly in cities—are much less likely to be seeing clinical psychologists. On the right axis and the dash line we see the rate of very high K10 scores getting higher with more disadvantage.

The X shape of the graph shows that, paradoxically, as the rate of disorders goes down in better-off areas, the rate of use of these mental health services goes up. Use of these services may be as much as nine times less proportionally to the number of people with mental health problems in the worst-off areas, compared with people in the best-off fifth of the country.

For example, we find double the specialist services in Melbourne's City of Bayside (IRSD band five) compared to Dandenong (IRSD band one) or in North Sydney (IRSD band five) compared with Blacktown (low in IRSD band three).

There are similar disparities, though differing in degree, for other Medicare-supported specialist psychological treatment services provided by different disciplines. GP mental health services, it is worth saying, are delivered somewhat more evenly.

Continued funding growth for mental health care is needed and welcome. However, we suggest more be done to ensure care gets to where it is needed most. This will not be simple: delivery models, mental health literacy, gap fees, funding and planning models all need urgent attention or reform.

This will require new levels of leadership and cooperation between governments, professional bodies and communities.

Source: Meadows, Enticott, & Rosenberg, 2018

Australia's inequality has been increasing

Given all these arguments we may be concerned about whether inequality and inequity are on the rise in Australia or not. This is a highly politically sensitive issue and the various indices are open to different readings. Income and wealth may behave rather differently and tracking the differences between the upper and lower quintiles and deciles, or the top 1% all may yield different results. We will not attempt to fully cover these issues but will note that if we simply go to the World Bank website (World Bank, 2019b) we can access a graph showing the Gini index for income in Australia. The Gini index is a measurement of inequality which varies from to notional extremes: 0, or no inequality where everyone has the same level of resources, and 100, where one individual or household has all the resources and no one else has any. Since the extremes are each never approached closely, even small changes in the Gini numerically can indicate considerable differences in disparities. Australia's Gini index in 1981 was 31.3, in 2000 it was 33.5 and the most recent number is 35.8, indicating that Australia has been becoming more inequitable, along with, it must be said, much of the world. But that may not be good news for mental health here or elsewhere.

Summary

What we know is that Australia has considerable inequality and arguably inequity in many of these risk factors. A social justice approach to how services should be targeted could sensibly be grounded either in the UN declaration proposition that medical care and necessary social services, adequate for health and wellbeing, should be a universal right, or as introduced earlier in a Rawlesian maximin framework, and taking into account the WHO proposition to progressive universalism. These together would indicate that Australian mental health care of adequate quality to be of substantial benefit should be delivered in ways accessible to the full range of Australian communities, adapted where necessary to meet local cultural, resourcing and geographic challenges. Here, the Australian system clearly is failing many and perhaps most people who have mental health problems. The treatment gap is much higher in some areas of the country than others. Regional and remote areas often fare badly but more people being poorly served live in poorer areas of cities (Meadows et al., 2019).

Developments in Australian and state level mental health care are discussed in Chapter 1.7. Key points about contemporary developments where considerations of relative and absolute inequity arise may be at least in the cases of the NDIS, delivery of state level services, distribution of Commonwealth-funded services including those funded by Medicare and through the Primary Health Networks. (See Chapter 1.7.)

1.2.7 COMMENTARY AND REFLECTION

GRAHAM MEADOWS & SEBASTIAN ROSENBERG

As should be clear from the above content, determinants of and influences on mental health come in many forms and operate at many different levels. Critically, Australia as the driest inhabited continent has much to be concerned about as climate change including global heating impacts. For some communities this can present threats of existential proportions; mental health services have important roles in responsiveness while constructive engagement with social action and environmental campaigning may be valuable strategies at personal, societal and environmental levels.

Through the course of the work of finalising this text, firstly the unprecedented 2020 bushfire season unfolded across much of Australia in January 2020 and then the COVID-19 outbreaks were declared a pandemic in March 2020. Preparedness, informed and agile responsiveness to such events, posing as they do threats to health and wellbeing as well as to the social and economic frameworks of the country, will be critical challenges for Australia as this century unfolds. Actions taking perspectives across the whole of society and whole of government are necessary to effectively respond to such challenges. Australia's political and health care system has qualities of fragmentation (see Chapters 1.5 and 1.7) which can impede such responsiveness.

Considering inequity in Australia, the UN and WHO policy documents that have featured heavily in this chapter would point us in the direction of social policy changes that would reduce inequality in society, but inequality in Australia has been trending up not down. This can exacerbate societal and personal impacts of natural disasters, anthropogenic ecological crises, and disease outbreaks. From the point of view of mental health service delivery we should be seeking to particularly target areas and groups with greater morbidity, providing services that might make a difference to their lives. But at present in better-off areas, we see people with mental health problems often receiving a much more comprehensive set of services than those in poorer areas. So Australia's services are in many cases not readily diverted to where public health or equity considerations might indicate they would do more good. In later chapters, we will consider how planning for areas service delivery (see Chapters 1.5 and 1.7) has capacity to address this but also addresses the challenges that rational planning in these areas, including potential barriers in the Australian Constitution. It may, however, be critical to find a way around these impediments in the coming years if we are hoping to bring down the rates of mental health problems in the community.

1.3

SPECIFIC COMMUNITY PERSPECTIVES IN MENTAL HEALTH

PAT DUDGEON, SABINE HAMMOND, GRAHAM MEADOWS, HELEN MILROY, SALLY MORRIS & SEBASTIAN ROSENBERG

1.3.1 INTRODUCTION

Mental health and mental illness are unique experiences, in that the way people feel is very individual. Indeed, it is dangerous, or inappropriate to make generalisations about the experience of mental illness. Despite this, there are some views and perspectives that often struggle to be heard or understood in relation to mental health. The aim of this chapter is to present some of these key views. We include sections which describe perspectives about mental health and illness from Indigenous and LGBTIQ people. This book could never fully reflect such a diversity of experiences. But we present these views in the hope that even in this summary form, they can provide readers with new understanding about these important perspectives.

As the Australian population grows it continues to diversify. Some of the issues pertaining to people from culturally and linguistically diverse communities are described in other parts of this book (see Section 1.6.5 and Section 2.1.12; see also Sections 2.3.4, 2.4.12, 3.2.5, 3.2.8, 4.6.6 and 4.9.10). There is a great deal to learn if we are to develop quality mental health care approaches which meet the specific cultural and social needs of Australia's diverse population.

1.3.2 WORKING WITH ABORIGINAL AND TORRES STRAIT ISLANDER PEOPLES: A SOCIAL AND EMOTIONAL WELLBEING PERSPECTIVE

HELEN MILROY, SABINE HAMMOND & PAT DUDGEON

1.3.3 INTRODUCTION

Understanding the historical context and continued disadvantage of Aboriginal and Torres Strait Islander peoples is critical for all mental health professionals. This section provides:

- A summary of who are Australia's First Peoples
- Historical background to Indigenous disadvantage and the health gap
- Indigenous conceptualisations of mental health and social and emotional wellbeing
- An outline of relevant frameworks, standards and guidelines
- Key considerations for supporting social and emotional wellbeing
- A discussion addressing the urgent crisis: Aboriginal and Torres Strait Islander suicide
- Conclusions and implications for practice in mental health.

This section of the book cannot address all the considerations and implications for working effectively with Aboriginal and Torres Strait Islander peoples. Instead, this chapter serves as an overview of important concepts, frameworks and considerations. Readers are referred to *Working Together: Aboriginal and Torres Strait Islander Mental Health and Wellbeing Principles and Practice* (2014) for in-depth consideration of respectful and effective knowledge and conceptual and practical work in this space.

WHO ARE AUSTRALIA'S FIRST PEOPLES?

Aboriginal Australians are recognised as the oldest continuous culture in the world, with a history of over 60 000 years or more (Langton, 2018). There are two distinct main cultural groups: Aboriginal peoples on the Australian mainland and the Torres Strait Islander peoples living on the islands in the Torres Strait off Northern Queensland. However, these two main groups include many diverse nations, cultures and languages, with estimates of over 250 separate language groups pre-colonisation (Behrendt, 2012; Hampton & Toombs, 2013; Langton, 2018; Pascoe, 2018). The books by these Indigenous authors provide an introduction to Aboriginal and Torres Strait Islander history and culture; and contribute to an understanding of the impact of colonial history in First Australians' health and wellbeing.

Terminology is important for showing respect and understanding of the diversity among Australia's First Peoples. The terms 'Aboriginal and Torres Strait Islander peoples' refers to persons of Aboriginal and Torres Strait Islander descent who identify, are recognised and accepted as Aboriginal and/or Torres Strait Islander people in their community. Aboriginal and Torres Strait identity is not about the percentages or skin colour but about being part of and contributing to the community (Behrendt & Fraser, 2012; Langton, 2018).

The term 'Indigenous' is a generic term that refers to over 370 million Indigenous peoples worldwide (see United Nations Declaration on the Rights of Indigenous Peoples, 2007; United Nations, 2007a). The United Nations (2013) has explicitly refrained from providing an official definition of 'Indigenous' given the diversity of Indigenous peoples. Many Indigenous peoples prefer to use other terms, including First Peoples, First Nations and First Australians. In Australia, the term 'Indigenous' refers to Aboriginal and Torres Strait Islander peoples. Aboriginal and Torres Strait Islander people typically identify the specific group(s) they belong to, such as Wurundjeri, Kabi, Kamilaroi, and so on. In this chapter, the term 'Indigenous' will refer to Australia's First Peoples, the Aboriginal and Torres Strait Islander people.

According to the 2016 Australian Census (Australian Bureau of Statistics (ABS), 2018a), the Indigenous population in Australia was 798 400 people, or 3.3% of the overall population of Australia, with 727 500 people (91%) identified as of Aboriginal origin, 38 700 people (5%) of Torres Strait Islander origin, and 32 200 people (4%) of both Aboriginal and Torres Strait Islander origin. The largest number of Aboriginal and Torres Strait Islander people lived in New South Wales (265 865), followed by Queensland (221 276), Western Australia (100 512), the Northern

Territory (74 546), Victoria (57 767), South Australia (42 265), Tasmania (28 537), with the smallest number in the Australia Capital Territory (7513). The Northern Territory has the highest percentage (30%) of Indigenous people compared with non-Indigenous populations, with all other states and territories below 5.5%.

The ABS data also show that the average age of the Aboriginal and Torres Strait Islander population is considerably younger than the non-Indigenous population (23.0 years compared to 37.8 years) and that the proportion of older people is much smaller due to higher mortality rates. This altered population age structure has implications for mental health due to the large numbers of children relative to adults. There is less support for families due to the relative loss of grandparents and Elders in the community and hence sometimes the burden of care rests with young people in the community. Over one-third (38% or 298 400) of Aboriginal and Torres Strait Islander people lived in major cities, 24% (189 400) lived in inner regional areas, 20% (161 800) in outer regional areas, 7% (53 500) lived in remote areas and 12% (95 200) in very remote areas around Australia. This data serves to illustrate that mental health workers are more likely to encounter Indigenous consumers and their families in urban and regional areas.

Historical background to Indigenous disadvantage and the health gap

Estimates of the Aboriginal and Torres Strait Islander population at the time of settlement in 1788 range from a low 315 000 to over 1 million (ABS, 2008). Many accounts of Australian history have focused on colonial history and have omitted the rich history and culture of Aboriginal and Torres Strait Islander peoples both pre- and post-colonisation. The colonial doctrine of '*terra nullius*' ('uninhabited land or land belonging to no one') was used to justify dispossession of Australia's traditional custodians from their lands and waters. Although Aboriginal and Torres Strait Islander peoples resisted invasion from the onset and continued to do so with the spread of colonialisation, the number of Indigenous people declined to 117 000 (and possibly as low as 60 000) people in 1900. Dispossession (including removal from lands), lack of resistance to introduced diseases and systematic massacres continued into the 1920s (Lydon, 2018, Nettelbeck & Ryan, 2018).

Beginning in the 1860s and continuing into the 1970s, policies under the guise of 'protection' of Aboriginal people were used to justify the forced removal of children from their families and placing them into institutions (Australian Human Rights Commission (AHRC), 1997; Behrendt & Fraser, 2012). The Report of the National Inquiry into the separation of Aboriginal and Torres Strait Islander children from their families conducted by the Australian Human Rights Commission (AHRC), concluded that 'forcible removal was an act of genocide' (Australian Human Rights Commission, 1997). The full magnitude of the colonial legacy must be considered in light of the ongoing issues of intergenerational trauma, grief and loss and the impact on mental health.

Self-determination and human rights

It has taken a long time to recognise Aboriginal and Torres Strait Islander peoples and their rights. The Australian Indigenous Human Rights movement started in the 1920s (Foley, Schaap, & Howell, 2014). The Australian Constitution was finally changed to grant citizenship status to Indigenous Australians following the 1967 referendum (Attwood & Markus, 2017; Gillespie, 2007). From 1972 to 1998, the Australian Government supported a self-determination policy for Indigenous affairs. The doctrine of *terra nullius* was only overthrown by the landmark 1992 Mabo judgment, which recognised Native Title in Australia for the first time (Brennan, Davis, Edgeworth, & Terrill, 2015).

From 1993, the AHRC published annual Social Justice Reports on the human rights performance of Australian Governments for Australia's Indigenous peoples. *The Bringing Them Home Report* (Australian Human Rights Commission (AHRC), 1997) demonstrated the extent of negative effects not only on the children who were forcibly removed, but also on their families, communities and descendants. The report highlighted both the individual suffering (abuse, maltreatment, low access to education), grief, cultural and community disintegration, the cutting of links to traditional lands and the ongoing issues (e.g. intergenerational trauma) resulting from this policy.

In 2008, the then Prime Minister Kevin Rudd issued an apology to the Stolen Generations—recognising the grief, suffering and loss that policies and laws had inflicted on Aboriginal and Torres Strait Islander peoples (Australian Government, 2019a). In June 2017, the *Uluru Statement from the Heart* called for a First Nations voice in the Australian Constitution (Parliament of Australia, 2017a).

In 2019, Ken Wyatt became the Federal Minister for Indigenous Australians, the first Indigenous person to hold this position. He raised the importance of Indigenous voice and self-determination (Wyatt, 2019). However, despite these positive steps forward, many Indigenous Australians remain concerned that their right to self-determination is still not acknowledged and supported adequately in laws, polices and services. Understanding this historical context and continued disadvantage for Aboriginal and Torres Strait Islander peoples is critical for all mental health professionals. For some groups who have had a positive Native Title determination, they have reported a positive impact on their wellbeing. This further demonstrates the interconnected nature of land, culture, identity and wellbeing.

A key concept for mental health practitioners to understand is the definition of Aboriginal and Torres Strait Islander identity (Dudgeon, Milroy, & Walker, 2014). Three criteria have replaced race-based definitions since 1981 and are now generally used to acknowledge Aboriginal and Torres Strait Islander status and identity:

1. being of Aboriginal and/or Torres Strait Islander *descent*,
2. *identifying* as an Aboriginal and/or Torres Strait Islander person and
3. being *recognised* and accepted as Aboriginal and/or Torres Strait Islander by the *community* where the person currently lives or has lived (Gardiner-Garden, 2003).

Carlson (2016) explores the complex and controversial considerations involving Aboriginal identity with respect to both government policy and the lived experience of Indigenous Australians. Oxenham (1999) provides another excellent resource that helps to understand Indigenous identity through in-depth personal discussions of issues central to contemporary Aboriginality among 10 Aboriginal leaders in the mental health and education area. Other resources include the Twitter handle Indigenous X (@indigenousx, 2020), where Aboriginal and/or Torres Strait Islander people discuss issues from their perspective.

The discussions in Oxenham (1999) include thoughtful reflection on constructions of identity, representation of Aboriginality, advantages and disadvantages of identification, problems of self-identification, sources of learning about Aboriginality, definition of community, status of traditional practices, internal and external racism. Understanding these nuances in the definition of Aboriginality and Aboriginal identity is of special importance for mental health professionals aiming to engage with Aboriginal and Torres Strait Islander consumers and carers—they need to challenge their assumptions of who is an Indigenous person, what Indigenous people look like and be aware how their responses may appear as racist and undermine consumers' trust and ability to engage, especially with a mainstream mental health service.

To this day, Aboriginal and Torres Strait Islander peoples experience significant inequalities and disadvantage in their health, life-expectancy, education and employment (Calma, Dudgeon, & Bray, 2017) and are overrepresented in rates of detention and imprisonment (O'Brien & Trudgett, 2018). The unacceptable disparity between Indigenous and non-Indigenous Australians is increasingly being acknowledged as long-term consequences of Australian colonial policies and the denial of Aboriginal and Torres Strait Islander peoples' human rights.

CONCEPTUALISATIONS OF MENTAL HEALTH AND SOCIAL AND EMOTIONAL WELLBEING

For Aboriginal and Torres Strait Islander people, mental health is holistic, reflecting the interrelationship of physical, mental, social, emotional, spiritual and cultural health (Hampton & Toombs, 2013; Ypinazar, Margolis, Haswell-Elkins, & Tsey, 2007). Parker and Milroy (2014) describe how the Indigenous holistic concepts of mental health, together with cultural factors (connection to country, kinship, sense of self), 'provided the optimal conditions for mental health and social and emotional wellbeing' (p. 26) for Aboriginal and Torres Strait Islander people and communities. For many Indigenous persons, the narrow definition of the term mental health does not fit their holistic concepts and may even denote mental illness and elicit negative associations with psychiatric hospitalisation.

The Social and Emotional Wellbeing Framework (Swan & Raphael, 1995; Gee, Dudgeon, Schultz, Hart, & Kelly, 2014) provides a full appreciation of this holistic concept of health and mental health. In this framework, social and emotional wellbeing (SEWB) is conceptualised as the experience and expression of connections to seven domains of wellbeing:

1 the body (physical)
2 mind and emotions
3 family and kinship
4 community
5 culture
6 country (land) and
7 spirituality/ancestors.

These seven dimensions need to be understood within the broader context of social, cultural, political and historical determinants (Zubrick et al., 2014). Nine guiding principles, first set out by Swan and Raphael (1995), have underpinned the SEWB framework since 2004 and have been reemphasised in the National Strategic Framework for Aboriginal and Torres Strait Islander Peoples' Mental Health and Social and Emotional Wellbeing 2017–2023. These principles include:

1 health as holistic
2 the right to self-determination
3 the need for cultural understanding
4 the impact of trauma and loss, including inter-generational trauma
5 recognition of and respect for human rights
6 the impact of racism, stigma and social disadvantage
7 recognition of the centrality of family and kinship
8 recognition of the diversity among Aboriginal and Torres Strait Islander peoples and
9 recognition of Aboriginal and Torres Strait Islander strengths.

Important additional elements focus on sustainability and a strength-based and capacity building focus of interventions, genuine partnerships, safe cultural delivery of programs and innovation, evaluation, community promotion and education.

Figure 1.7 A model of social and emotional wellbeing

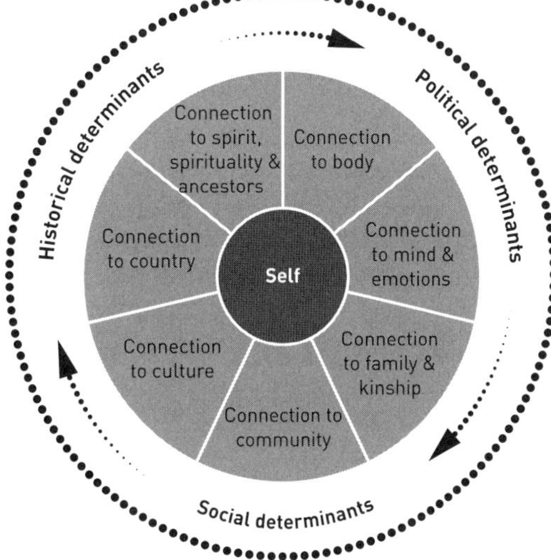

© Gee, Dudgeon, Schultz, Hart and Kelly, 2013

Using a SEWB framework does not mean ignoring mental health issues in Aboriginal and Torres Strait Islander people (Gee et al., 2014). Rather, this framework enables practitioners to understand domains of wellbeing (Butler et al., 2019) and mental health issues in a more holistic way (Balaratnasingam & Janca, 2019). The SEWB framework aims to prevent giving diagnostic labels and using individual-centred approaches, when the presenting issues may be better understood in terms of social determinants of health, the long-term effects of colonisation, racism and social disadvantage, trauma and grief.

Social determinants of mental health

Chapter 1.2 has introduced the concept of social determinants of mental health and the importance of understanding the contribution of social determinants such as social status, social supports, education and employment and access to health and social services, to the mental health and wellbeing of consumers (World Health Organization (WHO), 2019b). Racism is increasingly recognised as an important social determinant (Paradies et al., 2015). Understanding social determinants of health is especially important when working with marginalised and oppressed groups such as Aboriginal and Torres Strait Islander Australians and critical for case formulation, assessment and interventions. When working with Indigenous consumers, families and communities, mental health professionals should take a holistic view and consider the social determinants of social and emotional wellbeing (Zubrick et al., 2014).

Frameworks, standards and guidelines

Mental health professionals can obtain guidance on working with Aboriginal and Torres Strait Islander peoples from a range of policy documents, frameworks, standards and guidelines. Some of these frameworks apply to mental health service providers and settings, others to practitioners, others to both.

National Practice Standards for the Mental Health Workforce 2013

The National Practice Standards (Australian Government, 2013) were designed to complement discipline-specific practice standards or competencies. The Standards have been described in more detail in (see Sections 1.3.3 and 2.3.4). In revising the Standards in 2013, the working group agreed that a separate standard (Standard 4) was required to address the values, attitudes, knowledge and skills required for working with Indigenous people, families and communities. Standard 4 specifies 'By working with Aboriginal and Torres Strait Islander peoples, families and communities, mental health practitioners actively and respectfully reduce barriers to access, provide culturally secure systems of care, and improve social and emotional wellbeing' (p. 14) and identifies eight specific expectations of mental health practitioners for culturally sensitive and responsive practice (Australian Government, 2013; Walker, 2014).

National Strategic Framework for Aboriginal and Torres Strait Islander Peoples' Mental Health and Social and Emotional Wellbeing 2017–26

The National Strategic Framework (Australian Government, 2017) focuses on the importance of culture for the social and emotional wellbeing of Aboriginal and Torres Strait Islander people. The framework provides guidance and support for both health policy and practice by outlining a culturally appropriate model of care. The model embeds cultural considerations into practice and aims to ensure that Indigenous people can access care that is culturally responsive and safe. The model is applicable to specialised Aboriginal and Torres Strait Islander health services and to mainstream services. The framework complements the *Fifth National Mental Health and Suicide Prevention Plan* and the *National Aboriginal and Torres Strait Islander Health Plan 2012-2023*.

Gayaa Dhuwi (Proud Spirit) Declaration

The National Aboriginal and Torres Strait Islander Leadership in Mental Health (NATSILMH, 2016) is an Indigenous organisation established by senior Aboriginal and Torres Strait Islander people working in the areas of social and emotional wellbeing, mental health and suicide prevention. Most members of this group are based in, or associated with, national and state mental health commissions or other nationally important mental health bodies. The NATSILMH aims 'to help restore, maintain and promote the social and emotional wellbeing and mental health of Aboriginal and Torres Strait Islander peoples by advocating and providing advice and leadership in these areas. It also aims to reduce the high rates of suicide among Aboriginal and Torres Strait Islander people.' In August 2015, the NATSILMH developed the Gayaa Dhuwi Declaration as a framework for Indigenous leadership in mental health and suicide prevention. The five main statements in the Declaration have profound implications for mental health services and individual practitioners.

1 Aboriginal and Torres Strait Islander concepts of social and emotional wellbeing, mental health and

healing should be recognised across all parts of the Australian mental health system, and in some circumstances support specialised areas of practice.

2 Aboriginal and Torres Strait Islander concepts of social and emotional wellbeing, mental health and healing combined with clinical perspectives will make the greatest contribution to the achievement of the highest attainable standard of mental health and suicide prevention outcomes for Aboriginal and Torres Strait Islander peoples.
3 Aboriginal and Torres Strait Islander values-based social and emotional wellbeing and mental health outcome measures in combination with clinical outcome measures should guide the assessment of mental health and suicide prevention services and programs for Aboriginal and Torres Strait Islander peoples.
4 Aboriginal and Torres Strait Islander presence and leadership is required across all parts of the Australian mental health system for it to adapt to, and be accountable to, Aboriginal and Torres Strait Islander peoples for the achievement of the highest attainable standard of mental health and suicide prevention outcomes.
5 Aboriginal and Torres Strait Islander leaders should be supported and valued to be visible and influential across all parts of the Australian mental health system.

The Declaration also adopted the nine *Principles of Aboriginal and Torres Strait Islander Social and Emotional Wellbeing* that were first proposed in the 1989 National Aboriginal Health Strategy, expanded in the Ways Forward report (Swan et al., 1995), underpin the Working Together (Dudgeon et al., 2014) book, and are included in the National Strategic Framework for Aboriginal and Torres Strait Islander Peoples' Mental Health and Social and Emotional Wellbeing, including the current 2017–26 framework. The extensive focus on these principles is supported by the Aboriginal and Torres Strait Islander Suicide Prevention Project (Dudgeon et al., 2016) which found that programs that implement these nine principles are far more effective in addressing Indigenous mental health and SEWB than those not using the principles.

The role of cultural healing

The Gayaa Dhuwi Declaration sets out the importance of incorporating Indigenous knowledges of wellbeing and healing in health and mental health services. Cultural healing refers to therapeutic practices that are based on traditional Aboriginal and Torres Strait Islander knowledges. Traditional cultural healing, alongside mainstream approaches, 'has the potential to strengthen culturally safe practices and opportunities for self-determination, enhance health communication and to foster relationships that are built on trust and mutual respect' (Boot & Lowell, 2019, p. 3). *Working Together* (2014) describes several traditional healing systems from across Australia, including the Strong Spirit Mind Model, Red Dust Healing, the Marumali Program, the Djurruwang Program, Aboriginal offender rehabilitation programs, and loss and grief programs. There is a growing research base for these and other cultural healing approaches (McKendrick, Brooks, Hudson, Thorpe, & Bennett, 2014).

The Healing Foundation is a national Aboriginal and Torres Strait Islander organisation that aims to heal the ongoing trauma in Indigenous communities. The Healing Foundation has recently developed a theory of change for healing (2019). This theory outlines three domains that are critical success factors for positive and sustainable healing outcomes:

1 a supportive policy environment
2 healing networks, champions and organisations and
3 Indigenous community-led, trauma-informed quality healing programs and initiatives.

Central to these three domains is the restoration of connection to culture. Healing activities need to take place in 'safe places' and can include 'yarning circles, gatherings, healing camps, counselling, art, dance, song weaving, cultural ceremony and culturally safe referral pathways' (2019, p. 5).

Profession-specific frameworks, guidelines and supports

Information, frameworks and guidelines are increasingly available from both mainstream and Indigenous professional groups. The Australian

Indigenous Doctors Association (AIDA), the Australian Indigenous Psychologists Association (AIPA), the Congress of Aboriginal and Torres Strait Islander Nurses and Midwives (CATSINaM), the National Aboriginal and Torres Strait Islander Health Workers Association (NATSIHWA) and the Indigenous Allied Health Association (IAHA) all have websites with relevant information and helpful resources, and provide leadership on a national level. Professional associations also provide guidance to their members. For example, the Australian Psychological Society (APS) has developed specific guidelines for providing services for Aboriginal and Torres Strait Islander peoples (Australian Psychological Society (APS), 2015a). The Royal Australian College of General Practitioners has developed a National Guide to a Preventative Health Assessment for Aboriginal and Torres Strait Islander people (Royal Australian College of General Practitioners (RACGP), 2019).

The Dance of Life framework

The Dance of Life framework (Royal Australian and New Zealand College of Psychiatrists (RANZCP), 2019) outlines factors that can affect the mental health and social and emotional wellbeing of Aboriginal and Torres Strait Islander people. Developed by Milroy (2003) for the Royal Australian and New Zealand College of Psychiatrists, the Dance of Life matrix outlines physical, psychological, social, spiritual and cultural dimensions that health and mental health workers should consider in assessment and treatment. Hunter (2016) recommended that mental health workers following the RANZCP clinical practice guidelines for the management of schizophrenia and related disorders (2016) be guided by additional considerations, such as local knowledge, practices and relationships of trust.

KEY CONSIDERATIONS FOR SUPPORTING SOCIAL AND EMOTIONAL WELLBEING

Several other chapters of this book are relevant to work with Aboriginal and Torres Strait Islander people. We address these here briefly to create awareness of these areas for culturally safe and competent practice.

Cultural responsiveness and safety

There is increasing recognition that training in cultural awareness, responsiveness and safety is essential for professionals delivering care and support in mainstream health and mental health services (Laverty, McDermott, & Calma, 2017). The Australian Health Practitioner Regulation Agency (AHPRA) established an Aboriginal and Torres Strait Islander Health Strategy Group in 2017. A statement of intent signed by all health boards and accreditation authorities, AHPRA, and Indigenous leaders in the health sector is relevant to all mental health practitioners. The statement includes:

> a commitment to ensuring that Aboriginal and Torres Strait Islander Peoples have access to health services that are culturally safe and free from racism so that they can enjoy a healthy life, equal to that of other Australians, enriched by a strong living culture, dignity and justice. We also commit to ensuring that Aboriginal and Torres Strait Islander Peoples are actively leading the design, delivery and control of health services (AHPRA, 2017).

Many employers now offer or require that employees complete relevant cultural responsiveness training. There are many options and resources for developing relevant knowledge, including workshops and online courses (IAHA, 2015; 2019).

Advancing our knowledge in mental health care

Chapter 1.4 addresses this topic in detail. Ethical guidelines on research with Aboriginal and Torres Strait Islander peoples requires active involvement of Indigenous communities, leaders and/or Elders in research and evaluation projects. It also involves capacity building the local community people and other Indigenous researchers (NHMRC, 2018). Data sovereignty refers to the governance and authority of Indigenous people over the design, ownership, access to and use of data (Taylor & Kukutai, 2016). This concept is also relevant to Section 1.6.2, which discusses data, monitoring and reporting.

Health and mental health services

Chapter 1.7 outlines the policy context and mainstream services across the Australian states and territories. Many Aboriginal and Torres Strait Islander people may be reluctant to engage with these mainstream services, in part due to past experiences of racism and discrimination as well as other barriers including cost of service, lack of flexible appointments and lack of any services. Aboriginal Community Controlled Health Organisations (ACCHOs) are primary health services operated by local Aboriginal communities. ACCHOs play a significant role in providing culturally safe and holistic services to Indigenous consumers and their families (NACCHO, 2019). The National Mental Health Commission stated in its most recent report:

> Working to improve the health of Aboriginal and Torres Strait Islander people is a priority area for PHNs [Primary Health Networks]. The PHN Advisory Panel Report recommended that PHN funds for mental health and suicide prevention for Aboriginal and Torres Strait Islander people should be provided directly to Aboriginal Community Controlled Health Services (ACCHS) as a priority, unless a better arrangement can be demonstrated. The Senate Inquiry into the accessibility and quality of mental health services in rural and remote Australia also made a similar recommendation. PHNs should continue to work on formalising partnerships with ACCHS. The NMHC supports the recommendations made by both these reports and recommends that the Australian Government encourages PHNs to position ACCHS as preferred providers for mental health and suicide prevention services for Aboriginal and Torres Strait Islander people (2019, p. 14).

Workforce

Chapter 2.1 discusses providers of mental health care and support. Many Aboriginal and Torres Strait Islander clients would prefer to see an Indigenous health professional, but there remains a significant shortage of Indigenous general practitioners and psychiatrists, mental health nurses, psychologists, social workers, Aboriginal and Torres Strait Islander Health Workers and other allied health professionals, especially in rural and remote areas (Australian Institute of Health and Welfare (AIHW) 2019a). For the registered health professions, relevant statistics are published by AHPRA (2018) and the individual health boards.

Since July 2012, Aboriginal and Torres Strait Islander health workers have been a registered health profession under the National Registration and Accreditation Scheme. Their scope of practice is broad and tailored to the health care needs of the community (NATSIHWA, 2018).

Although building the Aboriginal and Torres Strait Islander mental health workforce is essential for success, in some cases, there needs to be a choice of practitioner. In small communities where very sensitive issues arise, some Indigenous people would prefer to see a non-Indigenous practitioner due to issues of confidentiality and relationship. Hence there is the need for upskilling of the mental health workforce to work competently within the cross-cultural context.

Role of cultural healers for the mental health workforce

As discussed in Section 1.3.3, the benefits of culturally safe traditional therapeutic approaches for Indigenous consumers are increasingly recognised as critical success factors (Healing Foundation, 2019). Cultural healers and Elders are trusted members of the community with oral knowledge and expertise in addressing health and mental health issues (Ngaanyatjarra Pitjantatjara Yankunytjatjara (NPY) & Women's Council Aboriginal Corporation, 2013). Possibly the best-known cultural healers are the Ngangkari healers, whose work since 1998 has led to a revival of traditional women's healing in Australia and been recognised internationally as a best practice culturally responsive approach to managing physical, emotional and spiritual wellbeing (Dudgeon & Bray, 2018).

Multilingualism and interpreters

For many Indigenous Australians, English may be a second, third or fourth language, and they may require working with interpreters (see Section 2.4.10). In our experience, many professionals are not aware of the linguistic diversity among Aboriginal and Torres Strait

Islander people, especially among consumers and their families from rural and remote areas. Thus, engaging and communicating effectively with consumers may be difficult due to language barriers (Dudgeon & Ugle, 2014). The Commonwealth Ombudsman (2016) reported continued issues with access to dedicated Indigenous interpreter services. Use of interpreters can raise ethical issues, especially in close-knit rural and remote communities, where few interpreters may be available, and family or friends may serve in that role.

Significance of mental health problems: epidemiology and assessment

A considerable challenge for providing services to Aboriginal and Torres Strait Islander peoples results from the limited evidence on the incidence and prevalence of mental health problems in the Indigenous population (Black et al., 2015; National Mental Health Commission (NMHC) 2019; Parker & Milroy, 2014). There is a lack of culturally valid diagnostic measures (Black, Toombs, & Kisely, 2018; Toombs et al., 2019) and there are limited numbers of screening measures for depression and definitions of depression as defined for Western populations need to be reconceptualised from an SEWB perspective (Balaratnasingam & Janca, 2019; The Getting it Right Collaborative Group, 2019). There are few measures of SEWB that have been designed and evaluated for Indigenous people (Le Grande et al., 2017; Newton, Day, Gillies, & Fernandez, 2015).

Recent studies have shown an extremely high prevalence rate for psychotic disorders in Indigenous populations in Northern Queensland (Gynther et al., 2019; Toombs et al., 2019) on the prevalence of mental health disorders among Indigenous Australians. Depression and anxiety have been found to be common (Nasir et al., 2018). Harmful substance use is a significant issue (Stephens, Bohanna, & Graham, 2017; Wilkes, Gray, Casey, Stearne, & Dadd, 2014). In addition, mental health practitioners need to be aware of how different symptoms develop in a cross-cultural context. For example, culture can influence the way symptoms develop, their meaning and their response to treatment. For Aboriginal and Torres Strait Islander people, the only way to assess whether a presenting problem may be culturally influenced or determined is through consultation with an Indigenous mental health practitioner, elder, healer or community member. It can take many years to develop a level of understanding of cultural influences in mental health to assist in assessment and recovery. Hence the need to have collaboration, partnership and connection between mainstream and Indigenous services. Many of the issues relevant to clinical practice are well described in *Working Together: Aboriginal and Torres Strait Islander Mental Health and Wellbeing Principles and Practice* (Dudgeon et al., 2014).

ADDRESSING THE URGENT CRISIS: ABORIGINAL AND TORRES STRAIT ISLANDER SUICIDE

Suicide was considered to be very rare for Indigenous peoples prior to the 1970s. There has been a significant increase in suicide rates, both worldwide (World Health Organization (WHO), 2019a) and in Australia (Dudgeon, Calma, & Holland, 2017). This increase has been considerably higher among Aboriginal and Torres Strait Islander peoples, especially among Indigenous youth. Today, there is increasing recognition of the importance of understanding the impact of colonisation, genocide and dispossession on Indigenous suicide and understanding it within a historical and cultural context.

In November 2018, delegates at the second Aboriginal and Torres Strait Islander Suicide Prevention Conference and the 2nd World Indigenous Suicide Prevention Conference called for a national suicide prevention and implementation plan designed specifically for and with Aboriginal and Torres Strait Islander people. Recommendations for the Implementation Plan included support for Aboriginal and Torres Strait Islander community empowerment and self-determination as non-negotiable Indigenous human rights, building the capacity and cultural competence of Aboriginal and Torres Strait Islander service providers, support for Aboriginal and Torres Strait Islander community-led and co-designed responses to suicide prevention developed in collaboration with governments, organisations and services, support for a broader Australian recovery and healing process based on truth-telling that recognises the events and impacts of colonisation including intergenerational trauma, disadvantage, marginalisation and neglect, support for a national Aboriginal and Torres Strait Islander suicide prevention research centre. The recommendations also included the need for a National Training Plan. This plan would focus increasing the Indigenous suicide prevention workforce to levels commensurate with need; ensuring a culturally safe and competent suicide prevention workforce; and embedding the role of Elders and cultural healers in mental health and suicide prevention services; and providing gatekeeper training in all Aboriginal urban, rural and remote communities. A National Data Plan would be part of the National Plan to protect Aboriginal and Torres Strait Islander community and other data sovereignty and to build local community capability for planning and evaluation of suicide prevention programs. Recommendations also highlighted the need for adequate funding for communities and Aboriginal Community Controlled Health Services and listening to the voices of the Elders, young people, the LGBTIQ+SB (denoting sister girl and brother boy) community and people with lived experience.

In early 2019, Indigenous leaders and communities called for urgent action in response to a high number of Indigenous youth suicides across Australia. Much is happening in Indigenous mental health and suicide prevention. The Australian Government has appointed a National Suicide Prevention Advisor in July 2019, with the aim to work towards zero suicides and the National Mental Health Commission (NMHC) has begun a connections tour to learn directly from the community about a *2030 Vision for Mental Health and Suicide Prevention* (National Mental Health Commission (NMHC) 2019).

The Centre of Best Practice in Aboriginal and Torres Strait Islander Suicide Prevention (CBPATSISP) was the continuation of the *Aboriginal and Torres Strait Islander Suicide Prevention Evaluation Project, Solutions That Work* (Dudgeon et al., 2016). This is based on core principles that are about establishing culturally responsive community, family and individual support systems and programs. These are to promote pathways to recovery through dealing with loss, grief and disconnection, trauma and helplessness, powerless and lack of control that are essential to reduce mental health issues, high risk behaviours and suicide. This in turn requires self-determination and community governance, reconnection and community life, restoration and community resilience.

The CBPATSISP website lists the relevant principles (as also outlined in the Gayaa Dhuwi Declaration) on the importance of culture, collaborative working relationships, and self-determination. In addition to a guide to implementing integrated suicide prevention the *Indigenous Governance Framework* (Dudgeon & Bray, 2018) focuses on collaborative mental health practice that acknowledges and values Indigenous self-determination. The CBPATSISP clearinghouse further provides a further report that highlights the important role of people with lived experience in suicide prevention (Dudgeon et al., 2018).

With respect to assessment, the CBPATSISP has developed a resource directory on screening and assessing tools for SEWB and mental health. It is recommended that mental health practitioners looking for appropriate tools refer to the guiding principles and frameworks for selection tools and consult with Indigenous colleagues about their relevance for the specific consumer and referral question.

In collaboration with the Menzies School of Health Research, CBPATSISP has recently published *Guidelines for Best Practice Psychosocial Assessment of Aboriginal and Torres Strait Islander People Presenting to Hospital Following Self-Harming Thoughts and Behaviours* (2019). The guidelines outline:

1 principles of cultural competence, including an understanding of the importance of social and emotional wellbeing and local Indigenous communities and cultures, and norms for interacting with Indigenous people
2 effective and appropriate engagement of Indigenous people in the assessment process, including initial

engagement, involvement of others, recommended approaches to communicating and interacting, managing refusal to take part in the assessment, and using structured assessment tools

3 elements of a comprehensive assessment
4 actions following the assessment
5 recommendations specific to young people. These Guidelines have been culturally validated and although they focus on suicide risk and self-harm, they provide helpful guidance for the health and mental health practitioners in conducting assessment in emergency department and general practice settings. These guidelines are being disseminated widely across Australia.

The CBPATSISP has updated and extended the evaluation of effective suicide prevention programs summarised in the ATSISPEP Solutions that Work report (ATSISPEP, 2016). Information on programs identified as promising practice and a range of evidence-based resources for mental health professionals and services is also available on the CBPATSISP website.

CONCLUSIONS AND IMPLICATIONS FOR PRACTICE

This section aimed to develop understanding in the mental health workforce that working effectively with Aboriginal and Torres Strait Islander peoples requires a significant conceptual shift.

First, mental health professionals need to develop an understanding of the historical, cultural and social determinants of Indigenous health and mental health. This includes examining their own beliefs and assumptions held about Australia's First Peoples. Cultural awareness and responsiveness training can feel challenging when cast in terms of decolonisation, white privilege and addressing racism. We believe that this understanding, which requires adopting a critically reflective stance, is a first and necessary step towards cultural awareness, responsiveness and competence.

Second, mental health professionals need to remain current in their work practices outlined in a range of relevant policy and practice frameworks. These have been outlined in the National Practice Standards of the Mental Health Workforce, with a separate standard for Aboriginal and Torres Strait Islander people. We have briefly summarised other relevant frameworks, standards and guidelines above and reiterate the importance of the Gayaa Dhuwi (Proud Spirit) Declaration in guiding mental health work.

Third, mental health professionals need to attend to the different understanding of health and mental health of Aboriginal and Torres peoples. They need to consider the historical background of dispossession, trauma and disadvantage in order to engage Indigenous consumers and their families effectively. Understanding how social determinants of health and intergenerational trauma contribute to mental health problems among Indigenous peoples is critical for case formulations. They need to be guided by the Social and Emotional Wellbeing Framework in their work. Within clinical skills development, practitioners need to have a good working knowledge of how culture impacts on the nature of distress, the onset of illness and the requirements for healing.

Fourth, self-determination, Indigenous governance and a collaborative approach ('Working Together') are critical success factors in all aspects of health and mental health, especially with respect to suicide prevention. This includes actively collaborating with Aboriginal Community Controlled Health Organisations, Elders and traditional Aboriginal and Torres Strait Islander healers. We have outlined solutions that work in our 2017 ATSISPEP report and on the website of the Centre of Best Practice in Aboriginal and Torres Strait Islander Suicide Prevention.

Finally, a focus on mental health problems, using Western conceptualisations of mental health, risks reinforcing the 'deficit dialogue' about Aboriginal and Torres Strait Islander people. It will also dismiss other important opportunities for healing. In order to provide effective services, we need to understand mental health issues from the holistic social and emotional wellbeing model and to adopt a 'strength-based' dialogue. This will allow mental health professionals to work from a perspective that appreciates the strengths of Australia's Indigenous culture and the wisdom that has underpinned Australia's First Peoples' care of country and its peoples for over 75 000 years.

REFLECTION AND SELF-ASSESSMENT QUESTIONS

- What are the implications for your practice of Standard 4 of the National Practice Standards for the Mental Health Workforce?
- What are the implications of the Gayaa Dhuwi (Proud Spirit) Declaration for mental health practice?
- What steps can you take to develop cultural awareness and responsiveness?
- Why is the SEWB framework important in assessment and interventions with Aboriginal and Torres Strait Islander people?
- What is the role of Aboriginal Community Controlled Health Organisations and traditional healers in working with Aboriginal and Torres Strait Islander consumers and their families?

SCENARIO

- At your service, you receive a referral for assessment and treatment of depression of an Aboriginal person.
- How do you know that it is appropriate for you to accept the referral?
- Where will you obtain guidance and feedback on culturally safe practice?
- What other service(s) may you consult with or refer to?
- What are key ethical and practice considerations for engaging with the person?
- How will you identify appropriate assessment tools?
- What is the best model to conceptualise the presenting problems? Why is a social and emotional wellbeing model indicated for Indigenous clients?
- How will you determine appropriate interventions?

RESOURCES FOR DEVELOPING CULTURAL AWARENESS AND RESPONSIVENESS AND FOR WORKING WITH ABORIGINAL AND TORRES STRAIT ISLANDER PEOPLE

- Working Together (Dudgeon et al., 2014)
- Centre of Best Practice in Aboriginal and Torres Strait Islander Suicide Prevention: www.cbpatsisp.com.au
- Australian Indigenous Health Infonet: https://healthinfonet.ecu.edu.au
- The Healing Foundation: https://healingfoundation.org.au
- AIATSIS: https://aiatsis.gov.au

Developing cultural awareness and responsiveness:

- *First Contact Clip*: a five-minute video depicting 'first contact' that challenges the deficit discourse: www.youtube.com/watch?v=bIrCovo_aCY
- The SBS series 'First Australians': www.sbs.com.au/ondemand/program/first-australians
- Cultural Responsiveness: Indigenous Allied Health Association (IAHA): https://iaha.com.au/workforce-support/training-and-development/cultural-responsiveness-in-action-training
- Griffith University, *Safer Health care for Australia's First Peoples*, a free online course, www.futurelearn.com/courses/first-peoples-safer-health care/1

1.3.4 THE MENTAL HEALTH OF LGBTIQ PEOPLE AND COMMUNITIES

SALLY MORRIS

UNDERSTANDING LGBTIQ PEOPLE AND COMMUNITIES

Key considerations of language

In Australia, the category of 'LGBTIQ' people and populations is now recognised by the Australian

Government in some federal legislation and policies, for example, in the *Aged Care Act 1997* (Cth). However there is a diversity of language used within Australia and across the globe. Within many communities, other letters and symbols are added to this collective initialism in an attempt to be inclusive of the vast diversity of identities and experiences found within these communities.

In reflection of current discourse within Australian society, for the purposes of this book, the acronym 'LGBTIQ' is used to refer collectively to people who are lesbian, gay, bisexual, transgender, intersex, and/or queer. It is clear that language within this space is continuingly evolving, and what is considered appropriate language is contextual, changes over time, and varies between locations and cultures. While there is certainly language that is offensive that should not be used, there is no single 'right' way for language to be used when talking about LGBTIQ people and communities. Given this, you will see a range of language used when talking about these communities, including different versions of the collective acronym. Undoubtedly the language used here will soon be considered dated.

It is vital to note that the use and acceptance of different words differs significantly from person to person. While the reclaimed term 'queer' has been used here to represent those who reject traditional sexual and gender identities, it is important to note that some find this term offensive due to historical use of the word as a derogative insult. Consequently, the term queer should be used with caution, particularly with older generations.

Unpacking the collective notion of LGBTIQ

The acronym 'LGBTIQ' does not represent a singular concept nor a homogenous group of people. Rather, LGBTIQ is a collective concept that encompasses several distinct but interrelated groups of people who share characteristics that fall outside of expected social and cultural sex, gender, and sexuality norms.

The use of a collective acronym to refer to a diverse group of people means that separate concepts of sex, gender, and sexuality, are routinely conflated into singular notion. However, it is important to understand the differences within and between these concepts as this works to highlight specific experiences and therefore health outcomes and support needs of different subgroups that make up the LGBTIQ population.

To help with this distinction, LGBTIQ will be broken down into three concepts, sex, gender and sexuality.

It is important to note that the understanding of these concepts changes over time and varies between cultures. This ongoing evolution demonstrates that concepts of gender and sexuality are in fact cultural constructs rather than concrete notions.

Sex is classification of a person's anatomical reproductive system as male or female. While the division of the population into male and female seems like a concrete foundational concept, sex is complex. Sex classification is based upon sex chromosomes, the types of gonads, the balance of sex hormones, internal reproductive anatomy, and external genitalia. Making up an estimated 1.7% of the population, *intersex* is a natural biological occurrence and refers to those with a biological sex that differs from medical definitions and cultural norms of 'female' and 'male' (IHRA, 2020). There is a number of intersex variations that involve a range of biological differences that relate to sex, including variations to sex chromosomes, genes, external genitalia, internal reproductive organs, hormones, or secondary characteristics. In contrast, *andosex* refers to those whose biological sex characteristics corresponds with a male or female classification.

Gender is the socially constructed roles, behaviours, activities, and attributes that are considered appropriate for men and women that are based on the sex of the person (WHO). Gender is demonstrated through dress, behaviour, and interpersonal interactions based on traditional gender roles of masculine and feminine. The term 'transgender' refers to people whose personal experience and identification of their gender and gender role in society does not align with their sex nor the gender that they would be expected to perform. This includes gender diverse or non-binary people whose experience of their gender does not fit social norms of male and/or female, but rather may sit outside the gender binary of male or female, and their gender is not exclusively masculine or feminine. In contrast, 'cisgender' refers to a person whose sense of gender corresponds with the sex they were assigned at birth and the gender that they are expected to perform.

Sexuality is the way that people behave and express themselves sexually, that involves physical, sexual, romantic, spiritual, and emotional feelings and behaviours. The terms 'lesbian' and 'gay' are used to describe a person's sexuality as being attracted to people of the same gender as themselves. *Bisexual* traditionally has been used to describe a person's sexuality as being attracted to both men and women. However, as the understanding of gender is broader than the binary male and female that the prefix *bi-* indicates, this term now includes any person who is attracted to people of more than one gender or to people regardless of gender. In response to the growing understanding of gender there is a diverse range of other identity labels used by many to describe their experience of their sexuality, such as pansexual, and queer. In contrast, 'heterosexual' refers to those who experience attraction to people who are of a different gender to themselves, and 'asexual' refers to a person's lack of sexual feeling or desires for others.

Population numbers

While it is assumed that LGBTIQ people represent a significant proportion of the population, it is important to note that most population research, including census data in Australia, does not consistently collect demographic data about intersex status, sexuality and gender identity.

There are numerous contributing factors to the lack of data. First, the most significant issue is an absence of any data questions pertaining to LGBTIQ people. This may be premised on the heteronormative assumption all people are heterosexual, cisgender and andosex and therefore there is no need to enquire.

While this may seem preposterous, it is only in recent years that research has started to include questions to identify LGBTIQ people, and this is still inconsistent.

Second, if questions pertaining to LGBTIQ people are included, which questions are asked will significantly alter the type of responses that are received. For example, if the question asks about identities a person holds it will collect different information than if it asked about what behaviours they are engaged in. There is also the tendency for research questions to conflate the subpopulations that make up LGBTIQ into a single category. Sex and gender in particular are likely to be confused and combined, which compromises data integrity (Ansara, 2016).

Third, as LGBTIQ people can only be counted through self-identification, the ability and willingness of an individual to identify themselves impacts on which data is collected. LGBTIQ people can make the choice to remain invisible when the environment around them is not safe, and the risk of harassment, prejudice, discrimination, violence and abuse is present (Gates, 2011, pp. 2–3).

It is vital to consider this lens when reviewing the data that is available. Census data on same-sex couples became available in 1996. It was obtained from responses to the 'relationship in household' question, where same-sex couples who were living together were counted. The 2016 Census counted just under 46 800 same-sex couples living together in Australia. This represents a 39% increase since the 2011 Census, which counted 33 700 same-sex couples (ABS, 2016). The increase in the reported number of same-sex couples may reflect the improvements in the rights of same-sex couples and therefore greater willingness by people to identify themselves as being in a same-sex relationship.

In 2016, the Australian census piloted an 'other' response option to the sex question to allow people whose sex/gender is not male or female to identify themselves, with 1260 providing a valid response (ABS, 2016). However, this was not a standard response option and respondents firstly needed to know this was available and then take extra steps to report their sex as other than male or female. Consequently, this count is not considered to be a count, due to limitations around the special procedures and willingness or opportunity to report as sex and/or gender diverse. People who have been treated with disrespect, abuse and discrimination because of their sex or gender may be unwilling to reveal their sex in an official document.

When considering data collected via population-based surveys, on average 3.5% of respondents identify as lesbian, gay or bisexual. The proportion of people who identify as bisexual is similar to the proportion that identify as lesbian or gay; however, bisexual people are more likely to be female. In all available research, there is a higher proportion of people who identify as lesbian, gay or bisexual in younger demographics compared to older populations (Gates, 2014). Those who report any lifetime same-sex sexual behaviour and any same-sex sexual attraction are substantially higher than the numbers of people who identify as lesbian, gay or bisexual. An estimated 8.2% of people have engaged in same-sex sexual behaviour and 11% acknowledge at least some same-sex sexual attraction (Gates, 2011).

An estimated 0.6% of adults identify as transgender; however, younger age groups are more likely than older age groups to identify as transgender (Flores, Brown, & Herman, 2016). Unfortunately, available data does not measure gender identity; however, there are suggestions that up to 2% of the population have strong feelings of being transgender (Gates, 2011).

Despite intersex variants being biological, there are still a range of barriers to accurate data collection, with many intersex people only coming to the attention of data collectors through chance or an apparent medical reason. Attempts to include intersex in data collection are often inadequate and often conflate intersex with gender identity or sex assigned at birth. Additionally, there is significant stigma around intersex variations that mean that someone may not know that they are intersex, or which may preclude someone from disclosing. While different types of intersex variations are more frequently occurring than others, Intersex Human Rights Australia suggests the use of a mid-range estimate of 1.7% of the population having an intersex variation (IHRA, 2020; Jones, 2016).

Components of sexuality and gender

Sex, gender and sexuality do not fit into strict binary categories of male and female or gay and heterosexual. Developed in 1948 the Kinsey scale (see Figure 1.8) was the first attempt to acknowledge the diversity of human sexual behaviour and that sexuality was a continuum. Kinsey also explored the concept that sexuality is fluid and subject to change over time (Kinsey, Pomeroy, & Martin, 2003).

Figure 1.8 Kinsey scale

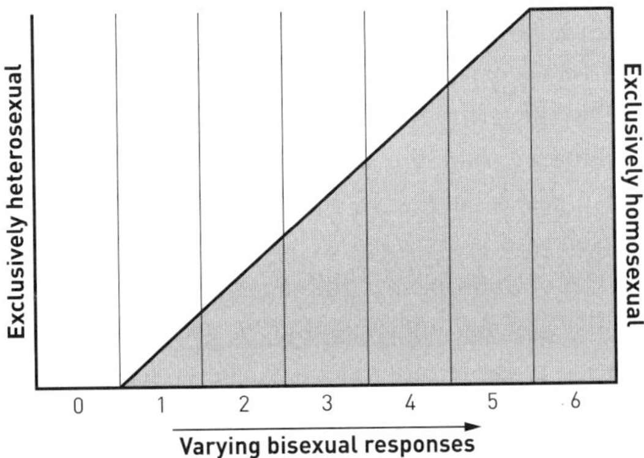

Importantly, the Kinsey scale also focused on sexual behaviour, rather than sexual identity which is often considered to define a person's sexuality. Building on this recognising that sexuality is not a single dimension, but rather is complex and multifaceted in nature (Laumann, Gagnon, Michael, & Michaels, 1994), proposed that there are three components of sexuality: sexual attraction, sexual behaviour and sexual identity (see Figure 1.9). Sexual attraction refers to the internal thoughts, feelings, desires that a person has. Sometimes this is split into physical attraction and romantic attraction. Sexual behaviour refers to the sexual interactions that a person engages in, while sexual identity is a self-ascribed word a person uses to describe and define their sexuality.

Importantly, these three components that make up a person's sexuality may not align with each other, and

Figure 1.9 Components of sexuality

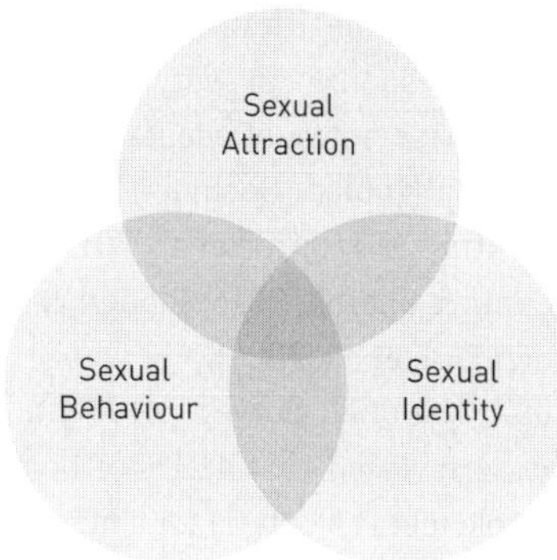

often do not align. For example, there may be a range of barriers that may prevent someone from acting on their same-sex attraction such as social obligations, opportunity, or risks of violence. Additionally, adopting a public non-heterosexual identity may have a range of negative consequences, including the expectation that they must behave and feel in particular ways that align with a specific identity.

Additionally, where someone sits along a heterosexual/homosexual continuum in each of these attractions, behaviour and identity components will often change and evolve over the course of an individual's lifetime. As Laumann and colleagues state: 'All these motives, attractions, identifications, and behaviours vary over time and circumstances with respect to one another–that is, are dynamically changing features of an individual's sexual expression'.

Sex and gender have also been explored through multiple components and continuums (see Figure 1.10), most notably by the Genderbread person (Killerman, 2015) which delineates between physical sex characteristics, sex assigned at birth, gender identity and gender expression.

Regardless of the anatomical sex characteristics a person has, even those with intersex variations whose bodies don't align with medical categorising of male and female, all people are usually assigned a legal sex of male or female on their birth certificate. (The ACT allows for a third sex option of 'unspecified/indeterminate/intersex' for infants and children, though it is unknown how many children have been allocated to this category.) In all states and territories, a person can apply to alter their legal sex categorisation as an adult, though there are varying requirements across jurisdictions in order to do so (such as having sex reassignment surgery), and not all states provide a third gender option.

Separate from our sex characteristics and legal sex categorisation, there is a person's internal experience of their own gender that can exist along a continuum between male and female. A person's expression of their gender through speech, appearance, dress, and mannerisms. This is how an individual intends their gender to come across to others.

Finally, there is the self-ascribed word that a person uses to describe and define their gender, which may or may not align with their gender, gender expression or legal sex categorisation. Those who consider their identity to fall outside of the traditional (and limited) woman-to-man spectrum and may use other language and labels to describe their gender identity.

Figure 1.10 Components of sex and gender

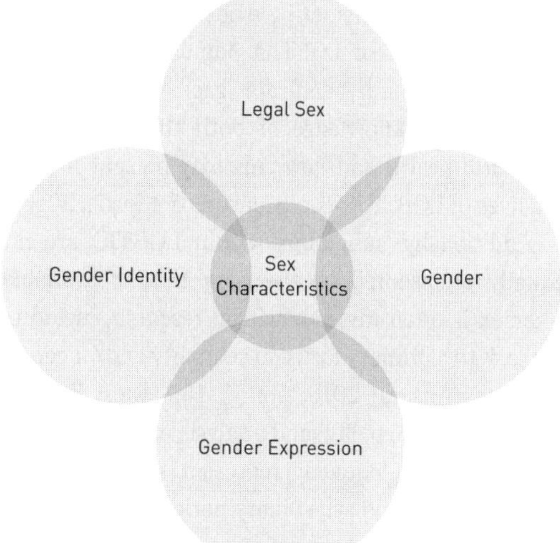

Whether discussing sex, gender or sexuality, identities are the words that a person themselves chooses in order to describe their experience of self. There may be peoples whose experiences align with the definitions of diverse sex, gender and sexuality diversity who may never use this language to describe or identify themselves. For example, not all gender diverse people will use identity-based language such as transgender or genderqueer to describe their experience.

The limitations of identity labels to adequately describe an experience is one reason why we are seeing a continuous evolution of language within LGBTIQ communities. The move towards the use of the word queer is because queer 'is less an identity than a *critique* of identity' (Jagose, 1996, p. 131, cited in Alexander, 1999, p. 301, emphasis in the original), and is often used by those who reject traditional sexual and gender identities and seek a broader and deliberately ambiguous alternative to traditional labels.

As humans, we have the desire to categorise into clearly defined (and often binary) boxes, and as such it is useful for us to notice and reflect upon our inclination to define, categorise and assign labels to the human experience.

MENTAL HEALTH OUTCOMES

Availability of data

As with data collection in relation to mental health generally, when considering evidence on the mental health outcomes of LGBTIQ populations it is vital to note there are significant gaps in data. There is insufficient knowledge of both the incidence of mental ill health and how this may present itself in the lives of LGBTIQ people (Jacobs & Morris, 2016).

Additionally, subgroups within LGBTIQ are not equally represented in the data that is available. Intersex is often invisible within research, including those with a primary focus on sexuality and/or gender diversity (Ansara, 2016, pp. 13–16; Jones, Hart, & Carpenter, 2016, p. 30), and analysis of collected data often fails to adequately represent the diversity of those falling outside the binary notions of gender and sexuality. These responses may either be collapsed into existing categories of male/female or gay/straight, or excluded from analysis completely (Ansara, 2016, pp. 7–9; Leonard, Lyons, & Bariola, 2015, p. 9).

While limited, current evidence has consistently demonstrated that LGBTIQ people have poorer mental health outcomes than the general population, including increased rates of depression, anxiety, suicide ideation, suicide attempts, and substance use. Rates of poor mental health vary across the LGBTIQ population in response to varying risk factors; however, as a rule rates of mental ill health are elevated in all subgroups (Boehmer, 2002; Jackman, Honig & Bockting, 2016; Kidd et al., 2016; King et al., 2008; McCann & Sharek, 2016; Plöderl & Tremblay, 2015; Schützmann et al., 2009).

The 2007 National Survey of Mental Health and Wellbeing revealed that 41.1% of homosexual/bisexual people met the criteria for a mental disorder and had symptoms in the last 12 months (Australian Bureau of Statistics (ABS), 2007).

Leonard and colleagues (2015) showed that 37.1% of lesbian, gay, bisexual and transgender people reported being diagnosed or treated for a mental disorder in the past three years. This research also revealed variations across the LGBTIQ population with women reporting higher rates of mental ill health than men (41.7% versus 29.7%). Mental health was reported to be poorer for transgender people (55.3% of trans men and 57.4% of trans women). Bisexual people report poorer mental health (50.6% of bisexual women and 34.1% of bisexual men) than gay and lesbian people, and lesbian women report higher rates of mental illness than gay men (39.1% versus 29.8%; see Figure 1.12) While data is lacking, Jones and colleagues (2016) show that that 41% of people with intersex variations describe their mental health as fair or poor (pp. 120–123).

Psychological distress

While the national average Kessler Psychological Distress Scale (K10) score is 14.5, indicating low levels of psychological distress and no presence of mental disorder, the average score of LGBT Australians (there is no available data on the K10 scores of intersex and queer people) is 19.6, revealing moderate rates of non-specific psychological distress and an increased likelihood of mental disorders (Leonard et al., 2015, pp. 15–17).

As with mental illness diagnosis, rates of psychological distress vary across the LGBTIQ population (see Figure 1.11). Notably the psychological

Figure 1.11 LGBT mean K10 scores

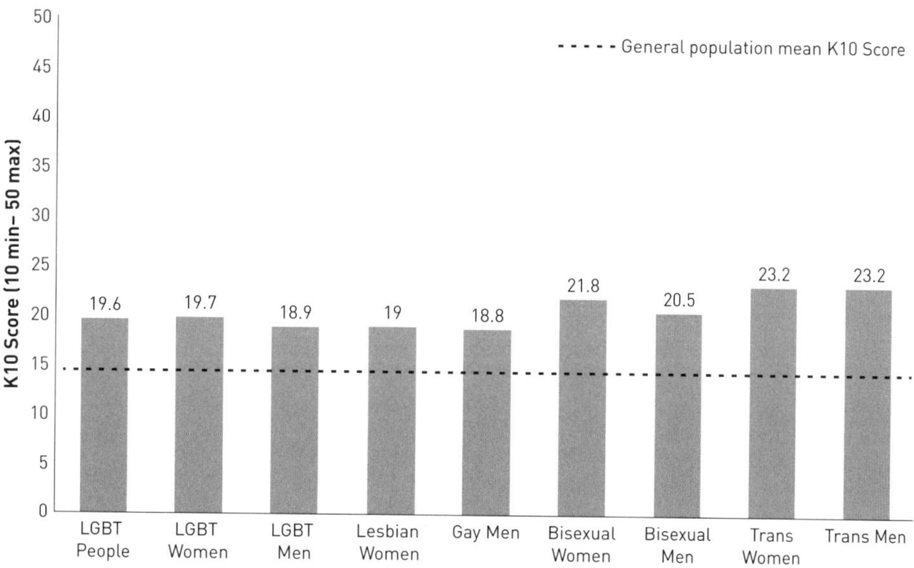

Source: Adapted from Leonard, Lyons, & Bariola, 2015, pp. 12–13

distress experienced by transgender people tips into the high range, as shown in Figure 1.11.

Suicide ideation and attempts

While not all people who experience poor mental health will be at risk of suicide, mental illness is nevertheless a significant risk factor for suicide, with mood disorders being present in 43% of suicide deaths in 2017 (Australian Bureau of Statistics (ABS), 2018a) (see Figure 1.12). Mood disorders are those that involve mood disturbance, such as depressive episode, bipolar affective disorder, and dysthymia. A depressive episode is a state of gloom, despondency, or sadness lasting at least two weeks (ABS, 2007).

Figure 1.12 Percentage of people with thoughts of suicide in the last 2 weeks to 12 months

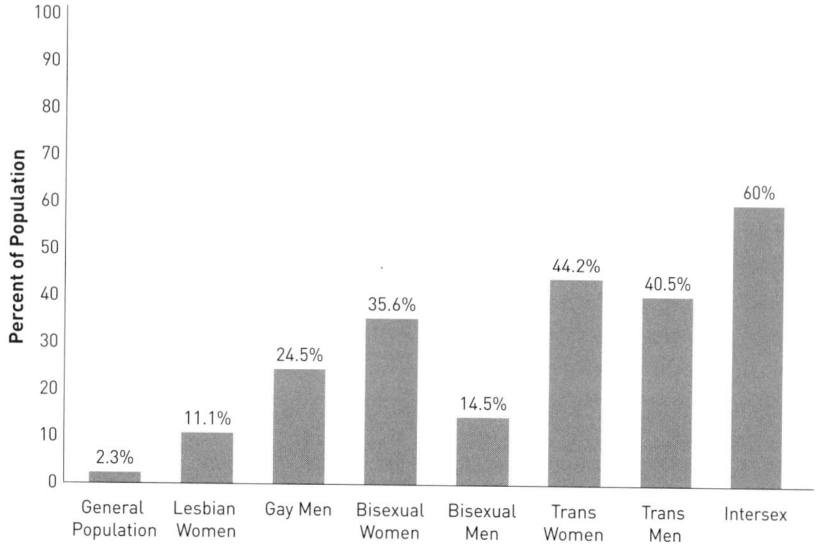

Source: Adapted from Australian Bureau of Statistics, 2007; Swannell et al., 2016; Hyde et al., 2014; Jones et al., 2016

While there is no data on the number of LGBTIQ people who have died by suicide, a literature review on the prevalence of suicidal behaviours in Australia concluded that LGBT people are at higher risk for suicidal behaviours, including suicide attempts, intentional self-harm, suicidal ideation, and suicide plans (Skerrett, Kõlves & De Leo, 2015). Furthermore, 60% of intersex people have had thoughts about suicide, and 19% had attempted suicide (Jones et al., 2016, pp. 120–123). An analysis of LGBT people identified in the Queensland Suicide Register showed that this cohort had a higher prevalence of major depressive episodes, generalised anxiety disorder, and post-traumatic stress disorder than non-LGBT suicides (Skerrett, Kõlves & DeLeo, 2014).

THE ROLE OF STIGMA AND DISCRIMINATION IN THE MENTAL HEALTH OF LGBTIQ PEOPLE

Understanding the role of stigma

Psychological distress and mental ill health are not characteristic of LGBTIQ individuals nor is this caused by sexuality, gender identity or intersex characteristics in and of themselves. Rather poorer mental health outcomes have a direct correlation to experiences of stigma, prejudice, discrimination, violence and abuse which cause stress and trauma that in turn result in mental ill health (Haas et al., 2011; Hillier, 2010; Jones et al., 2016; Leonard et al., 2015; National LGBTIQ Health Alliance 2016; Skerrett, Kõlves, & De Leo, 2016).

LGBTIQ people have endured a long and multifaceted history of social, cultural, and political exclusion, oppression, and persecution (Fone, 2000; Phelan, 2010; Willett, 2000). While all LGBTIQ people are immersed in a discriminatory environment that creates stress, those who encounter more incidents of harassment and abuse experience higher rates of psychological distress than those with fewer direct encounters (see Figure 1.13). The still high rates of psychological distress in LGBT people who have not directly experienced abuse demonstrates the impact that invalidating environments and structural stigma have on mental health (Plöderl et al., 2014, p. 1567).

This relationship was clearly demonstrated during the public debate that preceded and surrounded the Marriage Law Postal Survey conducted by the ABS at the end of 2017. Ecker and Bennett found that 80% of LGBTIQ people reported that they found this experience considerably or extremely stressful, and more than 90% of LGBTIQ people said that debate had a negative impact on them to some degree. Consequently, the number of LGBTIQ people

Figure 1.13 Mean K10 Scores of LGBT people who have experienced harassment and abuse compared to those who have not

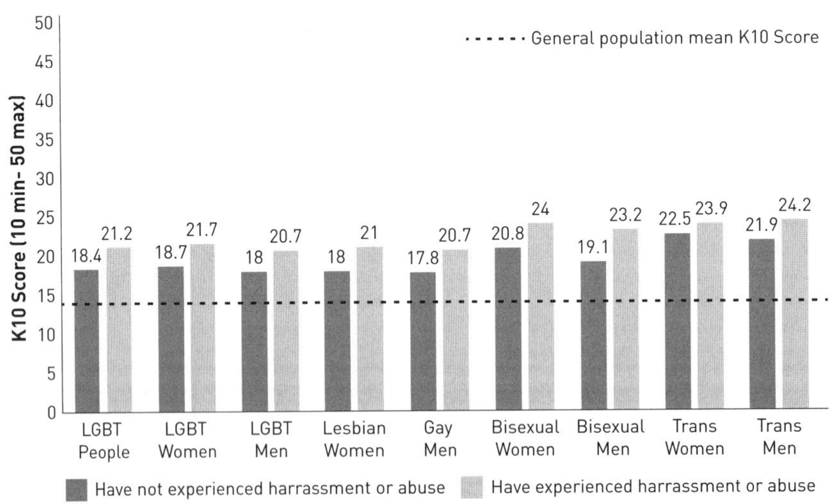

Source: Adapted from Leonard, Lyons, & Bariola, 2015, pp. 27–31

experiencing depression, anxiety and stress increased by more than a third after the announcement of the vote, compared to the six months before the announcement (Ecker & Bennett, 2017).

There are varying experiences of stigma and exclusion towards different identities and experiences within the collective LGBTIQ that are related to gender, gender expression and sexuality. Consequently, rates of mental ill health are not distributed equally across the LGBTIQ acronym with women, bisexual people, transgender people and intersex people being at particular risk. Additionally, other forms of marginalisation (such as that based on age, culture, location) can intersect with stigma related to being LGBTIQ, compounding the effects of discrimination. This results in subpopulations within LGBTIQ communities at increased risk of mental health problems.

In order to address the structural stigma and respond to the mental health of LGBTIQ people, it is important to understand the historical context of this stigma and how this still impacts mental health as well as creates barriers for LGBTIQ people in accessing mental health care and supports.

LGBTIQ stigma in law

Australia inherited British laws with colonisation, including criminalising homosexual behaviour. The states embarked on a process of legalisation of consensual sexual conduct between men between 1975 and 1997, with Tasmania being the last state to repeal this law after a UN Human Rights Committee ruling.

While law reform has led to broad improvements for LGBTIQ people's access to justice and human rights in Australia, problematic laws remain. This is due to the ad hoc nature of legal change, inconsistencies between jurisdictions and uncertainties regarding some areas of law. Rapid change also means that LGBTIQ people are often unaware of their legal rights and historic discrimination results in a deep mistrust of the government and the justice system. LGBTIQ people are significantly less likely than other victims of crime to report harassment or violence to the police. LGBTIQ people experience increased need for legal assistance in relation to discrimination, assault and harassment, as well as elevated demand for family law, family violence, end-of-life planning, medical treatment, and administrative law services (Law Council of Australia, 2020).

While sexual behaviour was no longer criminalised, systemic discrimination against same-sex relationships was still embedded in a range of laws. In 2009, following the Australian Human Rights Commission report *Same-Sex: Same Entitlements* and an audit of legislation, 85 Commonwealth laws were amended to eliminate structural discrimination against same-sex couples in area of tax, superannuation, social security, immigration, and child support.

SEX DISCRIMINATION ACT

In 2013, upon the implementation of the Sex Discrimination Amendment (Australian Human Rights Commission (AHRC), 2013), it was the first time in Australia that it was unlawful to discriminate against a person on the basis of sexual orientation, gender identity and intersex status under federal law.

The *Sex Discrimination Act* (SDA) maintains a number of exemptions, including sections 37 and 38 which state that 'religious bodies' and 'educational institutions established for religious purposes' can discriminate against people on the basis of certain attributes protected by the SDA including sex, sexual orientation, gender identity, intersex status. This means that it is not unlawful for faith-based organisations that are funded to deliver mental health services to discriminate against both staff and service users that are LGBTIQ. This does not mean that services provided by faith-based organisations will not be inclusive or accessible, indeed there are a vast number of proactive agencies who do. However, given this legal loophole, there is no clear way to determine which services are, nor any recourse if discrimination is experienced.

Same-sex marriage

Following a postal survey that showed that 61.6% of people who participated agreed that laws should be changed to allow same-sex couples to marry in Australia, The Marriage Amendment (Definition and Religious

Freedoms) Bill 2017 was passed. This amended the provisions of the *Marriage Act 1961* (Cth), bringing same-sex marriage into law on 8 December 2017.

Access to hormone therapy

In 2017 the Family Court ruled that transgender teenagers no longer have to front a courtroom in order to access Hormone Replacement Therapy (HRT) and instead just require the consent of parents and their health professional team. Prior to this ruling, transgender children under the age of 18 and their families would have to go to the Family Court in order to access the treatment, which was often a long, painful, and expensive process, which could be emotionally draining and psychologically harmful to the child in question.

Sex and gender markers

In 2011, when access to 'X' passports was formalised, and then in 2013, when the Australian Government issued guidelines to standardise sex and gender recognition by Federal Government departments and agencies, a third sex/gender marker has become available. Sometimes, the third classification is termed 'intersex', as is the case in the 2011 passport rules, the 2013 federal guidelines and, later, ACT birth registrations, which can refer to 'indeterminate/intersex/unspecified'.

LGBTIQ stigma in psychiatry and medicine

There has been a long and complex relationship between LGBTIQ people and the mental health system that has seen the pathologising of homosexuality, gender diversity and intersex variations. It is vital to consider how this impacts LGBTIQ people's perception of mental health professionals and their ability to access supports today.

Homosexuality was introduced as a diagnosis within the International Classification of Diseases (ICD) Version 6 in 1948 as a sexual deviation that was presumed to reflect an underlying personality disorder.

Even though homosexuality in and of itself was removed as a diagnosis from the IDC-10 in 1990, remnants that continued to pathologise sexuality remained until the release of the ICD-11 in 2018. Although not utilised by this text, the American Psychiatric Association Diagnostic and Statistical Manual (DSM) is still an influential diagnostic tool by psychiatry. It removed reference to homosexuality in 1973 but similar pathologisation of sexuality remained until the release of the DSM-5 in 2013.

Gender diversity has also experienced pathologisation, but with a slower transition, with 'Transvestitism' introduced as a diagnosis in ICD-8 in 1965. Although gender identity disorders was removed as a mental disorder from the IDC-11 in 2018, gender incongruence remains as a diagnosis under the newly created parent category of 'Conditions related to sexual health' due to evidence that being transgender or gender diverse is not a mental disorder. The DSM followed the ICD, introducing the diagnosis of 'transvestitism' in 1968, but continues to list gender dysphoria as a diagnosis in the DSM-5, used by psychiatry and the medical system to diagnose and treat gender diversity through counselling, cross-sex hormones, puberty suppression and gender reassignment surgery.

While this textbook has been designed to align with the ICD-11 as its diagnostic tool, many medical professionals will still be utilising the DSM-5. Transgender people often have little choice but to interact with the mental health profession to receive a diagnosis of gender dysphoria that will facilitate their access to cross-sex hormones and gender reassignment surgery, as well as to be provided with confirmation of their gender that allows for the changing of legal identification documents.

Medicalisation of intersex bodies

Intersex variations, often collectively termed 'disorders of sex development' have been long pathologised by the medical profession. Many intersex variations have a medical name to facilitate diagnosis, such as Kleinfelder's Syndrome, Turners Syndrome, Antigen Insensitive Syndrome, and Congenital Adrenal Hyperplasia. This has implications for intersex people whose bodies are considered 'disordered' males and females, who need to be 'normalised' through medical interventions.

While there may be the belief that unnecessary medical interventions are no longer practised on intersex babies and children, Intersex Human Rights Australia describes a lack of transparency about current clinical practices in Australia. Regardless, there is sufficient evidence that indicates the ongoing practice of normalising intersex bodies in Australia:

> Individuals born with intersex variations are routinely subject to so-called normalizing medical interventions, often in childhood. Often without medical need, but rather to minimizing family concern and distress, and mitigating the risks of stigmatization and gender identity confusion of atypical genital appearance–2013 Senate Inquiry on involuntary or coerced sterilization (Carpenter, 2018).

There is a significant amount of shame and stigma around intersex bodies (Jones et al., 2016). As intersex people's mental health is impacted by medicalisation and pathologisation of their bodies by health professions that view their bodies as 'disordered', needing to be fixed. Attempts to 'correct' bodies and socialise to fit male or female norms, creates a range of issues for intersex people around their gender and identity. Furthermore, intersex people's mental health can be impacted by hormonal and surgical medical interventions.

LGBTIQ stigma in religion

There is a long religious persecution of LGBTIQ people, and religion is often still used today as a justification for continuation of systematic discrimination towards LGBTIQ people. Religious groups have been core to vocal dissent against marriage equality for same-sex couples and the Safe Schools program. This program was designed to support schools to prevent and respond to discrimination against lesbian, gay, bisexual, transgender and intersex (LGBTI) students. However some in the community saw the program as 'political correctness' or promoting risky/ inappropriate behaviour.

Of particular relevance to mental health practitioners is the practice of conversion or reparative therapy which is often guided by particular interpretations of religious texts. Conversion therapy is any practice or treatment that seeks to change, suppress or eliminate an individual's sexual orientation or gender identity, and is founded on the beliefs that

- homosexuality is sinful
- homosexuality is a form of 'brokenness'
- 'same-sex attraction' results from childhood, developmental or family issues
- sexuality can be changed or overcome, or healed.

Despite these beliefs, not only is there is a lack of empirical support for the claim that sexual orientation or gender identity can be changed, evidence also indicates that attempts at changing this can be harmful, and affirming can make significant positive contribution to mental health (Australian Psychological Society (APS), 2015b).

In 2018, the Health Complaints Commissioner (HCC) conducted an inquiry into the practice of conversion therapy in Victoria that found long-term psychological harm and distress to people who have undergone conversion therapy/practices which result in ongoing mental health issues such as severe anxiety and depression (HCC, 2019).

The Australian Psychological Society (APS) strongly opposes any form of mental health practice that treats homosexuality as a disorder, seeks to change a person's sexual orientation, or any forms of mental health practice that are not affirming of transgender people (Australian Psychological Society (APS), 2015b). Christian Counsellors Association of Australia (CCAA, 2017) code of ethics state 'Counsellors shall not conduct therapeutic interventions aimed at modifying or changing the sexual orientation of clients, as distinct from treating recognised sexual disorders'.

While a person may feel distress at being LGBTIQ and may wish this to change, the APS recommends understanding the reason for the distress and psychological approaches that attempt to challenge negative attitudes, promote self-acceptance and develop affirming social supports. While religious ministries that promoted gay conversion therapy in Australia have closed down in recent years, this practice continues to be practised in more subtle and informal ways (Venn Brown, 2018). The HCC found that there are still psychologists, counsellors and counselling services offering conversion therapy/practices, despite the overwhelming evidence of the significant and long-term harm caused by these practices.

In February 2019, following the release of the HCC report that recommended the introduction of legislation to prohibit conversion therapy/practices, the Victorian Government announced its intention to bring in laws to denounce and prohibit LGBTIQ conversion practices (Victoria State Government, 2019).

Religious freedoms

In November 2017, following the introduction of the same-sex marriage equality amendment, an Expert Panel was formed to conduct a review of religious freedom in Australia, with its report being provided to the government in May 2018 (Department of the Prime Minister and Cabinet, 2017).

This review made a number of recommendations. It clearly demarcated between sexual orientation, gender identity as requiring different legal controls from intersex status, stating that intersex status should be protected from discrimination from religious bodies, whereas sexual orientation and gender identity should not.

The Australian Government's response, released in December 2018, highlighted existing religious exemptions for sexuality orientation, gender identity and relationship status in the *Sex Discrimination Act*, and stated that the Australian Government will introduce a Religious Discrimination Bill into Parliament.

Discrimination experienced by LGBTIQ people

Historical and current experiences of religious condemnation, legal restriction and medical pathologisation of LGBTIQ people has built a culture of stigma towards LGBTIQ people and communities that is deeply rooted in our communities. This perpetuates continuing inequality that continues today. Carroll and Mendos (2017) and Chiam, Duffy and Gil (2016) state that while there have been significant advances in human rights, LGBTIQ people still face significant unacceptable discrimination.

Much of this is entrenched in legal and medical systems, which then facilitate a culture of intolerance

Figure 1.14 Percentage of LGBTIQ people who have experienced heterosexist harassment, abuse, or discrimination

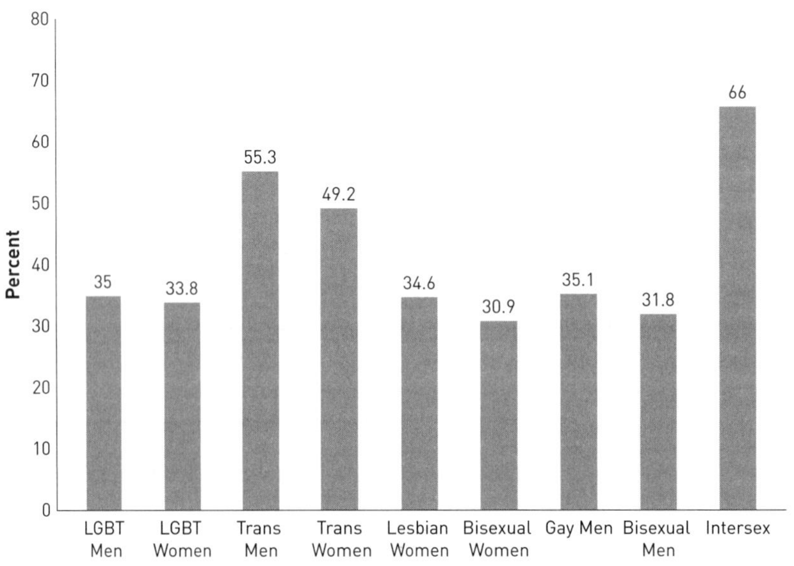

Source: Adapted from Leonard, Lyons, & Bariola, 2015, pp. 27–28; Jones et al., 2016

resulting in LGBTIQ people being subject to harassment, abuse, and violence (Australian Human Rights Commission, 2015, p. 14). This is demonstrated by 71.79% of LGBTIQ people experiencing violence, harassment, or bullying on the basis of their sexual orientation, gender identity, or intersex status (Australia Human Rights Commission, 2015, p. 16). Figure 1.14 shows how rates of discrimination vary, with transgender and intersex people being more vulnerable to abuse (Jones et al., 2016, p. 156; Leonard et al., 2015, pp. 27-28).

These changes reflect both emerging human rights standards and the lack of empirical evidence supporting the pathologisation and medicalisation of variations in sexual orientation expression.

For many there may be the perception that achieving marriage equality for same-sex couples was the final hurdle in LGBTIQ rights; however, there are still a range of legal, medical and social issues that remain barriers for LGBTIQ people in experiencing equality.

Certainly internationally, countries that have legislated same-sex marriage can still remain extremely dangerous for LGBTIQ people (Paletta, 2018).

Transition/gender affirmation

In addition to the relationship between stigma and mental health, for trans people there is an additional relationship between mental health outcomes and their ability to access medical support to transition, such as hormone therapy or surgery.

Although research has shown that accessing health services improves trans people's overall health and wellbeing–specifically through support and gender-affirming transitioning–in many countries the appropriate services are not available.

Trans young people in Australia and internationally have difficulty accessing health services that are appropriate and knowledgeable about trans issues.

Globally, trans people report negative experiences when attempting to access medical services, which contribute to poor mental health. Medical professionals serve as gatekeepers for hormone therapies and other medical interventions that trans individuals may pursue, and as such have a responsibility to help alleviate their clients' levels of discomfort and discrimination when accessing services. It has been argued that counselling services need to put the trans client's needs first, should accept their gender expression and diversity, and should not 'pathologise' their client. Moreover, counselling should be tailored for the needs of that individual, as trans populations are diverse

Trans people seek treatment from medical and mental health services for a number of reasons. General practitioners are often the first point of contact for a young trans person seeking help for mental distress or wanting to medically transition. While psychiatric services provide support for mental health issues, seeing a psychiatrist is often a requirement for obtaining puberty blockers, feminising or masculinising hormones and surgery. Endocrinologists provide hormone treatment. There are many trans young people who wish to access medical transition services within Australia but are currently unable to.

Generally, most trans people who take hormone therapy or undergo surgery report that it has a strongly beneficial effect on mood and wellbeing (Hyde et al., 2013). The proportion of people with clinically relevant depressive symptoms was lowest in those currently taking hormone therapy (39.8%) and in those who were not taking it, but either did not desire it, or were unsure if they wanted it (37.4%). In contrast, those with the highest proportion of clinically relevant depressive symptoms were participants who had not taken hormone therapy, but wanted to (58.4%).

FRAMEWORKS FOR WORKING WITH LGBTIQ PEOPLE

National strategic and political context

While the Australian Human Rights Commission has undertaken significant work on rights for LGBTIQ people, with no dedicated commissioner, or Commonwealth Ministers or government agencies that take primary responsibility for advancing issues that arise for LGBTIQ Australians, issues too often fall through the cracks of policy.

LGBTIQ populations have been relatively invisible in or excluded from national and state mental health policies and strategies. The absence of a strategic and coordinated approach to the wellbeing of LGBTIQ populations has resulted in insufficient investment and inadequate program responses (Jacobs & Morris, 2016, p. 9).

In recent years, there has been a slowly increasing recognition that LGBTIQ people and communities are unique subpopulations in terms of risk factors and therefore specific responses are required. A turning point in increased recognition was the 2010 report on suicide in Australia, *The Hidden Toll*, which clearly recommended that LGBTIQ populations be recognised as a higher risk group who should be provided with culturally sensitive and appropriate information and services.

While its predecessor made no reference to LGBTIQ populations, the Fifth National Mental Health Plan (released in 2017) recognised that LGBTIQ people have disproportionate experiences of mental health problems and mental illness. This Plan goes part way to redressing this by specifically including LGBTIQ people in Priority Area 6 on reducing stigma and discrimination against people living with mental illness.

Under the auspice of the Australian Government, in 2016 the National LGBTIQ Health Alliance released a National LGBTIQ Mental Health and Suicide Prevention Strategy. This paper provided Strategies for Action aiming to ensure that targeted responses adequately and appropriately support the needs of LGBTI people and communities.

Standards of care

Several standards of care guidelines are available to frame ethical work with LGBTIQ people:

- *Ethical Guidelines for Psychological Practice with Lesbian, Gay and Bisexual Clients* (Australian Psychological Society (APS), 2020a)
- *Ethical Guidelines on Working with Sex and/or Gender Diverse Clients* (Australian Psychological Society (APS), 2013)
- *Standards of Care, Version 7* (WPATH, 2012)
- Australian Standards of Care and Treatment Guidelines for Trans and Gender Diverse Children and Adolescents (Telfer, Tollit, Pace, & Pang, 2018).

Minority stress framework

To describe the correlation between stigma and mental health outcomes, the Minority Stress Model (Meyer & Frost 2013, Rood et al., 2016; see Figure 1.15) describes how stigma towards LGBTIQ people creates a hostile and stressful social environment that in turn leads to adverse mental health outcomes. This framework expands on the direct impact that encountering experiences of prejudice has on mental health, to describe how stress arises from the *expectation and anticipation* of encountering prejudice and negative responses from others. This anticipation leads to the maintenance of constant vigilance that rather than being innocuous keeps stress levels continuously high, which itself has a significant impact on both mental and physical health.

In response, many LGBTIQ people adapt their appearance, behaviour and language to conceal themselves, blend in, so as to avoid encountering negative stigma. Within a mental health context this sees LGBTIQ people delaying or avoiding accessing support, as well as censoring information they share about themselves to their health providers. A 2015 report found that 33.6% of LGBT reported usually or occasionally hiding their sexuality or gender when accessing health services (Leonard et al., 2015, p. 45–46). This can be particularly problematic as health care providers won't have adequate information to structure appropriate care that will meet the individual's particular needs.

The Darlington Statement

The Darlington Statement, released in 2017, is a joint consensus statement by Australian and New Zealand intersex organisations and independent advocates that sets out the priorities and calls by the intersex human rights movement. It calls for rights to bodily integrity, physical autonomy and self-determination.

1 We acknowledge that intersex people are the **experts** on our own lives and lived experience. Intersex people are experts in understanding the long-term effects of medicalisation and medical interventions.

Figure 1.15 Minority stress model for lesbian, gay and bisexual populations

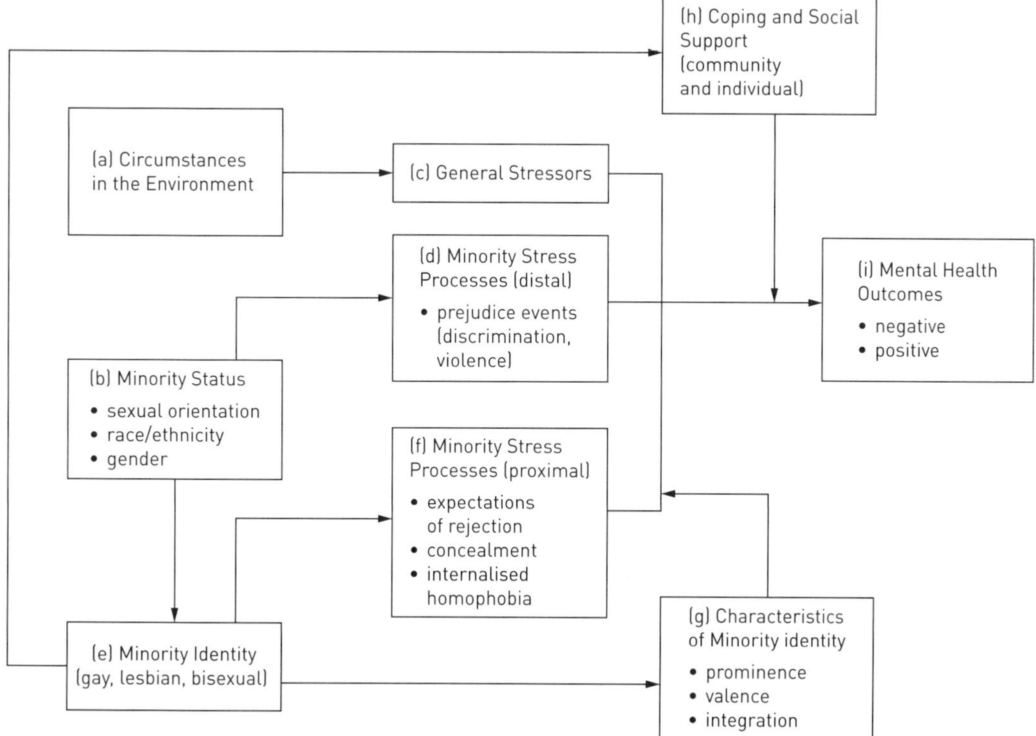

Source: Meyer & Frost, 2013

2 We recognise the fundamental importance and benefits of **affirmative peer support** for people born with variations of sex characteristics.

3 Our peer support organisations and other peer communities need resourcing and support to **build communities and networks** inclusive of all intersex people. No intersex person or parent of an intersex child should feel they are alone, irrespective of their bodily variation or the language they use.

4 We recognise the fundamental importance and benefits of **peer support for parents, caregivers, and families** of people with variations of sex characteristics.

5 We acknowledge the **long-term physical and psychological implications of harmful and continuing medical practices**, and limited access to support and peers.

6 We call for the immediate **prohibition as a criminal act** of deferrable medical interventions, including surgical and hormonal interventions that alter the sex characteristics of infants and children without personal consent.

7 We call for freely-given and fully informed consent by individuals, with individuals and families having mandatory independent access to funded counselling and peer support.

Source: Darlington Statement (IHRA), 2017

IMPLICATIONS FOR PRACTICE

Resilience

Because LGBTIQ people often do experience a lack of acceptance and varying degrees of discrimination, prejudice and trauma, they are often unusually resilient. They will have developed a set of unique personal strategies to deal with societal prejudice and to survive in a stressful environment

Belonging/social inclusion

In contrast to stigma being a risk factor, there are a range of protective factors that support the mental health of LGBTIQ people, with supportive social relationships and a sense of belonging being key.

Community participation is still associated with the mental health of LGBTIQ people. As Figure 1.16 demonstrates, positive impacts vary according to sexuality and gender (Leonard et al., 2015, pp. 49–54). For LGBTIQ people, alongside the benefit of social connectedness, a supportive and accepting community is believed to mediate the impacts that stigma has on mental health (Frost & Meyer, 2012; Pakula et al. 2016). 65% of intersex people report their wellbeing improved with intersex social group participation (Jones et al., 2016, p. 168).

Figure 1.16 Mean K10 Scores of LGBT people who have participated in LGBTIQ community compared to those who have not

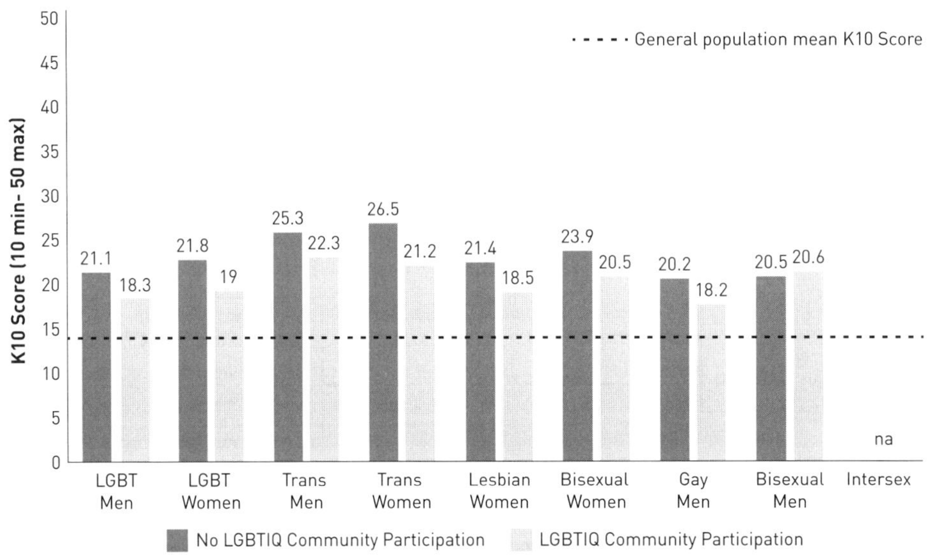

Source: Adapted from Leonard, Lyons, & Bariola, 2015, pp. 49–54

Seeking out supportive communities–individual and group support–is one of the key ways that minority group members develop a resilient response to discriminatory experience. However, in their efforts to remain self-contained and 'hardy', reaching out or help seeking skills may remain underdeveloped. Finding a balance between an internally generated sense of strength and having this validated through supportive others is sometimes difficult for LGBTIQ people. An exploration of these different internal and external strategies of resilience in clients' lives is an important part of developing an affirmative strengths-based assessment.

Key organisations provide information to help people working with LGBTIQ people. For example, the Australian Psychological Society provides information sheets that provide a broad overview of relevant terms, a discussion of the legal, practice and social contexts applicable to the lives of people who are not heterosexual or who do not identify with the sex assigned to them at birth, and information about stereotypes that should be challenged by psychologists and those they work with (Australian Psychological Society (APS), 2020b). There are also tips for psychologists and others working with LGBTIQ people available from the Australian Psychological Society (APS, 2020c; see also www.psychology.org.au/getmedia/78e53d5b-2d60-49ad-b55a-dfc8832fdd4c/APS-tips-for-psychologists-working-with-LGBTQI-amended.pdf).

1.3.5 COMMENTARY AND REFLECTIONS

Our inclusion of these perspectives is not merely some kind of democratic exercise or demonstration of inclusion. Our mental health system, the way decisions are made and services provided, needs to reflect this diversity if it is to meet the needs of our evolving communities. More importantly, these perspectives hold important and different ways of thinking about mental health and illness which can drive positive change in the mental health system more broadly. They have experiences we can learn from and approaches which understand the needs of their communities. These perspectives offer resources we need to consider.

1.4

ADVANCING KNOWLEDGE IN MENTAL HEALTH CARE

BRIDGET BASSILIOS, PHILIP BURGESS, AMANDA FAVILLA, ELLIE FOSSEY, FLICK GREY, BRENDA HAPPELL, MEREDITH HARRIS, BRETT INDER, MARLENA KLAIC, GRAHAM MEADOWS, FIONA MCDERMOTT, CATHERINE MCNAB, ALLAN PINCHES, JANE PIRKIS, FRANCES SHAWYER, SURESH SUNDRAM & YOLAND WADSWORTH

1.4.1 INTRODUCTION

FIONA MCDERMOTT, BRENDA HAPPELL, GRAHAM MEADOWS & ELLIE FOSSEY

SCOPE OF THE CHAPTER

We begin the chapter by sketching some of the issues fundamental firstly to research and then to evaluation in the mental health field. Ethical considerations are of central importance to both research and evaluation and these are then discussed. We proceed to explore the perspectives and interests of the many stakeholders in the mental health field as they relate to both research and evaluation. Then, contributions from different professions, disciplines and stakeholders describe how their research perspectives and approaches are applied. Often authors will draw on their own experience with projects in their areas of expertise and writing to illustrate key concepts and methodological issues. A range of perspectives also are captured in their application to evaluation. Examples of both research and evaluation studies illustrating these differing perspectives and approaches are provided. The final major section addresses the role of evidence in mental health research and evaluation, exploring this issue in relation to various perspectives and noting the existence of debate over what is understood as comprising evidence.

WHAT IS RESEARCH?

Research includes systematic collection and analysis of data or information to increase our understanding of a topic or question, including developing, testing and revising hypotheses to advance theory-based understanding. How we understand the nature and acquisition of knowledge is our epistemological position—researchers, either as individuals or groups with shared thinking, place themselves differently in epistemological terms according to how they define research questions, research designs and preferred methods.

Research usually follows a process that includes: posing a research question; conducting a literature review; collecting data; analysing and interpreting data; revisiting the original question with critique and discussion of it in the light of the findings; reporting and evaluating the results or findings.

There are at least five different approaches to research: the scientific method; quantitative research; qualitative research; action research; and consumer-led research.

- *The scientific method* can be widely defined (Chalmers, 2013). Here we refer to a structured process of observation, hypothesis formation to test the relationship between variables, an operational definition directing ways in which the variables will be measured, the gathering of data, analysis and interpretation of data, and testing and possible revision of the hypothesis posed.
- *Quantitative* research approaches use methods aimed at determining the causal connections between phenomena. Numerical data are collected and analysed using statistical methods.
- *Qualitative research* focuses on understanding the relationships rather than causal connections among phenomena. To that end, data are often text- and talk-based, and are analysed for emergent themes.
- *Action research* is characterised by an orientation towards using the research process itself as key to achieving change in, for example, the way phenomena are understood, or research is 'done', or how stakeholders are involved in the research are active in conducting it.
- *Consumer-led research* is an emergent, heterogeneous field which, as its name implies, is research designed and carried out by consumers themselves using a variety of methods appropriate to the question being asked. It is characterised by a diversity of approaches which reflect the different political, ethical and intellectual understandings of consumers.

Research approaches in mental health are wide-ranging and numerous, reflecting different epistemologies, methodologies and methods, the range of disciplines at work, and consumers and carers who contribute to the field. Research in one form or another as an activity leading to new knowledge is the primary tool of science. Science is commonly organised into broad themes. The natural sciences have a focus on the natural world, including processes of living organisms, while the social sciences are concerned with human behaviour and societies. Often science may also be considered in relation to orientation, which may be pure or applied.

In classifying research, be it natural or social and either pure or applied, in Australian universities eight broad categories are applied:

1. physical, chemical and Earth sciences
2. humanities and creative arts
3. engineering and environmental sciences
4. social, behavioural and economic sciences
5. mathematical, information and computing sciences
6. biological and biotechnological sciences
7. biomedical and clinical health sciences
8. public and allied health sciences.

Activity in all of these domains might take the form of scientific inquiry, perhaps with the exception of purely artistic research, and we may note that the organising term here does not use the word 'science', whereas others do.

Within research in mental health care we may find examples of almost all of the above categories. Not uncommonly, research may span more than one, sometimes several of these categories, especially in mental health care, where interdisciplinary research is very common. Most research in mental health care, however, would have at least some features either of the biomedical and clinical health sciences group or the social, behavioural and economic sciences group, even if this might not be the primary classification for a particular study or investigation.

As has been noted, a diversity of disciplines and key stakeholders are active researchers within the mental health field. In Table 1.3, we note their particular standpoint or perspectives, typical questions and methods likely to be used.

Table 1.3 Research stakeholder perspectives

Stakeholder group	Perspective	Examples of research interests/questions	Typical methods
Psychiatrists	As researchers, psychiatrists usually continue their clinical orientation, often with focus on understanding, better characterising or improved treatment of response to mental health problems.	Involvement in pharmaceutical trials; investigations of neurobiological, neurochemical or other fundamental mechanisms that can lead to disorder; trials of psychological or psychosocial treatments; research into models of training.	Collaborate on epidemiological surveys; trials of treatment approaches.
Mental health nurses	Research that identifies the unique contribution nursing makes to improved health outcomes for consumers of mental health services. Frequently work collaboratively with consumers in mental health research and promote consumer roles.	Nursing care of consumers experiencing a range of mental illnesses; professional issues having an impact on mental health nursing practice. Enhancing consumer and carer participation in mental health care, research and professional education. Role of clinical supervision in enhancing practice and practitioner satisfaction; nature of the practice environment itself, including the nurse–patient relationship; dealing with aggressive incidents; identification and prevention of suicidal actions.	Broad range of qualitative and quantitative approaches, co-production.
Psychologists	Strongly rooted in empirical research; predominantly couched within positivist paradigm.	Domains studied range from epidemiological to brain functioning to program effectiveness.	Full range of methodologies; typically, theories or models give rise to testable hypotheses, which are then subjected to empirical test, often involving comparison of groups or changes in experimental conditions; statistical methods used to describe the likelihood that the result may have arisen by chance, rather than from a real difference in the groups studied or the change in experimental conditions.
Consumers	Consumer perspective research is a subset of consumer research, which values lived experience as a *crucial* source of intellectual insight; tends to take a critical approach to research and has been described as delivering 'a coherent challenge to the research hegemony in mental health' (O'Hagan, 2009, p. i).	Evaluating services with regard to relevant issues *as defined by consumers*; generating research that reflects consumer priorities; may or may not even be framed within 'mental health', but may use other frames of reference, e.g. spiritual or political understandings of our experiences.	Qualitative research; hermeneutics as the study of meaning; interviews; participatory action research, including participating or collaborating in mental health research with other stakeholders.

Stakeholder group	Perspective	Examples of research interests/questions	Typical methods
Carers	Focus on carrying out research in order to provide carer insight into relevant research questions (Goodare & Lockwood, 1999), perhaps leading to strengthening culture of inclusion.	Significant focus on carer burden; research and evaluation of family interventions and psychoeducation current attention on carer participation in mental health services utilising an experience based approach; emerging research areas are: importance of family or carer resilience and recovery as key indicators of better outcomes for sufferers.	Qualitative and quantitative; carer involvement, as interviewers can lead to a higher number of respondents agreeing to take part and yielding more open responses.
Practitioner researchers	Practitioner (or practice) research is undertaken by practitioners most often working in clinical service delivery roles, e.g. practitioners from the range of mental health service providers in hospitals, clinics and community-based mental health services; practitioner research is embedded in the practice of the researcher rather than primarily an academic activity.	Questions address issues, problems and situations that practitioners encounter in their day-to-day practice or the programs they develop; identifying the evidence which supports or challenges their practice, perhaps prompting change (Fox, Martin, & Green, 2007); practice that challenges, surprises or perplexes them; evaluation of impact.	Primarily 'insider' research; typically small in scale and duration, varied in design and methods; with practitioners setting their own aims for their inquiry, focusing on their own or their peers' professional practice, or on aspects of service delivery or evaluation or practice-related organisational issues (Mitchell, Lunt, & Shaw, 2010), pp. 9–10). Insider research requires PRs to be mindful of ethical considerations and need to ensure rigour in data analysis (Chou, 2010; Shaw & Faulkner, 2006).
Social workers	Perspective emphasises context-bound nature of human action; importance placed on understanding person within his or her environment, conceptualised very broadly as including many 'levels' of action: intrapsychic, interpersonal and organisational; frequently adopt social constructivist perspective embedded in a critical theory approach, with focus on the meaning of action within context.	Particular interest in the experiences of vulnerable people, structural barriers to service access, impact of stigma or prejudice.	Qualitative and quantitative methods; participatory and collaborative research.

(Continues)

Table 1.3 Research stakeholder perspectives (Continued)

Stakeholder group	Perspective	Examples of research interests/questions	Typical methods
Occupational therapists	Research to develop knowledge and practice tools for understanding of lived experiences of daily life, and how consumers' and families' lives and activities may have been affected by experiences of ill health, restricted participation and social conditions. Perspective emphasises the interplay between meaning, performance and contextual factors that support or hinder what people have opportunity to do, and are able do in daily life. Research focused on articulating, developing and evaluating occupational therapy practices in mental health care and occupational therapy education.	Activity patterns and their links to meaning, satisfaction, recovery and wellbeing for individuals experiencing mental health issues, for families and carers. Experiences, barriers and enablers of participation and performance in particular occupations, such as work where issues addressed include: job seeking, managing personal information, work adjustments, and employment support. Development of practice tools, for example, focused on occupational histories, time use, consumer interests and concerns, and identifying strengths and difficulties in carrying out activities that a person wants or needs to do. Design and evaluation of individual and group interventions, for example, inpatient and community programs designed to support activity engagement and self-management of adults experiencing mental illness during their process of recovery; and home interventions designed to support carers to facilitate activity engagement of older persons with dementia.	Quantitative, qualitative, mixed methods, and participatory research approaches.
Health economists and Behavioural Economists	Systematic analysis of costs, benefits, management and consequences of health care; behavioural economics includes how psychological, and social factors may influence economic decision making.	Applies techniques of economics to service delivery and uptake questions regarding mental health care, from availability of drugs and other interventions, training of clinicians, shifts in public attitudes, to how decisions are made regarding prioritisation of all these issues, and how they may best be financed.	Analysis of data from randomised controlled trials, large service data bases, health insurance claims and medical records; often involves analytic or modelling approaches specific to economics.

RESEARCH AND EVALUATION

While there is often considerable overlap between activities described as 'research' and those described as 'evaluation', and many research methods are common to both, there are noteworthy differences. These differences often relate to the context in which research or evaluation takes place, evaluation generally requiring greater sensitivity to the political and organisational context and demanding the evaluator demonstrate awareness of the different needs of (often) multiple stakeholders.

Evaluation occurs within a social, economic and political climate, and thus can serve to meet a range of aims and be put to a variety of uses. It may be used to further political aims and objectives, for example, to keep an issue on or off the agenda. It is also important to bear in mind that the credibility and legitimacy that is given to particular approaches to evaluation is also a political factor. It may be that at different times and when different power brokers occupy influential positions, only some forms of evaluative activity will receive recognition and be used as the basis for policy making and decision making. For example, the current emphasis placed on evidence-based practice may seem to be in an ambiguous relationship with mental health policies that emphasise the need to hear the voices of consumers, which are often not accorded the legitimacy of being considered 'valid evidence'. Importantly, as Kirkhart (2010) points out, the cultural context in which an evaluation is undertaken is highly relevant. *Culture* refers to the values, beliefs and history of a program or of the stakeholders to a program. For example, we might think of the core values and locations in structures of power occupied by mental health consumers whose interests in the evaluation, whose participation in it and whose understanding of the purposes it is to serve are crucial to incorporate and study as key aspects of the cultural context in which the evaluation is being conducted, and thus central to ensuring validity of the evaluation itself.

Undertaking evaluation raises a number of issues for consideration and questions to be answered. They include:

- Who is it for?
- Who are the stakeholders?
- How are the values that form its basis arrived at?
- What is it for?
- Who is to do it?
- Can it (the issue, program or phenomenon) be evaluated?
- If not, can it be made so?
- Is the evaluation feasible, or how can it become feasible (politically, in terms of resources such as time, space, money, people and skills)?
- Is the evaluation ethical?
- Will the findings be acted upon?

Defining terms is helpful in order to link these definitions to these questions, thereby illustrating the extent to which answers to the questions may be influenced by the perspective being taken.

Defining terms

Evaluation

Evaluation refers to attempts to decide the value, worth, merit and/or significance of something. It is important to note the breadth of this definition and how much it is implicitly conditioned by value systems.

Stakeholder

The *Oxford English Dictionary* definition of 'stakeholder' includes 'a person or group with concern or interest in ensuring the success of an organisation, business, or system'. Many debates over proper conduct of evaluation are in effect debates over the relative status of different stakeholders being considered by evaluators. Defining who stakeholders are and gaining an understanding of their different positions in relation to the evaluation, is helpful in answering the above questions, including critically the final question—whether findings will be acted on.

Formative and summative evaluation:

This is often a very important distinction in evaluation practice.

> When the cook tastes the soup, that's formative.
> When the guests taste the soup, that's summative.
>
> *Robert Stake, 1991*

- *Formative evaluations* are used during the task of progressively forming a program or project. They are conducted with the intention of providing information that can be responded to reflexively within the program; information that is used to adjust or inform the conduct of the program. In other words, the focus of formative evaluation is upon *process*.
- *Summative evaluation* aims to summate information relating to a program. It is often aimed at assessing the overall value of a program or activity in question to inform judgements about *whether* or not it should continue. In other words, summative evaluations are about *outcomes*.

It has been argued that as the conceptual underpinning of evaluation develops, in some situations a developmental model of evaluation may be appropriate where the distinctions are less clear cut (Patton, 2010). Nevertheless in many settings there are clear punctuation points in a project where the distinction is very valuable. In these contexts the timing, correct conduct and dissemination of each kind of evaluation may be very different, and confusing the differing purposes of each may place the integrity of either approach at risk.

Often this issue (whether the evaluation is considered to be formative or summative) will have implications for many of the questions noted at the outset, and may affect judgements about access to information and ethics, as well as the use to which findings are put.

Reasons for doing evaluation

Evaluation is important:

- for accountability purposes: services and programs are accountable to funders, service users, service providers and the community in general, as well as the various professional communities
- to know what works in a situation, and what does not work
- to monitor what is being done
- to generate knowledge, especially in regard to value, merit, worth and significance
- to test out or verify what is known
- to keep a program responsive to changes in needs, attitudes or the priority given particular issues on the public agenda.

Individually or in groups, service providers may engage in evaluation because they want to:

- know about the efficiency of their own practice
- explore and understand their own experience
- participate in or play a part in effecting systemic or organisational change, or consider changes to existing treatment and intervention practices (Mark, Henry, & Jules, 2000).

While people may engage in many evaluation exercises out of curiosity, it is, however, very important to emphasise that evaluations need to be used; that is, an evaluation is incomplete unless the changes that emerge from it as rational recommendations are put into effect. This part of the evaluation cycle is sometimes omitted, for a variety of economic, political and historical reasons. However, without a commitment to implementing an evaluation's findings (and those from QI activities), the contributions of stakeholders appear to be disregarded, and the purpose of engaging in the evaluation process in the first place is diminished.

Generations of evaluation: A typology

Donaldson and Lipsey (2006) note that the 1940s saw the beginning of the modern evaluation movement, while the late 1960s and early 1970s mark the beginning of evaluation as a formal activity as we know it today. Guba and Lincoln (1989) argued for a developmental perspective on the growth of evaluation activity, considering that formal evaluation activity can be viewed as having gone through four 'generations' and having begun a move into a fifth generation. These generations represent changing views about the nature of evaluation. They are embedded in and reflect the continuing debates in the human sciences between the traditional scientific paradigm (positivism) and the 'new' or alternative inquiry paradigms (social constructivism, critical theory and postmodernism).

The first generation of evaluation

This was characterised by a focus upon measurement as evidenced, in the education field, by the use of aptitude and intelligence tests. The evaluator's role was that of technician, gathering data and administering tests. The results would then be used to evaluate a program's output.

During this generation, evaluation and measurement were synonymous. First-generation evaluation, then, can be seen as essentially outcome assessment. The ease of administering tests such as aptitude tests, relative to other forms of evaluation, has ensured its enduring popularity in economic- and production-focused evaluation methodology (Fox, 1997, p. 27).

While the first generation of measurement was notably successful in evaluating outcomes, it was unable to discern the factors that may have contributed to these outcomes. With regard to social programs, outcomes are important, but the means by which they are achieved are equally important.

The second generation of evaluation

In this generation, the problem in assigning change to causes was recognised. This led to a focus on the objectives of programs, and on describing patterns of strength and weakness that may impact on achieving objectives. Testing was retained in the new role of estimating the capacity of outcomes to match program intentions. According to Guba and Lincoln (1989), the evaluator's role in this second generation was that of a neutral observer who undertook the evaluation by beginning with a description of a program. This description was compared with the program outcomes until the most appropriate program description, which could account for the outcomes achieved, emerged. The role of the evaluator in this generation remained largely a passive one.

The third generation of evaluation

This subsumed the previous evaluator roles of technician and neutral observer, but added to it the role of judge. While less passive than in previous roles, the role of evaluator as judge is a powerful one. However, such a role was criticised frequently as belonging with a managerial, top-down perspective, heavily committed to the scientific paradigm of inquiry, with resultant difficulties in accommodating diverse values and perspectives.

Fourth generation evaluation

The problem of accommodating diverse values and perspectives required a 'complete reconstruction' (Guba & Lincoln, 1989, p. 31) of evaluation activity, from which emerged a fourth generation. Commonly called responsive or constructionist, fourth generation models were seen to take as their point of focus not objectives, decisions, effects or similar organisers, but instead the claims, concerns and issues put forth by various stakeholders with varying involvement in the evaluation, and thus potentially targeted by it.

The position of evaluation in the modern context has been and is the subject of debate. As Lincoln (1994) noted:

> Many social scientists now recognise that what is needed is many perspectives, many voices, before we can achieve deep understandings of social phenomena, and before we can assert that a narrative is complete. The modernist dream of a grand or master narrative is now a dead project; the recognition of the futility and oppression of such a project is the 'postmodern condition' (p. 303).

Fifth generation evaluation

The early to mid-1990s saw the emergence of fifth generation evaluation models. A fifth generation model, according to Caulley, can be seen to operate from an internal perspective: 'If evaluation is to make a difference, then there is a need to create in organisations a culture of ongoing monitoring and evaluation by program staff' (Caulley, 1994, p. 13). Fifth generation evaluation places emphasis on a managerial style characterised by assertiveness rather than an aggressive or authoritarian approach. Staff are encouraged to be reflective about their work and to take responsibility for their own quality control. Such organisational practices are considered to be empowering for staff, providing a force for motivation and consequently enhancing productivity.

Interestingly, in this collaborative and autonomy-valuing generation, the role of evaluator has become less discernible, and issues such as those relating to control, power and conflict appear to have moved to the margins.

The elements of the generations are summarised in Table 1.4, which includes instances of activities of each generational type.

Approaches to evaluation

Insider evaluation

In view of the foregoing comments, it is no wonder that service providers often feel that to evaluate their service or practice or program is difficult, requires expertise different from their own, may be costly and will undoubtedly raise anxieties. But it is also the case that service providers and service users have a great deal of knowledge and expertise about the relative merits of various interventions or strategies, and are frequently very well placed to evaluate what they know best. Action research and fourth (and fifth) generation evaluation have opened the way to recognise and legitimise the evaluation strengths of interest and stakeholder groups in order to generate trustworthy and usable knowledge for service and program development. Such 'insider' evaluations have in recent years become the focus of practitioner researchers (see Table 1.3). Insider evaluations are not without their challenges and difficulties, and have been subject to critique and debate (Shaw & Faulkner, 2006).

Evaluation as transdiscipline

In the early 2000s, a 'second boom' in evaluation occurred, with a more global perspective emerging, evident in a general embrace of such values as accountability and professionalism (Donaldson & Lipsey, 2006, p. 56). With this increasing demand for evaluation, new theories of evaluation practice, and new tools and methods, were developed to address a wider range of evaluation practice challenges. Evaluation began to be seen as a 'transdiscipline', with tools and techniques to support a range of other disciplines while remaining autonomous with reference to its focus on evaluation theory and on advancing knowledge about how to do evaluations. Interestingly, the debate over the role of theory in evaluation has continued to be contentious, with some arguing that the guidance that theory provides is essential to evaluation, although others suggest that evaluation can be done without theory, reflecting the 'sometimes chaotic conditions of the real world' (Donaldson & Lipsey, 2006, p. 57). Indeed in recent research into the degree to which evaluation theory is enacted in evaluation practice, it was found that there was 'little empirical evidence to buttress the numerous theoretical postulations and prescriptions put forward for most theory-driven evaluations' (Corryn, Noakes, Westine, & Schroter, 2011, p. 215).

ETHICAL CONSIDERATIONS IN RESEARCH AND EVALUATION

Ethical considerations inform all aspects of the research and evaluation process. Thus, ethics will be relevant from the very beginning, even in the choice

Table 1.4 Generations of evaluation

Generation	Key feature	An instance
First	Outcome measurement	Symptom measurement following a drug prescription
Second	Process and outcome combined	Prescribing and monitoring adherence as well as outcome evaluation
Third	Second generation, plus evaluator as judge	Collating information about a drug's performance, and recommending a specific prescribing policy
Fourth	Uses techniques from first to third generations, with the posture of empowerment of all parties	Engaging the consumers of a service, along with the providers, in becoming contributing parties to the prescribing policies of the service
Fifth	Evaluation as prevailing culture	Absorption of the lessons of the first four generations into the way people at all levels of an organisation conduct their practice

of questions to research or evaluate. It may be useful to draw attention to the specific mention of research in the *UN Declaration of the Rights of Mentally Ill Persons* (United Nations, 2003).

Clinical trials and experimental treatment shall never be carried out on any patient without informed consent, except that a patient who is unable to give informed consent may be admitted to a clinical trial or given experimental treatment but only with the approval of a competent, independent review body specifically constituted for this purpose.

Two central issues dominate the development and application of ethical principles for research and evaluation: the minimising of harm to those involved in the research or evaluation, and the assurance that participants give informed and voluntary consent to their involvement. Although these principles appear relatively straightforward, in practice researchers and evaluators need to think carefully about their implications. There are various forms of potential harm (see Section 1.5.2), such as physical, legal, psychological, emotional or social harm, that may be relevant to specific situations. For example, the trial of a new drug may incur unknown side effects, or the identification of people in certain categories, such as 'people diagnosed with mental illness', may be stigmatising and carry the risk of creating social harm to a participant. The onus is on researchers and evaluators to recognise these potential sources of harm and adopt strategies to minimise them, such as the provision of time for debriefing, encouraging participants to enlist support persons or making medical assistance available.

Again, the importance of obtaining informed consent from participants requires researchers and evaluators to consider the mental state of participants, or their capacity to read and comprehend information about the proposed research. The necessity to avoid any sense of coercion to take part in the research will suggest that researchers and evaluators need to be aware of the relationship between researcher and participant, doctor and patient (a sometimes subtle inequality), service provider and service user, and employer and employee. Above all, in consenting to take part, the participant in research or evaluation must know what he or she is 'in for' and must be free to participate or not, to withdraw or not from the research or evaluation without incurring any censure.

When we undertake research and evaluation in the mental health field, we must be keenly aware that people who experience mental health problems or psychiatric disabilities constitute a vulnerable group. As such, we must be very clear that any advantages to their participation will outweigh or, at the very least, not increase any possible disadvantages. Before embarking on any research or evaluation, it is important to consult the most recent *Ethical Guidelines for the Conduct of Research Involving Humans* (NHMRC & Universities Australia, 2018). Many health and welfare bodies have their own institutional ethics committees, which will provide advice, guidelines, and permission for researchers and evaluators to proceed.

PARADIGMS INFORMING RESEARCH

In parallel with the way that practitioners draw on different theoretical perspectives and discipline knowledge to guide practice, approaches to research and evaluation draw on differing philosophical perspectives. Each philosophical perspective represents a system of ideas about how the world can be understood, central assumptions, how knowledge is produced, and principles that underpin the methods used to observe, describe and measure the phenomena being studied (Neuman, 2003). These philosophical perspectives are often referred to as *research paradigms* (Kuhn, 1970). Paradigms may be considered commensurable or not dependent on whether communication between them is reasonably possible. An established paradigm will typically be defended by people schooled within it, often by process of a series of ad hoc modifications. Often it is not until an alternative body of theory or explanation offers an acceptable new interpretation of information that the old paradigm will be rejected. So paradigm-shifts are points where an established paradigm becomes so threatened by a body of contrary evidence that it must give way.

Three major research paradigms that inform the different approaches to research and evaluation discussed in this chapter include: an empirico-analytical research paradigm, that informs the use of hypothetico-deductive scientific methods; and interpretive and critical research paradigms, each of which place emphasis on seeking understanding of the meanings of human actions and experiences, and on generating accounts of their meaning from the viewpoints of those involved, but with some differences in how these meanings are framed and interpreted. Table 1.5 summarises some key characteristics of these three research paradigms that inform the different approaches to research and evaluation discussed in this chapter.

There may currently be a paradigm shift going on in mental health care internationally which while of a less major nature than shifting between the major paradigms in Table 1.5, may be very significant for mental health care delivery. It has long seemed an assumption of much mental health care research that if we only can extend provision of existing treatments to more and more of the population that benefit will accrue including eventually demonstrable impact on population prevalence. However evidence is accumulating that goes against this proposition internationally and here in Australia (Jorm, 2018; Jorm, Patten, Brugha, & Mojtabai, 2017; Meadows, Prodan, et al., 2019). As a result, new publications are querying whether this approach will achieve the desired result and whether reappraisal may be needed. In this the relatively mainstream medical literature is starting increasingly to accept propositions previously the domain of the recovery movement (see Sections 1.1.6, 1.5.2 and 2.6.2) and we may be at the point of seeing a paradigm shift that means these two domains of discourse may be becoming more commensurable (van Os, Guloksuz, Vijn, Hafkenscheid, & Delespaul, 2019).

1.4.2 NEUROSCIENCE

SURESH SUNDRAM

INTRODUCTION

The ancient philosophical split between the body and the mind finds a parallel in our understanding of the relevance of the brain to mental health. Historically, mental activity and illness has been understood and researched through intangible processes such as religious and spiritual beliefs and then more recently psychological and behavioural approaches. However, the intimate connection between the brain as an organ and its main outputs such as thinking, emotions and behaviour have compelled investigation into its mechanisms. This is the area of neuroscience research as it applies to mental health. The constraint has been the coarseness of the research tools in addressing the immense complexity of the brain. As these tools increase in sophistication it is increasingly possible to discover insights into mental processes and disorders, notwithstanding how embryonic this understanding. However, these technologies and tools, no matter how sophisticated, only permit us to ask 'how' questions to probe the mechanisms that underpin neural activity and outputs. The application of neuroscience research is, in the main, predicated upon the scientific method and relies on rigorous empirical approaches. This provides us with information on the mechanisms that underpin mental activity.

The challenges with using neuroscience in understanding mental phenomena and disorders though are numerous. They include the fleeting nature of thoughts and feelings, our profoundly endowed cognitive and language capacities compared to other animals, and the ethical prohibitions on sampling and examining the human brain. Therefore, approaches have needed to be indirect in contrast with most other biomedical research which has resulted in a slower rate of progress.

Table 1.5 Comparison of three major paradigms that inform social research

Key characteristics	Three major research paradigms		
	Empirico-analytical	**Interpretive**	**Critical**
1 Philosophical or theoretical origins	Positivism, natural sciences	Hermeneutics, phenomenology, symbolic interactionism	Marxist, feminist, psychoanalytic
2 Why conduct research?	To discover natural laws that enable prediction or control of events	To understand social life and describe how people construct social meaning	To uncover myths or hidden truths that account for social relations, and empower people to change society radically
3 What is the nature of social reality?	Social reality contains stable pre-existing patterns of order that can be discovered	Fluid definitions of situations created by people through their social interactions with others	Social reality is multilayered; events and relations based on hidden underlying social structures or forces that evolve in a historical context
4 What is the nature of human beings?	Self-interested and rational individuals shaped by external forces	Social beings who create meaning and constantly engage in making sense of their worlds	Creative, adaptive beings with unrealised potential, trapped by social forces that disempower or exploit
5 Role of common sense	Clearly distinct from and less valid than science	Powerful everyday theories that guide daily life; necessary to understand people; and no less valid than science	Raise beliefs that guide human actions, and contain myths that hide unequal control over power and objective conditions and resources
6 What constitutes an explanation or theory of social reality?	A logical, deductive system of interconnected definitions, axioms and causal laws stated in probabilistic form	A description of how a group's meaning system is generated and sustained; contains detailed contextual information and limited abstraction	A critique that reveals the underlying social structure of conditions, and helps people see the way to a better world
7 An explanation that is true	It is logically connected to causal laws and based on observed facts about social life	Resonates with or feels right to those who participated in the study	Is a resource that helps people understand their own experiences in historical context, and improve their own conditions and social world
8 Whose voices are privileged?	Researcher(s)	Participant(s)	Stakeholder(s)
9 What does good evidence look like?	Based on precise observations that others can repeat	Embedded in the context of fluid social interactions, in which meanings are assigned	Informed by a theory of what the social world is like that unveils myths or hidden truths
10 Where do social and political values enter into science?	Science is value free; values have no place, except when choosing a topic	Values are an integral part of social life; no group's values are presumed superior to others	All science must begin with a value position; some positions are better than others
11 What is the place of ethics in research?	Extrinsic; mechanisms guiding ethical conduct are external to the inquiry process itself	Intrinsic; participant values and personal nature of researcher–researched interactions are integral to the research process	Intrinsic; collaboration among participants and empowerment occur through the research process

Source: Adapted from Neuman (1994); Guba & Lincoln (1994); Fossey, Harvey, McDermott, & Davidson (2002)

BRIEF OVERVIEW

Within the parameters above, researching the brain may in the simplest way be arranged in an ascending order of size: genes and genetic processes; cells, in particular neurons, but also astrocytes and microglia; ensembles or assemblies of neurons; functional circuits and networks across brain regions; and brain regions and lobes (Kandel, Schwartz, & Jessell, 2013). In addition, to these modes of human research it is also possible to model components of mental activity and disorder using animals, non-human cells and in silico modelling.

RESEARCH APPROACHES

Genes and genetic processes are generally easily accessible through peripheral tissue where the genetic identity is identical between all cells in the one individual. Hence, it is possible to take a blood or saliva sample from an individual and sequence the whole or parts of the genetic code. By doing this for large numbers of people with a specific disorder (cases) and those without the disorder (controls), it becomes possible to compare and identify if whether there are genetic variations that predispose towards that disorder. These Genome Wide Association Studies (GWAS) have attracted much recent attention and funding for large multisite international collaborations. For example, recently a GWAS in major depression (Wray et al., 2018) included 135 458 cases and 344 901 controls and identified 44 gene loci that were associated with the disorder after statistical correction for multiple testing. These types of studies don't identify causative genes but rather, those more commonly associated with the disorder. This information can then be used by scientists to identify proteins and cellular pathways that may be involved in the pathology of the disorder, ultimately, to inform the development of biomarkers to indicate people at risk and even new target molecules for novel drug treatments.

Also of recent interest has been a growing understanding of how genes are regulated by environmental factors–epigenetics. Genes in every cell are tightly regulated by proteins called histones. They in turn are influenced by cell signals that respond to internal and external environmental stimuli. This gene regulation modifies the cell's behaviour and thus a mechanism is being understood that connects external factors with neuronal adaptations and function. These may be immediate and short-term but also influence early neural development resulting in long-term effects. The impact of early life adversity on the stress response through a protein, FKBP5, results in long-term brain changes and responses which predispose to the development of disorders such as major depression, post-traumatic stress disorder and schizophrenia (Matosin, Halldorsdottir, & Binder, 2018).

Understanding how neurons and other brain cells communicate chemically with each other has informed our current major hypotheses of mental disorders such as schizophrenia, major depression, bipolar disorder and attention-deficit hyperactivity disorder. Principally, this has been through identification of the protein and cellular targets of effective pharmacological agents such as antipsychotic and antidepressant drugs. However, in contrast to cells and tissue from most other parts of the body, human brain tissue and neurons are for the most part inaccessible from living people. Post-mortem tissue is available but is limited due to availability and the potential influence of confounding ante-mortem and post-mortem variables such as brain hypoxia. Nevertheless, these studies have identified changed levels of proteins or mRNA in brain tissue and now with advanced cell sorting and microscopy technologies are potentially able to be localised to specific neuronal types.

Major advances in stem cell biology have enabled the transformation of generic or pluripotent stem cells into neurons. This has enabled skin tissue to be collected from people with schizophrenia which is then transformed into neurons, plausibly carrying the same genetic and cellular machinery as affected neurons in the person's brain (Brennand et al., 2011). Thus, cellular processes actually altered in schizophrenia and now other neuropsychiatric disorders can be studied in real-time.

Neuroimaging has seen extraordinary progress over the last two decades from basic structural imaging and volumetric assessment of brain regions to integrated assessment of structure, function and connectivity between regions. This has been enabled through combining functional magnetic resonance imaging (fMRI), positron emission tomography (PET) and high resolution structural MRI. These methodologies have allowed visualisation of networks between brain regions not previously thought to be connected allowing a much more sophisticated construction of brain activity during mental processes both in health and disease (Kaiser, 2017). For example, a resting state fMRI study (Sheline, Price, Yan, & Mintun, 2010) of people with major depression showed higher connectivity, compared to controls, of three brain networks–the cognitive control, default mode, and affective networks. These networks linked much more in depressed people through the dorso-medial prefrontal cortex. Each network is associated with different symptoms in depression–decreased concentration, rumination, self-absorption, increased vigilance, and emotional, visceral, and autonomic dysregulation–and this increased connectivity explains how these different symptom domains associate and interact with each other. Understanding this allows people with depression to be classified according to which network may be more affected in any one person and this then may permit more specific targeting of treatment strategies. Ultimately, it may even be possible to develop pharmaceutical agents that target a specific network and tailor treatments at an individual level.

SUMMARY

Neuroscience research advances in light of the available technologies to answer how the brain is able to generate mental activity and how this is disturbed in mental disorders. The relative inaccessibility of the human brain to direct research has forced researchers to use animal models or indirect approaches both of which present limitations. Ultimately, each approach sheds light on a specific component of the brain machinery which then must be holistically integrated to understand the nature of the activity or dysfunction. This increasingly is becoming possible as newer technologies allow higher resolution imaging and modelling of neuronal function, which will then enable us to grasp how mental activity and disorder occurs and the opportunities for intervention.

1.4.3 EPIDEMIOLOGY

GRAHAM MEADOWS

THE STUDY OF DISEASE IN POPULATIONS

Epidemiology is the branch of medical science that deals with the incidence, distribution and control of disease in populations. General introductory and area-specific reference texts (Schneider & Lilienfeld, 2015; Tsuang, Tohen, & Jones, 2011; Prince, Stewart, Ford, & Das-munshi, 2020) provide information on concepts with specific usages in the field such as case, population, sample, risk, prevalence and incidence rates, also definitions of various properties of screening tests. We will not here attempt fully to survey this field or recapitulate these definitions–but many of the concepts and processes of epidemiological science are important to understand. Fairly obviously they are important in order to consider the conduct of, and findings from, epidemiological surveys (see Sections 1.4.11 and 1.6.4) and from studies of large health care data sets (see Sections 1.4.6, 1.4.11 and 1.6.5) as well as influences on populations of health care and other societal interventions (see Sections 1.4.11 and 1.6.6). Also these understandings may influence clinical and other practice. By way of an example of how some of these concepts apply in mental health we will consider a range of uses of one particular instrument, the Kessler 10 scale (K10).

DEVELOPMENT OF THE K10

Named after Ron Kessler, a Harvard-based epidemiologist who led its development, the K10 was developed to measure a dimensional concept termed 'psychological distress' and also includes items with features of categories of mental illness, particularly depressive and anxiety disorders. Developed using content from existing scales, using psychometric techniques to establish a good performing item-collection (see Sections 1.4.5 and 1.4.11), its extensive Australian use means we know a good deal about how it typically performs in Australian communities (Slade, Grove, & Burgess, 2011). You can explore the scale on various websites—for instance that of beyondblue. In Australia it is usually scored from 10-50, with a baseline of 10 (cf in the United States, 0–40.)

USE IN NATIONAL SURVEYS

The K10 was included in both National Surveys of Mental Health and Wellbeing (NSMHW; see Section 1.4.3) so we have information on associations of

Figure 1.17 Pre- and post-test probability

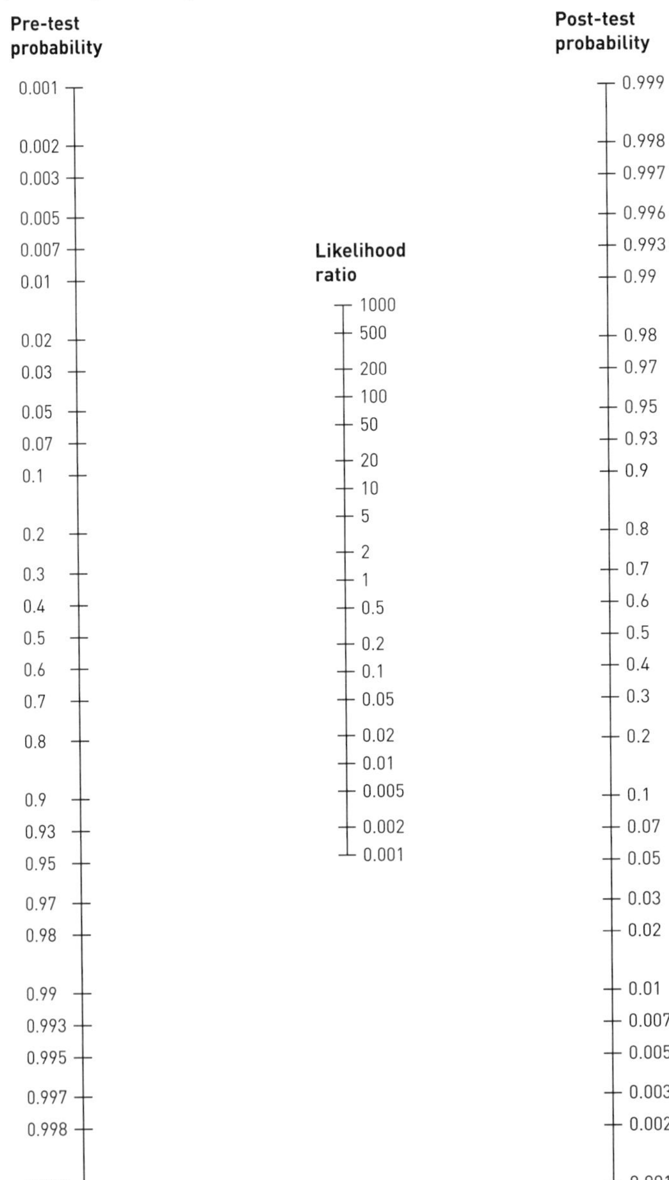

Source: Wikipedia, 2019

different K10 scores with rates of diagnosed mental illness according to an extensive interview for ICD-10 mental disorders (criterion validity). In the 2007 NSMHW where affective, anxiety and substance misuse disorders were assessed in the last 12 months it was found that the Positive Predictive Values (PPV—or the proportion of test-positive people who seem to have any of these conditions) of K10 score bands were: Low (10-15) 10.9%, Moderate (16-21) 32%, High (22-29) 57.1% and Very High (30-50) 79.6% (Slade et al., 2011). The K10 also has been included in regular national health surveys (see Sections 1.4.11, 1.6.1 and 1.6.2) and so provides our best source at present of information on changes through time in mental health problems in the Australian population, as well as area and income-specific differences (Enticott, Meadows, Shawyer, Inder, & Patten, 2016; Isaacs, Enticott, Meadows, & Inder, 2018).

SCREENING AND OTHER USE IN PRIMARY CARE

The K10 has come into regular use across the country in many primary care settings. Many GPs who have been trained up through the Mental Health Skills Training arm of the Better Access to Mental Health Care program (see Sections 1.4.11, 1.5.4 and 1.7.1) will be familiar with it for assessment and screening. Sensitivity and specificity are two terms applying to screening tests, or attempts to detect disease in populations: sensitivity is the proportion of cases correctly so identified by the test, and specificity is the proportion of non-cases correctly so identified by the test. A related statistic, the likelihood ratio, is the ratio of a positive screening test in cases as opposed to non-cases. Sensitivity and specificity are very unstable; these along with positive and negative predictive values (PPV/NPV) can change considerably as population frequency varies. The likelihood ratio, typically more stable, can be more useful for predicting probability of a problem given different pre-test frequencies. A 'nomogram' is typically used to assist this calculation (Streiner & Geddes, 1998). This works by using a straight edge from the pre-test probability (rate of the problem in the population where it is being used) through the likelihood ratio and then estimating from the crossing with the right hand line the Post-Test Probability (PPV).

This may mean for instance that in many general practice settings the performance of the K10 may be different from in the national surveys. Where the rate of mental health problems in the consulting population is higher than in the general community for instance, the PPVs may be higher than those found in the survey. However things may be further complicated by the fact that some items on the K10 can be scored positive based on symptoms of what may not be primary mental health problems, such as diabetes for instance (Schmitz, Lesage, & Wang, 2009). Use of the K10 in different settings then requires an understanding of its performance in surveys in relation to more extensive measures of mental health problems, and how that performance may vary in different settings based on coexisting medical problems and different underlying rates of mental health problems where it is being applied. These concepts and the nomogram apply across a wide range of detection and assessment issues. This discussion then provides an example of how some epidemiological concepts and techniques may be important in approaching what may seem a relatively simple matter of using a questionnaire to screen for possible mental health problems in one or other service setting.

1.4.4 CLINICAL TRIALS

FRANCES SHAWYER & GRAHAM MEADOWS WITH AMANDA FAVILLA

TRANSLATIONAL SCIENCE AS CONTEXT

The development of an evidence-based intervention is a complex undertaking involving many stages and the work is not complete until the intervention has achieved its highest level of potency and is fully implementable and available to the intended population (Onken, Carroll, Shoham, Cuthbert, & Riddle, 2014). The National Institutes of Health (NIH) Translational Science Spectrum outlines the key stages of translational research in a circular pathway, which has the patient at the centre (National Center for Advancing Translational Sciences, 2015). The model is nonlinear to denote that the stages are interactive and can take place in any particular order as long as it is based on sound scientific logic (Onken et al., 2014). The stages include: *basic research* that explores fundamental causal mechanisms; *preclinical research* that connects basic research with medicine and intervention development; *clinical research* that tests and refines interventions; *clinical implementation* that involves the adoption of interventions into routine care; and *public health* that looks at population health outcomes which may guide the development of delivery models. It has been argued that a further stage could be added which involves social structural reforms to address the social determinants of mental illness (Waldman & Terzic, 2010; World Health Organization and Calouste Gulbenkian Foundation, 2014). Sustainability is also a critical aspect for consideration and that is often not built into research design since data collection typically ceases when funding ends.

INTRODUCING THE RANDOMISED CONTROLLED TRIAL

Introduction

Clinical trials lie at the heart of the process of advancing evidence for interventions recommended for clinical practice. A clinical trial is an experiment designed to evaluate the effect of any new treatment or intervention. The *randomised controlled trial* (RCT) is considered to be the optimal design for a clinical trial. An RCT is a comparative study involving a control group and group exposed to the intervention of interest. The control group lets us know that any differential response is a result of the intervention rather than, for instance, spontaneous recovery (Everitt & Wessely, 2004). Randomisation helps ensure the intervention is the only systematic difference between the control and the intervention group. Participants are randomly (i.e., by chance alone) allocated to receive the intervention or not use, for example, a computer program or a random number table. To further minimise bias, the subject and the rater can be 'blind' to the intervention allocation; that is, they do not know the allocation and so cannot have their assessment of any effect influenced by this information.

The National Health and Medical Research Council developed a hierarchy to grade the clinical evidence for interventions (National Health and Medical Research Council, 2009). The single RCT provides the highest level of evidence for individual study designs and is second (level II) in the overall hierarchy of evidence for interventions. It provides more reliable evidence than other study designs, such as non-randomised and uncontrolled trials (Levels III–IV), because its methodology minimises systematic error.

The highest (level I) evidence for interventions are systematic literature reviews, which are based on synthesising and summarising evidence from multiple RCTs on a related topic. Including meta-analyses in such reviews increases the precision of the results (National Health and Medical Research Council, 2009). Traditionally, meta-analytic methods combine and analyse summary statistics (such as means) from multiple related RCTs. Increasingly, such methods are being applied to individual patient data ('individual patient data (IPD)' meta-analysis) which enables greater standardisation and consistency across included studies and therefore more reliable findings (Riley, Lambert, & Abo-Zaid, 2010). Alongside this development has been a shift towards making the sharing of deidentified individual participant data from clinical trials the norm in order to best progress research (Taichman et al., 2016; Taichman et al., 2017). Although data sharing is not yet mandated, journals that follow the International Committee of Medical Journal Editor's (ICMJE) recommendations for reporting now require that data sharing statements be provided alongside publications to specify the extent to which data will be shared. Data sharing may present some challenges. Unless data is also confidentialised, attempts to de-identify data through removal or alternation of potentially identifying data may still risk indirect identification of participants. As well, when done for the purpose of open access, the process of de-identification may result in lower data utility.

The CONSORT (*Consolidated Standards of Reporting Trials*) statement (Altman et al., 2001; see also Consolidated Standards of Reporting Trials, 2020) provides a checklist and flow diagram to assist researchers to design, implement and report RCTs to permit appropriate evaluation. Principles are also set out in conventional medical texts. To support research transparency, numerous national and international guidelines stipulate that trials be prospectively registered in an authorised registry. In Australia, this is the Australian New Zealand Clinical Trials Registry (ANZCTR, 2020). Trial registration is important for a range of reasons but particularly to counter publication bias, such as when only papers with positive results are published. If this occurs, the results of literature reviews and meta-analyses will be misleading because they will be based on a biased sample of all studies conducted (Song, Eastwood, Gilbody, Duley, & Sutton, 2000).

RCTs are designed to answer a specific question, for example, an evaluation of a pharmacological treatment. In such cases, it is feasible to conduct them in a tightly controlled experimental setting using so-called 'efficacy' or 'explanatory' studies. In mental health care, we are also interested in assessing more complex interventions. In attempting to maintain the ideal experimental conditions and the minimisation of bias to ensure internal validity, an efficacy study may be so different from what actually happens in real life that the study lacks external validity; that is, the results cannot be applicable to real-life settings.

'Pragmatic' or 'effectiveness' RCTs are designed to test treatments under conditions similar to routine clinical practice and allow the study of more complex interventions and settings. This focus on external validity (generalisability) provides a way of incorporating the diversity of clinical practice; for example, through the minimisation of exclusion criteria. Traditional RCTs may exclude comorbid conditions, yet comorbidity is the norm in clinical practice. Outcome measures in pragmatic RCTs are not merely there to minimise observer bias, but also to measure the participants' opinions and concerns, and thus have a subjective quality to them and attempt to measure functional outcomes (such as return to work), which are more practical indicators than just a specific reduction in symptoms.

Choice of comparator condition as an issue

The choice of the comparator (control) condition is an important consideration and depends on the question being asked and the stage of research. For example, researchers interested in the active components of treatments in efficacy trials may chose an 'active' psychological control therapy to rule out that the therapy is efficacious simply because of time spent with a therapist and expectancies. In reality however, people who do not receive an intervention will receive usual care. For pragmatic trials, this would be the most relevant comparison from the perspective of service delivery (Hotopf, Churchill, & Lewis, 1999), particularly if a health economic analysis is included (Hjelmgren, Berggren, & Andersson, 2001). An effect that may be important to consider in the use of a usual treatment control is 'resentful demoralisation', which is a bias that may arise in control group participants whereby the belief that they are not receiving a new, desirable treatment leads to disappointment and demoralisation, negatively affecting outcomes. The control condition in this scenario may acquire the properties of a nocebo, whereby negative expectations produce harmful effects (Pilcher, 2009). Thus, what look like promising findings may be due to relative deterioration in the control group rather than improvement in the treatment group.

Type I and type II errors

In biology and the life sciences generally, individuals show substantial interindividual variation. Hence, modelling of experimental evidence in mental health practice deals with probabilities of events; these models can make statements about probabilities but never entirely determine an issue. Somewhat arbitrarily, the threshold for reporting of positive findings in medical and psychological research is set by the conventional expression $p<0.05$. This means, in testing a hypothesis, including in an RCT, that there is less than a 0.05

probability (one in 20 chance) that the finding which seems to confirm the hypothesis would have occurred by chance even if the hypothesis were untrue.

This distinction in statistical testing between type I and type II errors relies on the idea of the 'null hypothesis'. In comparing outcomes in an investigation, the null hypothesis is that there is no difference between groups. Type I error, then, is the probability assigned by a statistical test to the event that the study findings, if they support the rejection of the null hypothesis, occurred as a chance event, given the way data tends to distribute in the findings of studies of this type. This is the probability level usually referred to in statistical testing, and by convention the level for acceptance of the findings of a test is set at a probability of 0.05: hence the common footnote of $p<0.05$ after positive statistical findings. This error level is the level of probability of 'type I error'. It estimates the chance that the findings are, in simple terms, a false positive finding. The level of this probability or 'significance' is set at $p<0.05$ only by convention, and there is no fundamental reason for choosing this level.

There is another important type of error, which is called type II error. This is the likelihood of accepting the null hypothesis based on the test that if the null hypothesis is false, so is the likelihood of a false negative. This may be important. If a new treatment or intervention is not found to be beneficial in an investigation, it is important to be aware of the likelihood that this particular data collection would yield this finding if there were a genuine difference. This can be quoted in terms of the degree of difference (often a measure known as effect size) a study was designed to detect, and the chance of detecting it with a positive finding, given that this size of effect was actually present. The type II error likelihood of a study is often also referred to as the 'power' of the study. Studies reporting negative findings of investigation, then proceeding to draw conclusions from them without making some satisfactory discussion of the issue of power, are to be treated with suspicion.

To take an absurd example of confusion between type I and type II errors, we might give two groups of five patients a drug or a placebo, find that three in the experimental (drug) group improved, and that two in the control (placebo) group did. We could do a type I error test for a difference here, and find that this set of events was quite likely even if there were no difference between the two treatments of drug and placebo. If we concluded, on the basis of a negative test to detect type I error, that there was no difference between the drug and placebo on the basis of this evidence, we might be rejecting a treatment that was actually half as good again as the placebo. Properly, such a conclusion should rest on estimation of power (type II) as well as conventional (type I) significance.

Novel designs

In usual clinical practice, consumers are, of course, not randomised to treatment. Here, most treatments rely on the motivation and compliance of the client and the client's motivation is typically a key determinant of choice of therapy (Everitt & Wessely, 2004; Hotopf et al., 1999). To better reflect real-world conditions, 'patient preference' trials have been proposed whereby participants who have a preference for a particular treatment are offered this treatment rather than being randomised, with randomisation limited to those without such preferences. The main disadvantage to this design is the loss of all the advantages of randomisation leaving open the likely influence for selection biases and confounding. Zelen's design is another variant to standard RCTs whereby participants are randomised prior to consent and treatment consent is obtained only from participants allocated to the active treatment. If participants decline, they receive usual care instead (but keep their original allocation for the data analysis). Advantages of this approach are that the sample is more representative of eligible participants and that participants in the control group are unlikely to be affected by resentful demoralisation since they are unaware of the active treatment. There are a number of significant disadvantages with this design however, including the ethical concerns of randomising clients without their consent, and challenges in collecting data from control group participants without alerting them to the study. Unless there was a very high risk of resentful demoralisation, Zelen's design would not be appropriate ethically for most clinical trials but may be useful for assessing population-based interventions such as screening (Torgerson & Roland, 1998).

CLUSTER RCTS

Overview

In clinical studies, the intervention is not always aimed at an individual but may have as its focus the wider community or service sector. An intervention aimed at educating GPs to detect depression better will likely have, as its unit of randomisation, groups of individuals attending a particular GP. The GP then becomes the unit of randomisation because the intervention is given at the level of the doctor, not the patient. This is called *cluster randomisation*. The individual patient of the doctor and the doctor form the cluster. This design permits the study of the relevant level of health service and minimises the risk of contamination between treatment and control groups. In cluster randomisation, the analysis of the results is different, because the patients attending a particular doctor are not independent of each other. That is, the group of patients seeing a particular doctor will have characteristics in common–such as their socioeconomic status–that they do not share with another group of patients who attend a different GP. Cluster designs usually require a larger number of subjects and specific analysis to ensure appropriate interpretation of results.

Parallel groups

The parallel cluster randomised trial (P-CRT) involves randomising clusters to intervention or control and these are both implemented over the same time period. An extension of the CONSORT statement is available to guide reporting for P-CRTs (Campbell, Piaggio, Elbourne, & Altman, 2012). An example of a psychiatric P-CRT is the REFOCUS study, which was trialled in the United Kingdom. In this large-scale study, a staff-training intervention designed to promote the personal recovery of consumers called REFOCUS was compared to usual care in 27 community mental health teams. The trial did not demonstrate any intervention effect on consumers based on the primary outcome measure of personal recovery (Slade et al., 2015).

Stepped wedge (PULSAR)

The stepped wedge cluster randomised trial (SW-CRT) is a novel design that is rapidly gaining in popularity (Hemming et al., 2018). Rather than randomising clusters to different treatment arms in parallel, all clusters are initially assigned to the control arm then progressively crossed over to the intervention until all clusters have received the treatment. The timepoint at which a cluster (or group of clusters) crosses over from control to intervention, which is called a 'step', is allocated randomly and staggered across study clusters. The term 'stepped wedge' was coined due to the stepped wedge appearance of the design when depicted diagrammatically (The Gambia Hepatitis Study Group, 1987, figure 2, p. 5784). Although this design is quite complex, it enables a method of evaluating service innovations with contemporaneous control groups as it is progressively rolled out across an entire service or even country, as in the original Gambia study (The Gambia Hepatitis Study Group, 1987). An extension of the CONSORT statement is available to guide reporting of SW-CRTs (Hemming et al., 2018).

An example of a psychiatric SW-CRT is the PULSAR specialist care project, which built on the work of REFOCUS. In PULSAR, a two-step SW-CRT design was used to evaluate a rollout of recovery oriented practice training to 190 staff across a large Victorian public and community mental health service sector (Meadows, Brophy, et al., 2019; Shawyer et al., 2017). Care delivery teams were grouped into 14 clusters which were randomly allocated to receive the training intervention at step one (year 1, 7 clusters) or step two (year 2, 7 clusters). The intervention led to a small but significant improvement in the recovery of consumers. The design made possible improvements in the training intervention from step one to step two. As a likely consequence of this, having a second step also enabled a stronger demonstration of the positive effects of the intervention compared to what might have been possible with a parallel group design. It might be noted that, although a SW-CRT was successfully implemented in specialist care services, this design involves a number of methodological challenges (Hemming et al., 2018). A similar design used in the PULSAR primary care project required downgrading to a pre- and post-intervention design due to challenges encountered when arranging for GPs to attend training in their allocated step (Enticott, Shawyer, et al., 2016; Enticott et al., Under review).

1.4.5 DIAGNOSTIC AND OUTCOME MEASURES

FRANCES SHAWYER, GRAHAM MEADOWS & CATHARINE MCNAB

INTRODUCTION

This summary, necessarily a selective one given the number of available measures, will introduce key principles to consider when selecting measures for use in mental health research and evaluation and give examples of instruments used to assess diagnosis and the status of depression and anxiety. More complete information is available for measures of depression (Nezu, Ronan, Meadows, & McClure, 2000) and anxiety (Antony, Orsillo, & Roemer, 2001) as well as psychiatric measures more generally (Baer & Blais, 2010; Rush, First, & Blacker, 2008).

Assessment instruments, though limited and imperfect in the context of varied and complex symptom profiles (Craddock & Mynors-Wallis, 2014; Garcia-Velazquez, Jokela, & Rosenstrom, 2017), are nevertheless important tools in research and clinical practice for efficiently gauging mental health status including changes over time. They should be administered clinically in line with ethical guidelines for professional practice (e.g., Australian Psychological Society, 2018) and, as part of broader assessment, interpreted in the context of other available information. In some usage settings guidelines for conduct of research will apply (National Health and Medical Research Council; Australian Research Council; Universities Australia, 2007, Updated 2018).

GENERAL PRINCIPLES AND PROPERTIES OF INSTRUMENT SELECTION

The process of selecting an instrument involves a number of considerations, starting with the intended setting for use. An organisation or project may have instruments already specified or the clinician or researcher may be in a setting where they are able to choose their own. In either case, practitioners need to become very familiar with the instruments they use. Completing the measure yourself is often a very useful way of immediately getting a sense of the items and overall suitability. Important formally measured instrument properties include *reliability* and *validity*. *Reliability* refers to the stability of measurement performance across various different situations, and *validity* refers to the extent to which the measure actually measures what it claims to. Souza and colleagues provide an in-depth discussion of how to use published measurement properties to help you choose the best tool (Souza, Alexandre, & Guirardello, 2017). Streiner and Goodes highlight key issues in relation to diagnostic and screening measures where quality is often assessed in relation to a 'gold standard' (Streiner & Geddes, 1998). Here some key properties to consider are: *sensitivity* (proportion of true positives so identified by the test), *specificity* (proportion of true negatives so identified by the test), *positive predictive value* (PPV; proportion of test-positive people who have the condition), and *negative predictive value* (NPV; proportion of test-negative people who do not have the condition). Sensitivity, specificity, PPV and NPV vary with how common the disorder is in the population of interest. The way this varies is determined by another key test characteristic, the likelihood ratio. There may be trade-offs to consider when weighing up formal measurement properties of an instrument with its pragmatic acceptability in regular and repeated usage. Factors here include burden of completion, type of administration (self-report vs clinician-rated), the presence of sensitive items and cost and copyright conditions.

DIAGNOSTIC MEASURES

A structured interview assessing psychiatric disorders must make precise operational definitions of sometimes imprecise diagnostic criteria, and differences between measures and resulting diagnosis may arise because of alternative ways of doing this. At time of writing, because ICD-11 is only newly released, the contemporary instruments that provide standardised diagnostic assessment do so according to ICD-10 (World Health Organization, 1992) and/or DSM-IV (American Psychiatric Association, 2000) or DSM-5 (American Psychiatric Association, 2013). Key examples include: the Schedules for Clinical Assessment in Neuropsychiatry (SCAN–Wing et al., 1990); World Health Organization World Mental Health Composite International Diagnostic Interview (WHO WMH-CIDI–Kessler et al., 2004; Kessler & Ustun, 2004), the Mini International Neuropsychiatric Interview (MINI–Sheehan et al., 1998) and the Structured Clinical Interview for DSM-5 (American Psychiatric Association, 2020a). We anticipate that updates corresponding to ICD-11 will unfold in the coming years. The use of diagnostic instruments typically require licensing agreements and/or training requirements. Practitioners may consider seeking training in these instruments if they are involved in research; beyond this though, learning how these instruments work and are administered can provide an interesting opportunity for clinical and other workers to extend and enrich interviewing and assessment skills.

SYMPTOM MEASURES

Depression and anxiety instruments can be divided into: measures of depression, measures of anxiety, and mixed symptom measures. One example of a brief self-report measure of depression with good measurement performance and pragmatic properties is the Patient Health Questionnaire-9 (PHQ-9–Kroenke, Spitzer, & Williams, 2001). The PHQ-9 has nine items based on the nine Criteria A symptoms for DSM-IV diagnosis of a major depressive episode and a tenth item assessing impact on functioning (Criterion C). PHQ-9 assesses symptom severity and includes an item related to self-harm thoughts, which usefully flags the need for further risk assessment. It can be used as a diagnostic screen for a major depressive episode according to DSM-IV (Lowe, Spitzer, et al., 2004) and DSM-5 [based on an unchanged symptoms list from DSM-IV (Blackwell & McDermott, 2014)], as well as a diagnostic screen for ICD-10 depressive episodes (Lowe et al., 2004). Our content appraisal of the relevant ICD-11 criteria suggests the PHQ-9 will continue to be suitable as a diagnostic screen for ICD-11 depressive disorder episodes. The PHQ-9 is free to use following agreement with its terms of use (Patient Health Questionnaire (PHQ) Screeners, 2020) and has an ultra-brief short-form (PHQ-2–Kroenke, Spitzer, & Williams, 2003).

The assessment of anxiety is more complex than the assessment of depression since 'anxiety' includes many specific disorders, and anxiety more broadly in what has been described as 'apprehensive anticipation of future danger or misfortune accompanied by a feeling of dysphoria or somatic symptoms of tension' (American Psychiatric Association, 2000, p. 820). The Panic Disorder Severity Scale (PDSS–Shear et al., 1997) is an example of the former while the Beck Anxiety Inventory (Beck, Epstein, Brown, & Steer, 1988; Beck & Steer, 1993) is an example of the latter. Measures of anxiety disorders can be understood within Lang's model of anxiety (Lang, 1968). This proposes that anxiety consists of three components: anxious cognitions; behavioural responses (particularly avoidance patterns); and psychophysiological responses. The measure of anxiety that is used will depend on the presence or absence of these different forms of anxiety in the disorder of interest. The PDSS, for example, would focus more on psychophysiological and behavioural responses than measures of generalised anxiety disorder, such as the Penn State Worry Questionnaire (Meyer, Miller, Metzger, & Borkovec, 1990), which focus on cognitions.

Depression and anxiety are very commonly comorbid and there are a range of instruments that assess both types of symptoms. Such instruments can be very useful to gauge overall mental wellbeing in the context of a broad range of mental and physical health conditions. The Kessler-10 (Kessler et al., 2002), for example (see Section 1.4.3), is a psychometrically strong 10-item measure of psychological distress that is widely used in Australia. It has been included in several state-based and national health surveys and is commonly used by GPs and other clinicians, being one of the outcome measures recommended by the Department of Health for use in relation to Medicare-funded mental health treatment. It has a six-item short-form, the K6 (Kessler et al., 2002).

1.4.6 MENTAL HEALTH ECONOMICS

GRAHAM MEADOWS & BRETT INDER

SCOPE OF THE FIELD

Health economics is concerned with the systematic analysis of costs, benefits, management and consequences of health care as well as working towards understanding the ways people make health decisions with economic implications. Mental health economics then applies the techniques of economics to the full range of service delivery and uptake questions regarding mental health care, from training of clinicians, shifts in public attitudes, availability of drugs and other interventions, to how decisions may be made regarding prioritisation of all these issues, and how they may best be financed. Introductory and reference texts of health economics (Drummond, Sculpher, Claxton, Stoddart, & Torrance, 2015; Glied & Smith, 2013) provide information on how these techniques can be applied and interpreted. In the interest of providing an illustration of how health economic findings may be useful in appraising mental health care at different levels we will take illustration of two different graphic approaches to health economic data presentation, the Cost Utility plane and the Concentration Index. In both cases we will draw on work the authors have been involved with.

THE COST UTILITY PLANE

Careful cost-counting is often an important aspect of health economic evaluation, with a critical element being the taking of a particular 'perspective'. This may involve counting for instance mental health expenditure only, all of health care or whole of society costs. For some evaluations multiple perspectives may be important. From whatever perspective(s) may be chosen, interventions can typically then be seen as having both costs and benefits for health. Measuring benefits is useful via the concept of Health-utility, where a value is assigned to different kinds of illness experience compared with a notional value of 1 for full health. This for different purposes may be expressed as Disability Adjusted or Quality-Adjusted Life Years (DALYs/QALYs). If we use a graphic display of costs (y-axis) and benefits (e.g. DALYs, x-axis) we can then estimate where a particular intervention falls on the Cost Utility plane compared with a studied alternative. Figure 1.18 is an example of this from work with Mindfulness-Based Cognitive Therapy as a targeted preventive intervention for depression (see Section 4.3.5; Shawyer, Enticott, Ozmen, Inder, & Meadows, 2016). A technique called 'bootstrapping' is used here to generate the range of likely estimates from the study, each with a separate dot. In this example, most of the estimates fall in the bottom right quadrant, which represents greater health gain and reduced cost, a part of the plane described as 'dominant'. This suggests the intervention dominates other alternatives in both the cost and benefits dimensions. This is an unusual outcome; more typically novel interventions have increased cost associated with any health gain (greater benefit). The findings can vary with perspective and setting–for instance in this study there was greater dominance where people were receiving specialist care rather than primary care.

MEASURES OF EQUITY

Elsewhere in this text we have given attention to the issues of inequalities and inequities in society (see Sections 1.2, 1.2.4, 1.2.5 and 1.6.3) and in mental health care delivery. Here we will say a few words about measurement of inequality. The most common measurement for comparing inequality across countries is the Gini index, which measures inequality of wealth or income varying from a level of 0 (everyone has the same amount) to 1 (one person has it all). Relatively small changes in

Figure 1.18 Cost utility planes for specialist care an primary care (mental health care perspective, intention to trust); the percentage of bootstrap iterations in each of the four quadrants is shown

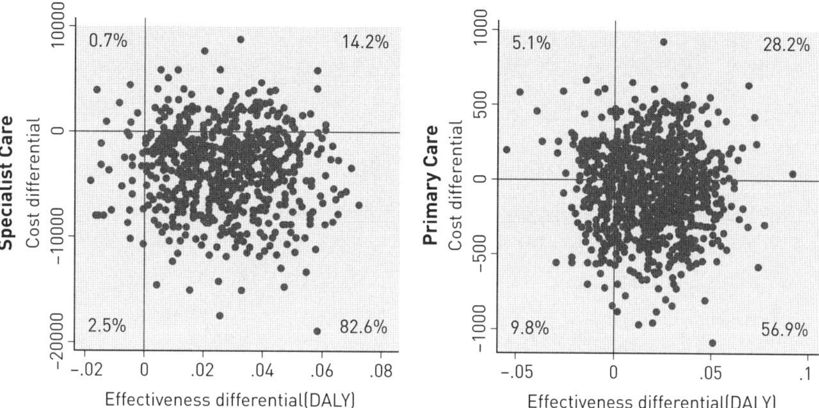

the Gini can have appreciable effects. Australia's Gini has increased through recent decades from around 0.28 to around 0.32, while still placing Australia as one of the world's less inequitable nations. An alternative approach to the Gini is to look at differences between income percentiles; for example, there is evidence that the income of the top 1% has been growing much more quickly than the lower 50% (Oxfam Australia, 2018).

A measurement that is a little like the Gini is the Concentration Index (CI) and this author with others used this to look at different rates of use of Medicare items for mental health care (Meadows, Enticott, Inder, Russell, & Gurr, 2015). Graphically the CI is represented by plotting cumulative frequencies of, say, population by socioeconomic deprivation of area, with cumulative frequency of use of specific services. The CI is obtained by measuring the area between the observed curve and the 45^0 line. Figure 1.19 presents some findings from this, showing that items for GP care (2702 and 2710) and GP shared care planning by psychiatrists (291) are more evenly distributed than the item for a typical psychiatrist's consultation (306). For 2702, 2712 and 291, the lines are fairly close to the 45^0 line that is suggestive of equity. Item 306 has a CI of below -0.2 and CIs are typically regarded as large above magnitude 0.2, which is the level at which the more affluent half of the population get twice the number of items.

The examples illustrate how health economics can provide us with valuable tools for understanding features of clinical and other interventions as well as broad-based issues for policy formation around equitable access to health services, along with many other areas of application.

1.4.7 QUALITATIVE RESEARCH

ELLIE FOSSEY

ORIGINS AND PERSPECTIVES

Qualitative research is a broad umbrella term for research that is concerned with developing understanding of the meanings of human experiences and interactions, and with how people make sense of their social worlds. Qualitative research has its origins within diverse disciplines, including anthropology, sociology and psychology, out of which differing qualitative research methodologies have developed, such as ethnography, grounded theory, and phenomenological research respectively. Nevertheless, some features of qualitative research include natural settings as the contexts for gathering information, commonly using individual interviews, focus group discussions and observations of naturally occurring interactions and practices (Fossey et al., 2002; Flynn & McDermott, 2016). In addition, qualitative research findings are generally presented as descriptive, textual, or narrative accounts. This does not preclude the use of enumeration. However, the primary intent is to

Figure 1.19 Concentration curves for key medical terms

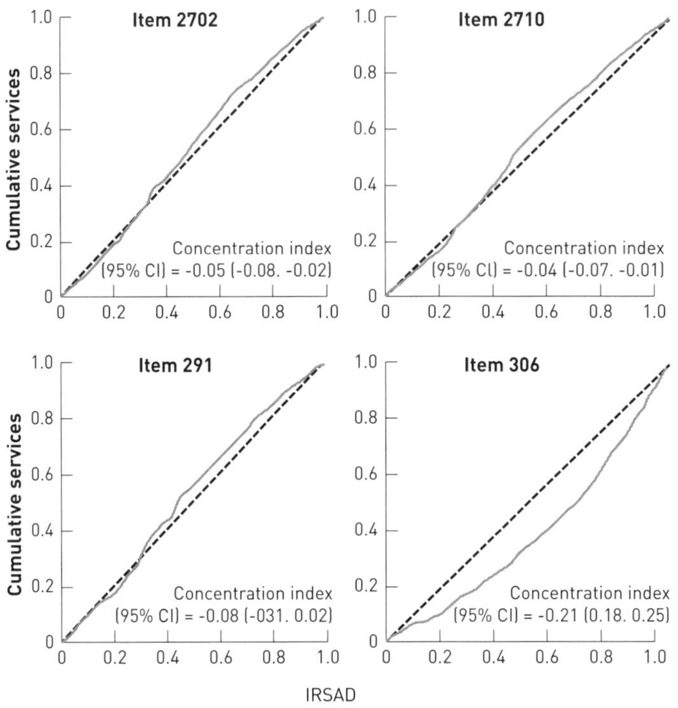

IRSAD = Index of Relative Socio-Economic Advantage and Disadvantage.
Item 2702 = general practitioner creation of a GP mental health treatment plan.
Item 2710 = GP review of a GP mental health treatment plan.
Item 291 = psychiatrist consultation for creation of a shared care plan, > 45 minutes.
Item 306 = psychiatrist consultation in rooms, 45–75 minutes.

illuminate the subjective meanings of the phenomena being studied; to represent the real world of those studied and in which their experiences are embedded; and to privilege the perspectives of research participants (Popay, Rogers, & Williams, 1998).

Qualitative research methodologies most often used in mental health research are typically informed by one of two philosophical perspectives: either an interpretive or critical research paradigm. Each places emphasis on seeking understanding of the meanings of human actions and experiences, and on generating accounts of their meaning from the viewpoints of those involved, but with some differences in how these meanings are framed and interpreted, as briefly described below.

INTERPRETIVE RESEARCH

Interpretive research addresses questions focused primarily on understanding and accounting for the meanings inherent in human experiences and actions. Most prominent in mental health research are ethnography, phenomenology, grounded theory, and narrative approaches, each of which addresses the issue of meaning from a differing standpoint. For example, in ethnography, description of the meaning of a phenomenon emphasises its particular societal and cultural context, and explores the way in which the phenomenon is understood within a particular community, or social group (Liamputtong, 2013). Phenomenological research, on the other hand, is concerned with the ordinary 'life world', the way in which people experience their world, and how best to understand their experiences (Fossey et al., 2002). The following two studies of deinstitutionalisation illustrate this difference in emphasis. An Australian ethnographic study by Newton et al. (2000) described how a group of long stay hospital residents moved and settled into supported community residences over a two-year period, focusing on their *shared social world* as an informal community, including how the residents got along with each other, with support staff, and with neighbours in the local vicinity. In comparison, Davidson, Hoge, Merrill, Rakfeldt, and Griffith (1995) similarly sought to understand the experiences of individuals returning to the community after extended hospital stays, but did so using a phenomenological approach to describe the *common elements of subjective experience* (for example, the importance of freedom and privacy) across the experiences of separate individuals.

CRITICAL RESEARCH

Critical research emphasises the *social and historical origins* and *contexts* in which meanings are constructed. It derives from sociopolitical and emancipatory traditions, in which knowledge is not viewed as discovered through objective inquiry but rather as acquired through critical discourse and debate (Fossey et al., 2002). It focuses on the critique of current social structures, relations, and conditions that shape practices within organisations, communities and societies by examining them within their historical, social, cultural, and political contexts, and in so doing seeks to uncover how issues of power and privilege are implicated in the dominant discourses and practices that shape people's lives (Neuman, 2003). Critical research then is not directed towards understanding for its own sake, but towards understanding as a means of practical action and transformation. Hence, research informed by a critical perspective is often concerned with issues of oppression, marginalisation and inequity; and aims to foster self-reflection, mutual learning, participation, empowerment and makes efforts to diminish the distinction between the 'researcher' and the 'researched' (Wadsworth & Epstein, 1998; Wallerstein & Duran, 2003). An example is the *Understanding & Involvement* project (Wadsworth & Epstein, 1998-2001) described in more detail later in this chapter. It aimed first to establish an exchange of experiences and ideas between consumers and staff in an Australian acute psychiatric unit about coming to, being in, and leaving the ward; and then to build consumer-staff dialogue into the organisational culture so that consumers' feedback could be routinely sought and heard, and consumers and staff could effectively collaborate to make changes within the service as a result. This study exemplifies the use of participatory processes to involve people of traditionally unequal power and status in research, and an orientation towards bringing about change in a practice setting, both of which are explicit features of critical research. It also highlights the possibilities of this type of research to amplify the consumer and carer voices and leadership in mental health research (see Section 1.4.1).

USEFULNESS OF QUALITATIVE METHODS IN MENTAL HEALTH RESEARCH

Qualitative research has a long history in psychiatry (Peters, 2010). Historical examples include Goffman's (Goffman, 1961) analysis of the social situation of people incarcerated in asylums, from which the impacts of institutions on individuals' lives, identities and self-determination came to be better understood, and Estroff and colleagues' (1981) research that offered one of the first accounts of life 'outside' psychiatric institutions through a two-year ethnographic study of the day-to-day existences of people with longstanding mental illness receiving community treatment in Madison, Wisconsin. This, and subsequent qualitative studies with similar populations, including in Australia, have drawn attention to the challenges to hope, agency, identity and connection faced when free neither from the institutional routines of mental health care nor the drawbacks of social and economic marginalisation (e.g., Davidson, 2003; Newton et al., 2000). Qualitative studies have also contributed much to highlighting the importance of understanding and valuing lived experience, as well as to developing knowledge of how recovery processes unfold, which in turn have influenced the shaping of contemporary recovery oriented mental health policies (see Sections 1.5.2 and 2.6.2). Indeed, given the emphasis that recovery places on the first-hand experience and perspectives of people affected by mental illness and distress, qualitative methods are increasingly useful in efforts to develop recovery-orientated practices and to improve experiences of care (Davidson, Ridgway, Kidd, Topor, & Borg, 2008).

Qualitative methods are important in advancing knowledge in mental health care (Peters, 2010).

Mental health issues are multifactorial and informed by understandings of the biological, psychological, social, cultural, ethical, and political dimensions of human lives generally, as well as the nature of human interactions, therapeutic relationships and service systems. Many of these understandings can at best be only partial where subjective perspectives are not included.

Some areas where qualitative research methods are being used to advance knowledge and practice in mental health care include:

- Subjective experiences of illness, health, and wellbeing. Examples include illuminating personal experiences of struggling with depression (Karp, 2017), lived experience of severe mental illness and recovering (Davidson, 2003; Kaite, Karanikola, Merkouris, & Papathanassoglou, 2015) gendered understandings of mental health issues (McKenzie, Jenkin, & Collings, 2016), and Indigenous Australians' views of mental health and disorders (Ypinazar, Margolis, Haswell-Elkins, & Tsey, 2007).
- Family experiences, such as how children of parents with mental illness experience their lives, and make sense of their parents' difficulties (Dam & Hall, 2016).
- Experiences of relationships with health professionals (Ljungberg, Denhov, & Topor, 2015) and of peer support (Walker & Bryant, 2013).
- Developing understanding of how specific interventions and services are experienced from consumer, family and practitioner viewpoints, such as mindfulness-based interventions (Wyatt, Harper, & Weatherhead, 2014), relapse prevention (Pontin, Peters, Lobban, Rogers, & Morriss, 2009); assertive community treatment (Krupa et al., 2005), care coordination (Schweizer et al., 2018) and Clubhouse programs (Kinn, Tanaka, Bellamy, & Davidson, 2018).
- Consumer experiences of housing support, and specialist supported accommodation services (Krotofil, McPherson, & Killaspy, 2018; Watson, Fossey, & Harvey, 2019).
- Work-related opportunities, challenges and needs for support among employees with common mental disorders (Thisted, Nielsen, & Bjerrum, 2018), and factors that contribute to finding and sustaining employment from the perspective of people experiencing persistent mental ill health (Fossey & Harvey, 2010).
- Developing, testing and implementing complex psychosocial interventions within mental health services, such as recovery-promoting practices, from consumer and staff perspectives (Le Boutillier et al., 2015; Slade et al., 2015; Wallace et al., 2016).
- Consumer-led and collaborative research to identify outcomes of services that are important to consumers themselves, so as to guide meaningful service evaluation and inform the development of tools that are responsive to consumer experiences of services (Waks et al., 2017).

As noted elsewhere in this chapter, qualitative methods are also well suited to practice-focused research and evaluation since they offer effective means to engage consumers, families and practitioners in asking questions that are meaningful to them, and obtaining not only their views but also their input in developing solutions to problems (see Sections 1.4.1, 1.4.8 and 1.4.9).

1.4.8 ACTION RESEARCH

YOLAND WADSWORTH

BACKGROUND

In action research, 'life itself is the laboratory' given that the experimental trialling of newly theorised action is being carried out by those within their own lived complex realities of everyday experience. Like all research and evaluation the methodology uses comparative analysis, observation and synthesis, but additionally must be strongly participatory in each of these, involving researcher, researched and 'researched for' in co-inquiring dialogue about the current situation in order to better understand it, develop new thinking and innovate action in situ.

The conditions and scale can vary enormously, from traditional small action research cycles of inquiry in naturally occurring investigation, to 'scaling them up' in larger more intentionally organised activities.

The latter taking of small-scale iterative emergent action research 'to scale' within large, complex, interdependent 'whole systems' is a more recent variant, and the experience of a sequence of action evaluation studies over a decade—known collectively as the 'U&I studies' (see later explanation of this 'You and I/Understanding and Involvement' naming under 'Common Assumptions')—will provide an exemplar of the operation of both small-scale studies (of which there were 35 identifiable), as well as systemic action research for 'whole systems change' at larger scale (Wadsworth, 2010; Wadsworth & Epstein, 1998, chapter 5). At the time when the U&I studies were being carried out (1990s), service user researchers explicitly rejected the language of 'patients' and 'customers' as disempowering, and chose the business language of 'consumers' to imply agency, and 'patient' or 'inpatients' where this was accurate to describe their current experience.

While the U&I project is now more than 25 years old, its recommended consumer consultants remains a feature of almost all mental health services to this day. It is also one of the internationally best known exemplars of small-scale action research evaluation taken to system-wide scale (see, for example, Burns, 2007).

The consumer perspective and staff-collaborative U&I studies, funded by the Myer Foundation, Royal Park Hospital, a medical research grant from VicHealth, and the State Health Department, were conducted between 1988 and 1996. They were auspiced by a state-wide peak consumer mental health organisation in Victoria in close collaboration with a willing large public mental health hospital and its state department area.

They set out to 'build in' empowering consumers to speak about their experiences, be heard by staff and have things change as a result. Staff did not only gain insights from this rich evaluative feedback about consumers' experiences of their acute admission, but collaborated with consumers to deepen understanding and trial modifications of acute psychiatric hospital practice to improve quality and reduce consumers' iatrogenic trauma. The project attracted strong local and international interest and has been extensively documented (McGuiness & Wadsworth, 1992; Epstein & Wadsworth, 1994; Wadsworth & Epstein, 1996b; Wadsworth & Epstein, 1996a; Consumer Participation Program Orientation and Job Manual—Mental Health Staff-Consumer Consultants, 1996; Wadsworth & Epstein, 1998; Wadsworth & Epstein, 1998, chapter 5).

CONTEXT FOR DEVELOPMENT

Action research's various 'strands, streams and variants' developed from 1920s work with disadvantaged urban women workers and then throughout the twentieth century, arising out of dissatisfaction with:

- traditional impersonal research methods, such as an over-reliance on reductionist fixed-choice questionnaire surveys, particularly where topics and questions were developed without the involvement of intended beneficiary 'subjects', or involved covert investigation that made incorrect or damaging interpretations independently of them
- the use of controlled experiments which distorted real-life conditions and did not seek properly informed consent, nor effectively empower participation for epistemic adequacy, and failed to ensure only ethically agreed new actions were trialled, or
- 'value free' research that did not realise what values it was inevitably enacting, or stopped at the relativities of 'difference of opinion' qualitative research, or at 'agreed facts' from comparative study, or at the drawing of conclusions without making recommendations, or failing to move to trial them in new observed practice.

In the mental health sector in Australia, these concerns coalesced from the early 1970s to produce both community mental health service evaluation devoted to examining what kinds of practical responses worked best to meet community needs (for example, (Lippmann, 1982), and 'community-of-practice' developmental evaluation, extending to include both staff and patients to achieve change.

ACTION RESEARCH AS RESEARCH

Action research, as 'full-cycle science', treats questions about 'how things are now' as no less scientific or research-like than questions about 'how things might better be' (Wadsworth, 2010, p. 78). Each is seen as sitting in logical relationship to the other in integrated cycles of research—with rigorous *induction* underpinning the *abduction* of new theory, followed by the subsequent *deductive* testing of innovation and change in new applied practice, going 'full cycle' to further observe using *retroductive* logic in audit-review evaluation and refinement, as well as being open to a new cycle of inquiry for further developmental evaluation.

To do justice to complex real-world experiential settings, action research utilises a particularly open-minded approach to what counts as data, methods and processes for the collection and interpretation of information by those involved. To this end numerous research methods, techniques, epistemologies and philosophies of science, can be mapped round the action research cycle (Wadsworth, 2010, Chapter 3, endnotes 24, 26, 36, 39, 43, 44).

In the U&I action evaluation research, this was expressed in the frequent field comment 'everything is data', and multiple methods were a feature, drawing on and further developing various ways of acquiring data, analysing it and planning new actions based on it, including:

- face-to-face individual and informal talk
- dialogue groups, which included the project management committee
- auto-ethnographic participant observation, written case storytelling and cartoons
- secondary analysis of written records, statistics and artefacts
- surveys, including a confidential questionnaire to all hospital staff and inpatients
- 60 interviews with representatives of all the different standpoints in the system (including consumers, carers, staff, managers, community and policymakers)
- analysis of other relevant consumer and other research and evaluation studies, sometimes with follow-up discussions with authors.

ACTION RESEARCH AS ACTION

Action research has its roots internationally in at least five streams of practice-based thinking (Selener, 1997; Wadsworth, 2010) responding to the social, economic and political changes of the late nineteenth and twentieth centuries:

- *local community development*—in disadvantaged inner-city and urban areas subsequent to the historic breakdown of strongly knit communities in the west and global 'north', and rural communities seeking to strengthen their local economies and cultures in the global 'south' (e.g. Participatory Research, participatory action research)
- *workplace relations and organisational development*—beginning with research and development (R&D) and moving to employee-management participation to improve industrial productivity in post second world war reconstruction (e.g. Action Learning)
- *education*, particularly focusing on teachers' practice research regarding their students' classroom learning needs (e.g. collaborative action research, group self-evaluation)
- *agriculture*, particularly with laboratory-based scientists learning to take their lead from the situated practice wisdom and needs of farmers rather than impose ecologically unsustainable techniques or chemicals (e.g. Rapid Rural Assessment)
- *health, human and community services*, particularly in Western countries, where applied social scientists and evaluators assisted quality assurance (QA) and quality improvement (QI) in services, particularly in response to consumer evaluation (e.g. Appreciative Inquiry, Open Space Technology, Deliberative Polling).

RECENT APPROACHES

Over recent years these have been joined by variants in user-centred co-design at all levels of government, non-for-profit community, industry and management; living system-centred architecture; client-centred rehabilitation or e-learning; customer focus, and plan-do-check-act (PDCA) cycles for QA and QI in Australian business and management, and in a transdisciplinary 'meta systems epistemology' applying to all (Wadsworth, 2010).

COMMON ASSUMPTIONS

All streams and variants of action research and developmental evaluation have in common a number of operational assumptions:

- *All human actors inquire*—no matter what their setting or status, people exercise conscious and unconscious inquiry into the circumstances in which they find themselves, gradually amassing and drawing on their own store of practical theoretical knowledge or conclusions about their situations in order to live their lives. *In the U&I work,* this was expressed in the use of strategic questioning that drew on all human inquiry capabilities of all participants to systematically propel the work 'full cycle' from existing undesirable situations to trialling preferred responses.
- *Collaboration through dialogue*—action research takes the next logical step of arranging the pooling and exchange of observations, agreed 'facts', differing opinions, insights, feelings and ideas to solve problems and enhance lives *between* all relevant parties or 'stakeholders' in collaborative co-research and dialogue (or multilogue) with and for the critical 'stake-owners' group. *The name 'U&I'*—an acronym for Understanding and Involvement—encapsulates the participatory and dialogic elements of the action research design, especially in its audible acronym, '*You and I*'. In progressively developing cycles of inquiry, the different parties to the U&I action research reflected together to generate alternative possible ways of working, then observed them in the hard test of new practice, refining them further *as part of the research* achieving better understanding and improvement for the 'critical reference/inquiry group' (Wadsworth, 2010; Wadsworth, 2011) of inpatients and consumers in collaboration with professional staff.
- *Theory and models*—Action research holds that 'there is nothing more practical than a good theory', and no better way of developing a powerfully accurate theory than by generating it within the field conditions of actual 'live' experimental practice. In this way, action research is able to generate/abduct new theory and creative solutions to the questions it has raised or problems the critical inquiry group may currently face, for testing in collective new action, using new models of practice. *In the case of the 'U and I' action research,* deep new explanatory theory was developed about the nature and form of the observed paradox in which staff both '*wanted* to hear from consumers', and at the same time seemingly 'did *not* want to hear from consumers'. In engaged face-to-face meetings, project members refined this analysis to construct a 10-component model of the conditions necessary for 'building in' and successfully sustaining feedback and staff-consumer communications. These included (a) multiple opportunities for staff-consumer collaboration—not only in committees but in daily decision making as well as in reflection-based dialogue away from busy daily practice; (b) a stronger infrastructure of managerial reward and staff peer support for patient-responsive consumer participation efforts; (c) the employment of consumer personnel as ongoing staff-consumer research consultants in teams of a minimum of two for strength; (d) a supportive network of staff including managers and consumers (both internal and external; e) funds to pay and support consumers for their work in the ways they needed; and (f) consumer-only groups to sustain their all-important consumer discourse.
- This new program theory and comprehensive implementation model for consumer evaluation of mental health services, contributed to the creation of a state policy on consumer participation and a funding program to employ consumers as service improvement consultants in every mental health service area in the State of Victoria—a policy-program that has continued to the present day.
- *Facilitating full cycles of unforced inquiry*—All the various streams of action research have observed that the use of coercion or control in research, evaluation or naturalistic inquiry, runs the risk of distorting complex self-organising processes, whether of individuals, groups,

organisations or communities. That is, coercion or manipulation risks blocking the transparency and collaborative 'discovery of truth' or the 'co-construction of people's multiple truth/s' if some parties are favoured at the expense of others, and thus risks inappropriate, narrow, damaging or even dangerous curtailing of observations, interpretations, analyses and solutions. *In the U&I work,* it proved critical to inquire organically throughout 'the system', building relationships and an organisational culture resilient enough to overcome the tendencies to respond to uncertainty and anxiety with disempowering personal and social 'defensive routines' (Argyris, 1993; Senge, 1990; Menzies, 1970).

- *Whole 'ecosystem' dynamics*—no particular individual or group of individuals are seen as able fully to achieve this 'full cycle' inquiry capability separate from other relevant parties. This approach has been articulated in a transdisciplinary theory of 'inquiry for living systems', bringing together sociology, psychology, bio-eco systems and epistemology. In part, this is a result of the U&I and a general hospital sequel study (Wadsworth, 2010), Ch. 5, U&I Exemplar 1, pp. 206-212; Lakeside Hospital Exemplar 3, pp. 219-21). *The U&I action research* found that, to alter systemically the experience of one inpatient on any single ward, it needed to start the dialogue there, and then build the conversations 'up and out' (bottom-up, laterally and top-down) to alter the implicated practices in all other wards, and then the policies and practices of the rest of the hospital, the area mental health service, the regional and central offices of the state department, and ultimately also professional education, service quality standards, and national government policies. To do this the U&I started small with a small group of people who facilitated the development of a research work team (including three consumer researchers and an external research design consultant). This core group in turn 'knit' a group of around 15 consumer research consultants who carried out various aspects of the research, participating in both a consumer-only group and, with around eight staff, in a 50/50 staff-consumer collaborative discussion committee that met for dialogue seminars. Consumers and staff operated also as consultants and co-researchers on other sub-projects—together overseeing the proliferation of 35 identifiable separate-but-connected mini action research QA and later QI projects across the hospital. A system-wide network of more than 300 people built from all those who took part in the project in these various ways, and was itself 'woven together' by use of short colourful monthly bulletins. The taped and transcribed dialogue meetings and butcher's-paper notes from sub-projects enabled feedback to further participants' reflection and thinking. Eventually quite organic and unexpected synergies began taking place to such an extent the U&I project felt more like 'a great big octopus' with many tentacles, or giant living organism that had got a 'life of its own', self-organising towards its own healthy culture-shift.
- *Action research for cyclic change*—following from this ecosystemic approach, action research is thus not (only) action that is researched, but research in action. That is, all action research routinely commences in current action, examines discrepant matters (either positively as in Appreciative Inquiry, or negatively as in critical theory) using close observation of the whole situation, reflection to develop meaningful grounded explanation and new theory, planning based on the logical consequences and implications of the new theory, and the taking of new experimental action which is again observed and responded to as feedback in an ongoing cyclic process. Past inquiry cycles have yielded what we already think, know and do now, and future cycles will yield new ways of thinking and knowing and doing. *In the U&I work,* identifying 'inquiry by and for whom, and for what purposes' ensured the critical reference group/critical inquiry group of consumers and inpatients: the end-beneficiaries of the mental health system, remained the driving impetus to retain the focus on the relevant end-goal, viz addressing iatrogenic trauma from acute hospital admissions—even when this was not always something on which all staff wanted to remain focused.

CONCLUSION

So while there have been numerous shifts in words and their meanings for these fields—for example from consumer participation to user-centred design, or from collaborative inquiry to co-design—the deeper purposes and learnings continue often to be shared despite changing contexts and situations. As new generations come to value *both* wanted change *and* chosen forms of stability (not just change or stability *per se*), new conversations will be possible drawing on these differing historical experiences and their discourses as a basis for potentially more life-giving futures.

1.4.9 CONSUMER-LED RESEARCH

FLICK GREY

SCOPE

Consumer-led research is an emergent, heterogeneous field. This is partly because it is emerging within (and in response to) diverse institutional and disciplinary contexts, for example, specific mental health services, psychiatric nursing, law or gender studies. The diversity within consumer-led research is also partly a result of different political, ethical and intellectual orientations among consumers.

Consumer-led research includes:

- consumer participation in research that is predominantly biomedical in orientation, for example, the Depression and Anxiety Consumer Research Unit at the Australian National University (Australian National University, 2020)
- service evaluation and quality improvement from a consumer perspective, for example, the collaboratively designed MH ECO Project—Mental Health Experience Co-Design—co-facilitated by the Victorian Mental Illness Awareness Council and the Victorian Mental Health Carers' Network (MH ECO, 2020)
- research that is framed entirely by the priorities and meaning-making of people with lived experience (for example, Dr David Webb's PhD research into the spirituality of suicide, the world's first PhD on the topic of suicide from the perspective of someone who has attempted suicide).

CONSUMER PERSPECTIVE RESEARCH

The starting point for consumer perspective research is our lived experiences: what actually matters in our lives. This ranges from concerns about the adequacy of information provision about medications and weight gain, to challenging the biomedical hegemony over explanations of mental distress.

The methodologies that we employ tend to be more exploratory than positivist, opening up the meanings people make of their experiences rather than engaging in statistical measurement. Cath Roper, a consumer academic, notes:

> We do not start off with the agenda tied up. We do not get involved in research that does not benefit our community. We make sure we are in constant touch with a critical reference group for our work, which means those people that the research is *for*—service users (Roper, 2009, p. 169).

Our research often embraces the inherently subjective nature of mental distress, in contrast to the objectifying relationships of 'evidence-based practice'.

Like the research efforts of other historically marginalised communities, there are many systemic and structural barriers to consumer perspective research. One of the main barriers is persistent marginalisation and underfunding of our research (O'Hagan, 2009, p. i), which tends to be self-perpetuating (it's challenging to get our research funded because we have less related research to cite in grant applications). Another barrier is the construction of consumers by ethics committees as 'a vulnerable population'. This erects frustrating barriers that inhibit grounded research with consumers, even when it is consumers conducting research into our own community!

Consumer perspective research has commonalities with research conducted by other historically marginalised populations, and can be contextualised within a broader research project of 'decolonising methodologies'. This is an epistemological shift, away from consumers being objects of study—effectively raw materials for others to construct theories about—to consumers being active creators of knowledge and theory. In many ways, it is comparable with Indigenous academic research, where 'the analysis has been acquired organically and outside of the academy' (Smith, 1999, p. 5). Sometimes, this involves 'researching back'—investigating the practices of non-consumers, of the mental health system, ethics committees and the non-mad community, from the perspective of consumers.

Several significant pieces of consumer perspective research were produced in the 1990s, sometimes involving non-consumer researchers. These include the U&I project (see Section 1.4.8), a result of collaboration between Yoland Wadsworth (a non-consumer academic) and Merinda Epstein (a consumer academic), and the *Lemon Tree Learning Project* (Epstein & Shaw, 1997)

Consumer perspective is often implicitly grounded in the question, 'What is it that only we can do?' Elsewhere, this has been called 'epistemic privilege': that we have privileged access to certain kinds of knowledge as a result of our lived experiences as consumers. Ultimately, consumer perspective research is underpinned by critical *political* questions:

> Whose research is it? Who owns it? Whose interests does it serve? Who will benefit from it? Who has designed its questions and framed its scope? Who will carry it out? Who will write it up? How will its results be disseminated? (Smith, 1999, p. 1).

Consumer perspective research is a growing field in Australia, with a growing number of consumer academics and consumer researchers; some are students, some hold academic positions within universities (often in Schools of Nursing, supported by clinical allies), some have connections with mental health organisations (e.g. the Consumer Led Research Network supported by the NSW Mental Health Commission), and some are independent or consultant researchers.

There is also a fledgling Mad Studies community in Australia, which significantly overlaps with but is not co-extensive with consumer perspective research. Mad Studies is 'a product of enquiry, knowledge production and political action' (LeFrançois, Menzies, & Reaume, 2013), grounded in the consumer/survivor movement, but drawing on research approaches from women's studies, queer studies, critical race studies and auto-ethnography (among others). Mad Studies simultaneously privileges the experiences of people who identify as Mad, psychiatric survivors, consumers, neuro-diverse, psychiatrically disabled, etc, while also unsettling and questioning identity labels. Internationally, Mad Studies is concentrated in Canada (e.g., LeFrançois et al., 2013), but includes contributors from many different countries, including Australia (e.g., Russo & Sweeney, 2016).

1.4.10 CONSUMER EVALUATION

ALLAN PINCHES

EMERGING THEMES

We will explore here a multiplicity of ways that consumer perspective knowledge can be regarded as a vital element in mental health service evaluation and development, as well as a resource for the wider society. Important themes will be of lived experience knowledge, social justice values and collaboration.

Consumer participation work over time tends to show that *carefully listening* to what consumers (service users) say about their experiences of mental health services, *engaging with them in shared discussion* about emerging lessons and *working collaboratively* towards a range of possible solutions, help create pathways towards service improvement and better lives for consumers.

This section picks up on some significant and emerging *consumer themes* from consumer-facilitated evaluation, research and project development over time, rather than focusing on techniques.

As a Consumer Consultant since 1996, in collaboration with consumer movement colleagues, service providers, academics, and other community allies, I have had significant involvement in the establishment of new consumer participation structures and processes in several large mental health services, both clinically based and community managed psychosocial disability support. I have researched and published on the mental health consumer movement's development and history. I draw upon these experiences here.

It is possible to envision services going further in utilising consumer perspective knowledge, seeking more effective, recovery-focused, and community-linked services. It also seems appropriate for consumer workers (recently termed as 'lived experience workforce members', including newer roles like peer support workers and consumer academics) to increasingly work in such multi-skilled, highly developmental, reflective and creative ways.

CONSUMER PERSPECTIVE KNOWLEDGE CAN BE REPRESENTED IN THREE MAIN LEVELS

The three levels of consumer perspective knowledge include:

- The lived experience of consumers of services, with their feedback/evidence/participation in discussions about experiences with services and beyond.
- The mental health consumer movement's large and diverse collective knowledge, theoretical base and philosophical approaches, from here and overseas.
- Desirably, systems and processes for consumers to communicate with each other, develop ideas, policies, and initiatives, and to be able to share with other parties, including service providers, government, organisations. Information sharing, opportunities for participation, coordination, reliable research and information, and well-facilitated discussion and development processes, with adequate resources, are important.

LOOKING AT SOME MENTAL HEALTH AND RELATED ISSUES THROUGH A CONSUMER 'LENS'

Increased efforts to incorporate principles highlighted by consumer perspective evaluation, research, project development, peer work, systemic advocacy and other key activities, could help guide the planning and implementation of a wide range of developments.

Some observations can be made from the service evaluation, research and development work of lived experience consumer workers, in collaborative projects, which may have a strong resonance for workers trying to promote major change, in a system resistant to change, with minimal resources.

A further possible aim to strengthen understanding of the broader lived experience of consumers in the community, beyond the immediate service settings, and tap into collective consumer-generated knowledge, including well-facilitated exploration of consumer thinking, could also help improve health and wellbeing outcomes for consumers. Consumer involvement in key discussions, in meaningful and nuanced ways, is clearly visible in favourable shifts within services around issues including dual-diagnosis, gender and sexuality, youth, peer support, recovery approaches, and cultural responsiveness with people from Indigenous and Culturally and Linguistically Diverse (CALD) communities (Davidson et al., 2005).

Questions about the medical model of mental illness/mental health and just what the most effective ways are to treat or respond to it, are a far from uncontested area, especially at a time when mental health services are struggling with overwhelming population demand for help. Among consumers, as well as the public, there is a wide spectrum of often strongly held beliefs about which approaches should be used. These are part of a wider debate beyond the scope of the current discussion.

The consumer movement arguably has much unexpended potential to contribute to mental health responses and solution seeking on many large-scale social and economic policy and practices on a wide range of contemporary issues. This may consider many complexities, the multifactorial nature of the issues, interconnectedness and many paradoxes involved. Several mental health service authorities and many consumer advocates have called for more holistic ways of providing mental health services–with a *whole of government, whole of community, whole of economy approach* (Victoria, State Services Authority, 2007).

BIG PICTURE PROBLEMS LINKED INTO MENTAL HEALTH OF SOCIETIES AND INDIVIDUALS

We live in a stressful world, with increasing social and economic competition and pressures, a widening gap between rich and poor, increasing social disadvantages in stark terms among many groups where some individuals bear the brunt of wider changes, and seemingly intractable conflicts, social dislocation and divisions are a staple daily problem. Key social institutions which were once seen as an influence for stability and cohesion, are now challenged on questions of relevance and legitimacy of authority.

Viewed in certain ways, mental health has a wide range of connections–virtually across the whole gamut of government portfolios, civil society, private enterprise and the lives of individuals.

A combination of powerful influences, including the pursuit of neoliberalist economics, globalisation, technological change, labour market and employment dislocation, population pressures, geopolitical conflicts, climate change and other environmental factors tend to create winners and losers, with increasing numbers of people subject to problems including poverty, unemployment and homelessness (Commission on Social Determinants of Health (CSDH), 2008).

In another historical overlay, the centrality of questions of sanity/madness in the human condition since time immemorial and the stigma and discrimination associated with this, has long been evident.

Thus, learning from the feedback and applied thinking of consumers, in collaborative conversations in the mental health field, offers many value-added factors to society, beyond a system becoming more efficient gatekeepers of treatment and support or arbiters of what is sane or normal or not.

POSSIBLE CONTRIBUTIONS OF CONSUMER PERSPECTIVE KNOWLEDGE

Consumer perspective knowledge can offer:

- A bridge between the lived experience of consumers and that of service providers, something like a 'rapporteur' role. i.e., facilitating discussions between parties aimed at evaluating and synthesising evidence at hand, seeking common understandings and developing action strategies for positive change.
- Ways for consumers, collectively and individually, to articulate about varied life circumstances and 'what happened', their own account of what they think about the causation of their mental health issues.
- Opportunities for consumers to demonstrate often marked abilities as problem-solvers on many levels.
- Synthesis of consumer knowledge based on lived experience, use of services, and thinking about what may or may not work within services–including lacks and gaps, ways to improve services or make them more helpful to people and to explore untried alternatives of 'potential'–both within services and the wider community.
- Potential contributions to solution seeking on many large-scale social and economic policy and practices on a wide range of contemporary issues, considering many complexities, multifactorial in nature, interconnectedness and many paradoxes involved.
- Ways to gauge, through various types of consultation, just how do consumers 'feel' about their experience of services, it being important to consider the actual words of consumers: i.e., concerning problematic effects which might be involved with the very act of diagnosis, grey-walled service environments, low expectations of consumer life possibilities, 'risk-management' and practices consumers often call *coercive*, which are often said to have counter-productive effects. Professional boundaries are sometimes perceived as a mask for indifference.

- Change or development in policy and practice, or method–whether it be in mental health treatments, organising of systems or quality improvement, smoking bans, trying to implement 'reforms' in the *Mental Health Act 2014* (Vic), with less than full service provider enthusiasm and engagement–is likely to result in unintended consequences (like 'side effects') even with originally good intentions. Considering consumer perspective evidence, discussion and thinking can help navigate towards new understandings.
- The mental health–physical health nexus has been a markedly under-recognised and under-resourced problem for a long time. Consumer advocates and researchers, with service provider 'allies' are becoming change agents in this area and efforts to address this issue are dramatically increasing.

MANY ASSUMPTIONS ABOUT CONSUMERS UP FOR CHANGING

Consumer perspective surveys and workshops have shown over decades that consumers want to be treated 'as human beings', with empathy, and that they who have a duty to treat, care, or support us can also 'walk a mile in my shoes'; to be spared being viewed as some 'other' lesser type of person; that we have enormous, yet unfulfilled human potential; that we are capable of learning and working effectively in many ways given the right opportunities; and having different or non-typical ways of viewing the world, which may sometimes sound strange, may somehow be a source of diversity in the world and may not necessarily equate with mental illness; and many consumers speak about unfavourable experiences related to stigma and discrimination both within the system and in the wider community.

Dr Daniel Fisher MD PhD is CEO of the National Empowerment Centre in the United States, a senior academic and a registered psychiatrist, has lived experience of serious mental illness and was a key developer of two consumer-led techniques, Open Dialogue and Emotional CPR. In his talks and books he speaks of hope and recovery through experiences of shared humanity. On a book jacket, he expresses hopes for consumers, including:

> Instead of being seen as threats to society, we will be seen as a source of wisdom that we have obtained through our recovery (Fisher, 2017).

1.4.11 MENTAL HEALTH POLICY AND EVALUATION

BRIDGET BASSILIOS, MEREDITH HARRIS, PHILIP BURGESS & JANE PIRKIS

The quality, effectiveness and efficiency of mental health systems are increasingly under scrutiny, not least because consumers, carers and other stakeholders are making themselves informed and are demanding systems that meet community need. Since its inception in 1992, the *National Mental Health Strategy* (the Strategy) has had a focus on monitoring and evaluation to achieve these goals, articulated in the themes of each of five National Mental Health Plans (Plans). This section provides a brief overview of the role of monitoring and evaluation in mental health policy in general, and the Strategy in particular. It provides two examples of monitoring and evaluation activities that have occurred within the Strategy–one in the specialised public mental health sector and one in the primary mental health sector.

MONITORING AND EVALUATION IN (MENTAL) HEALTH POLICY

Monitoring and evaluation are key mechanisms to enable governments to report to stakeholders on progress achieved under a policy or plan. Monitoring and evaluation have related but distinct functions. Monitoring the performance of a policy (or program) involves routine data collection and analysis to determine how well it is functioning, when compared against expected outcomes or processes (World Health Organization, 2013). Key performance indicators (KPIs; measures of input, output or outcome) are the basis for monitoring. Ideally, targets will also be determined for a given indicator, to enable judgements about whether intended aims have been achieved and whether adjustments in response to observed rates of progress are required. Various health performance frameworks exist that can be used to guide the development of indicators for health policy, systems or programs. For example, Australia's National Mental Health Performance Framework sets out a suite of 15 indicators organised according to the system performance domains of effectiveness, appropriateness, efficiency, responsibility, accessibility, sustainability, capability, safety and continuity (Australian Institute of Health and Welfare, 2015b).

In contrast, evaluation is a process of systematic, in-depth examination to determine the value or effectiveness of a policy (or program; see World Health Organization, 2013b). Evaluation should play a role in each stage of the policy cycle—from priority setting and the development of options or initiatives, to implementation, to evaluation. Evaluation frameworks guiding policy and program evaluation, including the World Health Organization's *Monitoring and Evaluation of Mental Health Policies and Plans* guidance, (World Health Organization, 2007) typically distinguish three categories of evaluation (described below) with a comprehensive evaluation ideally including all three:

Content evaluation is concerned with characteristics of the policy/plan itself and how it was developed. It focuses on the activities undertaken during initial stages of the policy cycle, however its findings can also assist in the design or interpretation of implementation and impact evaluations. Content evaluations take many forms, including: review of the alignment between policy elements and the evidence base or requirements the policy was designed to address; structured comparisons of policy elements with those of other relevant policies or best practices in policy development; the extent to which key stakeholders were involved in the development process; and program logic models to identify measures against which the policy may be monitored and evaluated (Centers for Disease Control and Prevention, 2014; World Health Organization, 2007).

Implementation evaluation is concerned with monitoring whether the options or initiatives outlined in the policy/plan were implemented as intended. Implementation evaluations are typically descriptive in design, and may include: mapping the extent to which initiatives have been implemented (as measured by, for example, the elements put in place, associated resources or expenditure, timeliness of implementation, and geographic or target population coverage); comparing variations in implementation across geographical areas or other meaningful units; and gathering qualitative data to explore factors that facilitate or hamper implementation or that contribute to variation (Centers for Disease Control and Prevention, 2014; World Health Organization, 2007).

Impact evaluation is concerned with assessing the objectives of the policy or outcomes of interest, and the extent to which these can be attributed to the implemented options or initiatives. Outcomes may be defined in terms of health-related characteristics in the target population or associated costs or cost-benefits. Examples of impact evaluations include: experimental and non-experimental studies that examine changes in measures of outcome over time or between groups (Centers for Disease Control and Prevention, 2014; World Health Organization, 2007).

MONITORING AND EVALUATION OF AUSTRALIA'S NATIONAL MENTAL HEALTH STRATEGY

The Strategy has been implemented via five National Mental Health Plans spanning the period 1993–2022 (Australian Government, 2017; Australian Health Ministers, 1992a, 1998, 2003, 2009). From 1993 to 2011, the *National Mental Health Report* (Department of Health and Ageing, 2013) was the key means of publicly monitoring and reporting progress towards agreed goals and initiatives under the Strategy. Data on Australia's mental health system are currently published in several other reports including: the *Mental Health Services in Australia* report series (Australian Institute of Health and Welfare, 2014a), prepared annually by the Australian Institute of Health and Welfare; the Productivity Commission's annual *Report on Government Services* (Productivity Commission, 2014), the National Mental Health Commission's *National Report Card on Mental Health and Suicide Prevention* (National Mental Health Commission, 2013), and the *Roadmap for*

National Mental Health Reform 2012-2022 (Council of Australian Governments, 2012). In addition to ongoing monitoring and reporting, the first three plans were subject to specific evaluations or reviews of varying scope (Grace et al., 2017), which have informed its ongoing directions.

Evaluation of the effectiveness and appropriateness of the First Plan (1993-1998; Australian Health Ministers, 1992) in 1997 involved review of the Strategy's impact in four local communities (including consumers, carers, mental health professionals and other professionals), consultation and survey views of national peak bodies (from 182 national organisations representing health professionals, consumers and carers), review of source data collected for the first *National Mental Health Report* (Australian Government, 1994) and expert review by the US Centre for Mental Health Services of appropriateness of national mental health policy settings (National Mental Health Strategy Evaluation Steering Committee, 1997). The evaluation reported improvements in the relative mix of inpatient and community services, and intersectoral links between mental health and housing and employment services (National Mental Health Strategy Evaluation Steering Committee, 1997). It also identified a need to expand the scope of reform from a focus on specialised mental health services to incorporating a broader population-focused approach, inclusive of primary care and less severe mental disorders (National Mental Health Strategy Evaluation Steering Committee, 1997). As a result, the scope of the Second Plan (Australian Health Ministers, 1998) was expanded to encompass a broader range of services (including mental health promotion, mental illness prevention and destigmatisation) and high prevalence disorders (depression and anxiety).

A two-stage review (Australian Health Ministers' Advisory Council, 2003; Thornicroft & Betts, 2002) of the Second Plan's (1998-2003; Australian Health Ministers, 1998) appropriateness, progress and effectiveness involved consultations with 350 stakeholders, including consumers, carers, non-government organisations, mental health professionals and their representative organisations, state, territory and Commonwealth officials, researchers, and a range of service providers. The first stage engaged international expertise (Thornicroft & Betts, 2002) and expert commentary from the United States and UK. The second stage involved national community consultation, a review of available data and a review of mental health in the Australian Health Care Agreements (Australian Health Ministers' Advisory Council, 2003). Evaluation findings presented a paradox. It reported both that significant progress had been made in mental health reform, but also that consumer dissatisfaction and unmet need were still high. The review also identified that further work was needed to ensure full and meaningful participation for consumers and carers, continuity of care, and a focus on priority populations, and, significantly, on service quality and monitoring. These findings led to the adoption of a population health approach in the Third Plan (Australian Health Ministers, 2003). which focused on reform in the areas of promotion and prevention, access and responsiveness (particularly for Indigenous populations, forensic populations and people with complex needs), strengthening service quality and fostering innovation (Australian Health Ministers, 2003).

Summative evaluation of the Third Plan (2003-2008; Australian Health Ministers, 2003) considered whether Australia had continued to make progress implementing the objectives of the Plan, and whether implemented programs or actions had affected reform of the mental health sector (Curie & Thornicroft, 2008). It involved a review of key documents, targeted consultations with 90 stakeholders about the effectiveness and appropriateness of the plan (Curie & Thornicroft, 2008). The evaluation made key recommendations for the development of the next mental health plan, including on workforce development, service models, consumer and carer participation, recovery orientation and a coordinated whole of government approach (Curie & Thornicroft, 2008). It also repeated calls for improvements in performance monitoring. Evaluation findings influenced the Fourth Plan which specified priorities for collaborative government action, identifying 34 reform actions to be undertaken across five priority areas, namely: social inclusion and recovery; prevention and early intervention; service access, coordination and continuity of care; quality improvement and innovation; and accountability (Australian Health Ministers, 2009).

There has not been a formal, public evaluation of the Fourth Plan (2008-2014; Australian Health Ministers, 2009).

In 2014 the National Mental Health Commission conducted a *National Review of Mental Health Services and Programmes* which examined the efficiency and effectiveness, and overall investment and spending, of Commonwealth-funded services and programmes (National Mental Health Commission, 2014c). The review recommended shifting funding priorities from hospitals and income support to community and primary health care services that increase service access to decrease preventable hospitalisations and support people to live contributing lives (National Mental Health Commission, 2014c). Consequently, commencing in July 2016, the Australian Government tasked its 31 Primary Health Networks (PHNs) with leading mental health planning and integration at a regional (area-based) level in partnership with state and territory governments and non-government organisations (Australian Government Department of Health, 2015). PHNs received a flexible funding pool to redesign the primary mental health system using a stepped care model intended to efficiently match service intensity with individual need (Australian Government Department of Health, 2015). Services are intended to target Aboriginal and Torres Strait Islander people, people at risk of suicide, people with severe and complex mental illness, and youth (Australian Government Department of Health, 2015).

The Fifth Plan (2017-2022; Australian Government, 2017) identifies eight priority areas influenced by the National Mental Health Commission's review (National Mental Health Commission, 2014) and the Australian Government's response (Australian Government Department of Health, 2015) to the findings of the review. The priority areas are: (1) achieving integrated regional planning and service delivery, (2) suicide prevention, (3) coordinating treatment and supports for people with severe and complex mental illness, (4) improving Aboriginal and Torres Strait Islander mental health and suicide prevention, (5) improving the physical health of people living with mental illness and reducing early mortality, (6) reducing stigma and discrimination, (7) making safety and quality central to mental health service delivery, and (8) ensuring that the enablers of effective system performance and system improvement are in place (Australian Government, 2017). Indicators for measuring change are described for each of the eight priority areas, but specific targets are not defined. The Fifth Plan indicates that the National Mental Health Commission will deliver an annual report on the Plan's implementation progress and 'performance against identified indicators once baselines have been established' (Australian Government, 2017, p.17). At the time of writing, 17 of the 24 indicators could be reported on in some form; the remaining seven are not currently reportable but could be potentially reported within the life of the Fifth Plan, contingent on investment and data development. The Fifth Plan also notes that it will be evaluated in its final year using annual reporting and targeted consultations with stakeholders (governments, consumers, carers, mental health sector; Australian Government, 2017).

MONITORING AND EVALUATION OF SELECTED MENTAL HEALTH POLICY INITIATIVES

Routine outcome monitoring and reporting in Australia's specialised public sector mental health services

From the outset, the Strategy sought to advance routine outcome measurement (ROM) and casemix classification as a means of monitoring the quality, effectiveness and efficiency of mental health services. Australia was the first country to implement ROM comprehensively within publicly funded mental health services.

In the late 1990s, under the Second Plan, bilateral agreements between the Australian Government and all states and territories were signed. These committed the states and territories to routinely collect and submit outcome and casemix data in their specialised public sector mental health services and the Australian Government to support the development of necessary infrastructure (Burgess, Coombs, Clarke, Dickson, & Pirkis, 2012). A National Outcomes and Casemix Collection (NOCC; Commonwealth of Australia, 2018) was progressively implemented in all inpatient and community-based services in this sector from 2001. The NOCC protocol specifies a suite of clinician- and consumer-rated measures to be completed at set points in the consumer's episode of care (i.e., admission, review and discharge), depending on the service setting (inpatient, residential and ambulatory), and the age group of the consumer (children and adolescents, adults and older persons). These arrangements are now firmly embedded; in 2012–13, 85% of services were collecting routine outcome data (Department of Health and Ageing, 2013).

Since 2003, the Australian Mental Health Outcomes and Classification Network (AMHOCN) consortium has undertaken data management, training and development, and analysis and reporting of the NOCC on behalf of the Australian Government. One area of focus has been the development of approaches to public reporting, informed by best practice principles (Burgess et al., 2012). AMHOCN regularly reports outcome data at national and jurisdictional (i.e., state/territory) levels, partitioned by age group and service setting. Reporting was initially via a suite of 'paper-based' standard reports and later via an online 'reports portal' which provides users with greater flexibility to tailor reports to their requirements. AMHOCN has supported states and territories to utilise their own outcome data and to benchmark against each other to identify opportunities for system improvement (Burgess et al., 2012). Given the complexity of the NOCC data, and the potentially sophisticated questions that can be asked of it, a Reporting Framework was developed to provide users with guidance on generating and interpreting reports at a local level. An online Web Decision Support Tool (wDST) provides a user interface to assist a greater range of stakeholders to query the NOCC data at national and state/territory levels. The wDST has evolved over more than a decade in response to the changing needs of users with respect to its functionality and utility. The most recent developments allow for the results of multiple queries to be displayed simultaneously. For example, scores on clinician- and consumer-rated measures can be displayed side-by-side, which provides an opportunity to promote engagement with the consumer/family around different perspectives on mental health status. (Details of these reporting approaches are at: AMHOCN, 2020; NOCC Reporting).

AMHOCN has also played a role in the monitoring of mental health policy through the development and operationalisation of KPIs measuring the effectiveness of mental health services (Burgess et al., 2012). For example, 'Change in mental health consumer's clinical outcomes (MHS KPI 1)' is one of the 15 KPIs developed under the National Mental Health Performance Framework (Australian Institute of Health and Welfare, 2018a) and is one of the 24 indicators (PI 14) for monitoring the Fifth Plan. For this indicator, pairs of baseline and follow-up scores on the Health of the Nation Outcome Scales are measured separately for adults, children and adolescents and older people. The key clinician-rated measures in the NOCC are classified as 'significant improvement', 'significant deterioration' or 'no significant change' using the effect size metric, and reported separately for three groups of consumers (consumers discharged from hospital, consumers discharged from ambulatory care, and consumers in ongoing ambulatory care). Such analyses have demonstrated that people in contact with public sector mental health services do achieve significant improvements, and documented how outcomes vary according to service setting and between collection occasions (Burgess, Pirkis, & Coombs, 2006).

Evaluation of Access to Allied Psychological Services (ATAPS)

Introduced under the Second Plan, Access to Allied Psychological Services (ATAPS) was the first national policy initiative to provide community access to government-funded primary mental health care. ATAPS operated from July 2001 to June 2016 and enabled GPs (and later other providers) to refer individuals with common mental disorders (anxiety or depression) to mental health professionals for free or low-cost, short-term evidence-based psychological treatment (Australian Government Department of Health and Ageing, 2012). Services were delivered Australia-wide through capped fund-holding arrangements that were administered by regionally based primary health care organisations (Australian Government Department of Health and Ageing, 2012). Due to the introduction of complementary primary mental health care policy initiatives (Better Access, which is larger in scale, and funded on a fee-for-service basis via the Medicare Benefits Schedule (MBS; Pirkis et al., 2011) and headspace targeting young people aged 12–25 years (Bassilios, Telford, Rickwood, Spittal, & Pirkis, 2017), new ATAPS sub-programs were introduced. These sub-programs targeted specific hard-to-reach groups or offered flexibilities service delivery (e.g., unlimited number of sessions, beyond in-person treatment options, sessions devoted to parents as part of treatment of children, leniency in requirement for formal diagnosis; Reifels et al., 2013).

From the outset, there was government commitment to evaluating ATAPS. The evaluation was unique in that it commenced with the introduction, and continued until the conclusion, of ATAPS. The evaluation focused on whether ATAPS had improved access to primary mental health services and, in turn, mental health outcomes for people with high prevalence disorders. The evaluation approach was both formative, assessing implementation processes or how the program operated, and summative, assessing the program's impact and outcomes to inform government decisions regarding the development of the program (Ovretveit, 1998). Consequently, the evaluation design was multifaceted, evolving in response to changes in the initiative and incorporating a range of data sources and analysis approaches. Quantitative program utilisation data from a purpose-designed national minimum dataset provided breadth of information and was complemented by qualitative data from stakeholder consultations to provide depth of information. Triangulation (Ovretveit, 1998; Patton, 1990) of the various data sources strengthened the evaluation by producing findings that pointed in a similar direction.

Evaluation showed that ATAPS was an integral part of the primary mental health care system in Australia. Its reach was substantial in the context of its capped funding with 530 000 treatment episodes (in 2.6 million sessions) provided from July 2013 to June 2016 (Bassilios, Nicholas, et al., 2017). Over one-third of treatment episodes specifically targeted hard-to-reach groups—for example, of the total patients reached, 33% were males, 64% on low incomes, 8% children, 7% Indigenous people, 34% received mental health treatment for the first time, 6% were at risk of suicide and 1% homeless (Bassilios, Nicholas, et al., 2017). Improving access for these subpopulations was facilitated by the previously mentioned service delivery flexibilities (Reifels et al., 2013) that are unavailable through its uncapped mainstream counterpart, Better Access. Finally, patient outcomes, which were available for around 11% of total treatment episodes, indicated statistically significant clinical improvement (Bassilios, Nicholas, et al., 2017).

Lessons learned from the evaluation of ATAPS, together with the 2014 *National Review of Mental Health Services and Programmes* (National Mental Health Commission, 2014), have influenced the previously mentioned PHN-led policy reforms in primary mental health that commenced in July 2016 including commissioning ATAPS-like services. For example, recommendations such as rationalising the number of outcome measures, comparing interventions introduced as part of the reforms to treatment as usual, and eliciting service experience feedback from consumers (Bassilios, Nicholas, et al., 2017) have been adopted in the evaluation of the new reforms (Department of Health, 2016).

IMPROVING MONITORING AND EVALUATION

Australia is a leader in the implementation of national outcome data collection systems, such as the examples described above. However, the quality of the data and ensuring its clinical utility could be enhanced (Whiteford & Buckingham, 2005). There is also a need to embed outcome data in robust processes of systemic quality service improvement. Furthermore, not all parts of the mental health system are routinely monitored; for example, national outcome data sets do not exist for all office-based private practice psychiatry and psychology including services provided through the MBS (Crome & Baillie, 2016). Addressing such gaps in monitoring could improve our overall understanding of the performance of Australia's mental health system and inform associated policy development.

The Strategy has evolved based on evaluation findings of the respective plans and has included KPIs, but a notable gap is the specification of targets that would facilitate measurement of whether objectives have been met. An analysis of policy success and failure in formal evaluations of the Strategy from 1992-2012 reported an overall improvement in the development and application of policy levers (e.g., organisation, regulation, finance, community education, payment) but highlighted variations in evaluation depth over time and difficulties matching indicators to specific reform objectives due to lack of correspondence between individual initiative and population level outcomes (Grace et al., 2017). Other analyses of Australia's approach to performance monitoring of mental health suggested there were gaps and problems, including the difficulty in establishing a link between outcome data and processes of quality improvement (Rosenberg et al., 2015; Rosenberg & Salvador-Carulla, 2017).

There have also been systematic attempts to identify policy-relevant gaps in mental health research including the extent of alignment of funding (and publications) with epidemiological evidence and stakeholder priorities, comorbid physical illness, digital mental health care and suicide prevention. Findings suggest that research publications and funding are not necessarily aligned with burden of disease and stakeholder priorities; for example, a study of these indicators in Australia in 2008 revealed that the areas of suicide and self-harm, personality disorders, anxiety disorders, childhood conditions and dementia were all insufficiently funded (Christensen, Batterham, Griffiths, Gosling, & Hehir, 2013). Using the World Health Organization Mental Health Action Plan 2013-2020 as a framework, an analysis of state and federal policies on mental and physical illness found that related policy attention had grown but policies and their implementation were inconsistent and insufficiently interconnected, therefore calling for a coherent national framework to guide system reform and address this shortcoming (Happell et al., 2015). Digital mental health interventions have rapidly proliferated over the past decade, accordingly, research focusing on policy development and implementation planning including issues such as financing and governance is needed (Meurk, Leung, Hall, Head, & Whiteford, 2016). A review of current and future priorities in Australian suicide prevention research from 2010-17, based on journal articles and funding, reported that epidemiological studies seemed to be a focus, but intervention studies had declined even though stakeholders had consistently deemed intervention studies to be the highest future research priority for real advancement (Reifels et al., 2017). These gaps have been addressed in the priority areas of the Fifth Plan to varying extents.

CONCLUSION

Monitoring and evaluation of mental health policy is vital to determine the nature of, and reasons for, its achievements as well as areas requiring improvement. Australia's National Mental Health Strategy has evolved in response to evaluations and reviews. Although KPIs have been a component of the Strategy, specific targets that could inform evaluation have been lacking. Under the Strategy, Australia has been a pioneer in establishing systems for the routine monitoring and evaluation of major mental health programs but processes of systemic service quality improvement are yet to emerge.

1.4.12 EVIDENCE-BASED PRACTICE

MARLENA KLAIC

DEFINITION AND ORIGINS OF EVIDENCE-BASED PRACTICE

The terms evidence-based practice (EBP) and evidence-based medicine (EBM) are often used interchangeably, but for allied health and non-medical professional groups, the term evidence-based practice is more commonly used. Guyatt and colleagues define EBP as the 'conscientious' and 'judicious' use of best evidence when making decisions about the care of consumers (Guyatt et al., 2000). It is both a philosophical approach to health care and a set of behaviours when applied in practice. The process of EBP involves integrating individual clinical expertise with the best available external clinical evidence derived from systematic research, with consideration to the consumer's values and wishes (Haynes, Devereaux, & Guyatt, 2002). EBP can be illustrated using a three-circle model (see Figure 1.20) with equal attention given to each of the three elements i.e. evidence-based clinical decision making is a result of the influence of the evidence, clinical experience of the health professional while also considering and incorporating the consumer's values.

Figure 1.20 The three-circle model of evidence-based practice

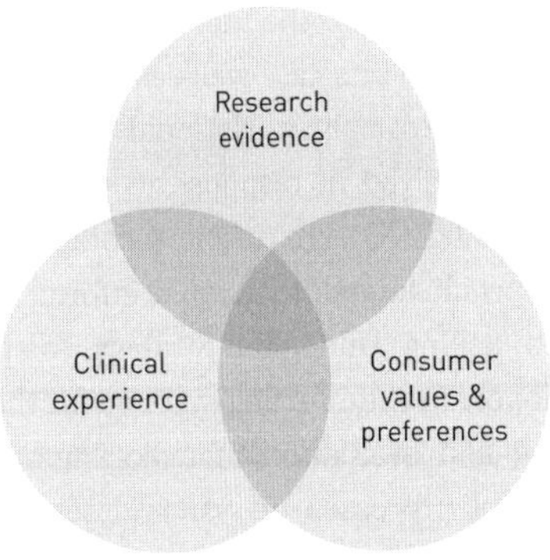

Source: Haynes et al., 2002

Evidence-based medicine was conceived of in the early 1960s at McMaster University in Canada (Smith & Rennie, 2014). This newly established academic facility introduced a medical curriculum called 'problem-based learning', which combined the traditional scientific studies in medicine with a focus on clinical problems gleaned from the bedside of health consumers. Simultaneously, David Sackett established the world's first department of clinical epidemiology and biostatistics and ensured that the new medical curriculum incorporated these subjects. Sackett subsequently developed a short course on critical appraisal of published literature. Thirty years later, Gordon Guyatt changed the medical residency program at McMaster University and based it on the critical appraisal methods developed by Sackett. The course was called 'evidence-based medicine'. Guyatt was a strong and vocal proponent for ensuring that medical students had the skills to consume, understand and apply research in clinical practice.

Both Gordon Guyatt and David Sackett have been recognised for their instrumental roles in the inception and further development of the evidence-based medicine model. Progression over the last 50 years can be measured by considering the increase in publications related to evidence-based medicine, from less than five in the late 1980s to almost 16 000 in 2017.

APPLICATION OF EVIDENCE-BASED PRACTICE IN A CLINICAL SETTING

Some ten years following introduction of evidence-based medicine, it was recognised that there was a significant gap between the evidence available, and application of this within clinical practice. In 2003, a group of international leaders in EBP convened a conference called 'Signposting the future of evidence-based health care' (Dawes et al., 2005). From this meeting, a consensus statement was published and included a clear description of the process of evidence-based practice and the necessary skills to implement it within clinical practice. The 5-step process of EBP was described as follows:

TRANSLATION OF CLINICAL UNCERTAINTY TO A QUESTION WHICH CAN BE ANSWERED

The first step to applying EBP requires the individual to develop a measurable question when confronted with a problem in clinical practice. One of the most popular methods is commonly known as PICO. This acronym provides a framework for developing a research question where the user must consider the following: P–population or patient or consumer; I–intervention; C–control or comparison intervention; O–outcome(s).

ACCESS AND RETRIEVAL OF THE BEST AVAILABLE EVIDENCE

The second step of EBP involves designing and executing a search strategy. This typically includes selection of appropriate search terms and databases. The evidence-based practitioner must also have some familiarity with the use of Boolean operators, such as 'and', 'not' and 'or' along with truncation symbols, to efficiently and effectively locate relevant evidence.

CRITICAL APPRAISAL AND ASSESSMENT OF THE EVIDENCE

The third step in applying EBP requires the ability to critically appraise the published evidence for quality, consistency, generalisability and applicability. There are a large number of tools and frameworks available to assist in appraising the quality of individual studies and appropriate selection is dependent on study type. Some examples include the PEDro scale which is used to assess quality of randomised controlled trials and the CASP checklist which is used to assess the quality of qualitative studies.

There are also a number of methods for assessing the overall strength of the evidence, although most appear to have similar criteria. In Australia, the National Health and Medical Research Council (NHMRC) developed a summary to guide interpretation of the evidence base, as illustrated in Table 1.6.

Table 1.6 Comparative levels of evidence

Level	Evidence
I	Systematic review of level II studies
II	Properly designed randomised controlled trial
III-1	Well-designed pseudo-randomised controlled trial
III-2	Comparative studies with concurrent controls and allocation but not randomised e.g. cohort studies, case control studies or interrupted time series with a control group
III-3	Comparative studies with historical control, two or more single-arm studies or interrupted time series without a parallel control group
IV	Case series, either post-test or pre-test and post-test

APPLICATION OF THE EVIDENCE IN PRACTICE

The fourth step to an evidence-based approach involves applying the findings to a clinical setting or in response to a research question. It is highly likely that this step will require engagement from numerous stakeholders including the broader multidisciplinary team and consumers.

INTEGRATION, ADAPTATION AND EVALUATION OF THE EVIDENCE

The final step in the EBP process involves evaluating the effects of applying the evidence in practice and adapting the evidence to the context. Evaluation may take a number of forms including consumer reported outcomes (pROMs), clinician outcome measures and organisation related measures of effectiveness. It is not uncommon for some adaptation to be required to meet the specific needs of the user and context.

ARGUMENTS FOR AND AGAINST THE EVIDENCE-BASED PRACTICE MODEL

Those in favour of the EBP model argue that it improves consumer outcomes and safety. Furthermore, effective evidence-based interventions can reduce the number of consumers re-presenting to health facilities and reduce the incidence of complications. Arguably, this can save funders of health care significant dollars and ensure consumers are not being exposed to ineffective treatments. Evidence-based practice aims to reduce variability in delivery of health care. In health care systems based on egalitarian principles, consumers expect to receive equal care, irrespective of who delivers the health care or where the health care is delivered.

Critics of the EBP model argue that there simply isn't adequate evidence or the evidence that is published is of low quality. Furthermore, application of the findings from research is viewed as being difficult, particularly when the findings are from a randomised trial with stringent inclusion criteria. Another argument relates to the requirement that clinicians must both obtain and maintain the skills necessary to undertake all 5 steps of the EBP process. They must also have access to computers, internet and most importantly, the time to complete the steps previously described. Critics of EBP argue that this approach to health care delivery is resource intensive. Finally, the most common argument against the 5-step EBP approach is that it is recipe-driven and cannot cater to the individual needs of a consumer and/or clinician. The Sicily Statement focuses solely on published evidence as the core skill set of the evidence-based practitioner and fails to adequately incorporate the consumer's values and needs and the context of health care delivery.

ALTERNATIVE APPROACHES TO THE EBP MODEL

A number of alternative models to EBP have been developed to support health professionals' engagement with and use of research evidence.

EVIDENCE-INFORMED PRACTICE

Evidence-informed practice is defined as the integration of evidence from multiple sources including qualitative studies, along with the health professionals' clinical experience while incorporating the consumer's values and preferences (Nevo & Slonim-Nevo, 2011). On the surface, evidence-based practice and evidence-informed practice appear to be interchangeable. However, the use of the term 'based' is a point of contention for those who argue for the term 'evidence-informed practice'. Evidence-based practice implies that clinical decisions must be 'based' on evidence primarily derived from scientific research. Evidence-informed practice implies that clinical decisions may be 'informed' by scientific research but equally, if none is available or the scientific evidence is weak, the clinician can and should rely on their own clinical expertise. Furthermore, evidence-informed practice does not rely on the 5-step model prescribed in the Sicily Statement, as this is perceived to be reliant only on published research. Rather, published evidence may be incorporated as part of the intervention but the process of finding and appraising the evidence should be based on the needs of the clinician and the consumer, rather than a prescriptive process (Epstein, 2011; Gambrill, 2008; Nevo & Slonim-Nevo, 2011).

PRACTICE-BASED RESEARCH

Practice-based research is an inductive approach to research that involves exploration of questions that emerge from a clinicians' critical reflection on their own practice (Epstein, 1996; see also Table 1.3). This approach to research began appearing in published literature more than 20 years ago and has featured primarily in studies within the field of social work. Irwin Epstein coined the term practice-based research and suggested it was an important, and sustainable, way for busy clinicians to integrate research within their own clinical context and practice. Clinical data mining is one example of practice-based research, where clinicians extract and analyse available clinical data to inform knowledge and decision making.

Practice-based research shows some promise for encouraging critical reflection on one's own practice and potentially maintaining EBP skills. However, this approach to engaging in research is typically small-scale and localised, thus the results are usually not disseminated more broadly for the benefit of other consumers, health care professionals and health care organisations.

PRACTICE-BASED EVIDENCE

Practice-based evidence is defined as the systematic and comprehensive collection of consumer treatment and outcome data, in order to determine effectiveness (Horn & Gassaway, 2007). Practice-based evidence has featured in published literature in health-related fields for the last 10 years, and appears to overcome some of the perceived limitations of the EBP model. Advocates of practice-based evidence argue that this approach offers the following benefits over and above EBP (Ammerman, Smith, & Calancie, 2014; Barkham & Mellor-Clark, 2003; Girard, 2008; Swisher, 2010):

1. Evidence is collected in a real-life setting. One of the major criticisms of EBP is that it is overly reliant on randomised trials (RCTs) and meta-analysis as the most important source of information to guide clinical decisions. The issue with data derived from RCTs is that it is difficult to generalise to consumers who rarely meet the eligibility criteria specified in the study. Practice-based evidence overcomes this by collecting data on every consumer that is being treated, rather than controlling for these confounding variables.
2. Evidence is collected within current resources. Evidence-based services and interventions that are published as best practice may be resource intensive and require additional equipment and training. This may prohibit use of the evidence in practice. Practice-based evidence works with the current resources, human and non-human, to generate research.
3. Evidence is collected as part of workflow. The most commonly reported barrier to EBP is the amount of time to undertake the 5 steps described in the Sicily Statement. Practice-based evidence involves a routinised approach to research generation and consumption, rather than a separate task requiring a separate set of skills.
4. Evidence is collected when there may be none available. A frequently reported barrier to the implementation of EBP in allied health is the lack of relevant published evidence. Practice-based evidence can overcome this by generating information on the treatments currently being provided and thus contribute to an evidence base.

The model of practice-based evidence typically involves larger groups of health professionals, both discipline specific and multidisciplinary teams. Therefore, practice-based evidence has the potential to expose many health professionals to research activities. Published studies have found that one of the strongest predictors of research utilisation is prior exposure to and engagement in research (Brown, Tseng, Casey, McDonald, & Lyons, 2010; Grimmer-Somers, Lekkas, Nyland, Young, & Kumar, 2007; Lyons, Casey, Brown, Tseng, & McDonald, 2010; Salbach, Jaglal, Korner-Bitensky, Rappolt, & Davis, 2007). Practice-based evidence appears to provide a means to bridge the research-practice gap.

SUMMARY

The benefits of providing health care utilising the three-circle model of EBP appear to be substantial and include improved consumer outcomes and better use of finite health resources. However, it is important to acknowledge that there are numerous issues related to the implementation of EBP in practice. Rapid development of medical innovations and health interventions over the last 50 years have significantly increased the body of knowledge. This increase in available evidence and knowledge does not automatically result in its actual use within everyday clinical practice. A number of alternative models have been proposed to assist health professionals with overcoming individual and contextual barriers. Although these models show some promise, there continues to be a sizeable research-practice gap which suggests there are ongoing difficulties with implementation of evidence into practice. The need to embed evidence in clinical practice remains a significant challenge for all health professionals.

CONCLUSION

GRAHAM MEADOWS AND FIONA MCDERMOTT

This chapter has necessarily been selective and some related themes are picked up elsewhere in the text. Having here given an overview of ethics in research, ethics in service delivery will be addressed further later (see section 1.5.2). Applications of neuroscience research will be further described in intervention and diagnostically focused chapters (see Chapters 2 and 3) while epidemiological principles will be seen in application through work in Australian epidemiological inquiry (see, for example, Section 4.1.3) and in some issues regarding service delivery and design (see Section 1.7.3). Clinical trial evidence of various kinds will feature extensively in this text as will considerations of systematic approaches to diagnosis and monitoring for outcomes (see Chapters 2 and 4). Further consideration in relation to service delivery will explore other health economic applications. Important and influential findings from qualitative and action research will be described later in the text. Consumer-led research and participation in evaluation feature heavily for instance in sections on Recovery (see Sections 1.1.6, 1.5.2, 1.7.2 and 2.6.7) while policy-related evaluations have been critical to decisions regarding service design and redesign in Australia (see Section 1.7.3), its states and territories. Applications of EBP are frequently discussed in this text (see Section 1.5.3). For instance, we will consider the issue that strength of evidence for treatment effectiveness is not necessarily evidence of strength of effect (see, for example, Sections 2.4.8, 2.4.9, 2.4.11 and 4.3.4). Discussion in the section on service delivery introduces the elaboration of the EBP concept into values based health care commissioning (see Chapter 2). Hence we hope that the concepts and content introduced here may usefully be returned to as the reader navigates or references later sections in the text.

1.4.13 COMMENTARY AND REFLECTIONS

GRAHAM MEADOWS & FIONA MCDERMOTT

This chapter has taken us through the range of approaches to carrying out research and evaluation in mental health. It is premised on the belief that 'good practice in mental health' relies not only on the trustworthiness of findings from research and evaluation studies but also on the capability of those working in the mental health field to understand the ways in which research and evaluations may be undertaken and their trustworthiness, validity and reliability assessed (see Section 1.4.16). As we have detailed here, the different perspectives, methodologies and expertise of all stakeholders (researchers, clinicians, policy makers, consumers and carers) provide a wide spectrum of approaches. These varying approaches, rather than 'undercutting' each other, instead offer opportunities for a richer understanding of the complexity and complicatedness of working with the challenges that mental health issues confront us with.

In later chapters of this text, you might consider how the principles of action research could apply to the work you do, for example, as a peer support worker (see Section 2.1.3) or whether a qualitative research method might further your understanding of consumers if you are a Mental Health Nurse (see Chapter 2.1.7). If as a psychologist you are working with people with mood disorders (see Chapter 4.3) you may find an understanding of how RCTs and clinical trials are conducted might influence the treatment approach you take. Again, if you work in the policy field in mental health, a grasp of the principles underpinning health economics and epidemiological research (see Chapter 1.7) will be of considerable value.

This chapter then, is to be thought about as a resource which you may return to in order to apply such research and evaluation skills to practice issues you confront, or at the very least, be confident that you understand the way results are arrived at from research and evaluation studies and can apply them in practice when relevant.

1.5

DELIVERING MENTAL HEALTH CARE

GRAHAM MEADOWS, SEBASTIAN ROSENBERG, ALAN WOODWARD, JOANNE ENTICOTT, JOHN FARHALL & MARGARET GRIGG

1.5.1 INTRODUCTION

GRAHAM MEADOWS & SEBASTIAN ROSENBERG

This text is written at a time of considerable change in mental health services in Australia (see Chapter 1.7). Difficult questions are being asked around existing service models (see Section 1.7.1). The accruing information for instance that expansion of traditional service models of mental health care does not seem to be having measurable impact on prevalence (see Section 1.5.10) should at least give us pause for thought that there might be other additional or alternative approaches that could give better results. Perhaps we are at one of those points of constructive perplexity that may constitute the prelude to a paradigm shift (van Os, Guloksuz, Vijn, Hafkenscheid, & Delespaul, 2019; Puras, 2018). While such time-points may be discomforting and potentially conflictual, they also may open up possibilities for dialogue between research, practice and policy that are closed in times when people are generally confident they know what the problems are and how they might best be fixed—times as it were of 'normal science'.

In a practical sense, this dialogue is manifest in several inquiries, commissions and reports into mental health. People are thinking now about better ways to design an organised response to mental illness. But these reports have been a common feature of mental health in Australia over past decades (Mendoza et al 2013). The issue has been less about the identification of opportunities for systemic improvement and more about the practicalities of change. What is it that people working at the coalface of mental health need in order to provide quality care? How can they be supported? How can this support take into account the complex, local context of care?

This chapter includes a section that considers health care ethics, given that ethical considerations intertwine with service delivery (including through laws). This section will have implications across much of the rest of this text. Some key UN statements will be introduced and the challenge presented by recovery orientation in practice will be discussed. We consider then how evidence and service delivery may connect and how mental health care may be funded. As first of several specific areas of focus we consider preventive interventions, then stepped care, disaster preparedness, services transformation towards recovery orientation, and teleweb or digital mental health services. In considering how an overall population mental health care system may be designed we introduce *The Lancet* Commission on Global Mental Health as being an important international statement with value in guiding mental health care development. A final section on simulation modelling as a way of considering whole of system design precedes some concluding comments.

1.5.2 ETHICAL UNDERPINNINGS OF HEALTH CARE DELIVERY

GRAHAM MEADOWS

INTRODUCTION

The health care system has an ethical dimension because its nature, including the incentives it presents to staff, consumers and other stakeholders (see Chapter 1.1), influences the prevailing ethical practice to be found in the system at all organisational levels. Some of these influences may be intended, some may arise out of properties of a complex adaptive system (see Section 1.1.1). So we begin the chapter considering the ethical assumptions of contemporary mental health care as developed through recent decades, for which we make use of four key reference points:

1. Some general background points on health care ethics.
2. United Nations Principles for the Protection of Persons with Mental Illness and the Improvement of Mental Health Care (UN Principles).
3. The implications of the development and increasing influence of what is termed 'Personal Recovery'.
4. Finally with exploration of the developing influence of the concepts articulated in the UN Convention on the Rights of Persons with Disabilities (CRPD).

Legislation and mental health care have a particular set of intertwined relationships and the operation of Mental Health Acts is more evident in mental health care than in many other branches of medicine. With considerations 1–4 as background and still in the context of ethical considerations then we will take an overview of the development of mental health legislation in the Australian states and territories.

PRINCIPLES OF MEDICAL ETHICS

Ethics in health care has a deep history, with the Hippocratic Oath being one of the early codifications of rules for how physicians should conduct themselves in their relationships with patients. The World Medical Association has issued a series of statements regarding medical ethics (Williams, 2009; World Medical Association, 2006) as has the World Psychiatric Association (World Psychiatric Association, 2011), and Australian medical colleges and other professional bodies, including for instance the RANZCP, have stated the rules that are seen as making for due professional conduct within a profession or discipline (The Royal Australian & New Zealand College of Psychiatrists, 2018). Practitioners should be aware of the codes of ethics of their particular professional body, and it may be helpful often also to be aware of the codes of practice of other disciplines in the multidisciplinary team.

Considerations of ethical practice feature in many parts of this text, reflecting some particular complexities of ethical practice in community mental health care. The structure of the system within which people work can influence opportunities and incentives for practice with varying ethical nature. Ethical practice, though standing in reference to professional rules of conduct, often cannot be reduced to acts of simple rule following, but rather represents a set of habitual styles of relating and reasoning frameworks that may be applied when ethical issues come clearly into the spotlight. The range of issues involved in ethical consideration can be likened to an iceberg (Seedhouse, 2009a); deep below the surface are ethics in the more general sense relating to our choices about how we live life and what we value in thought and deed. Just below the surface are persisting ethical questions regarding moral duties and rights as applying to general cases. Readily apparent above the surface are instances of dramatic or specific ethics involving evident ethical dilemmas as applying to particular situations. The modes of thinking identified elsewhere (see Chapters 1.1 and 2.3) as being important for the development of clinical decision making (i.e. skills of critical, reflective, complexity and dialectical thinking) will apply in the development of ethical decision making.

Beauchamp and Childress (2019) discuss the challenge of development of moral character in health professionals, with a fundamental orienting virtue of *caring* and five focal virtues important as providing a moral compass, being *compassion, discernment, conscientiousness, trustworthiness* and *integrity*. Commonly cited in consideration of medical ethics are four principles of medical ethics (Weise, 2016; Beauchamp & Childress, 2019; Gillon, 1986; Gillon, 1994; Gillon, 2003). Often decision making will involve weighing and balancing considerations between the decision drivers of the various principles:

1. *beneficience*, striving to bring benefit: where risk is also present, balancing decisions in favour of benefit
2. *non-maleficience*: working to avoid causing harm
3. *respect for autonomy*: a posture of respect for the choices and preferences of the autonomous person
4. *justice*: attendance to considerations of fairness as risks and benefits are distributed.

Psychiatry and mental health care present some particular challenges, and mental health care *systems* have at times and places in history become co-opted into roles in society that may later be seen as deeply abhorrent. Mental health problems can be seen as interfering with autonomy, indicating that the person so affected should have decisions made for them. Hence in many societies physicians with responsibility for mental health care are given far-reaching powers to deprive people of liberty and to impose treatment. These powers can become abused in sometimes terrible ways. Many of these examples, particularly of what above has been termed 'dramatic ethics', have been carefully reviewed and considered in the literature (Bloch & Green, 2009).

ELABORATIONS OF ETHICAL REASONING FRAMEWORKS IN HEALTH CARE

Another expression of an approach to ethical decision making broadly in health care can be found in Seedhouse's ethical grid (2009b). This model, established and refined over 20 years, uses as a support for reasoning in health care a diagram that assists the practitioner in balancing considerations of a fundamental respect for autonomy with considerations of widely valued rules to follow (deontological ethics) with considerations of the probability of outcomes given the range of decision options available (consequentialist ethics), and the realm of practical and societal considerations as constraining action in the real world. One outcome of a reading of Seedhouse's work, and considering how it might be supported in practice, is that it will involve a tolerance for careful thinking through of issues of a wide range of types of value system and a degree of sophistication in ethical thinking, as well as a tolerance through the reasoning process of evident uncertainty.

Common to both the four principles model and the ethical grid is a prominence for a notion of autonomy. In health care generally, an argument has been put forward that a shift is under way from an 'old school' model, where the target of health care is resolution of disease, illness or infirmity (described as 'Paradigm X'), to an orientation more towards health care as a support to personal freedom with freedom from illness only a part of that process ('Paradigm Y'; Seedhouse, 2009a, 2009b). One of the contexts where this comes to the fore in modern community mental health practice is in the consideration of redesigning services along 'recovery'-orientated practice. Just what this might mean in theory and practice is examined extensively elsewhere in this text (see Sections 1.1.4,

1.5.2 and 2.3.4), but clearly within this reorientation is a shift towards a greater prominence for respect for the autonomy of the individual.

With implications for the first three of the four principles and in the setting of beneficial consequences in Seedhouse's grid rests the concept of iatrogenesis, or harm resulting from treatment interventions. Commonly considered in a unidimensional way, iatrogenesis can be considered as having three dimensions, and some implications of knowledge of these for contemporary mental health care have recently been explored in the literature (Meadows, Prodan, et al., 2019a) in turn an account of concepts set out in Illich (1976).

- Clinical iatrogenesis is a regularly used concept. Here we may consider medication side effects, whether the nausea and sexual dysfunction commonly associated with serotonin specific reuptake inhibitors or the weight gain and metabolic disturbance associated with antipsychotics which may also be used in treatment of depression.
- Social iatrogenesis may occur where there is a clear expectation that people with some aspects of experience that become labelled as a mental disorder will seek help and primarily address those experiences through interactions with professional health care and the following of given advice. Specifically, this becomes iatrogenic if the following of this advice results in the reliance on an intervention that may on occasions be less effective than options for action otherwise in the repertoire of the individual or their community resources.
- Cultural iatrogenesis can be identified if we see cultural norms shifting such that certain kinds of human experience that might be classed as normal aspects of the human condition lose that validated status. Here we may consider the present-day functioning of social media with its encouragement to present a positive, buoyant picture of the self and where sharing normal human weaknesses and troubles may lead to ostracism and ridicule as forms of bullying.

The avoidance of iatrogenic harm can be seen as a target of quaternary prevention, to be discussed further in Section 1.5.5.

DEVELOPMENTS IN MENTAL HEALTH LEGISLATION

The most obvious expression of the ethical tensions in mental health is mental health legislation (Seedhouse, 2009a). Mental health legislation embodies the balance between autonomy and individual rights, paternalism and community safety. Hence a key consideration in proper conduct for practitioners in mental health care has to be compliance with mental health legislation. Ethics and law have been described as being inextricably intertwined (Stewart, Kerridge, & Parker, 2008), and it is most important that workers identify when an ethical issue that arises in their work has legal implications. Workers in mental health care systems and others involved with care of people with mental health problems should have familiarity with the act that applies in their jurisdiction. Mental health legislation in Australia is the task of the states and territories, and each has its own Act (Stewart et al., 2008). At the time of writing the oldest of these Acts is for the NT (1998) then NSW (2007), SA (2009), Tasmania (2013), Victoria and WA (2014), ACT (2015) and Queensland (2016). Readers making decisions on which the Acts bear should ensure their reference is to an up-to-date version. In many situations the relevant Act will provide a framework within which issues of dramatic and specific ethics need to be reasoned through and will create legal rights and duties. Typically these will cover issues of: defining mental illness for the purposes of the Act; consent and decision making regarding voluntary treatment; circumstances, criteria and processes whereby someone can be treated involuntarily; treatments that may be prohibited or specially regulated (within which psychosurgery, ECT and coma therapies may receive attention); regulation of seclusion and restraint; and provision of non-psychiatric treatment to mental health patients (Stewart et al., 2008).

In reviewing the changes in mental health legislation over recent times The Royal Australian & New Zealand College of Psychiatrists (2017) identified three major drivers of recent changes: the United Nations Department of Public Information (1991; the UN Principles), recovery oriented practice and the Convention on the Rights of Persons with Disabilities (CRPD; United Nations, 2007b).

The UN Principles for the Treatment of Persons with Mental Illness

The United Nations (UN) has over decades worked towards codifications of rights generally and as related to an increasing variety of specific circumstances. In 1991, the General Assembly ratified a UN position on issues related to people with mental illness (United Nations Department of Public Information, 1991). Since that time, the UN declaration has been influential in the way that subsequent mental health legislation has been drafted. The Principles have a strong emphasis on protection of the patient from potential abuses in the context of mental illness including through actions conducted as treatment. They remained grounded in a medical model of thinking around mental illness as deviation and deficiency, which more recently has been challenged by both thinking around recovery oriented practice and the CRPD.

Recovery oriented practice

Adopting a recovery agenda (see Section 1.1.4) involves a significant reorientation of approach, focus of attention, process of formulation and adoption of goals, a revision of what is to be valued and, perhaps most critically, a change in power relationships. There may be very real tensions in adopting such approaches in clinical service delivery systems that have strong imperatives to contain risk, and where existing team structures, relationships, accountabilities and procedures mitigate for more biomedical approaches (see Chapter 2.2).

The CRPD

This is based on a social model, that is to say one that holds that 'disability results from interaction between an impairment and social/environmental barriers'; a key aim of the CRPD is encouraging personal autonomy and independence. Included here is encouragement of freedom and independence in making active personal choices about treatment and other interventions. A challenge for the construction of law in this area if mental health problems are considered as constituting disability is that a critical point in the CRPD (Article 14) states that 'existence of a disability shall in no way justify a deprivation of liberty'.

1.5.3 CONNECTING EVIDENCE, POLICY, STRATEGY AND ACTIVITY

EVIDENCE-BASED HEALTH POLICY

GRAHAM MEADOWS & MARGARET GRIGG

As we have examined in earlier editions of this book, the text 'Evidence-based health policy' (Gibson, 2003) sets out the proposition that health policy is developed in a climate of tension, periodic competition and occasional concordance of three identifiable rationalities:

- Cultural rationality reflects societal values regarding what should be prioritised and considered correct when guiding health policy making. These, of course, may vary with time and in different sections of society; however, 'Of particular importance are the dimensions of the significance of health, the meaning and extent of solidarity or significance attached to universality, the value accorded to health and quality of life, and the importance of choice and opportunity for participation' (Gibson, 2003).
- Political rationality deals with power and the processes whereby power is gained, maintained and transferred, including shifts in power balance consequent on policy decisions and the influence they will have on policy making. 'It reveals the willingness of policymakers to have transparent processes and be accountable, the ability of interest groups to participate and influence policy processes and outcomes, and the role of communicators, be it media, experts or lobbyists, to define the context for policy making and comment on the possible consequences of policy' (Gibson, 2003).
- Technical rationality is typically dominated by positivist science, and is the primary product of the research community, often aiming and claiming to generate universally applicable findings. Commonly it accepts certain assumptions about what is already proven or demonstrated, and

has particular evidential rules. These notionally universal and evidence-based findings, however, may lack credibility to the health policy-maker facing decision making in a specific context and setting, and who may not agree that these rules of evidence have a valid claim to represent the only or preferred route to truth.

On occasions, the three rationalities will be compatible, and there are multiple examples through this work of policy initiatives where this has been the case. However, equally often the three rationalities are in tension, and dialogue between them arises because the questions being posed are different, reflect differing value systems or the paradigms underpinning them are not commensurable (see Chapter 1.4). Activities across the translational science spectrum can allow investigation of the influences of how these rationalities may be better informed (see Chapter 1.4). In an example of what might be seen as an attempt to increase the degree of worthwhile communication between these three rationalities, we can chart some increasing influence in Australia of the construct of Values Based Health care Commissioning (Victorian Agency for Health Information, 2019); the construct is well established as influential in services in the United Kingdom and in some sectors in the United States. At the core of this construct lies a proposition that health care should ensure prioritisation is given to securing outcomes that matter most to consumers or patients. Derived from this we can find tools, defined processes and accounts of experience that can be useful in pursuing this line of action. At time of writing, it seems this may be a term that will become increasingly influential in health care generally and in mental health care also. For instance, 2019 has seen the establishment of the Australian Centre for Values Based Health Care (Victorian Agency for Health Information, 2019; Gentry & Badrinath, 2017). The central ethos of the values based health care approach seems closely aligned with the key tenets of recovery oriented practice so we may anticipate that convergence between these two areas of influence on policy might well increase over time.

THE NATURE OF PROGRESS

In a consideration of mental health policy in the United States over time (Frank & Glied, 2006), the authors identified various ways in which progress can occur in mental health care (see Section 1.1.4). Familiar generally is the idea of adoption of innovations; that is, new or improved actions in care. Within this they identified two main kinds of change: efficacy advances, within which more beneficial forms of care become ascendant, and practice advances, where a new treatment may become adopted, not because it is more effective, but because it is better tolerated or easier to prescribe. The authors also coined the term exnovation, referring to the abandonment of outmoded or disproven treatments. Reviewing the history of changes in practice over the later part of the twentieth century based on a range of sources, the conclusion reached was that the major efficacy advances occurred earlier in this period; later advances were more dependent on practice advance and exnovation.

To summarise one example, in the case of schizophrenia: during the mid-part of the twentieth century the antipsychotics were introduced, bringing about a revolution in the responses available to schizophrenia. Later in the century, efficacy advances were more limited, featuring, for instance, the introduction of clozapine as an efficacy advance for people with resistant conditions, but without the same revolutionary impact. In contrast, practice advances were many, with, for instance, numerous better tolerated antipsychotics introduced. Exnovation played an important role, with the abandonment of insulin coma therapy and primary treatment with psychodynamic therapy for this condition as coming to be seen as techniques unsupported by evidence.

EQUITY ISSUES, TESTING THE BOUNDARIES OF MENTAL HEALTH POLICY MAKING

We have elsewhere (see Chapter 1.2) briefly described Wilkinson and Pickett's work on social determinants of health, including what we see as a reasonable inference regarding a causal relationship between the gaps between rich and poor in developed countries and rates of mental illness. So a measure that likely would positively impact mental health in Australia would be to reverse what seems to be a trend towards increasing inequality in this country (see Section 1.2.4). It would be in alignment with the UN Strategic Development Goals (see Section 1.2.3). But this would involve changes in taxation policy that would typically not be considered under the influence of mental health policymakers. It may be though that this could be a fundamental cause of why increased spending on mental health care is not achieving population health change. The capacity of increasing inequality in society to increase underlying prevalence may be simply overwhelming the effect achievable from mental care interventions, especially since there is good evidence that these are poorly targeted to those who through the effect of social determinants need them most (Meadows, Enticott, & Rosenberg, 2019; Meadows, Prodan, et al., 2019b).

1.5.4 FUNDING MENTAL HEALTH CARE

GRAHAM MEADOWS & MARGARET GRIGG

RESOURCE DISTRIBUTION

Health care is not typically regarded as an ideal market where individuals–as one party–might assess their needs and decide what they would purchase from a provider–as a second party. There is rather, typically seen as being a degree of intrinsic failure of a market model and a need for third-party payers through, for instance, private insurance or sometimes employers (Beauchamp & Childress, 2019). In Australia as in many countries the largest contribution to such funding flows is through government intervention in health care–which can be considered as having features of four major kinds of system (Frogner, Hussey, & Anderson, 2011):

- social insurance: where multiple insurance companies operate within the state-funded environment, typically from payroll taxes; the prototype here would be Germany
- national health service: centralised systems with direct provision, prototypically the United Kingdom
- national health insurance: centralised systems funding private provision, prototypically Canada
- private insurance: multiple insurance providers with relatively small involvement of government funding streams restricted to specific eligible groups; prototypically the United States.

Australia has something of a hybrid system (Duckett & Willcox, 2015) with features of a national health insurance scheme in the way that Medicare federally funds rebates for practitioners, with features of a national health service in the way that state and territory services operate as providers funded directly by government, and with supplementary private insurance encouraged with tax incentives.

One of the challenges for development and implementation of funding models in mental health care is to achieve reasonable levels of equity in access to care for different groups in society (Duckett & Willcox, 2015). Working towards more equitable mental health care (see Section 1.2.4) may involve trying to reduce the extent to which gender, income or location influence access and the relative quality of care received. A particular problem in mental health care is great variation in prevalence rates across areas. Some locations may involve more stress which might precipitate mental illness (*social causation*)–people with serious mental health problems often move into areas where rental accommodation, including accommodation suitable for single occupancy, is cheap and readily available–an example of *social drift*. This phenomenon was first demonstrated in Chicago the better part of a century ago (Faris & Dunham, 1939). This movement in turn can be into areas that are otherwise socioeconomically deprived, and where services and infrastructure may be proportionally lacking. The evolution of Australian cities has meant that poorer areas often are away from the central areas of the city, and may have poor associated infrastructure so isolation and poor access to social and care (O'Hanlon, 2018) where the lack of resources can add to the impact of socioeconomic deprivation as a determinant of mental health problems (see Section 1.2.4). Much of the health funding as administered by the Commonwealth is not well structured to ameliorating these inequities, since fee-for-item-of-service remuneration can be drawn upon anywhere and the permitting of co-payment can make practice in more affluent areas more attractive to practitioners. This pattern is very much in evidence in contemporary mental health care where for instance private psychological services—as heavily subsidised by Medicare—are concentrated in more affluent areas where there is less absolute need for those services (see Chapter 1.2). Where services are block funded, more along the lines of the NHS model above, it can be possible to estimate needs of areas and adjust resource levels accordingly. Often such needs assessment involves development of a Resource Distribution Formula (RDF)—see for instance Meadows et al. (1997)—which may include dimensions such as:

1 poverty, introduced above as a driver of urban drift
2 demographic structure of the population, which influences prevalence rates (see Chapter 1.6)
3 Indigenous persons, where these populations have need of special consideration
4 homelessness, within which context rates of disorder may be much higher
5 rurality, which can influence needs and costs.

This applies generally in state services and also to some federally funded initiatives such as ATAPS (see Section 1.4.11), and other services where block funding goes to PHNs. There are formulae for doing this to provide for transparency of distribution of resources between areas, and something like this approach has been used to distribute funds for ATAPS. The ABS produces a set of composite socioeconomic indicators for areas (SEIFA) which can be useful in such work. However, at the time of writing this approach is not, typically, explicitly and transparently adopted in Australian jurisdictions.

THE AUSTRALIAN NATIONAL MENTAL HEALTH SERVICES PLANNING FRAMEWORK

It was a commitment in the Fourth National Mental Health Plan 'to develop a national service planning framework that establishes targets for the mix and level of the full range of mental health services, backed by innovative funding models' (Australian Government, 2009a).The key output of work commissioned over several years to fulfil this commitment is a planning support tool (PST) designed mainly for hospital and other mental health service providers as well as Primary Health Networks. Despite the fact that the planning framework has been established as a commercial-in-confidence product, some elements of this PST have been made public (National Mental Health Service Planning Framework 2020). The tool requires considerable training for proficient use. Four key processes underpinning the PST include:

1 Estimating the number of people in a defined population with mental illness in a year, by age and levels of severity, and sets service demand targets for those who will require intervention (epidemiology);
2 Describing the full spectrum of interventions from self-help, digital and low intensity interventions to primary and specialist clinical treatment, to mental health community support services (taxonomy and staffing profiles);
3 Describing service needs within age and severity target groups, including types of intervention, intensity, provider and current funder (care profiles and funder type); and
4 Drawing on all of the above, produces resource estimates to deliver those interventions over a 12-month period.

A limitation of the PST, at least as it stands at time of writing this text, is that beyond some demographic influences it does not provide need estimates, as an RDF would, that take into account social determinants of mental health problems and their possible effect on population needs (see Section 1.2.4).

ACTIVITY BASED FUNDING

Considerable efforts at Commonwealth (Independent Hospital Pricing Authority (IHPA), 2020) and state levels have been going into development of Activity Based Funding (ABF) in mental health—a process whereby reimbursement relates to treated client/patient characteristics. In mental health care, cost drivers that consistently and desirably relate to clinical or other client characteristics have proved challenging to determine but it can be reasonably anticipated that ABF will gain influence through time in Australia, its states and territories. With greater movement towards ABF comes the challenge of ensuring that services are targeted towards those whose need is greatest and that they are more concentrated in areas where there are more such people. This then involves ideally some integration of work on RDF and ABF models and the largest flows of block funding in Australia are through state funding streams. At time of writing there is no Commonwealth-endorsed RDF that would augment the work on the National Mental Health Service Planning Framework PST (see Section 1.5.4). Since in any case the decision making lies with the states and territories it is unclear that such a formula would necessarily be consistently or widely adopted. To return to concepts introduced in Section 1.5.3 the considerations involve elements of cultural and political rationalities as much as technical aspects.

Within the Better Access initiative (see Section 1.7.2) as funded through the Commonwealth there is considerable specification of who may provide what kinds of care to people with which kinds of problems. Here, and in considering what may be eligible for ABF remuneration, again the development of funding models has reflected interchanges as much determined by political and cultural rationalities as technical ones. An important technical advance in distribution of health care was made when the Quality and Disability Adjusted Life Years (QALY/DALY) were introduced to support allocative decisions in health care (Glied & Smith, 2011). Mental health problems tend to more greatly affect time lived with reduced quality or greater disability than mortality so mortality-based approaches to resource allocation between major health care domains will typically determine less funding going to mental health care than will QALY/DALY based approaches that take into account time lived with reduced quality or with disability as part of the measure of the effect of the targeted problem. It might be argued that a technically optimised approach to resource distribution would involve a QALY/DALY based determination of what should be funded in mental health care which then informed area-specific estimation of need for the specific interventions and commissioning accordingly. Competing considerations in the other defined rationalities and the related role of values based commissioning (see Section 1.5.3) along with the fragmentation of the Australian Health Care system (see Chapter 1.7) mean that this technical solution seems unlikely to become a dominant or even common model in Australia's mental health care system.

1.5.5 PREVENTIVE MODELS

GRAHAM MEADOWS

INTRODUCTION

Preventive health care involves both actions that prevent disease occurrence and those aimed at eradicating, eliminating, or minimising the impact of disease and disability. If none of these is feasible, then the concept can extend to retarding the progress of disease and disability (Porta, Greenland, Hernán, dos Santos Silva, & Last, 2014). Prevention then is potentially a very broad concept which can be considered as an overarching framework for much of health and mental health care. In common use however it tends to focus attention on efforts to avoid development of risk factors, or incident disorder, along with interventions seeking to intervene earlier than might otherwise be the case in more routine clinical care. This account will focus on thinking around a categorical illness and disease paradigm but elements of such thinking also can be applied where a more dimensional construct of mental wellbeing and ill health is being applied.

LEVELS OF PREVENTION

One framework with longstanding influence in health care (Caplan & Felix, 1964) identifies prevention as primary, secondary, and tertiary; this has in recent times been expanded by other authors to include, bracketing these three, prevention considered as primordial, and quaternary

1 Primordial prevention (Porta et al., 2014), which can be seen either as separate or as a form of primary prevention, involves efforts to reduce the frequency with which adverse risk factors develop. Often targeting periods early in the life course, or even before conception, interventions may for instance address the role of nutritional or lifestyle factors in such risk factor development. This can involve action across a wide span of social policy including addressing social determinants of mental health problems (see Section 1.2.4).
2 Primary prevention, or alternatively within this, what is left after we have considered primordial prevention, aims to reduce incidence of health problems through collective or individual actions. Actions in this sphere are often classed also as health promotion. Through primary prevention it is sought to influence environmental exposures of different kinds and so to minimise the extent to which people's individual and collective risk factors combine causally with these influences so that a disorder episode occurs.
3 Secondary prevention aims to improve disease and disorder outcomes in terms of either earlier remission or improved experience through the course of the problem. Often this will involve seeking to detect and treat cases earlier when interventions may be more effective.
4 Tertiary prevention addresses reduction in longer-term impact of health including reducing suffering, improving quality of life, with reduction in impairment, disability, and handicap considered as features of disability. Traditionally classed as interventions under the framework of rehabilitation, in contemporary mental health care this indicates engagement also with the propositions around recovery and recovery oriented practice.
5 Quaternary prevention (Porta et al., 2014; Jamoulle, 2015). Here we address the occurrence and consequences of iatrogenesis, through practices and policies that can identify and intervene with people at risk at least of clinical iatrogenesis. Elsewhere in the literature (Meadows, Prodan, et al., 2019a) and in this chapter (see Section 1.5.2) we have argued that in the case of mental health at least the concepts of social and cultural iatrogenesis may also be important to consider as well as that of clinical iatrogenesis and there is a substantial, often quite polarising, critical literature proposing that over-medicalisation (Horwitz & Wakefield 2007) and over-medication are problems of contemporary mental health care.

A SPECTRUM OF INTERVENTIONS INCLUDING PREVENTION

A further influential piece of thinking around mental health care and prevention involves placing preventive actions within a wider framework of interventions (Mrazek & Haggerty, 1994; National Academy of Sciences, 2009) and so it is likely in the mental health literature that terms from this model will also be encountered. In contrast to the above grouping which concentrates on causality, this framework groups interventions around the target groups for this intervention and the nature of the intervention, so examples may be found across various combinations of categories 1–5. In this spectrum model, we can identify interventions grouped as follows:

Health promotion: preventive health care, with terms from the source documents in italics:

- *Universal preventive interventions.* Here the target may be the whole population or some specified subgroup but the strategy targets people whose risk is average.
- *Selective preventive interventions* aim their interventions at identifiable subgroups whose risk is understood to be above average, which may be considered over shorter or longer timespans.
- *Indicated preventive interventions.* Here the interventions are targeted at people who have some indications of disorder, where these are low-level at time of interventions but where these states are known to usefully predict transition to later disorders.

Treatment, including:

- *Case identification.* Self-identification and presenting for care here may be complemented by screening and identification by families or sometimes workers in other services (see Section 1.4.7).
- *Standard treatment for known disorders.* Here resides much of conventional health care which if practiced in alignment with Evidence-Based Practice principles or those of recovery oriented practice will combine professional understandings of relevant information about treatment options with collaborative decision making.

Maintenance, including:

- *Compliance with long-term treatment* with the goal of reduction in relapse and recurrence. This framing of longer-term care may be seen as rather dated now, and contemporary practice might rather emphasise consumer engagement and collaborative informed and the new terms are taken from source documents (National Academy of Sciences, 2009; Mrazek & Haggerty, 1994).
- Aftercare (including rehabilitation). Again a more contemporary framing would include attention to collaborative pursuit of recovery goals.

THE RANGE OF PREVENTIVE ACTIVITIES

Having introduced some of these key concepts around prevention, Figure 1.21 gathers together some thinking about current options for preventive activities. If we take a broad approach to consideration of these issues then some important risk factors to attend to in preventive activities involve social determinants of mental health problems (see Section 1.2.4). In this context, many actions that might be indicated either through preventive frameworks or through the approaches advocated by the WHO regarding these factors (World Health Organization and Calouste Gulbenkian Foundation, 2014), could be seen as involving large-scale social change where decision making lies well outside the conventional scope of mental health policy (see Chapter 1.2 and Section 1.5.3).

EVIDENCE AND INVESTMENT

The relative degree to which there should be investment in preventive interventions of various kinds involves complicated decision making in policy contexts. There is evidence that investment in preventive interventions may be cost effective, but the making of preventive investment may involve diversion or opportunity costs in regards to other parts of models described above. Often benefits of preventive interventions may be described in review papers as 'small' or 'modest' (Mendelson & Eaton, 2018; Arango et al., 2018). So the cost effectiveness of the preventive investment may need to be carefully considered in relation to the benefit forgone if other phases of care have resources withdrawn. Prediction of who may benefit from secondary, selected or indicated prevention or active case identification involves prediction of unmodified course and weighing up of the balance of positive and negative effects including the broad range of possible iatrogenic effects (see Section 1.5.2). So, put otherwise, active interventions of these kinds raise challenges us with consideration of quaternary prevention. The ethical considerations here are complex (see Section 2.3.15); sometimes active intervention to prevent an incident case in one person may necessitate some false positives who also receive the intervention but were not destined to have developed the disorder. They may have negative effects from stigma, internal or external, and other possible iatrogenic influences may cause them harm. This kind of trade-off has been explored in philosophy through the thought experiment of the 'Trolley problem' (Andrade, 2019). We should note that there have been examples where initially promising findings for preventive interventions have not been found to translate as these are scaled up (Fusar-Poli et al., 2019). This may involve the effects of the implementation cliff (see Section 1.4.18), or the implications of changed function of screening strategies as interventions (see Section 1.4.7) are moved out into less specialist health care settings.

Wide scale investment in preventive strategies involves anticipation of benefit in the future from actions taken now. In many cases the investment may be anticipated to have effects for the long-term, perhaps

Figure 1.21 Risk factors for mental disorders in sensitive periods of intervention

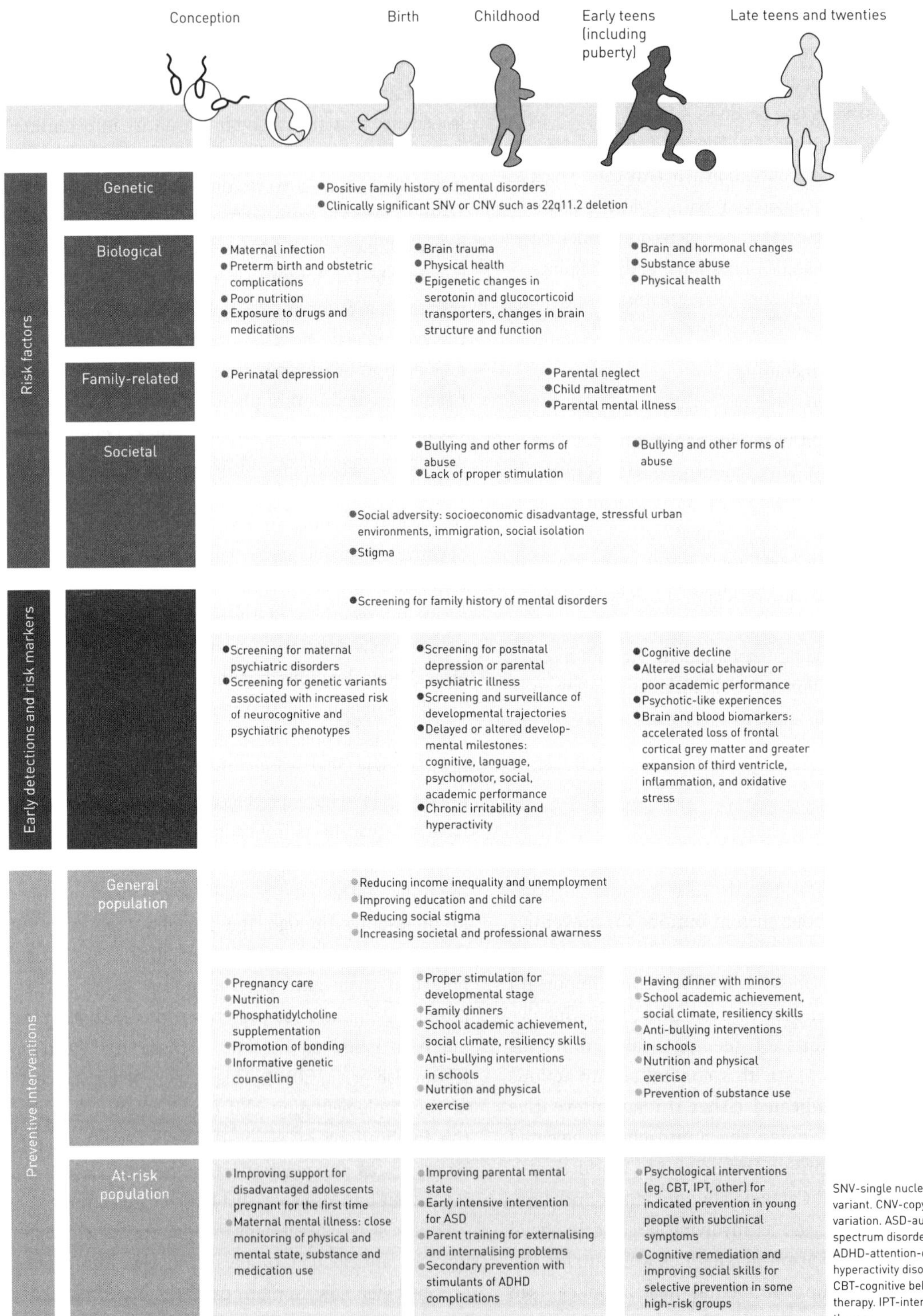

SNV-single nucleotide variant. CNV-copy number variation. ASD-autism spectrum disorders. ADHD-attention-deficit hyperactivity disorder. CBT-cognitive behavioural therapy. IPT-interpersonal therapy.

Source: Arango, 2018

several decades. Practically then the information about the intervention typically cannot be collected across such timespans before decisions about action need to be made. Support for such decisions then may involve forecasting tools and this is an increasingly sophisticated technology area (Long, McDermott, & Meadows, 2018; Lawton, 2019). Simulation modelling involving techniques such as Markov Models, Discrete Event Simulation, System Dynamics or Agent Based Models may all have application to contemporary quandaries about apportioning investment in preventive strategies. But these models are often complex to set up, and involve technical appraisal of likely validity that is different from the range of understandings typically held by health care professionals and many academics. Not uncommonly we can find assertions about financial gains or other benefits to be anticipated from a particular investment being claimed based on a model but with a duly critical eye we may find that the model is not clearly presented or described such that we have an opportunity adequately to consider its credibility to us. Different modelling approaches or parameter-setting choices can have substantial effects on outcomes, sometimes making the difference between something that looks convincingly worth substantial added or diverted investment, or with an alternative model, something that is unlikely to yield any really meaningful benefit (Atkinson et al., 2019). Simulation modelling is likely to have increasing influence over the coming years, so we devote some attention to this in Section 1.5.11. Full appraisal of the literature relevant to decision making about setting priorities in such areas will involve at least some ability to appraise publications of this type. When publications are in peer reviewed journals and cite adherence to key guidelines regarding preparation and presentation of such models (see Section 1.5.11) this presents some safeguard. Alternatively, if the reader comes across publications in reports that do not cite such guidelines or evidence of peer review, and where models are not well described either in their form or with attention to the information base supporting parameter-setting, then lack sensitivity analyses that might suggest what the uncertainty properties of modelling are, then there may be reasons to choose not to rely on the outputs of the model.

SUICIDE PREVENTION

One way in which preventive and service delivery considerations are brought together is the domain of concern of reducing suicide rates. Analyses of the problem typically identify that suicide has multiple contributing causes, many of which are not under direct control of mental health services, or even health services more broadly. Many people who suicide have not been in contact with mental health services in the period leading up to the act and among those who have attended, risk assessment in prediction of suicide acts is challenging and will always be an imperfect process (see Chapter 2.3). At time of writing, suicide rates in Australia have been rising for some years, returning towards very long-term norms (Jorm, 2019; Bastiampillai, Allison, Looi, Tavella, & Agis, 2020) and with evidence of widening social inequality (Too, Law, Spittal, Page, & Milner, 2018). There are real concerns that the effects of the COVID-19 pandemic as affecting Australia may negatively impact this further (see Section 1.2.5). Importantly, the effect of an event such as COVID-19 can be expected to be mediated by changes in social determinants including unemployment, financial stress and social isolation. So comprehensive approaches to addressing this problem involve actions at community levels and can be considered in relation to the approaches to addressing social determinants of mental health considered elsewhere (see Chapter 1.2). This has been a target of some applications of simulation modelling (see Atkinson et al., 2019; Section 1.5.11). For consideration of the actions that mental health services—along with other agencies—might take in this area, the following citations are examples of key strategy documents: Department of Health and Ageing, 2012a; Department of Health and Human Services, 2016; Mental Health Commission of NSW, 2018. Some examples of active programs in the area include The Hospital Outreach Post-suicidal Engagement (HOPE) initiative (State Government of Victoria, 2020; Department of Health and Human Services, 2016), and 29 national and state-based suicide prevention trial sites across Australia, comprised of 12 National Suicide Prevention Trials (Department of Health and Ageing, 2012b), 12 Victorian place-based trials (Department of Health and Human Services, 2016), plus one ACT and four NSW LifeSpan research trials (Black Dog Institute, 2020; Mental Health Commission of NSW, 2018).

1.5.6 STEPPED CARE

GRAHAM MEADOWS & SEBASTIAN ROSENBERG

An influential conceptualisation of how a mental health care system works in practice identified four filters (F1-4) and five levels (L1-5) through which a person with mental illness might pass (Goldberg & Huxley, 1980). First, among all people with mental health problems in the community (L1), self-recognition of having a problem and the decision to seek help (F1) influence whether symptoms are presented to any part of the health care system, and in the most general case the commonest place for such problems to be presented is in primary care, including general medical practice (L2). F2 is the effective recognition of mental health problems by the practitioner, leading to the opportunity for some service response in primary care (L3). F3 operates in referral to specialist care (L4) while F4 operates at the level of decision to admit to hospital (L5). So, hospital inpatients at L5 are very different in characteristics from typical people in the community with mental health problems (L1), having passed through four filters. The filters model has been influential in the development of 'stepped care' models, which can be considered as involving active manipulations of the filters.

In some stepped care work, the assumption has been that people firstly be offered a low intensity intervention and then stepped up to greater intensity if they do not respond to the first intervention. Commonly, recent presentations of the concept give greater weight to the idea that in a stepped care approach, a person presenting to the mental health system is matched to the intervention level that most suits their current need. An individual does not generally have to start at the lowest, least intensive level of intervention in order to progress to the next 'step'. Rather, they enter the system and have their service level aligned to their requirements. The implementation then shares common content with ideas of staging (see Chapters 2.3, 4.2) in mental health care.

The stepped care approach gained momentum in Australia in the Federal Government's response to the review into mental health care conducted by

Figure 1.22 Productivity Commission overview draft report

Estimated number of people requiring each level of care

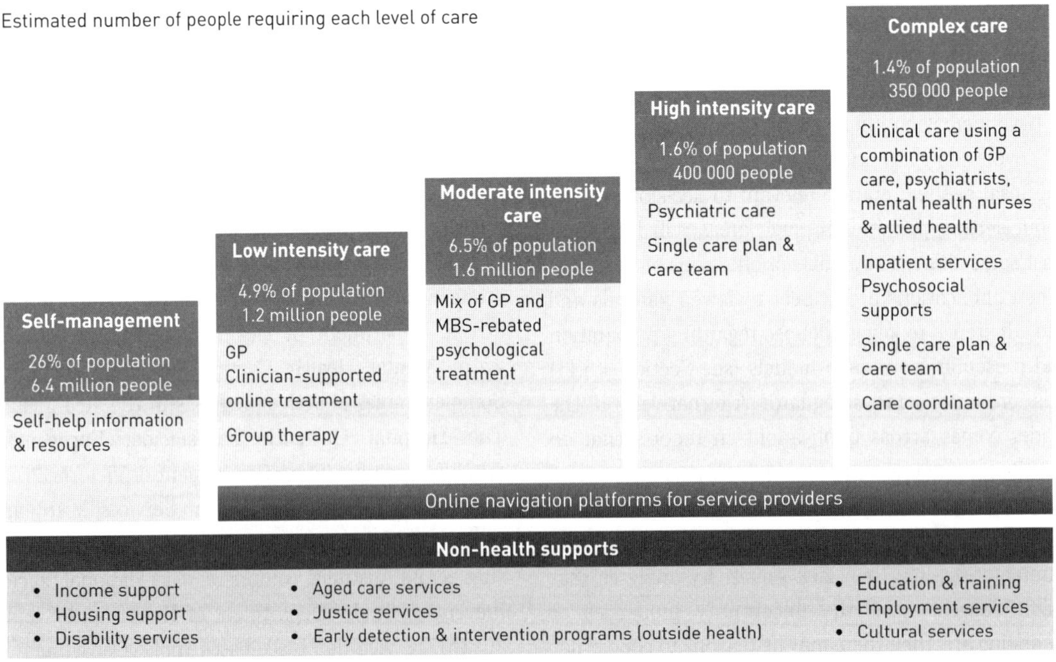

Self-management
26% of population
6.4 million people
Self-help information & resources

Low intensity care
4.9% of population
1.2 million people
GP
Clinician-supported online treatment
Group therapy

Moderate intensity care
6.5% of population
1.6 million people
Mix of GP and MBS-rebated psychological treatment

High intensity care
1.6% of population
400 000 people
Psychiatric care
Single care plan & care team

Complex care
1.4% of population
350 000 people
Clinical care using a combination of GP care, psychiatrists, mental health nurses & allied health
Inpatient services
Psychosocial supports
Single care plan & care team
Care coordinator

Online navigation platforms for service providers

Non-health supports
- Income support
- Housing support
- Disability services
- Aged care services
- Justice services
- Early detection & intervention programs (outside health)
- Education & training
- Employment services
- Cultural services

Source: Australian Government, 2019a

the National Mental Health Commission (Australian Government, 2015b). This response mandated stepped care as a preferred guiding strategy by which to plan and fund mental health. Stepped care has become highly influential in planning processes developed by the Primary Health Networks in Australia, which are constrained to follow directives from the Australian Government Department of Health (DoH). For these purposes, stepped care is defined (Australian Government, 2019b) as 'an evidence-based, staged system comprising a hierarchy of interventions, from the least to the most intensive, matched to the individual's needs.' It has been identified as including four core elements:

1 stratification of the population into different 'needs groups', ranging from whole of population needs for mental health promotion and prevention, through to those with severe, persistent and complex conditions
2 setting interventions for each group—this is necessary because not all needs require formal intervention
3 defining a comprehensive 'menu' of evidence-based services required to respond to the spectrum of need and
4 matching service types to the treatment targets for each needs group and commissioning/delivering services accordingly.

1.5.7 DISASTER PREPAREDNESS AND RESPONSE

GRAHAM MEADOWS & JOHN FARHALL

> Her beauty and her terror...
>
> *Dorothea MacKellar, 1908*

INCREASING RISKS

Any nation or community can face natural disasters but there are specific regional vulnerabilities. Australia, while for instance geologically relatively stable compared to neighbouring New Zealand or Indonesia, has other vulnerabilities. Over a century ago Dorothea Mackellar (MacKellar, 2016) characterised the country as 'of droughts and flooding rains' and of 'terror'—something recently particularly evident through global heating (CSIRO, 2018) and associated related increase in bushfire frequency and severity. So for this text the role of mental health services and clinicians in disaster preparedness and response will be considered through the perspective offered by response to bushfires. As a section in a general text, we will attempt here to cover this issue only briefly—readers actively involved in such response should usefully refer to key texts (e.g. Ursano, Fullerton, Weisaeth, & Raphael, 2017) but some points made from this consideration may also be more widely relevant.

PREPAREDNESS

While some aspects of disasters are not foreseeable, contingency planning can improve response times and the appropriateness of that response. Regional and rural areas hence need local planning to anticipate local risks and related plans. Mental Health Service involvement through both state-funded mental health *services* and Primary Health Networks here needs to involve a response across health sectors so represents a challenge for integrated planning processes (Australian Government: The Department of Health, 2018) as well as coordination with emergency services, Centrelink and even the Defence Force. Relevant here will be some of the issues raised in consideration of addressing social determinants in humanitarian relief settings (see Section 1.2.4).

RESPONSE

The narrative around development of strategies for disaster response is an interesting one from the point of view of Evidence Based Practice (EBP; see Section 4.4.9). A technique termed 'psychological debriefing', with a specific variant of 'critical incident stress debriefing' (CISD), gained popularity for some years and often involved inviting all who had experienced the event to a group single-session intervention supporting reconsideration of the events within a proposed processing model. But as evidence accumulated

(Wessely, Rose, & Bisson, 2000), it became apparent that the technique could have negative effects of 'serial revivification and heightened arousal' along with unhelpful pathologising of symptoms (Devilly, Gist, & Cotton, 2006) and greater risk of PTSD (see Section 4.4.4) rather than having the intended prevention benefit. Further multi-session interventions seeking to reduce risks of PTSD in those exposed to trauma have not accumulated convincing evidence, based on a further Cochrane review (Roberts et al., 2019) which noted deficiencies in the research including the common failure of a lack of attention to negative effects. A more contemporary view of mental health needs in the face of disaster response is that most people will not require any specialist intervention because natural coping processes and supports will do their job and can be supported (Wade, Forbes, Nursey, & Creamer, 2013). Principles of response can perhaps be well summarised as:

> Successful responses will generally deal with practical and instrumental needs ... provide structure and continuity, validate concerns and provide a sense of presence and care, and take measures to ensure that any in need of specialised attention are recognised and receive timely referral to appropriate avenues of effective intervention (Devilly et al., 2006).

In 2009, the Black Saturday fires in Victoria led to the greatest ever loss of life from an Australian bushfire. Findings of a Royal Commission into the fires led to substantial changes in emergency management advice and practice and the 2020 catastrophic fires which affected a larger area were accompanied by much less loss of life. In terms of lessons for mental health services following the 2009 fires there was a substantial state government led response which was able to make use of learnings from the literature around psychological debriefing and attend to quaternary prevention by avoiding widespread use of psychological debriefing. The response, developed with support from a rapid literature review (Hawe, 2009) followed a clearly set out psychosocial recovery framework (State of Victoria: Department of Human Services, 2009) and involved Australian adaptation of a training package termed Skills for Psychological Recovery (Wade et al., 2014) developed in the United States. Some key principles from the state framework were that:

> Recovery from extreme experiences is facilitated when the resilience of affected people is recognised and is accompanied by information about associated health issues including: the impacts, effects and normal responses of such experiences; indicators of stress and strategies for managing this; the importance of using existing support networks; and information about how and when to access other services for additional support (State of Victoria: Department of Human Services, 2009).

Key processes in the intervention involve consideration of: information and prioritising, problem-solving skills, positive activities, managing reactions, helpful thinking, and healthy connections (Wade et al., 2013). This led to a multilevel intervention strategy which usefully encapsulates how mental health workers and planners might understand mental health disaster responses to address the range of needs (Wade et al., 2013; Wade, Forbes, Nursey, & Creamer, 2012).

1 Psychological first aid to reduce initial distress and to promote adaptive coping and connection with wanted others. This should be followed by community development programmes to bring people together around re-building
2 Help for persisting mild and sub-clinical conditions via trained primary care and community workers, with the aim of wide dissemination of Practical Skills for Psychological Recovery
3 Psychological interventions for diagnosable mental health conditions—required for a significant minority

Follow-up findings from a long-term study emphasised the resilience of communities affected but also the increased incidence and prevalence of mental health problems and the need to work to identify people at higher need of specialist input who might need more rapid 'stepping up' (see Section 1.5.6) with important risk factors identified as 'living in a high impact community, fear of dying at the time of the disaster, loss of someone close (including friends and community members), separation from family members at the time of the disaster, experiencing major life stressors after the disaster, intense anger, and living alone'.

1.5.8 RECOVERY TRANSFORMATION

GRAHAM MEADOWS

To transform services towards this agenda will require intervention at multiple levels in this service system. Slade and colleagues have identified seven key actions involved:

1 lead the process
2 articulate and use values
3 maximise pro-recovery orientation among workers
4 develop specific pro-recovery skills in the workforce
5 make role models visible
6 evaluate success in relation to social roles and goal attainment
7 amplify the power of consumers (Slade, Johnson, Oakley Brown, Andrews, & Whiteford, 2009).

In relation to these actions, a substantial research project reported in 2019 (Meadows, Brophy, et al., 2019) on work that took place with an Australian adaptation of work from Mike Slade's team. Using a cluster RCT methodology with an adaptation known as a stepped wedge design, and spanning multiple specialist mental health care providers, the study identified positive changes at level 6 based on interventions targeting at least actions 2-5. So this gives some encouragement that this transformation is at least possible.

Embedding such change though would also require changes in key performance indicators (KPIs). To give an example, services regularly have to report on variables such as readmission and seclusion rates, while there is usually no such formal accountability in place regarding social roles or a recovery orientation. While of necessity any attempt to construct KPIs for large-scale use in organisations risks a simplification of subtle underlying constructs, it would be an interesting shift of set in relation to these accountabilities if some novel KPIs came into use. In the last edition of this text we suggested a possible recovery KPI. This was the proportion of people who endorse 'strongly agree' among a range of response options to this regular questionnaire item: 'In the last year, the staff of this service have regularly discussed my values, treatment preferences and my individual strengths with me while working to identify my goals and help me to meet these'. This still might represent a minimal approach to gathering some useful information but to our knowledge it has never been trialled. There do however exist questionnaires that capture something of the recovery experience (Neil et al., 2009; Williams et al., 2015) including having had some psychometric work done (Argentzell, Hultqvist, Neil, & Eklund, 2017).

1.5.9 TELEWEB MENTAL HEALTH SERVICES

ALAN WOODWARD

IMPETUS FOR TELEWEB

TeleWeb, or digital services in mental health, have emerged in the past 50-60 years as components of the wider mental health service system. These services utilise technologies for contact and communication between people, in contrast to personal or 'face-to-face' interactions.

Another term often used for technology oriented service provision is eMental Health (eMH). This term was adopted by the Australian Government in 2012 with the launch of the first national eMental Health Strategy. A definition of eMH is 'the delivery of services targeting common mental health problems through online and mobile phone interactive websites, apps, sensor-based monitoring devices and computers' (Australian Government: Department of Health, 2012). The term also extends to telephone crisis lines and online crisis support services. eMH services are delivered in real-time through multiple settings, including the home, the workplace, schools, and through clinicians' workplaces.

Their development reflects the movement of new technologies into wider society, firstly with the telephone in Western countries to a more common place in individual and family lives, through to the arrival of personal computers in the 1980s and the internet from the 1990s. More recently, the introduction of social media and mobile device applications has changed again the nature of the technologies associated with 'teleweb' to the extent that a more current definition of technology operated mental health services would be 'digital mental health services'. This term was reflected in the Australian Government announcement in 2016 of an online Digital Mental Health Gateway to encourage community and professional use of these services (this is now known as Head To Health). Many services also now refer to themselves as digital mental health services and the related service improvement terminology of Digital Transformation and Digital Access has been more widely seen.

Digital Mental Health Services have particular attributes and benefits associated with technology-based communications. They also have limitations and challenges. It is not fruitful to attempt to directly compare these services with face-to-face services; each mode of communication has benefits and pitfalls. Rather, it is useful to consider the circumstances, audiences and intended service outcomes that best match particular modes of communication.

Their emergence and acceptance to a large extent across the population reflects the modern reality in Australia and globally that interactions between people are now occurring through mixed modes of communication and in increasingly different and more dynamic ways. The potential benefits therefore for mental health and wellbeing outcomes, as well as suicide prevention, to be addressed through a wider range of options for service delivery has been a fundamental motivation for the development of teleweb and digital mental health services. It is important for mental health consumers, professionals and workers, as well as policy makers and funding agencies, to be familiar with the range of and applications for digital mental health services.

CONSUMER USE OF DIGITAL MENTAL HEALTH SERVICES

It is not surprising that the increased use of technology enabled contact and communication in Australian society has been matched with uptakes in use of digital mental health services and related supports and suicide prevention resources. Australians are known for their early adoption of technologies; telecommunications have featured in our lives and have been used to overcome the vast distances and geographic spread of the Australian population. In many respects, the use of these technologies for our mental health and wellbeing may be seen as aligned to directions in the delivery of all services in Australia.

Australian population use of all mental health services has been examined through the ABS National Mental Health and Wellbeing Survey data (see Section 1.6.2). A key result from this survey is that 11.9% of the general Australian adult population make use of any services for mental health problems in a 12-month period. For those who meet a criteria for a mental disorder, the survey results show only approximately one-third of people (34.9%) in that category do so (Burgess et al., 2009). More recent data analysis to model the proportion of people with mental health problems that access services in Australia has found that the estimated population treatment rate for mental disorders in Australia increased to 46% in 2009-10 (Whiteford et al., 2014). Despite this increase, the statistics reflect a substantial unmet need in the Australian population for mental health services and supports.

The ABS survey data also records that 3.7% of Australian population in 2007 reported having used telephone counselling for problems with mental health in their lifetime. Of those who had used telephone counselling, about one-quarter (24.6%) had done so in the past 12 months. So, around 1% of the Australian population used telephone counselling in the past 12 months (Bassilios, Harris, Middleton, Gunn, & Pirkis, 2015). This survey data is now somewhat dated—more than 10 years since collected—yet it demonstrates that digital mental health services feature in the overall mix of services being used by Australians.

The potential for use of digital mental health services for particular population groups is greater. Research undertaken through the Young and Well Co-operative Research Centre found the following:

Young people reported using the internet to connect with other young people (76.9%; 1464/1905) and to seek information about a mental health problem, regardless of whether they had a problem themselves (38.8%; 735/1894). Twenty per cent of young people (398/1990) had personally experienced a mental health problem in the previous 5 years; when these people were asked about sources of information used for this problem, 30.8% (70/227) reported searching the internet (Burns, Davenport, Durkin, Luscombe, & Hickie, 2010).

Digital Mental Health Services may attract persons who otherwise will not seek or access mental health services, thereby suggesting that technology enabled service provision can perform a significant role in population level mental health promotion and prevention. This is relevant at a population level given the under-use of mental health services by those who would benefit from these services. It is particularly pertinent with regard to younger persons, given the emergence of mental health disorders before the age of 24 years, and because younger persons—notably males—are even less likely to access mental health services through conventional means. The ABS National Survey of Mental Health and Wellbeing (2007; see Section 1.6.2), for instance, records that while 26.4% of those aged between 16 and 24 years had a mental health disorder, only 13.2% of young males and 31.2% of young females used a clinical mental health service to address their mental health problems (Burgess, Pirkis, Slade, Johnston, Meadows, Gunn. 2009).

Moreover, the potential for technology enabled services to offer evidence-based treatments has been established, especially with regard to CBT and other depression and anxiety treatments, signalling a role beyond simply getting people through the door to one of actual intervention and recovery support. In this respect, digital mental health services offer an alternative mechanism for service provision that can overcome workforce availability and geographic limitations which are well-known limits to the provision of face-to-face services in Australia (see Section 1.7.5), especially in rural areas.

As an example, MindSpot, which offers a range of digital psychoeducation, support and treatments for anxiety and depression, has identified service users who have not engaged—or have ineffectively engaged—with conventional services for treatment of their mental disorders. Analysis of data from assessments completed by a total of 23 235 service users in 2015 and 2016, showed that 33.2% of non-Indigenous and 31.6% of Indigenous users had never spoken to a mental health professional; 42.8% of non-Indigenous and 46.8% of Indigenous users had previously spoken with a mental health professional and yet were seeking digital services (Titov, Schofield, Staples, Dear, & Nielssen, 2019). These findings suggest that large numbers of people with mild to moderate anxiety and depression may use digital services ahead of seeking face-to-face treatments, with the potential for significant population level benefits in the increased treatment of these disorders.

Research on the help-seeking behaviours of persons who have attempted suicide has also shed light on the importance of digital mental health services: in a study undertaken through the Black Dog Institute, persons surveyed reported contacting hospitals and emergency services most frequently following a suicide attempt (40%) while few contacted mental health professionals (less than 5%). A visible proportion (10%) of survey respondents stated telephone and online support services as a point of contact (NHMRC Centre of Research Excellence in Suicide Prevention, 2014). This is reflected in operational data from services such as Lifeline Australia, which reported that 22% of all contacts to the telephone helpline warranted a suicide safety assessment (Spittal, et al., 2014).

Into this mix is the question of the extent that non-clinical support services which are offered digitally can work in a complementary way to the provision of clinical and professional services through conventional means. In a major study of the callers to Lifeline Australia, Burgess and others identified many of those callers experienced mental health issues at clinically significant levels, with average scores on depression and anxiety symptoms being 5.7 (SD¼2.4) and 6.3 (SD¼2.2), respectively. Similarly, half of respondents reported experiencing a panic attack in the past four weeks while 57% indicated experiencing a social phobia (Burgess, Christensen,

Leach, Farrer, & Griffiths, 2008). In the same study, it became apparent that many of the Lifeline service users were also receiving professional assistance for their mental health issues: 30% reported that in the previous month they had seen a counsellor, 12% a case-worker, 11% a psychologist and 28% a psychiatrist. In addition, 33% of respondents were currently taking antidepressant medication. Consumers appeared to use both a telephone support service and access conventional mental health professional services.

Interestingly, not much is known from research or data analysis on consumer experiences and use of digital mental health services, but what is known suggests that there are perceived unique benefits and situational factors that surround consumer choice to access these services, especially with regard to mental health issues and suicide prevention.

Early research in the United States by David Lester and others identified common themes in consumer choice to use telephone based services when seeking support on mental health issues. In particular, several unique qualities of telephone based services are identified by Williams and Douds, based on their thematic analysis of a series of research studies:

1 *Client Control:* Entry to conventional services requires disclosure, effort and attendance, with the therapist in control. Use of telephone services puts the control with the caller, who can simply hang up if the process is not working and who decides when they will call.
2 *Client Anonymity:* 'being able to hide one's identity may facilitate greater self-revelation and openness on the part of a patient.' Feeling safe and secure is important for disclosures. Anonymity reduces the fear of being ridiculed or abused in a situation.
3 *Bridging Geographic and Personal Barriers:* From transport issues to mobility difficulties, getting to help may be hard for some people especially those from lower socioeconomic backgrounds. Also, some people living with mental health issues withdraw from social and interpersonal contacts (Williams & Douds, 2002).

Each of these features of digital mental health services suggest an alignment to consumer needs and preferences for accessing services and support–on their terms rather than necessarily through arrangements designed primarily to suit service providers. The nature of mental health issues, and when and where help is often needed, means that this dimension of service provision may enable help-seeking and personal engagement in addressing mental health issues. Disclosures of mental health struggles and symptoms, as well as suicidality, may be more forthcoming and allow more rapid and effective service responses. These aspects of consumer experiences of digital mental health services may be seen as part of the overall solution to the fundamental challenge of attracting more people with mental health issues to use services that can address their needs.

An additional element has emerged in recent times through the introduction of online counselling, chat and text based services–all of which provide contact and communication by word, not voice. Consumer feedback obtained suggests that some people have preferences for the use of word based modes over voice based modes of communication when seeking help or disclosing personal issues surrounding their suicidality, mental health and wellbeing. The 2013 study of the Lifeline Online Chat Service (which provides real-time, one-on-one service) included a survey of a sample of users and found that 30% of those surveyed stated an explicit preference for the word–online chat–mode of contact. Qualitative data from this cohort showed two frequently nominated reasons:

a difficulties expressing intense emotions using speech and challenges talking about things that are highly distressing (word mode seems to discount the barrier in these circumstances)
b safety and privacy concerns regarding use of voice based services because someone may overhear the communication (Net Balance, 2013).

Studies by other services, such as the Veterans Crisis Line in the United States and the Online Counselling Service in Israel, have identified similar preferences for a word-based interaction by some people (Predmore, et al., 2017; Gilat & Shahar, 2007). There appears to be evidence that the actual mode of communication matters and the main distinction is drawn across voice or text dimensions, rather than a commitment to a particular platform or type of technology. Accordingly, there is a sound argument in terms of whole of population access to teleweb mental health services for there to be options for voice or word-based interaction. Some people will not use voice.

DIGITAL MENTAL HEALTH SERVICE DEVELOPMENT IN AUSTRALIA

The telephone services were the first obvious form of technology based services for mental health and suicide prevention in Australia. In the post-world war era, the telephone became a fixture in many family homes and the use of the telephone grew as a normalised form of communication. In 1963, the Lifeline helpline was established in Sydney, NSW, as an innovation in the use of the telephone. Anyone could contact this service at any time of the day on any problem or issue they were facing. The Lifeline helpline reflected similar services that were established in the United Kingdom (Samaritans) and the United States (Los Angeles Suicide Prevention Centre). The use of the telephone for helplines and related information or therapy lines grew considerably in the 1970s and 1980s, to the point that by the time of the first major review of teleweb services in Australia, undertaken in 2002 by Urbis Keys Young consultants, there was estimated to be 171 services identified as 'appeared to provide telephone counselling, telephone support or a "helpline" free or at token cost' (Urbis Keys Young 2002). The majority of these services were found to have operated for more than 10 years.

Most of the telephone services examined in the Urbis Keys Young review were specialised around particular audiences (e.g. young people) or issues (e.g. domestic violence, cancer treatment/recovery, mental health issues, family relationships). Some were purely information-oriented rather than providing therapy or counselling services. The review examined the nature of services offered and found four service types: information, referral, counselling and empathic listening. Most services offered several of these service types to some extent. Only a few were for national audiences; most were geographically oriented towards certain regions or states/territories. The range of purposes and approach shows the flexibility with which telephone based services can operate and their capacity to be tailored to particular needs as well as offered as population level generalist services.

Table 1.7 Examples of Telephone Helplines in Australia

Service	Phone Number	Website
Lifeline	13 11 14	Lifeline.org.au
Mensline	1300 789 978	Mensline.org.au
Kids Helpline	1800 55 1800	Kidshelpline.com.au
1800 RESPECT	1800 737 732	1800respect.org.au
Beyondblue Support Line	1300 22 4636	Beyondblue.org.au

Online or web services followed the telephone services as the technology surrounding personal computers and the internet prompted greater use in the wider community of these modes of communication. By the time of the Urbis Keys Young review in 2002, it is noteworthy that 78% of telephone services also had a website and online presence (although mostly these were static sites providing information and referral only). The introduction of interactive services using online platforms has been relatively recent. Those that offered online interaction in the early stages were mostly question-and-answer style formats, less likely to be conducted in 'real time' and more often used to supply referral information to other services.

The first online counselling service in Australia was through the Centre for Mental Health Research at Australian National University. There, a suite of online services were trialled through research studies. These included Mood Gym, which offered psycho-education and CBT treatments for depression;

eCouch, which was oriented for young audiences also addressing depression; and Blue Pages which offered 'forum' interactions to enable peer support on depression in an online context. Another early online service offering treatments was This Way Up, which pioneered anxiety treatments. The first attempt to list online therapies and services that held a research and clinical standard of practice was through the website Beacon, which was operated by the Australian National University.

The early forms of online interaction for mental health services were in the form of chat rooms or similar settings, where a person would register to be able to communicate with other registered users in a structured environment. The structures and management of the operating environment was seen as important for mental health service provision because the management of the online interactions could address safety and supervision considerations. A critical distinction between the approach for online (word-based) and telephone (voice-based) modes of communication in mental health services was drawn at this stage–the former generating a written record through the interactions that would require storage management, privacy protections and oversight for supervision and accountability purposes. The telephone mode had been substantially free of these considerations–no records of service processes were created. Interestingly, as technology has advanced to enable voice recording and as consumer expectations of records of service for accountability purposes have grown, the distinction between word and voice mode requirements for management of access, use and service processes has become far less apparent.

Email counselling was another form of word-based technology communication that has been used for counselling and mental health services. The Kids Helpline was the first major national provider in Australia to offer contact by email to service users. This communication mode was seen as potentially very useful in the 1990s as the use of email generally expanded in Australian business and community communications. However, by the mid-2000s, email was being less utilised in comparison to the emerging 'quicker and easier' mobile device SMS text and messaging modes. Moreover, email faces two difficulties as a mode of communication for mental health services:

1. Confidentiality and security of information transferred by email is very difficult to address given the uncontrolled nature of email transmission and the potential for these transmissions to be intercepted by other parties.
2. Email can operate without boundaries on size of text content and length of material sent-this unregulated characteristic in a counselling or disclosure environment can result in large amounts of communication that cannot easily be responded to or managed.

Of interest, however, is the parallel development of phone-based SMS or text messaging as a mode of communication for mental health services. The growth of mobile telephone use in the 1990s saw an unexpected consumer preference for the brief text-based format that SMS offered because of the simplicity, the comparatively low cost and the ability to use this mode even when mobile reception was poor. However, it has been in relatively recent times that this text or messaging facility has been studied as a viable mode of contact and communication for mental health and suicide prevention services (Berrouiguet, et al., 2018; Sindahl, et al., 2019). Further exploration of this mode of communication is likely to occur.

Interestingly, there are now few service organisations in the digital sector that provide services using one mode of communication only. The majority offer telephone (voice) and chat/text (word) based interactions to consumers. This possibly reflects the convergence of the technologies where a mix of voice and word interactions occurs in wider Australian society across business, personal and social communications on an increasingly routine basis. For instance, telephone contact may precede or follow a word/text-based contact. Online word interactions may expand on service contact initiated by telephone. Urgent or after hours contact services may use telephone as the gateway to rapid assessment and responses, while word/text-based services can be useful for quick 'check-ins' after an earlier service contact. It is likely that the trend will continue towards a seamless set of multiple interactions with consumers across word and voice modes.

One mode that has not received as much attention, to date, is video conference or 'face-based' interactions. However, some services are moving towards the integration of this communication mode to service delivery. Mens Line and Veterans Counselling Services, which are operated by the organisation On The Line, have been pioneers in video conferencing at scale in Australia. The contexts and effectiveness of this form of service provision remains to be established, although the potential for enhanced communication using body language may be appealing in some situations. Some government agencies, notably South Australia Country Health, have invested in video conferencing technology and training of health professionals to provide specialist services to remote areas by video link. These experiences will undoubtably inform service development more widely.

Another mode of digital mental health service is the fully automated self-help program which operate without the involvement of a service worker, such as a counsellor. These services use technology to facilitate self-directed interaction through a series of questions or options that are presented automatically in response to the nature of the user's contact. An example of automated self-help is the Next Step feature in ReachOut.com, which enables a user to disclose the issues they are concerned about regarding their mental health and wellbeing, and then presents the user with questions to explore the issue further based on decision trees and algorithms. The program can then provide insights and raise the user's awareness of the nature of their situation and supports the user in finding referrals to other suitable services. Current development of automated services includes 'bot' type interactions: the Australian Government Head to Health online site incorporates a chat bot to assist users identify the mental health issues that they are concerned about and guides the user in finding suitable other information, service and referral resources.

TELEWEB SERVICE TYPES

The range of services and programs through TeleWeb operations in Australia has flourished over the past 20 years. In a paper prepared in 2014 by the eMental Health Alliance (a group of Digital Mental Health Service Organisations that formed an informal network to advocate for service promotion and development), the following five types of service or programmes were described representing a 'point in time' stock take of the service environment:

1. *Health promotion, wellness promotion and psycho-education.* Examples of these programs include BluePages, beyondblue, ReachOut.com, KidsMatter, MindMatters, HeadsUp, Man Therapy.
2. *Prevention and early intervention.* Examples of these programs include BiteBack, Kids Helpline, BraveOnline, beyondblue's Support Service.
3. *Crisis intervention and suicide prevention.* Examples of these programs include Lifeline, Healthy Thinking and ibobbly.
4. *Treatment.* Examples of these programs include MindSpot, myCompass, eCouch, MoodGYM, This Way Up, eheadspace.
5. *Recovery and mutual/peer support.* Examples of these programmes include BlueBoard, an online internet support group for people with depression, or telephone support lines staffed by mental health consumers (eMental, 2014).

In the early stages of development of digital mental health services in Australia, it was common to have services operating within larger organisational structures as contained service or business units. At the time of the Urbis Keys Young review, only half of the teleweb services surveyed were 'stand-alone' organisations. Many tele-web mental health services were developed within academic institutions (MoodGym, Anxiety Online, This Way Up/CRuFAD), which reflects the innovation and research-based testing of services that occurred. The other common organisational arrangement in the early stages was non-government or charitable organisation (Lifeline, Kids Helpline, SANE Support Line). Although in more recent times, government has taken a greater interest in the provision of tele-web mental health services, including their promotion, practice improvement and quality assurance, it has retained an arm's length' from service provision by tendering or contracting for service provision only. The health and family/community portfolio areas within governments have been most active in funding Digital Mental Health Services.

Table 1.8 Key government-funded digital mental health services

Service name	Website
Head to Health	Headtohealth.gov.au
MindSpot	Mindspot.org.au
Health Direct	Healthdirect.gov.au
eHeadspace	headspace.org.au/eheadspace

The workforce for digital mental health services reflects the diversity of organisational arrangements in their provision. The Urbis Keys Young review found half of those surveyed reported use of volunteers-almost always specially trained-for service delivery. This has continued with some services in Australia continuing to utilise volunteers (e.g. Lifeline, SANE Australia, Q-Life, Griefline) and some focusing on a peer support dimension (e.g. ReachOut.com, eCouch, Mates In Construction helpline). There is some research evidence to suggest that for those services seeking to engage empathetically with people who are seeking emotional support and a safe place for disclosure of suicidality, sexual assault or other personal issues, there are intrinsic benefits to service character if volunteers, non-professional or peer workers are involved (Mishara, et al. 2016).

POLICY ENVIRONMENT ON DIGITAL MENTAL HEALTH SERVICES

Australia has been thinking about strategies for e-mental health for more than a decade with a major Federal Government initiative to address the policy and program issues for mental health occurring in 2002 with a commissioned review on telephone and web counselling services in Australia by Urbis Keys Young. This review provided a national perspective on the scope, characteristics and challenges facing the digital mental health services. The review found that digital mental health services had been operating for more than 40 years in Australia and had grown largely at the state/territory and regional levels. It noted that the range of service types extended beyond 'counselling' and that there was no national coordination of their activities or the policy context in which they should develop and operate.

The 2006 National Action Plan on Mental Health developed by the Council of Australian Governments was a turning point in national involvement in digital mental health services. This reform package established the following:

- a national TeleWeb funding program for services through the Federal Department of Health
- a mental health specification for the National Health Call Centre Network (coordination of health telephone and online information services through states/territories)
- a national eMental Health Advisory Group to the Federal Department of Health to examine the various issues surrounding growth and development of Digital Mental Health Services.

Other milestones in the Australian policy environment for digital mental health services are as follows:

- **2008:** Australian Quality Framework for TeleWeb Services was developed with the Federal Department of Health and more than 20 digital mental health services.
- **2011:** eHeadspace established with Federal Government funding to provide a digital service accompanying conventional delivery of headspace youth mental health services throughout the country. This service offered telephone and online contacts for young people.
- **2012:** Young and Well Co-operative Research Centre established with Federal Government funding as a research partnership across academic institutions, consumer advocates and end-user service organisations to investigate the application of technologies to young person's mental health and wellbeing.
- **2012:** eMental Health Strategy in Australia released. This represented the first national

strategy for the development, promotion and quality assurance of tele-web mental health services. It has guided the Federal Government's investments in building the capacity of the digital mental health services in three key ways:

- *Online Portal on Digital Mental Health Services,* developed to provide information and promote access to a range of quality services in Australia, making it easier for consumers and professionals to find about these services and use them. This became known as *Mind Health Connect* and operated from 2013 to 2017.
- *Support Program for Digital Mental Health Services*, developed to coordinate development of quality improvement and practice guidance, to address workforce training and liaison with professionals in conventional services on knowledge and understanding of digital services. This became known as *eMHPrac (eMental Health Practice Project)* and continues to provide resources and capacity development for those involved in digital mental health services and those operating in conventional services with regard to their referral and use of digital services.
- *Virtual Clinic*, developed to increase the telephone and online availability of evidence based treatments for anxiety and depression. This became known as *MindSpot* and has operated since 2014.

- **2016:** An additional initiative occurred: the establishment of *Head to Health* as an online 'digital mental health service gateway' to replace the *Mind Health Connect* site. This represented a greater investment in national coordination of digital mental health services. *Head to Health* was co-designed through a series of intensive research and consultation processes. The site uses technology for continual improvement and refinement to adjust to emerging consumer preferences for information about digital mental health services.

The *Fifth National Mental Health and Suicide Prevention Plan* (2016) sits as the latest strategic policy statement in Australia, with Digital Mental Health Services addressed as part of the overall five year directions for mental health and suicide prevention.

FUTURE DIRECTIONS FOR DIGITAL MENTAL HEALTH SERVICES

The inclusion of Digital Mental Health Services in the Fifth National Mental Health and Suicide Prevention Plan in Australia represents an extension of the fundamental shift that occurred in 2006 under the COAG Mental Health Reforms to recognise digital services in inter-governmental agreements on mental health and suicide prevention. Accordingly, the place of digital mental health services in the policy and program environment for mental health and suicide prevention seems assured.

However, future challenges surrounding the growth of these services and their propagation by other providers will need to be addressed in detail through policy and quality assurance measures. It is likely that there will be growth in the provision of digital mental health services, including greater private sector investment as their potential and performance is increasingly established through research and the evaluation of ongoing operations. While growth is welcome if it provides for more services, wider choices and innovation, mechanisms to ensure that consumer interests are upheld in these services will need to be active. This is a challenge given consumers can choose digital services internationally, not just domestically. A strength in digital mental health services to date has been their ability to boost consumer control in their use and enhance consumer experiences of self-directed engagement and empowerment on their mental health. Principles and practice of meaningful co-design and continual improvement in digital services need to be upheld for those operating in mental health.

There also remains ongoing work in the promotion and explanation of digital mental health services to professionals and organisations working in conventional service delivery, to maximise the promotion and use of digital services appropriately. A divide remains in Australia between the digital and non-digital worlds in terms of access to technologies and internet connectivity and in terms of affordability and cost of data services, with use of mental health digital services being no exception. Greater understanding and skill is required for individuals, organisations and governments to fully realise the potential for these worlds to operate more seamlessly, in an integrated and complementary fashion. This will not occur without effort and investment, but the benefits would seem to be substantially worthwhile.

1.5.10 GATHERING THESE STRANDS TOGETHER INTO A SYSTEM

IDENTIFYING DESIRABLE COMPONENTS OF A MENTAL HEALTH CARE SYSTEM

Having introduced some key elements of thinking about contemporary mental health care we now progress to thinking about how to gather these together into a health care system for a population. While acknowledging that the reality is that this is a complex adaptive system (see Section 1.1.1) that will in important ways create its own behaviour, sometimes in surprising ways, we can influence things substantially and hopefully for the better by design approaches. We can seek to fund specific identifiable programs, or create entitlements for particular insurance claims in line with funding model principles for instance. The choices we make here are vitally important. *The Lancet* Commission on Global Mental Health And Sustainable Development (Patel et al., 2018) proposed services components we might expect to see provided in low, medium and high resource settings. The Commission grounded its considerations in the UN Sustainable Development Goals which will be in place until 2030 so we anticipate that the Commission's work should have some relevance for and influence on service directions through the 2020s.

THE LANCET COMMISSION ON GLOBAL MENTAL HEALTH AND SUSTAINABLE DEVELOPMENT

The Lancet has a history going back two centuries while a specialty journal *Lancet Psychiatry* was established in 2014; both are highly ranked among global journals. *The Lancet* has a manifesto which explicitly embraces research translation as including:

> Increasing the social impact of science. We recognise that a great research paper is not enough and that it requires development, mobilisation, and exposure. So we promise to set agendas, create context, inform leaders, start debates, and advocate for the idea that research can and will make a difference' (*The Lancet*, 2019).

In 2007, *The Lancet* published an influential series on global mental health, and subsequently Patel and colleagues (2018) published one of its Commissions, this time on Global Mental Health and Sustainable Development. The term 'sustainable development' here refers directly to the United Nations Sustainable Development Goals (SDGs; see Section 1.2.3). The Commission report is a wide-ranging and often masterful summary of key challenges in delivery of mental health care, and no less relevant to agenda setting in Australia by virtue of its international scope and inclusion of issues facing developing nations. The report proposes indeed that 'all countries can be thought of as developing countries in the context of mental health'. Issues summarised in the report include historical considerations of the development of the Global Mental Health agenda, staging approaches (see Section 1.2.4), the role of social determinants (see Section 1.2.4), preventive approaches (see Section 1.5.5) and research priorities (see Chapter 1.4). In terms of considerations of delivery of mental health care directly the Commission present proposed mental

Figure 1.23 Mental health service components relevant to low-, medium- and high-resource settings

Low-resource settings

Community
(provided across relevant sectors)
- Basic opportunities for occupation/ employment and social inclusion
- Basic community interventions to promote help-seeking
- Range of community-level suicide prevention
- Early childhood and parenting intervention programmes
- Basic school-based mental health programmes
- Promotion of self-care interventions
- Integration of mental health into community-based rehabilitation and community-based inclusive development programmes
- Home-based care to promote treatment adherence
- Activating social networks

and

Primary health care
(provided by general primary care workers)
- Case identification
- Basic evidence-based psychosocial interventions
- Basic evidence-based pharmacological interventions
- Basic referral pathways to secondary care

and

Secondary health care
(provided in general hospitals)
- Training, support and supervision of primary care staff
- Outpatient clinics
- Acute inpatient care in general hospitals
- Basic referral pathways to tertiary care

and

Tertiary health care
(provided by mental health specialist services)
- Improve quality of care in psychiatric hospitals
- Initiate move of mental health inpatient services from psychiatric hospitals to general hospitals
- Initiate close of long-stay institutions and develop alternatives in community settings
- Establish means of licensing all practitioners treating people with mental disorders, including non-formal care facilities
- Range of evidence-based psychological treatments
- Ensure compliance with relevant human rights conventions
- Initiate consultation-liaison services in collaboration with other medical departments and improve physical health care of people in mental health services

Medium-resource settings

Community
Services as provided in low-resource settings and:
- Coordinated opportunities for occupation/employment and social inclusion
- Coordinated community interventions to promote understanding of mental health
- Coordinated interventions to reduce stigma and promote help seeking
- City-wide and district-wide coordination of integrated mental health care plans
- Attention to mental health in policy across all sectors
- Range of independent and supported accommodation for people with long-term mental health disorders
- Drug and alcohol use prevention programmes
- Range of services for homeless people with mental or substance use disorders
- Community-based rehabilitation for people with psychological disabilities

and

Primary health care
Services as provided in low-resource settings and:
- Equitable geographical coverage of mental health care integrated primary care
- Coordinated collaborative care across service delivery platforms
- Comprehensive mental health training for general health-care staff

and

Secondary health care
Services as provided in low-resource settings and:
- Multidisciplinary mobile community mental health teams for people with severe mental disorders
- Integration of mental health care with other secondary health care (eg maternal and child health, HIV)

and

Tertiary health care
Services as provided in low-resource settings and:
- Consolidate move of mental health inpatient services from psychiatric hospitals to general hospitals
- Basic range of targeted specialised services (eg, for children and young people, older adults, forensic settings)
- Consolidate consultation-liaison services

High-resource settings

Community
Services as provided in low-resource settings and:
- Intensive opportunities for occupation/employment and social inclusion
- Intensive community interventions to promote understanding of mental health
- Intensive interventions to reduce stigma and promote help seeking
- Full range of independent and supported accommodation for people with long-term mental disorders
- Range of evidence-based services in community platforms (eg in schools, colleges and workplaces)
- Intensive drug and alcohol use prevention programmes
- Intensive childhood and parenting intervention programmes (life skills training)
- Intensive community-level suicide prevention programmes (eg reduce access to means of self-harm, media training)

and

Primary health care
Services as provided in low-resource settings and:
- Full geographic coverage of mental health care integrated in primary care
- Collaborative care model with specialists supporting primary care practitioners

and

Secondary health care
Services as provided in low-resource settings and:
- Full range of evidence-based psychosocial interventions delivered by trained experts
- Full range of evidence based pharmacological interventions available

and

Tertiary health care
Services as provided in low-resource settings and:
- Complete move of mental health inpatient services from psychiatric hospitals to general hospitals
- Full range of targeted specialist services (eg, for early intervention for psychoses, for children and young people, older adults, addictions, and forensic settings)

Source: Patel et al., 2018

health service components relevant to countries at different income levels.

DEVELOPING CHALLENGES

The Lancet Commission is a useful summary of contemporary thinking around mental health service delivery. While very broad ranging in its construction it remains strongly connected to what can be described as an 'evidence-based group-level symptom-reduction model as the organizing principle for mental health care' (van Os et al., 2019). This is in turn receiving some challenges based in part on the findings that neither in Australia (Meadows, Prodan, et al., 2019a) or internationally, at least in the anglophone countries (Jorm, Patten, Brugha, & Mojtabai, 2017), does increased expenditure in mental health care seem to have brought prevalence of mental health problems down. It is possible that we need a differently focused system to achieve this, with, for instance, suggestions (van Os et al., 2019) that:

> The mental health service of the 21st century may be best conceived of as a small-scale healing community fostering connectedness and strengthening resilience in learning to live with mental vulnerability, complemented by a limited number of regional facilities. Peer support, organized at the level of a recovery college, may form the backbone of the community. Treatments should be aimed at trans-syndromal symptom reduction, tailored to serve the higher-order process of existential recovery and social participation, and applied by professionals who have been trained to collaborate, embrace idiography and maximize effects mediated by therapeutic relationship and the healing effects of ritualized care interactions. Finally, integration with a public mental health system of e-communities providing information, peer and citizen support and a range of user-rated self-management tools may help bridge the gap between the high prevalence of common mental disorder and the relatively low capacity of any mental health service.

Internationally, the UN Special Rapporteur on mental health has raised concerns about over-application of medicalised interventions (Puras, 2018). From Australia, this author, with others, has put forward a testable model drawing on possible iatrogenic mechanisms (see Section 1.5.5) with implications that would bring a greater attention to equitable service delivery and to more widely recovery oriented practice, emphasising:

> This framework for considering pathogenic influences would lead us to seek practice models that acknowledge risks of harm from therapeutic interventions; support attention to consumer-defined goals; avoid unhelpful biomedical labelling of normal life experiences; support social, educational and vocational participation; and encourage people to apply themselves energetically to self-help and other active strategies in their pathway through experiences of mental health problems. Our interventions should encourage, not replace or subvert, autonomy, independence and active coping.

1.5.11 SIMULATION MODELLING

JOANNE ENTICOTT & GRAHAM MEADOWS

INTRODUCTION

In a final section we extend consideration of a contemporary and developing approach to developing and monitoring funding strategies introduced in the prevention section. That approach is of simulation modelling. Setting up models of health care systems can help us in linking together key concepts introduced in the chapter. Software-based models resting on best available data can help us to consider complex processes including emergent properties and feedback (see Section 1.1.1) as a feature of mental health care systems. Both the process of developing these models and then making use of them can help us understand whether and how funding strategies may be achieving the aims set out in ethical frameworks (see Section 1.5.2), operationalised through service delivery and transformational models (see Chapter 1.5), guided in varying degrees by linkage with translational research (see Chapter 1.4).

COMPLEX SYSTEMS

In complex systems, the number of components is usually large and conventionally deterministic descriptions (e.g. involving a series of differential equations) do not adequately map the system because the overall behaviour of the system may not be predicted by the behaviour of the individual components. Complex Adaptive Systems (CAS; see Section 1.1.1) also have a degree of adaptive capacity, where the components simultaneously affect and are shaped by the other components and overall system. The CAS approach is a way of thinking about and analysing health care and other systems by recognising complexity, patterns and interrelationships rather than focusing on simple cause and effect. Mental health care, especially the Australian model with multiple organisational inputs, needs to be considered as a CAS; open, embedded, with nested components, fuzzy boundaries, self-organisation, sensitivity to initial conditions and historicism.

Systems modelling tools can provide evidence suited to addressing complex problems and consist of computer simulation (system dynamics, agent based and discrete event) techniques. These system models have the capacity to simulate aspects of CAS such as feedback loops, non-linearity, phase changes and emergence. Computer simulation provides a platform for integrating evidence sources into an analytic tool that can allow researchers and policy makers to explore in a robust, risk-free and low-cost way the likely impacts of different intervention scenarios over the short and longer term, and can be used to conduct virtual experimentation where real-world studies are not feasible. Systems modelling has been applied extensively in engineering, defence, aviation, economics, ecology and business to simulate and help solve complex problems, and optimise the use of limited resources (see Section 1.5.4). Their value in helping to solve complex problems in the health sector is being increasingly recognised, with local and international applications for the prevention of infectious and chronic diseases, reduction in alcohol related harms, and prevention of childhood obesity

There are efforts and progress in using systems modelling tools to support complex public health problems. For example, a recent dynamic simulation model focusing on diabetes in pregnancy in Australia has been built. The model was built using participatory methods with local, national and international experts in endocrinology, public health, primary health, diabetes education, health economics and simulation modelling. It combines a range of data sources and modelling methods, including System Dynamics, Agent Based and Discrete Event modelling. This means that the model is used to explore questions at different scales ranging from 'below the skin' dynamics to health service utilisation to population-based interventions. Dynamic systems modelling such as this also supports analysis of the combined effects of interventions and emergent behaviour of systems.

SIMULATION MODELLING IN MENTAL HEALTH

A recent systematic review of simulation modelling in mental health identified 160 studies. However, only a minority (6%) applied to health system planning, supporting recommendations for expansion of their use to answer pressing policy questions. This systematic review also recommended the use of epidemiological data to underpin service simulation models in mental health.

An example of a relevant and pressing mental health system planning issue requiring such an investigation using systems modelling tools is as follows. As discussed elsewhere in this text, depression, anxiety and substance use disorders affect one in five Australians each year. Reducing prevalence is paramount as these disorders account for 24% of the burden of disability in Australia, almost on par with the highest (25%) from musculoskeletal conditions (Australian Institute of Health and Welfare, 2019). There should be a causal connection between greatly increased expenditure and lowered rates of mental illness in the population. But despite doubling of Australian expenditure on mental health services over two decades (see Section 1.2.5), there has been no reduction in the prevalence of either psychological distress or mental disorders (Australian Institute of Health and Welfare

2019). This is a paradox. Systems modelling tools of computer simulation can be applied to address this complex problem; modelling components of the system or the entire system. Exploring, identifying and quantifying the factors contributing to the complex and dynamic nature of possible casual mechanisms in this paradox can only be done with computer simulation. A computer simulation model of common mental disorders (CMD) could be developed with a focus on the emergence of CMD clusters in the population. Computer simulation modelling methods can be used to forecast the likely impact of actual or hypothetical scenarios (for example, a hypothetical intervention delivered by GPs to increase active self-help strategies and exercise levels) for CMD prevention and recovery. The model could capture both individual- and population-level dynamics of CMD behaviour.

Agent Based Models (ABMs) are a class of computational model that provide powerful tools for simulating human behaviour due to their ability to capture the interacting influences of individual characteristics, social networks, local context, and the broader sociocultural, economic and policy environment that are important drivers of CMD. In practical terms, agents (individuals) in the model are given key characteristics and exposures that reflect those in the real world. Conditional transition rules are articulated (for example, relating to probabilities of engaging in suicidal ideation, planning, and attempts, and conditional on such behaviours in other individuals in the population network) that specify how simulated individuals act and interact. Resulting population-level behavioural patterns and outcomes emerge from millions of stochastic interactions, patterns which are iteratively tested and validated against empirical data. This type of model can contribute new knowledge regarding the complex interplay of factors influencing the emergence of CMD in regions (through the iterative process of hypothesis building and testing), and provide a risk-free environment for testing new intervention strategies before they are implemented in the real world. Outputs from the proposed model can be validated against the empirical data from national surveys to establish plausibility of the model to ensure it is a valid representation of the 'real-world' system. The resulting validated model can then be used as a 'what-if' tool to test the likely impacts of counterfactual situations and different combinations of the priorities strategies (or interventions).

A validated computer simulation model can be used to test the likely impacts of the prioritised strategies and interventions in a safe and timely way, before it is implemented in the real world. Such models allow the investigation of the potential impact of modifying interventions based on a range of different scenarios relating to the: (1) frequency; (2) content; and (3) mode of dissemination of the intervention among the population network. For example, it could be possible to investigate the effectiveness, or otherwise, of different modes of delivery of the intervention, including: the optimal frequency with which GP care (or other care) need to be deployed; the most effective location of new primary mental health care services; and those sentinel individuals to target who are receptive to that particular care type. Results can estimate the potential number of people whose CMD is averted over a forecast period (expressed as a preventive fraction) in regional and non-regional groups under the baseline scenario of 'no intervention' compared to counterfactual scenarios.

ASSESSING SIMULATION MODELLING PUBLICATIONS

Simulation modelling is likely to have increasing influence over the coming years. Full appraisal of the literature relevant to decision making about setting priorities in such areas will involve at least some ability to appraise publications of this type. When publications are in peer reviewed journals and cite adherence to key guidelines regarding preparation and presentation of such models–such as this protocol for Agent Based Models–this presents some safeguard. Alternatively, if the reader comes across publications in reports that do not cite such guidelines or evidence of peer review, and where models are not well described either in their form or with attention to the information base supporting parameter-setting, then lack sensitivity analyses that might suggest what the uncertainty properties of modelling are, then there may be reasons to choose not to rely on the outputs of the model.

1.5.12 COMMENTARY AND REFLECTIONS

GRAHAM MEADOWS & MARGARET GRIGG

The Australian health system involves a complex distribution of responsibilities between the Commonwealth, the states and territories, and public and private funding arrangements. Traditionally, states and territories have had responsibility for the public health system, including mental health services, while the Commonwealth has been largely responsible for primary care, private fee-for-service specialist doctors (including psychiatrists), pharmaceuticals and aged care. The system as it stands in Australia carries imprints of its development in the context of shifting tensions in Australia's system of government as a federation. Very broadly, the existing health care system in Australia has been in place since the introduction of Medibank in 1975, becoming Medicare in 1984. Hence, while this was introduced in the adult lifetime of most of the baby boomer generation, three subsequent generations, often typified as Generations X, Y and Z, have grown up with the expectations and implied understandings of rights as established with the introduction of Medicare. These commonly may be taken for granted. However, the system as it stands represents only one of many possible solutions to the challenge of delivery of affordable, accessible and high quality mental health care. Internationally, of course, we can find many health care systems with radically different designs.

Finally we acknowledge that, as noted at the start of the chapter, the existing paradigms are under some degree of challenge. There are suggestions in major journals that we need to go about things in potentially very different ways if we are to actualise personal recovery goals for people, families and carers in their communities. So it seems that the decade of the 2020s will be one in which the challenge should be addressed of developing and implementing service delivery models and systems that are capable of making some desirable difference to population prevalence of mental health problems.

1.6

INFORMATION ON AUSTRALIAN MENTAL HEALTH AND ITS MENTAL HEALTH CARE SYSTEM

GRAHAM MEADOWS, JOANNE ENTICOTT, CAROL HARVEY, VERA MORGAN, FRANCES SHAWYER & SEBASTIAN ROSENBERG

1.6.1 INTRODUCTION

GRAHAM MEADOWS

AIMS

This chapter has three aims:

- to provide information on the Australian population and within that the distribution of people with mental ill health of different kinds
- to describe some of the characteristics of the services that are in place to respond to the needs of people with these disorders
- to describe the extent to which needs of people with mental health problems are being met, or not, by those services

Within these three major sections, a range of sources of information will be used to sketch a picture of what is known about these issues. The aim then is both to provide information most current at time of writing and to inform the reader as to how to access and understand key resources that will serve over time to update that picture more frequently than is possible in a text like this one.

AUSTRALIA, ITS DEMOGRAPHICS AND PHYSICAL STATISTICS

Australia includes a vast island continent and surrounding islands stretching from temperate zones to the tropics. As the sixth largest country, it makes up 5.2% of the global land mass. Much of the country is managed in some form of cultivation, though low rainfall and poor soils make for very poor productivity for much of the land area.

The estimated population in mid-2019 was 25.4 million people (Australian Bureau of Statistics, 2019b), about 0.3% of the world population. With its land area of 7 682 300 square kilometres, this creates an overall population density of 3.3 persons per square kilometre. However, this population density is quite different from the life experience of most Australians, 67.4% of whom live in the capital cities. In mid-2016 (Australian Bureau of Statistics, 2016a), when the latest census available at time of writing was conducted, 18.7% of the population was under 15, and 15.8% was over 65. For every 100 females there were 97.2 males. The age distribution is changing, becoming more aged; for instance, the proportion of the population over 65 was 12.9% in 2005, 14.0% in 2011 and 15.8% in 2016.

The population has had very substantial expansion in the years since World War II, initially with white European migrants, then, more recently, a wider variety of migrant groups. In 1945 the population was around 7.5 million, roughly doubling to nearly 15 million by 1980, with a further 10 million added since then. Lately the population has been growing steadily at 1.6% per annum, the majority of which growth is due to migration. The 2016 statistics show that 67% of the population is native born; of the 33% (7.7 million people) foreign born, 26% were born in English-speaking countries. The United Kingdom-born group is the largest migrant group, with 3.9% of the total population. After this, the rest of the top 10 countries of birth for non-Australian-born are New Zealand, China, India, the Philippines, Vietnam, Italy, South Africa, Malaysia and Sri Lanka (Parliament of Australia, 2018).

Current life expectancy from birth is estimated at 80.5 years for males and 84.6 years for females (Australian Bureau of Statistics, 2018a). According to World Health Organization (2016) estimates, this is fourth highest in the world. Median weekly personal income in 2016 for people aged 15 years and over was $662, which had increased by 15% since 2011 (Australian Bureau of Statistics, 2016a). There is an average of 1.8 motor vehicles per dwelling. The Gini index, as a measure of income inequality (see Chapters 1.2, 1.4) is 0.34, compared with an OECD average of 0.32 (University of New South Wales, 2018).

INFORMATION AND MENTAL HEALTH IN AUSTRALIA

The first systematic and representative national population mental health survey in Australia, in 1997, was the *National Survey of Mental Health and Well-being* (NSMHW 1997). This program of research included a household survey concentrating on high prevalence disorders (Andrews, Anstey, Brodaty, Issakidis, & Luscombe, 1999; Australian Bureau of Statistics, 1998), another study concentrating on lower prevalence disorders (Jablensky et al., 2000) and one targeting issues of childhood and adolescence (Sawyer et al., 2001). A later household survey (NSMHW 2007) was conducted in 2007 (Australian Bureau of Statistics, 2008b), while a further survey collecting information on lower prevalence disorders, the Second National Survey of Psychosis (or Study of High Impact Psychosis (SHIP) was conducted in 2010 (Morgan et al., 2011). A third household survey is planned. These surveys then are not held on a particularly regular or frequent basis, with a 10-year gap between the first two and 13 years between the second and third. Changes that may occur in instrumentation and other features of the surveys mean that, while they have had important influences on mental health care planning in Australia, they do not serve well to monitor population mental health, or ill health. So we need to look elsewhere for that. And what we do have to work with is information on psychological distress as gathered with a questionnaire (see Chapters 1.2, 1.4) within the regular (three-yearly) National Health Survey program. As we will see below, this does give us some useful information including somewhat finer-grained information about area characteristics and something about time trends.

As regards national information on mental health services, instigated with the First National Mental Health Plan (see Section 1.7.1), a series of National Mental Health Reports described developments in services across the country. These ceased in 2013 and so contemporary information now is sourced from the Australian Institute for Health and Welfare which regularly produces the web report 'Mental Health Services in Australia'.

THE AUSTRALIAN SURVEYS OF HIGH AND LOW PREVALENCE DISORDERS

The *National Survey of Mental Health and Well-being* (NSMHW 1997; Andrews, Anstey, et al., 1999; Australian Bureau of Statistics, 1998) used computerised administration of a field questionnaire, with interviewers carrying laptop computers into the homes of participants. It was designed to detect in the community the disorders with prevalence rates around 1% or more. For this, a sample size planned as approximately 10 000 people was chosen. This is large enough to give estimates for population rates with reasonable precision for disorders with prevalences as low as 1%.

The 2007 household survey was similar in overall design to that conducted in 1997 (Australian Bureau of Statistics, 2009; Slade, Johnson, Oakley Brown, Andrews, & Whiteford, 2009; Slade, Johnston, et al., 2009), though for some important differences see the next section. Many disorders of interest to mental health practice, however, occur at lower frequencies than the 1% level for which this approach can give helpful information. For disorders such as these, a different methodology is necessary. In 1997, the NSMHW was separated into two major arms:

1. The High Prevalence Survey, already introduced, being a community sample with an intended sample size of about 10 000
2. The Low Prevalence studies, a series of four studies with a different methodology for studying disorders, such as schizophrenia, that have expected prevalences of well below 1% (Jablensky et al., 2000).

A decade later, the Second Australian National Survey of Psychosis (Morgan et al., 2011), a study similar to the NSMHW Low Prevalence Survey, was conducted some three years after the household survey.

The next two sections outline the key findings of, first, the high prevalence disorders surveys; and second, the low prevalence disorders surveys.

1.6.2 THE NSMHW HOUSEHOLD SURVEYS OF HIGH PREVALENCE DISORDERS

GRAHAM MEADOWS

THE FIRST SURVEY: SAMPLING AND RECRUITMENT

In 1997, the Australian Bureau of Statistics (ABS) identified 13 600 households as representative of the Australian population. Interviewers visited each household several times, if necessary, to try to find a respondent at home (Australian Bureau of Statistics, 1998). To the person who answered the door they asked who in the house was the person with the next birthday, then arranged, where possible, to interview that person. Non-clinical interviewers, recruited and trained by the ABS, administered the field questionnaire. The field questionnaire was designed to detect and describe psychiatric morbidity, associated disability, service use and perceived need for care. It included a demographics section, and a specially prepared and modified version of the Composite International Diagnostic Interview twelve-month form, the CIDI 2.1 (World Health Organization, 1994; Wittchen, 1994). Then followed measures of general psychological symptoms (Goldberg & Williams, 1988), disability and physical health (Ware, Kosinski, & Keller, 1996) followed by a section collecting recall of service utilisation, and perceived needs for care (Meadows, Burgess, Fossey, & Harvey, 2000).

From the initial identification of 13 600 households, completion of the field questionnaire was achieved in 10 641 cases, a response rate of 78.2%. Participation was voluntary. Interviewing, on average, took less than an hour with each participant. The ABS used the demographic characteristics of the surveyed sample to estimate weightings for use in estimating true population rates from the sample. These were based on the relative frequencies of the sociodemographic characteristics of the sample, as compared to those derived from the relevant census of the Australian population. A decade later, the conduct of the NSMHW 2007 household survey (Australian Bureau of Statistics, 2009; Slade, Johnson, et al., 2009) was in overall design similar to the 1997 survey, but there were some important points of difference.

THREE SURVEYS COMPARED

An important difference between the two surveys conducted to date lies in the instrument used to assess presence and diagnosis of mental health problems. For several reasons, the twelve-month version of the CIDI (CIDI Auto 12) was selected as the basis for the 1997 field interview. Among considerations that weighed here were: (a) for service planning, recent episodes are of greater relevance than lifetime ones; and (b) the twelve-month interview, while exploring key diagnostic criteria for disorders experienced in the last year, could be briefer, so, it was hoped, increasing compliance and reducing respondent burden.

By the time of construction of the 2007 survey design, a multinational wave of studies including one in New Zealand (Wells, Oakley Browne, Scott, McGee, Baxter, & Kokaua, 2006; Wells, Oakley Browne, Scott, McGee, Baxter, Kokaua, et al., 2006) had used a different instrument, Version 3.0 of the CIDI. The CIDI 3.0 was specifically designed to increase likelihood of accurate recall of episodes throughout the lifespan, with changes in ordering of questions designed to maximise capture of this information. Once lifetime history was established, then the question was asked in the CIDI 3.0 as to whether the respondent had experienced some of the symptoms of the disorder in the last year (Kessler & Ustun, 2004). Typically analyses of the survey reporting prevalence rates are based on this report, rather than ascertaining whether they had clearly met the threshold for one or more diagnoses in the last year. So the 2007 survey, based on the CIDI 3.0, has the advantage of an estimate of lifetime prevalence of disorders but the disadvantage of lower face validity to its regularly used estimates of recent experience of disorder; diagnostic comparisons are not typically valid between the 1997 and 2007 surveys. The field interview for 2007 was longer than 1997, around 90 minutes. The response rate in 2007 proved to be lower than in 1997, nationally around 60%. The total sample was smaller, at 8841 individuals.

The next national mental health epidemiological project was announced in August 2019 as part of a larger initiative, the Intergenerational Health and Mental Health Study. It generally will be referred to as a study rather than a survey and this may serve to distinguish it by an important feature. This national Australian survey is for the first time intended to have a longitudinal dimension, with surveys planned across three years on aggregate, allowing study of course and outcomes of mental health problems. This time a design decision has been taken to keep much of this instrumentation common with the 2007 survey so putting aside the problems with validity of the CIDI 3.0 introduced earlier, there should at least be better instrumental comparability between the 2007 and the next surveys. However no such large exercises are exactly comparable in terms of sample selection and response biases. Early then in the course of the life of this edition of *Mental Health in Australia*, the first findings from the next survey will become available. This can be expected firstly to happen in the way of an ABS report, then publications based on further analyses. These are made possible by release of Confidentialised Unit Record Files (CURFs) to researchers who then can carry out analyses directly on a version of the study data set. These typically begin to flow into journal publications a couple of years after the survey is conducted. In the case of this longitudinal study there will likely continue to be a flow of relevant publications through the mid- to late 2020s.

INTERVIEWING AND RESPONSE

Presentation of NSMHW 2007 results

As will be clear from the introductory material above, there are strengths and weaknesses to both the

NSMHW 1997 and 2007 results. The NSMHW 1997 results have been highly influential in Australia, and often quoted in formulation of policy nationally and at state level. The NSMHW 2007 findings do include lifetime prevalence, and in this way represent an advance over the NSMHW 1997 findings, although validity of this information based on self-report can be criticised (Andrews, Hall, Teesson, & Henderson, 1999), and modelling approaches suggest recall failure can be appreciable (Patten, 2003; Patten, Gordon-Brown, & Meadows, 2010). Based on the way the questions were posed (see above), the estimates of one-year prevalence would appear to be likely to set the threshold for case identification (p. 174) lower than in 1997. This in turn is likely to be lower than the criteria by which a clinician and also the consumer affected might wish to agree that such a disorder was present. Clinical diagnosis usually goes along with significant distress or disability associated with the symptoms, and other features that mitigate for help-seeking or other ways of presenting to care. It by no means follows from identification as a 'case' in one of these surveys that a person would have had a diagnostic label assigned by a clinician, or that as a consumer they would have wished to accept such a label, or that this would have necessarily been of benefit to them. With the above caveats in place, we will from here forward concentrate on prevalence findings from the NSMHW 2007. When the next survey results become available these may make for more up-to date figures, and possibly some information on trends, though this will depend on how the survey goes in the field. The 2007 survey had considerably lower response rated than the 1997 survey. Fatigue regarding surveys in the workforce and increased apartment or gated-community living which makes establishing contact more difficult may both have contributed to this. It will represent a challenge for the implementation of the next survey to see how much these influences can be overcome.

PREVALENCE FINDINGS

Overall prevalence

Based on the NSMHW 2007 data (Australian Bureau of Statistics, 2009; Slade, Johnson, et al., 2009) it was found that 45.5% of the population had at some time in their lives had a mental disorder. Twenty per cent of the population has had symptoms of their disorder or disorders in the last year, and 10% in the last 30 days. Considering the three major disorder groups assessed in this household survey of affective, anxiety and substance use disorders, the findings were as listed, in order from most to least common:

Anxiety disorders:

- lifetime prevalence 26.3%
- twelve-month symptoms 14.4%
- thirty-day symptoms 7.7%.

Substance use disorders:

- lifetime prevalence 24.7%
- 12-month symptoms 5.1%
- 30-day symptoms 1.8%.

Affective disorders:

- lifetime prevalence 15.0%
- 12-month symptoms 6.2%
- 30-day symptoms 2.4%.

The occurrence of disorders together constitutes comorbidity of mental disorders. It is common: 8.5% of the population had more than one mental disorder; 3.4% had multiple disorders from the same group; while 5.1% had disorders from multiple groups. The prevalences of the major mental disorder diagnostic groups and associated comorbidities with other mental disorders are given by way of a Venn diagram, one each for males and females as shown in Figure 1.24 (Teesson, Slade, & Mills, 2009).

Moving from these broad diagnostic classifications into specific disorders, rates for these, as assessed both for lifetime history and by presence of symptoms in the last year are set out in Table 1.9.

Age and mental disorder: Findings

Figure 1.25 shows how the overall rates of all mental disorders declines with age, from the rate of 26% of all people with a mental disorder in the age range 16–24 to 5.9% among those aged 75-85 years. However the picture here is very different for different disorder groups, as is clear from Figure 1.26. Substance use disorders peak in early adult life, while anxiety and affective disorders peak in the middle years.

Figure 1.24 (a) Prevalence (percentage) of single and comorbid affective, anxiety and substance use disorders among Australian subjects in the previous 12 months (b) Prevalence (percentage) of single and comorbid affective, anxiety and substance use disorders among Australian female subjects in the previous 12 months

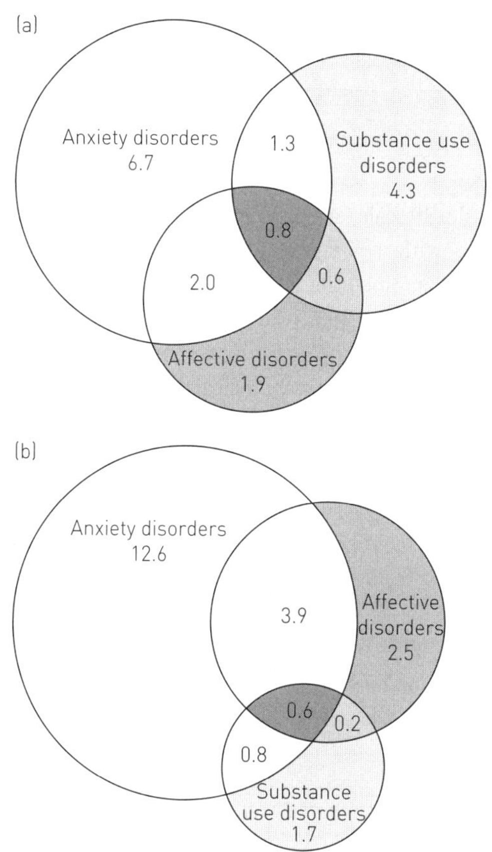

Source: Adapted from Teesson et al. 2009; Australian and New Zealand Journal of Psychiatry 2009

What more recent information do we have?

The information from the 2007 NSMHW is the most recent detailed information we have on mental disorders in the Australian population until the next survey becomes available. These specific surveys are a long way apart and not committed to as part of a regular program, so there is no guarantee even for instance that there might be another such survey in 2030. It would be useful then if we had some other survey information that would tell us something about trends in mental disorders in Australia over time. Indeed there is such a data source, within a regular survey conducted by the ABS on the nation's health, a description of which forms the next section.

1.6.3 AUSTRALIAN NATIONAL MENTAL HEALTH DATA COLLECTION: THE AUSTRALIAN NATIONAL HEALTH SURVEY

JOANNE ENTICOTT & GRAHAM MEADOWS

INTRODUCTION

These country-wide household surveys, typically with samples around 20 000, are conducted regularly every

Table 1.9 Lifetime and one-year prevalence rates, common mental disorders

Mental disorders: prevalence rates: population percentages as assessed by the NSMHW, 2007							
		Persons		***Males***		***Females***	
		Lifetime	**12 months**	**Lifetime**	**12 months**	**Lifetime**	**12 months**
Anxiety disorders	Post-traumatic stress disorder	12.2%	6.4%	8.6%	4.6%	15.8%	8.3%
	Social phobia	10.6%	4.7%	8.4%	3.8%	12.8%	5.7%
	Agoraphobia	6.0%	2.8%	4.1%	2.1%	7.9%	3.5%
	Generalised anxiety disorder	5.9%	2.7%	4.4%	2.0%	7.3%	3.5%
	Panic disorder	5.2%	2.6%	4.6%	2.3%	5.8%	2.8%
	Obsessive-compulsive disorder	2.8%	1.9%	2.3%	1.6%	3.2%	2.2%

(Continues)

Table 1.9 Lifetime and one-year prevalence rates, common mental disorders (*Continued*)

Mental disorders: prevalence rates: population percentages as assessed by the NSMHW, 2007							
		Persons		*Males*		*Females*	
		Lifetime	**12 months**	**Lifetime**	**12 months**	**Lifetime**	**12 months**
Substance use disorders	Alcohol harmful use	18.9%	2.9%	28.1%	3.8%	9.8%	2.1%
	Drug use disorders	7.5%	1.4%	10.2%	2.1%	4.8%	0.8%
	Alcohol dependence	3.8%	1.4%	5.2%	2.2%	2.4%	0.7%
Affective disorders	Depressive episode	11.6%	4.1%	8.8%	3.1%	14.5%	5.1%
	Bipolar affective disorder	2.9%	1.8%	3.0%	1.8%	2.7%	1.7%
	Dysthymia	1.9%	1.3%	1.5%	1.0%	2.4%	1.5%

Source: NSMHW, 2007

three years by the Australian Bureau of Statistics (ABS) At time of writing the latest of these is the 2017-18 National Health Survey (NHS). Information collected bears on: prevalence of long-term health conditions; health risk factors and demographic and socioeconomic characteristics. Importantly for this purpose a measure of psychological distress, the Kessler 10 scale (see Chapters 1.3 and 1.4) is collected along with self-report of anxiety and depressive problems. Since the K10 has featured in all surveys this century (2001, 2004-05, 2007-08, 2011-12, 2014-15 and 2017-18), we have some information on how prevalence of psychological distress has changed (or not), in this country through this time. The K10

Figure 1.25 12-month mental disorders—Prevalence rates by age

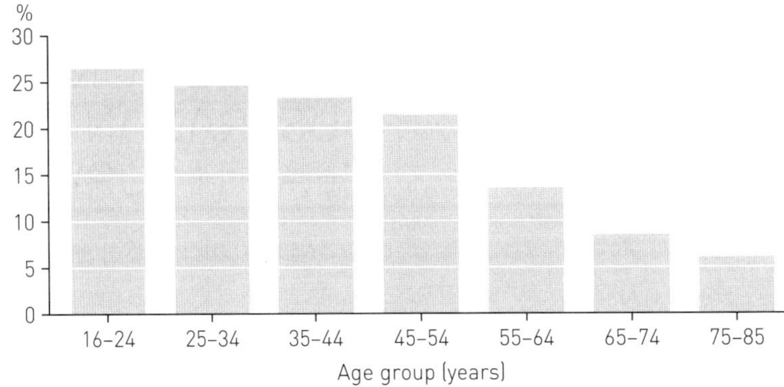

Source: NSMHW, 2007

Figure 1.26 12-month mental disorder symptoms—Major disorder group and age

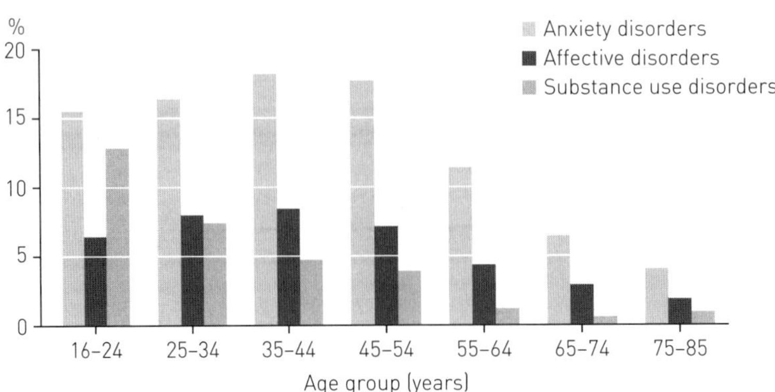

Source: NSMHW, 2007

scores can be used to assign survey participants into bands, commonly calculated as ranging between 10 and 50, with score bands of low (10-15), moderate (16-21), high (22-29) and very high (30-50). These score bands have reasonably consistent relationships with rates of mental disorders. Findings from the 2007 NSMHWB were that for people with very high scores, 80% met 12-month criteria for a mental disorder while for people with low scores 11% had a mental disorder (Slade et al., 2011). There is no clear reason to believe these associations would have changed much in the intervening years (see Chapter 1.4). For this purpose the important score levels are the very high scores, and in some measure the combined high and very high score bands. The NSMHWs are voluntary in nature, and as mentioned above, low response rates can be a problem. In contrast, the NHS is carried out under the Census Act and so participation for selected individuals is required. Because the response rate of this survey is reasonably high (e.g. 76% in the 2017-18 survey) and because the sample is large (21 315 in 2017-18), with sophisticated sampling, we can make more use of these data for information on regional and other distributions associations with mental health problems than has been possible with any of the NSMHWs. The NHS gives us two things that the NSMHW program so far could not:

1 The ability to track the rates of mental health problems through time in the Australian population.
2 The ability to examine with some precision associations of higher levels of psychological distress, a reasonable proxy measure for mental disorders, with important social determinants of mental health and illness.

We will now consider what information is available to us on these questions.

MENTAL HEALTH THROUGH TIME IN THE AUSTRALIAN POPULATION

In Chapter 1.2, we reproduced a graph of changes in the K10 scores from 2001-14 (Meadows, Enticott, & Rosenberg, 2018) analysed with careful comparative methods (Harvey et al., 2017). This showed an essentially flat line, not increasing but not decreasing either as might have been hoped for given increased mental health spending. The analytic process used in this work including population standardisation has not been applied to comparisons with the latest survey but the headline figures from the 2017-18 NHS are concerning. The 2017-18 survey (Australian Bureau of Statistics, 2018c) found 13.0% of adult Australians with high or very high K10 scores, increased from 11.7% in 2014-15. Fewer people had low scores in 2017-18 (60.8%) than in 2014-15 (68.0%). Confirmation as to whether this change might be due to demographic shifts is needed but these initial findings raise concern that despite efforts towards better treatment and prevention, mental health may be getting worse. We will return to this issue at the end of the chapter.

ASSOCIATIONS OF MENTAL ILL HEALTH WITH IMPORTANT SOCIAL DETERMINANTS

Psychological distress in 2017-18 had higher frequency among women than men (14.5% versus 11.3% respectively). Between 2017-18 and 2014-15 there seemed to be a greater proportion of 55-64-year old women with high or very high K10 scores (16.9% versus 12.3%).

Associations have also been examined with socioeconomic disadvantage of area and with income levels (Isaacs, Enticott, Meadows, & Inder, 2018). These are summarised in Table 1.10. We have noted elsewhere in the text taking a life course perspective how relative and absolute socioeconomic deprivation increases a range of risk factors for mental health problems including: unemployment, homelessness, being a victim of domestic violence and other crime (see Section 1.2.4). There then is the challenge of coping with these where there is deficient social capital and infrastructure. The table then sets out the magnitude of the relationships with these factors, both using the composite census indicator of the Index of Relative Socioeconomic Disadvantage (IRSD; see Section 1.2.5) and income levels. Using these findings we have calculated and elsewhere

Table 1.10 Prevalence of psychological distress across Australia, separated by capital cities and balance of state

Number of 18- to 64-year-olds		Greater Capital City Statistical areas ASGS 2011							
		K10 high/very high distress				K10 very high distress			
		Capital cities n=6,904 %(95%CI)		Balance of state n=5,428 %(95%CI)		Capital cities n=6,904 %(95%CI)		Balance of state n=5,428 %(95%CI)	
Australian population		11.0	(10.2, 11.8)	11.4	(10.2, 12.5)	3.4	(2.9, 3.9)	4.0	(3.3, 4.6)
Gender	Male	8.8	(7.6, 9.9)	9.9	(8.3, 11.5)	2.5	(1.9, 3.2)	3.8	(2.6, 4.9)
	Female	13.3	(12.0, 14.6)	12.8	(11.1, 14.6)	4.3	(3.4, 5.1)	4.1	(3.2, 5.1)
Age group (years)†	18–24	12.2	(9.9, 14.6)	11.4	(7.7, 15.1)	2.5	(1.1, 3.9)	4.1	(1.8, 6.3)
	25–34	11.4	(9.6, 13.2)	9.9	(7.5, 12.2)	3.2	(2.2, 4.2)	2.0	(0.8, 3.2)
	35–44	10.3	(8.7, 11.9)	12.3	(9.9, 14.7)	2.8	(2.0, 3.6)	4.1	(2.3, 5.9)
	45–54	11.3	(9.6, 13.0)	11.8	(9.3, 14.2)	5.1	(3.9, 6.3)	5.4	(3.6, 7.1)
	55–64	9.9	(8.0, 11.7)	11.4	(9.1, 13.8)	3.4	(2.5, 4.3)	4.0	(3.6, 5.5)
Income quintiles	(rich) 1	5.2	(4.0, 6.5)	6.5	(4.3, 8.7)	1.3	(0.7, 2.0)	1.6	(0.5, 2.8)
	2	8.4	(6.7, 10.1)*	4.7	(3.1, 6.3)	2.2	(1.0, 3.3)	0.8	(0.3, 1.4)
	3	10.8	(8.7, 12.8)*	8.8	(6.5, 11.0)	2.6	(1.5, 3.7)	3.9	(2.2, 5.5)
	4	17.4	(14.5, 20.4)*	17.8	(14.7, 21.0)*	6.7	(5.0, 8.5)*	6.9	(4.7, 9.0)*
	(poor) 5	24.9	(20.9, 28.8)*	28.4	(22.9, 33.9)*	9.7	(7.5, 12.0)*	12.8	(9.0, 16.6)*
IRSD quintiles	(rich) 1	7.0	(5.4, 8.5)	6.5	(3.9, 9.2)	1.6	(0.9, 2.2)	2.5	(0, 4.9)
	2	8.9	(7.3, 10.5)	7.0	(4.4, 9.6)	3.1	(2.2, 4.0)	2.9	(0.9, 5.0)
	3	12.1	(10.1, 14.2)*	11.7	(9.2, 14.3)	3.9	(2.4, 5.3)*	3.5	(2.0, 4.9)
	4	14.3	(11.9, 16.7)*	12.0	(9.9, 14.1)*	4.5	(3.0, 6.0)*	3.6	(2.4, 4.7)
	(poor) 5	16.9	(14.1, 19.7)*	15.2	(12.0, 18.4)*	5.4	(3.5, 7.4)*	6.1	(4.6, 7.7)

Source: Adapted from Isaacs, et al., 2018

Notes: IRSD: Index of Relative Socioeconomic Disadvantage; CI: confidence interval; ABS: Australian Bureau of Statistics; K10: Kessler 10. The K10 *very high* distress category represents a score of 30 or higher. Combined *high/very high* distress category represents a score of 22 or higher. CI: Confidence Intervals are based on replication-based standard error estimation. ABS weighting was used to produce population estimates. *K10 percentages had significant differences between quintile 1 and the quintile indicated ($p < 0.05$), indicating less distress in quintile 1 (richest areas of Australia).

presented (Meadows et al., 2019) that within all adults with very high psychological distress, 30% have areas of residence in the most disadvantaged quintile of Australian areas while 9% come from the most advantaged quintile. Considering personal income, in the lowest quintile for this measure, a quarter of people have high or very high distress; in the least disadvantaged quintile it is one in 20.

HOUSEHOLD IMPACTS OF COVID-19 SURVEY

As noted elsewhere (see Section 1.2.5), the final stages of the preparation of this text coincided with the advent of the COVID-19 pandemic. The ABS has responded with an extraordinary range of information to help understand the effects of this for the nation. Much of this is based on regularly available data sets, but there also has been the innovation of a regular community survey, including data collection on mental health. So, from early April 2020, and (at time of writing) twice a month, the ABS has been conducting a voluntary telephone survey involving over 1000 Australians, with rapid public reporting. The cohort sample was designed to be nationally representative except for very remote locations and analysis used population weighting to maximise the accuracy of the estimates for the Australian population. So far, response rates have been around 90% which is extremely high for such surveys. Targets of the survey data collection have been: 'financial stress; stimulus payments received and how used; changes to job situation; feelings of emotional and mental wellbeing; and contact with family and friends' (Australian Bureau of Statistics, 2020). Elsewhere in this book we have highlighted the influences that financial and job stress can have on population mental health and the importance of occupation and social connectedness in recovery journeys (see Chapters 1.2 and 2.6).

At the point of the latest survey, the ABS highlights from the survey were: 'Nearly a third of Australians (31%) reported that their household finances had worsened due to COVID-19; one in four Australians aged 18 years and over (28%) reported receiving the first one-off $750 economic support payment from the Commonwealth Government; and compared to the 2017-18 National Health Survey almost twice as many adults reported experiencing feelings associated with anxiety, such as nervousness or restlessness, 'at least some of the time' (Australian Bureau of Statistics, 2020). The instrument used to assess mental health and wellbeing was an abbreviated version (six items) of the Kessler-10 questionnaire (see Section 1.4.3). Of course, feelings of anxiety in the context of a disease outbreak unprecedented in the lives of almost all Australians are not necessarily pathological or an indication for specific or specialist mental health care. Some level of anxiety is necessary probably to prompt what also were reported as very high rates of engagement with social distancing instructions. But there likely will be a time-course for some of those experiences that will lead to need for mental health care and the survey estimate was that around 10% of Australians had discussed feelings of psychological distress with a doctor or other health professional. To date, the survey is not showing definite increases in feelings of worthlessness or hopelessness that would be more distinct indicators of depressive disorders, but application of experiences from disaster management would suggest that such sequelae can typically take longer to develop than the relatively brief time-window so far elapsed.

1.6.4 THE SECOND NATIONAL SURVEY OF PEOPLE LIVING WITH PSYCHOTIC DISORDERS

CAROL HARVEY & VERA MORGAN

TWO SURVEYS

The Second *Australian National Survey of Psychosis* (Survey of High Impact Psychosis (SHIP)) took place in 2010. It built on information gained in the first survey in 1997-98, the *Low Prevalence (Psychotic) Disorders Study* (Jablensky et al., 2000; Jablensky et al., 1999) with a substantial collection of new and updated information using a much-expanded interview and assessment package. The second survey aimed to extend and deepen our understanding of clinical presentation, living circumstances, social and economic participation and needs of people with a psychotic disorder, as well as identify factors associated with better outcomes (see further details in Morgan et al., 2011; 2012). For the first time, the survey included people with a psychotic disorder who were solely in contact with non-government organisations funded to support people with mental disorders in recognition of the growing and important contribution of this service sector.

SECOND SURVEY DESIGN AND METHODOLOGY

Population coverage

The 2010 survey was conducted at seven mental health service sites in five Australian states. The geographical regions covered by the survey were the catchment areas of each site. They were: Hunter New England and Orange services in New South Wales; West Moreton in Queensland; Northern Mental Health in South Australia; North West Area Mental Health Service and St Vincent's Mental Health

Service in Victoria; and Fremantle, Peel, Rockingham and Kwinana Services in Western Australia. These sites covered a total area of 61 682 square kilometres and an estimated resident population aged 18–64 years of 1 464 923 people, or approximately 10% of the Australian population in the same age range. The survey included people who were 18 to 64 years of age, resident in the catchment sites and in contact with designated services: public specialised mental health services (inpatient, outpatient, ambulatory and community services and clinics—hereafter abbreviated to public mental health services) and non-government organisations supporting people with mental disorders. Unlike the 1997–98 survey, the 2010 survey did not cover people with psychotic disorders who were being treated only in the private sector or by their general practitioner, and screening did not include contact points for homeless people. This should be kept in mind in making comparisons between the two surveys.

Census month and interview period

The census of people with psychosis was in March 2010. Interviewing took place from April to December 2010.

Design

Two phases

A two-phase design was employed (Morgan et al., 2011; Pickles, Dunn, & Vázquez-Barquero, 1995). This design was chosen as appropriate for estimating the prevalence of relatively uncommon disorders, and was also efficient in identifying those likely to meet diagnostic criteria for whom the full interview schedule was relevant.

Phase 1: Screening

Phase 1: Screening in the census month identified three mutually exclusive groups: (a) people in contact with public mental health services in the census month; (b) people not in contact with these services in the census month but in contact with non-government organisations supporting people with mental disorders in that month; and (c) people not in contact with public mental health services or non-government organisations in the census month but in contact with public mental health services in the 11 months prior to census.

A psychosis screener was used to identify individuals likely to meet criteria for formal diagnosis. The screener was developed for the first national psychosis survey (Jablensky et al., 1999; 2000) and pilot tested prior to the second survey, which led to minor modifications (see Morgan et al., 2012). Mental health inpatient and outpatient administrative records were scanned to identify people with a recorded diagnosis of psychosis and in contact with public mental health services in the 11 months before the census but not in the census month. People with the following diagnoses on administrative records were within scope for the survey: ICD-10 schizophrenia (F20); schizotypal disorder (F21); persistent delusional disorder (F22); acute or transient psychotic disorder (F23); induced delusional disorder (F24); schizoaffective disorders (F25); other and unspecified non-organic psychotic disorder (F28, F29); manic episode with psychotic symptoms (F30.2); bipolar affective disorder with psychotic symptoms (F31.2, F31.5); severe depressive episode with psychotic symptoms (F32.3); recurrent depressive disorder with psychotic symptoms (F33.3); or at least two admissions with a drug- or alcohol-induced psychosis (F10–F19: .5 and .7 only).

Phase 2: Interviewing

In phase 2, 7955 people who were screened as positive for psychosis and met eligibility criteria were randomised for interview at each site, stratified by age group. Equal numbers were targeted in two age strata (18–34 years and 35–64 years) to ensure adequate coverage of younger as well as older age participants. People were excluded from the interview phase if (a) they had insufficient English or a communication or cognitive impairment affecting their capacity for informed consent or completion of a valid interview; or (b) they were unavailable for interview because of residence in a nursing home or prison. In total, 1825 screen-positive people were interviewed.

Assessment

The interview schedule consisted of 32 modules and over 1500 items covering:

- sociodemographic characteristics, including income, education, housing, activities of daily life, employment, child and other caring responsibilities
- psychopathology and general cognitive ability
- physical health conditions, smoking, alcohol and drug use, nutrition and exercise
- health and other services used for physical and mental health problems, covering hospital admissions, emergency department attendances, outpatient and community mental health care, rehabilitation programs, contact with case managers, visits to general practitioners and contact with non-government organisations supporting people with mental disorder
- medications used for mental health problems and their side effects
- family contact, social participation, crime, offending and personal safety.

Questions from the 1997–98 psychosis survey were included to enable an assessment of change over time. In addition, questions from the 2007 *National Survey of Mental Health and Well-being* (Australian Bureau of Statistics, 2008a; Slade, Johnson, et al., 2009) and Australian Bureau of Statistics national surveys facilitated comparison with population norms. There were a number of embedded instruments (see Morgan et al., 2012). Physical health information was also collected through a physical examination and blood sample.

Diagnostic assessment was based on a semi-structured clinical research interview, the *Diagnostic Interview for Psychosis* (DIP-DM; Castle et al., 2006) which was first used in the 1997–98 survey. The DIP-DM contains selected interview questions and probes from the WHO Schedules for Clinical Assessment in Neuropsychiatry (Wing, Babor, Brugha, & Burke, 1990) mapped on the 94 diagnostic items of the OPCRIT (McGuffin, Farmer, & Harvey, 1991). The DIP scores serve as input to a computer algorithm that provides a diagnostic classification in accordance with ICD-10 and DSM-IV criteria, thus reducing substantially subjective bias in the interpretation of the scored symptoms and signs. The DIP interview was administered by mental health professionals who had undergone extensive training.

Participant response

The response rate among the 4189 people who screened positive for psychosis and were randomised and contacted for interview was 44%. A further 2107 people had been randomly sampled for interview but not asked to participate, because (a) they could not be traced or had died in the period since screening (57%; b) case managers had assessed them as not mentally well enough or, in some cases, had neglected to pass on the request (21%); or (c) interviewers judged them to be too unwell physically or mentally to provide consent (22%). Comparison of screening data for interviewed participants and those selected for interview but not participating for any reason indicated no systematic selection biases (see Morgan et al., 2012, for further details).

RESULTS

Estimating the number of people with psychotic disorders treated by public specialised mental health services

In March 2010, the estimated treated prevalence of psychotic disorders ascertained in a one-month period for people aged 18–64 years was 3.5 people per 1000 population, distributed as 3.1 people per 1000 population in public mental health services and 0.4 people per 1000 population in non-government organisations (NGOs) supporting people with mental disorders. The prevalence of psychotic disorders was higher in males than females (3.7 per 1000 compared to 2.4 per 1000; see Figure 1.27). Prevalence was also estimated for the twelve-month period at 4.5 people per 1000 population. Scaled to the national level, this suggests that almost 64 000 people aged 18 to 64 years have a psychotic disorder and are in contact with public specialised mental health services in a year.

At 3.1 people per 1000 population, the one-month treated prevalence of psychotic illness in

Figure 1.27 Estimated national one-month treated prevalence of ICD-10 psychotic disorders in public specialised mental health services by sex

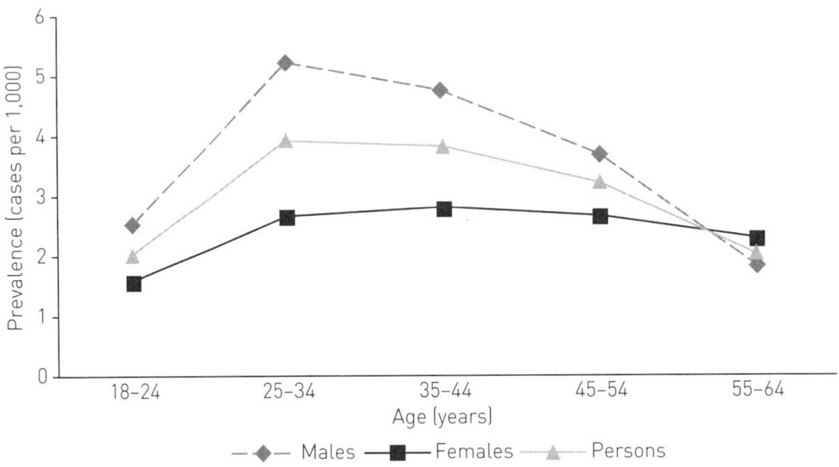

Source: Morgan et al. 2011. Used with permission.

public mental health services in 2010 is similar to the 1997-98 rate of 3.3 people per 1000 population. However, these estimates do not take account of people with psychosis being treated solely in the private sector or those not receiving any treatment. Combining data from all treatment sectors across the two surveys (public mental health services, NGOs and private treatment services) gives an overall estimated one-month treated prevalence of approximately 4.9 people per 1000 population, with a further 0.4 people per 1000 population in homeless settings. The population prevalence will be somewhat higher as this figure excludes people who have the diagnosis but are not in contact with any services.

The interviewed sample

The interviewed sample consisted of 1825 people. Three-fifths (59.6%) of people being treated for psychosis in the public mental health system were male, and a similar proportion (57.6%) were aged 35-64 years (see Table 1.11).

Two-thirds (66.4%) were using public mental health services in the census month; 11.2% were only using NGOs supporting people with mental disorders in that month; and a further 22.4% had not used public mental health services or non-government agencies in the census month, but had been using public mental health services in the 11 months prior to the census month.

Demographic characteristics of people living with psychotic disorders in Australia

Many people living with psychotic disorders experience disadvantages that, largely because of onset of illness in late adolescence and early adulthood, have an impact upon their educational outcomes. One-third (33.7%) of people with psychotic disorders had not attained a school certificate, compared with 24.9% in the general population (Slade, 2011). Almost one-quarter (22.5%) had left school before Year 10. Another third (31.5%) had completed their Year 12 qualification or leaving certificate. About half (47.1%) of participants had completed a TAFE or trade certificate or higher post-school qualification (see Table 1.11). Compounding their difficulties, almost one in five people with a psychotic disorder (18.4%) reported difficulty with reading and/or writing. Despite these disadvantages, one-fifth (20.8%) were enrolled in formal studies in the previous year.

People with psychotic disorders experience very high rates of unemployment and low rates of labour force participation (see Table 1.11). Government pensions were the main source of income for 85.0%. One-third (32.7%) had been in paid employment over the past year, and one-fifth (21.5%) in the week prior to interview. By comparison, 72.4% of the general working age population (15–64 years) were employed in July 2010 (Australian Bureau of Statistics, 2010). Three-quarters of those participants who were employed (74.8%) were in open, competitive employment; 7.6% were self-employed; and 17.1% were in sheltered, non-competitive employment. Of those employed, the majority (69.0%) were working part time and over a quarter (27.5%) would have preferred more hours.

At the time of interview, one-half (48.6%) of all survey participants were living in rental accommodation, with 26.8% in public rentals and 21.8% in private rentals. While two-fifths (39.8%) would prefer to be living in their own home or unit, only 13.1% were doing so at the time of interview. Almost one in four (22.7%) were on a public housing waiting list. There is a greater risk of homelessness among people with psychotic disorders. Some 5.2% were homeless at the time of the study, and 12.8% had experienced periods of homelessness over the previous year (see Table 1.11). A specific subgroup at risk of homelessness is those who are admitted for acute inpatient treatment. Half (52.8%) had discussed accommodation needs before their most recent hospital discharge, but 6.9% reported they had not been given any assistance and were homeless on discharge from hospital.

Table 1.11 Key socioeconomic and demographic characteristics

	Proportion (%)		
	Males	**Females**	**Persons**
Older age group (35–64 years)	55.3	63.7	57.6
Sex	59.6	40.4	–
Born in Australia	83.3	80.6	82.2
Currently married or in de facto relationship	12.1	24.5	17.1
Own children (any age)	25.9	56.2	38.1
Dependent children living at home, including stepchildren	5.5	23.6	12.8
Education			
Left school with no qualifications	36.1	30.2	33.7
Completed Year 12 education	31.0	32.1	31.5
Post-school qualification	43.3	52.6	47.1
Enrolled in formal studies (past year)	16.7	26.7	20.8
Income and employment			
Main source of income: government payment	85.6	83.7	85.0
In paid employment (past year)	33.6	31.3	32.7
In paid employment (past 7 days)	21.2	22.0	21.5
Homelessness and housing			
Living in supported accommodation (currently)	14.4	6.0	11.0
Homeless (currently)	7.3	2.0	5.2
Homeless (past year)	15.4	8.9	12.8

Source: Morgan et al. 2011. Used with permission.

Diagnosis, symptoms and nature of the disorder

The most common psychotic disorder was schizophrenia (47.0%), accounting for the majority of males (56.3%) and one-third (33.2%) of females (see Figure 1.28 for further diagnostic details). Two-thirds (64.8%) of people experienced their first episode before the age of 25 years.

One in 12 people (8.1%) had experienced just one episode of psychotic disorder, while the majority (61.5%) had experienced multiple episodes with periods of good or partial recovery in between (29.7 and 31.8%, respectively; see Figure 1.29). Many people (30.5%) have continual chronic disorder, with or without deterioration. The most common symptoms of psychotic disorder are delusions and hallucinations: 41.3% experienced delusions currently, with a corresponding figure for hallucinations of 37.5%. The majority of participants (59.8%) reported symptoms of anxiety, and just over half (54.5%) reported one or more symptoms of depression over the past year.

Physical health, trauma and at-risk behaviours

People with psychotic disorders receiving public mental health services have poorer physical health than the general population and are more at risk because of their high levels of obesity, smoking, and alcohol and drug use. Almost half (45.1%) of people with psychotic disorders were obese. One-half (49.9%) met criteria for metabolic syndrome and one-quarter (24.0%) were at high risk of cardiovascular disease or already had cardiovascular disease. Two-thirds

Figure 1.28 ICD-10 lifetime diagnosis by sex

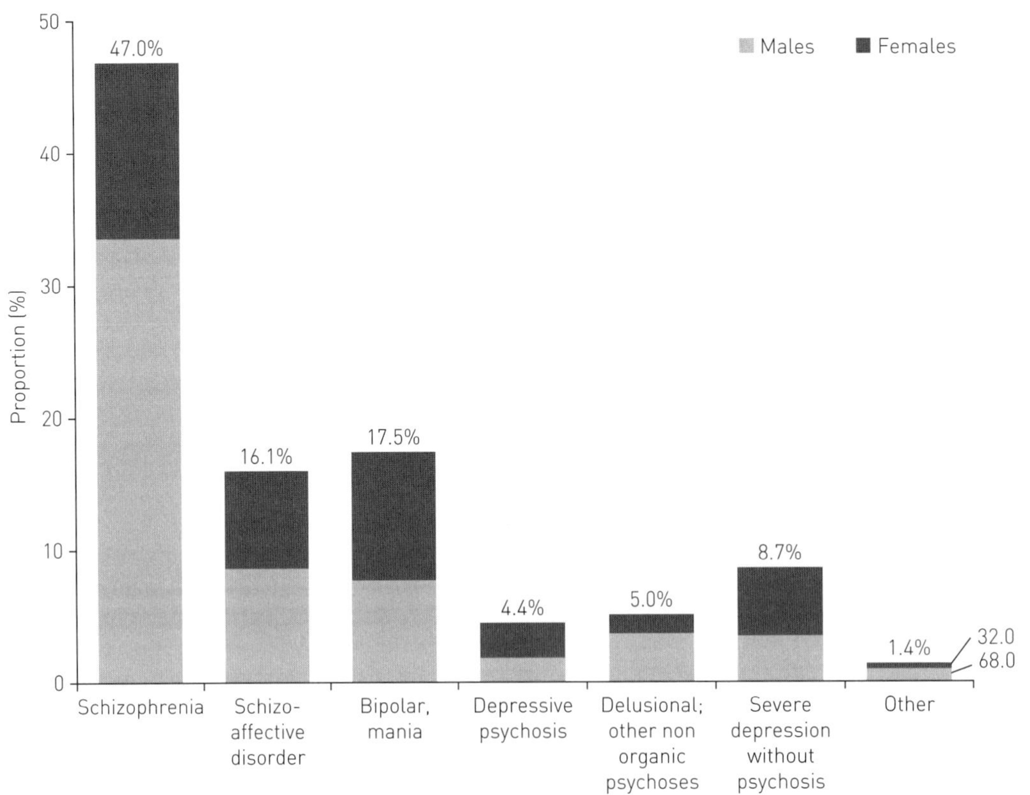

Source: Morgan et al. 2011. Used with permission.

Figure 1.29 Course of illness

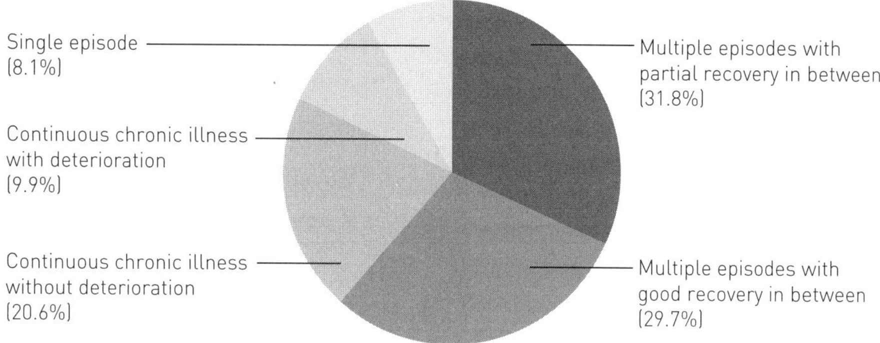

Source: Morgan et al. 2011. Used with permission.

(66.1%) of people with psychosis smoke, and they smoke an average of 21 cigarettes per day. By contrast, only one in four (25.3%) of the general population are smokers (Slade, 2011). Alcohol abuse was high, with 58.3% of males and 38.9% of females assessed by interviewers as consuming alcohol at levels that constitute abuse or dependence at some point in their lifetime (compared with 35.3% of males and 14.1% of females in the general population; Slade, 2011). Rates of lifetime use of cannabis or other illicit drugs were very high, with 63.2% of males and 41.7% of females assessed by interviewers as using at levels that constitute abuse or dependence (compared with 12.0% of males and 5.8% of females in the general population; Slade, 2011). However, only 12.9% of people with psychotic disorders were participating in drug and alcohol treatment programs.

Over half (57.2%) of people with a psychotic disorder reported experiencing a distressing or traumatic event in childhood, with 16.1% reporting having been sexually abused. People with psychosis are also far more likely to think about and attempt suicide than the general population. Just over one-tenth (11.5%) of people reported that they were thinking about suicide at the time of interview. Half (49.5%) reported they had attempted suicide at some point in their lifetime, compared with only 3.7% in the general population (Slade, 2011).

Relationships and social support

People with psychotic disorders are often isolated by their symptoms, and this isolation can be exacerbated by recurrent episodes of disorder, periods of hospitalisation, as well as stigma and discrimination that make maintenance of family and social contacts more difficult. For instance, two-thirds of participants (63.9%) reported good social functioning before the onset of first symptoms, whereas a similar proportion (63.2%) were assessed as having a significant level of dysfunction in their capacity to socialise over the year before the survey. Only one in five people with a psychotic disorder (17.1%) had a partner (married or de facto), compared with two-thirds in the general population (ABS 2009). Nevertheless, many people with psychosis are carers for children and others. As many as one-half (56.2%) of females in the survey had children of any age, with one-quarter (23.6%) having dependent children living with them. The proportion of males with children was much lower, at 25.9%, and only 5.5% had dependent children living with them. In 14.7% of cases, participants were providing care to another person because of a disability, long-term disorder or due to old age.

Nearly one-quarter (22.4%) of people with psychosis reported feeling socially isolated and lonely, and of these, two-thirds (69.3%) said their disorder made it difficult to maintain close relationships. Although the majority of people had at least one friend (86.5%), 13.3% had no friends at all. Nonetheless, many participants had frequent contact with family. Most (96.1%) had at least some contact with a family member over the last year. For many (65.4%) this was almost daily, and another 18.2%

had at least weekly contact. One-quarter (24.5%) of participants had a carer. For 40.8% of these people, this was their mother, for 25.7% it was a partner and for 5.4% it was their child. Overall, with regard to support to function, just over half (56.4%) of people with psychotic disorders reported receiving no or minimal support from any source.

Service and medication use

The majority of people with psychotic disorders used a wide variety of health services for both their mental and physical health problems (see Figure 1.30). Almost all (95.3%) had used services for their mental health problems, and 81.0% had used services for their physical health problems. Most people with psychotic disorders (88.2%) had visited a general practitioner in the past year, averaging nine visits a year. One-quarter (28.8%) averaged over 12 visits in the past year. This compares to a general population average of six visits a year (Australian Institute of Health and Welfare, 2018c).

43.7% of all participants reported at least one inpatient admission in the previous year, and one-third (34.8%) of all participants had had one or more psychiatric admissions in this same period. Most people (82.2%) had used outpatient or community clinics and ambulatory health care services for mental health problems in the past year. More than two-thirds (69.2%) had a case manager in the past year. This service was provided by public services for 61.6% of the total sample, and by non-government organisations for 20.2%. Around two-thirds of people were very satisfied with their case manager (62.2% for case managers from public services and 69.6% for those from non-governmental agencies). Three in ten (29.8%) people with psychotic disorders received mental health services through non-government organisations in the past year. Almost one-quarter (22.4%) had attended a group rehabilitation program run by a non-government organisation. With regard to one-on-one support provided by non-government organisations, two-thirds (68.6%) of people received counselling or emotional support, and many were helped to access other community services (45.4%) or link with other mental health services (36.6%).

Figure 1.30 Health service use in the last year by people living with psychotic disorders

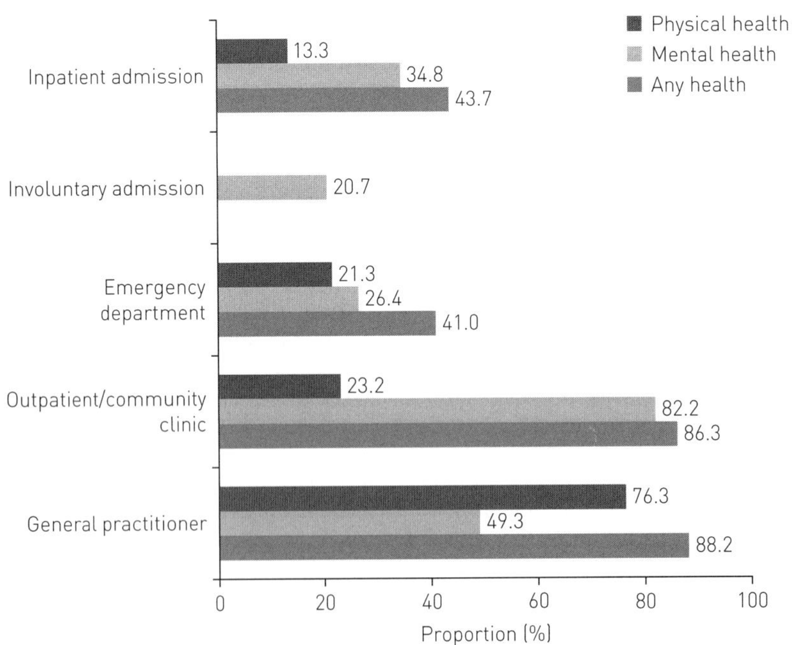

Source: Morgan et al. 2011. Used with permission.

One in five people (20.7%) had at least one involuntary inpatient admission and one-fifth (19.2%) were under a community treatment order in the past year. Most people (91.6%) were taking prescribed medications in the previous four weeks, with four-fifths (81.6%) taking antipsychotics. The majority of people were on atypical psychotics (74.0%). Only a minority of participants (38.6%) reported that they had received any psychosocial therapies in the previous 12 months, fewer still if evidence-based criteria were applied to these reports (Morgan et al., 2017).

About one-half (55.5%) identified unmet needs in relation to their treatment. Almost one-third (30.5%) reported the need for assistance in other areas of their lives including, but not limited to, housing, finances, employment, legal assistance and practical assistance. Financial matters, social isolation and lack of employment were noted as the biggest challenges over the next 12 months by participants. However, in spite of the difficulties facing them, 77.4% of people believed their circumstances would improve over the coming year.

HOW THINGS HAVE CHANGED SINCE 1997–98

Since the first national survey, there have been major changes in mental health service delivery, particularly affecting public specialised mental health services. The first and second Australian national surveys of psychosis present a rare opportunity to assess change over time as they had similar aims, employed the same two-phase design and methodology and used the same core instruments. However, there were some differences in coverage. In addition to screening in public specialised mental health services, the 1997-98 survey included private psychiatric and general medical practices and contact points for homeless people, while the 2010 survey included NGOs. To ensure comparability, in this section comparisons across the two surveys have been restricted to those people using public mental health services in the census month. This subsample included 1211 participants from the 2010 survey and 687 participants from the 1997-98 survey. The proportions of male participants, older participants and participants with schizophrenia or a schizoaffective disorder were similar in both subsamples.

There appear to be some changes in the course of disorder people experience. The majority of people had multiple episodes of disorder, but more people experienced periods of good recovery in between episodes (29.3% compared with 21.3% in 1997-98). The proportion of people experiencing deterioration because of chronic psychotic disorder had halved since 1997-98 (11.3% compared to 23.6%).

Changes in service use are consistent with changes in mental health service delivery (see Table 1.12). For example, hospital admissions for mental health reasons decreased by 35.9%, and involuntary admissions decreased by just over one-quarter from 31.4% to 22.7%. There was a 60.7% increase in the use of community rehabilitation or day programs. One-quarter (26.5%) of people received mental health services from non-government organisations, compared with 18.9% in 1997-98. The proportion of people with a psychotic disorder who had a case manager increased from 71.9 to 78.1%. Also, general practitioners continue to be major providers of services, with the proportion visiting general practitioners increasing from 76.7 to 87.8%. There was a large increase in the proportion of people taking atypical antipsychotics: 78.4% in 2010 compared with 37.1% in 1997-98.

Table 1.12 Use of health services in the year prior to interview by people with psychosis in contact with specialised mental health services in the census month, 1997 and 2010

	Proportion (%)	
	1997	**2012**
Inpatient: any admission	62.9	45.6
Mental health	58.7	37.6
Physical health	7.9	12.6
Involuntary admission	31.4	22.7
Emergency department attendance	47.6	43.0
Outpatient/community clinic contact	75.3	92.8
Community rehabilitation/day program	22.9	36.8
Case manager	71.9	78.1
Non-government organisation for mental health	18.9	26.5
General practitioner visits	76.7	87.8

Source: Morgan et al. 2011. Used with permission.

More people were in their own home or rented accommodation (61.5% compared with 49.0% in 1997–98), and the proportion in supported group accommodation had doubled to 10.9%. The proportion of people who had been homeless at some time in the previous 12 months was more than halved (5.0% compared with 13.0% in 1997–98). Smoking rates remained very high, and lifetime alcohol and drug abuse or dependence increased markedly, both rising from around 30% to just over half having these disorders.

CONCLUSION

The Second National Survey of Psychosis provides a comprehensive picture of multiple facets of the lives of people living with psychosis. Many data elements are unique, in that they have not been collected previously in the context of such a large, representative sample. Comparison of screening data with interview data suggested no systematic biases in the data, despite some participant refusal and the inability to interview some very ill people which, if anything, would result in underestimation of the disability and disadvantage faced by people living with psychosis in Australia. The survey shows some encouraging improvements since 1997–98, principally related to the ongoing shift to community-based care with patterns of service use generally reflecting increased proportions of people with psychosis treated in the community and more people experiencing recovery from episodes of disorder. However, major challenges remain. These are elaborated, together with the detailed findings underpinning them, in an update paper (Morgan et al., 2017). This is organised according to the biggest challenges faced over the next 12 months as reported by Australians living with psychosis. In brief, the observed changes in service use and location do not appear to have translated into improvements in living well, such as higher rates of employment, decreased isolation or indeed improved physical health. Since gains in living well matter and are likely in turn to reduce morbidity, concerted actions are required to enable people with psychosis to pursue meaningful employment, education and relationships and thus overcome the many disadvantages they currently face, including financial difficulties. The importance of factors outside the delivery of good clinical practice for those experiencing severe mental illness is a major identified issue (Mulder, 2017). In addition, many areas requiring special attention have been highlighted, including but not limited to, better supporting people living with psychosis as parents, tackling challenges posed by experiences of trauma, poor physical health, smoking and substance use and providing better support to the families of people with psychosis. The implications for future policy and service initiatives, within and beyond health services, and incorporating strategies aimed at improving socio-structural and sociodemographic circumstances are summarised in Table 1.12 (Morgan et al., 2017). Considering the continuing challenges, a third national survey of psychosis is warranted to review progress in a rapidly changing landscape, including the establishment of Primary Health Networks and the rollout of the National Disability Insurance Scheme. Preliminary planning for such a survey is underway.

1.6.5 REFUGEE MENTAL HEALTH

INTRODUCTION

GRAHAM MEADOWS

This chapter concentrates on presenting data illustrating the impact of mental illness on different communities. There is some useful data in relation to refugees. The study in question is known as the Building a New Life in Australia (BNLA study). This is important because it provides one of the best sources of information internationally about the mental health of settling and settled refugees. Also it provides an example of a longitudinal, or cohort, study. One significance of this is that the forthcoming NSMHW, introduced earlier (see Section 1.6.1) will also have a longitudinal design element. Taking a look then at the BNLA study may illuminate the mental health experience of people with a refugee background and also give the reader some idea of what kind of publications are likely to emerge when for the first time we see successive waves of data from a national Australian survey.

THE BNLA STUDY

FRANCES SHAWYER

Background

The United Nations High Commissioner for Refugees (UNHCR) defines a refugee as a person outside of their country of nationality due to a well-founded fear of persecution for reasons of race, religion, nationality, particular social group membership or political opinion and is unable or unwilling to avail themselves of the protection of their country or return to it (UNHCR, 2015). According to recent UNHCR reporting, 2018 saw 70.8 million people forcibly displaced continuing the annual trend of being the highest level on record (UNHCR, 2019). As a result of the Syrian conflict, which began in 2011, the Syrian Arab Republic continued to head the list of refugee source countries in 2018 reporting (6.7 million). It has held this place since 2014, ahead of Afghanistan (2.7 million) which had previously occupied this position for over 30 years (UNHCR, 2015, 2019).

In Australia, protection for refugees is offered through the Humanitarian program. In 2018, 12 706 refugees were resettled in Australia. This intake gives Australia the third highest rate of UNHCR humanitarian resettlement globally behind Canada and the United States, an index of contribution often claimed by politicians. The Refugee Council of Australia, however, has criticised this claim as misleading because only 0.4% of refugees get access to resettlement globally. They further note that if recognition of refugee status is added to resettlement figures as the index of contribution, Australia recognised or resettled 23 002 refugees in 2018. This represents 1.39% of the 1.65 million people globally who had their refugee status recognised or were resettled that year with an associated ranking of 14 (or 60 relative to GDP; Refugee Council of Australia, 2019).

Refugees are known to be at particular risk for mental health problems due to the physical and psychological stress associated with their displacement, as well as during transition and on arrival in the host country including for some a long period of uncertainty about their visa status and inability to work. While mental health has been shown to affect resettlement over the short- and long-term (Beiser & Hou, 2001; Steel, Silove, Phan, & Bauman, 2002), rates of mental illness can be expected to vary considerably across different refugee populations and across gender and time. The Australian Government has many policies and programs to assist refugees and it is critical that information risk factors for mental illness in different refugee groups be available to help guide effective practices. This includes understanding any impact on mental health after assistance reduces, which occurs generally 12 months after arrival.

Conceptualisation and design

Funded by the Australian Government, the Building a New Life in Australia (BNLA) survey is a longitudinal, population level, cohort study into the mental health needs of refugees. The study initially aimed to collect five annual waves of national-representative data following refugees through 2013 to 2018 (De Maio, Silbert, Jenkinson, & Smart, 2014); however, data collection is now continuing beyond Wave 5. Participants include offshore permanent humanitarian visa holders who arrived in Australia between May and December 2013 or onshore permanent protection visa holders who received their visa during the same time period.

This project is being conducted by the Australian Institute of Family Studies (AIFS) with the aim of identifying factors that affect the successful settlement of humanitarian migrants in Australia. The BNLA includes data relating to employment and income, language proficiency, education, housing, health and life satisfaction. Thus, it includes key government target areas often termed the three E's (English language proficiency, Education and Employment) and Accommodation. Most critically, the K6 (Kessler et al., 2002) and the PTSD-8 (Hansen et al., 2010) are included as mental health screening measures for psychological distress and PTSD respectively.

The BNLA project is a well-designed and comprehensive national study with a sampling framework that helps ensure the findings of the survey represent the populations of interest (Enticott et al., 2017). This gold-standard survey has no equal worldwide that we could find and provides an outstanding opportunity for analysis of how time-varying factors may influence critical elements of refugee settlement in Australia. Around 2400 individuals and families have been recruited to the study via the Australian Settlement Database, which has contact details for refugees coming to Australia. Australia is one of only a few countries using government immigration records as a sampling frame for such research.

Table 1.13 Results from generalised linear mixed models using 'severe mental illness' as positive outcome. OR=odds ratio. p=p-value. CI=confidence interval. AIC=Akaike's Information Criteria. BIC=Bayesian information criteria. S.E Asia=South-East Asia

		Model 1			**Model 2**		
Variable	***Response***	***OR***	***P***	***95%CI***	***OR***	***p***	***95%CI***
Survey wave	*1*	-	-	-	-	-	-
	2	0.67	0.060	[0.45–1.02]	0.59	0.095	[0.32–1.10]
	3	1.09	0.691	[0.72–1.66]	1.09	0.741	[0.65–1.83]
Gender	*Male*	-	-	-	-	-	-
	Female	1.51	0.010	[1.10–2.08]	1.73	0.012	[1.13–2.64]
Region of birth	*Middle East*	-	-	-	-	-	-
	Central Asia	0.57	0.003	[0.39–0.83]	0.60	0.024	[0.39–0.94]
	Southern Asia	0.29	<0.001	[0.15–0.58]	0.47	0.065	[0.21–1.05]
	South-East Asia	0.14	0.002	[0.04–0.49]	0.24	0.114	[0.40–1.41]
	Africa	0.51	0.042	[0.27–0.97]	0.53	0.084	[0.26–1.09]
Housing contract	*No/temporary contract*	-	-	-	-	-	-
	Short-term lease	0.51	0.066	[0.25–1.05]	0.55	0.181	[0.23–1.32]
	(<6 months)	0.43	0.018	[0.22–0.87]	0.48	0.086	[0.20–1.11]
	Long-term contract (>6 months)						
Number of financial hardships	*0*	-	-	-	-	-	-
	1-2	1.97	0.003	[1.26–3.10]	1.80	0.035	[1.04–3.11]
	3-4	4.00	<0.001	[2.13–7.49]	3.69	<0.001	[1.83–7.43]
	5-6	3.50	0.011	[1.33–9.18]	2.75	0.119	[0.77–9.81]
Has a chronic health condition	*Yes*	*	*	*	-	-	-
	No	*	*	*	0.57	0.034	[0.34–0.96]
Overall health past 4 weeks	*Excellent–Good*	-	-	-	-	-	-
	Fair	3.78	<0.001	[2.40–5.95]	2.58	0.002	[1.41–4.71]
	Poor–Very Poor	13.3	<0.001	[7.38–23.9]	7.92	<0.001	[3.81–16.46]
Discrimination	*Yes*	-	-	-	-	-	-
	No	0.48	0.033	[0.24–0.94]	0.55	0.161	[0.24–1.27]
Selected loneliness as stressor	*No*	*	*	*	-	-	-
	Yes	*	*	*	2.07	0.007	[1.23–3.49]
Selected finances as stressor	*No*	*	*	*	-	-	-
	Yes	*	*	*	1.72	0.042	[1.02–2.91]
AIC Criteria		**3632**			**3191**		
BIC Criteria		3751			3327		
Number of observations		5563			4829		

Some illustrative findings

At the time of writing, 34 publications in the grey and black literature were listed on the AIFS library catalogue. The informational value of studies such as BNLA and the primary agency reports from them can be added to significantly by academic researchers. For example, a study by Cooper, Enticott, Shawyer, & Meadows (2019) using the first three waves of data found a high prevalence of mental illness over the first three years of resettlement. Having a high risk of severe mental illness based on the K6 Table 5 and a positive PTSD screen were both associated with females, Middle Eastern birthplace, having a chronic health condition, poor self-rated health, and more financial hardships. K6 high risk scores had additional associations with unstable housing and discrimination. Of note, PTSD had additional associations with older age, increasing traumatic events and, unexpectedly, having like-ethnic social support (see Section 4.4.4). These findings suggest tangible opportunities for screening, intervention and further investigation.

Further work

Other national data sets from non-refugee populations as have been described will potentially provide important sources of comparative data. However, when refugee group statistics are compared with national data, it is important to take into account the influence of factors other than refugee status on findings—here including particularly age and gender. There may also be arguments for analyses including controlling for key socioeconomic factors. Large areas of variance can be removed by accounting for the variation of these factors that are associated with different rates of mental illness. For example comparing refugees in a local study with a socio-demographically matched Australian-born group of people sampled in the 2007 National Survey of Mental Health and Wellbeing showed that the relative risk of mental ill health for refugees reduced from 3.83 (unmatched) to 3.16 with matching (Shawyer, Enticott, Block, Cheng, & Meadows, 2017).

1.6.6 AUSTRALIA'S MENTAL HEALTH SERVICES

JOANNE ENTICOTT, GRAHAM MEADOWS & SEBASTIAN ROSENBERG

AVAILABLE NATIONAL INFORMATION SOURCES

A central tenet of the National Mental Health Strategy over decades has been accountability. To this end, each national policy or plan has made commitments to the enhancement of Australia's capacity to assess the progress of mental health reform. As the strategy proceeded, the emphasis of this reporting evolved, shifting from a focus on purely health outcome data to a broader consideration of social, economic and other outcomes. The aim was to produce an increasingly clear picture not just of the mental health care and services provided to people, but also on the actual impact these services had on quality of life. Issues like employment, housing and education emerged as worthy of inclusion in national reporting but have yet to be implemented specifically as they affect people with a mental illness.

Information on mental health services had been published in a series of National Mental Health Reports (Department of Health 2013), instigated by the First National Mental Health Plan. These Reports developed by consultants working for the Australian Government, described developments in services across the country between 1993 and 2013. Unfortunately, these reports have ceased.

There are now two main sources of national information illuminating progress in mental health reform.

The first is the annual Report on Government Services (ROGS; Productivity Commission 2020). This report relies on data provided to it by all Australian states and territories.

The second key source of data is the Australian Institute for Health and Welfare (AIHW) which regularly produces the web report 'Mental Health Services in Australia' and an annual companion hardcopy publication called Mental Health Services in Brief (Australian Institute of Health and Welfare, 2018a).

Both ROGS and the AIHW rely entirely on data supplied to them by all governments. Given the need to ensure the data is clean and accurate, there is some delay between the provision of data and its eventual publication. For example, the 2020 ROGS report refers to the financial year 2017-18. And both sources depend on governments agreeing to collect information at the same time, in the same way. How this is organised and which data items are prioritised for collection is in the hands of government health officials. Their priorities may not always match those of researchers, providers, consumers, carers or the community more generally.

Both ROGS and the AIHW provide a valuable overview of the first 25 years of the National Mental Health Strategy. However, overall, it is reasonable to suggest that sources of information by which to monitor and report on the progress of mental health reform are narrow and remain largely health-focused. Each of the eight Australian states and territories has its own organisational approach to health service delivery and, to a substantial degree, an autonomous set of financial management systems. Organisational structures and lines of accountability differ. Within the aims and imperatives of a national mental health policy, it is necessary to impose some standardisation on collection of data across these disparate service environments. From the 1990s onwards, this has been achieved in Australia, first through the vehicle of the *National Survey of Mental Health Services* (Department of Health and Ageing, 2005) and now facilitated by the AIHW as custodians of various data sources and creators of the online report *Mental Health Services in Australia* including the National Mental Health Establishments Database (Australian Institute of Health and Welfare, 2016-17a) and National Hospitals Data Collection (Australian Institute of Health and Welfare, 2018b; Australian Institute of Health and Welfare, 2019).

An important source of data for reporting mental health service usage is found in the information collected for the administration of Medicare. For the purpose of managing remuneration, the Commonwealth must effectively collect data that can be used to describe the number of service providers drawing on this medical benefit scheme for reimbursement, and the volume and, to some extent, the type of work that they do. The Medicare-subsidised mental health-specific services are reported in the *Mental Health Services in Australia* report for annual periods between 1984-85 and 2017-18 (Australian Institute of Health and Welfare, 2017-18a).

Since July 2016, transfer of responsibility occurred for a range of Australian Government mental health and suicide prevention activities to the newly created Australian Government's Primary Health Networks (PHNs). There are 31 PHNs in Australia and their role includes leading mental health planning and integration with states and territory, non-government organisation, private sector, Indigenous, drug and alcohol and other related services and organisations (Australian Government, 2015c).

A staged implementation of the National Disability Insurance Scheme (NDIS) began in July 2013 (Buckmaster & Clark, 2018). People with a psychosocial disability who have significant and permanent functional impairment are eligible to access funding through the NDIS. The full scheme is intended to be delivered in 2020, however significant concerns and tensions have been emerging including criticism of the application process, which is viewed as complicated particularly for those from special needs populations. In addition, there is concern that the capacity of the NDIS will be insufficient, as it is planned to support approximately 64 000 people living with severe mental illness, which is far fewer than the estimated 230 000 Australians who are living with such illnesses (Rosenberg, Redmond, Boyer, Gleeson, & Russell, 2019). Arrangements for funding the NDIS are complex, with approximately half of the revenue pooled from the Commonwealth and remaining half from state/territory governments (Dickinson, 2019; NDIS, 2019).

Most of the information that follows derives from the Mental Health Services in Australia online reports (since 2013) and the National Mental Health Reports (1993-2013), though some items come from other sources cited that will be mentioned at the end of the section.

SERVICE DELIVERY

Spending on mental health care delivery: An overview

In 2017-18 (AIHW, 2020), the Commonwealth spent $3.3 billion on mental health, the states and territories $6 billion, and $0.5 billion was spent by private insurers. Overall, mental health expenditure was $399 per capita. The per capita amount had increased by an annual average of 1.1% between 2013-14 and 2017-18.

State and territory expenditure for 2017-18 was:

- New South Wales: $1.85 billion
- Victoria: $1.45 billion
- Queensland: $1.14 billion
- Western Australia: $0.8 billion
- South Australia: $0.5 billion
- Tasmania: $0.12 billion
- Australian Capital Territory: $0.1 billion
- Northern Territory: $0.07 billion.

Australian Government expenditure for 2018-19 was:

- Medicare-subsidised mental health-specific services: $1.3 billion
- Subsidised mental health-related medications services: $0.54 billion
- National programs and initiatives: $1.3 billion.*

*2017-18 data

People working delivering public mental health care services

As regards medical primary care overall, we can say that in 2017-18 there were approximately 36 000 general practitioners working in Australia (Australian Government, 2015) and almost all (97%) had provided a Medicare-subsidised mental health-specific service (Australian Institute of Health and Welfare, 2017-18b). The number of other providers of Medicare-subsidised mental health-specific services were psychiatrists (2923), clinical psychologists (6055), other psychologists (13 014) and other allied health providers (2436). Percentage increases for these Medicare services for each provider type since 2008-09 were as follows: general practitioners (126%), psychiatrists (45%), clinical psychologists (193%), other psychologists (111%) and other allied health providers (239%).

Statistics used here regarding public specialist services come primarily from the National Mental Health Establishments Database (Australian Institute of Health and Welfare, 2016-17b) and National Health Workforce Data Set (Australian Institute of Health and Welfare, 2017a). In 2016-17:

- in public sector specialist services, there were 7175 inpatient psychiatric beds, or 29.4 per 100 000 population
- the total public sector workforce was 32 573 people, or 13.36 per 10 000 adult population
- there were 3475 medical staff in the public sector (1.43 per 10 000 population)
- there were in total 3244 psychiatrists providing self-reported full-time clinical equivalence (public and private) of 10.8 per 100 000 population
- there were 13 723 nurses in public mental health work (6.81 per 10 000 population)
- there were 5107 diagnostic and allied health staff (2.59 per 10 000 population)
- there were 1087 other personal care staff (0.5 per 10 000 population)
- there were 167 consumer and carer workers (0.1 per 10 000 population)
- there were 4931 administrative and clerical staff (2.02 per 10 000 population).

Work settings for delivery of services

Of the public sector workforce in 2016-17 (Australian Institute of Health and Welfare, 2016-17b):

- 14 675 were in inpatient services (45.1%)
- 12 346 were in ambulatory services (37.9%)
- 2092 were in community residential services (6.4%)
- 3459 were in organisational overhead (10.6%).

The private sector plays a key role in overall service delivery. By 2016-17, the sector provided 29.6% of total psychiatric beds and employed approximately 10% of Australia's mental health workforce.

STATE AND TERRITORY TRENDS

Figure 1.31 presents the distribution of recurrent spending on mental health services by source, providing for comparison between the amounts put into GP remuneration, prescribing budgets and specialist services, public and private.

Figure 1.32 provides for sequential comparison of expenditure in the various states and territories. The central bar chart shows, after a drop in 2012–13, a progressive increase thereafter. The picture in individual states varies somewhat.

Figure 1.33 provides for sequential comparison of expenditure expansions in the Medicare Benefits Scheme for mental health-related services. Since 2006 psychologists and relevant allied health providers have been eligible to provide Medicare-subsidised services under the Better Access to Mental Health Care Scheme when requested by a GP.

Relative budget expenditure is not the only meaningful comparison between the states. The first plan set an agenda of developing community-based services with reduction in stand-alone and other institutional settings. To capture evidence of this planned structural shift we also can consider the employed workforce in community settings as a rate per 100 000 population in the states and territories. The change in these numbers overall and in the states and territories can be found in Figure 1.34.

ACCESSING FURTHER INFORMATION

There are other sources for information about mental health service provision. Prominent among these are other materials produced by the Australian Institute of Health and Welfare (AIHW), accessible via its website. The Medicare website also can be valuable, and includes the capacity to generate item-related reports that may be of value in tracking specific Commonwealth-funded initiatives. For primary care, the Primary Health Networks host some useful resources. The NDIS is administered by the National Disability Insurance Agency (NDIA) and its websites might also become a source of relevant information, as the full rollout of the scheme is achieved. These various websites

Figure 1.31 How 2016–17 spending was distributed

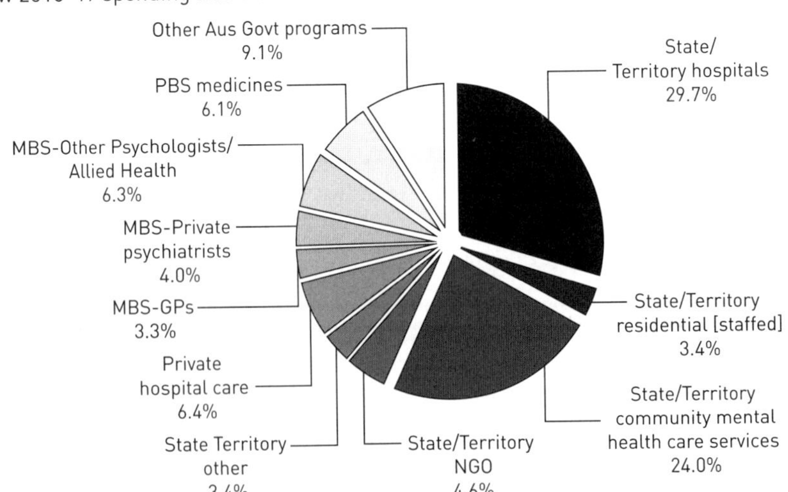

Source: Mental Health Services in Australia

Figure 1.32 Per capita expenditure by state and territory government (2016–17 dollars). National averages are shown in the central bar charts.

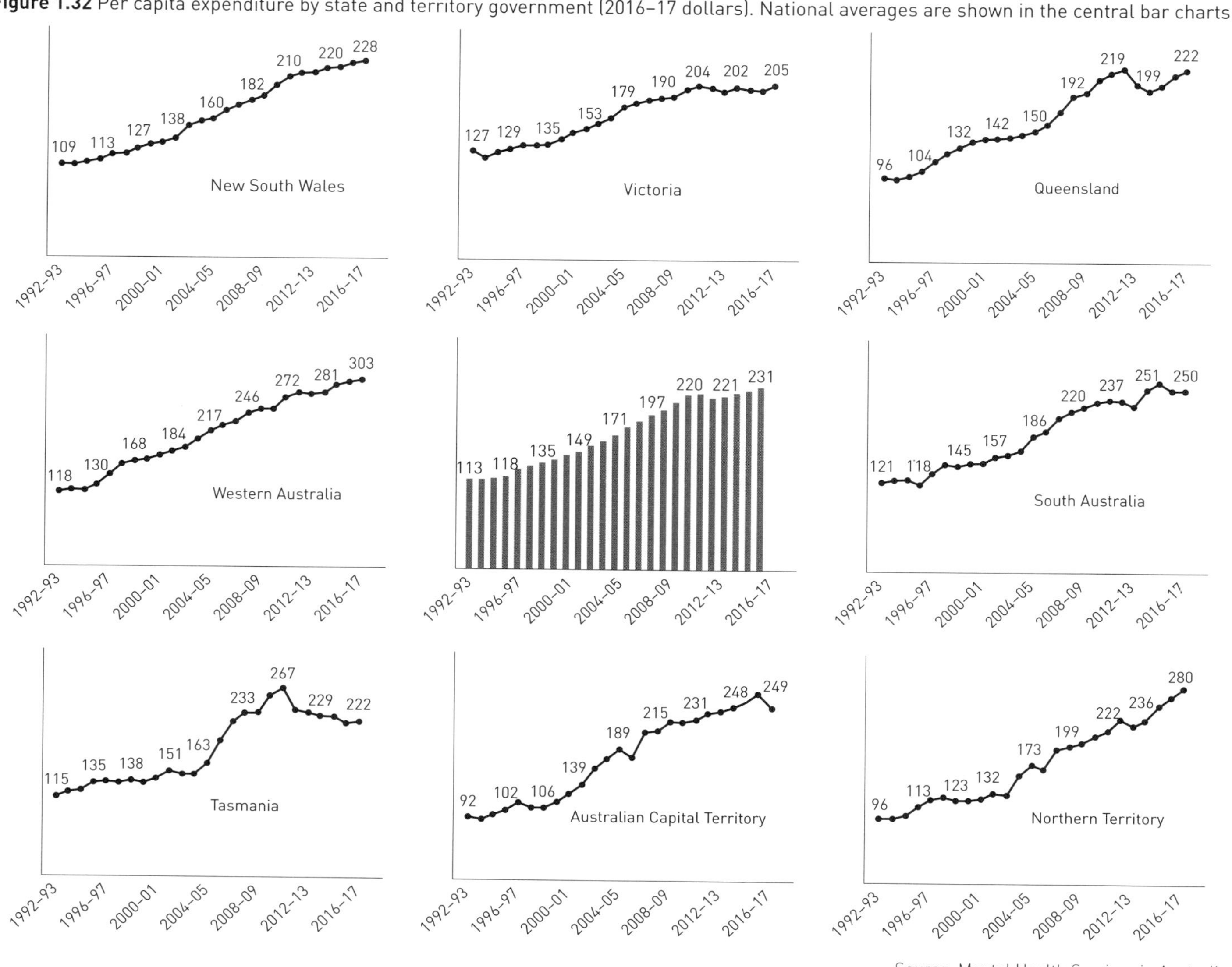

Source: Mental Health Services in Australia

Figure 1.33 Public access to government mental health services (%)

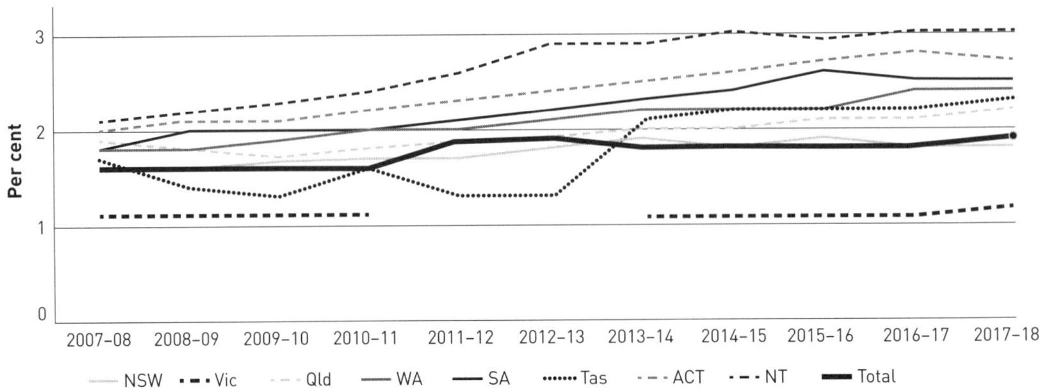

Source: Mental Health Services in Australia, Key Performance Indicators

Figure 1.34 Per capita expenditure by Medicare Benefits Scheme (2016–17 $)

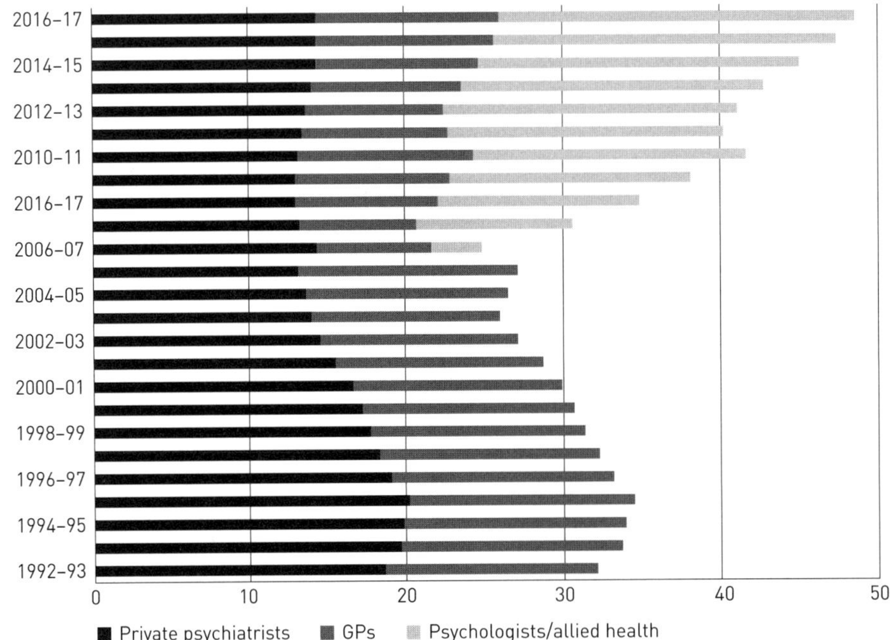

Source: Mental Health Services in Australia

and the *Mental Health Services in Australia* online reports, which go into great detail around various aspects, are valuable further sources of information. Collectively, these sources hold a wealth of detailed information on service delivery across the nation, its states and territories.

While Figure 1.35 demonstrates the steep increases in government mental health spending, less clear is the impact on the rate of access to care. Figure 1.36 suggests that the national rate of access to government mental health services has proven stubborn to shift. It has been between 1.5% and 2% for a decade.

Figure 1.35 Full-time equivalent (FTE) clinical staff per 100 000 population employed in community mental health care services, 1992–93, 2007–08, 2016–17

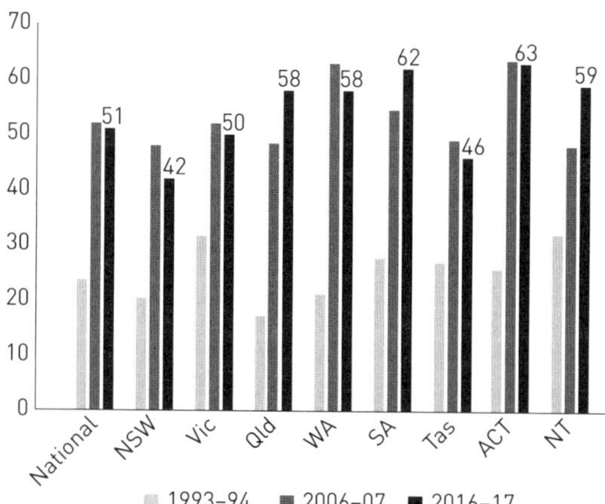

Source: Mental Health Services in Australia

Figure 1.36 12-month prevalence of all disorders, as related to perceived need and service use

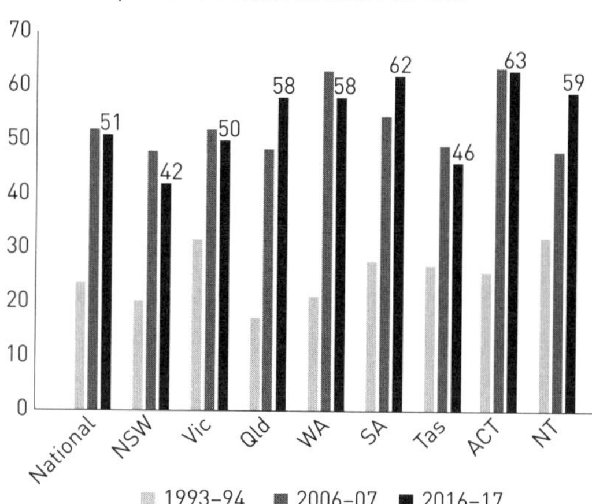

Source: NSMHW, 2007

1.6.7 MEETING OF NEEDS FOR CARE OF PEOPLE WITH MENTAL HEALTH PROBLEMS

GRAHAM MEADOWS

INTRODUCTION

Having set out something of what we know about mental disorder and psychological distress in Australia, we now consider what we might know at a population level about service responses to mental health problems and to what extent those services might be meeting particular needs for mental health care. Here we return to the studies introduced in the first section of the chapter and particularly the 2007 NSMHW. The next study, at least will add and update this information. Until that time this is the most recent available information, while from around 2021-22 it would be expected that there will be ABS and journal publications emerging with updated information. At that point this should serve as a guide for information on the earlier (2007) work as baseline, and also what to look for in publications. The ABS reports are a good place to start but in the last two surveys some of the important analyses of this and other parts of the study findings have been found in the journal papers that follow. For instance much of the important information regarding service use and perceived need from the 2007 survey was published (Burgess et al., 2009b; Meadows & Burgess, 2009) among a set of papers on the 2007 NSMHW set together in a 2009 edition of the *Australian and New Zealand Journal of Psychiatry.*

HOW MANY OF THOSE WITH DISORDERS ARE IN CONTACT WITH SERVICES?

The NSMHW 2007 provides us with some information on this. The field questionnaire asked survey participants to report their numbers of contacts with various health service providers in the last year, if any. Along with an estimate of the number of these contacts, the participant was asked directly to identify use of services for mental health problems; 11.9% of the population used services for a mental health problem in the year before the survey (Burgess et al., 2009a).

The relationship between lifetime history of an ICD-10 diagnosis, symptoms in the last year and mental health service use:

- 7.0% of the population had a lifetime history of mental disorder, with symptoms in the last year, and also used services for a mental health problem
- 13.0% of the population had a lifetime disorder, some symptoms in the last year, but made no use of services for a mental health problem

- 2.4% of the population had a lifetime history of disorder without symptoms in the last year, and used mental health services
- 2.6% had no apparent lifetime history of mental disorder based on the CIDI, and used mental health services in the last year.

The mental health services used by the total population are as follows:

- GP: 8.1%
- psychologist: 3.5%
- psychiatrist: 2.3%
- mental health professional: 2.2%
- other health professional: 2.4%.

WHAT DO PEOPLE THINK ABOUT THEIR NEEDS FOR MENTAL HEALTH CARE?

The Perceived Need for Care Questionnaire (PNCQ)

The instrument to assess this was derived particularly for this survey program in 1997 and extended for use in 2007. The four-stage design of the Perceived Need for Care Questionnaire (PNCQ), as used in the national survey, mimics a conversational exploration of the topic of perceived needs. Five categories of perceived need are each assigned to one of four levels of perceived need. These categories are:

- *information:* 'information about mental illness, its treatments and available services'
- *medications:* 'medicine or tablets'
- *counselling:* includes 'psychotherapy–discussion about causes that stem from your past'; 'Cognitive behaviour therapy–learning how to change your thoughts, behaviours and emotions'; and 'Counselling–help to talk through your problems'
- *social interventions:* help to sort out housing or money problems
- *skills training:* help to improve your ability to work, look after yourself and your home, or use your time in other ways.

An overall classification of perceived need can be obtained by a set of logical coding rules. The levels of perceived need are:

- *no need:* no endorsement of any of the options for being in need
- *unmet need:* perceived need and no service response to this need
- *partially met need:* perceived need and some service response to the need, but not judged as satisfactory
- *met need:* perceived need with a satisfactory service response.

The NSMHW field questionnaire in 2007 was designed to deliver the PNCQ to people who met CIDI criteria for a diagnosis, who used services for a mental health problem or who otherwise identified themselves as having a mental health problem.

PERCEIVED NEED, DIAGNOSIS AND SERVICE USE

Some outputs of this questionnaire for the full sample can be found in Table 1.14. The Venn diagram in Figure 1.37 shows findings from the survey in terms of:

1. any perceived needs
2. any diagnosis based on twelve-month symptoms of an identified lifetime disorder
3. any service use for a mental health problem.

From a consideration of Table 1.14 and the Venn diagram in Figure 1.36, we can observe that overall 13.8% of the population saw themselves as having a need for mental health care. The most common kind of need expressed is for some form of psychological treatment in the item labelled *counselling*. Second is *medication*, with 7.7% of the population, then lower figures for information, *social interventions* and *skills training*. Needs for medications are most likely to be seen as fully met. The majority of needs for *counselling* and *information* also are rated as met, less so for *social interventions* and *skills training*. The figure provides some insights into relationships between these three sets of responses. Most people identified in the community as having symptoms of a disorder in the last year (*Any diagnosis* in the Venn diagram) and who do not use services in that time do not identify themselves as having needs for mental health care. Indeed only 1.9% of the population have such symptoms, no service use and perceived need.

Table 1.14 Perceived need for different kinds of mental health care in the total Australian population

Perceived needs for mental health care in the Australian population: 12-month estimates					
	Need level				
	No need	Any need	Need not met	Need partially met	Need fully met
All perceived needs	86.2%	13.8%	2.5%	5.1%	6.2%
Information	92.5%	7.5%	2.3%	1.3%	3.9%
Medication	92.3%	7.7%	0.5%	0.7%	6.5%
Counselling	89.4%	10.6%	2.7%	1.6%	6.2%
Social intervention	95.8%	4.2%	2.7%	0.4%	1.1%
Skills training	96.0%	4.0%	1.9%	0.5%	1.6%

Source: NSMHW, 2007

Figure 1.37 12-month prevalence of all disorders, as related to perceived need and service use

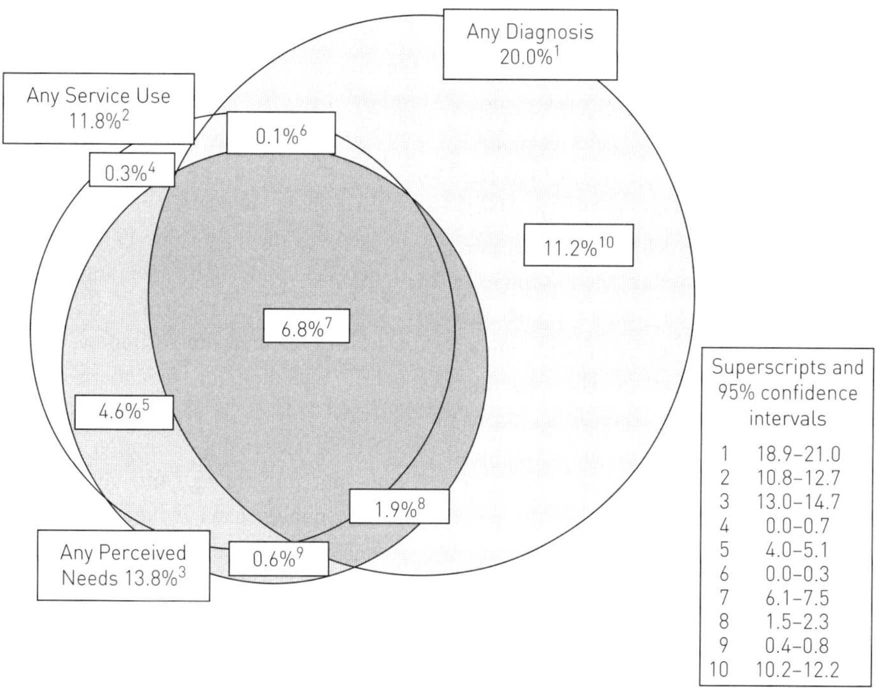

Source: NSMHW, 2007

COMPARISONS BETWEEN 1997 AND 2007

Following directly on from this last observation that 1.9% of the population had unmet need associated with symptoms of a lifetime disorder in the last year and no service use, looking back to 1997, the closest comparable figure would be the number of people with a CIDI diagnosis who had no service use and unmet need. In the NSMHW 1997 this figure was 3.6%. This could be an encouraging observation, representing almost a halving of this gap between community perceived need for care and delivery. Met needs also typically seem to have increased between 1997 and 2007, as follows:

- all perceived needs: 5.7-6.2%
  - *information*: 2.2-3.9%
  - *medication*: 4.9-6.5%
  - *counselling*: 4.9-6.2%

- social interventions: 1.0–1.1%
- skills training: 0.4–1.6%.

There are many possible sources of bias in these comparisons as already introduced. Nevertheless, if the analyses are restricted to specific subgroups of service users, and other forms of correction used, then many of these biases can be controlled for (Meadows & Bobevski, 2011). The findings from these comparisons were that overall perceived needs among service users seemed to have increased, and where people identified needs they identified more of them, a set of findings compatible with increased mental health literacy (p. 260) and improved clinical case identification. Unmet need has apparently declined generally. For instance, unmet need for counselling declined from 19.9% of service users in 1997 to 12.5% in 2007. In contrast, the proportion of identified need that was rated as met remained relatively constant (for example, Counselling: 1997: 79% compared with 2007: 80%). So while the impression from the findings is of improved engagement with care, there is less to suggest that the care delivered has become much more effective in the eyes of the consumers. The PNCQ is to be maintained without significant changes between the 2007 survey and the next one, so as long as the sampling strategies for the upcoming survey prove adequate, some further comparisons will be possible after more than a decade of further changes in Australian mental health care.

1.6.8 COMMENTARY AND REFLECTIONS

SEBASTIAN ROSENBERG & GRAHAM MEADOWS

Successive Australian mental health plans and policies have promised more and better accountability. So far, this has largely manifested in a suite of administrative datasets which provide an impressive amount and diversity of information, focusing mostly on different aspects of service utilisation and cost. There have also been some important surveys of population mental health, against which to assess both the demand and the supply of services available. Our federal system makes establishing national consistency in data collection challenging. There are typically significant delays between data collection and reporting. For example, in 2020 the most recent published data on mental health expenditure relates to the 2017-18 financial year. Governments want to ensure data is cleaned and accurate before publication. This can make it difficult to develop policy in a timely fashion. While the focus on administrative data reporting is not unhelpful, Australian has so far failed to develop the capacity to obtain and report genuine consumer and carer experiences of care, particularly reflecting the broader social determinants of mental health.

Available data indicates that while mental health's share of overall health spending has not changed significantly since 1992-93, there has been an increase in per capita spending.

Unfortunately that extra spend does not seem to be leading to measurable improvements in mental health, including in reduction of psychological distress. This is a cause for some concern and is getting increasing attention in the literature. Issues put forward as contributing to this include possible quality gaps in key areas of development (Jorm, 2018). While the situation is not unique to Australia (Jorm, Patten, Brugha, & Mojtabai, 2017), it does raise questions about whether there should be more dramatic reconfigurations of services than have been achieved to date (van Os, Guloksuz, Vijn, Hafkenscheid, & Delespaul, 2019), or whether issues of inequity in Australian service delivery need more effective action if we are to see population mental health improve (Meadows et al., 2019; see also Chapter 1.4).

1.7

MENTAL HEALTH SERVICES ACROSS AUSTRALIA

STEPHEN ALLISON, EDDIE BARTNIK, TARUN BASTIAMPILLAI, MALCOLM BATTERSBY, RICHARD BENJAMIN, LISA BROPHY, BRETT EMMERSON, VALERIE GERRAND, MARGARET GRIGG, AARON GROVES, CATHERINE LOUREY, GRAHAM MEADOWS, MARY MORRIS, SEBASTIAN ROSENBERG, JAMES SCOTT, BRUCE SINGH & SEBASTIAN ROSENBERG WITH PEGGY BROWN AND BERNARD HUGHSON

1.7.1 INTRODUCTION

SEBASTIAN ROSENBERG

Australia has had a federal system of government since 1901 which delivers autonomy to Australia's eight states and territories in relation to the management and delivery of health care, including mental health care. A national referendum and constitutional change in 1946 giving the Commonwealth (i.e. federal or national) government permission to get involved in health care also constrained what forms that involvement could take (Commonwealth of Australia Constitution Act, 2013). So there is some tension, even at times confusion, about the respective roles to be played by Australia's nine major governments in the organisation and delivery of mental health care, with responsibility for different aspects of mental health care split between the Commonwealth and the state and territory governments.

In the early 1990s the Burdekin Report (Burdekin, Guilfoyle, & Hall, 1993), named after the Human Rights Commissioner who conducted it, made for a critical juncture in Australian mental health care. Conducted in response to increasing national concern regarding mental health care in Australia, the inquiry, conducted by the Australian Human Rights Commission, gained considerable publicity, both during the hearings and when tabled in Parliament. It anecdotally reported widespread abuse of the UN Principles on the Rights of the Mentally Ill to which Australia was a signatory.

As the inquiry proceeded, federal, state and territory governments advanced the establishment of a framework for reform by releasing two landmark documents that initiated the National Mental Health

Strategy. These were the National Mental Health Policy and the National Mental Health Plan.

Australia has had a National Mental Health Strategy since 1992, with two national policies and five national plans. We will describe the evolution of this planning process here and explore the tensions arising between different critical jurisdictional levels (state and territory; and Commonwealth).

This chapter includes contributions from authors from every state and territory across Australia. We asked them to prepare short summaries of the mental health system where they live, by answering two key questions:

- What do mental health services look like in your jurisdiction?
- What makes them unique?

This chapter presents these responses, providing some understanding about the variation between places.

And of course, mental health care is not just provided or funded by governments. Australia has a significant private mental health service sector. It also has a non-government sector, including large charities and myriad community organisations providing particularly psychosocial support services.

> Our similarities bring us to a common ground; our differences allow us to be fascinated by each other.
>
> *Tom Robbins*

Our aim is to acquaint readers with this complex landscape. A recurring theme is that while Australia is not short of mental health policies and plans, the enduring challenge is about implementation of sustained change.

It is also worth noting by way of introduction that, like in so many parts of mental health, a clear understanding of change and progress is severely hampered due to the paucity or limitations of data. For example, almost no data is available on the mental health and psychosocial services provided by the non-government sector. The data currently reported as 'community mental health services' is in fact dominated by outpatient services provided through public hospital services. Our view is restricted.

Nevertheless, considering the various jurisdictions as complex adaptive systems (see Chapter 1.1) there are both examples of commonly emergent properties as well as interesting differences. As we have explored elsewhere, the type and quality of mental health care available to Australians depends a lot on where you live (see Chapters 1.2, 1.5). Some of the authors of this section have been active in researching issues of social justice, efficiency and effectiveness in Australian mental health care (see Chapter 1.2) and we suggest that in approaching this reading, some points for reflection in the process (see Chapters 1.1, 2.3) may include: Is the variation affecting mental health similar to other areas of health care? Is this acceptable? Is this situation generating a culture of systemic quality improvement?

1.7.2 OVERALL POLICY CONTEXT

SEBASTIAN ROSENBERG, VALERIE GERRAND & GRAHAM MEADOWS WITH BRUCE SINGH

DEINSTITUTIONALISATION, INQUIRIES, POLICIES AND PLANS

As was typical of the English-speaking world at least, through most of the twentieth century Australia's mental health care system was structurally dominated by large institutions (see Chapter 1.1; Vrklevski, Eljiz, & Greenfield, 2017). But a momentum developed, internationally and in Australia, through the later part of the twentieth century away from care provision through major stand-alone psychiatric hospitals to other service solutions. Drivers for this included: shifting social values related to these institutions (see Chapter 1.1); increasingly effective psychotropic medications (see Chapters 1.1, 2.5); concerns regarding safeguarding human rights in psychiatric care including in such institutions; values based preferences for less restrictive environments (Office of the High Commissioner for Human Rights, 1991); and developing evidence related to community mental health care. This included influential Australian work (Hoult, Rosen, & Reynolds,

1984; see Chapter 1.1). Many of these international trends were influential in the forming of the UN Principles for the protection of persons with mental illness and the improvement of mental health care (Office of the High Commissioner for Human Rights, 1991), passed by the UN General Assembly in 1991.

The deinstitutionalisation process as it had unfolded through the 1970s and 1980s had created community concerns including that as people had left the institutions, they had transitioned into living environments that were in different ways problematic. The Burdekin inquiry (Burdekin et al., 1993) demonstrated serious inequities and deficiencies in Australia's response to mental illness, and spurred reform. In 1992, influenced by these concerns and against the conceptual backdrop of the UN principles, Australia was one of the first countries to develop a national mental health policy. This policy was backed up by initial strategy documentation released in 1993.

Enquiries such as that led by Brian Burdekin in 1992 have, in truth been a recurring feature of Australia's mental health reform landscape. There were 32 separate statutory inquiries into mental health just between 2006 and 2012 (Mendoza, Rosenberg, & Griffiths, 2013). The Parliamentary Inquiry Report *From Crisis to Community* was published in 2006 (Parliament of Australia, 2006). Countless hearings have occurred and recommendations made, by parliamentary and other bodies. The National Mental Health Commission conducted an important review (2014). The Australian Government Productivity Commission (2020) and a Victorian Royal Commission (State of Victoria 2019) have both provided draft reports, with final recommendations due for publication in 2020–21. The consensus of all these reviews has been to suggest that too often people fall through the cracks in our mental health system. Most inquiry reports suggest current problems are widespread and grave. The term 'crisis' is often used.

Back in 1993 however, there was some concerted attention and effort directed towards mental health reform. Funding was provided by the Commonwealth to the state and territory jurisdictions for a range of related activities, not least of which was to encourage the closure of psychiatric specialist institutions. The provision of these incentives was to some extent successful. Mental health services previously provided in 'asylums' shifted into mental health units in general public hospitals.

Australia has now had five National Mental Health Plans. The original 1992 policy was also updated in 2008. This national policy and planning activity has often been replicated by each state and territory. In addition to policies and plans in relation to mental health, there are also similar documents aiming to influence the direction of a range of related areas such as suicide prevention, addictions, Aboriginal and Torres Strait Islander health and so on. There has also been a National Action Plan for Mental Health produced by the Council of Australian Governments in 2006, which also produced a ten-year Roadmap for National Mental Health Reform (2012). Australia is not short of policies and plans.

EVOLUTION OF THE NATIONAL MENTAL HEALTH STRATEGY

The National Mental Health Strategy launched a national mental health reform agenda, agreed to by all Commonwealth, state and territory health ministers, in recognition of the significant impact of mental health problems and mental disorders on individuals, their families, the wider community, as well as on the Australian health system (Australian Health Ministers, 1992). The shifting pattern of mental health service provision from institutional to community orientated care was also recognised as placing increasing demands on other community services, as well as specialist mental health services. The National Mental Health Strategy has been articulated in a sequence, albeit sometimes an interrupted one, of major documents:

- The National Mental Health Policy (Australian Health Ministers, 1992), defining the broad aims and objectives to guide reform
- The National Mental Health Plan (Australian Health Ministers, 1992), describing a five-year plan for implementing these aims and objectives
- The Mental Health Statement of Rights and Responsibilities (Australian Health Ministers,

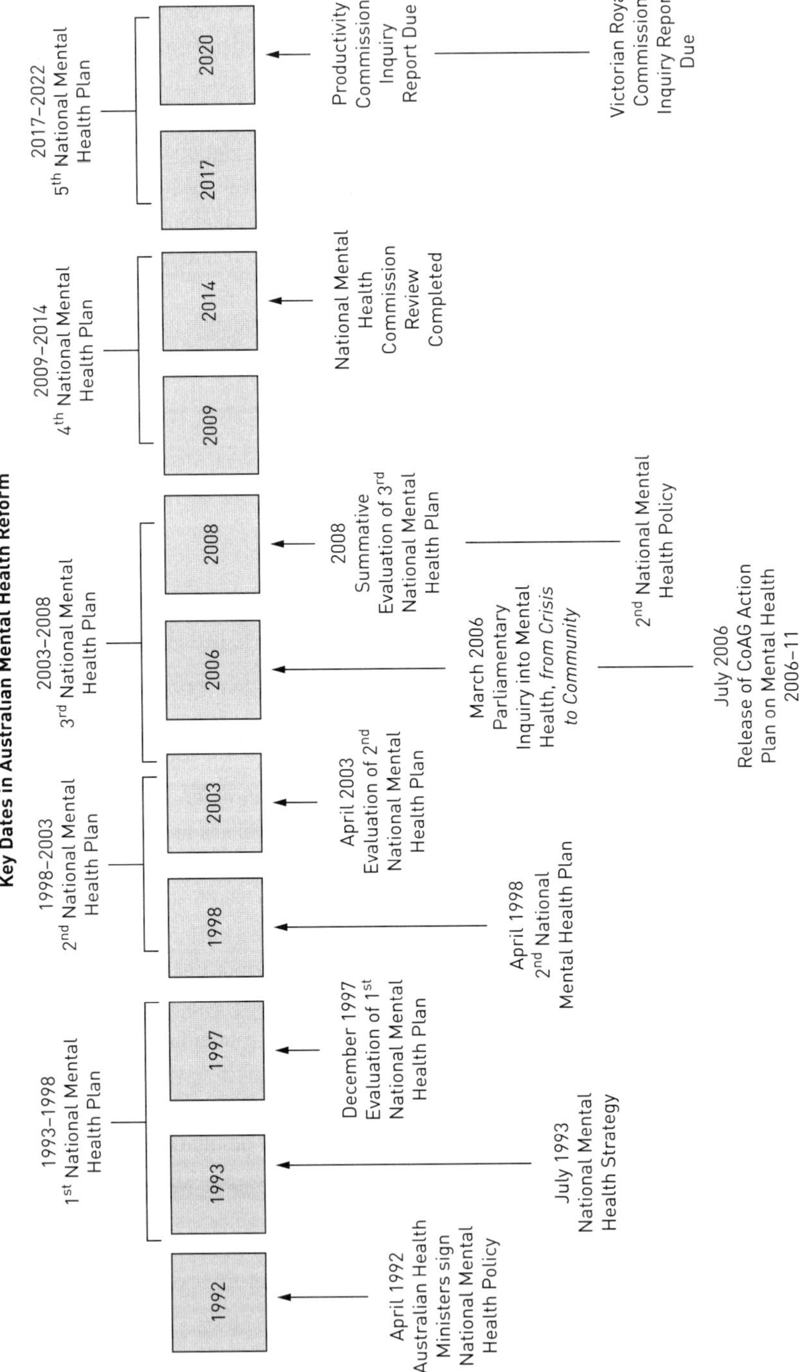

Figure 1.38 Key dates in Australian mental health reform

1991), outlining the civil and human rights framework underpinning the strategy

- The Medicare Agreements, which discussed funding arrangements to support the reform agenda
- The Second National Mental Health Plan that followed covered the years 1998-2003; then another from 2003-08
- In 2006, the (Council of Australian Governments (COAG), 2008) released a separate national plan called the National Action Plan on Mental Health 2006-2011
- The National Mental Health Policy 2008, published in March 2009, replaced the 1992 National Mental Health Policy (Australian Government Department of Health, 2009)
- The Fourth National Mental Health Plan running from 2009-14
- The Fifth National Mental Health Plan 2017-22.

THE NATIONAL MENTAL HEALTH POLICY 1992

This was an innovative document. The priority areas for reform identified in the National Mental Health Policy (Australian Health Ministers 1992) related to consumer rights; relationships and linkages between mental health, general health and other community services; service mix; promotion and prevention; primary care services; carers and non-government organisations that provide support services; mental health workforce; legislation; research and evaluation; standards; and monitoring and accountability. The National Mental Health Policy also articulated key underlying principles that provide the policy framework for service planning and development in mental health care:

- services should be provided in a multifaceted and interdisciplinary manner to achieve good outcomes for persons with mental health problems, or mental disorder
- people with mental disorders have potential for personal growth and the right to opportunities that support this growth
- every person with a mental disorder should have the same civil, political, economic, social and cultural rights as everyone else in the community
- the community and individuals within it have a justifiable right to protection
- positive consumer outcomes are the first priority in mental health policy and service delivery
- priority should be given to those with severe mental health problems and mental disorders
- the quality and effectiveness of mental health services are enhanced when they are responsive to consumers and their communities, and create opportunities for their participation in decision making about service developments, and services for individuals
- mental health service systems should be responsive to the varying needs of particular groups in the community
- positive consumer outcomes depend on informed and well-trained mental health staff, and strong support from carers and advocates.

Based on this policy, Australia's nine governments then agreed to (what has become) a series of mental health plans. Initially, the timing of these plans coincided with the broader Medicare Agreements, covering five-year arrangements for health funding between the Commonwealth and the states and territories.

THE FIRST NATIONAL MENTAL HEALTH PLAN (1993–98)

Content and implementation

The aims of this first plan (Australian Health Ministers 1992) were:

- the promotion of mental health of the Australian community and, where possible, the prevention of the development of mental health problems and disorders
- reduction of the impact of mental disorders on individuals, families and communities
- the assurance of the rights of people with a mental disorder.

The plan expressed commitment to deinstitutionalisation, and formalised this in the two overarching principles of mainstreaming and integration:

- mainstreaming refers to the process of moving psychiatric services into the mainstream of general

health; in particular, co-locating psychiatric units with general hospitals
- integration refers to the coordination of hospital and community components of a mental health service so that together they provide a seamless continuity of care.

These processes were no longer to be considered optional 'good ideas' to be implemented or not, depending on the whim of the government in power, but rather, as basic human rights to conform to the UN principles to which Australia had agreed.

The First National Mental Health Plan recognised:

- the need to give mental health a higher priority
- the need to have a national focus and approval
- the goals of customer service and greater efficiency (therefore microeconomic reform)
- the relative responsibilities of the Commonwealth and state governments.

The National Policy and Plan required that traditional attitudes and work practices of the mental health workforce undergo considerable change, as both mainstreaming and integration required greater cooperation and flexibility than asylum-based practice.

Introduction of the first plan also included a cross-jurisdictional government process for oversight of implementation. This responsibility lay with the Australian Health Ministers' Advisory Council (AHMAC), and in particular its Mental Health Working Party.

This group consisted of all the directors of mental health from the states and territories, together with bureaucrats from the Commonwealth Department of Health with responsibilities from mental health to suicide prevention. Some version of this intergovernmental, bureaucratic oversight, now called the Mental Health Principal Committee (MHPC), has existed throughout all five National Mental Health Plans.

Evaluation

The evaluation of the strategy by an independent team in 1997 (National Mental Health Strategy, 1997) showed the following positive trends:

- substantial changes had occurred in the structure and mix of public mental health services
- there was broad consensus that the range and plurality of services had improved substantially, and that they were now more responsive and community orientated and better integrated with general health care
- funds provided by the Commonwealth had been critical in catalysing changes
- intersectoral links with housing and employment services had improved.

The evaluation report noted that changes were patchy across the country, with some places moving faster than others. The emphasis on serious mental illness was disenfranchising many consumers and carers, and general practitioners still complained about the insularity of the mental health system.

THE SECOND NATIONAL MENTAL HEALTH PLAN (1998–2003)

Key elements of content

The Second National Mental Health Plan (Australian Health Ministers, 1998) aimed to build on the achievements of the first plan and expand its focus within the original policy framework. The consumer focus of the Second National Mental Health Plan was expanded to cover a broader range of people with high-level needs. This plan acknowledged that the intent of the first plan to give priority to people with serious mental illness had in places been wrongly interpreted as only to include those with a psychotic diagnosis. The Second NMH Plan explicitly declared that the remit of public mental health services should be broader than this. In particular, it emphasised a focus on depression. Specified priority areas for reform included:

- mental health promotion, including community education, in which the attitudes of mental health workers and mental health literacy within the community are targeted
- mental illness prevention through early intervention, and population level measures
- development of partnerships in service reform, planning, delivery and evaluation between service

providers, consumers and carers, and between mental health, general health, primary care, welfare, disability support, community support and other government services
- quality and effectiveness of service delivery, including accreditation of services based on National Standards for Mental Health Services, the use of evidence-based practice, the development of measures of effectiveness and mental health workforce education and training initiatives.

Evaluation

Evaluation of the Second NMH Plan was a two-stage process. A mid-term review was undertaken in 2001 by Professor Graham Thornicroft, a senior UK psychiatrist, and Professor Virginia Trotter Betts, a US health policy advisor with a mental health nursing background (Thornicroft & Betts, 2002). Their observations were then incorporated into a comprehensive evaluation released in March 2003 (Australian Health Ministers, 2003i).

This evaluation noted that, although the Second NMH Plan provided clear directions for change, effective implementation was lacking because of insufficient commitment and funding. For instance, although mental health expenditure increased over the five years of the Plan, this increase really only mirrored an overall growth in health expenditure. Weaknesses in implementation are a recurring theme throughout all the plans, after the first.

A key finding was that structural reforms were largely complete, with the scaling down and closure of many psychiatric institutions. This is certainly true, though it should be noted that in 2017-18, out of total state and territory spending of $6 billion on mental health care, $565 million was still spent on services provided by psychiatric specialist hospitals. These facilities still exist in several states.

The evaluation found that most public mental health services were now managed by the general health system and community-based clinical services had undergone significant expansion. However, this pattern was not uniform across Australia. Further, growth in the non-government sector had not kept pace with the increased expectations of its contribution. Another important finding was that the mental health agenda now encompassed a broader range of mental health problems and mental illnesses, including comorbidity, with an emphasis on depression and on the key role of general practitioners. Improvements in mental health literacy were also noted, especially through school-based programs.

The evaluation identified areas for further attention. These included better access to services, more involvement of consumers and carers in treatment planning, better continuity of care and more adequate data collection to enable service monitoring. In addition, particular population groups with special needs still lacked adequate service access and responsiveness. Examples given included Indigenous people, those with complex needs and forensic populations. The authors called for development of a new plan in order to continue the reforms.

THE THIRD NATIONAL MENTAL HEALTH PLAN (2003–08)

Key content

The Third Plan in the sequence (Australian Health Ministers, 2003ii) endorsed a population health framework as the basis for policy (see, for example, p. 60), and then set out some principles and priority themes. Most of the principles were familiar, such as 'all people in need of mental health care should have access to timely and effective services, irrespective of where they live', and 'the quality and safety of mental health care must be ensured'. However, a new principle reflected the contemporary emphasis on recovery, noting that 'A recovery orientation should drive service delivery'.

The priority themes for the plan were also familiar from earlier NMH documents:

- promoting mental health and preventing mental health problems and mental illness
- increasing service responsiveness
- strengthening quality
- fostering research, innovation and sustainability.

These were then followed with 24 outcomes and associated key directions. The general tone of the document was more one of encouragement and aspiration towards desired outcomes rather than specific commitment to concrete structural reforms or to goals or targets regarding population health. This was in line with the absence of any allocation of Commonwealth funds for the plan's implementation, beyond those of the Medicare agreement with the states and territories. This contrasted with the first two NMH plans, which attracted Commonwealth funding for their execution.

Arguably, because this plan was more aspirational and less concrete, and because it lacked significant presentation of either the stick and/or the carrot, it had little influence on service developments at state levels. This case has certainly been presented in the Australian literature: 'While all strategies are again possible, no government is required to deliver on any specific items in the plan within any given time-frame' (Hickie & Groom, 2004). This related to calls for a body external to government that might monitor progress towards desired service reforms, along the lines of the Mental Health Commission, which seemed to have been successful in this role in New Zealand (Rosen et al., 2004).

Evaluation

The Third Plan was evaluated by Charles Curie, a US health consultant with a social work background, and Professor Graham Thornicroft, the senior UK psychiatrist who had co-authored the interim evaluation of the Second Plan (Curie & Thornicroft, 2002). Overall, the aspirational tenor of the plan was seen as helpful for maintaining reform momentum. However, the authors observed that the plan did not specify actions to meet key directions or outcomes, so lacked the detail needed to guide implementation and gauge its success. They reported that many of those interviewed during their consultations expressed frustration at this lack of specificity. Moreover, in July 2006, the plan was overtaken, and in effect sidelined, by the release of the COAG National Action Plan on Mental Health 2006. The Action Plan introduced a wide range of initiatives, with the Commonwealth allocating $1.9 billion for their implementation.

THE NATIONAL ACTION PLAN ON MENTAL HEALTH (2006–11)

Novel and different engagement from the Commonwealth

The National Action Plan (NAP) on Mental Health was unusual in several ways. It was released halfway through the life of the NMH Plan 2003–08, and unlike the previous plans, was the product of a highly politicised process. An important Australian Parliamentary Inquiry into Mental Health was completed in 2006 (*From Crisis to Community*, Parliament of Australia 2006). The peak body for the mental health sector, the Mental Health Council of Australia had also just published its seminal work, *Not For Service* (MHCA 2005), in conjunction with the Australian Human Rights and Equal Opportunity Commission in 2005. *Not For Service* was a comprehensive investigation into the performance of each jurisdiction against the National Mental Health Service Standards (National Mental Health Strategy 1996). The report demonstrated countless stories of poor quality and dangerous care, and a mental health system in crisis. Politically, there was sufficient concern about mental health to lift the issue from the responsibility of health ministers to first ministers (i.e. the state and territory Premiers and the Prime Minister). This also reflected recognition that solutions would need to look outside of health care. The NAP emerged into an environment of unprecedented attention on the issue of mental health and widespread community concern.

On this basis the Council of Australian Governments (COAG) agreed to a new National Action Plan, promising new coordinated action in five key areas, as follows:

1. promotion, prevention and early intervention
2. integrating and improving the care system
3. participation in the community and employment, including accommodation
4. coordinating care
5. increasing workforce capacity.

However, on 5 April 2006, Coalition Prime Minister Howard unilaterally announced new Commonwealth funding of $1.9 billion for a range of mental health initiatives. In doing so, he recognised the need for sustained action:

> Reform of mental health services cannot be achieved through a quick fix–it will require a sustained contribution...from both the Commonwealth and the states and territories to ensure long-term fundamental improvements in services for the mentally ill. Together, our investment in mental health will support reform of the system and ensure that it remains sustainable into the future.

In practice, and in accordance with their constitutional rights, each jurisdiction had complete autonomy over how they spent any associated funding. Detailed joint design of a national response to mental health by all governments was not undertaken. Rather, there was some significant variation between jurisdictional efforts across these five areas. The Action Plan, released later in July that year, included all the new Commonwealth-funded initiatives as well as commitments by each of the states and territories. Many of the latter were already underway, and some involved one-off capital projects rather than expanded service provision. For example, NSW spent most of its NAP contribution on building a new forensic jail at Long Bay Prison. Overall spending on mental health under the NAP over the period 2006-11 totalled more than $5.5 billion with the Commonwealth's share just under $2 billion. The great majority of all spending was directed towards action area 2, integrating and improving the care system.

The Commonwealth's contribution included:

- Funding for mental health nurses to be employed in private psychiatrists' offices and general practice 'to assist patients with serious mental illness to receive better coordinated treatment and care'.
- Personal Helpers and Mentors (PHaMS) program: funding to non-government agencies to employ workers to assist people living with a mental illness in the community to access the range of treatment, support, employment and accommodation services they need. Nine hundred PHaMS were to be employed across Australia.
- Support for Day-to-Day Living in the Community: funding for an additional 7000 places in programs to assist people with a mental illness improve their daily living skills and social participation.
- An extra 650 respite places for families and carers of people with a mental illness or an intellectual disability, with priority to elderly parents looking after an offspring with a mental illness or an intellectual disability.

The Commonwealth's most significant commitment however, was the Better Access to Mental Health Care program, under which for the first time, psychologists, social workers and occupational

Figure 1.39 Growth in Medicare psychology services under the Better Access Program

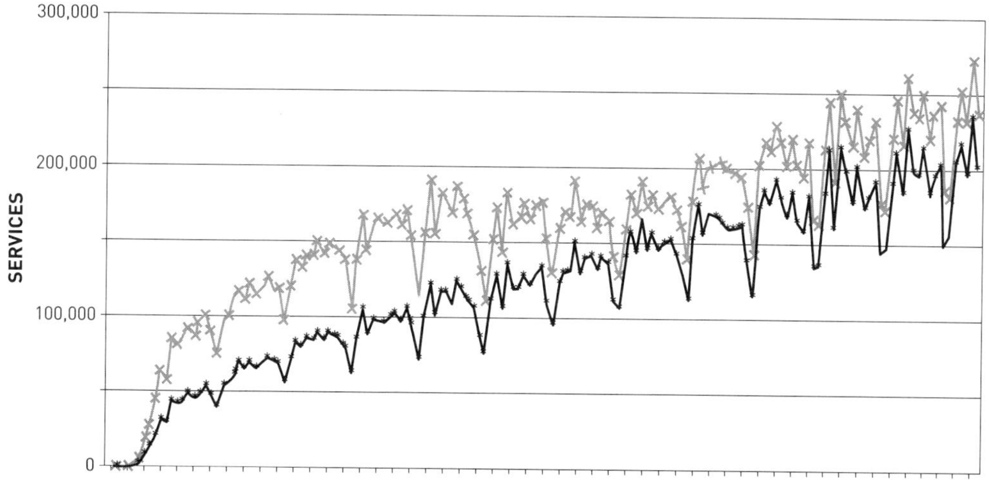

Source: Medicare Benefits Item Reports, http://medicarestatistics.humanservices.gov.au/statistics/mbs_item.jsp

therapists in private practice could register as Medicare Providers, and their clients could receive Medicare rebates for a set number of individual or group sessions of 'focused psychological strategies'.

The clients had to be referred by a GP or psychiatrist who had formulated a mental health plan. Client progress was supposed to monitored by the GP through a review after the sessions were complete. It became clear that only half the plans written were ever reviewed (Rosenberg & Hickie, 2019). Despite some changes limiting the number of sessions per client per year, the Better Access Program has continued to grow very strongly, as shown in Figure 1.39.

In 2018-19, more than five million psychology services were provided under Medicare costing more than $10 million weekly. Evidence has been published suggesting this investment has had a very significant impact on overall rates of public access to mental health care (Whiteford et al., 2014). At the same time, there has also been considerable debate regarding accountability under the Better Access Program, and the extent to which it is really helping people (Rosenberg & Hickie 2019) or making a difference to overall rates of prevalence of mental illness across the Australian community (Jorm, 2018 and Meadows, Enticott, Inder, Russell, & Gurr, 2015).

An alternative way of delivering primary mental health care from allied health practitioners was already in place. Called Access to Allied Psychological Services (ATAPS), this program was introduced in 2001 with funding of around $50 million per year. With funding administered through General Practice Divisions, ATAPS had demonstrated the capacity to improve access to psychological services for groups disadvantaged by low income, age or living in rural and remote locations. Funding was capped and the program had shown good value for money (Bassilios et al., 2016). After intensive lobbying by the relevant professional organisations, the Howard Government opted for the Better Access Program. This was administratively simpler, relying on existing fee-for-service payment arrangements under Medicare, whereas ATAPS services were funded under separate contracts.

NATIONAL MENTAL HEALTH POLICY (2008)

The Council of Australian Government's National Action Plan did contribute to a shift in thinking in relation to mental health, to see the issue in broader terms more aligned with the social determinants of health than just as health issue. Issues like housing, education and employment were given more prominence than before.

This was further articulated in the second national mental health policy which emerged in 2008, which gave a vision for mental health in Australia:

> ... a mental health system that enables recovery, that prevents and detects mental illness early and ensures that all Australians with a mental illness can access effective and appropriate treatment and community support to enable them to participate fully in the community (Commonwealth of Australia, 2009i).

THE FOURTH NATIONAL MENTAL HEALTH PLAN (2009–14)

This broader perspective carried over into the next national plan in the sequence (Commonwealth of Australia, 2009ii). This plan had five key priority areas:

- social inclusion and recovery
- prevention and early intervention
- service access, coordination and continuity of care
- quality improvement and innovation
- accountability–measuring and reporting progress.

However, perhaps because of the concurrent investments being made under the COAG NAP, this Fourth Plan had few dedicated resources. This meant that while the plan enunciated more than 30 sensible mental health reform ideas, governments, professionals and the mental health sector needed to rely on existing resources to drive change. Implementing change is difficult even with resources. Without, even well-argued policies and plans look increasingly gestural.

It should also be noted that one of the sensible suggestions made was to conduct a rigorous evaluation of the Fourth National Mental Health Plan. No such evaluation has occurred.

Mental Health Commissions

Seven of Australia's nine governments have chosen to invest in a new form of administrative leadership in mental health–the Mental Health Commission. As stated by Rosen et al. (2004), these organisations vary in scope and mission (see Table 1.15). Type 1 Commissions generally focus on individual cases and operate more like a complaints commission. Type 2 Commissions typically have a more strategic or systemic remit, aiming to influence broader policy and funding decisions or priorities.

The most significant difference between these bodies is that the WA Commission is the only one to hold the budget for mental health and thus exercise all the powers and responsibilities of a government department. The other commissions attempt to influence the shape of reform through policy, strategy and agreement. All the Type 2 commissions above have produced a jurisdictional strategic plan.

Some criteria have been established by which to assess the impact these organisations have had on mental health reform (Rosenberg & Rosen, 2012) but this kind of broad evaluation is yet to be undertaken. The need to evaluate their own performance is part of the legislation which underpins some of these commissions. At this stage, it is not possible to easily demonstrate that mental health commissions have materially progressed mental health reform across Australia.

Table 1.15 Mental health commissions across Australia

Jurisdiction	Commenced	Commission type	Established under specific legislation	Fundholder
WA	2009	Type 2—Strategy/Systemic	N	Y
National	2012	Type 2—Strategy/Systemic	N	N
NSW	2012	Type 2—Strategy/Systemic	Y	N
Queensland	2013	Type 2—Strategy/Systemic	Y	N
Victoria	2014	Type 1—Complaints Commission	Y	N
SA	2015	Type 2—Strategy/Systemic	N	N
ACT	2018	Type 2—Strategy/Systemic	N	N

National Mental Health Commission Review (2014)

In 2013, the Federal Government asked the National Mental Health Commission to conduct a review into mental health. The Terms of Reference aimed to permit assessment of the efficiency and effectiveness of programs and services, particularly federally funded services, in supporting individuals experiencing mental ill health, and their families and other support people, to lead a contributing life and to engage productively in the community.

This took more than one year with the report completed in November 2014. This Review focused largely on the Commonwealth role in mental health and overall, identified that services and programs:

- often are not well linked or integrated (to each other and to the states/territories)
- are administered by separate Commonwealth departments
- are delivered through short-term funding arrangements, which limits operational certainty, workforce stability and continuity of service delivery
- do not explicitly enable service coordination and integration
- often target similar population groups and/or provide similar types of supports
- do not appear to be planned for or designed with integrated whole of government, whole-of-life outcomes objectives in mind.

The Commission concluded that currently 'instead of a 'mental health system'– which implies a planned, unitary whole–we have a collection of often uncoordinated services that have accumulated spasmodically over time, with no clarity of roles and responsibilities or strategic approach that is reflected in practice' (Australian Government Department of Health, 2015, p. 5; see Chapters 1.1 and 1.5). The review found opportunities for positive change. It made 25 recommendations across eight key areas (see Table 1.16). These seem to bring together many of the challenges and imperatives for Australian mental health care even a few years later and may well do so for some time—so they are reproduced here for reference and reflection.

The findings of the Review were eventually made public when they were leaked in April 2015. A formal government response was issued later that year (Australian Government Department of Health, 2015). The initial government response, at the time the report was leaked, focused on media attention associated with recommendation 7. This suggestion had upset some professional groups, who saw this recommendation as a direct attack on the bed-based services provided in acute public hospitals. Despite the fact the Commission was suggesting the

Table 1.16 National Mental Health Commission Review Recommendations, 2014

1.Set clear roles and accountabilities to shape a person-centred mental health system
Rec 1. Agree the Commonwealth's role in mental health is through national leadership and regional integration, including integrated primary and mental health care.
Rec 2. Develop, agree and implement a National Mental Health and Suicide Prevention Plan with states and territories, in collaboration with people with lived experience, their families and support people.
Rec 3. Urgently clarify the eligibility criteria for access to the National Disability Insurance Scheme (NDIS) for people with disability arising from mental illness and ensure the provision of current funding into the NDIS allows for a significant Tier 2 system of community supports.
2. Agree and implement national targets and local organisational performance measures
Rec 4. Adopt a small number of important, ambitious and achievable national targets to guide policy decisions and directions in mental health and suicide prevention.
Rec 5. Make Aboriginal and Torres Strait Islander mental health a national priority and agree an additional COAG Closing the Gap target specifically for mental health.
Rec 6. Tie receipt of ongoing Commonwealth funding for government, NGO and privately provided services to demonstrated performance, and use of a single care plan and eHealth record for those with complex needs.
3. Shift funding priorities from hospitals and income support to community and primary health care services
Rec 7. Reallocate a minimum of $1 billion in Commonwealth acute hospital funding in the forward estimates over the five years from 2017–18 into more community-based psychosocial, primary and community mental health services.
Rec 8. Extend the scope of Primary Health Networks (renamed Primary and Mental Health Networks—PMHNs) as the key regional architecture for equitable planning and purchasing of mental health programmes, services and integrated care pathways.
Rec 9. Bundle-up programmes and boost the role and capacity of NGOs and other service providers to provide more comprehensive, integrated and higher-level mental health services and support for people, their families and supporters.
Rec 10. Improve service equity for rural and remote communities through place-based models of care.
4. Empower and support self-care and implement a new model of stepped care across Australia
Rec 11. Promote easy access to self-help options to help people, their families and communities to support themselves and each other, and improve ease of navigation for stepping through the mental health system.
Rec 12. Strengthen the central role of GPs in mental health care through incentives for use of evidence-based practice guidelines, changes to the Medicare Benefits Schedule and staged implementation of Medical Homes for Mental Health.
Rec 13. Enhance access to the Better Access programme for those who need it most through changed eligibility and payment arrangements and a more equitable geographical distribution of psychological services.

Rec 14. Introduce incentives to include pharmacists as key members of the mental health care team.

5. Promote the wellbeing and mental health of the Australian community, beginning with a healthy start to life

Rec 15. Build resilience and targeted interventions for families with children, both collectively and with those with emerging behavioural issues, distress and mental health difficulties.

Rec 16. Identify, develop and implement a national framework to support families and communities in the prevention of trauma from maltreatment during infancy and early childhood, and to support those impacted by childhood trauma.

Rec 17. Use evidence, evaluation and incentives to reduce stigma, build capacity and respond to the diversity of needs of different population groups.

6. Expand dedicated mental health and social and emotional wellbeing teams for Aboriginal and Torres Strait Islander people

Rec 18. Establish mental health and social and emotional wellbeing teams in Indigenous Primary Health Care Organisations (including Aboriginal Community Controlled Health Services), linked to Aboriginal and Torres Strait Islander specialist mental health services.

7. Reduce suicides and suicide attempts by 50% over the next decade

Rec 19. Establish 12 regions across Australia as the first wave for nationwide introduction of sustainable, comprehensive, whole of community approaches to suicide prevention.

8. Build workforce and research capacity to support systems change

Rec 20. Improve research capacity and impact by doubling the share of existing and future allocations of research funding for mental health over the next five years, with a priority on supporting strategic research that responds to policy directions and community needs.

Rec 21. Improve supply, productivity and access for mental health nurses and the mental health peer workforce.

Rec 22. Improve education and training of the mental health and associated workforce to deploy evidence-based treatment.

Rec 23. Require evidence-based approaches on mental health and wellbeing to be adopted in early childhood worker and teacher training and continuing professional development.

9. Improve access to services and support through innovative technologies

Rec 24. Improve emergency access to the right telephone and internet-based forms of crisis support and link crisis support services to ongoing online and offline forms of information/education, monitoring and clinical intervention.

Rec 25. Implement cost effective second and third generation e-mental health solutions that build sustained self-help, link to biometric monitoring and provide direct clinical support strategies or enhance the effectiveness of local services.

redirection merely of growth funding, the Federal Government were quick to reject any suggestion that funding for hospitals would be 'cut'.

The full government response to the Review did not attempt to address the specific recommendations made by the Commission. Instead, and drawing on advice from an 'expert reference group', it made new commitments towards increased regional planning of mental health, using a model described as stepped care (see Section 1.5.6). It also committed the Australian Government to work with the states and territories on a Fifth National Mental Health Plan.

THE FIFTH NATIONAL MENTAL HEALTH AND SUICIDE PREVENTION PLAN (2017–22)

This plan (Council of Australian Governments 2017) made more explicit reference to suicide prevention, in line with evolving government priorities and as reflection of the stubbornly high rate of suicide (see Figure 1.40).

The plan also continued to emphasise the interest of governments in more regional approaches to planning and budgeting for mental health. It suggested that overall responsibility for this

Figure 1.40 Standardised death rate per 100 000 persons for intentional self-harm, 2009–18

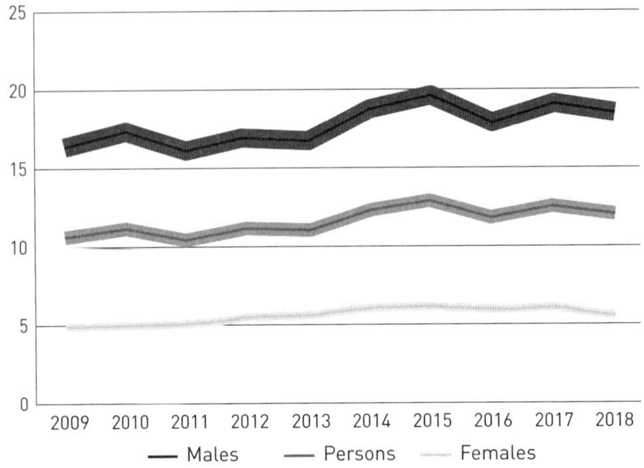

25
20
15
10
5
0
2009 2010 2011 2012 2013 2014 2015 2016 2017 2018
Males Persons Females

Source: Australian Bureau of Statistics, 2018

planning should rest on cooperation between the state/territory managed Local Health Districts (also called networks) and the 31 Commonwealth-funded Primary Health Networks (PHNs). However, in emphasising the primacy of this association between state and federal health agencies, the Fifth Plan does not carry the same focus on social determinants as some of its predecessors. This Fifth Plan is a health plan. There was no additional funding associated with the plan or its implementation.

It should be noted that the MHPC continues to have general oversight of the Fifth Plan.

STATE AND TERRITORY PLANS

It should also be noted that accompanying this national activity are myriad state and territory mental health policies and plans, explaining how each jurisdiction intends to shape their response to mental illness and promote mental health. Each jurisdiction generally also has a suicide prevention plan, a drug and alcohol plan, a plan in relation to the health of the Aboriginal and Torres Strait Islander populations, young people, Culturally and Linguistically Diverse populations and so on.

ACCOUNTABILITY

Despite this plethora of plans and policies, accountability for mental health has been elusive. It is difficult to assess the impact of care provided. Australia has invested in the collection of Health of the Nation Outcome Scores—among other measures—across different service settings. This work is managed by the Australian Mental Health Outcomes and Classification Network. However, it does not appear as if this data is commonly used as part of a framework of systemic quality improvement.

Indeed, Australia lacks any such framework. The need for improved accountability was an issue first raised in the original 1992 Policy which plainly stated the urgent need to overcome poor accountability and to closely monitor the progress of reform:

> There needs to be greater accountability and visibility in reporting progress in implementing the new national approach to mental health services. Currently mental health data collection is inconsistent and would not be adequate to enable an assessment to be made of the relative stage of development of the Commonwealth and each state/territory government in achieving the objectives outlined in the National Mental Health Policy (Australian Health Ministers Advisory Council, 1992).

Data collection systems have improved over time, but these have generally focused on health and hospital administrative data. Data collection from community and non-government services is patchy, often missing. Data outside of the health sector, reflecting social determinants like education, housing or employment (see Chapter 1.2) are not specifically collected, or rely on information drawn from broader data collections from general health surveys. There have been to date, only two specific surveys of mental health and wellbeing, in 1997 and 2007, with another scheduled for 2020.

This situation means that despite repeated policy rhetoric, accountability for mental health in Australia remains weak (Rosenberg & Salvador-Carulla, 2017). The National Mental Health Commission Review pointedly found a 'lack of outcome-based evaluation data and accountability mechanisms' (National Mental Health Commission, 2014b).

Sources of data in Australia have become narrower. From 1993, to support the National Mental Health Strategy, the Commonwealth Department of Health commissioned consultants to produce a series of 12 National Mental Health Reports. These reports were designed to specifically reflect the impact of mental health reforms. This series halted in 2013.

The main sources of information now are the Australian Institute of Health and Welfare's (Australian Institute of Health and Welfare (AIHW, 2019a) *Mental Health Services in Australia* website and the mental health chapter of the Report on Government Services (ROGS) produced annually by the Productivity Commission. Neither of these sources obtain primary or original data. They are both reliant on data supplied to them by governments. There is often a considerable delay here, with data needing checking and cleaning. This is a process managed by the Mental Health Principal Committee (MHPC). In 2020, both these reports refer to mental health data relating to 2017-18.

Data provided by these organisations, while useful, does not always reflect key policy goals or intent. For example, the data presented as 'community mental health' by both the AIHW and the Productivity Commission in fact blends outpatient hospital services and those services not provided in a hospital, out in the community. The inability to differentiate creates confusion. Attempting to alter the way data is collected or add new data items has proven to be a cumbersome and difficult exercise, again under the bureaucratic oversight of the MHPC.

EXPENDITURE ON MENTAL HEALTH

The AIHW Mental Health Services in Australia website is nevertheless an informative resource. It provides a range of publicly accessible graphs, tables and other information, such as is shown in Figure 1.41, where they demonstrate the increase in mental health spending since the First National Mental Health Policy in 1992-93.

Figure 1.41 AIHW Mental Health Expenditure, 1992–93

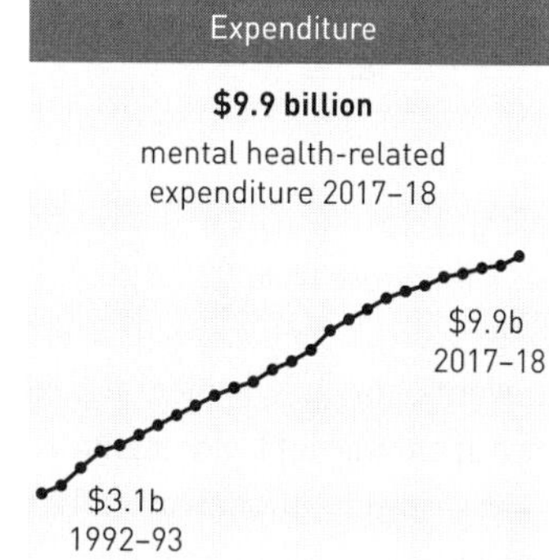

The AIHW then report that mental health experienced a 1.1% annual average increase in the real per capita spending between 2013-14 and 2017-18, a per capita increase from $382 to $400. However, further examination of the expenditure shows that mental health represented 7.25% of total health spending in 1992-93 and 7.63% in 2017-18. This rate of spending should be considered in relation to the burden of disease for which mental illness is responsible. In Australia, mental and substance use disorders were estimated to be responsible for 12% of the total burden of disease in 2015, placing it fourth as a broad disease group after cancer (18%), cardiovascular diseases (14%) and musculoskeletal conditions (13%; AIHW 2019b).

As shown in Figure 1.42, while mental health-related expenditure has doubled over 20 years or so (see Chapter 1.5) the trend line for mental health spending as a proportion of health expenditure is practically unchanged over nearly 30 years, despite the plethora of mental health inquiries, recommendations, policies and plans.

Figure 1.42 Mental health's share of total health expenditure, 1992–2017

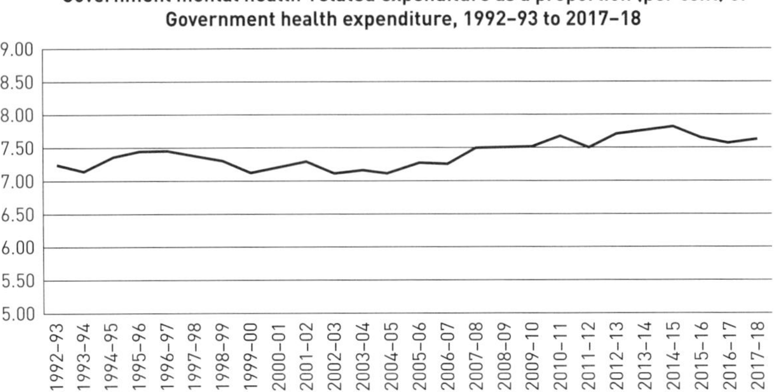

And according to the AIHW again, total health spending per capita rose from $7157 to $7485, a 1.2% annual average increase between 2013-14 and 2017-18. In other words, not only is mental health's share of total health spending not fundamentally changing, it is growing at a slower rate than overall expenditure on health care.

Of the $9.9 billion in spending, 60.6% was provided by state and territory governments, 33.9% by the Australian Government, and 5.5% by private health insurance funds. This distribution has remained steady over the past five years. Spending on state and territory specialised mental health services totalled $6.0 billion for 2017-18. The largest proportion of state and territory expenditure was spent on public hospital services for admitted patients ($2.6 billion); this was closely followed by expenditure on community mental health care services totalling $2.3 billion. Again, as stated earlier, it is likely that much of this 'community' spending is outpatient services provided in hospitals or in community clinics run by hospital institutions, rather than outreach services. In 1992-93, funding to NGOs represented just over 2% of total spending by the states and territories. In 2017-18, it had risen to 7.25%. So spending on psychosocial and other services typically provided by non-government organisations remains a very small fraction of overall mental health spending, and hospital-sourced mental health care remains a dominant locus of provision for many people with serious mental health problems.

SUMMARY

Australia has a comprehensive history of National Mental Health Plans and policies. These have often set aspirational direction for change. However, particularly after the second national plan, there was little if any national investment in implementation and change. Services and programs already under pressure from unmet demand for mental health care struggle to find from existing resources the capacity to drive desired reforms.

The scope of mental health reforms has grown and shrunk over time, with more recent iterations of National Mental Health Plans re-emphasising health services over a broader conception of mental health and its social determinants. The current strong reform trend focuses on greater regional autonomy in mental health planning, policy and funding. This will require considerable thinking and investment in the skills and resources necessary for each region of Australia to undertake this task successfully. These regional reforms reinforce the need to establish useful accountability and benchmarking. These tools can drive systemic quality improvement.

The stewardship of mental health policy by the Mental Health Principal Committee has remained constant. Members of this Committee are largely responsible for hospital-based mental health care, which itself is under critical pressure. Perhaps this is another reason why lasting alternatives have struggled to emerge.

1.7.3 THE AUSTRALIAN GOVERNMENT AND THE NATIONAL SETTING

SEBASTIAN ROSENBERG

INTRODUCTION

The first of the nine jurisdictional roles to be described here concerns the Australian Government (sometimes called the Commonwealth or Federal Government). This section will describe how their role has evolved in relation to mental health, focusing in particular on Medicare, Pharmaceutical Benefits and, latterly, the National Disability Insurance Scheme (NDIS). Aspects of the national mental health reform program will also be dealt with, for example in relation to suicide prevention.

This discussion will occur while attempting to respond to the two key questions posed in relation to all these jurisdictional reports:

- What do mental health services look like in your jurisdiction?
- What makes them unique?

Overall, the role played by the national government in mental health could be split into three phases. The first phase saw their main role focus just on funding. Australia's federated system of government means responsibility for health care largely rests with the states. However, it is the role of the Federal Government to fund the states for hospital care, to fund primary care through Medicare, and also to provide access to drug treatments under the Pharmaceutical Benefits Scheme.

The second phase of Australian Government action in relation to mental health saw it begin to become more engaged in the provision of services, particularly community mental health services, through a range of programs like Personal Helpers and Mentors and Partners in Recovery.

The third and current phase sees the Australian Government largely return to its historic role as funder. Greater emphasis on regional responsibility for planning and organising mental health care has meant national leadership has diminished.

This last phase leaves mental health at an interesting and important junction. There is a need to determine what aspects of mental health are best decided nationally and what should be local. Systems of benchmarking and quality improvement require national and coordinated action. The extent to which the Australian Government is prepared to drive this process will be considered.

WHAT DO AUSTRALIAN GOVERNMENT MENTAL HEALTH SERVICES LOOK LIKE?

As stated, the historic role of the Australian Government is that of funder. In 2017-18, mental health spending by the Australian Government totalled just over $3.3 billion as shown in Table 1.17.

Four main agencies provide mental health programs and services; the Department of Health, the Department Social Services, the Department of Veterans' Affairs and the Department of Defence. The focus of the last two agencies is the mental health and welfare of military or ex-military personnel and their families. This has been subject to several recent parliamentary and other inquiries (Parliament of Australia, 2017b).

The Department of Health's mental health spending is mostly directed towards Primary Health Networks, which operate regionally to determine spending priorities. However, Health also funds some specific programs, like headspace, Kidsmatter, Mindframe among others. Health also provides funding to some organisations operating in the mental health sector, such as Mental Health Australia.

Health also take responsibility for an Indigenous mental health program and a program aimed at suicide prevention (both costing around $50 million). The Australian Government also provides around $70 million for mental health research, largely

Table 1.17 Australian Government Spending on Mental Health 2017–18

Funded item	$'000
Mental health specific payments to states and territories	0
National programs and initiatives (Department of Health managed)	754 074
National programs and initiatives (DSS managed)*	234 276
National programs and initiatives (DVA managed)	209 710
Department of Defence funded programs	52 340
Indigenous social and emotional wellbeing programmes	47 788
National Mental Health Commission	7 738
National Suicide Prevention Program	55 942
Medicare Benefits Schedule—psychiatrists	358 300
Medicare Benefits Schedule—general practitioners	299 181
Medicare Benefits Schedule—psychologists/allied health	584 199
Pharmaceutical Benefits Scheme	519 852
Private Health Insurance Premium Rebates	164 016
Research	69 441
Total	**$3 356 857**

administered through Health. The Department of Social Services are funding a program aimed at improving the employment of people with a mental illness. They are also providing some support enabling access to psychosocial mental health services for people ineligible for the National Disability Insurance Scheme.

The Australian Government fund Medicare, the national public health insurer, to provide mental health care. This cost more than $1 billion in 2017-18, split between psychiatrists, psychologists and general practitioners. It should be remembered of course that health professionals often charge more than the fee Medicare pays them. This becomes an additional 'out of pocket' expense borne by patients. Pharmaceutical treatments are also subsidised under the national Pharmaceutical Benefits Scheme, meaning patients can access their medication easier.

The Federal Government has been a very strong supporter of private health and private insurance. The rebate provides some incentive for people to take out private insurance.

As described earlier in this chapter (see Section 1.7.2), the Australian Government provided some specific financial incentives to the states and territories to close psychiatric specialist institutions under the First National Health Plan in 1993. Since that time however, this kind of incentive to drive change has been rare. Instead, the Commonwealth chose to focus on its own spending and programs, particularly under Medicare.

However, part of the rationale for the 2006-11 Council of Australian Governments National Action Plan on Mental Health was to see a much greater involvement in Commonwealth spending on mental health programs and services. Programs such as Personal Helpers and Mentors, Partners in Recovery, Activities of Daily Living and Carer Respite began, led by Health or Social Services. Often these services were delivered by non-government organisations (NGOs). Spending on NGOs as a proportion of total spending in mental health rose from around 7% in 2007-08 to 9.6% in 2014-15. This increase has now ceased, since the advent of the NDIS.

By way of comparison, New Zealand allocate between 20 and 25% of their total spending on mental health towards services provided by NGOs. This has resulted in a greater range of service options in that country, both psychosocial and clinical, in comparison to Australia. The peripheral role funded for NGOs in mental health care leaves Australia very dependent on mental health care provided by the predominantly hospital-based public services run by the states and territories, and the health professional services funded under Medicare.

THE NATIONAL DISABILITY INSURANCE SCHEME (NDIS)

There are around 4.3 million Australians who have a disability. Beginning in 2013, the NDIS is a new public insurance scheme designed to meet the needs of around 500 000 Australians with a disability aged under 65. Once it is fully enrolled, it is estimated that the Scheme will cost $22 billion a year. The initial focus of the Scheme was to attend to the care needs of people with permanent and significant disability. Mental health was a reasonably late inclusion in the Scheme. For many people, notions of permanent disability jar with the hope and expectation of recovery from mental illness. Many people with severe mental illness often experience problems episodically. Again, notions of permanence and chronicity don't easily translate between some physical and mental disabilities.

Under the NDIS, it is expected that at full enrolment, 64 000 people with psychosocial disability will be covered. As at September 2019, there were 25 864 NDIS participants with psychosocial disability as the reason, representing 9% of all NDIS participants. Spending on the NDIS in 2018-19 had reached $10 billion.

The impact of the NDIS has been considerable. As stated earlier, the investment in the psychosocial services, provided mostly by NGOs, was never significant, even as the Commonwealth increased its funding under the National Action Plan. In setting up the NDIS, both the Commonwealth and state/territory governments transferred the funding associated with support for people with a disability to the new NDIS. The underpinning philosophy of the NDIS is to enable personal choice and autonomy in decision making for people with a disability. In practice, this meant that the traditional block funded contracts between governments and NGOs ended. Under the NDIS, services would be purchased directly by consumers and NGO services would be dependent on individuals choosing their services. An already fragile psychosocial sector has now been significantly affected. Organisations have struggled to offer staff ongoing employment contracts. Rare psychosocial expertise has been lost (Smith-Merry et al 2018). The Department of Social Services are maintaining, for now, some funding to enable 'continuity of support' for some mental health clients not eligible for ongoing support under the NDIS.

Beyond these practical considerations, the NDIS raises fundamental questions about the role to be played by psychosocial services as part of Australia's overall response to mental illness. Even if it is agreed that this is important, the NDIS suggest they are prepared to provide this type of care to only a small proportion of the nearly 700 000 people in Australia with severe mental illness (see Figure 1.43). How people with 'milder' conditions access this kind of assistance is unclear.

The NDIS is essentially a funding mechanism. It provides people with mental illness little if any guidance regarding any 'preferred' model of care or support. This is consistent with the primacy the scheme places on choice and autonomy. The NDIS has also been carefully drawn to avoid any confusion with other funding arrangements. There is supposed to be clear demarcation separating health services and NDIS services. However, this can be difficult to enforce and is not clearly monitored. For example, psychologists provide mental health services for clinical improvement under Medicare but also mental health services for functional improvement under the NDIS.

COMMONWEALTH MENTAL HEALTH INFRASTRUCTURE

The current approach to mental health planning and funding as described in the Fifth National Mental Health Plan (Council of Australian Governments, 2017) points to an increased role for regions in decision making. This is as opposed to a more centralised approach, decided by either national or state/territory governments. In theory, this approach permits more localised, tailored approaches to the needs of communities. In the past, essentially the nine departments of health across Australia would use a variety of tools to allocate

Figure 1.43 National Mental Health Commission estimates of prevalence of mental illness

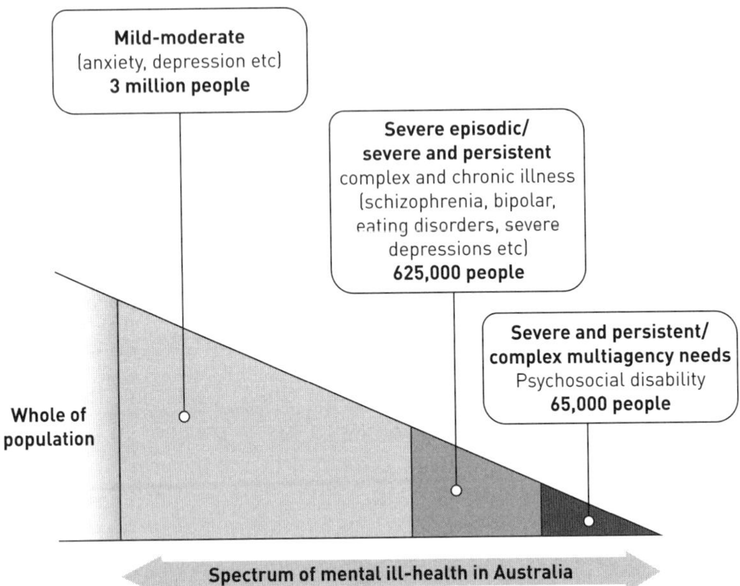

resources for mental health. Often these were based on historic usage. More recently, some jurisdictions relied on casemix style planning and funding arrangements. The Commonwealth developed a National Mental Health Casemix Classification system (Independent Hospital Pricing Authority (IHPA), 2017) to assist with this but it is yet to be widely applied.

Similarly, the Commonwealth has recently invested considerable resources in a National Mental Health Service Planning Framework (NMHSPF, 2017). Derived from a resource allocation formula first developed in NSW, this Framework has been further developed by the University of Queensland, to incorporate not only acute care, but outpatient, primary and psychosocial care (see Section 1.5.4). The Framework operates as a commercial-in-confidence product, with planners buying licences and training. Its underlying assumptions, about how many of which services are needed to meet the needs of regional populations, are not open to public scrutiny though extracts of some key documents were published recently including Care Profiles, Service Element & Activity Descriptions and several Technical Appendices (NMHSPF 2020). Overall, the Framework focuses on health services.

It is not designed to address the broader social determinants of mental health, meaning at this stage, issues such as housing, education, social inclusion and employment are not dealt with. Nevertheless, the Council of Australian Governments have mandated that the Framework be used to drive regional mental health planning efforts. The Commonwealth is continuing to invest in further development of the Framework, to increase its applicability and capacity to reflect local circumstances.

The Commonwealth has built other national mental health infrastructure elements. A second edition of National Standards for Mental Health Services was produced in 2010 (National Mental Health Strategy, 2010). The extent to which mental health services meet these standards is one of the key mental health indicators reported by the Australian Institute of Health and Welfare. However, there appears to be some disconnection in that 85% of all mental health services are accredited as meeting level 1 of these Standards yet reports of service failure are common. There is a question as to the extent to which these Standards really drive systemic quality improvement or are primarily gestural.

Similarly, a national framework for recovery oriented mental health services was developed in 2013 (Australian Health Ministers' Advisory Council (AHMAC), 2013). However, there is no regular reporting regarding the extent to which services operate according to this framework.

The Commonwealth provides funding to support Mental Health Australia (MHA), the peak body representing the mental health sector. In turn, MHA provide support for the National Mental Health Consumer and Carer Forum, which has links to consumer and carer organisations operating at the state/territory level. Many consumers and carers do not see this as ideal. They would prefer their views are expressed autonomously, through their own consumer and carer organisations. MHA also manage the Embrace project, designed to develop mental health tools and services aimed at assisting Australia's many multicultural communities.

WHAT MAKES AUSTRALIAN MENTAL HEALTH SERVICES UNIQUE?

The Federal Government is solely responsible for primary care. It provides primary health through Medicare and drug treatments through the Pharmaceutical Benefits Scheme. It provides the funding and sets the policy. Under Australia's federal system, the Australian Government is probably the only jurisdiction with a realistic prospect of providing national leadership. This is a task beyond individual jurisdictions. It is reasonable to say that while there seemed a willingness to embrace this role in the early days of the National Mental Health Strategy, subsequent plans have seen this diminish. The current emphasis on regional planning and funding brings this into sharper focus. While this local control may be sensible and desirable, systemic quality improvement will depend on the continued development and implementation of National Standards, frameworks, benchmarking and reporting. And even when a national government is willing to invest in this infrastructure, the states and territories have clear rights, roles and responsibilities which mean that national leadership is not axiomatic (Smullen, 2016). Incentives, sanctions, persuasion and persistence are necessary. It is complex and the national government has many competing priorities. So, while the capacity for national mental health leadership is probably unique to the Australian Government, its exercise is by no means certain or consistent.

1.7.4 AUSTRALIAN CAPITAL TERRITORY

SEBASTIAN ROSENBERG, BERNARD HUGHSON & PEGGY BROWN

WHAT DO MENTAL HEALTH SERVICES LOOK LIKE IN THE ACT?

Growth of a small country town

From 1908, when the site for the national capital was selected, until early in the 1960s, Canberra was little more than a small country town. There were no public mental health services and, indeed, no private specialised service until the end of this period. The first Mental Health Acts were pieces of Commonwealth legislation allowing the transfer of involuntary patients to NSW hospitals. Most such patients were admitted to Kenmore, one of the major psychiatric hospitals in NSW, although when a census was conducted in 1986, smaller numbers were also found in all of the psychiatric hospitals in that state.

Early in the 1960s, the government of the day made the decision to relocate Commonwealth Government departments progressively to Canberra, and rapid growth followed. By the end of the decade, the city population was approaching 100 000. A psychiatry ward, opened at Canberra Community Hospital, admitted voluntary patients, and there was a weekly half-day clinic at the same hospital providing some medical care for patients discharged from Kenmore. A child guidance clinic was established, and a Sydney child psychiatrist visited monthly. However, there were no other services in the city or in the neighbouring region, and increasing community dissatisfaction with the inadequacies led to inquiries, first by Dr E Cunningham Dax and later by Professor WA Cramond.

The first organised public mental health service was the result, with Dr Brian Hennessy appointed in 1968 to head and develop this service.

This history explains some of the differences in the way services developed in Canberra compared with other parts of the country. The absence of a psychiatric hospital was in part an advantage, but it also meant that there was no pool of financial or staff resources for redirection to alternative services. The demography of the city was also very different from that in the other urban centres. The immigrant population was heavily weighted towards young adults, who came from all parts of the country to work in the public service. A mental health community survey around this time demonstrated relatively high levels of minor disorder associated with adjustment to life change, but low levels of psychosis. The service that developed in response to population needs was notable for its focus on family and child problems, and was staffed predominantly by social workers, psychologists and a group of social health visitors from various backgrounds, whose mental health training was 'on the job'. As the city continued to grow through the 1970s, a second psychiatry ward was opened at the new southside Woden Valley Hospital, but involuntary patients were still removed 100 km to Kenmore Hospital in NSW. Community-based services were extended, and longer stay residential care established. Much of this was innovative, at least in the Australian context.

Critically, in the early 1970s, the Federal Government permitted the establishment of Calvary Hospital in the north of Canberra, a private facility operated by the Little Company of Mary and offering acute, emergency and other hospital care.

DEVELOPING SELF-SUFFICIENCY

By the early 1980s, the transfer of government departments to Canberra was complete and the growth rate was slowing. The demography of the population (and, with it, an increased prevalence of major psychiatric illness) was approaching Australian norms, and this determined the need to change service provision to better meet the needs of those with mental illness. The increase in prevalence of serious illness was reinforced by the increasing tendency of patients from the surrounding New South Wales region to seek admission at Canberra hospitals rather than travel the extra distance to Kenmore. In 1994, a new Mental Health (Treatment and Care) Act provided for involuntary care locally, social health visitors were replaced with community mental health nurses, and training schemes were established in mental health nursing, psychiatry and clinical psychology.

Territory self-government was enacted in 1989. The new Territory Health Department entered into arrangements with Calvary Hospital for the provision of public health services, including in relation to mental health. Calvary's mental health services have since become an important element in the Territory's overall mental health system, though the casemix at Woden Hospital (now the Canberra Hospital) tends to be more acute. Having a private provider play such a key role is unique.

This was put into sharp focus in the mid to late 1990s when the ACT Government chose to implement the purchaser/provider model of health care (Aulich, 2002). This left a small rump central department as a purchaser of services from three separate organisations: Calvary Hospital, the Canberra Hospital and an agency called ACT Community Care which brought together a range of public community health service providers. The aim of these arrangements was to encourage greater accountability and better planning. This experiment ceased after a few years but has recently been reinstated, with the policy arm of the ACT Health Directorate now split from Canberra Health Services.

Beyond mental health, Canberra has generally sought to become self-sufficient in terms of health care. The local health services provide most procedures, even some transplantation. This level of service is possible and viable largely due to the role played by the Canberra Hospital as the major tertiary hospital operating between Sydney and Melbourne. In this context the ACT Health system plays an important regional role, beyond the 420 000 ACT residents to the broader population estimated to be around one million. Complex cross-border negotiations ensure that the ACT is compensated by surrounding jurisdictions, mostly NSW, when their residents receive care in Canberra. This 'income' is a vital part of supporting self-sufficiency.

It is an anomaly therefore that this regional role does not apply to mental health. ACT mental health services, apart from in extreme emergency situations, generally exclude non-ACT residents who must seek services in their own home states. One contributing factor here may be the confusing set of competing legal arrangements which see different legislation apply across each jurisdiction. But the impact of this situation is that the ACT mental health system operates largely just for ACT residents, unlike all other parts of the Territory's health service.

ACT MENTAL HEALTH SERVICE OVERVIEW

The key parts of the ACT public mental service are:

- The Adult Mental Health Unit (AMHU) provides short-term individualised care. Located at the Canberra Hospital, the purpose-built facility contains 37 beds and offers a range of amenities including individual rooms, a gymnasium and spiritual room. Ward 2N is an adult mental health unit in Calvary Hospital Bruce.
- The Mental Health Short Say Unit (MHSSU) provides admissions for a maximum of 48 hours and may be voluntary or involuntary.
- The Adult Mental Health Rehabilitation Unit (AMHRU) is a specialist mental health rehabilitation unit located at the University of Canberra Hospital. The unit provides care and support for people with a primary diagnosis of mental illness who require a longer hospital stay between 3 and 12 months to complete a rehabilitation program.
- Dhulwa is a secure forensic mental health unit located adjacent to a nature reserve in Symonston. The unit provides 24-hour care for patients in a secure, structured and safe environment. The facility includes both acute and rehabilitation mental health programs. People are generally admitted to the unit from the criminal justice system under the *Mental Health Act 2015*. A small group of people may be admitted from other mental health services under the *Mental Health Act 2015*.
- The Extended Care Unit is located within the Brian Hennessy Rehabilitation Centre on the grounds of Calvary Hospital, Bruce. The unit provides medium term, residential care for people with complex and long-lasting mental health issues.
- There is a Child and Adolescent Mental Health Service (CAMHS) and a Specialist Youth Mental Health Outreach Team.
- There are five adult community mental health teams that are located throughout Canberra in the major town centres of Belconnen, City, Gungahlin, Woden and Tuggeranong. These multidisciplinary teams include doctors, nurses and other health care professionals.
- In 2018 the ACT established an Office for Mental Health and Wellbeing (2020), operating with a remit akin to a Mental Health Commission, aiming to drive strategic change and reform.
- The Capital Health Network (2016) recently completed their mental health needs analysis and found key gaps, including:
  - early intervention and prevention services
  - management of comorbidities, particularly metabolic disorders in the community
  - psychological services for people with moderate to severe presentations
  - integration between primary and tertiary services, and with the NDIS
  - multidisciplinary services for some key demographic groups, including transgender population, homeless people and Aboriginal and Torres Strait Islander population
  - need to build workforce skills in relation to trauma-informed care
  - need for follow-up community support after discharge following a suicide attempt, including better GP support
  - need to build network of peer support services.

The recently completed Integrated Mental Health Atlas (Furst et al., 2018) reported that the key ACT gaps were:

- acute and sub-acute residential care
- day care

- employment related services and
- CALD services.

UNIQUE FEATURES OF THE ACT SYSTEM

While staff shortages in mental health are not unique, in the ACT they are critical. There has been particular concern, including in relation to public psychiatry, from both the community and in the media (ABC News, 2018; Burdon, 2017).

Reflecting Canberra's small size and commitment to public community mental health care, the Australian Institute of Health and Welfare report that the ACT has the highest rate of community contacts of any jurisdiction per 1000 population (Australian Institute of Health and Welfare, 2020a).

In addition to these public services, traditionally the ACT has also invested in a range of psychosocial services provided by non-government organisations. In 2014-15, average per capita spending on these services was $18.13 but in the ACT it was $47.74 (Australian Institute of Health and Welfare, 2020). While this created a vibrant community mental health sector, the extent to which NGO service providers could work in partnership with public mental health services was unclear. And now, as described elsewhere in this chapter, the impact of the National Disability Insurance Scheme has been to reduce funding. By 2017-18, per capita spending by the Territory on NGO mental health services was down to $20.55. The ACT has built valuable expertise in psychosocial services. It will be important these are not lost as a result of shifts in mental health funding (Rosenberg et al., 2019).

The most obvious unique feature of the ACT is that it operates as both a fully fledged Health Department with policy and oversight functions, but also as a 'health district', organising and providing regional health services. This combined role offers the potential for coordination and efficiency.

The ACT has also enjoyed some continuity in relation to primary care. The ACT was covered by one Division of General Practice, then one Medicare Local and now one Primary Health Network—Capital Health Network (CHN). The alignment between federally funded PHN and the Territory health services opens unique opportunities for integrated planning. A recent example of this potential is the ACT Regional Mental Health and Suicide Prevention Plan 2019-2024 which brought together not just the CHN and the Territory service providers, but also non-government organisations, consumers and carers in a joint effort to describc priorities for mental health reform (Capital Health Network, 2019).

One of the main challenges for the Office of Mental Health and Wellbeing will be whether it can help to capitalise on the natural advantages of scale and resources which apply to the ACT. Canberra is growing. There is pressing need to develop and design new, coordinated approaches to mental health care involving a range of stakeholders.

1.7.5 NEW SOUTH WALES

CATHERINE LOUREY

New South Wales is the largest jurisdictional provider of mental health services in Australia. The breadth, distribution and complexity of the mental health system means that no one community has identical services. This is a function of historical patterns of service development, of workforce recruitment challenges and how innovation and alternative approaches have been pursued to meet local needs.

In 2017-18, NSW had the highest number of beds in specialist psychiatric units in public hospitals per 100 000 population of any jurisdiction in Australia. (Australian Institute of Health and Welfare (AIHW), 2020a). NSW had 34.8 beds per 100 000 population, higher than the national rate of 27.9 beds and almost double the lowest rate recorded, the Northern Territory at 17.4 per 100 000 population. NSW also had the highest rate for mental health hospital beds in general services and in child and adolescent services.

Staffing in specialist mental health services in 2015-16 was over 10 600 full-time equivalent (FTE) positions (NSW Government, 2018-22). The emerging peer workforce is a growing presence across public mental health services, integrated care models and the community managed organisation (CMO) sector.

The rollout of new Commonwealth-funded initiatives and programs, delivered through both the public and private mental health sectors (including private practitioners and general practitioners), is also important in understanding what the NSW mental health system looks like. Or, more specifically, what NSW people can expect from their local public mental health services.

All NSW government agencies are expected to deliver on their state outcomes. There are five state outcomes for health for 2019-20 (NSW Government, 2020). One is specifically on related to mental health:

> Mentally healthy communities: Strengthening health care for people with mental illness, their families and carers, including through better access to community mental health services and improved quality of care and patient safety.

One other state health outcome refers to mental health and the role of the NSW Mental Health Commission:

> Continuously improving health care: Improving health care through the Health Care Complaints Commission that acts to protect public health and safety, and the Mental Health Commission responsible for monitoring, reviewing and improving the mental health system.

The 2019-20 budget investment for Mentally Healthy Communities was $2.1 billion, which provided the operational budget for mental health services and programs and included the first year of a $700 million Mental Health Infrastructure Program, $19.7 million to support initiatives to reduce suicides in NSW (NSW Government, 2020) and four-year funding of $23 million to expand the capacity of Lifeline and Kids Helpline (Taylor, 2019).

The overarching strategic direction for mental health in NSW is outlined in *Living Well: The Strategic Plan for Mental Health in NSW 2014-24* (NSW Mental Health Commission, 2014). This takes a whole of government, whole-of-sector and whole-of-person approach. It places people with lived experience at the heart of the strategy to improve outcomes across the domains of their lives, and across the system to improve the mental health and wellbeing of the community. The role of the Mental Health Commission is to monitor, review and report on how the Living Well strategic plan is progressing.

WHAT DO MENTAL HEALTH SERVICES LOOK LIKE IN NSW?

Public mental health services and programs in NSW are funded at around $2.1 billion annually, to deliver emergency mental health services, hospital interventions when people are acutely unwell, and recovery support services in hospital settings and the community. It also funds community mental health services, the mental health access line to assist people to connect with the service or support they may need, as well as funding to supporting crisis lines and a range of housing and accommodation support initiatives (HASI) and community living supports (CLS).

The Ministry of Health manages the distribution of these funds and the performance and governance arrangements for the public mental health system. The funding extends to suicide prevention initiatives and specific programs, such as perinatal services provided through non-government organisations. The Ministry works with Local Health Districts (LHDs), the Justice Health and Forensic Mental Health network and the Sydney Children's Hospital Networks in planning and delivering mental health services and supports.

The public system alone does not provide all the services to meet the mental health needs of the community.

Mental health services and programs are also provided through partnerships with other agencies, such as the Departments of Education and of Communities and Justice, to fund programs in schools and courts. The public mental health system also works within the wider mental health system including the community managed sector and Aboriginal Community Controlled Health Services (ACCHS). In NSW, there are approximately 117 community managed organisations providing mental health services (Mental Health Coordinating Council (MHCC), 2020a) and 38 ACCHSs that support the social and emotional wellbeing of their community.

Child and adolescent services are provided through specialised community teams, the Sydney Children's Hospitals' Network (SCHN) and local child and adolescent mental health services. The SCHN provides specialist tertiary clinical consultation services and telehealth services. In NSW, child and adolescent counselling programs are provided through schools and funded by the Department of Education. Program such as GOT IT are jointly funded by both Health and Education.

Mental health services for adults are provided in community mental health services, emergency departments and hospital units, responding the mental health needs that are severe and complex, acute or where people can 'step down' to recovery rehabilitation services. General practice, private psychologists, psychiatrists and social workers provide mental health treatments and support via Commonwealth-funded programs. Likewise, Primary Health Networks (PHNs), also Commonwealth-funded, provide mental health supports as well as suicide prevention interventions.

Older persons' mental health services provide specialist mental health services for people aged over 65 years, and where appropriate they can include people aged under 65 or Aboriginal people aged over 50 years. These specialist services are provided across multidisciplinary community services, acute and non-acute hospital settings, and in partnership with specialist services and residential aged care services.

Forensic mental health services are provided at the Forensic Hospital and secure and medium secure units located in a number of Local Health Districts along with community forensic services.

COMMUNITY MANAGED ORGANISATIONS

There are approximately 117 community managed organisations (CMOs) in NSW providing mental health services (Mental Health Coordinating Council (MHCC), 2020). The Ministry of Health funds the CMO sector to provide psychosocial rehabilitation, recovery and disability support services. These include key government programs that support people to live well in the community:

- Housing and Accommodation Support Initiative (HASI) and HASI+
- Community Living Supports (CLS)
- Pathways to Community Living Initiative (PCLI)
- Family and Carer Mental Health Program.

There are also three mental health non-government organisations (NGOs) in NSW that play a peak or advocacy role. While these NGOs can receive grants from a range of sources, the NSW Mental Health Commission provides their operating grant:

> Being, which is the peak organisation that represent and advocates for people with lived experience of mental health issues, and brings the voice of lived experience into the planning and consideration of issues that affect people with mental illness.

These include Mental Health Carers NSW, which is the peak advocacy body for families and carers of people living with mental health issues, and WayAhead, which focuses on promoting mental health and wellbeing and reducing stigma and discrimination through community education and forums.

WHAT MAKES THEM UNIQUE?

Across NSW, Local Health Districts are responding to the specific health needs of their communities. Some provide state-wide specialist services in specific locations, others are the sites of pilot programs or local initiatives. This may not be a unique approach across Australia, but it demonstrates a commitment and attempt to make service availability unique to the needs of that local community.

- Your Experience of Service (YES) survey: NSW is only one of three jurisdictions that has implemented this survey for people using public mental health services, allowing direct and anonymous feedback to services. This brings the experience of care directly into considerations of service accountability and responsiveness, and quality improvement. In 2017–18, NSW scored the highest positive response at 68.7%, with Victoria recording 50.4% and Queensland 47.1% (Australian Institute of Health and Welfare (AIHW), 2019b).

- Peer workforce: peer worker numbers are growing in NSW, in hospital and community settings. The rate of consumer peer workers has grown in NSW from 31.6 per 10 000 mental health care staff in public mental health services in 2011–12 to 40.0 per 10 000 staff in 2017–18 (Australian Institute of Health and Welfare (AIHW), 2020a). What is also emerging is the inclusion of peer workers in multidisciplinary teams, especially those examples of integrated care models that work in partnership with a LHD, Primary Health Network (PHN), a CMO and a General Practice.
- The Resolve Program: this is a seven-year pilot community program in Western NSW and Nepean Blue Mountains LHDs (Social Ventures Australia, 2020). It uses a peer workforce to provide support for people with frequent mental health hospital presentations to manage their mental health in the community and stay connected with family, friends and social networks while reducing the need for frequent hospital admissions.
- Gold Card Clinics: this is a program to better identify and treat people with personality disorders so they receive the right care quicker (Mental Health Commission of NSW, 2020). It provides practical, evidence-based, therapeutic techniques for people when they go to hospital in psychological distress. As part of the clinic process, a Gold Card is given to the person when they arrive in the ED, so specially trained mental health teams can work to prevent further distress for them and their family or carer.
- LikeMind: this is a trial model that co-locates clinical and psychosocial services and supports provided by CMOs (LikeMind, 2020). The pilot services aim to streamline access to services through an integrated care approach providing a single point of contact for assessment, triage and treatment.
- Interagency models: such as the Mid-North Coast Communities and Justice Department and LHD collaborative peer worker role. Here, the peer worker is co-located with the Communities and Justice team.
- Project Air for Schools: this is a partnership program between the Department of Education, the Ministry of Health and Wollongong University, to increase the capacity and knowledge of teachers and staff to respond to students with complex mental health issues (Project Air Strategy, 2020).
- Djirruwang Program: this is the only Bachelor's Degree program in NSW for Aboriginal and Torres Strait Islander people that leads to a Bachelor of Health Science (Mental Health). Provided at Charles Sturt University, the Djirruwang Program (Insight, 2020a) the course is both unique and critical to building and supporting an Aboriginal and Torres Strait Islander workforce and future leaders across the health and social and emotional wellbeing area (Insight, 2020b).

There are other unique aspects in mental health at the state strategic level.

The establishment of the NSW Mental Health Commission in July 2012, the first such Commission in Australia established under legislation. The Act set out the central place of people with lived experience of mental illness, their families and carers. It also gave the Commission scope to work across mental health and wellbeing of the community.

Under the *Mental Health Commission Act 2012*, the Commission has a role to monitor and report to improve the mental and wellbeing of the community of NSW. Under its functions it also delivered to the government a state mental health strategic plan that took a whole of government approach. This 10-year strategic plan, Living Well, was adopted by the NSW Government in November 2014.

The central place of lived experience and growth of the peer workforce is increasing.

The meaningful adoption of lived experience as the driver for service planning, co-design and review is evident in NSW. In 2018, the Mental Health Commission released its Lived Experience Framework (Mental Health Commission of NSW, 2018). A year later, in 2019, the Agency for Clinical Innovation developed a suite of consumer-led practice guidelines (NSW Government and Agency for Clinical Innovation, 2019).

The drive to increase peer workers is a game changer in how mental health services and supports are provided to people with mental illness and psychosocial disability. The number of peer workers in the public mental health services and in innovative interagency services is increasing. Likewise, the community managed sector is showing leadership in recruiting and growing their peer workforce.

The mental health system in NSW is exploring and leading innovation; this now needs to be built upon and scaled up.

1.7.6 NORTHERN TERRITORY

MARY MORRIS

SETTING AND CONTEXT

The Northern Territory accounts for approximately 17% of Australia's total land mass but has an estimated population of 250 000 people. This is less than 1% of the total Australian population. With a population density of 0.16 people per kilometre, the NT is one of the least populated states in the world (Australian Bureau of Statistics (ABS), 2018d). Darwin (population 135 000) is considered more multicultural than Australia as a whole, with 30% of people born overseas. While Aboriginal and Torres Strait Islander people represent just over 3% of the national population, in the NT they are 25.5% of the total population. As the Aboriginal and Torres Strait Islander population has a higher birth rate and a lower life expectancy compared to the general population, the demographic profile in the NT is relatively young. Outside of Darwin and the satellite city of Palmerston, most of the NT is considered remote or very remote with many people living on cattle stations, in mining towns or in Aboriginal communities. Over 43% of the NT population resides in remote or very remote areas of which 70% are Indigenous people residing in one of over 600 communities or outstations. Larger towns, such as Alice Springs (29 000 people), Katherine (11 000), Tennant Creek (3000) and Nhulunbuy (2000) provide essential services to surrounding areas. As such, the geographic spread of the population and the significant trauma and disadvantage experienced by a large proportion of the Aboriginal population contribute to the complexity and unique challenges of delivering mental health services in the Northern Territory (Northern Territory Mental Health Coalition & Queensland Alliance for Mental Health, 2018).

The estimated gap in life expectancy between Aboriginal and non-Aboriginal Australians in the NT is 16.4 years for males and 16.1 years for females, which is considerably higher than the national average (National Indigenous Times, 2017). In part due to social disadvantage, people living in the NT have a disproportionately higher burden of disease across a range of conditions. Premature mortality rates in the NT are the highest in Australia, with diseases such as cancer, diabetes, kidney disease, cardiovascular disease, respiratory disease and suicide all contributing significantly to these statistics. Underlying factors such as high alcohol consumption, smoking rates and poor nutrition are associated with these poor statistics, as are high levels of socioeconomic disadvantage and the related poor social determinants of health. The ability to address these factors is further complicated by the challenges of distance, and fragmentation of the health system (Northern Territory Primary Health Network, 2018).

WHAT DO SERVICES LOOK LIKE IN THE NT?

Health services are primarily provided through six public hospitals. The Royal Darwin Hospital (367 beds), Palmerston Regional Hospital (116 beds) and Alice Springs Hospitals (183 beds) are the largest. Smaller regional hospitals are Katherine District Hospital (60 beds), Gove District Hospital (32 beds) and Tennant Creek Hospital (20 beds). Primary health care is provided across a range of clinics, 74 Primary Health Centres and on Aboriginal communities in partnership with Aboriginal Community Controlled Health Organisations (ACCHOs; Northern Territory Health, 2018). Darwin private hospital, a day surgery centre in the Casuarina Health Precinct and many non-government organisations also provide services in the NT.

The NT Mental Health Strategic Plan recognises that the best health outcomes occur with early intervention, holistically and close to the person's home and community. Further, it suggests a mental health system should focus on a health-promoting environment and the promotion of self and community care.

The NT mental health service system

Mental health service delivery in the Northern Territory is divided into five main regions–Darwin, Alice Springs/Central Australia, Barkly, Katherine and East Arnhem regions, with each centre providing services to large geographic areas. Specialist outreach services, through the Medical Outreach Indigenous Chronic Disease (MOICD) program, provide services to over 80 communities across the Northern Territory to complement and extend local services.

Top End Mental Health Services (TEMHS) forms part of the Top End Health Service and provides specialist services to children, adolescents and families through the Children and Adolescent team. The adult teams provides service through the on-call team, inpatient services and youth services. Teams are based in Darwin, Katherine and Nhulunbuy. TEMHS operates a 30-bed inpatient unit at the Royal Darwin Hospital which consists of Cowdy Ward (16 open beds), Joan Ridly unit (8 secure beds) and a 6-bed youth inpatient program.

Central Australia Mental Health Services (CAMHS) forms part of the Central Australian Health Services and has community teams based in Alice Springs and Tennant Creek. It operates the 12-bed acute mental health unit, and another unit consisting of six sub-acute beds and two supported accommodation beds at Alice Springs Hospital. The Barkly team, based in Tennant Creek, supports residents in the Elliott, Ali Curong, Epenarra, Canteen Creek and surrounding areas. The remote team travels throughout Central Australia and services 28 remote and very remote communities. It works closely with remote health centres, NGOs and the Royal Flying Doctor Service. Other specialist teams include Forensic, Community Care, Crisis Assessment and Triage and Child and Youth Mental Health (Yffer, 2017).

Around 30 non-government organisations operate in the NT, including Team Health, Mental Health Association of Central Australia, Northern Territory Mental Health Coalition, Mental Illness Association of Australia (NT) and headspace (Northern Territory Government, 2020). These organisations provide sub-acute care, supported accommodation, psychosocial rehabilitation services and mental health promotion activities.

Aboriginal Community Controlled Health Services

The aim of the Indigenous Australian's Health Programme (IAHP) is to provide Aboriginal and Torres Strait Islander people with access to high quality health care services in urban, regional, rural and remote locations across Australia. Wherever possible and appropriate Aboriginal Community Controlled Health Services (ACCHS) are used, although mainstream services delivering comprehensive, culturally appropriate primary health care are also employed. Indigenous mental health funding is specifically quarantined to improve access to culturally appropriate mental health services for Aboriginal and Torres Strait Islander people which is in accord with the Australian Government Response to Contributing Lives, Thriving Communities–Review of Mental Health Programmes and Services (Australian Government, 2019b). This funding aims to increase access to culturally appropriate and safe mental health services for Aboriginal and Torres Strait Islander peoples (PHN Mental Health Tools and Resources, 2019). There are 12 services addressing the social and emotional wellbeing and mental health in Aboriginal Australia in the NT (Australian Government Department of Health and Ageing, 2020a).

The Aboriginal Medical Services Alliance Northern Territory (AMSANT) is the peak body for Aboriginal community controlled primary health services. It is a not for profit organisation that receives funding from the Australian and NT governments as well as from a range of charities and not for profit organisations. AMSANT supports Aboriginal health services by advocating for the right of local Aboriginal communities to control their own primary health care services and to have those services adequately funded.

Aboriginal and Torres Strait Islander health workers and health practitioners make a vital contribution to health care in Australia in both specialised service delivery and in a wide range of mainstream health care role. Their roles may include enhancing the amount and quality of clinical services provided to Aboriginal and Torres Strait Islander people clients, facilitating communication with Aboriginal and Torres Strait Islander people and communities, and practice administration and management (Bird & Henderson, 2005).

Tele and eHealth

The Australian Government recognises the potential benefit of telehealth to deliver mental health services, especially to people in rural and remote areas. On 1 November 2017, the Better Access initiative was expanded to include telehealth consultations to improve access to mental health services for people in regional, rural and remote Australia. A telehealth service is a psychological therapy service that is delivered via video conference where both a visual and audio link has been established between a patient and their treating allied health professional. Telehealth services can be delivered by psychologists, social workers and occupational therapists that are registered with Medicare. Eligible patients are required to have a Mental Health Treatment Plan and be located in a rural and remote area, namely, Modified Monash Model areas 4–7. From 1 September 2018, further changes to Medicare took effect so that eligible patients in rural and remote areas have the option of accessing all of their Better Access sessions via videoconference.

System summary

There is a range of complex, interrelated factors that impact the accessibility and quality of mental health services in rural and remote communities in the Northern Territory. However, as noted in a Joint Senate Submission report to the (Northern Territory Mental Health Coalition & Queensland Alliance for Mental Health, 2018) while advances have been made in relation to the accessibility and quality of mental health services they cannot be considered in isolation from the significant socioeconomic disadvantage and intergenerational trauma experienced by many Aboriginal and Torres Strait Islander communities in the Northern Territory. Factors such as poverty, unemployment, AOD use, family violence, chronic disease and ongoing grief and loss are central to the disproportionately high rates of suicide and psychological distress experienced by Aboriginal and Torres Strait Islander people in the NT (Northern Territory Mental Health Coalition & Queensland Alliance for Mental Health, 2018). This attests to the need for culturally appropriate and accessible mental health services.

In terms of service provision, the mental health system is skewed towards high-intensity services which are required to provide mental health care across large, isolated regions. In many remote communities low intensity prevention and early intervention services are largely unavailable. To this end, as noted in the Joint Senate Submission (2018), the scarcity of services across the spectrum of low to high intensity is a significant cause of low access rates among rural and remote communities in the NT (Northern Territory Mental Health Coalition & Queensland Alliance for Mental Health, 2018).

Factors that are unique to the NT

Without doubt, Territorians are experts in living and working in tropical, arid and remote locations. They are innovative and self-reliant, with broad skills and a unique outlook created through necessity. However, health and mental health care in the NT is not without its unique challenges.

Workforce

The NT faces quite unique challenges in this area due to its geographic location and distinct demography. Recruitment to remote areas continues to be challenging, with high turnover of staff and unfilled positions for lengths of time. In part this may be due to the deficient extrinsic motivation factors. As noted by Campbell, McAllister, and Eley (2012), 'while it is clear that the intrinsic incentives which contribute to job satisfaction are present, they appear insufficient to mediate for the burden of the extrinsic disincentives which contribute to excessively high turnover'. While the majority of research focuses on ways to increase retention it is also necessary to identify factors that lead to health professional departure. For example, rural and remote practitioners may experience inadequate housing, excessive travel, personal security concerns and issues with taking annual leave (Campbell et al., 2012; Onnis & Pryce, 2016), issues with schooling for their children and a lack of professional development opportunities. While the recruitment strategies tend to relate directly to the unique aspects of rural and remote health care practice, there is also the reality that the climate can be harsh and there is limited communication in some areas, as noted by Hall and Mattick (2007). Recruitment needs to be accompanied by a caveat that people may need to work hard in a climate that is sometimes difficult, often with limited communication, inflexible working arrangements and with management that can be constantly changing and perceived as unsupportive.

Many non-government organisations in regional communities highlight the significant costs in attracting and retaining staff while uncertainty around government funding of contracts added to this challenge. Job insecurity necessitates employees to seek alternate employment creating additional costs to the provider. While many government programs quickly respond to specific community needs (such as the impacts of flood and drought) by investing in additional staff, without ongoing funding it is not possible to embed these professionals in those regions (Northern Territory Mental Health Coalition & Queensland Alliance for Mental Health, 2018).

In summary, the Territory workforce is faced with climactic, geographic, cultural and professional challenges. In order to attract and retain staff in remote and regional areas issues such as professional isolation, professional support and building the Indigenous workforce need to be addressed.

In contrast to rural and remote areas, Darwin has become increasingly attractive as a career choice in mental health through growth in population and services, the expansion of the Menzies School of Health Research and the continued development of Charles Darwin University. Other higher educational advances are the continued growth and diversification in medical education at the Northern Territory Medical School, now affiliated with both Flinders University and James Cook University, and the new NT Rural medical school (Nagel, 2007).

Aboriginal health workers play a key role in the provision of health services to Aboriginal and Torres Strait Islanders and additional support is needed to develop and support the profession. There is often a lack of incentives and support for housing for Aboriginal health workers, with the result that recruitment to positions is very difficult and retention rates extremely low. Indigenous health workers also continue to encounter stigma in workplaces dominated by non-Indigenous staff which impacts on levels of satisfaction and retention rates for Indigenous workers. This suggests a need for compulsory cultural awareness training for non-Indigenous health workers, perhaps as a core requirement of service industry orientation programs.

Rural and remote health services need greater emphasis on multidisciplinary teams, with individuals from a variety of health disciplines working together. This has important implications for how health professionals are educated and trained, and for the infrastructure that needs to be provided for their work. The variety of successful service arrangements already in place in rural and remote areas provides some evidence of how workforce reform should proceed in Australia and should encourage further developments in interprofessional education and professional development (National Rural Health Alliance Inc., 2008).

Culture

There is no doubt that mental illness was present in Aboriginal and Torres Strait Islander culture prior to European colonisation of Australia but was, most likely, a fairly rare occurrence (Parker & Milroy, 2009). However, post colonisation, factors such as discrimination and racism, grief and loss, child removals, unresolved trauma, life stress, social exclusion, economic and social disadvantage, incarceration, family violence, substance use and physical health problems have been linked to higher rates of mental illness, suicide, substance abuse and psychological distress (Northern Territory Mental Health Coalition & Queensland Alliance for Mental Health, 2018). Some experts argue that there is a lack of 'fit' between Aboriginal and Torres Strait Islander concepts of social and emotional wellbeing and mainstream concepts of mental health and illness which have informed mental health service provision.

In rural areas there can often be apprehension around help-seeking and a fear of the stigma sometimes associated with mental illness—particularly in smaller communities where individuals are more visible, and confidentiality may be less assured.

Furthermore, at odds with the unrealistic expectation to deliver outcomes within a short timeframe, it takes time to earn the trust of Indigenous people living on communities before they feel comfortable engaging with a mental health professionals. It is not 'a single process or set of activities but an ongoing process or conversation that builds trust and relationships' (FaHCSIA, 2012). As the NT Mental Health Coalition reported to the recent Senate Inquiry into rural and remote mental health, the Northern Territory perspective is that 'a well-trained, well supported and well-resourced Aboriginal mental health workforce is critical to the delivery of equitable, culturally engaged mental health care for Aboriginal people in the Northern Territory' (Northern Territory Mental Health Coalition & Queensland Alliance for Mental Health, 2018).

Housing

A lack of residential mental health services means that community members have to rely on visiting specialist services or are required to travel, often quite large distances, to communities or towns where the service is available which increases stress and denies the patient an important source of social support. A lack of accommodation is also an issue for visiting service providers as well as for the patients, their families and carers. Further, the major cost of transport and accommodation is a further barrier to early intervention and continuing care (AIHW, 2017). As noted by a remote area service provider in the submission:

> One of the main reasons we can't get services to come out here is lack of accommodation. The few places there are to stay are booked up, and they are also expensive. It costs more to stay out here than it does to stay in town. Who is going to pay accommodation prices like that for this sort of place. If we had more accommodation at decent rates, we might be able to attract some more services to come out here.

Internet access

Internet access is another critically important part of health service delivery in remote areas. The advancement of information technology has exponentially improved communication via email, videoconferencing and computerised information systems reducing the isolation for some rural and remote areas (Nagel, 2007). While a significant advancement in the provision of care, there is little point providing telehealth services if internet accessibility is fragile and continuous connection is unreliable.

Furthermore, there is a lack of internet access for most Aboriginal and Torres Strait Islander people living in remote communities. The Telstra coverage map shows the vast majority of the NT has no mobile coverage. Any strategy for delivering more telehealth services would need to address the challenge of providing these services in remote Aboriginal and Torres Strait Islander and other isolated communities. There is great potential for these services to improve access to mental health services in regional and remote locations. Telehealth for Aboriginal patients in remote areas is an ideal model of culturally safe care as it enables a patient to use a health care service in their own environments and in the company of their family and trusted health care providers (Quilty, Bachmayer, & Congdon, 2015). However, cultural and linguistic diversity, coupled with limited access and uptake of web-based services, limits the potential of widespread use of digital therapies in regional and remote areas of the NT.

SUMMARY

The challenges for mental health services in the Northern Territory continue to be the vast distances needing coverage, the multicultural nature of its community and difficulty in recruitment and retention of staff. These are complicated by well-recognised social disadvantage with high rates of substance use, violence and chronic disease. A number of new initiatives and services have been, and continue to be, implemented through the Department of Health (Australian Government, 2019b). Comorbid illnesses are being addressed by a joint Mental Health and Alcohol and Other Drug Service in Darwin, the implementation of hospital-based interventions in Royal Darwin Hospital and Alice Springs Hospital, a focus on screening and early intervention within the Chronic Conditions Prevention and Management Strategy Implementation Plan (2010–12) and through implementation of the Mental Health and Palliative Care initiative to improve recognition and treatment of mental health problems experienced by people with a terminal illness.

Local research capability has grown through the continued growth of Charles Darwin University and the expansion of the Menzies School of Health Research, with its strong national and international collaborations and partnership with the Department of Health. The Menzies-based Aboriginal and Islander Mental Health initiative seeks to address mental illness by identifying the tools and methods people and communities need to stay socially, spiritually, emotionally and mentally strong. Its focus is on two-way communication promoting access and engagement of Indigenous people to mental health treatment and care, and developing the skills of Indigenous researchers (Menzies School of Health Research, 2019).

In an attempt to address workforce shortages the 'Welcome to the Territory' incentive is an initiative of the Northern Territory Government to boost and retain the Territory's population by attracting interstate workers in priority occupations. $17 million over seven years has been committed to attract around 2600 people to the Territory from interstate and retain them for at least five years (The Territory Boundless Possible, 2020).

The incentive incorporates: New Territorian Relocation Bonus (up to $8000 for a couple with two children), Local Spending Benefit (up to $1250) and a 5-Year Retention Bonus (up to $8000 for a couple with two children).

1.7.7 QUEENSLAND

ASSOCIATE PROFESSOR BRETT EMMERSON AM & ASSOCIATE PROFESSOR JAMES SCOTT

OVERVIEW

Mental Health Services (MHS) in Queensland are provided by the Queensland Government, Non-Government Organisations (NGOs) and the private sector. The Queensland Government MHS are provided through the Hospital and Health Services (HHS). The Mental Health Alcohol and Other Drugs Branch of the Department of Health funds a growing range of NGOs who provide disability support, housing and rehabilitation services. Private psychiatrists, psychologists and other allied health deliver community-based services while there are a growing number of private psychiatric hospitals/ wards throughout the state.

PUBLIC SECTOR MHS

Since 2012, public sector mental health services have been devolved and are run by 16 HHSs with an independent Board, while the Department of Health acts as the system administrator via the Mental Health Alcohol and Other Drugs Branch. Mental health services exist in all the HHSs and their organisation varies. In the bigger centres of Brisbane, Sunshine Coast, Toowoomba and Townsville, the MHS are run by the Executive Director/Service Group Director and have a designated budget and report either directly to a Chief Executive (CE) or a Chief Operating Officer (COO). In some smaller centres, the MHS have been combined with other health services in a divisional structure where they lose their identity, budget and ability to influence the HHS. This has been disastrous in some with a slow return to direct reporting to a CE/COO. In others such as West Moreton and Gold Coast the MHS has had other non-related areas added such as prisons or specialised health services which is far from ideal as it takes the focus off mental health. Under the executive directors, most MHS work on a co-chair model with an operations/service director and clinical/medical director jointly running the service.

Queensland has had acute adult inpatient mental health beds based on a planning ratio 20:100 000 per population. Since 2012, new acute inpatient units have been built at Logan, Caboolture, Gold Coast, Sunshine Coast and Mackay. Step Up, Step Down units have existed at Cairns and Logan for several years with new units in Mackay, Gladstone, Bundaberg and Nundah (North Brisbane) based on the Victorian Prevention and Recovery Centres (PARCS). They are either co-managed with health staff or managed entirely by an NGO.

The two remaining stand-alone psychiatric hospitals at Wacol and Toowoomba have been closed except for their medium and high secure wards.

The psychiatric hospitals have been replaced by a further eight community care units (CCU) in Cairns, Mackay, Rockhampton, Bundaberg, Sunshine Coast, Toowoomba. Logan and Bayside. While the original CCUs are staffed by full-time HHS staff, some of the newer CCUs are either co-managed or managed by an NGO.

There are also medium secure units re-titled Secure Mental Health Rehabilitation Units (SMHRU) at Wacol, Toowoomba, Chermside, Caboolture and Townsville with a further unit planned at the Gold Coast which will be relocated from the now 30-year-old Toowoomba unit. The SMHRUs while officially for severe long-term rehabilitation suffer from role confusion in that they were originally meant to provide short-term containment for aggressive consumers as well as long-term rehabilitation. However, the mix was seen as non-compatible and the former group has now been officially blocked and their care has been relegated to existing acute High Dependency Units.

Adult community MHS are organised into Acute Care Teams (ACT), Continuing Care Teams (CCT), Mobile Intensive Rehabilitation Teams (MIRT) and Homeless Health Outreach Teams (HHOT). In some services Resource Teams have evolved which provide specialist consulting services to the other adult teams which include dual-diagnosis, multicultural, forensic and Indigenous services. All adult MHS have now introduced a single state-wide telephone number 1300MHCALL (1300 642 255) to assist consumers to access adult MHS anywhere in Queensland. This has been introduced with no new resources. Our ACT have seen their role change over the last five years with the government preoccupation to avoid people staying in emergency departments for more than four hours. Unfortunately, our ACT have now become emergency department responders as a priority, rather than assessing and treating people in the community and keeping them away from emergency departments. Consultation Liaison (CL) psychiatry services are provided to all medium and large hospitals through either dedicated CL teams or by staff from the ACT.

Child and Youth Mental Health Services (CYMHS) are generally provided by the catchment area MHS apart from the Brisbane metropolitan area where the services are provided by Children's Health Queensland. CYMHS have generic teams as well as specialist services for high risk populations including children living out of home (Evolve Therapeutic Services), children whose parents have a severe mental illness (COPMI/KOPING), specialist forensic, day programs and consultation liaison services. Rural areas are supported by a state-wide video consultation (E-CYMHS) and visiting fly-in services. Acute Mobile Youth Outreach Service (AMYOS) has recently been established to provide intensive acute support to a small number of complex adolescent and young adult consumers in the community.

New state-wide acute inpatient children's beds have been built as part of the new Lady Cilento Children's Hospital at South Brisbane which was completed in 2015. This new facility combines the resources of the Royal Children's Hospital from Herston and the Mater Children's Hospital at South Brisbane. It is the only inpatient unit for children, with eight beds.

The number of acute adolescent inpatient beds has grown substantively with new beds opening in Toowoomba, Townsville and the Sunshine

Coast joining existing beds at Lady Cilento, Royal Brisbane, Robina and Logan Hospitals. The only long stay adolescent unit–Barrett Centre–was controversially closed in 2014 with no replacement. Three consumers died by suicide after being discharged following the Barrett Centre closure resulting in the current Queensland Government, while in opposition, promising a Royal Commission into the closure. A Commission of Inquiry occurred and in 2016 recommended a new longer stay facility be built. Planning is now well underway to rebuild the Adolescent Extended Care Unit at a cost of $49 million on the grounds of The Prince Charles Hospital which will be run by Children's Health Queensland. In the international literature, there is no evidence supporting the effectiveness of long stay adolescent units in providing care and in Queensland, there is little support by mental health professionals that this facility is needed with AMYOS and two new Step Up, Step Down facilities at Logan and Caboolture.

Forensic services have continued to expand and are organised around five clinical programs:

1. Court Liaison Service
2. Community Forensic Outreach Service (CFOS) which provides specialist forensic opinions to adult MHS
3. Prison MHS
4. High Secure Inpatient Services via 90 beds at the Park Centre for mental health and
5. Queensland Fixed Threat Assessment Centre (QFTAC).

There is still controversy between the general adult psychiatrists and forensic psychiatrists over Queensland's current policy of having serving prisoners treated on adult mental health wards in general hospitals instead of having dedicated prison mental health inpatient beds. There is agreement that these consumers deserve treatment, but it is the setting that is the issue. The negative reaction of consumers and their families to having serving prisoners on our wards is commonplace. The need to have dedicated acute inpatient beds for serving prisoners in South-East Queensland is gaining momentum.

Alcohol and drug services are now all aligned administratively to HHS MHS. Previously most sat with Primary and Community Health Services. In 2010, the Corporate Policy Alcohol and Drug teams merged with the Mental Health Branch to become the Mental Health Alcohol and Other Drugs Branch (MHAODB).

Specialist older persons mental health services (OPMHS) are provided in the larger MHS, while in a smaller service this population is treated by the general adult MHS. In most Queensland MHS, the Older Persons Team treat only new presentations over the age of 65 years. In only two services do all the consumers over the age of 65 years receive care from the OPMHS.

All HHS MHS have a close working relationship with GPs via primary care liaison officers, shared care programs, GP patient liaison schemes and GP psych opinion clinics.

The relationship with the new Primary Health Care Networks continues to evolve. Some HHSs having a very mature working relationship and carry out joint planning and commissioning of new services

SERVICE PLANNING

The MHAODB role is state-wide policy and planning and the administration of the *Mental Health Act 2016*.

In 2007 the Queensland Plan for Mental Health 2007-17 was released. It committed $617 million new funding for 140 new beds, 193 community-based staff, expanded consumer and carer services and additional NGO services for 2007-11. This expansion represented the largest single commitment ever by a Queensland Government. Unfortunately, with the global recession and 2011 spate of natural disasters, the Queensland Government's commitment to fund the 2011-17 parts of the Plan disappeared. With the election of the Campbell Newman LNP government in 2012-15, and the resultant massive cuts in the public sector, mental health services suffered disproportionately.

With the unexpected election of the Palaszczuk Labor Government in January 2015, funding for mental health has again become a priority. The new government introduced the Connecting Care to Recovery 2016-2021 Plan for Mental Health and the Alcohol and Drug Services which provides $25 million of new funding every year for four years (total of $100 million recurrently).

While this additional new funding is welcome, the focus on specialist mental health services (MHS) and not on core community MHS across child, adult and older persons services has been of concern. There has not been any expansion of community MHS since 2011 and over this time the lack of adequate community team staffing has become a major risk. This has occurred at a time of a major increase in complexity and risk of people treated by a community MHS, population growth, increased amphetamine use, lack of affordable housing, increasing public expectation and increased reporting burdens for staff (outcome measures etc.).

Also, the new National Mental Health Service Planning Framework showed a major gap between recommended and existing Queensland community mental health staffing. In early 2018, this led to major lobbying about this issue to the re-elected government from the Mental Health Commission, Royal Australian and New Zealand College of Psychiatrists (RANZCP) and the HHS Chief Executives. Pleasingly, in the June 2018 Budget the government announced an additional $26.5 million each year for the next four years to expand community mental health staffing levels (total $106 million recurrently).

In May 2015, the Minister for Health and Ambulance Services established a state-wide clinical review to examine fatal mental health events in Queensland. The Mental Health Sentinel Events Clinical Review was conducted over 12 months and the final report 'When mental health care meets Risk: a Queensland Sentinel Events review into homicide and public section mental health service' was released in April 2016. The Review made 63 recommendations including how forensic MHS are provided, more focus on family engagement, improved clinical assessments, new three level violence risk screening and staff training, improved partnerships with other agencies and the establishment of a state-wide Mental Health Quality Assurance Committee. By August 2018, 39 of the 63 recommendations have been completed with the others well underway. The response from the MHS has largely been supportive, although a level of scepticism exists over whether the Violence Risk Framework will make the intended difference, as there is limited evidence risk screening tools are effective.

Suicide prevention has been another priority for the MHAODB who have adopted the Zero Suicide Methodology, introduced to Queensland by the Gold Coast MHS. The Branch has established a Collaborative of 11 MHSs to implement the model across Queensland.

NON-GOVERNMENT SECTOR

The non-government (NGO) sector in Queensland is not as well-resourced as those in Victoria and New Zealand. This has meant the community mental health teams have had to take on disability support services as well as providing treatment services. Until recently Queensland has had two distinct NGO programs:

a Housing and Support Program (HASP) provides packages of care for complex consumers in the community, especially people discharged from our community care units, secure mental health units and the psychiatric hospitals.

b Mental Health NGO programs, which allocates $34 million annually to NGOs to provide support persons at risk of homelessness, people leaving the justice system, individual support and group based peer support.

With the introduction of the National Disability Insurance Service (NDIS), HASP have been cashed out as part of the Queensland Government commitment to the NDIS. It is too early to know yet whether the NDIS will be a successful model for dealing with psychosocial disability.

The Commonwealth Government has funded 21 headspace centres in Queensland. Headspace are early intervention mental health services delivering care to 12-25-year-olds. The centres have been implemented across Australia and in Queensland, and are located in major cities as well as in rural and remote locations such as Mt Isa and Warwick. They have been shown to be accessible for young people though their integration with other existing mental health services varies. This has led to a significant disjunction in the continuity of care in some regions though other headspace centres have integrated well with the state MHS. This highlights the challenges in integration and coordination that can arise when services are funded by different levels of government.

MENTAL HEALTH ACT 2016 (QLD)

A new Mental Health Act was proclaimed in 2016 (*MHA 2016*) and began operation on 5 March 2017. The key changes involved strengthening patient rights by utilising a capacity test for a Treatment Authority, utilising Advanced Health Directives, better access to second opinions and legal advice, appointment of Independent Patient Rights Advisors, strengthening of the role of support persons and additional safeguards and monitoring for the use of seclusion and mechanical restraint.

The Emergency Examination Order (EEO) under the previous *MHA 2000*, which enabled police and ambulance to bring people to hospital for an assessment, has been transferred to *Public Health Act 2005* and became Emergency Examination Authorities (EEA). This change has seen intoxicated individuals who did not require MHS involvement managed by the emergency departments.

The *MHA 2016* continues with the Mental Health Court and the role of Forensic Orders but limits their use for serious charges such as murder, attempted murder, arson and rape. Less serious charges are now able to be dealt with by the Magistrates Courts, who are assisted with a greatly enhanced Court Liaison Service.

The Mental Health Review Tribunal (MHRT) role has also been strengthened. The MHRT reviews all Treatment Authorities and Forensic Order applications for ECT and deep brain stimulation and interstate transfer of forensic patients. Free legal representation is now provided for ECT hearings, fitness for trial hearings and all matters involving minors.

The Office of the Chief Psychiatrist has also been enhanced and has also developed a series of Chief Psychiatrist Policies to guide the new Act.

The initial response to the *MHA 2016* from psychiatrists, public and private mental health services and consumers has been largely positive.

WORKFORCE

Like all states, the Queensland mental health workforce is ageing. There is currently no state-wide mental health workforce strategy, which means workforce becomes a major risk for this state. With the new community mental health enhancements ($106 million) over four years, there is no clear recruitment strategy other than recent new graduates (grow your own) or interstate and international poaching. Major improvements in terms and conditions about 10 years ago for all clinical staff have helped attract and retain staff.

The Queensland Centre for Mental Health Learning provides education packages for both existing and new staff.

One area of significant expansion over the last five years has been the employment of consumers and carers with the lived experience as peer support workers, consumer and carer consultants and Director of Recovery in the two Brisbane Hospital and Health Services. This workforce is being seen increasingly as cost effective and beneficial for our consumers' recovery. The peer workforce is employed by both the HHSs and NGOs. The consumer and carer consultant and the two Directors of Recovery also provide the public MHS with consumer and carer advice on policy and planning, participate with recruitment of senior staff and provide education for MHS staff on recovery. There continues to be an argument that once a consumer is 'employed' they are no longer independent. This concern has also led one of the larger MHS to have a Consumer and Carer Engagement Group to advise on policy and planning, review complaints and sit on the MHS Executive Group.

Queensland has had a long-term maldistribution of mental health staff, especially psychiatrists in our non-metropolitan areas. Pleasingly, the maldistribution is slowly improving with most major non-metropolitan areas now employing a critical mass of psychiatrists. Psychiatric Registrars and Occupational Therapists remain a scarce resource.

QUEENSLAND MENTAL HEALTH COMMISSION

One of the current trends cross Australia and New Zealand is a Mental Health Commission (MHC). The Bligh Labor Government announced it was establishing a Queensland MHC (QMHC) in late 2012 and it came into effect on 1 July 2013.

It was established as an 'independent statutory body to deliver ongoing reform towards a more integrated, evidence-based, recover-oriented mental health and substance misuse system'. The act also established the 'Queensland Mental Health and Drug Advisory Council to provide advice to the Commission' and 'a Mental Health Commissioner to manage the Commission and its function'. The QMHC was not to be a fund holder like the WA Mental Health Commission.

The impact of the QMHC over its first few years is debatable. Firstly, the Commission failed to have any member of the Council from the public sector and showed disinterest in public MHS. Then when the Newman Government (2012-15) sacked 14 000 public servants and MHS staff were disproportionally affected and then ordered the locking of the doors in all acute inpatient units, the MH Commission failed to speak out publicly. After a review, a new MH Commissioner was appointed in July 2017 and the QMHC has successfully re-engaged with the public MHS and has a new Strategic Framework 2018-2023 to achieve better outcomes for people living with mental health issues or substance misuse. The key strategies to achieve this include a whole-of-government approach, research and awareness and prevention.

One new key focus is to commence a rational informed discussion about the risks and benefits of taking a health response rather than a criminal justice response to persons who use and/or are in possession of small amounts of illegal drugs, similar to Portugal and other countries.

INFORMATION

The state-wide mental health information system—CIMHA (Consumer Integrated Mental Health Application) continues to be upgraded and essentially is a mental health electronic medical record, used for all community patients and for some inpatient units. With the roll-out of the Cerner ieMR for inpatient notes, it is unclear how CIMHA and ieMR will relate. Whether they will be two separate systems or a technical solution can be found to enable the two systems to be integrated, has yet to be worked out. The benefits of a single electronic mental health record, available to mental health services across the state, cannot be underestimated and sets Queensland apart from some other states.

A unique innovation is the Queensland Mental Health Clinical Collaborative, which is the state-wide mental health benchmarking consortium, consisting of the 16 adult MHSs. It began operating in 2007 within Metro North Mental Health and has successfully benchmarked a range of indicators including schizophrenia length of stay and readmission rates, 1-7 Day post discharge follow-up, seclusion indicators, metabolic monitoring and now-smoking cessation. On each of these indicators, there has been improvement in the indicator and clinical care.

Three of these indicators have attracted payments under the Queensland Clinical Practice Improvement Program (CPIP) in which the treating service/team attracts a cash payment if they reach the threshold for the indicator. These payments can be used for education and training by the service/team and have been a positive benefit to improve indicator compliance.

MENTAL HEALTH RESEARCH

Research in mental health and neurosciences has matured and expanded in Queensland. Traditionally, Queensland was known internationally for studies conducted in fields of epidemiology, developmental neurobiology and genetics. The last five years has seen a rapid expansion of collaborations between universities and health services, which has enabled new research enterprises such as clinical trials and neuroimaging studies.

Multicentre clinical trials in psychosis have been successfully completed through the Cadence Clinical Trial Platform (Cadence, 2015). This collaborative enterprise has enabled the large HHS in South-East Queensland to successfully recruit participants with psychosis to studies of pharmacological and psychosocial interventions. Concurrently, in response to the Commonwealth Government's Department of Health and Aging 2013 Strategic Review of Health and Medical

Research, the Brisbane Diamantina Health Partners (BDHP) was established in 2014 of which Brain and Mental Health is a leading theme. This academic health science centre has formalised partnerships between health services, universities and primary care in order to support large-scale research trials. Sustainable collaborations are still under development, with the BDHP yet to reach its potential in the field of mental health.

The Queensland Centre for Mental Health Research (Queensland Centre For Mental Health Research, 2020), originally established in 1987 as the 'Clinical Studies Unit', has a broad research program which is well established. While it is located at Wacol, West of Brisbane, it supports research groups at the University of Queensland in The School of Public Health, the Centre for Clinical Research and the Queensland Brain Institute. The Herston Imaging Research Facility (Herston Imaging Research Facility (HIRF), 2020) opened in 2015 and is one of only a handful of imaging research facilities in Australia and the first to be devoted entirely to clinical research. It has arisen from a partnership between the University of Queensland, Queensland University of Technology, the QIMR Berghofer Medical Research Institute and Metro North Hospital and Health Service.

These are some of the examples of universities partnering with health services to provide the necessary infrastructure for the continued expansion of research in mental health. In spite of the capital investment and the alliances that have formed, bedding research into health services is an ongoing challenge.

There is a substantial translational gap between what is investigated in academic facilities and the clinical care delivered to patients. Health service research and implementation science is urgently needed in Queensland mental health services so that consumers can directly benefit from the large investment in medical research.

QUALITY AND SAFETY

There is an emphasis on the quality and safety of clinical care in the public and private mental health services. In the public sector, this is governed by policy from the Mental Health Branch, and in both private and public sectors, services are accredited by the Australian Council of Health Care Standards. In general, the standard of care is good, although there is a large administrative requirement that accompanies the provision of clinical care in the public sector. This has an inevitable impact on the efficiency of the delivery of care, but is one of the unintended costs of maintaining and monitoring good standards of clinical care.

There is an innate risk in providing care to mental health patients with serious mental illness in the least restrictive settings.

Tragically, serious adverse outcomes (serious self-harm, aggression and suicide) occur in this clinical population. Queensland Health mandates that all serious incidents or death are reviewed by either Mental Health Mortality Review or Critical Incident Committees who can also order a Root Cause Analysis (RCA). The risk of these reviews is that clinicians sometimes feel blamed for outcomes that are outside of their control. Also, these reviews are time consuming and sometimes costly changes are recommended even though, from a clinician perspective, they do little to improve clinical care or reduce risk. The delivery of efficient, quality and safe clinical service to the high-risk population is a challenge that Queensland shares with many other jurisdictions around the world.

QUEENSLAND MENTAL HEALTH SERVICES: WHAT MAKES THEM UNIQUE?

The models of mental health care across public, private and non-government services are similar to most other jurisdictions. Queensland has copied a lot of its public mental health models and services from Victoria. Where Queensland is unique is that it has had mainstream mental health inpatients much earlier than most other states. Its state-wide clinical information system CIMHA and the achievement of the Queensland Mental Health Clinical Collaborative utilising practice improvement payments are other unique features. Queensland is Australia's most decentralised state and over the last five years all the major new metropolitan areas have managed to recruit and retain a critical mass of public sector psychiatrists for the first time in the state's history.

1.7.8 SOUTH AUSTRALIA

TARUN BASTIAMPILLAI, MALCOLM BATTERSBY & STEPHEN ALLISON

INTRODUCTION

There is a major mental health policy debate in Australia, as to whether we can significantly disinvest from hospital care, and divert these resources specifically into residential beds and community mental health care. In their 2014 review of Australia's mental health system, the National Mental Health Commission specifically recommended a 10% reduction in (federally funded) growth funding to acute hospital care. They recommended this funding be redirected over coming years to fund increases in both primary care, residential beds and community mental health care (National Mental Health Commission, 2014a). This amounted to a proposed funding transfer of $1 billion from acute hospitals to community-based programs over five years.

This policy position was not accepted by the Federal Government and the Royal Australian New Zealand College of Psychiatrists also expressed their concerns about the impact of this funding shift.

However, between 2007 and 2014, South Australia had already effectively implemented this exact policy agenda as part of the *Stepping Up* Report recommendations (South Australian Inclusion Board 2007). While this section refers to SA, it also contends that understanding the outcomes of the SA policy experiment is important to inform future mental health policy and planning in Australia.

Hospital key performance indicators (KPIs) reveal the extent of the current crisis facing Australian acute mental health services. There is currently significant concern Australia-wide about mental health patients waiting for extended periods in emergency departments (ED), a problem which is worsening due to increasing ED demand. Our key concern is that there has been no increase in public psychiatric inpatient capacity to adjust for this increased ED demand (AUstralasian College of Emergency Medicine, 2018; Allison et al., 2015, 2018i, 2018ii, 2019; Benjamin et al., 2018). Indeed, severe problems with ED mental health care is one the most visible aspects of the crisis in mental health services that has spurred major current inquiries (Australian Government Productivity Commission, 2020b; State Government of Victoria, 2019).

In this section, we examine the observed outcomes of the major SA mental health reforms between 2007 and 2017 on the functioning of the hospital mental health care system. The primary focus is state government reforms, which were based on a stepped model of care.

The central hypothesis was that increased community care could reduce the need for hospital care. The first period covers the Stepping Up reform period (2007-14), which reduced non-veteran, general adult acute psychiatry beds by 23% (45 beds), while significantly increasing general adult residential beds (45 beds) and community mental health resources. These shifts are shown in Table 1.18.

However, these reforms did not have the expected outcomes, and a second period of major reform was required between 2015-17, to address the subsequent ED access block for mental health patients, which had reached a peak in 2014.

After the Stepping Up reforms, thousands of SA mental health patients waited for more than 24 hours in ED for an acute general adult psychiatry bed (Allison et al., 2018iii), resulting in the introduction of a Ministerial 24-hour target for maximum ED length of stay for mental health patients. Meeting this target required a significant increase in general adult acute psychiatric beds and a major reversal in policy. This section has a particular focus on the issue of ED mental health demand and the general adult (ages 18-64) service continuum required to meet this demand.

The first part of this analysis will look at international benchmarking for psychiatric bed numbers, the existing evidence for what is the optimal number of psychiatric beds, and a brief discussion of using observed real-life outcomes and

Table 1.18 Changing patterns of mental health spending in SA

Area of mental health spending	2007–08		2014–15	
	$ million	% of spending	$ million	% of spending
Public psychiatric hospital services	80 601	29	59 335	14
Specialised psychiatric units or wards in public acute hospitals	60 245	22	108 692	25
Community mental health care services	98 702	36	182 709	43
Residential mental health services	6337	2	28 952	7
Grants to non-government organisations	24 487	9	39 703	9
Other indirect expenditure	5662	2	10 439	2
Total SA expenditure on mental health	**276 033**	**100**	**429 830**	**100**

key performance indicators, to determine optimal psychiatric bed number requirements.

The second part of the analysis will summarise the Stepping Up Report recommendations with particular reference to the replacement of general adult acute care beds with general adult sub-acute residential care beds.

The third part of the analysis will draw on data provided by the Australia Institute of Health and Welfare (AIHW; Australian Institute of Health and Welfare, 2019a) describing the changes that took place in primary care, supported housing, non-government organisation (NGO) grants, community mental, general adult residential and general adult acute and non-acute beds between 2006-07 and 2013-14, and the impact these had on ED mental health performance.

The fourth part of the analysis will summarise the SA policy response to the ED mental health access block crisis between 2015 and 2017.

Finally, we will provide a conclusion outlining Australian mental health planning and policy recommendations based on the SA reform experience between 2007 and 2017.

PSYCHIATRIC BED NUMBER REQUIREMENTS: WHAT DOES THE AVAILABLE EVIDENCE TELL US?

There are various methods used to calculate optimal psychiatric bed numbers (Torrey, 2008), including expert consensus, normative approaches, population health approaches and observed outcomes approach.

Expert consensus

The Treatment Advocacy Center (Torrey, 2008) in the United States collated the view of expert clinicians who recommend a target of 50 public sector beds per 100 000 population with no clear description of the methodology utilised to describe how this was reached.

Normative approach

The normative approach considers that countries with similar health care systems will require approximately the same number of beds. The OECD average for psychiatric beds is 69 beds per 100 000 population in 2016-17 with the median being 62 beds. The OECD bed count does not include residential bed numbers (Organisation for Economic Co-operation and Development (OECD), 2020). The World Health Organization psychiatric bed median for European countries is 50 beds per 100 000 population and the median for high income countries is 48 beds per 100 000 population, not including residential bed numbers (World Health Organization, 2017).There is however marked variation within the OECD. Germany, Norway, Netherlands, Switzerland and France have over 80 psychiatry beds per 100 000 population, down to 9 beds per 100 000 population in Italy. Anglosphere countries (UK, Australia, New Zealand, US and Canada) are mostly in the bottom third of psychiatric bed numbers (World Health Organization, 2017a; Tyrer et al., 2017), ranging from 42 beds per 100 000 population in Australia to 21 beds per 100 000 population in the United States. Australia has 42 psychiatric beds per 100 000 population with 29.4 public sector beds per 100 000 population and 12.3 private sector beds per 100 000 population in 2016–17 (AIHW 2019a), ranking 23 out of 36 OECD countries in terms of overall psychiatric bed provision (see Figure 1.44). Australia is 39% below the OECD average and 32% below the OECD median for overall psychiatric bed numbers (public and private bed numbers).

Population health approach

A population health approach evaluates the population prevalence and severity of mental illness and then applies algorithms and modelling to calculate psychiatric bed and community requirements. The Australian National Mental Health Services planning framework (NMHSPF 2017) uses a population health approach. The framework's psychiatric bed requirements for Australia have not been officially released.

Observed outcomes approach

We suggest there is an alternative approach, based on the fact that varying numbers of psychiatric beds might lead to observable effects on health care systems and populations, as measured by hospital KPIs and population outcomes (O'Reilly et al., 2019). Our literature review of hospital and population outcomes revealed 16 metrics that, when used in combination, could be powerful measures of the adequacy or otherwise of mental health bed numbers. The identified KPIs are listed below, and explained in full within our article. We propose that there are thresholds for the number of psychiatric beds, below which adverse clinical and population health outcomes begin to appear.

Summary of bed numbers

The OECD specifically commented on Australia's low inpatient psychiatric bed numbers, and the impact on hospital KPIs in 2014:

> that Australia has a large number of community services available for mental health care—e.g. crisis and home treatment, early intervention, and assertive outreach—but Australia should ensure that services are sufficient to meet population need. Without sufficient high quality community care, and with low inpatient psychiatric bed numbers, patients with severe mental illness risk worsening symptoms, more stays in emergency settings, and more hospital readmissions. Australia should pay attention to getting the tricky balance of care provision right (OECD, 2014).

Figure 1.44 OECD psychiatric beds per 100 000 population

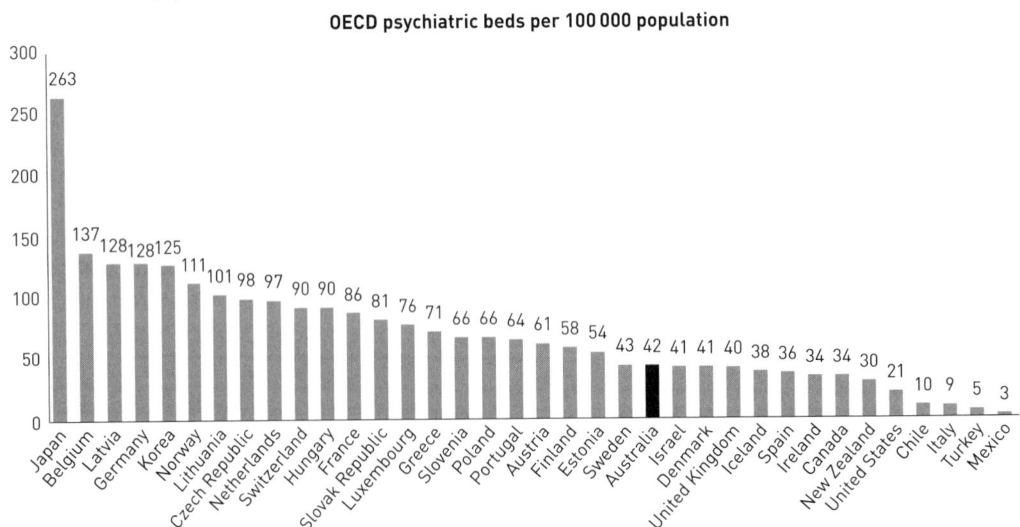

Table 1.19 Hospital KPIs and population outcomes

Hospital KPIs	Population outcomes
Out of area placements	Rates of homelessness among people with severe mental illness
Boarding in emergency rooms	Rates of people with severe mental illness in homeless shelters
Involuntary admission rates	Rate of all-cause mortality
Occupancy rates in psychiatry units	Rates of suicide
Average length of stay in psychiatric units	Rates of crime committed by people with severe mental illness
Level of acuity on inpatient wards	Rates of incarceration among people with severe mental illness
Discharge to homelessness	Rates of people with severe mental illness in jails
Readmission rates	Burden on carers

Largely in response to the OECD's warning, we have conducted an extensive literature review on this topic and based on a combination of expert consensus, normative approaches (OECD and WHO psychiatric bed averages) and an observed outcomes approach (incorporating Scandinavian mental health registry data).

On this basis, we specifically recommend that a minimum of 50–60 public sector psychiatric beds are required (Allison et al 2018iii) to prevent adverse consequences such as out of area placements, boarding in ED, high occupancy rates in psychiatric units, high 28-day readmission rates, homelessness, suicide rates, incarceration of the mentally ill and carer burden (Siebert, 2017). Australia currently only has 29 public sector psychiatry beds per 100 000 (AIHW, 2019a), much lower than our recommended benchmark, and patients are at risk of the adverse effects noted by the OECD.

SA STEPPING UP REFORMS (2007–12)

In the context of community concerns about the mental health system, the then SA State Premier, Mike Rann, referred mental health reform to the Social Inclusion Board in August 2005. The Chair of The Social Inclusion Board, Monsignor Cappo, then laid out a 5-year reform agenda between 2007 and 2012, known as *Stepping Up: A Social Inclusion Plan For Mental Health Reform 2007-2012* (South Australian Social Inclusion Board, 2007). In total there were 41 recommendations. One of the key recommendations that specifically aligned with the National Mental Health Commission (2014a) was the proposal to significantly invest in sub-acute general adult residential care beds, known as intermediate care (recommendation 12) and disinvest from the acute general adult inpatient beds. These intermediate care beds were to be placed in a community residential setting, designed as either a Step Up option from the community to avoid acute hospitalisation, or a Step Down option from an acute general adult inpatient ward.

The specific proposal was to reduce SA non-veteran general adult acute inpatient beds by between 32 and 62 beds, from 252 beds (not including 24 veterans mental health beds as these are funded by DVA and usually allocated to the private sector) to between 190–220 beds and increase general adult intermediate care beds from zero to somewhere between 80–92 beds.

At the time of the Stepping Up Report in 2006-07, SA had 26.7 general adult acute inpatient beds, compared to the national average of 24.7. The Social Inclusion Board (2007) specifically aimed for Victorian general adult acute inpatient bed numbers of 19.9 beds per 100 000 population, which was the lowest among the Australian states at that time.

Stepping Up recommended the continuation of already planned decreases in general adult non-acute beds from 129 beds in 2004-05 (13.5 per 100 000 population, 35% higher than the national average of 10 per 100 000 population) to 40 secure care rehabilitation beds. This reduction of general adult non-acute beds was to be substituted with between 60 and 80 community rehabilitation residential beds.

Stepping Up made specific recommendations for marked increases in social housing levels which were significantly below the national average in 2006-07 with 7.2 supported houses per 100 000, in comparison to the national average of 20.2 supported houses per 100 000 population).

Stepping Up emphasised community mental health as the new centre of the service system. However, it did not make any specific recommendations to increase community mental staffing levels, noting that SA was already above the national average in this staffing category. In 2006-07 SA had 54.7 FTE per 100 000 in community mental health (all service components) compared to the national average of 51.4 FTE per 100 000. At the time of the report SA also had a sub-specialised general adult community mental health service with three distinct teams—Assessment and Crisis Intervention Teams, Continuing care teams and Mobile and Assertive care teams. The Stepping Up Board cautioned against a restructure of these functional teams at that time.

CHANGES ARISING FROM STEPPING UP (2007–14)

The data presented here summarises the impact of the Stepping Up reforms, based on information provided by the AIHW (2019a).

- SA state mental health total expenditure increased by 17% in real terms from $220 per capita in 2006-07 (national average $195 per capita) to $256 per capita in 2013-14 (national average $225.50). SA was 13% above the national average in 2006-07 and was 14% above the national average in 2013-14. Per capita spending on acute hospital inpatient care in SA was $70 in 1992-93 when the National Mental Health Strategy began, rising to $97 in 2007-08 but by 2010-11 had fallen to $87 in SA (Department of Health and Ageing 2013). **Stepping Up made no specific recommendation about increasing overall state mental health expenditure.**
- SA state general adult mental health expenditure (acute and non-acute beds, residential, community mental health) in real terms increased by 21% from $213 per capita in 2006-07 (national average $173 per capita) to $258 per capita in 2013-14 (national average $198 per capita). SA was 24% above the national average in 2006-07 and was 31% above the national average in 2013-14 servicing the general adult population aged between 18-64. **Stepping Up made no specific recommendation about increasing overall general adult mental health expenditure.**
- The Federal Government increased access to psychology-allied health services (Better Access) for the treatment of anxiety and depression with population coverage in SA increasing from negligible population coverage levels in 2006-07 to 3.9% population coverage in 2013-14 (national average 4.1%). SA was 5% below the national average in 2013-14 for this Medicare service for psychology/allied health access for mental health.
- SA supported housing places significantly increased by 269% from 7.2 per 100 000 population (national average 20.2 per 100 000) in 2006-07, to 26.6 per 100 000 in 2013-14 (national average 23.2 per 100 000 population). SA was 180% below the national average in 2006-7 and 15% above the national average in 2013-14. **The Stepping Up supported housing target was achieved.**
- SA increased NGO funding by 21% from $20.31 per capita in 2006-07 (national average $12.95) to $24.54 per capita in 2013-14 (national average $17.20). SA was 56% above the national average in 2006-07 and was 42% above the national average in 2013-14 for NGO spending. **Stepping Up supported increases in NGO service provision and funding (though it should be noted that the NGO share of overall mental health expenditure in SA was unchanged over this period at 9%.**
- SA Community mental health staffing for all age groups increased by 31% from 46.4 FTE per 100 000 population in 2006-07 (national average 42.5 FTE per 100 000 population) to 60.9 FTE per 100 000 in 2013-14 (national average 46 FTE per 100 000 population). SA was 9% above the national average in 2006-07 and was 32% above the national average in 2013-14 for community mental

health staffing levels. Most of this difference is located within the general adult community mental health sector which has 66.9 FTE per 100 000 population compared to the national average of 50.1 per 100 000 population (34% above the national average based on 2016-17 data). **Stepping Up did not specifically recommend increasing community mental health or general adult community mental health staffing.**

- SA changed its general adult community mental health model of care from three sub-specialist teams consisting of assessment and crisis intervention teams, contusing care teams and mobile assertive care teams to a single integrated team model in 2011. **Stepping Up Report did not specifically recommend this, but this was the outcome of another report done shortly afterwards.**
- SA proportion of population receiving community mental health care increased by 28% from 1.8% population coverage in 2007-08 (national average 1.8%) to 2.3% population coverage in 2013-14 (national average 1.8%). SA was at the national average in 2006-07 and 28% above the national average in 2013-14 in terms of community mental health population coverage. **Stepping Up goal of increasing community mental health care provision (population coverage) was achieved.**
- SA community mental health contact rate increased by 36% from 290 contacts per 1000 population in 2007-08 (national average was 303) to 395 per 1000 population 2013-14 (national average 374). SA was 4% below the national average for community mental health contact numbers in 2007-08 and was 6% above the national average in 2013-14. **Stepping Up goal of increasing community mental health care provision (community contacts) was achieved.**
- SA general adult 24 hour residential beds increased by 137% from 5.1 beds per 100 000 population (national average 5.3 beds) in 2006-7 to 12.1 beds in 2013-14 (national average 6.8 beds). SA was 4% below the national average for this bed type in 2006-07 and was 78% above the national average in 2013-14.
- SA intermediate care beds for general adults commenced in 2011, with 45 beds operational between early 2012 and 2013-14 (36% of the total 125 general adult residential beds). **Stepping Up recommended a target of 80–92 intermediate care beds and therefore this recommendation was only partially achieved.**
- Community rehabilitation residential beds doubled from 30 beds in 2006-07 to 60 beds in 2013-14. **Stepping Up target for Community rehabilitation residential beds was achieved by being between 60—80 beds for this bed type.**
- Non-veteran general adult acute beds decreased by 45 beds, from 258 beds in 2006-07 to 213 beds in 2013-14. This represented a 22% decrease from 26.7 non-veteran general adult acute psychiatry beds per 100 000 population (national average 24.7 beds) to 20.7 non-veteran general adult acute psychiatry beds (national average 24.2). SA was 8% above the national average for this bed type in 2006-07 and was 14% below the national average in 2013-14. **Stepping Up target for non-veteran general adult acute psychiatry beds was achieved by being between 190–220 beds for this bed type.**
- SA general adult acute inpatient average length of stay increased by 1.5% from 13.4 days in 2010-11 (national average 13.8 days) to 13.6 days in 2013-14 (national average 12.9 days). SA had 3% reduced average length of stay in 2010-11 compared to the national average which changed to being 5% above the national average for average length of stay in 2013-14. **Stepping Up Report forecast and intended that sub-acute residential care (intermediate care centres—45 beds) would significantly reduce general adult acute average length of stay which did not eventuate.**
- General adult non-acute beds decreased by 57, from 96 beds in 2006-07 to 39 in 2013-14. General adult non-acute beds decreased by 62%, from 9.8 beds per 100 000 in 2006-07 (national average 9.6 beds) to 3.8 beds per 100 000 in 2013-14 (national average 9.1). SA was 2% above the national average for general adult non-acute psychiatry beds in 2006-07 and was 58% below the national average

in 2013-14. **Stepping Up target for general adult non-acute psychiatry beds was achieved by being between 30-40 beds for this bed type.**

In summary then in SA, the period 2006-07 to 2013-14 saw:

- a 3.9% increase in population coverage in primary care (psychology)
- a 17% increase in overall state funding for mental health
- a 21% increase in general adult mental health funding
- a 269% increase in supported housing
- a 21% increase in NGO funding
- a 31% increase in community mental health staffing levels
- a 137% increase in general adult residential beds
- significant changes to the general adult community mental health model of care in 2011.

Did these investments and changes reduce SA ED mental health-related presentations?

The SA Government increased all components of non-hospital care between 2006-07 and 2013-14 and was also significantly above the national average in every category of non-hospital care funding and service provision described above, with the exception of Federal Medicare related psychology services (5% below the national average in terms of population coverage).

It was anticipated that the above combination of significantly increased primary care, residential care community mental health investment, endorsed and recommended by Stepping Up would result in a significant reduction in ED related mental health presentations.

SA ED related mental health presentations were 91 per 10 000 population in 2006-07, which was 5% above the Australian average of 87. SA ED related mental health presentations increased by 29% (after accounting for population growth), between 2006-07 and 2013-14, rising to 117 ED presentations per 10 000 population, which was 12% above the Australian average of 105. The majority of mental health presentations to the ED were within the general adult (ages 18-64) population.

Did the reduction of general adult acute beds substituted with intermediate care beds reduce ED visit times for mental health patients?

In 2011, prior to the commencement of the intermediate care beds (45 beds) and the reduction of general adult acute beds (45 beds), ED visit times for all mental health patients was 10 hours (CENA 2020). However, the reduction of 45 non-veteran general adult acute bed numbers which was 7% above the national average in 2010-11, to being 15% below the national average in 2013-14, contributed to ED visit time increasing rapidly by 60% every year reaching 16 hours in calendar year 2014 (Allison, 2018iii).

The average ED admission stream visit times (waiting for acute beds) for mental health patients in 2014 was 34 hours, which contrasted with non-mental health waiting times of 9 hours (AIHW, 2019a). In fact, 2450 mental health patients waited more than 24 hours in ED in 2014 (AIHW, 2019a). The majority of patients waiting more than 24 hours in ED were in the general adult (ages 18-64) population. The introduction of 45 intermediate care beds in SA between 2012 and 2014 did not substitute for the loss of 45 general adult acute beds, leading to significant ED access block for patients requiring general adult acute beds. The average length of stay in general adult acute psychiatry wards had not improved as a result of the introduction of intermediate care beds as intended, with a marginal deterioration in average length of stay of 1.5%.

SA policy response to emergency department access block (2015–17) and outcome

In the context of the ongoing rise in ED mental health-related presentations and the accompanying dramatic deterioration in ED visit times for mental health patients, the SA mental health system was in a major crisis. The ED visit times for mental health were the worst SA had ever seen in 2014 with 2450 patients waiting for more than 24 hours in the ED, and some patients spent several days in the ED, waiting for an acute bed. There were significant concerns being expressed by multiple professional groups (CENA, 2020) about the distressing situation confronted by mental health patients having to wait for prolonged periods in the ED.

Major reforms were required to resolve this mental health systems crisis and major changes were initiated between 2015 and 2017. The process of reform first began with an in-depth analysis of the available data and an international review of the literature (Siebert, 2017). This analysis was accompanied by a KPMG external review (KPMG, 2015), leading to the development of two major reform areas: 1) Leadership, system oversight and governance reform 2) Increased general adult acute bed supply and localised ED based bed management systems.

LEADERSHIP, SYSTEM OVERSIGHT AND GOVERNANCE REFORM

The political leadership decided to move away from the theory of stepped care, and resolved to increase psychiatric bed numbers to directly address a hospital KPI: ED length of stay. This policy change had significant Ministerial sponsorship, with the Minister of Health Jack Snelling announcing a Ministerial 24 hour ED target in late 2014, with specific aim that no SA mental health patient should routinely wait in ED for more than 24 hours by 1 January 2016 (Allison et al., 2018iii). Accompanying this Ministerial target there was enhanced Department of Health, Local Health Network Executive, and clinical oversight of ED mental health demand management. To assist in the reform process there was enhanced use of data analytics, to understand and accurately benchmark mental health system performance and guide specific policy and commissioning directions. A major governance reform also ensured that the Clinical Director had overall leadership and strategic oversight of area mental health services, resulting in a single point of accountability at the area (Local Health Network) level.

Increased general adult acute bed supply and localised ED based bed management systems

The in-depth analysis of the international literature (Allison et al., 2018iii), analysis of the AIHW mental health data and the operational SA health data with respect to ED and inpatient flow analysis led to a number of major changes in policy direction. The major decision was to commission extra general adult acute beds to specifically meet local ED demand and efficiency expectations. Mental health bed management moved from a state-wide centralised bed management system to a localised ED based bed management system, significantly reducing the need for inter-hospital transfers. In parallel to the localisation of bed management, extra general adult acute psychiatry beds were commissioned aiming to at least reach the Australian average for this bed type. Non-veteran general adult acute beds increased by 53 beds, from a baseline of 213 beds in 2013-14 to 266 beds in 2016-17. This represented a 24% increase from 20.7 non-veteran general adult beds per 100 000 population in 2013-14 (national average 24.2 beds) to 25.6 beds in 2016-17 (national average 24.5 beds). This increase in non-veteran general adult acute beds moved SA from being 14% below the national average to being 4% above. Of the extra non-veteran general adult acute beds, specifically 17 extra short-stay psychiatry beds for 48-hour crisis related admissions, were specifically commissioned in four out of the six major metropolitan teaching hospitals, based on the in-depth data analysis, which revealed a shortage of this particular bed type.

In addition to the above an extra 10 forensic beds were commissioned, taking SA from 3 per 100 000 population forensic beds in 2013-14 (national average 3.4) to 3.7 in 2016-17 (national average 3.5). SA is the only state to commission forensic residential beds having 10 of these beds.

The original intent of Stepping Up was to increase intermediate care beds to between 80 to 92 beds. SA only achieved 45 intermediate care beds, but further increases were not actioned, as the results indicated they were not reducing ED mental health-related presentations, reducing ED visit times and they were not reducing general adult acute inpatient length of stay. Therefore a decision was made to reduce this intermediate care bed type from 45 to 30 beds. SA's overall general adult residential beds reduced by 13% from 12.1 per 100 000 population in 2013-14 (national average 6.8) to 10.5 in 2016-17 (national average 7). SA was 78% above the national average for this bed type in 2013-14 and was 50% above the national average in 2016-17.

No changes were made to general adult non-acute beds between 2013-14 and 2016-17 and SA remained 60% below the national average for this bed type at 3.8 beds per 100 000 population (national average 9.5).

It is important to note that SA has one of the lowest private sector bed numbers in Australia with 5.2 private sector beds per 100 000 population, being 58% below the national average of 12.3. Therefore SA still remains below the national average with respect to total psychiatry bed numbers available to the general adult population when you factor in the significant lack of private sector beds (see Figure 1.45).

What impact did these reforms have on ED visit times for mental health patients?

The system oversight and governance reforms in combination with localising bed management and significantly increasing general adult acute capacity by 24% were specifically intended to significantly reduce ED visit times. In 2016 the ED mental health visit times reduced by 40% from 16 to 9.6 hours, the lowest it had been in SA since data collection recorded in 2004 (see Figure 1.46). This major reduction in ED visit time occurred despite ongoing increases in ED mental health presentations between 2013-14 and 2016-17. ED mental health-related presentations increased by 19% from 118 presentations per 10 000 population in 2013-14 to 137 in 2016-17. SA remained 20% above the national average for ED mental health-related presentations in 2016-17 (national average 114). The increases in general adult acute beds was also accompanied by 32% reduction in average length of stay from 13.6 days in 2013-14 to 9.3 days in 2016-17 (lowest length of stay in Australia, with national average being 11.5 days).

CONCLUSION: SA MENTAL HEALTH REFORMS (2007–17) AND NATIONAL POLICY IMPLICATIONS

SA had one of the highest combined investments in supported housing, NGO, general adult community mental health and general adult residential care, but this investment had no impact on reducing ED mental health presentations, which have consistently been the highest in the nation for some time. The increasing rate of SA ED mental health-related presentations may have been partially related to the dissolution of sub-specialist community mental health teams in 2011-12. The mental health system is planning to revert back to sub-specialist community mental health teams with the re-establishment of assessment and crisis intervention teams and continuing care teams, but these have yet to be operationalised. It will be important to evaluate whether these reformed

Figure 1.45 Australia and SA: Mental health beds—general adult, forensic, veterans, private sector

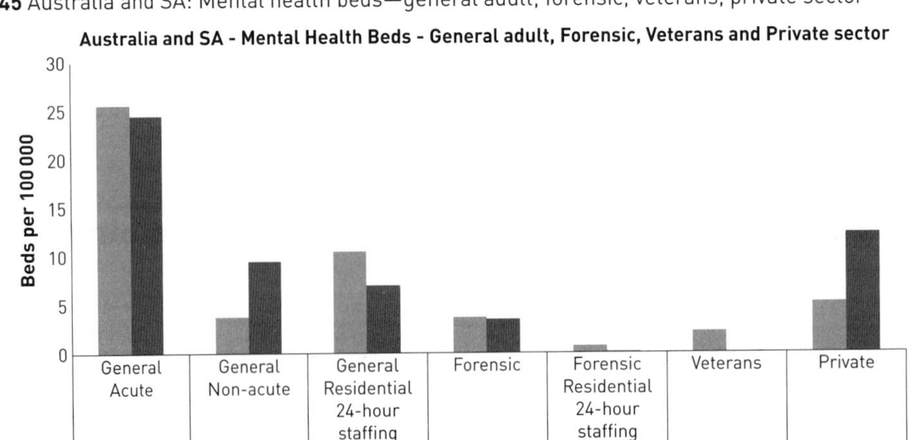

	General Acute	General Non-acute	General Residential 24-hour staffing	Forensic	Forensic Residential 24-hour staffing	Veterans	Private
SA	25.6	3.8	10.5	3.7	0.7	2.2	5.2
NAT	24.5	9.5	7	3.5	0.1	–	12.3

Figure 1.46 General adult community mental health reform—loss of sub-specialist teams

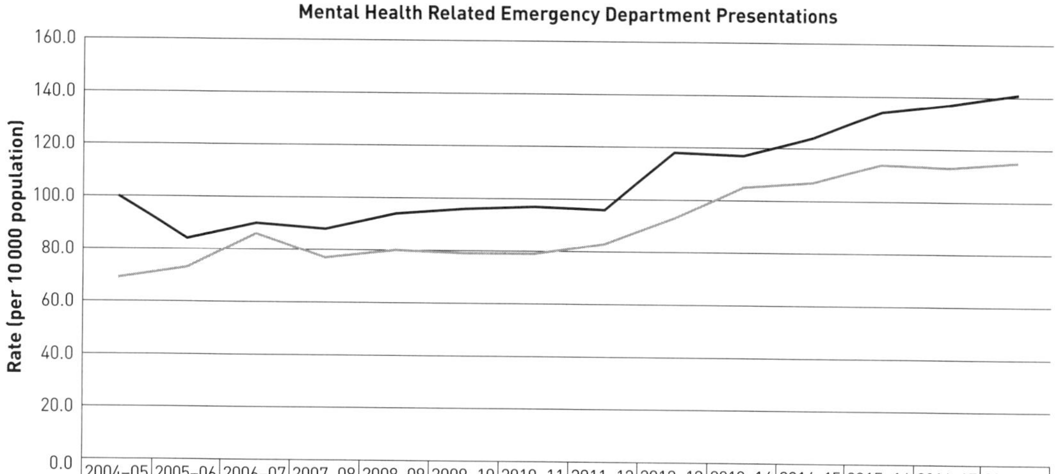

Mental Health Related Emergency Department Presentations

Rate (per 10 000 population)

	2004–05	2005–06	2006–07	2007–08	2008–09	2009–10	2010–11	2011–12	2012–13	2013–14	2014–15	2015–16	2016–17	2017–18
—SA	100.7	84.1	90.7	88.4	94.3	95.8	97.0	96.2	118.1	117.4	124.7	134.8	137.4	140.9
—NAT	69.2	73.6	86.6	77.4	80.1	78.9	79.4	83.8	93.3	105.1	107.8	114.0	113.6	115.9

sub-specialist teams will have an impact on reducing ED mental health-related presentations in SA.

It is clear, based on the SA experience, that intermediate care beds were not a substitute for general adult acute beds, which was a key reform agenda for the Stepping Up reforms (Tyrer, 2011). The reduction of 45 general adult acute beds and increase of 45 sub-acute residential beds led to a dramatic rise in ED visit times from 10 hours in 2011 to 16 hours in 2014. The subsequent commissioning of 53 general adult acute beds and reduction of 15 intermediate care beds led to a 40% reduction in ED visit times from 16 hours in 2014 to 9.6 hours in 2016. This suggests that Australian policy makers should be very cautious in trying to reduce general adult acute beds below 25 general adult acute beds per 100 000, even if they increase investment in residential and community mental health staffing. It may well be that once you go below a certain number of acute beds then further increases in community

Figure 1.47 Mental health-related emergency department presentations

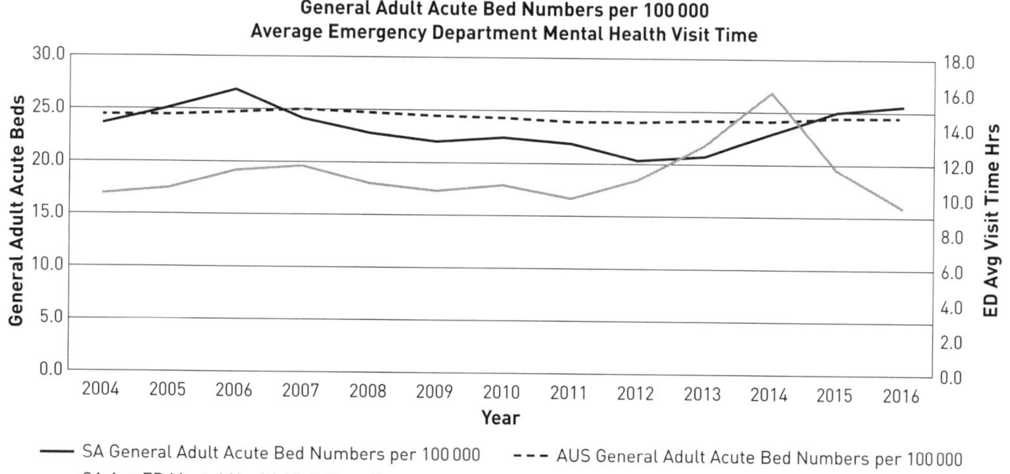

or residential care may not compensate for further reductions in acute bed numbers (Australasian College of Emergency Medicine, 2019).

It is important to note that Australia has a very low number of overall psychiatric beds by OECD averages. It is unlikely that Australia will be able to further reduce its psychiatric bed numbers based on the SA experience and current significant acute demand pressures across Australia. There are nationwide problems with regards accessing acute psychiatric beds, due to increasing ED demand, and a failure to match this increasing demand by adjusting the acute and non-acute psychiatric bed supply. There is international evidence to support the idea of 50–60 public sector psychiatric beds per 100 000 population, which is much higher than Australia's current overall level of 29.

The Australasian College of Emergency Medicine has seen the value of SA's 24 hour Ministerial target for ED mental health care. They have made this a key recommendation of addressing ED access block issues for mental health patients. They have specifically recommended that 'All 24 hour waits should be reported to the Health Minister regularly, alongside any CEO interventions and mechanisms for incident review.' This recommendation has also been endorsed by the Royal Australian College of Psychiatrists.

Further research and national debate is required on this important area of public policy to make better evidence-based decisions and prevent the current ED access block crisis for mental health patients in Australia. SA's experience between 2007 and 2017 has important lessons for national policy planners.

1.7.9 TASMANIA

RICHARD BENJAMIN & AARON GROVES

BACKGROUND

Not long after the first European settlement in 1803 of Van Diemen's Land as a penal and defensive colony of the British Empire, a 'very humble Invalid Barracks' was built in New Norfolk (Gowlland, 1981). Most of those who were treated there were transported convicts who had fallen ill as a result of poor living conditions and associated disease. In 1827, Governor Arthur ordered that 'Invalids' from around the state be sent to the Barracks at New Norfolk.

Those travelling from Hobart were initially sent by open boat, a difficult journey, often in inclement weather, that took up to three days. It quickly became clear that the available facilities were totally unsatisfactory, and, by the early 1830s, a new hospital had been erected that housed approximately 100. A high proportion of the Invalids were classed as 'Lunatics' and the hospital increasingly specialised in this type of patient; for several decades in its early history the facility was known as the 'Lunatic Asylum'.

The institution went through many iterations over the next 170 years, growing substantially in size. Many men, women and children were accommodated. Figures from a report to the Tasmanian Parliament in 1988 indicated that, on average, approximately 930 residents were housed there during the 1960s (Mental Health Services Commission, 1988), and, throughout the twentieth century, by far the majority of the state mental health budget was spent on inpatient care there. The facility, ultimately known as the Royal Derwent Hospital, was, however, repeatedly criticised for overcrowding and poor or even appalling conditions and treatment, and by the turn of the millennium its doors were closed, although a painful legacy remains for many who had been admitted there, and for their families.

A description of service development in Tasmania until the mid-2000s was completed for the Third Edition of this text, and this chapter will focus on more recent challenges and developments. It should be noted though that the history of service development in Tasmania occurred subsequent to de-institutionalisation and the gradual closure of Royal Derwent Hospital, the mainstreaming of services and the development of community services, as in mainland states. However, a number of relatively unique local issues are worthy of mention.

First, Tasmania, although geographically a small state, is sparsely populated. Approximately 45% of the approximately 520 000 population live in the Greater

Hobart area, with the remainder living in a range of smaller cities and towns, often with limited service provision across many domains; economies of scale are difficult to replicate under such circumstances. To assist with service delivery, Tasmania is generally split into three regions, South, North and North-west.

Second, although there have been notable improvements, Tasmania struggles in comparison with the rest of the country on a number of health and social indices, including with higher rates of chronic disease, smoking, obesity, and poor nutrition, and with lower physical activity levels (Department of Health and Human Services, 2016). In addition, Tasmania also has lower levels of literacy and health literacy, secondary school retention rates and per capita income, higher unemployment levels, and difficulties with both affordable housing and public transport. These factors in combination contribute to not only some of the worst population health outcomes in Australia, they also contribute to poorer mental health outcomes. Finally, there is a growing recognition of the tragic history of Tasmania's Aboriginal population, the Palawa people, present some 40 000 years before European settlement. Violence between colonists and Aboriginals, known as 'the Black War', disease and dislocation from land led to almost total obliteration of this group of Tasmanians in the early nineteenth century. Over the last 40 years, however, advocates have worked tirelessly to increase awareness of local Aboriginality and to ensure cultural identification and safety. Today, more than 4% of Tasmanians identify their Aboriginal heritage.

Service structure and set-up

The overarching health service structure in Tasmania has recently changed, as has the structure within Mental Health Services. Importantly, a three region generic health system was unified, and in 2018 the *Tasmanian Health Service Act* was proclaimed, making the Tasmanian Health Service directly accountable to the Secretary of the Department of Health, to streamline governance activities and to support local decision making.

The Mental Health, Alcohol and Drug Directorate was formed in 2013 as part of a national strategy for health reform. The Directorate provides a key role in implementing both state and national strategic direction in relevant areas. The Office of the Chief Civil and the Chief Forensic Psychiatrist has overall responsibility for ensuring that the objects of the Mental Health Act (Tasmanian Government, 2013) are met in respect of involuntary patients and voluntary patients in both civil and forensic settings.

The Mental Health Services restructure has led to the delivery of clinical services through six separate streams: Child and Adolescent Mental Health Services, Adult Mental Health Services, Older Persons Mental Health Services, Alcohol and Drug Services, Forensic Mental Health Services and Correctional Health Services. Because of the different sizes of each stream and because of the population distribution across the regions, operational and clinical governance lines remain complex.

The make-up of each public sector service is similar in many ways to those in other jurisdictions. A number of variations are, however, noteworthy. A Mental Health Helpline, based in Hobart, provides a triage and advice service for the entire state, across all subspecialty groups. In addition to the usual acute inpatient mental health units in the three major public hospitals, stand-alone inpatient units also provide services for those requiring extended inpatient stays, for older people, for forensic patients and for those requiring detoxification; all of these facilities are, however, in the south of the state.

There are no dedicated inpatient beds for child and adolescent patients in Tasmania; however, medical inpatient units are currently being constructed at the public hospitals in both Hobart and Launceston that will cater solely for adolescent patients, and these units will provide care and treatment for those experiencing mental illness. Younger children who require admission are cared for in paediatric units.

For reasons relating to population size, other specialised teams seen in more populous states, catering for those with Early Psychosis, Eating Disorders, Borderline Personality Disorder or Intellectual Disability, for example, are not available, although there is an increasing awareness that such specialist services are required. A consultation liaison style perinatal mental health service is available in the south of the state.

The next stage of redevelopment of the Royal Hobart Hospital, the state's leading teaching hospital, first announced in 2006, is scheduled for completion in 2019, at a projected cost of $689 million. The redevelopment required the demolition of facilities that previously accommodated acute psychiatric inpatients. During the redevelopment process, people with acute mental illness requiring admission have been accommodated in a temporary demountable facility in the hospital's forecourt, known as J Block. It is expected that the Mental Health Inpatient Unit in the new K Block will be commissioned by 2019.

'Rethink Mental Health'

The problems that affect the delivery of mental health services in Tasmania are in many respects like those throughout Australia, and relate to philosophy and culture of service delivery; service capacity; integration of services; and workforce training, recruitment and retention. Following in the footsteps of the Bridging the Gap Review (Department of Health and Human Services, 2004) and the Tasmanian Mental Health Services Strategic Plan 2006–2011 (Department of Health and Human Services, 2006), 'Rethink Mental Health—Better Mental Health and Wellbeing' was a substantial project undertaken by the Tasmanian State Government in partnership with the local peak body for the community managed sector, the Mental Health Council of Tasmania, to establish a 10-year vision for mental health service provision, from 2015 to 2025 (Mental Health Alcohol and Drug Directorate, 2015). The process involved a lengthy and comprehensive stakeholder consultation.

The resulting plan noted that the local mental health system had become 'complex, disjointed and confusing to navigate' (Mental Health Alcohol and Drug Directorate, 2015). The plan also noted that a range of issues in service delivery had become apparent, including: the need to put the consumer at the centre of their care, and to broaden the focus to wellness, as opposed to illness; to be more inclusive of consumers, families and carers; to increasingly recognise the 'lived experience' of consumers via peer support models and peer workers; and, to reduce service fragmentation.

The plan included ten key directions for reform with associated key actions. The following is a list of the report's recommendations for key actions:

1 To establish a single state-wide public mental health system.
2 To establish a peer workforce in public mental health services to complement the existing workforce.
3 To establish early referral pathways especially following a suicide attempt or self-harm.
4 To strengthen mental health services for infants, children and young people and their families and carers.
5 To develop stepped models of mental health support in the community.
6 To support primary mental health to be the 'front end' of mental health care in Tasmania.
7 To develop a joint workforce strategy for the public mental health services and the private mental health sector, including the establishment of joint psychiatrist positions.

The remainder of this chapter will focus on a number of these recommendations, and two broader issues of current priority for reform.

An integrated Tasmanian mental health system

During the Rethink consultation process, concerns were repeatedly raised with respect to fragmentation between inpatient services and community teams, and variations in models of care across regions. General Practitioners have also provided feedback that the primary care sector is often excluded from care planning decisions, and the tender processes for the community managed sector have brought about confusion, as 'who provides what service to which group for how long with what resources' has not been transparent.

As a result, it was felt that the establishment of the Tasmanian Health Service presented a significant opportunity to also establish a single, integrated state-wide public mental health system. The aim was to create a system 'where mental health care and support is seamless, smooth and easy to navigate'

(Mental Health Alcohol and Drug Directorate, 2015). The key, it was thought, was to view the process from the perspectives of both service users and service providers. Better integration of critical components of the system, public mental health services, primary care, and the community managed sector, was thought to be particularly important.

The Tasmanian Government further acknowledged that the mental health system is complex, and that collaboration with a broader range of stakeholders was crucial, so that private providers, alcohol and drug services, housing, services for children and youth, and the education sector, also needed to be involved. Important integration strategies recommended included the creation of single care plans across multiple agencies, shared information systems, joint service provision through multi-agency teams, cross-training of staff, and formal interagency collaborative agreements. Following the re-election of the State Government in 2018, the Government committed to the formation of a Mental Health Integration Taskforce for Southern Tasmania. This Taskforce met regularly throughout 2018 to develop appropriate recommendations for that region. It is envisaged that, if the recommendations are endorsed by government, they may also act as a model for implementation in the North and North-west of the state.

Moving towards a more fully integrated mental health system, the Government has also committed to an important philosophical change for the sector, the need to fully embrace the concept of a person-centred, recovery approach. 'An integrated Tasmanian Mental Health System ... will ensure that design and delivery of programs and services are underpinned by the principle that each person brings with them their own circumstances and life experiences... It will listen to people with a lived experience together with their families and carers about what helps and what interferes with their recovery' (Mental Health Alcohol and Drug Directorate, 2015). The full adoption of this principle, enshrined in National Standards for Mental Health Services for many years, will require cultural shift, dedicated organisational support, and associated staff re-training.

Stepped models of mental health support in the community

One of the Rethink's major reforms involved 'shifting the focus from hospital-based care to support in the community', in line with community sentiment and in order to reduce the level of demand on inpatient services. Both the primary care sector and the community managed sector play critical roles in such a shift in focus. Providing support for consumers in the community enhances autonomy, is more convenient and comfortable, allows consumers to stay in much closer contact with family and friends, supports families and carers, and improves recovery. Step Down services from acute inpatient beds, 'step-up services' from the community, and high-level supported accommodation options for those who have been hospitalised for protracted periods may all be of benefit.

In Tasmania, however, demand for inpatient services has increased significantly, as it has across the nation. Between 2013 and 2018, mental health presentations to emergency departments in Tasmania increased by 50% (internal statistics). As a result, occupancy rates in the three acute inpatient units are high and lengths of stay in emergency departments have increased. Particular problems have been evident in the South, compounded by the closure of the 42 bed inpatient unit during the Royal Hobart Hospital Redevelopment; occupancy rates in the current temporary 32 bed unit are now 98% or above, with lengthy waits for beds (internal statistics).

The local Adult Mental Health Service in the South has long provided a stepped care model, including community mental health team care, crisis components of community mental health teams, residential respite care, Step Up and Step Down care, acute inpatient care, and extended inpatient care. Over more recent years, additional community support has been made available via the community managed sector and from funds sourced through the National Disability Insurance Agency. To address the acute inpatient crisis at the Royal Hobart Hospital, however, the State Government has responded with an additional range of commitments. These now include the introduction of a Mental Health Hospital in the Home Unit and new community beds.

The Hospital in the Home Unit will provide an alternative to acute inpatient care for 12 consumers. Services will be provided by a seven day a week multidisciplinary team offering intensive support. Twenty-seven additional community beds will also be built in two different locations. It is envisaged that these facilities will be commissioned as integrated service centres and will include community mental health services, the community managed sector, housing and disability support. The addition of these services to the local pool will enhance the stepped model of care already available, and, once functional, it is expected that they will significantly impact upon the demand for inpatient beds. If successful it is also envisaged that similar facilities will be developed throughout the state.

Suicide prevention

A national report in 2018 concluded that, 'Despite ongoing work to improve suicide prevention, there has been no significant reduction in the suicide rate over the last decade' (National Mental Health Commission, 2018). The issue is particularly relevant in Tasmania where statistics show that the rate of suicide has been consistently high. Recent rates peaked in 2016 at 17 per 100 000 people, while the national average was 11.7 (Australian Bureau of Statistics, 2018).

Fully cognisant of the problem, the Tasmanian Government has taken a comprehensive approach to suicide prevention that is reflected in a number of policies that were launched in 2016. These include a state-wide prevention strategy, a youth suicide strategy and a workforce development and training plan. Central to these policies are the need to 'start' early, by focusing on resilience, mental health and wellbeing of children, parents and families, and the need to empower young people, their families and their communities to talk about suicide and to respond to suicidal behaviours. Also critical is the need to create a responsive, coordinated health service system for people experiencing suicidal thoughts and behaviours, and to increase the capacity of clinicians to respond to suicidal ideation and behaviours.

Concrete steps taken in these endeavours have included tendering of aftercare services for those presenting to public hospital emergency departments with suicidal ideation and behaviours, and training large numbers of staff cross-sectorally in a contemporary suicide mitigation program, 'Connecting with People: Mental Health and Suicide Prevention Training'. This training is designed to reduce stigma and to improve clinicians' ability to compassionately respond to those in suicidal distress or to those who have self-harmed. The Tasmanian suicide rate in 2017 was lower, at 15.6 per 100 000 (Australian Bureau of Statistics, 2018); preliminary figures, and it is hoped that the range of policies and actions put in place by government will lead to further reductions.

Mental health legislation in Tasmania

Tasmania's first Mental Hospitals Act was proclaimed in 1858. The next relevant piece of legislation, proclaimed 105 years later, in 1963, established a Guardianship Board for those who could not manage their own affairs, and made changes to the language used to avoid offensive terminology in an effort to change public attitudes. The 1996 Act introduced a greater degree of oversight, and the most recent Act, proclaimed in 2014, after an exhaustive seven-year consultation and drafting process, introduced model mental health legislation into the state by adopting the presumption of capacity as a central principle. Oversight roles were significantly enhanced and treatment decisions for involuntary patients, previously made by the local Guardianship Board, were brought under the jurisdiction of the Mental Health Tribunal. A series of Amendments introduced in 2017 improved the applicability and the efficiency of the Act. The Office of the Chief Psychiatrist is currently preparing a Plain Language Guide to the Act, and is revising Approved Forms, Standing Orders and Clinical Guidelines. The Minister of Health is required to complete a formal review of the operation of the Act by 2020, and this process is anticipated to commence in the first half of 2019.

Trauma-informed care and practice

In Tasmania, mental health services are increasingly expected to develop greater competence in consumer, family and carer-centred approaches, as well as adopting the recovery concept. However, it is increasingly recognised that Tasmanian mental health services will also need to focus on Trauma-informed Care and Practice (TICP; Benjamin, Haliburn, & King, 2019). This paradigm shift acknowledges that most of those who present to public mental health services have experienced abuse or trauma, and that this trauma can have significant effects on mental, physical, social, emotional and spiritual wellbeing. These subsequent effects of trauma are often the reason why people present to mental health services; however, the trauma often goes unrecognised. Rather, the mental health focus on symptom reduction, risk and referral in an often-busy service tends to further obscure a person's individual story and its relevance to the presenting problems.

In Tasmania, the adoption of TICP is vitally important given the occurrence of child abuse, both familial and institutional, and domestic and sexual violence. However, it is of particular relevance given the context of the local Aboriginal population, a series of bushfires starting with the catastrophe in 1967 that claimed 62 lives and destroyed nearly 1300 homes, the massacre that took place at Port Arthur in 1996, and the history of the many people with mental illnesses who were taken away from their families to New Norfolk.

TICP, as a strengths-based approach that understands and responds to the impact of trauma, is a critical component of a reformed mental health system for Tasmania. Avoiding retraumatisation, particularly via restrictive practices in inpatient settings, is particularly important in this consumer group. The Hospital in the Home service that is currently being developed for people experiencing acute mental illnesses in the South of the state will be the first service in Tasmania to formally adopt all contemporary mental health principles into policy and clinical practice, including TICP. Importantly, there will be a focus on the consumer and their personal narrative.

The future of mental health care in Tasmania

The Tasmanian public mental health system is currently undergoing substantial change. More modern principles and practices are being embraced, the broader system is being restructured and remodelled, and new services and treatment approaches are being introduced, with more envisaged. It is expected that substantial improvement will follow, but there will be a need for those in leadership positions to keep contemporary principles of mental health care at the forefront throughout the journey.

1.7.10 VICTORIA

GRAHAM MEADOWS, LISA BROPHY & MARGARET GRIGG

WHAT ARE SERVICES LIKE IN VICTORIA?

Understanding how services in this state are shaped may be helped by knowledge of some history. In this chapter, we briefly summarise material from the last edition of this text (Ash et al., 2012), which covered up to 2010.

In the mid-1990s, the state services administration determined a general framework for adult mental health services which drew on international work and models in place in Victoria. The Framework (Human Services Victoria Mental Health Branch, 1994; Meadows & Singh, 2003), included 24-hour crisis teams (Community Assessment and Treatment Teams or CATs), mobile assessment and treatment services (providing assertive case management) and continuing care teams (CCTs; developed from community clinics already established). Acute inpatient units and continuing care units for long-term residential stays complemented these community services. Commonwealth National Mental Health Plan funds discussed earlier in this chapter provided important transitional support to the community services before revenue and capital expenditures could be freed from the hospital closures. An area-based funding model drew on census variables to guide funding allocation at regional levels. Funding was increased to the NGO sector, and this sector came to provide most of the day care provision available, since this was not a component in the Victorian service framework. The Framework was followed closely in most urban areas, at least initially, while across the rural areas, services moving out from a hospital base tended to negotiate an integrated model, which worked better in the less densely populated parts of the state. The model was referred to as integrated, both because it merged components such as CATs and CCTs, and because it drew on work from Ian Falloon from the United Kingdom, who had elsewhere described his 'integrated care' approach (Falloon & Fadden, 1993).

The advent of mainstreaming, with closure of all the large stand-alone institutions by 2000, brought community mental health services under the charge of general hospitals; not always an easy cultural or organisational innovation. Harsh budget cuts in the early 1990s were followed by progressive restoration of funding to around 1993 levels by 2000, but with a different service mix, less being spent on institutions and more on NGOs. Through this time there was an increase in the use of Community Treatment Orders (see Section 2.4.13) resulting in many case managers (alongside medical staff) needing to combine care and control dimensions to their practice in the community, a situation many were ill prepared for (Brophy, Campbell, & Healy, 2003). Furthermore, an emphasis on a sometimes inflexibly interpreted model of case management served often to reduce the scope for exercise of specialist skills and the delivery of more specialist interventions to some clients. However, by the end of the first national plan period, and as Victoria moved forward into the new century, a reasonably consistent model of service delivery, reasonably consistently resourced, was seen as in place across the state.

THE NEW MILLENNIUM IN VICTORIA

In 1999, in the context of a new Labor administration, the Health Department made the first substantial addition to the Framework, establishing primary mental health and early intervention services (PMHEIS) in each mental health service area. These small teams, typically of three to five full-time equivalent staff, had a broad brief to provide consultation, education and support to the primary care sector and to facilitate early interventions. Establishment built in part on previous experience with GP shared care pilots (Meadows, Harvey, Joubert, Barton, & Bedi, 2007). Further initiatives introduced through time included specific initiatives to support hospital emergency departments including Emergency CATT (ECATT) Services, specific programs for recurrent attenders at emergency departments, as well as community-based discharge planning positions addressing transfer to primary care, and, more recently, designated early intervention services and the Prevention and Recovery Care Services (PARCS). These, in turn, reflected overall substantially increased spending.

While each of these service additions has evident merits and addressed a valid problem, service managers have been faced with the challenge of coordinating these various add-ons to the main framework structure, often being of teams of small size with a number of different ways in which they could be best linked with other parts of the service system. Many services through much of the twenty-first century so far have not succeeded in running inpatient units within their allocated budget, which has often been perhaps unrealistic, so there has been diversion of community funds to support the inpatient units, squeezing the provision of continuing care case management resources and staff. This sometimes has restricted the capacity of community services to avert admissions, with consequential stress on the inpatient units that become more difficult to keep within budget: a potential example of positive feedback loop (see Section 1.5.11). Area-based funding has not been so clearly pursued since the late 1990s, particularly where this would involve decisions to move funds away from relatively better resourced services. Victoria's population has increased and for example Melbourne as the largest city has had major structural and demographic changes (O'Hanlon, 2018) so it has become increasingly unclear whether the initially calibrated distribution of resources according to need has been maintained as funding levels have changed.

The early 2000s provided for some consolidation of the structures set in place in the 1990s. A period without major structural reform, it provided some time for stabilisation of work practices and policies, and for clinicians to gain confidence in their practice and their capacity as seniors to supervise. In 2009, the Honourable Lisa Neville, Victoria's first Minister for Mental Health, released the Victorian Mental Health Reform Strategy, Because Mental Health Matters (Department of Human Services, 2009). This strategy identified six reform areas; however, it was the strong focus on early intervention that has led to the most significant structural reform, the redesign of specialist child and youth services within the 0-25-year-old framework. Other key flagship projects included the introduction of a twenty-four-hour mental health support line and the development of care coordination models for people with complex needs.

THE DEVELOPING TWENTY-FIRST CENTURY IN VICTORIAN MENTAL HEALTH CARE

Politically, the teen years of this century break roughly into two halves, the Liberal National administrations led by Premiers Baillieu and Napthine to December 2014, then the Andrews Labor administration, current at time of writing. The funding environment for public health services in Victoria under the Liberal administration from 2010 to 2015 was adverse, with funding levels not keeping up with inflation, or where they did, being associated with substantial additional commitments so not representing real increases. These impacts were magnified with the rapid population growth, particularly in the outer ring of Melbourne and the Barwon-South-West region, resulting in significant maldistribution of resources with communities with substantial levels of socioeconomic disadvantage, such as Western Melbourne, particularly disadvantaged. Real expenditure declined from $204 per head in 2010-11 to $202 in 2015-16, while other states and territories in that time typically (Tasmania excluded) had increases of around 5-20% (Productivity Commission, 2019). Funding has been increasing since then under a Labor administration. For most of the last 10 years as reviewed by the Productivity Commission, Victoria has had the lowest per capita expenditure on mental health of any Australian state or territory, sometimes lagging 50% behind the leading state (Productivity Commission, 2019) Victoria consistently reports the lowest proportion of the population receiving public sector mental health care at 1.1%; other states and territories report between 1.6% and 3.0%. Concurrently the number of people on compulsory Community Treatment Orders (CTOs) in Victoria continued to rise until the state was identified as having the highest rate in the world, with 98.8 per 100 000 population compared, for example, to 30.2 per 100 000 population in Tasmania and 46.4 per 100 000 in NSW (Light, Kerridge, Ryan, & Robertson, 2012).

Policy developments through this period have been guided by documentation that carried forward from the earlier decade (Department of Human Services, 2009) and product of the then Labor administration, more recently by a 10-year plan from 2015 (Department of Health and Human Services, 2015). The *Mental Health Act 2014*, superseding the 1986 Act, aimed to support recovery oriented practice and introduced legal mechanisms that could enable supported decision making and a stronger emphasis on human rights, including Advance Statements and Nominated Persons (Brophy, Kokanovic, Flore, McSherry, & Herrman, 2019; Vine & Judd, 2019). The Act has contributed to efforts in Victoria to reduce the use of coercion and restrictive interventions in the community and in inpatient services (Brophy et al., 2019; Fletcher et al., 2017). An independent mental health advocacy service has been established and the state now has a Mental Health Complaints Commissioner. In her most recent analysis of the data available, Edwina Light has now found that rates of CTO use in Australia range from 40.0 per 100 000 population (in Western Australia) to 112.5 per 100 000 (in South Australia). The rates of people subject to CTOs fell in Victoria to 76.4 (Light, 2019). Some have argued that, considering a lack of increased investment in services, this decrease says more about reduced access to care rather than a realisation of human rights, so this finding needs to be considered with caution (Vine & Judd, 2019).

Many of the changes indicated in the Act will require improved resourcing levels which in many areas are only recently becoming evidently available.

Even so, some innovation in services delivery has occurred, in particular through continued expansion of Prevention and Recovery Care (PARC) services. Almost all area mental health services now include a residential sub-acute service that supports people to either avoid an inpatient hospital admission (Step Up) or leave hospital early (Step Down). PARCS are based on a partnership between public mental health services and mental health community support services, offering a strong emphasis on integrating clinical mental health care with intensive recovery-focused psychosocial input. The model has been extended to Youth PARCS and women's only services (Fletcher et al., 2019; Harvey et al., 2019).

A one-off investment in mental health research was made through a $10 million Mental Illness Research Fund (MIRF) program but since that time the Victorian Government has not directly funded competitive research grant rounds directed at mental health.

In 2015, the then Victorian Government introduced a major reform of mental health community support services (MHCSS), the part of state-funded provision in the NGO sector. This process was seen as necessary to deal with a longstanding need for reform and also to assist the sector to prepare for the much larger transition process of having all MHCSS funding rolling into the National Disability Insurance Scheme (NDIS) by 2019. Referred to as 'recommissioning', this made for an 'extended period of uncertainty' (Silburn, 2015). Recommissioning involved the establishment of new catchment areas, centralised intake and assessment processes, and a reduction in the number of providers. Many small services lost their funding altogether and larger services had both losses and gains that required considerable adjustment. For example some services were allocated to other providers and staff and clients needed to transition from one provider to another. This resulted in a long and difficult transition period. The costs to the sector were considerable. Agencies had to make staff redundant and also explain to consumers why they were no longer going to provide services to them.

MHCSS sector clients are categorised into three tiers, consistent with NDIS categorisation. To be eligible for a service, clients have to have a permanent disability associated with a mental illness. Once clients are deemed eligible they are then categorised based on the severity of the disability and/or their current needs. This means that clients with high levels of disability, but who are otherwise stable/doing well (and therefore might have low levels of need) might get the same level of priority as someone who has a lower level of disability and a high level of current need. People in this group can include people experiencing their first psychosis or life circumstances like deterioration of their support networks, who with early intervention may not become dependent on the MHCSS system. The system has therefore lost significant capacity for prevention for this group of clients (Silburn, 2015).

With the advent of the Better Access initiative (see Section 1.7.2) there was a perception that care for people with high prevalence disorders was better resourced. This along with general funding constraints has led to the whittling away and unusual disappearance of the PMHEIs earlier mentioned. Unfortunately the delivery of psychological services through 'Better Access' is highly uneven across the state (Meadows, Enticott, & Rosenberg, 2018) and the functions of the PMHEIs in terms of capacity building and secondary consultation are not substituted for through Commonwealth provision. The reduction in state investment in primary care has perhaps been a false economy and primary care providers often find themselves less well supported by state-funded services than they were a decade ago.

Broad community concerns have related to events that threatened community safety, including the Bourke St car-attack tragedy in which a man in a psychotic state murdered six people and injured 27 others. In this context, Victoria's prison incarceration rates increased from just over 4000 in 2009 to over 8000 in 2019. The majority of the increase has been in remand populations with some evidence that it has resulted in an increase in the imprisonment of people with mental health issues, effectively becoming new institutions (see Chapter 1.1; Australian Bureau of Statistics, 2019).

Overall, innovation has been limited and resources stretched such that there has been broad recognition that Victoria's mental health services are not coping with demand and the quality of services is in decline. An election promise from the ALP has led to the establishment of a Royal Commission into Victoria's Mental Health System with final reporting due in 2020.

WHAT MIGHT BE DISTINCTIVE ABOUT SERVICES IN VICTORIA?

So how does this history help us understand the current shape and composition of services in Victoria? While some services in metropolitan areas retain the structure set out in the Framework with its separate teams attending to different phases and intensities of care, along with the tiered residential elements, elsewhere there has been some blending of these functions. These transitions have not necessarily been comprehensively evaluated and may have led to some compromise to the diversity of treatment delivery profiles which could be reliably delivered in the Framework setting (State Government of Victoria, 2019). Many services have been through strained times in the recent past, with substantial funding reductions that have impacted morale and function. However in many areas there has also been a sense of recent growth funds having impact such that services which had been well below establishment funding for some years now seeing returns to more like reasonable staffing levels. Nevertheless in much of the public mental health services compulsory treatment runs at very high levels. Emergency department presentations for mental health problems are a challenge across much of the state, which may reflect composite influences including changed demographics, increased community demand and reduced capacity in the MHCSS and primary care sectors.

Victoria has a number of progressive developments under way (Department of Health and Human Services, 2018). In some cases, for instance a Place-Based Suicide Initiative, there is sensible attention to strategic developmental processes with piloting and evaluation intended to precede systematic implementation across the state if indicated. As a result of the MIRF and the PULSAR project (Meadows et al., 2019) Victoria has generated the only study internationally to date to demonstrate the impact of staff training on consumer-rated recovery outcomes. This finding has received international interest but locally it will require considerable investment and ongoing translational research to lead to sustained improvement in practice.

One challenge that Victoria faces along with other states is that of working towards integration of Commonwealth and state-funded services. Victoria's private sector provision, in line with a pervasive national problem, is heavily concentrated in affluent inner-city suburbs, conspicuously in Melbourne in two large inner-city facilities in Richmond and Southern Melbourne. The degree of collaboration between Primary Health Networks and Local Health Networks is presently variable. Within Fifth Plan implementation timelines (see Chapter 1.7) are some for development of collaborative plans (Integrated Regional Planning Working Group, 2018a, 2018b)—and this should be unfolding from 2020, which offers some hope that this issue might see some serious attention.

The current Royal Commission into Victoria's Mental Health Services (State Government of Victoria, 2019) has strong governmental support and may provide a helpful push forward for funding and development. An interim report (State Government of Victoria, 2019) has suggested some bed increases as well as focus on Indigenous mental health and the peer workforce and establishing a translational research centre, but at time of writing the impact the Commission will have on longer-term planning in Victoria is unclear.

1.7.11 WESTERN AUSTRALIA

EDDIE BARTNIK

HISTORICAL CONTEXT TO 2010

It is possible to describe the history of the development of mental health services in Western Australia as occurring in several phases.

DECLINE OF THE ASYLUM

Early services (as across Australia and the world) were stand-alone psychiatric hospitals. Claremont Hospital for the Insane had the central role in the mental health system, opening in 1908 to replace the Fremantle Asylum and growing to a peak population of 1500 patients in 1954. Heathcote Reception House was opened in 1929 and in 1972, Claremont Hospital was separated into two hospitals: Graylands Hospital and Swanbourne Hospital. Although there were inpatient units in the three tertiary general hospitals in Perth, Graylands and Heathcote were the only hospitals with approved beds under the *Mental Health Act 1962* (WA) for the treatment of involuntary patients.

Swanbourne Hospital closed in 1983, Heathcote Hospital in 1994 and Graylands Hospital is still in operation, albeit with greatly reduced bed numbers. Services for people with intellectual disabilities were transferred from Swanbourne to community hostels and group homes under the new Division for the Intellectually Handicapped and the other adult and older adult services into purpose-built services on general hospital sites.

GROWTH OF COMMUNITY SERVICES

The first community-based mental health services in Western Australia began to spring up in the late 1960s and early 1970s with the establishment of metropolitan clinics and visiting psychiatrist services to major regional centres.

These were followed by the development of purpose-built community mental health clinics on site with general hospitals throughout the metropolitan area, and the growth of visiting and then progressively local services to a number of regional centres.

Despite a number of attempts to replace the 1962 Mental Health Act to complement the shift in practice, it was not until 1996 that new legislation was finally passed, bringing Western Australia into line with other national and international jurisdictions.

MENTAL HEALTH BECOMES PART OF HEALTH

In 1984, the Mental Health Department was amalgamated with Public Health and Hospitals and Allied Services to form the Health Department, with a Directorate of Psychiatric Services. In the late 1980s, the growth and development of mental health services began to gather pace with the establishment in 1989 of the metropolitan Psychiatric Emergency Team and YouthLink was set up with a focus on enhancing the mental health and wellbeing of marginalised and disadvantaged youth.

MAINSTREAMING AND INTEGRATION

The National Mental Health Strategy began in the early 1990s. The funding for reform that followed saw the development of early intervention in psychosis services, the growth of community-based and child and adolescent services and the development of the Independent Living Program. Telepsychiatry services were commenced and in the early 1990s academic chairs were established in child and adolescent psychiatry, older adult psychiatry and forensic psychiatry. Forensic services were expanded including the development of a new purpose-built forensic unit.

GROWTH OF RURAL SERVICES

It was not until the late 1980s that the first locally based service outside Perth was established in the Kimberley. This was followed by the establishment of services in the mid-west and south-west of the state and then community-based services in all the major regional centres and many of the larger towns, with visiting services to the smaller communities.

In 1998, the first inpatient units outside the metropolitan area were established in Bunbury (South-west) and Albany (Great Southern), and these were followed by a unit at Kalgoorlie (Goldfields) in 2002.

PRIVATE MENTAL HEALTH

Private psychiatry was slow to develop in Western Australia. It was not until the 1990s that this began to change with the development of private psychiatric hospitals in Perth and a vigorous private sector.

Some factors which make the WA mental health sector unique

Western Australia's population, geography challenges and mining boom/bust cycles create some substantial and unique challenges:

- Western Australia is Australia's largest state, with a total land area of 2 529 875 square kilometres. The capital city Perth has an estimated population of 2.14 million people and the state's regional and remote areas are home to some 500 000 people.
- The cyclical mining 'boom and bust' cycles and fly-in, fly-out culture, create very significant challenges for mental health services throughout the state but especially in regional and remote areas.
- The WA Health Sustainability Review Interim report (Government of Western Australia, 2018b) notes that salaries for staff within the WA health system, particularly doctors and nurses, are among the highest in the country while key services in WA have significantly lower capacity than the national average. For example, there are significantly fewer general practitioners (GPs) and residential aged care beds per capita than the national average and there is a maldistribution of GPs in rural and remote areas (Government of Western Australia, 2018b, p. 6).
- Providing culturally appropriate mental health services to Aboriginal people and their families throughout vast geographical areas.

Western Australia's isolation however has also been a breeding ground for innovation as traditional solutions have often been a poor fit for the WA landscape. For example:

- As part of the state government mental health reform strategy and building on evidence overseas, a Minister for Mental Health was appointed following the 2008 state election and in March 2010, Western Australia's (and Australia's) first Mental Health Commission came into effect.
- Western Australia faces unique challenges of supporting people and their families and communities in country Western Australia. In the late 1980s through its Disability Services Commission, the state developed a world-first methodology around developing personalised support solutions for people through a state-wide system of Local Area Coordination and individualised funding (Bartnik & Chalmers, 2007). The early work of the Mental Health Commission through the Individualised Community Living Support Program engaged the sector in this new methodology which was an excellent precursor to the new National Disability Insurance Scheme (NDIS).
- On 12 December 2017, the Commonwealth and Western Australian governments agreed that WA would join the Australia-wide NDIS. This announcement meant that the WA State Government would no longer deliver the NDIS (which used to be known as WA NDIS).
- As part of the whole of WA government 'Delivering Community Services in Partnership policy' (2011), additional funding was provided to establish the sustainable basis for community services in WA and this complemented moves by the Mental Health Commission to grow a strong and sustainable community sector in addition to public mental health services. This dual approach supported the rapid development of the community sector mental health services in the period since 2010.

Some key developments during the period 2010–2018

Significant changes were made during this period both in the administrative arrangements for the mental health system overall and also the delivery of mental health services in WA.

The administrative arrangements for mental health and drugs/alcohol in WA were significantly changed with the establishment of the Mental Health Commission (MHC) in 2010. The scope of the WA Mental Health Commission remains unique to this day. Of Australia's seven mental health commissions, WA is the only one to hold the budget for mental health. The Commission has the aim to be a world class commissioning organisation (Bartnik, 2013).

To create this role in 2010, the budget and resources of the previous Mental Health Division in the Department of Health (DoH) was transferred to the MHC, leaving little dedicated system coordinating capacity within Health to support the individual Health Services.

In 2013 following the Stokes Review (see below), a small Office of Mental Health was established within the DoH with a strong focus on Stokes Review Implementation. In 2018, this now operates as the Mental Health Unit (Government of Western Australia, 2018a) and has a role in the coordination, review and reform of public mental health services.

On 1 July 2015, the Mental Health Commission amalgamated with the Drug and Alcohol Office to deliver an integrated approach to helping people with mental health, alcohol and other drug problems, recognising that these problems commonly coexist.

The new organisation, still called the Mental Health Commission, is accountable to the Minister for Mental Health. The Commission plans and purchases mental health, alcohol and other drug services through government, non-government and private sector service providers. The Commission also directly provides some alcohol and other drug treatment and support services.

A core objective of the amalgamation is to help individuals who experience both mental health, alcohol and other drug issues to access integrated care (Mental Health Commission Annual Report 2012/13; Government of Western Australia, 2012–13)

The Commission's strategic direction is guided by the *Western Australian Mental Health, Alcohol and Other Drug Services Plan 2015–2025: Better Choices. Better Lives* which was released on 7 December 2015.

The early work of the Commission was guided by the three key reform directions set out in the State's 2013 strategic mental health policy, *Mental Health 2020: Making it Personal and Everybody's Business*:

- Person-centred supports and services—recognising that there is no 'one-size-fits-all' approach to mental health care.
- Connected approaches—recognising that everyone has a role in delivering good outcomes for people with mental illness.
- Balanced investment—ensuring that money is spent on the right mix of supports and services (Mental Health Commission, 2019).

The 2015 integrated 10-year plan estimates the optimal mix, level and type of mental health, alcohol and other drug services required to meet the needs of our population over the decade. By comparing these estimates with existing service levels, the plan identifies gaps in the current system, and explains where new investment needs to be targeted to build a comprehensive and contemporary service system (Mental Health Commission Annual Report 2015/16; Government of Western Australia, 2015–16).

A range of improved commissioning practices have been systematically implemented with the launch of the Commission's Quality Management Framework in December 2014 and the introduction of Special Purpose Accounts which offer a more transparent view of the funding the Commission provides to public mental health services and how it is spent by ensuring all funding provided by the Commission must be expended on mental health services (Mental Health Commission Annual Report 2014/15; Government of Western Australia, 2014–15).

On the 30 November 2015, the new *Mental Health Act 2014* (WA) commenced, as the Commission supported the transition from the *Mental Health Act 1996* (WA). As part of this change the Commission assumed responsibility for providing support and staff to the following independent entities: the Office of the Chief Psychiatrist, the Mental Health Tribunal and the Mental Health Advocacy Service.

Following extensive consultation, key changes in the new legislation were in line with national directions and included:

- stronger recognition of the important roles of families and carers
- processes that encourage supported (rather than substitute) decision making
- more frequent review of involuntary status

- a Charter of Mental Health Care Principles, which promotes recovery oriented practice and service delivery, and a positive culture within services and
- a requirement that, to the extent that it is practicable and appropriate in the circumstances, services involve Aboriginal or Torres Strait Islander mental health workers and significant members of the person's community (including elders and traditional healers) in the assessment, examination and treatment of people who are of Aboriginal or Torres Strait Islander descent (Mental Health Commission Annual Report 2014/15; Government of Western Australia, 2014–15).

Stronger consumer, advisory and network mechanisms were established during this period, including significant developments such as establishing the Mental Health Advisory Council, developing an association for mental health consumers and recruitment of a dedicated consumer advisor position at the Commission. A stronger collaboration was also established with the non-government sector through the Commission's increased funding and partnership with the WA Association for Mental Health. These new arrangements complemented the important collaboration with traditional roles such as the Chief Psychiatrist, and the heads of the Mental Health Review Board and the Council of Official Visitors.

The new Mental Health Network was launched in October 2014 to provide a forum for consumers, families and carers, service providers and other stakeholders to contribute to improving the State's mental health system (Mental Health Commission Annual Report 2014/15; Government of Western Australia, 2014–15).

In July 2012, Professor Bryant Stokes delivered a report to the Western Australian Government into admission, transfer and discharge practices in public mental health services within Western Australia (Stokes, 2012). This review was jointly commissioned by the Mental Health Commission and the Department of Health in November 2011, with a view to ensuring that effective services, policies and practices are in place and consistently implemented.

The principal recommendation was for the development of a joint plan which was subsequently named the *Western Australian Mental Health, Alcohol and Other Drug Services Plan 2015–2025: Better Choices. Better Lives* (Mental Health Commission, 2019).

Modernising and locating mental health hospital beds closer to communities

The extensive hospital capital works program in WA since 2010 had many highlights including the opening of the new Broome Hospital Inpatient Unit, modernisation of Albany and Kalgoorlie Hospitals in the regions and the new Rockingham, Fiona Stanley, Midland and Perth Children's Hospitals in the metropolitan area. The State's first dedicated inpatient service for youth was opened at Fiona Stanley Hospital and a further youth unit was opened at Bentley Hospital.

The period since 2010 saw the building of a more comprehensive range of contemporary community-based services:

- The state's first sub-acute units were established and progressively developed including the first 22 bed unit in Joondalup (May 2013) and Rockingham (10 beds, October 2016). Planning, design and procurement activity was underway throughout 2017–18 to establish additional Step Up, Step Down services, providing a further 48 beds over the next four years in regional Western Australia. The Mental Health Commission's 2016/17 Annual Report cites evidence that Joondalup has been highly effective in both avoiding hospitalisation in the first instance and then hospital re-entry after discharge (p. 23).
- The state-wide Specialist Aboriginal Mental Health Service (SSAMHS) was established in 2010/11 to address the mental health needs of Aboriginal people in Western Australia. The program involves specialist Aboriginal mental health teams working with mainstream services to support Aboriginal people with severe and persistent mental health issues. SSAMHS funding provides 59.3 full-time equivalent staff across the state—including psychiatrists, Aboriginal health workers, clinical nurses, social workers, psychologists and coordination staff—many of whom are Aboriginal

people. Staff are employed through the Department of Health and the Kimberley Aboriginal Medical Services Council.

- The State's first multidisciplinary Mental Health Court Diversion Program was established in 2014, comprising the Adult Start Court and the Links Clinical Assessment Team in the Perth Children's Court. In 2017 enhancements included the addition of a dedicated Diversion Officer to provide assessment and referral to AOD treatment providers from the Start Court.
- The Individualised Community Living Strategy (ICLS) was established in 2102 with an initial target of 100 places to unblock hospital beds and helps people with severe mental illness to live in their community in their own homes throughout the state. This new and highly innovative initiative was based on the principles of self-directed support including a personal recovery plan, personal budget, choice of housing and choice of support provider. The holistic support offered through the ICLS is made possible by extensive collaboration between the Commission, the Department of Health, the Department of Housing and the numerous non-government mental health and housing organisations (Bartnik, 2015).
- The 2015 establishment of a Police and Mental Health co-response service in the north-west and south-east metropolitan districts.
- Youth mental health services continued to be strengthened during the time of the new Commission, building in the metropolitan area on Youth Link and Youth Reach South to include Youth Axis, Youth Hospital in the Home and 12 dedicated youth beds at Fiona Stanley Hospital. In 2015/16, the Commission allocated $1.8 million for a youth mental health service for people aged between 16 and 24 years of age in regional Western Australia including programs in the Pilbara and South West as well as a specialist youth clinical consultation and liaison service throughout regional Western Australia.
- A Western Australian Recovery College Expert Panel was appointed in 2017 to progress the co-design of a comprehensive, evidence-informed Model of Service for Recovery Colleges, that addresses the particular needs of Western Australians who experience mental health and co-occurring AOD issues (Mental Health Commission Annual Report, 2017/18; Mental Health Commission, 2018).

Looking forward

A key overall challenge underpinning implementation of the *Western Australian Mental Health, Alcohol and Other Drug Services Plan 2015–2025* (Mental Health Commission, 2019), remains to be the resourcing of sufficient intensity of community-based services to offset the urgent demand for emergency departments and inpatient hospital beds—thereby establishing the sought after balance of investments across the spectrum of prevention, community and acute hospital-based services.

A recent inquiry conducted by the State Auditor General (2019; Office of the Auditor General, 2019), found that while the Plan's articulation of the goals and targets for change are clear, WA still faces massive challenges in shifting the focus of its mental health system. For example, of the 212 000 people reported by the Auditor as having received mental health care between 2013 and 2017, just 10% of these used 90% of the total state-managed mental health hospital care and almost 50% of emergency and community treatment services. The proportion of hospital-based care increased from 42% to 47%, moving further away from the optimal 29% spend the MHC aimed to achieve by the end of 2025. The Auditor found that proportion of funding towards community treatment services remained the same at 43%. However, the proportion of funding for both prevention and community support had decreased instead of steadily increasing (3% to 1% and 8% to 5% respectively).

On this basis, the Auditor reported that the 'current mix of mental health services has not changed significantly and does not work as intended for some people' (p. 24).

The Fifth National Mental Health Plan and increased role of Primary Health Networks in regional commissioning provides an excellent opportunity for more integrated planning and commissioning alongside the WA Mental Health Commission.

The progressive funding of the optimal levels of psychosocial disability support for those people eligible under the NDIS also provides an unique opportunity to model the optimal mix of clinical services and start to demonstrate this in a targeted regional area, for example. The NDIS experience also provides for learning as to how self-directed support could be applied more broadly within the overall mental health system (as in the United Kingdom and the United States for example; Croft, Battis, Isvan, & Mahoney, 2020).

As public mental health services operate within the broader Department of Health system, the issue of mental health system clinical governance and overall financial sustainability continue to be a strong focus and challenge.

Further key challenges include planning for the decommissioning of Graylands Hospital (Mental Health Commission Annual Report 2017/18; Mental Health Commission, 2018), stabilising and reducing the number of suicides through the State Suicide Prevention Strategy against a national backdrop of a near 10% increase in the 2017/18 year and maximising the unique opportunities of the amalgamated mental health and drugs/alcohol capability in the Mental Health Commission.

PART 02

PRINCIPLES FOR COLLABORATIVE COMMUNITY PRACTICE

Part 2 explores the principles and approaches that inform the rapidly evolving, and increasingly complex landscape of community mental health practice. It brings our attention to the building of a recovery-oriented culture in mental health services, in which the lived experience, knowledge and insights of people with mental health issues and their families must be at the heart of what services do, so as to ensure high quality care and support.

Chapter 2.1 introduces the reader to the backgrounds and perspectives of a range of people who contribute to community mental health and may potentially be involved in supporting people experiencing mental health issues in their recovery—including experts by experience, family and carers, and mental health practitioners.

Chapter 2.2 explores collaboration, co-production and partnerships in complex systems for delivering community care and support, including: working collaboratively with people who have accessed services; with families and carers; within teams and networks of services; and with partnership and collaboration in cross-sectoral work.

Chapter 2.3 focuses on the conceptual, procedural and interpersonal aspects of assessment practice in mental health care. Beginning with consideration of assessment from a consumer perspective and the importance of reflective, critical, complexity and dialectical thinking, this chapter outlines processes for undertaking assessment, including awareness of diversity, principles of trauma-informed care and recovery-oriented practice. Discipline-oriented assessment from general practice, nursing, occupational therapy, clinical psychology and social work perspectives are also presented.

Chapter 2.4 examines case management, and the evolving nature of its practice in community mental health care within an Australian context. The centrality of developing and sustaining respectful and supportive working relationships with consumers, families and others; supported decision making and advance statements as practices central to supporting consumers in directing their own recovery; and contemporary implications in policy and law for involuntary treatment in the community are each highlighted.

Chapter 2.5 considers medications as one of the treatment options in mental health care, their uses, effectiveness and clinical practice guidelines.

Chapter 2.6 presents a range of approaches focused on social, occupational, psychological and physical dimensions of health and wellbeing that can contribute to promoting recovery and. It begins by highlighting how a recovery orientation, person-led approach and rights-based practice need to inform how these approaches are practised to promote self-determination, recovery and wellbeing.

Chapter 2.7 explores how families are affected by experiences of mental health issues and mental health services; the involvement of families in mental health care; and a range of family inclusive practices, including substantial evidence demonstrating the effectiveness of family interventions for improving family outcomes.

2.1

WHO PROVIDES MENTAL HEALTH CARE AND SUPPORT?

ELLIE FOSSEY, CATH ROPER, HAMILTON KENNEDY, RORY RANDALL, ANNETTE MERCURI, LOUISE STONE, GRANT BLASHKI, DAVID HUPPERT, KYLIE BOUCHER, FIONA BEST, JOHN FARHALL, MARILYN CUGNETTO, JUSTIN SCANLON, BANI AADAM, MELISSA PETRAKIS & HARRY MINAS

2.1.1 INTRODUCTION

CATH ROPER & ELLIE FOSSEY

Mental health care is an evolving field, and so the range of people in the mental health workforce is both diverse and constantly developing. In this chapter, we consider the perspectives of a range of people who may potentially play roles in supporting people experiencing mental health issues in their recovery–including peers, family and mental health practitioners. Recovering is often described as a personal journey of healing and growth, of 'living well' and being in control of one's life choices and decisions, while being supported, cared for and having a sense of someone 'being there' are often spoken about as important in promoting recovery (Davidson, Rowe, & Tondora, 2009). In other words, relationships with family, friends, peers and professionals can potentially support persons in recovery, but the quality of these relationships is crucial in whether or not they are recovery-promoting. Mutually respectful, hopeful and growth oriented relationships are highly prized by people in recovery. See Part 1 for further discussion of 'recovery', the origins of the recovery movement as a civil rights movement, and its significance as a driving force in recasting mental health policy and mental health services in Australia and internationally (see Sections 1.1.4, 1.1.6, 1.5.2, 1.5.8 and Chapter 1.7).

The lived experience, knowledge and insights of people with mental health issues and their families are at the heart of a recovery orientation to mental health practice and a recovery-oriented culture in mental health services (Australian Health Ministers' Advisory Council, 2013). Hence, this chapter begins with a focus on the lived experience perspectives and expertise of people living with mental health issues. This is followed by considering the perspectives of families and carers, and how a range of health practitioners view their potential contributions in offering mental health care or support to people experiencing mental health issues.

2.1.2 CONSUMER LIVED EXPERIENCE WORKFORCE

CATH ROPER

Contemporary mental health services are rapidly evolving, with workforces extending beyond the conventional professional disciplines. A significant proportion of this workforce now has lived experience of mental health issues. For example, people in this workforce are employed as consumer consultants, advocates, researchers, educators, and peer support workers. The balance in the workforce between experts by professional training and experts by lived experience is shifting; and roles for peer practitioners—both people in recovery, and families and carers—are expanding (Australian Health Ministers' Advisory Council, 2013). For mental health practitioners, this does not mean that their particular knowledge bases have no value or relevance, but it does mean that traditionally dominant knowledges in mental health services are insufficient in, and of themselves, to fully understand experiences of mental distress or how to support recovery (Slade, 2009a). Furthermore, it means that mental health services need to be founded on 'personal recovery', in which peers have a central place (Slade, 2009a).

2.1.3 PEER SUPPORT WORKERS

HAMILTON KENNEDY & RORY RANDALL

WHAT IS PEER SUPPORT?

The concept of peer support, broadly speaking, refers to the process of a person with a particular lived experience engaging in a supportive partnership with someone who might be experiencing something similar (O'Hagan, 2011). In mental health contexts, most commonly, this refers to the lived experience of using mental health services and experiencing challenges related to mental health. This is where peer support work is distinct from traditional support roles, it is a form of support that relies on a peer relationship based in equality and mutual support (Mead & Macneil, 2006).

Within peer support partnerships, both parties are assumed to have experiential knowledge and unique worldviews, exploration of which might involve respectful challenging, and can contribute to reciprocal learning, support and potentially new ways to conceptualise their experiences. Peer support work also makes no assumptions of deficits and the relatively non-hierarchical nature of the relationship, in contrast to traditional helpee/helper relationships, can empower people to advocate for what they want in their care and in understanding what they want their recovery to look like.

Peer support work might look different when it takes place in mainstream mental health organisations than it does in independent peer-led contexts; however, a consistent set of values and principles is central to the work. These include that the work should be:

- mutual
- hopeful
- empowering and encouraging of self-determination
- recovery-focused (where recovery is defined by the individual)
- person-led
- avoiding of assumptions
- avoiding stigmatisation of people
- challenging of power relationships and be empowering of consumers
- voluntarily engaged in
- encouraging of accountability/responsibility
- strength based
- trauma-informed (Centre of Excellence in Peer Support, 2011; Western Australian Association for Mental Health, 2014).

Peer support workers not only provide support for consumers (service users), but their particular set of values, skills and approach can prove useful for clinical staff in understanding ways to connect and work with consumer. These perspectives and their influence on culture and discourse have the opportunity to promote a focus on human rights that may have been lost or impinged upon in risk-averse services and public policy.

Mental health peer support occurs in a broad variety of contexts. These contexts are contingent upon the peer support worker's particular lived experience, which makes them a peer in that setting. Some examples of the settings in which peer support takes place include:

- community peer support work
- inpatient peer support work–Step Up-Step Down services
- residential services
- vocational peer support work
- alcohol and other drugs and dual diagnosis peer support work
- forensic peer support work
- peer-run crisis hotlines
- carer peer support work
- LGBTIQ peer support work.

ENTERING THE PEER WORKFORCE

While a lived experience qualifies one to be a peer support worker, as the field expands, so do the options for formal training in peer support work and minimum requirements for roles. This has manifested in many jobs requiring formal qualifications and training and in the recent creation of the Certificate IV in Mental Health Peer Work. This has been met with mixed reactions from peer workers and their employers. Some have suggested that the person's lived experience itself is the qualification required to undertake peer work, while others have expressed that formalising the workforce is important to ensuring that the workforce is consistent in its approach. Some of the available trainings for peer support work include the intentional peer support, or the one- and five-day peer support trainings from Mind Australia. These are excellent entry level trainings for individuals looking to start work in the field. Another option for entry to the peer support workforce is through volunteer experience. Many non-government organisations run volunteer peer support programs that also include access to subsidised or free relevant training.

It is important to note that someone does not need to be 'cured' of their experiences of mental health challenges to be an effective peer support worker; the key competency for the role is a capacity to meaningfully reflect upon one's experiences.

PEER WORK IN PRACTICE

Identity

Being a peer support worker in mental health explicitly signals having previous, or ongoing experiences of mental illness. This can come with difficulty for the peer support worker as it can mean defining oneself by that lived experience and associated clinical labels. Revisiting this identity on a daily basis, or even just working in service settings where one might have memories of difficult experiences, can often prove retraumatising for the peer support worker. On the other hand, engaging in peer support work can be experienced as supportive by workers themselves (Mead & Macneil, 2006).

Tensions in peer support work

There can often be a tension between lived experience and other staff due to differences in values, or where services request peer support workers to perform tasks that are incongruent with peer support work principles.

Peer support is not intended to be a therapy, although it can be therapeutic. It is also not intended to be used in the conduct of assessments, outcome measures or to be complicit in restrictive or prescriptive practices. For example, undertaking an assessment of symptomatology would fall into the category of staff 'doing to' a consumer, as opposed to a mutually agreed upon and undertaken task, and be considered in contradiction with the principles of peer work. Similarly at odds with the principles of peer support work is the tendency for services to capitalise on a peer support worker's unique ability to form meaningful relationships as the means to elicit information from the people with whom service providers are working. To obtain information for the purposes of sharing with other colleagues, without permission from the consumer, would again transgress the values that underpin peer work.

The values, principles and practice of peer support work can complement traditional mainstream mental health care and contribute to the provision of recovery-oriented services and the reduction of stigma and discrimination (Mahlke et al., 2014). However, for the roles to be successful, employers have the responsibility to ensure access to supports. Critical issues for the implementation of peer support roles within mainstream services include that roles are well designed, job descriptions are clear and effective organisational support strategies are in place (Mahlke et al., 2014). Peer support workers need regular access to discipline-specific supervision or supervising staff who have a clear understanding of intentions of peer support work and training and work arrangements are necessary to mitigate what can be stressful employment for the peer workforce (Mahlke et al., 2014; Walker & Bryant, 2013). Barriers to the effectiveness of peer support from the perspective of workers themselves include the lack of perceived credibility for their work, negative attitudes from staff, poor organisational arrangements, and inadequate overarching social and mental health policies (Vandewalle et al., 2016).

2.1.4 CARERS AND CARER WORKFORCE

ANNETTE MERCURI

WHO IS A CARER?

Carers do not necessarily identify themselves as carers as they more usually think of a carer as a person who is paid to care/support someone. Unpaid or informal carers usually see themselves as a member of the family: a mother, father, sibling, son or daughter, aunt, uncle, grandparent, partner or friend. According to the Australian Government's *Carer Recognition Act 2010* (Cth), an individual is not a *carer* merely because of either being a person's partner or family member, or because of living with a person who requires care and support, but a carer can be anyone who is in a 'care relationship' with another person. Hence, 'a carer is an individual who provides personal care, support and assistance to another individual who needs it because that other individual has a disability; or has a medical condition (including a terminal or chronic illness); or has a mental illness; or is frail and aged' (Australian Government, 2010). While mental health legislation varies between the state jurisdictions in Australia (see Chapter 1.3), a carer may be similarly defined. For example, Victoria's *Mental Health Act 2014 Handbook* defines a carer as 'a person, including a person under the age of 18 years, who provides care to another person with whom he or she is in a care relationship but does not include a parent if the person to whom care is provided is under the age of 16 years' (Victoria State Government, 2018).

Approximately 240 000 informal carers were supporting people with mental health issues in Australia in 2015, representing an estimated economic contribution of $14.3 billion to community mental health care (Diminic et al., 2016). So, 'family caregivers are an irreplaceable resource for the mental health services system and the pillars on which the system currently rests' (Shankar & Muthuswamy, 2007, p. 302). Yet, caring is also stressful and many carers, especially young carers, are unrecognised, unsupported, and expected to manage on their own (Gray, Robinson, & Seddon, 2008; Wilkinson & McAndrew, 2008). Having someone in the family diagnosed with a mental illness is often extremely traumatic for the carer/family, as well as the consumer, and may impact relationships with all family members, as well as children's development (State of Victoria, Department of Premier and Cabinet, 2017). Carers may also feel they have no choice but to take up the caring role, with the majority seeing it as a family responsibility that they cannot deny. As a result, carers are at risk of poorer mental and physical health, as well as financial impacts of caring (see Chapter 2.7).

To address some of these issues, carers need to be recognised, respected for their knowledge and expertise, and included as partners in care with access to information to support the caring role and support for themselves (Australian Government,

2010c; Worthington & Rooney, 2010). When clinical mental health services focus predominantly on the relationship between patient/consumer and mental health practitioner, carers may be overlooked and need to overcome unhelpful staff attitudes and communication barriers in trying to access information on how to assist the consumer (Rowe, 2012). In addition, misunderstandings about confidentiality, what can be shared and when represents one of the biggest barriers to effective communication between mental health practitioners and carers, which in turn limits carers being able to support the consumer (Wynaden & Orb, 2005), as well as address their own and the families' wellbeing (Pagnini, NSW Health, & Carers NSW, 2005).

Carers and families may support consumers in a variety of practical ways, including providing encouragement and motivation, managing crises, paperwork, bills, medication support, self-care and household tasks, as well as by providing emotional support, advocacy and liaising with health professionals. They also have long-term knowledge of the consumer, his or her life experiences and behaviours pre-mental illness and those that reflect symptoms (Froggatt, Fadden, Johnson, Leggatt, & Shankar, 2007). An abundance of research highlights overwhelmingly that working in partnership with family/carers results in better outcomes not only for consumers but also for carers and indeed for the community at large (Worthington & Rooney, 2010). (See Chapter 2.2.)

A carer workforce with lived experience and knowledge related to carer needs, carer peer support, advocacy and service development is evolving in the mental health sector (Paton & Sanders, 2011). This includes carer consultants, carer peer support workers and carer advocates.

Carer consultant

A carer consultant is a person with lived experience of caring/supporting someone with mental illness, who is employed by mental health services to provide both a personal and a broader carer perspective to service delivery and development. With lived experience of caring for someone with mental illness, the carer consultant brings experience of many of the barriers to accessing support from mental health services, and can identify where the service can improve in its collaborative practice to provide better outcomes not only for carers, but also for consumers, which is the ultimate goal of the carer. The role is predominantly a systemic advocacy role that informs the executive and professional development of the service, with the aim of improving service responsiveness to the needs of families and carers (Paton & Sanders, 2011). Some carer consultants over the years have provided carer peer support as well.

The carer consultant role has been pivotal in highlighting the need for carers to be supported in their caring role and involved in the treatment partnership wherever possible. Part of the work has also involved educating mental health practitioners about how to work in partnership with consumers and carers and how to overcome the perceived barriers that impede this work. The carer consultant role has expanded significantly since its inception, shifting from a largely isolated role that essentially ensured a service met its policy requirement for carer participation to an integrated Lived Experience discipline providing education to mental health practitioners and carers, running carer advisory groups, and developing and overseeing a team of carer peer support workers.

Carer peer support worker

The carer peer support worker is a person with carer lived experience who is employed by a mental health service to engage with carers/family on a peer-to-peer level to support them in their own recovery journey. While the consumer may have a whole treating team to support them on their recovery journey, the carer very often is isolated and trying to manage as best they can. Carer peer support workers can assist carers to identify their own self-care needs and focus on their own wellbeing, as well as being a willing ear with whom the carer can speak openly and confidentially, without fear of saying the wrong thing or prompting negative responses from the consumer or treating team. Carer peer support workers can facilitate linkages for family/carer support both within the service and wider community, so as to provide support and information to family/carers about mental illness, navigating the mental health system, dealing with challenging situations, as well as their rights and responsibilities. They also provide peer education and facilitate the collaboration between the mental health practitioner, consumer and family/carer, however it is also important to understand carer peer support is a separate adjunct to clinical services and not an avenue for mental health practitioners to access further information about the consumer. There are explicit boundaries to carer peer support work, in which confidentiality for the carer is upheld and information only shared with mental health practitioners when the carer has given explicit permission for doing so, or in situations where there is a duty of care to disclose.

Carer advocate

A carer advocate is a person with carer lived experience and advocacy training who works independently of mental health services. Carers have identified that navigating the mental health system, including service complaints systems, is difficult and daunting (Paton & Sanders, 2011). Carer advocates can assist carers to identify issues/complaints and accompany carers to discussions/meetings with mental health services. They provide carers with individualised support to address issues, such as being excluded or not being listened to by the service providers, or concerns about how they or the consumer may have been treated by the mental health service. Carer advocates can also support carers who have made complaints to the Mental Health Complaints Commission in meetings with the mental health services to ensure the carer's voice is heard, complaints/issues are acted upon and resolved wherever possible.

2.1.5 THE ROLE OF GENERAL PRACTITIONERS IN MENTAL HEALTH CARE

LOUISE STONE & GRANT BLASHKI

For the vast majority of people who seek professional treatment for a mental illness, the first port of call will be a general practitioner (GP) (Australian Bureau of Statistics, 2016c; Australian Institute of Health and Welfare, 2018b). Australian general practitioners are pivotal to the provision of mental health care in the community, with more than 11% of GP consultations involving a mental health problem (Britt et al., 2010).

GPs provide assessment, management and coordination of care to a diverse patient population with a range of mental health needs. They are in a unique position to do so, because they are reasonably accessible to most consumers. GPs provide care in rural and remote communities, in institutional settings such as nursing homes and correctional facilities, and within other settings targeting specific populations, such as Aboriginal medical services and in refugee health centres. GPs also provide important mental health services for vulnerable communities who may have reduced access to other services (Australian Institute of Health and Welfare, 2010, 2011a).

GPs are uniquely placed too because they assess people in the early stages of illness, when consumers may not recognise that they have a mental disorder. Mental illness often presents with a complex mix of physical and psychological concerns that can make the diagnosis more difficult (Clarke, Piterman, Byrne, & Austin, 2008; Stone, 2013, 2015). The very nature of general practice, including care of physical disorders and understanding individuals' past medical histories, means that GPs are well placed to integrate what are often very complex intertwined clinical presentations.

Most early deaths of people with mental health disorders are due to physical illness (Lawrence, Hancock, & Kisely, 2013) and there is increasing interest in the physical health needs of consumers (National Mental Health Strategy, 2017). GPs provide long-term continuity of care, which is essential for people who are experiencing mental disorders, especially in the context of comorbid physical illness. GPs also manage stressful life events that may trigger the onset of mental illness, such as birth, injury, the diagnosis of serious illness or end of life care. GPs can also provide consumers and carers with resources and strategies to navigate the mental health care system and reach their recovery goals.

People at risk of mental health disorders can also be screened in the GP setting. This often offers a low-stigma option (Komiti, Judd, & Jackson, 2006) for people including carers, veterans and refugees (Wang & Du, 2019; Hodson & McFarlane, 2016; Farley, Askew, & Kay, 2014), as well as people with strong family histories of mental illness. GPs in rural settings may also manage whole communities at risk, especially after trauma such as natural disasters (Edwards, Gray, & Hunter, 2015; Farley et al., 2014; Rigby, Rosen, Berry, & Hart, 2011).

BARRIERS TO MENTAL HEALTH CARE IN GENERAL PRACTICE

General practice does present some significant barriers for people accessing mental health care (Gunn et al., 2012). Perhaps the greatest difficulty is the perennial competing demands that are unavoidable in a generalist clinical setting (Cheshire et al., 2017). Mental health care is only one of a number of priorities, which include care of chronic physical illnesses, prevention of disease and health promotion, and acute care (Gunn et al., 2012). This broad range of clinical responsibilities not only impinges on the time available for mental health care, but it also affects the GP's relationships with patients (Stone, 2014). The GP's role is often shifting, at times ambiguous, and may include other roles, such as certification of fitness to work (Gunn et al., 2012).

The fee-for-service billing system can also blur clinical responsibility. In Australia, a consumer can see a number of GPs, and it is easy for continuity to lapse (Hofer & McDonald, 2019). Australia's fee-for-service system also rewards short consultations and procedural practice, rather than long mental health consultations (Duckett, Swerissen, & Moran, 2017). Disadvantaged communities have lower access to other mental health services, increasing the burden of care for GPs and making access to longer consultations more challenging (Meadows, Enticott, Inder, Russell, & Gurr, 2015).

DIAGNOSING MENTAL HEALTH PROBLEMS IN GENERAL PRACTICE

Much has been made in peer-reviewed literature over the last few decades about missed diagnoses by GPs, particularly of depression (Carey et al., 2014). In these studies, GP diagnoses are usually compared with validated psychiatric questionnaires and tend to conclude that the GPs have missed a significant proportion of the mental disorders among their patients. To some extent, this says more about the philosophical underpinnings and culture of this type of research than about GPs' clinical skills (Lampe et al., 2012). That is, whether or not a psychiatric diagnosis is made in general practice is much more complex than a symptom count or a list of criteria.

For people who are distressed with a mental disorder, what they choose to disclose to the GP, how they conceptualise their distress, and indeed whether or not they are amenable to the idea of a mental disorder, are as important as the specific nature of their symptoms (Berry, Hogan, Owen, Rickwood, & Fragar, 2011; Reavley, Cvetkovski, Jorm, & Lubman, 2010). In general, the diagnosis of mental disorder in general practice is something that emerges over time and multiple consultations, as a shared understanding between the GP and the consumer. It is also fair to say that the diagnostic processes are intimately bound up with the person's beliefs, and their background, the perceived stigma around mental illness and their perceptions of possible treatment options (Jimenez, Bartels, Cardenas, Dhaliwal, & Alegría, 2012). Recovery-oriented practice requires an understanding of these beliefs and an open and frank dialogue about the way in which a consumer may choose to conceptualise their distress. Early in the illness, this may take some time.

Diagnosis is also complicated by the prevalence of somatisation (see Chapter 4.6) in the GP setting. Somatisation, or the tendency to 'experience and communicate somatic distress in response to psychosocial stress' (Lipowski, 1988), is more common in Australian general practice than depression or anxiety (Clarke, Piterman, et al., 2008). However, it is not the only way that mixed emotional and physical symptoms can present. It is common for GPs to need to manage mental illness triggered by certain medications. It is also common for people to experience mental illness as part of another chronic illness, such as hypothyroidism, anaemia and some forms of cancer. Similarly, conditions such as cardiac arrhythmia can present predominantly with anxiety. Consumers with existing major illness commonly experience depression, but may present differently from people with depression occurring without concurrent chronic illness (O'Keeffe & Ranjith, 2007). Symptoms of physical disease, side effects of physical treatment and associated disability can all have an impact on the assessment and management of mental illness in the setting of chronic disease (Clarke, Cook, Smith, & Piterman, 2008; Stanners, Barton, Shakib, & Winefield, 2012).

MENTAL HEALTH CARE REFORMS IN AUSTRALIA

In 2001, the Australian Government recognised the high burden of common mental health disorders and the poor integration of medical and psychological care for consumers. In acknowledgement that psychological treatments were not accessed evenly across the population, the Better Outcomes in Mental Health Care initiative was introduced (Pirkis, Kohn, Morley, Burgess, & Blashki, 2004). The scheme was designed to provide time-limited, evidence-based, non-pharmacological treatments for common mental health disorders, and enabled GPs to access subsidised psychological services for their patients.

Now called the Better Access initiative, it incorporates the key elements of assessment and planning by the GP, subsidised allied health services and additional GP mental health training. The scheme is available to anyone with a mental health disorder 'who would benefit from a structured approach to their mental health care needs' (Medicare program, 2019). At the core of this initiative is the mental health treatment plan, a document shared between consumers, carers and health service providers to enhance coordination and integration of care. Most GPs under this scheme undertake mental health skills training, while some GPs undertake extended training to provide 'focused psychological strategies' under the scheme. This additional training is designed to assist GPs with an interest in extended mental health care to utilise evidence-based strategies for the treatment of common mental health disorders. Training is usually based on cognitive behavioural therapy and interpersonal therapy models.

Better Access delivered over 18 million services between 2015 and 2016 with over 10% of Australians accessing Medicare-subsidised mental health services in 2017-18 (Australian Institute of Health and Welfare, 2018b). This represents a doubling of services when compared with 2007-2008 (Pirkis et al., 2011). Nevertheless, access to mental health services is unevenly spread across the country, and while assessment options have expanded with the implementation of telepsychiatry and fly-in, fly-out services, GPs can still struggle to access specialist care that is accessible and affordable for their patients.

GPs navigate a complex mix of acute mental health services, community-based state-funded services, non-government organisations, Primary Health Network commissioned services and private practitioners to coordinate care for their patients. The constantly changing landscape of services and funding arrangements is a continuing struggle for GPs, consumers and carers alike. Consumers in rural and remote settings have greater difficulty accessing services, and this means rural GPs need additional skills. Management of mental health emergencies is particularly challenging, especially when patients require sedation for safe transport (Bishop, Ransom, & Laverty, 2017; Ellis & Philip, 2010).

GP as prescriber of pharmacological treatments

An important role for GPs is the prescription of psychotropic medications. Common medication classes that GPs prescribe include the antidepressants, anxiolytics, hypnotics and the antipsychotic medications. GPs prescribed over 90% of psychotropic medication in Australia in 2016–17 (Australian Institute of Health and Welfare, 2018b), although some of these medications are undoubtedly initiated by psychiatrists, or administered with psychiatrist advice.

GPs need to consider the severity of illness, co-existing physical or mental illness, likely side effects, potential for abuse or overdose and the consumer's health beliefs and cultural background when commencing or continuing to prescribe psychotropic medication. Consumers and carers may be concerned about a range of side effects, including the potential for addiction, and may also be concerned about the stigma of taking a psychotropic medication (Reavley & Jorm, 2011). Careful, targeted patient education material and a strong therapeutic alliance can assist both the consumer and families to make well informed decisions about initiating or continuing medication (Stacey et al., 2017; Thompson & McCabe, 2012).

A plethora of psychotropic medications and brands exist, from which the GP can choose. Pharmaceutical companies have strong vested interests in encouraging GPs to prescribe their brand, and can overemphasise the differences and advantages of their recommended medication. The marked increase in psychotropic prescribing in the last decade suggests that extensive marketing of certain medications has been effective (Stephenson, Karanges, & McGregor, 2012).

A sensible approach for GPs is to become comfortable and familiar with two or three medications in each class, so as to develop a feel for its particular effects on patients, and also the likely side-effect profile, interactions and problems that can occur (De Vries et al., 1994). Guidelines, such as those developed by the Royal Australian College of Psychiatrists (Malhi et al., 2015), can assist GPs to make rational prescribing decisions.

A central aspect of monitoring of mental illness is monitoring of medication. Some medications require very specific monitoring regimes, such as the prescription of lithium or clozapine. Monitoring should also include checking for common physical disorders associated with medication. For example, some antipsychotic medications have been associated with raised levels of lipids and glucose. In the case of the antidepressants, by far the most commonly prescribed psychotropic medication, caution is also required when reducing or ceasing the medication, as withdrawal syndromes are common.

GP as coordinator of mental health care

Traditionally, GPs have been responsible for care coordination, but this can be challenging in mental health. Communication between the various service providers is often problematic (Fuller et al., 2011). Carers and consumers often differ in their understanding, expectations and choices during decision making (Jacob, Munro, Taylor, & Griffiths, 2017). There are also issues when care plans intersect. The person with chronic illness, for instance, will often have several teams involved in his or her care, and intersecting guidelines for the management of the various conditions. For consumers, carers and GPs, this can be confusing, frustrating and even dangerous. Consumers with the continuous care of a GP and a well-planned, integrated and multidisciplinary collaborative care plan receive better care and better health outcomes (Mitchell et al., 2015).

For people who are isolated, either through geography, language and cultural barriers or disability, the GP can coordinate mental health care in different ways to overcome these barriers. For example, telepsychiatry services and e-health options for education and intervention are expanding, and evidence for positive outcomes is growing (Langarizadeh et al., 2017; Reynolds, Griffiths, Cunningham, Bennett, & Bennett, 2015). These distance treatments and sources of advice for GPs will expand over time (see Sections 1.2.5, 1.5.9).

GP as the first point of call for crisis

GPs manage more than mental health disorders. Other common and distressing life events and circumstances can adversely affect mental health and benefit from identification and treatment. Trauma, through accident, injury or assault requires a coordinated approach to care (Wade, Howard, Fletcher, Cooper, & Forbes, 2013). Victims of sexual violence (Tarzia et al., 2017; Taylor, Pugh, Goodwach, & Coles, 2012) or intimate partner violence (Hegarty,

Forsdike-Young, Tarzia, Schweitzer, & Vlais, 2016; Hegarty & O'Doherty, 2011) are often managed in the GP setting. Life crises, such as bereavement (Breen, 2011), infertility (Alesi, 2005), palliative care (Armitage & Trethewie, 2014; Mitchell, 2014) and the advent of serious illness (Thistlethwaite, 2009) all require sensitive mental health care and preventive strategies. Bereavement is often particularly complex following suicide (Spillane, Matvienko-Sikar, Larkin, Corcoran, & Arensman, 2018). In rural and remote areas, the GP may be the central health professional managing the consequences of natural disasters or other community-wide issues with mental health consequences, such as drought (Carnie, Berry, Blinkhorn, & Hart, 2011; Hart, Berry, & Tonna, 2011).

Doctors' health and wellbeing

It is also important to recognise that GPs experience high rates of suicide, depression, anxiety disorders, substance abuse and self-medication (Beyond Blue, 2013; Lemaire & Wallace, 2017). Recent attempts to address these concerns have led to local and national programs to address the mental health of doctors. Peer support programs and access to safe, confidential mental health services are critical to raise awareness and improve management of mental illness in the medical community (Rowe & Kidd, 2018).

2.1.6 MENTAL HEALTH AND EMERGENCY RESPONSE SERVICES

DAVID HUPPERT

ROLE OF TRIPLE ZERO EMERGENCY SYSTEMS AND TELEPHONE TRIAGE

Triple zero (000) is the Australian emergency number designed to be the central point of contact for calling police, ambulance or fire services. The triple zero service triages calls to one of the three emergency services. Trained personnel continue the process and trigger a response that is usually determined by an organised decision-making process.

Local public health and mental health triage services provide an additional form of access to the emergency response to that of triple zero. These local telephone triage systems typically connect to a local mental health service, which has the capacity to mobilise a community mental health response to mental health crises.

The process of triage by various services is usually undertaken by senior staff and enables an efficient and effective way of determining the next requirement for consumers. Poor triage can be associated with morbidity and poorer outcomes.

Immediate responses in the community: ambulance

In Australia, ambulance services mostly provide urgent medical responses with various service delivery systems in place depending on the geography and population density. Practices in city settings can differ significantly from rural settings. Volunteer ambulance services are often in place in smaller communities, and have a greater knowledge of their local population compared with services in metropolitan communities. Sometimes significant rural distances make access to specialist medical or mental health services more difficult (for example, transport to acute mental health inpatient units after local assessments may take many hours).

The role of the ambulance services with regard to mental health may vary widely. Other than the provision of emergency care, the ambulance service may also provide transport of mental health patients for initial evaluation. Rural, metropolitan and air ambulance responses also differed more profoundly across geographic and ambulance transport types. Various legislative requirements in state and territory Mental Health Acts guide processes and care. Sedation guidelines are evolving for use by ambulance personnel to manage acute behavioural disturbances. These are not always aligned with emergency department and mental health sedation guidelines and will be an area of discussion and review in coming years. In New South Wales, ambulance services have the same powers as police under the *Mental Health Act 2007* (NSW) (New

South Wales Government, 2007), that is, they may detain and transport a person due to risk, for the purpose of taking an individual to a medical practitioner for a mental health evaluation.

Ambulance emergency responses systems are the most utilised service by the community for transport to hospital emergency departments (EDs). They frequently manage a very broad range of acute and diagnostic issues that increasingly include mental health and substance use.

Immediate responses in the community: police

Police interaction with people with mental illness and behavioural disturbance in the community may be triggered by triple zero calls, or during police day-to-day activities. As with ambulances, the type of police response may depend on the different service systems in place across states and geographic areas.

When people with mental health problems demonstrate a need for attention or exhibit abnormal or dangerous behaviour in a public place, police services are often called. Their capacity to respond rapidly means they are often on the scene before any other emergency service. They may not be familiar with the person or his or her background history. They are often required to make a judgement call on what risks exist and what should occur next.

Specific police work related to mental health care will also include a range of other functions. These include emergency response, apprehension under mental health legislation, locating mental health patients who abscond from involuntary inpatient care, support to community mental health services in assessment and management of risk in community assessment and treatment, and support to mental health inpatient services in containment of violence and investigation of violence or assault on inpatient units.

A police officer's training, attitude and experience will sometimes influence his or her decision as to whether to charge an individual or seek resolution and health interventions. Health and mental health strategies that help police to attain their imperatives can be useful in de-escalation techniques, provision of specific information as the first-on-the-scene observers for health providers, and a frame of understanding individuals they might frequently encounter with complex psychiatric, personality and physical issues.

Police emergency response services are often involved in social welfare and safety in their duties. They regularly encounter substance and mental health issues in their day-to-day activities and frequently rely on specialist mental health services to complete formal assessment of individuals they believe to be at risk.

EMERGENCY AND CRISIS MENTAL HEALTH SERVICES

The onset of a severe mental health crisis, as we have noted, brings into action both emergency and mental health services. In light of this, various service configurations have developed in Australia and other countries in an attempt to provide a coherent and coordinated response in such situations.

Many states and territories in Australia have similar systemic issues with bed access and with ED and police mental health interface with the community mental health teams who perform acute or outreach functions. These teams are known by a variety of names, for example, Acute Care Team (ACT) in Queensland and NSW and Crisis or Community Assessment and Treatment Team (CATT) in Victoria. They are connected in various ways to community mental health clinics, acute mental health wards and ED mental health service personnel, as well as mental health triage services.

The role of these teams is to provide alternatives to hospitalisation or assist with early discharge from acute units. However, their ability to respond to police requests for mental health evaluation has become limited with their increased involvement in sub-acute home care and a subsequent reduced capacity to provide urgent unplanned response. This shift, and a corresponding differing expectation of the police and public regarding the role of crisis mental health services, has led to some adverse public perceptions. The Victorian Auditor-General Report (2009) report on *Responding to Mental Health Crisis in the Community* describes this issue and the gaps in care.

Deinstitutionalisation has led to increasing mental health resources being delivered in the community and the evolution of community-based emergency and urgent response teams. This is a trend that will likely continue with the types of services designed to suit the city or region that operate within.

Mental health care in emergency departments

Over the last 30 years, there has been considerable change in the mental health and emergency services interface. This has been the result of a number of factors such as change in bed access and location. Changes in the configuration of mental health acute services and deinstitutionalisation, which decommissioned many stand-alone psychiatric asylums and established integrated mental health facilities within general health organisations.

EDs have grown and evolved in recent decades. Typically, 5% of patients attending the ED will have mental health issues, including patients with comorbid medical conditions (Alarcon Manchego, Knott, Graudins, Bartley, & Mitra, 2015). ED design often does not take into consideration the behaviourally disturbed person and the arrival of police. Gun storage, secure rooms for evaluation and access to specialist mental health expertise in the emergency department are some of the issues that complicate the work of ED staff and police.

With a general increase in demand in EDs and a filtering of non-urgent cases to nearby super-clinics, the number of acute cases presenting is amplified with the most unwell people presenting to ED. There are periods of time when EDs have excessive demand and access to inpatient beds (including acute mental health) is limited. This has led to delays in moving patients from ED to acute inpatient beds, and sometimes mental health patients are caught up in this system-related issue. Delivery of acute mental health care to patients waiting for beds precipitates a new set of challenges, with a high-stimulus environment and poor privacy.

Security services have become a more common feature of large emergency departments. The reliance on such personnel to assist in the care of the mental health or behaviourally disturbed individuals can be complex. Training and education of ED staff and security providers are important in order to facilitate safe and effective care.

There has been a trend for increased use of EDs by patients with mental health and substance issues. It places increased and different demands on EDs that require systems adjustments and improved collaboration between mental health and emergency services.

Mental health clinical streams in emergency departments

Some service systems have mental health staff assigned to emergency departments for 24 hours a day, seven days per week, and provide services through a consultation liaison model. In other health services, there is direct psychiatric care in specific mental health units co-located with, for example, Brisbane EDs Psychiatric Emergency Centre (Frank, Fawcett, & Emmerson, 2005). Mental health clinicians working in these types of services are usually highly experienced and work mostly autonomously. They also have significant connection to acute inpatient mental health services as well as community mental health services.

To increase flow through ED and change the health system's acute care options, short stay units (SSU) have become a growing service element in many large emergency departments, particularly in metropolitan and larger cities. These SSUs are designed to allow sub-acute care for a limited period of time (usually less than 24 hours) as an alternative to prolonged stay in ED or formal admission to a typical acute health bed. Acute behavioural disturbance and significant risk (suicide, self-harm and harm to others) are contraindications. Such units are usually staffed by ED staff and are co-located with EDs.

In recent years, new models have emerged in EDs or adjacent to EDs, to manage the changes in demands. These include new initiatives such as PECC (NSW), HOPE teams (Vic) and Crisis hubs (Vic).

Psychiatric Emergency Care Centres (PECC) have evolved in NSW (Brakoulias, Seymour, Lee, Sammut, & Starcevic, 2013) as 4–6 bed SSUs adjacent to the ED that allow for 48 hour stays. These units are often managed directly by mental health with separate governance structures to EDs.

The Way Back Support Service (Beyond Blue, 2018), a new initiative in various states, and the Hospital Outreach Post-suicide Engagement (HOPE) teams (Department of Health and Human Service Victoria, 2018a) are new services that build on the experience of clinicians working with individuals who attend ED with suicide attempts. The latter team provides clinical and nonclinical care and practical support for 3 months following an ED presentation for attempted suicide.

Mental health and addiction crisis hubs are a new initiative in Victoria (Department of Health and Human Service Victoria, 2018b). They seek to extend the role of ECATT and combine a 28-day brief follow-up function to mental and addiction issues that present to ED. As a specialist stream within ED, they will bring further resources and amenity to EDs.

MENTAL HEALTH AND POLICE PARTNERSHIP MODELS

The number of police, ambulance and criminal justice partnership models in Australia and around the world has increased in recent years. There is acknowledgement that combining the expertise of various agencies that have overlapping areas of activity can lead to improved outcomes for individuals with mental health and addiction issues. The extent and type of partnerships are broad and may include education and combined primary response as well as secondary and tertiary responses.

The Mental Health Intervention Team (MHIT) has been operating since 2008, and seeking to improve mental health awareness of police officers in New South Wales (NSW Police Force, 2008). Mental Health First Aid Training (Mental Health First Aid Australia, 2018) provides for more intense education for organisations frequently in contact with individuals with mental health needs.

The Police Ambulance Crisis Emergency Response (PACER) team is a novel police and mental health partnership model that has been trialled in metropolitan Melbourne since 2007 (Huppert & Griffiths, 2015). Many similar teams now operate around Australia in metropolitan and regional areas. These teams typically have a mental health clinician and police officer working together as a team and closely link to local police and public health service mental health and EDs. They seek to intervene early in the community and improve the pathway of care, reducing unnecessary ED admissions and the risk of behavioural escalation in the community.

Fixated Threat and Assessment Centre (FTAC) teams were first created in the United Kingdom in 2006 (Metropolitan Police Service, 2018) and have recently been established in Australia. These teams are a partnership between police, counter terrorism and mental health services that offer support to local mental health, addiction and police services through expert assessments of risk, treatment and management strategies. They focus on individuals with fixation on for example, public official, royalty, and parliamentarians, as well as on individuals with pathological grievances. Individuals who are part of terrorist groups are excluded as they are dealt with by other services.

These cooperative partnership models between police and mental health services seek to identify at an early stage individuals with mental health and/or drug and alcohol issues who may be amenable to health care interventions that can reduce the risk.

FTAC, PACER and other partnership models seek to harness the combined knowledge and expertise of police and mental health services, to deliver person-centred safe and effective care as well as reduce the risk to individuals and community.

2.1.7 MENTAL HEALTH NURSES

KYLIE BOUCHER

Mental health nursing is a branch of nursing that focuses on working with people with mental health concerns. In Australia, the usual pathway to begin working in mental health nursing is the same as for other nursing fields, the completion of a 3-year degree for registered nurses or a diploma of nursing for enrolled nurses. Many services offer mental health specific graduate programs to new nurses to aid in their transition from student to mental health nurse. Many services and industrial agreements then expect or require that nurses will get further qualifications in mental health nursing, such as a postgraduate diploma or masters, before gaining permanent employment in mental health nursing or promotion to higher levels of responsibility. The Australian College of Mental Health Nurses (ACMHN) is the peak professional mental health nursing body in Australia. The ACMHN states that 'a Mental Health Nurse is a registered nurse who holds a recognised specialist qualification in mental health' (Australian College of Mental Health Nurses, 2010, p.5), though there are nurses practising solely in mental health who have not acquired those specialist qualifications.

THE MENTAL HEALTH NURSING WORKFORCE

Both registered nurses (RNs) and enrolled nurses (ENs) can work in mental health. In 2016 almost 7% of all nurses employed in Australia worked primarily in mental health and 85% of these were registered nurses (Australian Institute of Health and Welfare, 2018). Mental health nurses are mainly employed in the public sector in hospital and community health settings (Australian Institute of Health and Welfare, 2018b; Victorian Government Department of Health, 2011). There is a shortage of mental health nurses, partly attributable to the ageing workforce (Victorian Government Department of Health, 2011).

Mental health registered nurses can become nurse practitioners (MHNPs). MHNPs have specialist skills and training and are endorsed to work autonomously and in advanced clinical roles.

Practice Standards

A number of legislative standards guide mental health nursing practice. As for all nurses, mental health nurses must renew their registration with the Nursing and Midwifery Board of Australia (NMBA) each year, in a process is managed by the Australian Health Practitioner Regulation Agency (AHPRA). Nurses must meet the NMBA professional stands which include codes of conduct, standards for practice (previously called 'competency standards') and codes of ethics.

The ACMHN has published Standards of Practice for Australian Mental Health Nurses that 'specify the minimum level of performance required for a registered nurse practising in any mental health setting' (Australian College of Mental Health Nurses, 2010, p. 5). In 2013 the ACMHN also published *Scope of Practice of Mental Health Nurses in Australia* which broadly describes the parameters that guide mental health nursing practice (Australian College of Mental Health Nurses, 2013). In summary the Scope of Practice of MH nurses is 'nested within a holistic theoretical and clinical framework..., distinguished by person-centred and consumer-focused therapeutic approaches..., characterised by engagement..., underpinned by personal and professional reflection' (Australian College of Mental Health Nurses, 2013, p. 12).

The *National Practice Standards for the Mental Health Workforce* (Victorian Government Department of Health, 2013), as described in Section 1.3.3, also suggest ways of working. These standards outline the values and attitudes that should inform mental health practice, including nursing practice, and the required skills and ways of working. To complement these various practice standards, we also have a *National Framework for Recovery-Oriented Mental Health Services—Guide for Practitioners & Providers* (Australian Health Ministers' Advisory Council, 2013) which lists 17 capabilities grouped into five domains of recovery-oriented practice. The document describes values, knowledge, behaviours, and practice of mental health practitioners and providers that reflect recovery-oriented practice.

THE WORK OF THE MENTAL HEALTH NURSE

According to the ACMHN, the *Scope of Practice of Mental Health Nurses in Australia* 'encompasses a wide range of nursing roles, functions, responsibilities, accountabilities, activities and creativities, modalities and innovations' (Australian College of Mental Health Nurses, 2013, p. 13). MH nurses work across the settings described in this text and their work will also be setting dependent. In 2016, 93.9% of full-time equivalent mental health nurses reported they worked as clinicians, 3.1% as administrators and 2.2% as educators. Most worked in hospitals (63.7%), 21.0% in community settings and 4.8% in residential facilities (Australian Institute of Health and Welfare, 2018). Within each of those larger setting categories the range of teams and roles for MH nurses is also varied. For example, hospital settings can include acute inpatient units, adolescent settings, units that cater to specific conditions such as eating disorders, dual diagnosis beds, emergency department MH roles or consultation liaison work. Community work for MH nurses can involve assessment and triage work, early intervention teams or assertive community treatment.

The way an individual mental health nurse will practice is dependent on a number of factors, of which the setting is just one. Other factors include skill, experience, competence, and also the individual's personality and ethical framework. To do the work of mental health nursing as described in the standards previously requires a significant utilisation of self so a nurse's personality and ethics significantly contribute to the way they work. The *National Practice Standards for the Mental Health Workforce* list respect, advocacy, recovery, working in partnership and excellence as the values that underpin the work of mental health practitioners (Victorian Government Department of Health, 2013).

All states and territories in Australia have individual legislation that allows compulsory treatment in specific circumstances. Registered nurses sometimes play a role in enacting that legislation. In public inpatient settings, the nurse-in-charge is often the person responsible for authorising or supervising the use of restrictive interventions such as restraint or seclusion. Mental health nurses work within a system that utilises compulsory treatment but also need to develop therapeutic relationships in order to be able to promote recovery and autonomy. The existence of these two contrasting ways of working produces a tension that must be acknowledged and challenged. How do nurses build trust and collaborative relationships with consumers who may be receiving treatment against their will? How do nurses support social inclusion within a locked unit? How do nurses provide holistic treatment when their job requires them to administer medications that have significant physical health side effects?

The section below describes three different ways of framing the work of the mental health nurse. These three frames are not necessarily mutually exclusive and there is overlap and intersection between them. But there are also points of conflict and contrast, and a strong adherence to one way of thinking or practising will necessarily mean challenges to other ways.

'Getting the job done'

This is presented as a task-oriented view of the role of the mental health nurse. As an example, the role of a mental health nurse within an acute inpatient unit can be very busy and include looking after five or six patients on one shift. Some of this work may include: working through admission processes of newly admitted patients; administering medications prescribed for both physical and mental health purposes; monitoring the effects and side effects of medications; measuring and monitoring physical health indictors, such as vital signs, food intake, blood sugar levels, sleep habits and urinary output. Further, it may involve engaging individually with each allocated patient to perform and document 'mental state examinations' and risk assessments; implementing interventions based on risk assessments, for example completing regular 'visual observations'; accompanying patients on escorted leave; and contributing to discharge planning. With skill and genuine intent, some of these listed tasks may possibly be performed in a way that respects and promotes autonomy, for example facilitating access to treatment that contributes to an individual's stated recovery goals. Yet, many competing factors make this difficult, such as workload and having to administer medications that the consumer may not want. Nurses are also involved in the implementation of a number of restrictive practices, particularly within inpatient settings and especially with involuntarily admitted consumers. These can include seclusion, restraint and the forceful administration of medications, but also the implementation of community treatment orders (see Section 2.4.11).

'The therapeutic use of self'

A popular theoretical basis to mental health nursing concerns the therapeutic use of self. Hildegard Peplau is an early nursing scholar who emphasised that the nurse-patient relationship and interactions were the foundation of the work of a nurse (Peplau, 1952). In 1971, Travelbee defined the therapeutic use of self as 'When a nurse uses self therapeutically she consciously makes use of her personality and knowledge in order to effect a change in the ill person' (Travelbee, 1971, p. 19). This perspective emphasises the personality and psychotherapeutic skills of the nurse in significantly contributing to the improved mental health of the consumer through support, engagement and empathy. Many mental health nurses acknowledge that their interpersonal skills significantly contribute to their work with consumers whether in inpatient settings or otherwise.

Many characteristics of recovery-oriented practice can align with this approach. For example, a therapeutic relationship provides space to engage to understand the person's preferences and to promote self-advocacy. Nevertheless some nurses might build therapeutic relationships, yet practise from a 'best interests' perspective, utilising this relationship to promote care and treatment that they believe is best for the consumer. This differs from a truly human rights based approach to MH nursing.

Building a therapeutic relationship requires trust and honesty. It is therefore challenging, and perhaps impossible, for MH nurses to build truly therapeutic relationships with consumers being treated involuntarily. MH nurses are in a position of considerable power and working within a system that can impact on individual human rights and self-determination and autonomy. How genuine can this relationship be when the two parties do not come to it with equivalent agency?

'A human rights approach'

As discussed earlier in Section 1.5.2, Australia is a signatory to the United Nations Convention on the Rights of People with a Disability. In 2014, the United Nations made clear that according to this convention 'both the abolition of substitute decision-making regimes and the development of supported decision-making alternatives' is required (United Nations Committee on the Rights of Persons with Disabilities, 2014). Despite this, all states and territories in Australia retain provision for substitute decision making in their respective mental health legislation. Therefore, while not obligated by Australian legislation to ensure adherence to the concepts of supported decision making, MH nurses who wish to position their practice within a broader human rights framework might strive to understand and practise supported decision making.

Supported decision making focuses on and prioritises the consumer's preferences, and providing support to assist the consumer in determining and communicating their will (see Section 2.4.3). Examples of supported decision-making practice that could be performed by MH nurses include: working with consumers to support them in identifying their goals and priorities; and working with consumers to utilise tools such as advance statements and directives to communicate their preferences. MH nurses could also identify people trusted by the consumer to communicate their preferences in the event that they may not be able to themselves, advocating for the consumer's identified preferences and building the consumer's decision-making capacity. Much of this work requires a trusting relationship with the consumer but, rather than a 'therapeutic' relationship, this is a respectful relationship where the nurse vigilantly maintains an approach that places the consumer's rights, priorities and agency at the fore. The focus is squarely on the promotion of the consumer's own preferences and priorities, not what anyone else might believe is in the consumer's best interests.

Practising within a human rights framework and supporting the decision making of consumers is a change of focus for mental health nurses and poses particular challenges for those working within legislation that has breached the human rights of consumers and allowed for substitute decision making.

The three frames for conceiving of the work of the mental health nurse as discussed above are not exhaustive but meant to illustrate a variety of approaches. This breadth and lack of specificity around the role of the mental health nurse should not be seen as a failure to define, and therefore value, the role. Instead, it suggests that the work of the MH nurse can adapt along with changes in the MH system, in a future where the status quo of the dominant medical model may be challenged and the expertise of lived experience truly embraced.

2.1.8 PSYCHIATRISTS

FIONA BEST

PSYCHIATRY: A MEDICAL SPECIALTY

Psychiatry is a clinical discipline of medicine that defines and treats disorders of the mind. The underlying cause of those disorders can be obscure and may not be linked to an underlying metabolic, endocrine, constitutional or genetic vulnerability. More often disorders of the mind in fact are occurring within the interplay between an environment and the individual. We may consider for instance individuals with significant developmental trauma histories who go on at times of personal adversity to develop problems such as mood disorders, anxiety or fear-related disorders–and where the environment provided the immediate cause exposing the vulnerability, leading to expression of mental illness. Similarly psychotic disorders may develop in the setting of an underlying brain or genetic vulnerability and/or substance abuse, and/or trauma. For at least 40 years now (Engel, 1977; Engel, 1980), it has been argued in psychiatry that disorders of the mind are multifaceted in origin and have biological, psychological, social and cultural determinants (see Chapters 1.1 and 1.2).

There is often confusion among the public about the clinical discipline of psychiatry and it is often confused with psychology. Many psychiatrists will relate to the question 'what's the difference between a psychiatrist and a psychologist?' Indeed, unless an individual has cause to seek out the services of a psychiatrist, it is often poorly understood that psychiatry is a medical specialty and that psychiatrists are medically trained. The reasons for this confusion are unclear, but it may be something to do with psychiatry not being seen as a medical discipline that requires biological treatments as well as psychological ones. Importantly however, psychiatrists are potentially uniquely placed to treat individuals from both of these perspectives.

ON BECOMING AN PSYCHIATRIST

The Australasian Association of Psychiatrists was founded initially in 1946, subsequently becoming the Royal Australian and New Zealand College of Psychiatrists (RANZCP) in 1977. Prior to 2010, the College was governed by a General Council and an elected Board of Directors oversaw the affairs and activities of the College. In 2010, following review of governance models the General Council was replaced by a smaller governing body (the RANZCP Board) with a new governance model being implemented at the College's Annual General Meeting in May 2013. Established in 1985, the Australian Medical Council Ltd is a national standards body for medical education and training and is the accrediting body for the RANZCP.

Individuals who wish to train to become a psychiatrist must have first completed medical training and obtained a medical degree. General medical registration is also a prerequisite. Registration as a medical practitioner and specialist status is determined nationally by the AHPRA whose operations are governed by the *Health Practitioner Regulation National Law Act 2010* (Cth), which regulates 16 health professions under the National Registration and Accreditation Scheme. Registration as a specialist or consultant psychiatrist is required by the Commonwealth Department of Health for private billing purposes via the Health Insurance Commission.

The RANZCP sets the standards for psychiatry training and provides the curriculum, examinations and certification process for local (Australian trained) applicants. Overseas psychiatrist qualifications may also be wholly, substantially or partially recognised by the RANZCP for those psychiatrists moving to Australia from overseas and the RANZCP provides a pathway for overseas psychiatrists to become Fellows of the RANZCP by a tailored Substantial Comparability Assessment Review Panel (SCARP) pathway for international medical graduates. In 2013 there were 3599 Consultant Psychiatrists registered as working in Australia and New Zealand (Royal Australian & New Zealand College of Psychiatrists, 2014). Of these almost one-third were working in major cities of Australia, one-third exclusively in public work, one-third exclusively in private work and one-quarter of psychiatrists registered as working in both public and private practices.

Training

On completion of a medical degree (five or six years as an undergraduate or four years in a graduate medical program), medical practitioners seeking to embark on psychiatrist training must first undertake at least one year of internship as a resident medical officer to achieve general registration with AHPRA before applying to the RANZCP to join the psychiatry training program. Psychiatry training is a postgraduate medical course for doctors, and doctors who complete the training program are eligible to become Fellows of the RANZCP. In 2012 the RANZCP made changes to their curriculum for training and adopted a Competency Based Fellowship Program based on the CanMEDS educational framework. The Royal College of Physicians and Surgeons of Canada CanMEDS Physician Framework (Jurd et al., 2015), underpins the development of the RANZCP Competency Based Fellowship Training, in which seven key roles expected of contemporary psychiatrists are defined:

1 Medical experts: psychiatrists perform comprehensive, culturally appropriate psychiatric assessment of patients.
2 Communicators: psychiatrists communicate effectively with patients, families, carers, colleagues, and other health professionals.
3 Collaborators: work with other psychiatrists effectively.
4 Managers: psychiatrists contribute and work within clinical governance structures.
5 Health advocates: advocate for individual patients, families and carers.
6 Scholars: psychiatrists demonstrate lifelong commitment to learning and critical appraisal.
7 Professionals: psychiatrists demonstrate ethical conduct and practice.

To be selected for training, applicants need to demonstrate a commitment to join psychiatry training and in reality, very few applicants move from internship straight to psychiatrist training as they are unable to demonstrate sufficient commitment (by way of previous psychiatry experience) or consultant psychiatrist references to support an application at post-graduate year 2 stage. To fulfil the selection criteria, increasingly applicants are applying later to enter psychiatry training and may have achieved specialty training in other fields of medicine before applying. In recent years, psychiatry training is becoming increasingly popular and the number of applicants generally exceeds the number of places available for trainees. The selection process is two-pronged in that applicants must first be selected to the RANZCP training program and then be selected by an area mental health service to work in an RANZCP accredited psychiatry training post. The RANZCP Fellowship Program takes a minimum of 60 months full-time equivalent (FTE) to complete. Training is provided by the area mental health services and trainees work in RANZCP accredited posts in hospitals and clinics where they are supervised by RANZCP accredited supervisors. Training is undertaken in three stages, each stage introducing a new element of experience. By completion, trainees will have worked in general psychiatry and a range of subspecialty psychiatry roles. Assessments are work based and centrally administered. The work based assessments comprise a process of formative work based assessments, summative professional activities and in-training assessments. The centrally administered assessments comprise two written exams, a practical clinical exam, a psychotherapy written case and a scholarly project of original research. In addition trainees undertake an RANZCP accredited formal education course (usually a Masters of Psychiatry or equivalent), usually in the first three years of training.

Roles

Psychiatrists play a key role in mental health care in Australia and New Zealand and undertake a wide range of roles to do this. In line with the CanMEDS roles adopted by the RANZCP, psychiatrists may work in a combination of private, public, or academic practice. They can also be involved in research, teaching and undertake administrative roles associated with mental health care. They may be involved in advocacy for patients and service improvements, leading teams and also collaborating with other medical specialties or with other mental health disciplines in order to care for their patients. Of course, the key and paramount role of the psychiatrist is treating patients with mental illness, emotional disturbance and/or abnormal behaviour and this is done by careful examination of the mental state, history taking, formulating and implementing treatment and management plans and making a diagnosis. Treatments may vary from psychotropic medication, psychotherapy, and other interventions. In recent times a patient-centred recovery model has been adopted in Australia. Following this model, the psychiatrist seeks to empower the patient to achieve control about their mental health care by encouraging informed decision making, instilling hope and meaning, and fostering personal autonomy. Psychiatrists are expected to adhere to the RANZCP Code of Ethics, which lays down expected ethical standards and professionalism in psychiatry.

2.1.9 PSYCHOLOGISTS

JOHN FARHALL & MARILYN CUGNETTO

Psychology as a scientific discipline addresses both 'normal' and 'abnormal' human behaviour. As a profession, psychologists aim to apply this knowledge to improve the wellbeing or performance of individuals, organisations or communities.

THE PROFESSION

In Australia, professional psychologists must have a 'general registration' with the Psychology Board of Australia (PBA) to practise; some advance their qualification and obtain an 'endorsement' (specialisation) in one of nine areas of psychological practice. Clinical psychology is a specialisation that aims to understand and ameliorate mental health problems and disorders. In public mental health settings, most psychologists are endorsed clinical psychologists; however, a small number of endorsed clinical neuropsychologists are also employed specialising in assessment and rehabilitation of thinking and behaviour difficulties caused by measurable brain dysfunction. Both general and clinical psychologists can be found in non-government organisations (NGOs) and in private practice, with general psychologists predominating in these sectors. As of December 2018, there were over 36 700 registered psychologists; one-third in NSW, one-quarter in Victoria and one-fifth in Queensland, with about 22% 'endorsed' as clinical psychologists (Psychology Board of Australia, 2019).

Standards of practice and training for the profession are set both by the Australian Psychological Society (APS) and by the PBA, overseen by AHPRA, the Federal Government body regulating most health professions. 'Psychologist' and 'Clinical Psychologist' are legally protected titles that require the practitioner to be registered with the PBA. The introduction of the Better Access initiative in 2006 by the Australian Department of Health (Australian Government Department of Health, 2018) allowed psychologists to provide Medicare-subsidised services. The Health Insurance (Allied Health Services) Determination 2014 stipulates Medicare reimbursement and allows clinical psychologists to offer a broad range of psychological therapy health services at a higher rate of remuneration than generalist psychologists who are authorised to provide 'focussed psychological strategies' including psychoeducation and cognitive behaviour therapy (Office of Parliamentary Counsel, 2018). Recent improvements include items for telehealth sessions for rural consumers and an increased number of sessions per year for individuals diagnosed with an eating disorder.

Training

Registration as a psychologist involves either attainment of a professional postgraduate degree or additional study and/or supervised practice that is entered into following four years of undergraduate study of general psychology. Postgraduate training choices include a one-year Master of Professional Psychology program, which prepares the practitioner for generalist registration, and a two-year Master's program that prepares the practitioner for practice as a Clinical Psychologist, clinical neuropsychologist or other 'area of practice endorsement'. Alternatively, a three- to four-year Doctor of Psychology program allows the student to gain greater depth in research and clinical training than is possible with a two-year Master's degree; and there are opportunities to combine a PhD research program with clinical Master's training. Registration following completion of a four-year undergraduate degree plus two years of supervised practice is being phased out.

Trainees seeking an endorsement to practise in a specialist area such as clinical psychology must firstly have completed a postgraduate course comprising study of assessment and treatment theory and methods, development of clinical skills by training and supervised practice, and completion of a substantial independent research project. Following attainment of general registration, completion of a 'registrar program' is required to obtain endorsement as a Clinical Psychologist. The registrar program includes psychological practice, Board-approved supervision and continuing professional development (CPD) over a period of one to two years. During their careers, many clinical psychologists seek further specialist training, for example, in family therapy or in specific therapies for disorders such as post-traumatic stress disorder or borderline personality disorder. Documented CPD, including supervision, is a requirement for annual renewal of registration.

WHAT IS THE UNIQUE CONTRIBUTION OF PSYCHOLOGISTS?

Perhaps the clearest defining theme of clinical psychology is that of the 'scientist-practitioner' (Martin & Birnbrauer, 1996). Not only is the practice of clinical psychology primarily based upon knowledge from theory building and empirical investigation, but up to one-third of psychologists' university study is devoted to research training and practice. This knowledge and skill is reflected in psychology practice in four main ways. Firstly, in routine clinical practice, psychologists are likely to seek 'data' to test out hypotheses about consumers' presenting concerns; for example, supporting a consumer to self-monitor mood, or administering a delusions rating scale before, during and after implementing an intervention. Secondly, their scientist-practitioner background means that psychologists can understand the science behind the 'evidence-based' interventions published in clinical practice guidelines and review articles in scientific journals, and thus be in a good position to choose appropriate therapies. Thirdly, understanding the theoretical and empirical bases of therapies enables psychologists to tailor their work to the individual while implementing the *principles* underpinning the treatment. Finally, the 'scientist' background can also be valuable at the team or organisation level, for example, in interpreting the significance of a change in symptom ratings or test scores, devising a behavioural observation chart that can provide reliable data, or designing an effective program evaluation with colleagues.

A further defining feature of professional psychologists that complements the scientific orientation is the use of self-knowledge in clinical practice (Teyber & Holmes McClure, 2011). Psychologists are ethically required to be sufficiently self-aware of their beliefs and accumulated life histories to ensure these do not adversely affect their professional work with consumers and colleagues, particularly during therapy (Australian Psychological Society, 2007). Furthermore, this self-knowledge can serve as another form of 'data' when conceptualising a consumer's presenting concerns (for example, do other people in the consumer's life react in a similar manner as the clinician did?) and devising a potential intervention (for example, responding to the consumer in a way that differs from others in their life). Continued self-reflection is woven into CPD requirements for registration.

Variation in roles

The roles of Clinical Psychologists in public mental health settings vary according to service type and local traditions. For example, psychologists working in inpatient units tend to be more involved with assessment, behavioural management and brief therapeutic interventions, whereas those in specialist teams such as crisis assessment teams, or dual diagnosis (substance use and mental illness) teams, may share a largely generic assessment and support role with other professionals, though some are intervention specialists. However, even within the one service type, the roles may differ widely. In some community mental health teams, psychologists spend most of their time in general case management practice; in others, the role is predominantly as a therapist.

Therapist

The central skill of a Clinical Psychologist, and of many generalist psychologists, is that of individual therapy. The aim of therapy may be to assist clients to cope better with symptoms of a disorder, resolve problematic life issues or build a stronger or more adaptive sense of self. A minority of clinical psychologists have psychodynamic training (that is, originating from the psychoanalytic theories of Sigmund Freud), but most have cognitive behaviour therapy (CBT) as their core skill. CBT is best understood as a family of related therapies that incorporates interventions founded in traditional behaviour modification (e.g. strategies such as desensitisation and contingency management), 'cognitive' theory (techniques based upon the power of thoughts and language in shaping our emotions), and mindfulness (ways of changing how we observe and act in relation to internal experiences, particularly emotions). The subject matter discussed in cognitive therapy may be automatic thoughts (for example, 'I can't stand it any longer!'), attributions ('They're persecuting me because I'm different') or core beliefs. These may be about the self ('I'm useless'), or others ('People are critical'), and the world ('It's unsafe') (Barlow, 2014) (see Chapter 2.6 for more details).

Other important therapies offered by psychologists in mental health settings include interpersonal therapy for depression (Bleiberg & Markowitz, 2014), dialectical behaviour therapy (DBT) for borderline personality disorder (Linehan, 2015), and acceptance and commitment therapy (ACT) (Hayes, Strosahl, & Wilson, 2012). Chapter 2.6 introduces the major psychological therapies. In addition to therapies directed at diagnosed disorders, some of a psychologist's work may be: counselling to aid adaptation in the face of stress; or skills development, such as interpersonal communication, mindfulness or other skills in order to improve one's life, or performance, or to live better with a disability.

Test-based assessor

This traditional role of psychologists has diminished since the 1970s, in adult mental health services, as therapy has become a more important use of psychologists' time. At the same time, the breadth and depth of available psychological assessments has widened. These cover domains of diagnosis, intelligence, personality and neuropsychological function. A fuller introduction to this role of psychologists and to the main tests in current use is presented in Chapter 2.3.

Program evaluator and measurement consultant

While usually employed as clinicians, some psychologists spend time in data-based planning and service evaluation for their local or area mental health service, or NGO. Whether as part of quality-assurance exercises, funding justifications or service planning, the methodological and statistical background of psychologists is often sought for this work; for example, a psychologist may work with staff and consumers to construct a client satisfaction questionnaire for a program and analyse the results.

In both private practice and mental health service settings, organisations and funders may require practitioners across disciplines to use disability rating scales, routine outcome measures or to provide statistical data (for example, the Health of the Nation Outcome Scales (HoNOS); Wing et al., 1998). This requirement has drawn psychologists into roles of educators and evaluators about such instruments, for example, advising on the clinical significance of scores or developing data-based arguments.

Behavioural consultant

Helping clients to manage behavioural disturbance (for example, persistent intrusion into others' rooms in a residential setting, or shouting in public settings) has been a traditional role of clinical psychologists. In this approach, the analysis of behaviour and supporting its change is based on principles of conditioning and modelling. Following monitoring, the psychologist and client collaborate around change goals, rewarding successive approximations to the target behaviour via praise, progress charts or more tangible rewards, such as celebratory outings. The psychologist's role may be as a consultant to other staff in assessment and program design, or as the therapist who designs and implements the program.

Some issues and directions

The roles outlined above are largely specialist roles utilising professional competencies expected of clinical psychologists. However, psychologists may also spend significant time in generic roles, such as case management, program coordination, staff development, service administration, professional and student supervision, and service planning and development.

A continuing issue for some clinical psychologists in public mental health services has been the emphasis of their training on treatment of mild to moderate depression and anxiety disorders, rather than the psychotic disorders and complex personality and mood disorders that predominate in these settings. The knowledge base of empirically supported psychological treatments for these disorders is developing rapidly. This especially includes treatments such as recovery-focused CBT for people with persisting psychosis (Hazell, Hayward, Cavanagh, & Strauss, 2016; Morrison, 2017; Steel, 2012); specialist therapies such as DBT for people with borderline personality disorder (Linehan, 2015); and relapse prevention interventions for schizophrenia and bipolar disorder (Gumley, Braehler, Laithwaite, MacBeth, & Gilbert, 2010; Gumley et al., 2003). These marry the therapeutic training of psychologists with the needs of consumers in public mental health settings, but are not yet taught by all university training programs.

A difficult issue for psychologists and policy-makers is the extent to which the general case manager role in community-based services is a cost-effective use of the expertise of psychologists, particularly those with doctoral-level training (Goldberg, 2000). Some services interpret the 'multidisciplinary team' ideal as meaning that all team members perform the same work (see Section 2.2.6). Such a team ethos may include a view that the most important work to be done is relatively non-specialist, such as monitoring of medication compliance, crisis care, personal support and practical assistance (for example, with social security benefits). This can leave little time for psychologists to work directly with clients to redress emotional disturbance that may be complicating their recovery, build resilience and direction in life, or to develop ways of noticing early signs of impending relapse. With sensible planning and resourcing, access to psychological therapies in public sector settings is both possible and beneficial to consumers (Johns et al., 2019).

Psychologists' skills are well-suited to utilising advances in technology to better meet mental health needs and reduce barriers to treatment. This includes implementing and supporting consumer use of web-based interventions. Practitioner-supported online therapies are serving a range of consumer needs from parents at high risk of child maltreatment (the Triple P interactive web-based program) (Love et al., 2016) to improvement of social functioning in youth who are at Ultra High Risk of developing psychosis (Álvarez-Jiménez et al., 2018). The latter, known as MOMENTUM, utilises a model that combines an online, interactive, personalised psychological intervention along with a social media platform. Psychologists provide guidance and serve as moderators. Online service provision is growing as the expectations of younger generations (including vulnerable populations) include such technologies (Richardson & Simpson, 2015), and online therapies reach some people who would not attend a face-to-face therapy.

2.1.10 OCCUPATIONAL THERAPISTS

JUSTIN SCANLON & ELLIE FOSSEY

Occupational therapy is concerned with enabling people to participate in occupations that bring meaning and satisfaction to their everyday lives; that enable people to participate in socially valued roles; and in turn support health and wellbeing (Hancock,

Honey, & Bundy, 2015; Kielhofner, 2009; Krupa, Fossey, Anthony, Brown, & Pitts, 2009).

The term 'occupation', from which occupational therapy takes its name, is broader than simply referring to one's vocation or employment. 'Occupation' refers to what people do to occupy themselves in daily life, their occupations, including the range of paid and unpaid ways in which we look after ourselves, connect with others, find enjoyment and contribute to our communities socially and economically (Townsend & Polatajko, 2013). Occupations are not only those performed in workplaces, but also in our homes and the places where we learn, socialise and participate in recreation. They describe engagement in everyday activities that may sometimes be taken for granted but bring rhythm to daily life, allow meaningful use of time, assumption of life roles and participation in the social world (Taylor, 2017). Hence, occupation is a complex concept that requires consideration of the meaning, temporal and contextual dimensions of participation, not solely how tasks may be performed (Christiansen & Townsend, 2010).

Occupational therapy is informed by an occupational perspective of health; that is, a perspective from which participation in everyday occupations is understood as a fundamental human need, an important determinant of mental, physical and social wellbeing, and an agent for restoring and maintaining health (Townsend & Polatajko, 2013). The origins of this perspective of health are intertwined with historical efforts to understand mental illness, and to develop treatment approaches for those experiencing mental illness.

OCCUPATION, HEALTH AND ILLNESS

During the late eighteenth and nineteenth centuries, the 'moral treatment' movement emerged in psychiatry, one element of which, regular participation in occupations, was advocated to restore dignity and encourage people to regain some control over their disorders and lives in settings thought to mimic the world beyond the asylum (Kielhofner, 2009; Wilcock, 2001). Its advocates observed that lack of organised occupation exacerbated symptoms of mental illness and contributed to continuing disorganised behaviour in asylums; and argued that participation in occupations could divert attention, provide respite from the distress, and strengthen underdeveloped capacities and existing skills (Kielhofner, 2009; Paterson, 1997; Wilcock, 2001). The occupations deemed most useful were reflective of their Quaker philosophy: patients being directed towards work, religious education, healthy exercise of mind and body, and restoration of self-restraint and moral behaviour in daily life (Foucault, 1967; Wilcock, 2001). While moral treatment was abandoned for social and political reasons, the use of occupation continued in asylums, and the organisation of patients' labour in domestic, trades and outdoor work actively contributed to the running of these institutions. Hence, its use undoubtedly took an exploitative turn, despite the humanitarian rationale initially advocated (Paterson, 1997; Wilcock, 2001).

In the early twentieth century, Dr Adolf Meyer sought to understand how mental illness develops and manifests within the everyday contexts of people's lives. Often thought of as one of occupational therapy's founders in the United States, Meyer viewed mental illnesses as multifaceted 'problems in living', rather than solely existing as separate disease entities; and emphasised seeking to understand patients as persons with biographies, everyday lives and social worlds, as well as their biology (Davidson, Rakfeldt, & Strauss, 2010). His key ideas about occupation and health may be summarised as follows:

- humans maintain themselves in the world of reality through being actively engaged in occupations that bring meaning, purpose and pleasure to the use of time
- occupation engages and exercises the mind and body in an integrated fashion
- a balance of occupations involving being, thinking and doing is essential to health, so that health in occupational terms is reflected in the pattern and organisation of one's use of time in daily life
- enforced idleness (or lack of occupation) results in demoralisation, breakdown of habits, physical deterioration and loss of abilities, but so too activity imposed by others without the person's choosing

may be detrimental to mental health and wellbeing
- specific physical and social contexts may contribute to difficulties in everyday living, but are also adaptable to create possible solutions, or a better fit between the person and the demands of the environment
- the healing and restorative potential of occupation comes from *opportunities* to discover interest, try out and engage in freely chosen occupations–not specific prescriptions of what to do or how to act in life (Davidson et al., 2010; Meyer, 1922/1977; Kielhofner, 2009).

From these foundations, occupational therapy practice has grown and developed several different models for psychosocial practice and a supporting evidence base. These models support the occupational therapist's understanding of the unique interplay between the person's capacities, interests and motivations, their roles and desired occupations and the contexts within which they engage in occupations. One such model with a substantial impact on occupational therapy practice in mental health is the Model of Human Occupation (Taylor, 2017).

The key ideas in the Model of Human Occupation (MOHO) are used to explain how the inner processes of choosing (*volition*), organising (*habituation*) and enacting occupations (*performance capacity*), in interaction with the environment, contribute to what a person does. Further, occupation is seen as an organising force for health, development and adaptation because our *participation* and development of *skilled performance* of occupations shapes and sustains our sense of who we are (*identity*) and what we are capable of (*competence*) over time (Kielhofner, 2009; Taylor, 2017).

What occupations individuals choose to engage in are influenced by their values, interests and their own view of their own capabilities. These elements, referred to as *volition*, are considered to be the driving force behind engaging in occupations. However, volition can be disrupted when people's sense of competence is undermined, when access to meaningful occupations is restricted, when occupational engagement no longer provides pleasure or satisfaction or when individuals, typically through lack of exposure, are unable to identify occupations that are meaningful to them.

Habits and *routines* serve to structure daily life. Habits and routines are deeply connected with occupational role identities: routines demonstrate occupational roles, but at the same time, loss of occupational roles can significantly impact on individuals' routines. In addition to volition and habituation, *performance capacity* is the third major element of MOHO. This construct covers individuals' capacities (e.g., musculoskeletal and cognitive capacities) as they relate to engaging in occupations.

The environment in which occupations are undertaken is also important. Physical and social environments can each support performance by affording opportunities to participate in occupations, or create barriers to involvement in occupations (Taylor, 2017). For example, people experiencing mental health issues may experience restricted options for engaging in occupations, or their participation may be constrained or excluded by inadequate resources, such as transport, finance and services, or by lack of social supports to sustain involvement.

Our cumulative experiences of participating in occupations over time contribute to creating an occupational identity based in how we view ourselves, what we are capable of and what we envision for ourselves in narrative terms (within a life story), and in turn guides how we seek to enact occupational lives. Similar processes of constructing or realising one's identity through everyday acts of doing, and re-crafting a positive identity and sense of competence by participating in meaningful and satisfying occupations are also frequently described features of the processes involved in *recovering* (see Section 1.1.6 and Chapter 2.6).

Occupational therapists then are concerned with addressing challenges in everyday living, in particular issues of choice, meaning, balance and routine that are interconnected with health, wellbeing and recovery (Doroud, Fossey, & Fortune, 2015; Moll et al., 2015). In broad terms, these challenges include: restricted access to sources of meaningful and satisfying occupations; isolation, loneliness and powerlessness resulting from unmet occupational needs; stresses associated with patterns of time use that constrain involvement in occupations necessary to maintain wellbeing; and limited involvement in occupations resulting from social exclusion and disadvantage (Fossey & Krupa, 2016; Krupa et al., 2009). These types of occupational issues are raised in many first-person accounts and qualitative studies describing lived experiences of mental health issues as problems that hinder recovery, or further disrupt everyday life, health and wellbeing.

OCCUPATIONAL THERAPY IN MENTAL HEALTH PRACTICE

Occupational therapists work in a wide range of mental health settings in Australia (Hardaker, Halcomb, Griffiths, Bolzan, & Arblaster, 2011; Hitch, 2012; Lloyd & Williams, 2010). This includes the spectrum of primary care, acute care, residential care and community services providing case management, psychosocial rehabilitation, housing support and assistance with return to employment and education.

Occupational therapists aim to facilitate clients' engagement in meaningful occupation directly, or to address environmental barriers (physical or social) that restrict their participation. They do so by collaborating with clients to identify occupational issues that impact their participation, and then work together to create opportunities or overcome barriers to their involvement in occupations chosen by or of interest to the client (Townsend & Polatajko, 2013). Broadly speaking, then, the focus is on creating opportunities for participation, enabling skill development, collaborative problem solving and use of strategies to make environmental adjustments (whether physical and/or social) with the intended outcome of enabling people's participation in occupations that support recovery, health, wellbeing and social connectedness (Kielhofner, 2009; Krupa, 2016). Described below are some contributions of occupational therapy in mental health services in Australia.

Enabling participation

At the time of de-institutionalisation, 'skills training', whereby occupational therapists supported individuals to develop skills required to live independently, became a prominent feature of occupational therapy practice. While helpful in many ways, this process sometimes led occupational therapy practice towards a focus on what individuals 'should' be doing rather than on what they wanted to be doing. More recently, occupational therapists have adopted a more person-centred approach to focus on those occupations that individuals wish to make part of their daily lives. This requires collaborating with people and supporting them to find ways of participating in those everyday activities that are personally meaningful. In this enabling role, occupational therapists seek to facilitate clients' participation in real-life occupations. The ultimate aim is to enable people's engagement in everyday living, and participation in daily occupations of benefit for fostering health, wellbeing, development of capabilities and inclusion in society (Townsend & Polatajko, 2013).

The primary emphasis of this role is on experiential learning, skill building and personal development *through* active participation in relevant occupations in real-life contexts wherever possible, rather than 'training'. People develop, practise and maintain capacities and skills through actively taking part in real-life occupations, rather than by therapists doing things to or for them (Mattingly & Fleming, 1994; Taylor, 2017). So occupational therapists working alongside clients may use processes such as guiding, coaching, information sharing, prompting, consulting and reflecting to support skill building. These 'enabling' processes also create the means and opportunity for clients to participate actively in their own learning, problem solving and personal development, whether focused on enabling participation in self-chosen occupations at home, in social or community activities or individualised support in education or employment (see Chapter 2.6). The term *enabling*, then, is used to reflect this participatory and action based orientation, and more recently to also make explicit the consideration of client choice, risk and responsibility, collaboration and power sharing in occupational therapy's practice approach (Townsend & Polatajko, 2013).

Facilitating groups

While facilitating groups can be undertaken by a range of mental health staff, occupational therapists are recognised for their skills in this area and their valuing of the benefits provided by groups. Occupation-focused groups typically have goals oriented more towards *doing* and engaging in activities than other 'talking'-based groups. Groups facilitated by occupational therapists can be quite diverse, but they generally have a focus on engaging participants in meaningful activity and fostering connection and cooperation between participants through the use of group dynamics (Cara, 2013).

Aims of occupation-focused groups often centre around aspects such as:

- engagement in natural, everyday activities
- fostering a sense of enjoyment and mastery
- scaffolding cooperation, sharing and mutual support
- providing opportunities to use existing skills or develop new ones
- learning about and applying coping skills to improve everyday life and
- supporting a sense of autonomy and self-efficacy through making choices, goal setting, shared learning and supporting others.

In facilitating groups, occupational therapists often draw on their skills in grading and adaptation of activities to promote engagement of a wide variety of individuals. Doing this supports providing individuals with the 'just right challenge' to promote enjoyment and skill development.

Supporting self-management

While not specifically focusing on occupational engagement, another important role of the occupational therapist is to support individuals to develop self-management approaches to manage consequences of mental and physical health difficulties and how to manage effects of treatment. This often involves the exploration and practising of various strategies to manage these difficulties and then supporting the individual to embed these strategies into daily life activities. Examples include the use of sensory modulation activities to reduce anxiety or distress, or to optimise arousal to engage in desired activities (Scanlan & Novak, 2015); adaptive strategies and supports to overcome challenges associated with cognitive difficulties (Cairns, Hill, Dark, McPhail, & Gray, 2013); and strategies to lessen the impact of persistent symptoms that cause distress and assist individuals to manage the unpleasant effects of medication (Gibson, D'Amico, Jaffe, & Arbesman, 2011).

All of these interventions aim to maintain the focus on reducing barriers to optimal occupational engagement and performance. By supporting individuals to develop self-management skills, the intent is to enable their engagement in activities that will promote enjoyment, personal meaning, social connectivity and wellbeing.

2.1.11 SOCIAL WORKERS

MELISSA PETRAKIS & BANI AADAM

WHAT IS SOCIAL WORK?

Social work is a profession that is committed to the pursuit of the wellbeing of people and communities. The consensus definition of social work agreed to in 2001 by the International Federation of Social Workers, representing practitioners, and the International Association of Schools of Social Work, representing the educators of students in the field, is:

> The social work profession promotes social change, problem solving in human relationships and the empowerment and liberation of people to enhance wellbeing. Utilising theories of human behavior and social systems, social work intervenes at the points where people interact with their environments. Principles of human rights and social justice are fundamental to social work (Australian Association of Social Workers (AASW), 2010, p. 7).

Social work has stated aims to 'maximise the development of human potential and the fulfillment of human needs' (AASW, 2010), p. 7), particularly through commitments to:

- working with Australia's First Peoples
- working with and supporting people to achieve the best possible levels of personal and social wellbeing

- working to address and redress inequity and injustice affecting the lives of clients, client groups and socially disadvantaged
- working to achieve human rights and social justice through social development, social and systemic change, advocacy and the ethical conduct of research.

How do social workers practise?

Social work typically operates at points where there is an interface between people and their physical, social and cultural environments. It is a discipline interested in joining with people at times and points when they experience strain, stress, distress, discrimination, hardships and challenges. It is an empowerment-oriented discipline.

Typical social work practice involves interpersonal practices, and these may include: casework or case management, counselling and clinical interventions. The work may be with individuals, families, people in partnerships, communities and groups of people. There is an advocacy component to what social workers do and how they practise. The engagement in social action is of interest to social workers, to address both personal difficulties and systemic issues (Petrakis & Lethborg, 2018). Some social workers also undertake research and engage in critical analysis and commentary to influence social policy (AASW, 2010).

Social workers may work in human services in management, consultancy, education, training, supervision and evaluation roles. They are trained to be systemic thinkers, and often engage in practice development and service improvement activities, so that:

> In all contexts, social workers maintain a dual focus on both assisting human functioning and identifying the system issues that create inequity and injustice (AASW, 2010, p. 9).

THE ROLE OF MENTAL HEALTH SOCIAL WORK

In contemporary mental health social work there is a tension between professional aims, values and principles on the one hand and pragmatic roles and functions in services and systems on the other. This is a tension between being a recovery-oriented practitioner, and so an ally in aid of personal choice and empowerment led by consumers, and yet being an agent of the state, tasked with monitoring compliance with medical regimes, social security paperwork and expectations, forms and procedures for access to housing and social services.

While it is important that mental health social workers develop a keen grasp of the medical approach to managing mental illness, the preferred biopsychosocial approach is increasingly supported by colleagues and in mental health law. Furthermore, the developing understanding of recovery suggests that while remission of symptoms is a desirable goal for many, the process of personal, social and functional recovery is as important if not more so for most (Early Psychosis Guidelines Writing Group and EPPIC National Support Program, 2016; Leamy, Bird, Le Boutillier, Williams, & Slade, 2011).

Being ethical in mental health practice involves doing right by the people using social work services (Aadam & Petrakis, 2020). Questioning structures and processes, using good practice models and being morally courageous are three ingredients to being a good ethical social worker.

Questioning structures and processes

Social work practice is political by its very nature since it examines social structures as a means to improve people's lives (Maylea, 2016; Maylea, 2017; Davidson, Brophy, & Campbell, 2016; Ramon, 2009). As stated by Bland et al.:

> The domain of social work in mental health is that of the social context and social consequences of mental illness. The purpose of practice is to promote recovery, restore individual, family, and community wellbeing, to enhance development of each individual's power and control over their lives, and to advance principles of social justice. Social work practice occurs at the interface between the individual and the environment (Bland, Renouf, & Tullgren, 2015, p. 9).

This tension is exacerbated because social work practice operates within a political health system that engages with the contradictions of its emancipatory values and the controlling interventions enacted on people by Australia's mental health service systems (Aadam & Petrakis, 2020; Maylea, 2016 2017; Davidson et al., 2016; Ramon, 2009). The challenge then is to remain '... consistent with...ethical principles while also... balancing the care and control dimensions of practice' (Brophy & McDermott, 2013, p. 3). Or, as opposed to some form of coercion and compliance to diagnose and treat, to collaborate actively by genuinely including people in the planning and implementation of their health plans (Maylea, 2017; Brophy & McDermott, 2013).

On a broader level, taking on the role of a social worker means understanding and speaking up about wider structural injustices and wider structural inequality that contributes to disadvantage, and how this disadvantage can trigger or exacerbate mental illness. The AASW's (2010) Code of Ethics outlines how social workers should enable people to reach their full potential by supporting individuals. It stipulates how social workers should work in, and with communities, to identify system issues that create or perpetuate inequities and injustices. According to the AASW then, social workers are not only concerned with the inner life and biology of the individual, but with the context the individual lives in. Social work is therefore concerned with issues of inequality; stigma and discrimination; political freedoms and civil rights; promoting access to necessary treatment and support services; and promoting consumer and carer rights to participation and choice in mental health services (Bland et al., 2015). Questioning systems and processes that impinge on the principles of human rights and social justice is hence fundamental to social work practice (Fronek, 2012; AASW, 2010).

Using good practice models

The second element in being a good ethical social worker is identifying and using good practice models that have been tested and are evidence based. Two such models are recovery-oriented practice and strengths-based practice.

Recovery-oriented practice

Recovery as a guiding philosophy for practice emerged as a reaction and from the ruins of deinstitutionalisation and the anti-psychopharmaceutical revolution (Braslow, 2013). It challenges the perceptions of 'experts' and their understanding of people with severe psychosocial challenges as 'irrational' (Ramon, 2009), p1616) and 'passive recipients of treatment' (Hyde, Bowles, & Pawar, 2014, p. 6). While there is little consensus on what the concept of recovery is, it has nevertheless become ubiquitous across community, public and private settings and a central feature of mental policy and practice aims and objectives (Davidson et al., 2016; Hyde et al., 2014; Ramon, 2009). In Australia, for example, this is evident in the *National Framework for Recovery-Oriented Mental Health Services* (Australian Health Ministers' Advisory Council, 2013) as well as state mental health policies (see Chapter 1.7).

A brief critical analysis of recovery-oriented practice as currently practised by social workers includes the acceptance of recovery as a given through 'mainstreaming', which has been argued to 'dumb down opportunities for critical practice' (Pilgrim, 2008). Secondly, the discourses of recovery tend to focus too much on the individual while ignoring both the structural experiences that bring about distress, inequalities and injustices (Harper & Speed, 2012; Davidson et al., 2016). It is only when recovery is seen more broadly that recovery can claim to create something 'substantive' in areas like: participation, parity of opportunity, informed consent and autonomy. This broader vision can be achieved through the social model of disability, to which social work subscribes, and which argues that psycho-disability is caused by the way that society is organised, rather than by a person's impairment or difference, or through the framework of human rights, which promotes equality of opportunities (Day & Petrakis, 2018).

It is surprising then that the practice of the recovery has been uncritically accepted by practitioners working in the field (Davidson et al., 2016), as well as by people who have themselves experienced acute psychological distress and have received recovery-style support. It could be because recovery allows people their own choice around treatment and support, people who have historically been stripped of their power and ability to make any decisions for themselves, enabling agency and allowing people to feel invested in their own recovery. This *ownership* creates responsibility and accountability, empowering people as they self-direct 'in devising their own lives and values' (Gillon, 2003, p.310). Recovery-oriented practice is a framework to provide a supportive and empowering experience, especially compared to the medical model of recovery and other alternative treatment methodologies in mainstream treatment practices. Fundamentally then, recovery is aspirational, with the idea of living life well, the way one wants, with or without the presence and experiences of mental health distress.

For a social work practitioner, recovery-oriented practice is firstly, about listening; or better still, privileging lived experience voices and narratives. The goal is to learn what people want and to provide hope. It is also about including people in developing their health care plans, to empower through supporting their preferences and helping with system navigation. This potentially gives freedom and space for people to make decisions, to aid in their sense of and growth in autonomy. The hope is to be responsive and allow some flexibility to offer compassion. Ideally, this will allow space for mistakes, via trial and error, to facilitate positive risk taking. It is sometimes referred to as 'personal recovery' because it is a more personalised way of working with people, and to distinguish it from the medical concept of medical recovery—the idea that one is genetically and biologically wanting, and whereby severe and persistent psychological distress is seen as one of pathology and dysfunction (Fulford, 1989).

Recovery-oriented practice for the social work practitioner then means to go beyond pathological and deficit-based perspectives and to view persons as complete and autonomous individuals with self-determination. It should also consider the person within their socioeconomic context and focus on social inclusion and stigma reduction strategies (Ramon, 2009). In the context of the valuable role of peer support in recovery-oriented practice, social workers are emboldened by a longstanding commitment to empowerment and principles of self-determination. This focus assists social workers to work collaboratively with peer support workers (Carpenter, 2002; Brophy, Bruxner, Wilson, Cocks, & Stylianou, 2015).

Strengths focused practice

Strengths focused practice is a feature of social work that fits very comfortably with, and can be argued to be a key component in, the overarching recovery-oriented practice framework for mental health care (Australian Health Ministers' Advisory Council, 2013). Essentially, a strengths-based outlook invites social workers to look at individuals as people with possibilities and the potentiality to continue to grow and change (Petrakis, 2015; Tse et al., 2016), rather than looking at problems the people face—and them by extension—as 'deficits' to solve. Social workers do this by exploring with individuals what interests, skills and assets they have.

Assets can be tangible, like a home, which facilitates a smoother and quicker transition back to ordinary life (rather than staying in the system longer than they need to because they are waiting for accommodation). Assets can also be intangible like one's confidence in their ability to speak to different people, which will be useful when meeting different clinical staff members. Knowing that one has this asset (confidence when talking with clinicians), social workers can shape a recovery plan that incorporates this asset in their recovery, ultimately aiming to empower the individual and assist their recovery. The implication here is that a social worker should ask people about their interests, skills and assets (Petrakis, 2015), but some things may not be stated and it is up to the social worker to notice those things through their conversations and interactions with the individual. Moreover, it means that the relationship between social workers and consumers are then more genuine and substantive, beyond mere clinical inquiries.

Rapp and Goscha (2006) established a guiding text for strengths focused practice in case management (see Section 2.4.6). As Patricia Deegan, a leading consumer researcher, noted:

> In this model, strength is not constructed as some superheroic state of invulnerability. Rather, we learn that even when people present with obvious vulnerabilities, they also have strengths. Their strengths are in their passions, in their skills, in their interests, in their relationships, and in their environments. If mental health practitioners look for strengths, they will find them. After strengths have been identified, the practitioner and the service user can begin to co-create help that is helpful (Rapp & Goscha, 2006, p. viii).

The selection of the word 'strengths' for the model rings true, in practice, to consumers and social work practitioners alike as a self-respecting way to see ourselves, and a respectful way to engage another person. This word was selected so very deliberately, it is worth pausing to really think about what it means to move away from 'The Dominance of Deficits' in how we assess, and therefore how we *see* people and can move away from 'The Damage Model' and from 'Blaming the Victim' (Rapp & Goscha, 2006). Personal models of recovery differ, and need to be distinguished both from pejorative medical framings of mental disability that locate distress within 'an individual disease framework', and from disease and disorder framings of mental health challenges that 'construct psychological, emotional, and behavioural conditions as innate, biological, pathological states independent of socioeconomic, cultural, and political context' (Burns, 2009).

Being morally courageous

Ethical reasoning in a professional context can assist social workers in fulfilling their responsibilities to the people they work with, the organisation they work for and their profession. Four useful ethical approaches may assist social workers in decision making (Adams, Dominelli, & Payne, 2009) and moral courage: being normative, contextual, rational and interpersonal.

Ethical reasoning should be used to always ask oneself how a professional should act in a certain situation and how one can improve workplace protocols that support professional practice. In this *normative* approach, the practitioner uses rules or guidelines in their workplace to support the people whom they are serving. If these conventions do not support the people served, then they should be changed (Paalanen & Hopia, 2017). Questions that can assist services in exploring solutions to ethical dilemmas encountered, and provide moral justifications for changes include: 'How will this decision or action affect people?' 'How can a service minimise harm to the person it seeks to treat?' and 'What will create the least inconvenience to the person the service is working with?'

That being said, ethical decisions may not be ethically feasible for every person in every situation. So, it is always necessary that the social worker takes into account the milieu of the consumer. This *contextual* approach needs social workers to discern the situation of the individual and service setting. Questions about family, culture and religion; whether the person is experiencing symptoms acutely; what assets and strengths are brought to the table; and what past treatment has contributed to their recovery, can all be part of the conversation with the consumer and other practitioners to explore treatment and support strategies.

Ethical decisions should always be logically consistent, compatible with the facts concerning the situation and well-grounded in evidence (Paalanen & Hopia, 2017). This *rational* approach does not give space to one's beliefs and assumptions. One's instinctual feelings are not enough to disregard ethical boundaries (or practice and validate ethical exploitations). Questions of evidence-based treatment and the impactfulness of services and programs exist as features to this ethical line. Finally, the *interpersonal* approach in formulating decisions dictates that ethical practice is found in the interaction or the interpersonal activities that occur between people. Therefore, ethically sound decisions transpire through the interaction and subsequent effects on others around them. From this perspective, actions that affect only the actor, that is the social worker, are ethically extraneous (Paalanen & Hopia, 2017). Questions about how we should each interact with people who seek our assistance are at the forefront of this ethical technique.

To conclude, the mental health sector is a dynamic, multidisciplinary, rapidly changing environment that places competing demands and responsibilities on social workers, who advocate for the interests of the people and communities they work with, as well as accommodating the fiscally conservative governments and risk-averse organisations in which they work. A question then is how does one ethically balance this spectrum of needs and focus? Adopting recovery and strengths focused models will assist in implementing work practices that are appropriate and evidence based; and promoting their universal implementation will ensure a genuine regard to ethical practice and the hopes, needs and wants of people experiencing mental ill health.

2.1.12 INTERPRETERS

HARRY MINAS

The interpreter is a crucial member of the mental health team. Mental health legislation and policy require that communication or cultural barriers do not prevent immigrants and refugees from gaining access to mental health services.

Several Australian universities offer Graduate Diploma and Master level courses in translating and interpreting, however it has long been recognised that interpreting in mental health settings (mental health interpreting) requires specialised skills. Yet, there is little specific training for this role. Guidelines for mental health interpreting, including an online resource for practitioners, are freely available from the Victorian Transcultural Mental Health Unit (VTMH, 2019).

Interpreters are professionals whose task is to facilitate effective communication and, where language and culture are an issue in assessment and treatment, they are essential members of the clinical team. Interpreting practice is governed by The Australian Institute of Interpreters and Translators professional code of conduct.

An interpreter is someone who renders messages verbally between parties. A translator is someone who translates written documents. An interpreter may or may not also be a translator. If you require written text to be explained to clients, you may ask the interpreter to sight translate the document–read it into a language other than English. It is important to note that a sight translation is not the same as a standard translation, and may not accurately translate the document with exact style, register, and complexity. An interpreter may suggest that a sight translation is inadequate, or that the text is too complex to sight translate. If this is the case, you may need to arrange for the document to be translated by a translator.

The National Accreditation Authority for Translators and Interpreters is responsible for setting and monitoring standards for the translating and interpreting profession in Australia through its system of certification, which is designed to evaluate whether an individual is competent to practise as a translator or interpreter. It does this by setting minimum standards of performance across a number of areas of competency. The required competencies may be found at NAATI (2020). Certification is available in a large number of languages, including Auslan (Australian Sign Language), the sign language of the Deaf community in Australia.

It is strongly recommended that mental health interpreters be accredited at a professional level, and that they receive additional training specific to mental health interpreting. Nevertheless, there is a lack of accreditation in many languages and dialects spoken in Australia; there is also a shortage of professional level interpreters in many languages. This results in the common situation where clinicians must work with the assistance of paraprofessional interpreters in mental health. This presents some significant challenges for the professional and client, and professionals should be aware of the level of certification and experience of the interpreter with whom they are working.

Views vary among health professionals and among interpreters about whether interpreters should be regarded as a source of information about cultural issues. Interpreters may have considerable knowledge of a particular culture, and it may be useful to ask for information from them on religious or cultural practices or historical or political events. In some situations, interpreters may be able to provide information about whether a particular behaviour is common or socially acceptable in the country of origin. However, information that is clinically significant may be more appropriately obtained from bicultural clinical staff in mental health services.

Clinicians should be circumspect about relying on language interpreters (and bicultural clinical staff) for cultural information or interpretation of the possible meaning of a client's behaviour. All cultures are heterogeneous and change (sometimes substantially) over relatively short time frames. There are many possible reasons that the interpreter may in fact know little about the culture of the client. For example, even though an interpreter may come from the same country or cultural group as the client, the interpreter may have arrived in Australia many years before the client, during which time the culture of origin has significantly changed. In addition, the interpreter and client could be from different cultural or religious sub-groups within a country; and either the client or the interpreter could have rejected important elements of the culture of origin. Therefore, the clinician should not assume that because the client and interpreter share the same language, they are also ethnically and culturally 'matched', or that they have a good cultural understanding of each other. The clinician must take responsibility for eliciting and understanding potentially relevant cultural information through discussion with the client and, where this is appropriate, with the client's family. It is the clinician's responsibility to determine the clinical relevance of a client's experience, beliefs, values, appearance, body language and behaviour. Interpreters are not trained to interpret specific behaviour, although they may be able to offer general comment on cultural practices. Interpreters are also not trained mental health professionals, and so interpreters should not be asked to assess the symptoms of clients.

2.1.13 COMMENTARY AND REFLECTIONS

ELLIE FOSSEY

This chapter considered the perspectives of a range of people who may contribute to supporting people experiencing mental health issues in their recovery—including peers, family and carers, and mental health practitioners. What these diverse perspectives share is the goal of putting people with lived experience at the heart of what services do in order to achieve high quality care.

As articulated in the *National Framework for Recovery-Oriented Mental Health Services* (Australian Health Ministers' Advisory Council, 2013), recovery-oriented mental health care encompasses each of the following practices addressed in subsequent chapters:

- recognising the possibilities for recovery and wellbeing created by the inherent strength and capacity of all people who experience mental health issues (see Chapters 2.2, 2.3 and 2.4)
- maximising self-determination and self-management of mental health and wellbeing and use of person-centred, strengths-based and evidence-informed approaches (see Chapters 2.3, 2.4 and 2.6)
- acknowledging the diversity of people's values, as well as being responsive to their gender, age and developmental stage, unique strengths, needs, preferences and beliefs, families, culture and circumstances (see Chapter 2.3)
- understanding that people with lived experience of unresolved trauma struggle to feel safe, consider the possibility of unresolved trauma in all service settings, and incorporating the core principles of trauma-informed care into service provision (see Chapters 2.3 and 2.4)
- addressing factors, including social determinants, that impact on the wellbeing and social inclusion of people experiencing mental health issues and their families, including housing, education, employment, income, geography, relationships, social connectedness, personal safety, trauma, stigma, discrimination and socioeconomic hardship (see Chapters 2.3, 2.4 and 2.6)
- assisting families or support people to understand lived experiences of mental health issues, recovery processes and how to assist persons in recovery, while also addressing their own needs for counselling, therapy, education, training, guidance, support services, peer support and advocacy (see Chapter 2.7).

2.2

WORKING COLLABORATIVELY

BRENDA HAPPELL, CATH ROPER, GRAHAM MEADOWS, LOUISE BYRNE, HELENA ROENNFELDT, ANNETTE MERCURI, FLICK GREY, LAURA COLLISTER, BRETT SCHOLZ, NOEL RENOUF, FIONA SMITH & LISA BROPHY

2.2.1 INTRODUCTION

BRENDA HAPPELL & GRAHAM MEADOWS

Just as the needs of people accessing mental health services are complex, so too is the system of service delivery itself. Chapter 2.1 demonstrates the numerous professionals and other stakeholders involved in service delivery. Ensuring the various compartments of the system work together collaboratively is paramount. The consumer is at the centre of service delivery and this fundamental premise must be achieved for effective service delivery. Teamwork is the basis whereby the respective knowledge and skills each discipline brings contributes to meeting the needs and achieving the goals of consumers. Whether working with individuals, families, networks, groups, organisations or service, we may conceptualise a collaborative partnership in which the worker and consumer work as equals, each with areas of strength and expertise, each with the ability to exercise autonomy and choice. The quality of this collaboration has the most profound effect on the nature of the work. Effective partnerships between workers and clients is an essential element of effective practice, while open communication and respectful collaboration are recognised as crucial parts of the process of recovery (McCloughen, Gillies, & O'Brien, 2011).

National mental health policy directions, standards and recommendations are increasingly explicit in their promotion of collaboration and partnership at many levels (e.g., Australian Government, 2010b; Council of Australian Governments, 2017). For instance, mental health workers, consumers and families are encouraged to work as partners in direct care and to collaborate actively in service planning, delivery and quality improvement within and across differing parts of a service. Furthermore, the development of partnerships with primary care and other community services is promoted, and the need for greater cross-sectoral collaboration and 'joined-up' approaches to issues such as housing and employment is increasingly recognised. This chapter explores some of these differing contexts for working collaboratively: with consumers in consultant, advisory and educator roles; with families, carer consultants and advocates; within teams and networks of services; and partnership and collaboration in the community sector and in primary care.

2.2.2 WORKING COLLABORATIVELY WITH PEOPLE WHO HAVE ACCESSED SERVICES

LOUISE BYRNE & HELENA ROENNFELDT

In Australia in the 1980s and 1990s, a series of reports (see Chapter 1.7) uncovered significant human rights abuses in our mental health system and consequently poor outcomes for people accessing services. Urgent reform was recommended and the reform agenda in Australia has progressively insisted on a move from the existing paradigm, towards a person-directed mental health system This person-directed approach has been informed increasingly by the participation and perspectives of people with a 'lived experience' of accessing mental health services. Most recently, the Fifth National Mental Health Plan states an intention to ensure the longstanding motto of the lived experience movement 'Nothing about us without us' is realised more fully than ever before (Council of Australian Governments, 2017; see Section 1.7.1.)

The push towards greater lived experience perspective/participation has led to the development of 'lived experience' mental health roles in both paid and voluntary positions. Lived experience perspective is acknowledged as broader than simply experiences of diagnosis, encompassing experiences of marginalisation; loss of social status/citizenship, damage to or loss of relationships, for many loss of or reduced employment/finances and for some loss of safe housing. These experiences, in addition to reduced autonomy, often associated with hospitalisation and particularly involuntary treatment, have been found to contribute to people feeling 'other' or 'less than'. People employed in lived experience roles possess understanding of their own experiences of service use, loss of identity and place, and are also grounded in the collective understandings of the wider lived experience movement, including the concepts and shared perspectives of the movement (Mead & MacNeil, 2006).

Box 2.1: Regarding language

Multiple terms are used to describe people with a mental health diagnosis, including 'consumer', 'person accessing services' and 'service user'. Similarly, various terms describe job roles designed specifically to employ people with a personal or 'lived' experience of mental health diagnosis, service use and periods of healing.

Box 2.2: Lived experience roles

People are employed across the mental health sector and beyond in a variety of positions in government, not for profit and private organisations. Job roles include provision of direct support, systemic advocacy, executive level governance, research, training and education. Job titles include: experts by experience, peer support workers, consumer consultants, peer or lived experience management, consumer or lived experience academic, peer or consumer representative and a range of other titles.

Box 2.3: Umbrella terms

In describing the workforce as a whole, a number of umbrella terms are employed. In Australia the collective workforce is most commonly referred to as the 'lived experience', 'peer' or 'consumer' workforce. In other countries the term 'survivor' is also commonly used to describe both individual roles and the collective workforce.

While having a variety of terms can create confusion, integral to person-directed service delivery is the need for people to describe and define their experiences in a way that is comfortable and accurate to *them*. Therefore, it is perhaps unsurprising the lived experience movement embraces multiple perspectives, including the use of language.

For the purposes of this work, the term 'lived experience' will be utilised to encompass the workforce collectively and to describe the perspective/participation of people with a lived/living experience.

As the workforce has developed, research has identified substantial and diverse benefits as a result of lived experience employment. Research has also identified significant challenges in the implementation and design of individual roles and the larger workforce.

Benefits and challenges

Benefits and challenges in this context are often opposite sides of the same coin. For example, when lived experience roles are poorly accepted, professional defensiveness from colleagues in traditional roles reportedly leads to lack of collaboration and isolation (Happell et al., 2015). Conversely, when lived experience positions are well understood and supported to work from their unique 'lived' perspective, diverse benefits are identified for organisations, colleagues in traditional roles, and people accessing services (Byrne, Roennfeldt, O'Shea, & Macdonald, 2018). Similarly, research suggests people in lived experience roles are exposed to higher than usual levels of discrimination/prejudicial attitudes, but are also the most effective means of decreasing these prejudicial attitudes towards service users and others with a lived experience. The presence of people in lived experience roles not only reduces negative attitudes but has also been found to enhance workplace culture in a number of ways. Lived experience staff impact positively on the recovery understanding and practice of other staff and the recovery orientation of the organisation. However, this increased understanding and orientation towards recovery only occurs when the orgnisation embraces the potential role of lived experience as 'change agent' and allows that transformational change to occur (Bennetts, Cross, & Bloomer, 2011). Lived experience roles are commonly cited as providing authentic, empathetic connection as well as fostering deeper empathy, thus improving therapeutic relationships between traditional service providers and people accessing services. Other frequently reported benefits include fostering and providing an example of hope, creating more equitable and mutual relationships with people accessing services, and decreasing the cost of service provision by decreasing relapse and days spent in hospital (Trachtenberg, Parsonage, Shepherd, & Boardman, 2013).

Best practice strategies

Workplace preparedness including the attitudes of all staff is essential to the success of lived experience roles (Gillard et al., 2017). This preparedness needs to build workplace culture in which there is willingness to collaborate and a clear sense of what lived experience roles bring that is unique and complements the work of other disciplines rather than threatening or duplicating existing roles. Further, the more recovery orientated an organisation or service is or is willing to be, the easier it is for people in lived experience positions to be authentic in their roles (Byrne, Happell, & Reid-Searl, 2016).

Meaningful and appropriate recruitment strategies that consider the role lived experience will play in the organisation are critical to the success of roles. Clear and well thought out job descriptions are also crucial. In relation to ongoing supports, lived experience supervision is deemed particularly important as it allows ongoing reflection, debriefing, feedback and enhances role clarity (Davis, 2015).

Co-production has been described as organisations intentionally aiming to 'work with' as opposed to 'doing for' people with a lived experience and involves partnership during planning, design, delivery and evaluation phases (Roper, Grey, & Cadogan, 2018). Within co-production, the relationship between people with a lived experience and 'allies' often requires a willingness on the part of allies to hand over or at least share power (Happell & Scholz, 2018). See Section 2.2.3 for further information about co-production.

An effective means of providing both ongoing supervision/role clarity as well as ensuring power is shared, is provision of leadership roles for people with a lived experience. Increasingly having lived experience roles in management and executive governance roles is being prioritised and promoted (Byrne, Stratford, & Davison, 2018).

As lived experience roles are better understood and supported within the workplace, the already significant benefits are likely to expand and be felt further by people accessing services, their family, friends and communities.

2.2.3 WORKING COLLABORATIVELY WITH FAMILIES AND CARERS

ANNETTE MERCURI

The benefits of working collaboratively with carers and families of people with mental ill health have been well documented (see Chapter 2.7). Working in partnership is advantageous as it leads to better outcomes for consumers, carers and families, as well as having benefits for mental health practitioners (Leggatt, 2011). For instance, when working collaboratively, consumers and family/carers are informed about the illness, aware of the recovery plan and ways to support the consumer where necessary. This can lead to an increased likelihood of the identification early warning signs and subsequent crisis aversion. In addition, as consumers and family/carers learn more about the illness, relevant coping strategies, and early warning strategies they are more likely to feel respected, heard and supported. This can lead to greater satisfaction for all involved as well as better outcomes for the consumer, the family/carer and the likelihood of less intense work required by the clinician over the medium to long term.

The importance of collaboration with families and carers in mental health care is recognised in both federal and state mental health policies and legislation. At a national level, working in partnership with consumers, families and carers is integral to both the current mental health plan and the national framework for recovery-oriented care (Australian Government, 2013; Commonwealth of Australia, 2017) as well as being expected of mental health services at individual and organisational levels (Department of Health, 2010). Carers' rights to be recognised and respected as part of the care relationship are endorsed in legislation, as are their rights to have their views and needs listened to, heard and taken into account, and to be involved in care planning decisions when the decision or outcome will impact on them or other family members. (See Chapter 1.3 for further information about the Carer Recognition Acts and Mental Health Acts.) Carers also have the right to agree to take on the caring role or not and this could change at different points along the caring journey. The impact of caring can be traumatic, life altering, life threatening and often relentless for many carers and families, so that not being appropriately supported either in this choice or in their caring roles adds to carer and family stress (see Chapter 2.7).

Despite the endorsement of working collaboratively in policy and legislation, carers are often taken for granted in practice, and their rights are not routinely acknowledged (Gray, Robinson, Seddon, & Roberts, 2008). Carers/family have known the consumer before the onset of symptoms and have important and relevant information to share that can add to a holistic understanding of the consumer, yet their opinions are routinely not sought despite research findings suggesting that carer opinions about the severity of consumer symptoms are reliable (Wooff, Schneider, Carpenter, & Brandon, 2003). Indeed, mental health professionals tend to view their work as focused on working with the consumer and, for the most part, give less consideration to working with carers/families as part of their role (Gray et al., 2008), except to obtain collateral information about the consumer. Consequently, carers may be overlooked or excluded from the care team, and often lack information about care plans, medication and complaints procedures (Rowe, 2012). In addition, carer support is frequently seen as the role of specialised external community services either because mental health practitioners do not know how to work in a three-way partnership with carers (Mind and Helping Minds, 2016) or may not see it as part of their role. Hence, there needs to be a culture shift in mental health services towards seeing the whole family as impacted when a family member experiences mental health issues, not solely the consumer, and working jointly with those affected (Worthington, Rooney, & Hannan, 2013).

Best practice indicates that carers/families need to be identified (preferably as early as possible), recognised for the support they give, and involved in the treatment continuum wherever possible, and especially at critical times of admission, transition points and discharge (Mind and Helping Minds, 2016; Worthington et al., 2013). Carers/families require information about how mental health services can support them in their caring role; they need assistance in understanding mental illness, supports to manage behaviours and relationship difficulties created by the illness, as well as supports to make sense of their experience and take care of themselves (Stanbridge & Burbach, 2007). When engaged and included in treatment, carers are better able to support consumers' recovery. They can assist in identifying the early warning signs of possible relapse and, through a working partnership with the mental health team, can facilitate access to additional care and support before a crisis point is reached for the consumer and potentially avert hospitalisation. In addition, carers and families may need other supports or interventions, such as support for children or obtain assistance in family violence situations (see Chapter 2.7).

Families and carers currently face many and varied difficulties and barriers to accessing the information, assistance and support that they require when supporting a family member with mental health issues. Becoming aware of and addressing these barriers is central to enhancing collaborative ways of working.

Barriers to working collaboratively with families and carers

Confidentiality is a key barrier to working collaboratively with family/carers. A lack of clarity and consistency in mental health practitioners' understanding and interpretation of confidentiality and privacy requirements results in caregivers being excluded from carer planning and participation (National Mental Health Consumer & Carer Forum, 2017; Wynaden & Orb, 2005). This can leave the carer to manage on their own, without any understanding of what the problem is and how best to support the consumer. The challenge is to balance the consumer's right to privacy with the carer's right to be supported in their caring role. This requires mental health practitioners to have a clear understanding of:

- the carer's right to receive support for themselves and their family without consent of the consumer and the role of mental health services in providing this
- how to work in a tripartite relationship in ways that promote transparency and collaboration and minimise confidentiality issues
- the nature of general information that may be shared with family/carers without breaching a person's privacy
- what information requires explicit agreement with the consumer to share with other persons, such as specific family/carers and
- when a consumer's mental health information must be disclosed, according to mental health legislation, such as when a decision will directly affect the carer or the care relationship, or when it is required for a carer to be able to perform, or prepare for, their caring role (see Chapter 1.3 for more details).

Staff attitudes towards engaging with carers and families can also be a barrier to collaboration. When staff focus solely on consumer issues, lack commitment to engaging family/carers or lack empathy in their communication with them, this contributes to the lack of support and disempowerment felt by carers and families (Rowe, 2012). Carers who persist in their efforts to be involved or access information may be seen as the problem (Gray et al., 2008), not taken seriously or even ignored by mental health practitioners (Lyons, Hopley, Burton, & Horrocks, 2009).

Language is a perennial challenge faced by family/carers. Mental health services use a lot of technical language to describe diagnosis, symptoms, treatment options and to name services, which is often unfamiliar and confusing for families and carers, and particularly for those from Culturally and Linguistically Diverse (CALD) communities (see Chapter 2.3 and Sections 2.3.4 and 2.4.10). Adding to the challenge of language, differing cultural understandings of mental health also impact how families interact with a family member who experiences mental illness, as well as their interactions with the mental health system (see Chapter 2.7 for more detail).

Challenging or disturbing behaviours that may be associated with mental health issues are also be difficult for families, and can potentially lead to the breakdown of family relationships or sometimes even violence within the family (Shankar & Muthuswamy, 2007). If family/carers are not included in discussions about the impact of mental illness on the family early in the treatment continuum, carers/families/children can find themselves 'at risk' and not know how to manage or to find support (Wynaden & Orb, 2005). This situation is very stressful, meaning carers can be at greater risk for mental distress and mental illness, and may sometimes even feel so hopeless or desperate as to contemplate suicide (Stansfeld et al., 2014).

Thus, it is important that mental health practitioners understand consumers' relationships and family contexts, so as to enable conversations with family/carers from early contact onwards and to provide information about mental illness, how to respond to disturbing behaviours, and how to access practical assistance and community supports.

Strategies to foster working in partnership

The practice of working in partnership with family/carers is increasing in mental health services and, with clear guidelines, better collaborative practice and better outcomes for all can be achieved.

Central to collaborative practice is the concept of the 'triangle of care' in which mental health practitioners, consumers and carers/families are viewed as a three-way partnership. Originating in the United Kingdom, the triangle of care recognises that while the link between practitioner and consumer often defines the nature of the service, the relationships between consumers and family or carers generally pre-existed and many carers wish to also be active partners in the care team (Mind and Helping Minds, 2016). In Australia, the six key standards for the implementation of the triangle of care have been proposed to guide improvement to collaborative practices in mental health services (Mind and Helping Minds, 2016). These partnership standards include:

- Carers and the essential role they play are identified at first contact, or as soon as possible thereafter.
- Staff are carer aware and trained in carer engagement strategies.
- Policy and practice protocols regarding confidentiality and sharing of information are in place.
- Defined staff positions are allocated for carers in all service settings.
- A carer introduction to the service and staff is available, with a relevant range of information across the care settings.
- A range of carer support services is available.

Strategies to promote these kinds of collaborative practice involve working at individual and organisational levels within services, and across areas that include education and training, policy and service development.

The key to collaborative practice is ensuring that the family carer and consumer workforces are involved in equal partnership at all levels of service development. Using approaches to service design, such as Experience-Based Co-Design (EBCD), actively reduces the power differentials between stakeholders (e.g., consumers, family/carers and staff), actively involves all in identifying and creating a plan, initiative or service that reflects common goals, and ensures that the outcomes are mutually acceptable to all stakeholders (National Mental Health Consumer & Carer Forum, 2017; Point of Care Foundation, 2018). Examples include the Mental Health Experience Co-Design (MH ECO) project bringing consumers and carers together to co-design quality improvement in services, and using EBCD to develop carer involvement in mental health services (Chisholm, Holttum, & Springham, 2018; Palmer et al., 2019).

Education of staff is also a pivotal component of working in partnership. Experienced members of the family carer workforce (and consumer workforce) who are aware of the broad range of lived experiences, as well as having an understanding of mental health practice, need to be involved in the development and delivery of education for staff in mental health services. For example, the carer (and consumer) lived experience perspectives need to be interwoven throughout education sessions. Education sessions also need to address barriers to collaborative practice that create gaps in practice for families, carers and consumers, as well as to increase mental health practitioners' confidence in practising inclusively.

A Carer Advisory Group within a mental health service provides a further means to promote the carer lived experience voice. These advisory groups comprise groups of carers, ideally with differing cultural backgrounds and caring experiences (e.g., as partners, parents, siblings of persons with varied diagnoses), who are passionate about making systemic change. Reporting to the service organisation's executive, a carer advisory group can provide carer leadership, perspectives, advice and recommendations about strategic directions, service improvement, how to work in partnership with family/carers, and carer specific activities. For advisory groups to be effective, the organisation needs to be prepared to work in a collaborative manner, to value carer participation, and to integrate the carer perspective in service development, delivery and staff education. The organisation also needs to actively identify opportunities for collaboration in projects in which carer advisory group members can be actively involved, and thus the carer perspective is included. It is also important that their contributions are acknowledged with appropriate remuneration, working conditions and resources, and that appropriate peer supervision and peer networks are available to carers in these roles (Lived Experience Workforce Strategies Stewardship Group, 2019).

Family carer workers and carer advisory groups may partner with mental health services to develop guidelines that aim to promote engagement with families and carers at different points along the treatment continuum. These guidelines should be clear and simple and include practical points on how to engage family/carers and promote respect, collaboration, flexibility, acknowledge diversity, and uphold the rights of all involved (Waters, 2016). Some important points might include:

- exploring with carers what has been happening and how services can help
- exploring carers' need for information, support and the options available
- discussing how to work and share information
- discussing plans for treatment and support, including discharge and transition plans.

Similarly, guidelines can be developed with family/carer and consumer workers, along with carer and consumer advisory groups, about information sharing with family/carers within services to facilitate better understanding of privacy, confidentiality and information sharing among mental health practitioners. The National Mental Health Consumer & Carer Forum (2011) is a useful document to inform the development of such guidelines within services. It emphasises the need for open communication processes to reduce the potential for misunderstandings around information sharing; better dissemination of information to consumers, carers and staff about privacy and confidentiality legislation, as well as the development of practical local guidance to support informed decisions about information sharing.

Carer peer support programs also have the potential to identify gaps in service for carers and can work as an interface between carers and mental health practitioners to advocate for more collaboration and information to support the caring role when required. They also provide important support to the family/carer, including the provision of general education about mental illness, how to navigate the system, and links to community supports (see Section 2.7.8).

2.2.4 CO-PRODUCTION

CATH ROPER & BRENDA HAPPELL

WHAT IS CO-PRODUCTION?

One way to think about co-production is that it's a method of doing work–a way of putting into practice the principle: 'nothing about us without us'—a type of process where the people who use a service or product, are actively and genuinely involved in the planning, design, delivery and evaluation phases. Figure 2.1, adapted from Roper and colleagues (2018, p. 2) shows how all phases need to be developed collaboratively in co-production. While collaborative activity can be a feature of any of these phases independently, co-production cannot occur unless there is collaboration across all of the phases (Roper et al., 2018).

Figure 2.1 What does co-production involve?

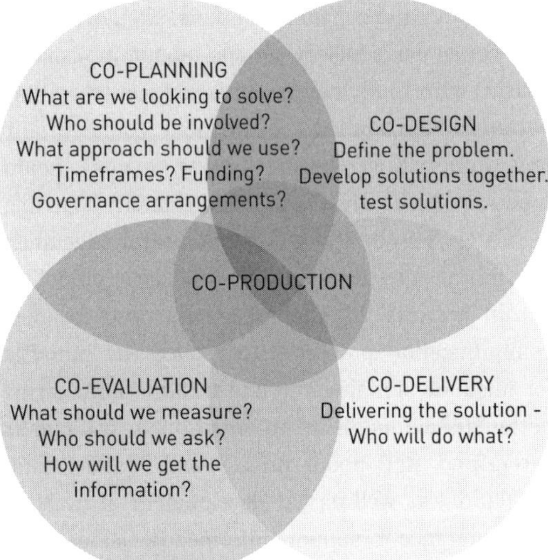

When reading about co-production you will sometimes see the term used to describe a collaborative 'therapeutic' relationship between an individual consumer and health care professional but this is a confusing use of the term (Roper et al., 2018). Rather, such individual relationships are more usefully described as informed by either shared or supported decision making (depending on whether decisions in the therapeutic relationship are shared or led by the consumer) (Roper et al., 2018).

What can be co-produced?

Any project or initiative can be co-produced, from service planning, design, delivery and evaluation to research processes where the topic, design, implementation and dissemination phases are co-produced. There has been growing interest in co-production in the past decade, largely stemming from the United Kingdom where partnerships between governments, services, service users and communities are formed in the commissioning and development of health and community services (Boyle, Harris, Foundation, & National Endowment for Science, 2009). Rationales for co-production in this context include enabling people's democratic rights to shape the services they use and acknowledgement that the people who use services can provide unique knowledge and skills essential to developing and delivering quality services (Roper et al., 2018).

In Australia, as in other developed countries, mental health services have often led the way regarding consumer and family/carer involvement in service development and delivery. However, involvement should not be confused with co-production: 'Co-production raises the bar for working with consumers, shifting from seeking involvement or participation after an agenda has already been set, to seeking consumer leadership from the outset so that consumers are engaged in the initial thinking and priority-setting processes' (Roper et al., 2018, p.2). These authors identify three core principles in the context of co-production partnerships with mental health consumers:

- consumers are involved in setting priorities from the very beginning for their leadership, thinking and expertise
- power differentials need to be deliberately acknowledged, explored, and addressed which may mean that more powerful partners will need to step back and facilitate empowering environments for those with less power and
- consumer leadership and capacity needs to be developed as part of any project or enterprise.

Co-production involves actively shifting mindsets, developing a culture that embraces exploration and learning, and authentically valuing consumer knowledge and expertise (Roper et al., 2018). Creating such partnerships is not straightforward and often involves an 'emotionally charged process of reciprocal change' (Durose & Richardson, 2016, p. 35) and 'a struggle because the process entails a shift in status that may be embraced or resisted' (Cahn, 2000, p. 31). The process of co-production takes time to think through how to work together, build trust, and make decisions; however, a positive consequence of investing in co-production is the tendency for the processes to lead to 'profound and sustainable change' (Spencer, Dineen, & Phillips, 2013, p. 7).

Co-production: A practical example

An example of co-production was the development of a mental health consumer academic position at the University of Melbourne. Successive mental health policy plans had articulated the importance of consumer participation in the development and delivery of services yet clinicians' attitudes had been identified as impeding its progress (Happell & Roper, 2009). The then Director, Professor Brenda Happell, established a partnership between the Centre for Psychiatric Nursing, University of Melbourne, and the Melbourne Consumer Consultants' group to seek funding for a consumer academic role intended to promote consumer perspective in teaching, training and research activities (planning phase). Through this partnership funding was obtained from the Commonwealth Government to implement this position. Two representatives from each of the organisations worked together to develop the position description, recruit to the position and subsequently to support the implementation of the position. The role and initial activities to be undertaken were not set in stone but developed in partnership between the incumbent and members of the original partnership, by then operating as a reference group for the role (design phase). Activities undertaken in the role included: provision of consumer perspective in the education and training of clinicians, training for consumers developed and delivered in partnership with Victoria's peak consumer organisation (Victorian Mental Illness Awareness Council), and the further articulation of consumer perspective as a unique discipline through the interdisciplinary Psych Action and Training group 'think tank' and consumer-led/co-produced research and policy development (delivery phase). While the co-produced nature of the role itself has not been formally evaluated, activities undertaken such as the impact of consumer-led teaching on nurses' attitudes, and conditions required for role success have been articulated (Happell & Roper, 2009).

How can I support co-production?

Respecting the valuable contribution consumer perspective brings to all aspects of mental health service delivery and research is a necessary precursor for co-production. Meeting policy requirements by having a consumer in the room is insufficient and the associated attitudes would present a major barrier to co-production (Roper et al., 2018). Health professionals need to comprehensively understand the principles of co-production, refer to them continually and allow their learning to be led by their consumer colleagues. Because co-production starts at the beginning or planning stage, health professionals must be prepared to consider ideas and possibilities that take the focus from their original starting point, and allow the fundamental ideas to be shaped through the partnership. This can be very challenging particularly given the hierarchical nature of knowledge which preferences the professional over the consumer (Happell et al., 2018a). Co-production is therefore not easy and requires the professional to continually reflect on and challenge their own views and beliefs. Particularly importantly it requires exploration of power. As described above, power differentials clearly exist and must be acknowledged. In relation to research, it has been suggested a declaration of power would be helpful to identify and address these issues (Happell et al., 2018b).

Practice points

The following questions or reflections might help you to decide if co-production is appropriate for this work and if the resources are available to support it:

- Do we know what consumers/family carers think about this? How might we go about learning more? Where will funds to pay for expertise come from?
- Is having consumers/family carers on a committee the best/only way to add value? Are there stronger, better supported, more effective ways to involve people?
- Do we have all the people we need around the table?
- Do consumers/family carers have opportunities to drive this initiative, be there from the start, shape it?

2.2.5 CONSUMER-LED SERVICES

FLICK GREY

Internationally, people with experiences of using (or avoiding) mental health services have been establishing and running our own services, drawing upon our own understandings of the kinds of responses and spaces people in distress most need. For some, the emphasis is strongly on creating alternatives outside of mainstream psychiatric services, while others have collaborative or complex relationships with non-consumer-led services.

In 1977, the National Empowerment Centre (USA) published Judi Chamberlin's book *On Our Own: Patient-Controlled Alternatives to the Mental Health System* (Chamberlin, 1978), which has become a classic text, inspiring many consumers/survivors around the world to dream about and create our own services. Chamberlin's work is grounded in collective political activism and consciousness raising—the mental patients' liberation movement (today known as the consumer/survivor/ex-patient movement). Chamberlin and her fellow activists railed against the harms caused by institutional psychiatry, coming together to create alternative supports. Their work passionately rejected the psychiatric system, founded in an unwavering commitment to self-determination and collective liberation. The most famous example of a consumer-led (or rather, survivor-led) service that continues to have strongly anti-psychiatric roots is the long-running Berlin Runaway House (Germany). Here, residents are supported, often over an extended period of time (months or even years) to move through altered states without the use of psychiatric medication or any form of restraint, chemical or otherwise (see also Hartmann & Bräunling, 2007).

Today, there is a huge diversity of consumer-led services, internationally and within Australia. Different services have different emphases, perspectives, language and relationships with mainstream services. All place a high value on mutual support and the value of insights gained through lived experience.

The Western Massachusetts Recovery Learning Community (WMRLC) in the United States is an example of an elaborated and (relatively) independent consumer-led service, combining peer-to-peer support, access to alternate healing practices, a crisis respite, peer support telephone line, learning opportunities and advocacy. The RLC emphasises community and 'recognizing and undoing systemic injustices such as racism, sexism, transphobia and psychiatric oppression' (Western Mass Recovery Learning Community (WMRLC), 2019). The WMRLC has also pioneered peer support groups for people struggling with suicidality—Alternatives to Suicide—which has gained some traction in recent years in Australia, particularly in Western Australia. Funding for the WMRLC comes from the Massachusetts Department of Mental Health and private foundations. WMRLC offers a multilayered response to being described as 'anti' (anti-psychiatry, anti-medication or anti-medical model), arguing that they see themselves a 'more 'pro': pro-information, pro-sharing of resources, pro-informed choice, pro-control over your own story and path, pro-change, pro-empowerment, pro-community, pro-human rights, pro-questioning *everything*.' They also staunchly argue that 'we are all human beings living together in our communities' (Western Mass Recovery Learning Community (WMRLC), 2013).

Closer to home, another example of a consumer-led service is Piri Pono (2019), a peer-run crisis alternative service in Aotearoa New Zealand, staffed by peer workers, as well as some nurses, working in collaboration with the local District Health Board. Piri Pono offers an alternative to hospitalisation in a homely environment and a holistic approach to wellness for those experiencing acute mental distress.

In Australia, there are many consumer-led services, ranging in scale from small community-led initiatives, to services employing dozens of staff. Some examples of smaller consumer-led services in communities across Australia include:

- Recovery Rocks, which began in 2012, located just outside of Perth Western Australia. Recovery Rocks is an entirely volunteer-run community of 'people with lived experience of mental health challenges who are choosing to live a life of Recovery and Wellbeing' (Recovery Rocks Community Inc., 2019). The community offers each other peer support, social gatherings, recovery education and an annual retreat.

- Also started in 2012, Echoes is an independent bi-weekly peer support group based in Melbourne for people who experience dissociation or multiplicity. Based on Hearing Voices groups, Echoes offers an opportunity to connect, share common experiences and feel understood. The group is not intended to be a therapy group, intentionally offering 'something unique—a way to support and be supported by others who may in many ways be in the same boat' (3CR 855 AM community radio, 2016).
- In 2017, the Cairns and Hinterland Consumer and Carer Advisory Group (CHCCAG) began a Warmline, with funding from the local Primary Health Network. The CHCCAG Warmline offers callers a warm listening ear: 'The aim is to listen. A warm line does not aspire to be a counselling service. It is an understanding ear when understanding can be hard to find' (CHCCAG Warm Line, 2017). The Warmline is staffed by consumers, carers and 'students with tertiary level interpersonal skills accreditation.'

Larger consumer-led services in Australia include:

- Brook RED, established in 2002, a 'peer-managed and operated community mental health organisation' in Brisbane (Brook RED, 2019), offering peer support, groups, 'an active recovery environment' as well as consultations to the sector. Brook RED has grown from one site to multiple sites and services.
- Established in 1995, the Victorian Self Help Addiction Resource Centre (Self Help Addiction Resource Centre (SHARC), 2019) offers another way of thinking about consumer-led services, from the Alcohol and Other Drugs (AOD) sector. SHARC is led by people with a lived experience of AOD struggles, right up to the CEO and Board level, but professional qualifications (in addition to lived experience) are also highly valued and integrated. SHARC includes people with lived experience working in clinical roles, peer support roles, and various volunteer positions across the organisation (Self Help Addiction Resource Centre (SHARC), 2019).

There are also countless consumer-led services who occupy what Arnstein (1969) describes as a position of 'delegated power'—consumer-led but nested within larger (non-consumer-led) clinical or community services. An example of such a service is Voices Vic, a state-wide specialist service led by people with a lived experience of Hearing Voices, an initiative of Prahran Mission, offering peer support, training and support for Hearing Voices groups across the state.

In addition to the passion and commitment that often drives the establishment of consumer-led services, there is also a growing evidence base for their effectiveness (Grey & O'Hagan, 2015).

2.2.6 THE ROLE OF ALLIES

BRENDA HAPPELL, BRETT SCHOLZ & CATH ROPER

WHO IS AN ALLY?

The term ally describes people, generally health professionals, who do not identify as consumers of mental health services, and who promote, support and advocate for consumer roles in academia and service settings (Happell & Scholz, 2018). Allies are often in leadership positions, which afford access to resources to facilitate the development of leadership positions for consumers (Roper, 2016b; Slay & Stephens, 2013).

The role of allies

Although until recently there has been almost no literature addressing the topic of allies of the mental health consumer movement, there have always been people who do not identify as consumers who have used their influence to argue for and assist the development of consumer leadership roles.

As in other social justice movements, the term 'ally' can be contentious. For example, some critique the way some individuals might claim the term 'ally' for themselves without really contributing to the goals of the movement (Ostrove & Brown, 2018). Indeed, others have suggested that although some claim to be 'allies' it might be 'accomplices' who are working together with a movement to undo the power structures that are entrenched and that keep marginalised people and groups oppressed (Yull & Wilson, 2018).

One practical strategy for confronting issues of power present in relationships between allies and consumers is to acknowledge these relationships are not equal and cannot be equal. In practice, this means starting by shifting the focus away from trying to reach equality, to a commitment to continually articulating what inequalities are present, before trying to address them.

Seeking equity not equality

While equality seeks to treat everyone in the same way, equity means ensuring that different individuals or groups have what they need. Strategies for equity, therefore, focus on removing systemic obstacles rather than trying to fix individual differences. In relation to the consumer movement, this might include addressing fundamental differences in influence and access to resources: including the limited number of senior positions for consumers; and the difference in status afforded to knowledge based on lived experience compared to that of health professionals. Well-intentioned allies may dismiss these concerns with statements like 'we are all equal', which unfortunately is likely to widen inequities rather than reduce them. A declaration of power has been suggested as an important starting point in identifying and addressing these differentials (Happell et al., 2018c).

Characteristics of an effective ally

Roper (2016b) writes 'our allies are prepared to disturb the status quo. They work with us to promote consumer perspective and they help make space for it. They create agency for us, provide mentorship when we need it and create opportunities for us to lead....Our allies want to know our agenda. They know that consumer perspective is unique and has much to teach others' (p. 208). Given the way that true allies can champion equality together with the consumer movement, they can contribute to attitudinal change in others. One important way they might do this is by challenging stigma and assumptions—including those held by health professionals—about consumers lacking capacity and value. As such, allies can play a vital role in realising consumer leadership of mental health services (Scholz, Bocking, & Happell, 2018).

Allies must respect the uniqueness and autonomy of consumer knowledge, which by definition restricts the role of ally to one of support and facilitation. Although they may be called upon to do so, allies must not speak on behalf of consumers, but instead, refer others to consumer leaders and/or consumer knowledge. Four main characteristics of effective allyship have been identified:

Nothing about us without us

Consumers must be involved in all discussions and decisions that concern them. This may seem obvious, however it is not always put into practice. For example, it is not uncommon for mental health textbooks to be written or for research to be conducted that does not include consumer knowledge and activity as part of the team. On the other hand, there has recently been growth in the mental health peer workforce and consumer leadership roles in mental health services. This will lead to greater opportunities for allies to continue to involve and support the consumer workforce to be involved in all aspects of service design, delivery and evaluation and to do what they can to ensure such roles are not tokenistic.

Confidence to express views

Consumers must be able to express views without censorship. Allies must respect these views even when they are hard to hear. This means allies need to learn to sit with their own discomfort at times.

Acknowledge and respect consumer knowledge

Consumer knowledge is central to the facilitation of consumer leadership. It must be acknowledged and respected for its uniqueness and its origins. Recovery is a prime example of consumer knowledge. It was developed by the consumer movement as a form of resistance to the medical focus of mental illness on diagnosis, symptoms and illness. Recovery is based on having self-determined choices and the idea that people can live satisfying lives regardless of symptoms (Anthony, 1993; Deegan, 1988), Over time recovery has been adopted earnestly by mental health professionals, frequently without collaboration with or even acknowledgement of its origins in the consumer/survivor movement (Walker, Emmens, & Simpson, 2012).

Wear only one hat

Allies may well have lived experience of mental distress, and may be asked to provide a consumer perspective on occasions. However, allies are not employed in consumer positions and so cannot provide the specialist knowledge and expertise consumers bring to their roles in addition to their lived experience. Just as a consumer who may also be a social worker should not be asked to provide a social work perspective.

Oppose the one-size-fits-all approach

Like all groups of people, consumers are heterogenous and should be included in roles based on specific expertise, not solely on being the 'token' consumer in the room. For example, a project on reducing restrictive interventions in inpatient settings should include expertise from consumers who have experienced inpatient settings and coercive practices.

2.2.7 WORKING COLLABORATIVELY IN TEAMS

FIONA SMITH, NOEL RENOUF, GRAHAM MEADOWS & LISA BROPHY

TEAMWORK IN RECOVERY-ORIENTED PRACTICE

The task of providing a comprehensive service is beyond the capacity of any one discipline or area of expertise so mental health teams are important. Teams often comprise members of different disciplines working together, including people with lived experience expertise, as a way of increasing the range of possible coordinated responses to the various needs of consumers and families. A well-functioning mental health team is one through which core and specialist assessments, support and interventions are provided in an integrated manner, in partnership with consumers, family carers and other service providers. Collaborative teamwork is a complex undertaking which should not be taken for granted. Interdisciplinary collaborative practice, which Bailey and Campling (2012) suggests is essential to mental health service delivery teamwork, enables paying attention to issues of power, culture and inclusiveness.

For recovery-oriented practice, a person-centred approach enabling individual choice and control in relation to 'treatment and care' is crucial (Bailey & Campling, 2012; Leamy et al., 2016; Pilgrim & McCranie, 2013). Adopting recovery-oriented practice requires rethinking structures, functions and purposes of teams—supporting people in their recovery journey with less emphasis on 'doing to' and more emphasis on 'doing with' (Asad & Chreim, 2016; Australian Health Ministers, 2013; Leamy et al., 2016; Department of Health, 2010; Woody, Baxter, Harris, Siskind, & Whiteford, 2018). Peer support workers have been found to assist with this shift to recovery-oriented practice through their contribution of the lived experience (Asad & Chreim, 2016; Gillard & Holley, 2014; Health Workforce Australia, 2014). Ensuring positive outcomes for consumers requires visionary leadership, shared values, clarity of purpose, and an atmosphere of trust in which all team members have a voice (Nancarrow et al., 2013).

When we talk about mental health teams, words such as 'multidisciplinary' and 'interdisciplinary' are often used interchangeably. It can be useful to distinguish among teams more carefully. Choi and Pak suggest the following:

- *multidisciplinary* refers to different disciplines working on a problem in parallel or sequentially, and without challenging their discipline boundaries

- *interdisciplinary* teams bring about the reciprocal interaction between disciplines necessitating a blurring of disciplinary boundaries, in order to generate new common methodologies, perspectives, knowledge, or even new disciplines
- *transdisciplinary* teams involve participants from different disciplines and other stakeholders, and through role release, and role expansion, transcend the disciplinary boundaries to look at the dynamics of whole systems in a holistic way (Choi & Pak, 2006, p. 359).

In contemporary mental health practice in Australia with the inclusion of peer workers, carer consultants and others with lived experience expertise, *transdisciplinary* may be the most useful description of how teams are evolving. Despite this, the majority of current mental health literature refers to *interdisciplinary* practice, therefore this term will most often be used.

In Australia, the main professions contributing to clinical mental health team membership are psychiatry, psychiatric nursing, psychology, social work and occupational therapy (State of Victoria, 2013). Peer support workers comprise one of the most rapidly growing components of the mental health workforce (Health Workforce Australia, 2014). Non-government psychosocial rehabilitation and community support services do not usually employ the same range of professionals. In these residential and individual support service settings, teams can form with less emphasis on professional composition and greater emphasis on different types of expertise, including, and in particular, the lived experience (Davies, Gray, & Butcher, 2014). In the context of personalised service delivery funded by the National Disability Insurance Scheme (NDIS) for people with psychosocial disability in Australia. This team composition, and mental health practitioner roles, continue to evolve.

In mental health settings team members perform a range of overlapping core shared tasks, such as establishing and maintaining a therapeutic relationship, complemented by specific specialties, such as assessments, practice orientations and treatments requiring specific expertise. Even where core work is shared, professional differences can be valuable. Different professions—and indeed different individuals—each bring their particular knowledge and skills to shared tasks in teams (Bailey & Campling, 2012; Ndibu Muntu Keba Kebe, Chiocchio, Bamvita, & Fleury, 2019; Payne, 2000). For example, many teams organise most of their work through a system of case management, care coordination or key working (Brophy, Hodges, Halloran, Grigg, & Swift, 2014). In such situations, the approach taken by a social worker may differ from that of a psychologist, for example, because of differences in professional knowledge and skill. Careful and thoughtful allocation of work is required to match workers with consumers in a way that acknowledges individual variations in expertise, views and consumer preferences. An essential element of team functioning is clarity about the respective roles of team members, including an awareness of the nature and limits to individual roles (Nancarrow et al., 2013). A clear (but humble) appreciation of what each person on the team can offer is a sound basis for negotiation about the distribution of roles. The complex communication and coordination required to successfully bring these disparate individuals and perspectives together necessitates thoughtful and committed leadership (Bailey & Campling, 2012; Nancarrow et al., 2013; Wenger, 2000).

Working with people who are experiencing mental distress necessitates going beyond psychiatric symptoms to include attention to physical problems, housing, income security, employment, recreation, family relationships, and emotional, psychological and spiritual issues (Davidson, Brophy, & Campbell, 2016; Leamy et al., 2016; Pilgrim & McCranie, 2013; World Health Organization and Calouste Gulbenkian Foundation, 2014). Meaningful peer workforce participation is an essential element in achieving optimal outcomes (Asad & Chreim, 2016; Gillard & Holley, 2014; Stanford, Sharland, Heller, & Warner, 2017; Vandewalle et al., 2016). Taking into consideration the requirements of funding bodies and the shift to personalised service delivery, team composition has to be responsive to need, not simply oriented to historical staffing patterns and local expedients. Meaningful peer workforce participation is now an essential element of achieving this responsiveness (Asad & Chreim, 2016; Gillard & Holley, 2014; Stratford et al., 2019; Vandewalle et al., 2016).

POWER, RESPONSIBILITY AND ACCOUNTABILITY IN TEAMS

The authority, power and status differentials inevitably present in teams and organisations need to be recognised and understood. Some of these derive from structural requirements (e.g. requirements of leadership, accountability, legal responsibilities), some are 'earned' (e.g. due to recognised knowledge and skills; (Bailey & Campling, 2012; Nancarrow et al., 2013; Onyett & Campling, 2002; Payne, 2000). In mental health teams, other differentials derive from variances in the 'language and models professional groups use to understand and describe mental distress' (Bailey & Campling, 2012, p.20; see also Maddock, 2015; Stacey et al., 2016). Some may be associated with wider social patterns of power, such as class, gender and race (Payne, 2000). Among the professions, tensions may exist regarding differences in education, and the often wide variations in financial remuneration, conditions of work and status. Leadership requires recognition of such tensions and their impact on team performance (Bailey & Campling, 2012; Nancarrow et al., 2013; Probst, 2012).

Some of the most contentious issues in teams relate to accountability and responsibility: *responsibility* being 'a set of tasks that an employing authority, professional body or court of law can legitimately demand of a practitioner', and *accountability* 'the relationship between that practitioner and the authority' (Onyett, 1995, p. 281; see also Bailey & Campling, 2012; Onyett & Campling, 2002). All team members have certain responsibilities, and teams are part of systems which demand professional accountability.

Clinical responsibility or professional responsibility generally refers to duty of care, attention to all the relevant factors and established and expected standards. Such responsibility rests with every member of the team, each of whom is accountable for their own professional conduct and the care provided. Psychiatrists, alone among the professions, sometimes carry 'vicarious responsibility' for the work of other team members, but because each carry personal responsibility for the standards of their work, the concept of one individual having ultimate or overall responsibility is not justified (Herrman, Trauer & Warnock, 2002; Payne, 2000). In practice, different team members may have varying degrees of responsibility for work with a particular client depending on their specific circumstances. For example, recent changes to the *Victorian Mental Health Act 2014* (Victoria State Government, 2014) apportion responsibility for key aspects of clinical practice among a range of mental health professionals and members of the Mental Health Tribunal (Maylea, 2017).

In practice one or more team members may assume responsibility for the allocation of work, coordination of assessments and treatment, and 'ultimate' decision making about certain matters. Team leaders and managers have responsibility for establishing and maintaining the conditions necessary for team functioning and decision making. Supervisors have responsibility for the supervision they provide. Psychiatrists may have particular responsibilities under mental health law. All members of the team have responsibilities to their colleagues, such as the requirement to share information properly. In well-functioning teams all responsibilities will be explicit and clear. Team leadership needs to be based in an agreed and sanctioned operational policy to assist the team achieve its goals and objectives. There should be agreed systems for coordination within the team (e.g. a case management system in a community mental health service), and systems to provide supervision and professional development appropriate to each member's responsibilities (Bailey & Campling, 2012; Nancarrow et al., 2013; Payne, 2000).

Neoliberal concerns about risk often dominate mental health service delivery, policy and law contributing to a risk-averse environment in which primary concern relates to fear of adverse outcomes (Davidson et al., 2016; Stratford et al., 2017). Such outcomes may include consumers harming themselves or others. Some argue such fears are over-emphasised and inconsistent with the recovery paradigm, respect for autonomy and the 'dignity of risk' (Carroll & McSherry, 2015; Davidson et al., 2016; Marsh & Kelly, 2018; Pilgrim & McCranie, 2013; Sawyer, 2008; Sawyer & Green, 2013; Wand, 2015). Carroll and McSherry (2015) provide a rationale for teams and individual practitioners to adopt a promotional rather than preventative focus to the risk of harm to self or others, which 'is intended to promote longer term recovering but, in the short term at least, may increase the risk of harm' (p. 2). Further, to enable greater respect for consumer autonomy and to reduce the need for individual practitioners and teams to engage in coercive and controlling practices Carroll and McSherry (2015) propose a three-step process of collaboration, clarification and communication.

Individual team members may have formal accountabilities to their employer, professional body and a state and/or federal registration authority, e.g. Australian Health Practitioner Regulation Agency (AHPRA). Team members will also be accountable to consumers, families and colleagues; will have legal accountabilities; and may hold *themselves* accountable in relation to religious, moral or ideological positions. Organisations often have different 'lines' of accountability: to a discipline senior (e.g. the senior nurse) for matters such as professional standards, training, recruitment and effectiveness; and to a team leader or manager for matters related to time, money and efficiency and adherence to organisational policies and procedures. Professional supervision may be provided by a team leader or by someone with relevant expertise outside the team. While serving important purposes, such multiple accountabilities require clear communication and a shared understanding of responsibilities. Regular feedback to individual team members and the team as a whole facilitate achievement of shared objectives.

GETTING THE BEST FROM TEAMS: ACHIEVING THE RIGHT BALANCE OF CORE AND SPECIALIST WORK

Effective teamwork requires that each team member have a sound professional foundation. However, when working in teams, the focus can sometimes be on being a 'good professional' (e.g. doctor, nurse, social worker, peer support worker), forgetting that effective team work demands effort and skill in working with others. Fortunately, many professional education programs now seek to prepare graduates for interdisciplinary or transdisciplinary work. Holtman and colleagues describe 'interprofessional professionalism' thus:

> Professionalism, as defined within disciplinary 'silos', can be misused to justify unchallenged autonomy and can inhibit cooperation across professional boundaries. Interprofessional professionalism, in contrast, is a transcendent phenomenon that works across the professions to support coordination in communication and care for the benefit of patients, clients, and families (Holtman, Frost, Hammer, McGuinn, & Nunez, 2011, p. 383).

As the professions possess their own training and expectations, they may view effective interdisciplinary teamwork quite differently (Bailey & Campling, 2012; Miller, Freeman, & Ross, 2001; Nancarrow et al., 2013; Tomizawa, Shigeta, & Reeves, 2017; Woody et al., 2018). Choi and Pak (2006) encourage a transdisciplinary approach which, in a mental health context, supports the rejection of paternalistic approaches of 'doing to', and facilitates 'doing with' by incorporating other stakeholders in a way that transcends disciplinary boundaries. Without the presence of peer workers and others with lived experience the real interests and voice of the consumer and the family may become lost due to preoccupation with other issues within the team. In contemporary service delivery systems it is expected that these interests be incorporated through the presence, within teams, of peer workers. It is essential the team structures its activities in order to keep its focus firmly on its primary task or function, and in this an explicit binding philosophy can be essential. To this end the team must have a meaningful, clearly defined and achievable task, explicitly expressed and understood, and must be committed to finding ways to collaborate directly with the consumer so that their views and interests are heard (Asad & Chreim, 2016; Health Workforce Australia, 2014).

Practice within teams may be adversely affected by incommensurable professional paradigms or theoretical approaches, differences in value systems, principles, moral language and definitions of what constitutes good practice. For example, varying understandings of what constitutes 'recovery' may be held by members of different professions (Leamy et al., 2016; Maddock, 2015; Pilgrim & McCranie, 2013). Avoiding or glossing over significant differences in language and perspective can easily reduce the level of communication to a common denominator, with a subsequent loss of depth and clarity in formulation and conceptualisation. Openness to the different perspectives of colleagues, consumers and other stakeholders leads to richer communication and understanding, the essence of good teamwork.

Team members' roles and tasks are both shared and specialised, as are their knowledge and skill. In the theoretical and conceptual foundations of the team's work existing differences must be valued – 'celebrated, not homogenised' – and practice based on a certain amount of 'ideological middle ground' (Onyett, 1999; Choi & Pak, 2006; Stacey et al., 2016; Woody et al., 2018). Teams tend to be most effective when individual members develop an attachment and commitment to the team without risking their professional identity (Mitchell, Parker, & Giles, 2011). Paying explicit attention to a shared value base of the different professions is one way of strengthening the common ground of the team (Bogg, 2010). For example, a recovery-oriented approach in which the consumer is the central active participant in treatment requires a distinctive service ethos, which in turn affects the way the team needs to function (Bee et al., 2015;). Genuine engagement with the complexity of problems and needs of consumers and their families requires a very high level of cooperation and coordination within teams and across service networks.

SOME DYNAMICS OF TEAMWORK

It is useful to think of the team as having two sets of functions. The first and most obvious is as a mechanism for providing comprehensive mental health care in a specific organisational context. Secondarily, the team functions as a vehicle and arena for its members to share and deal with workplace issues, including stresses and anxieties associated with the work.

Workplace stress may result from many sources, e.g. responsibility, difficulties in carrying out work roles, inadequate resources, and challenging work conditions (King, 2009; Salyers et al., 2015). Much of the work in the mental health field is inherently stressful as it involves a human encounter between a professional and a person experiencing great pain and suffering. This will inevitably be personally affecting, sometimes in ways not consciously recognised. Connections between work experiences and painful and conflicted personal experiences, present and past, can be all the more powerful for remaining unconscious and unacknowledged. Individual ways of dealing with work-related anxieties often come to the surface within teams.

The sustaining and energising potential of the team can be a vital source of support in the face of difficult work problems such as excessive workloads, the quality of supervision, and challenging working conditions. It is often within teams that effective professional practice is developed. Much of the process of developing professional resilience, and hence greater job satisfaction, relies on implicit learning that is 'embedded' in workplace interactions (Fleury, Grenier, Bamvita, & Chiocchio, 2018). Informal workplace interactions support coping strategies in managing challenging work situations and are invaluable in learning to thrive as effective and committed professionals (Carson, King, & Papatraianou, 2011).

By contrast, difficulties associated with team dynamics may have a debilitating effect on team members and their work. For example, the practical and emotional demands of teamwork may be so heavy team members feel overworked despite spending little time on direct client work (Galvin & McCarthy, 1994). Strong feelings expressed in the team setting may contribute to team dynamics that foster an atmosphere of pervasive discomfort characterised by confusion, frustration and bad feeling, unproductive overt and covert conflicts, overwhelming hopelessness or its opposite, manic unrealistic optimism. Sometimes the team seems to just avoid the work. Under these circumstances the team may tend to act in irrational ways, impeding rather than facilitating the thoughtful collaboration of experts. Not uncommonly the real decisions are then made outside the team's formal decision-making processes, with considerable team time and energy expended instead on discussions that cannot result in decisions, at least not ones capable of implementation. Sometimes individual team members may seek to exempt themselves from the team's activities and requirements (Norman & Peck, 1999). Even positive experiences may hinge on an artificial sense of togetherness and cohesion as a refuge from the pressures of work and a defence against possible conflicts (Stokes, 1994). Dynamics can be so powerful that team members can momentarily forget the real purpose of the work. This is not a new phenomenon. Freud was one of the first to describe, strongly and cogently, the 'group mind' or what these days might be called 'group-think':

> A group is extraordinarily credulous and open to influence, it has no critical faculty, and the improbable does not exist for it. It thinks in images, which call one another up by association and whose agreement with reality is never checked by any reasonable agency. The feelings of a group are always very simple and very exaggerated. So that a group knows neither doubt nor uncertainty (Freud, 1985 (1921), pp. 104–5).

Team members need to develop the reflective capacity and conceptual tools for understanding and working with such dynamics.

2.2.8 SPIRITUALITY AND THE TEAM

GRAHAM MEADOWS

Historically, concerns grounded in a religious outlook were very much within the foundations of moral treatment (see Chapter 1.1) during the period when the asylums were established in the United Kingdom, and for teams of mental health workers as they existed at that time. While the medical paradigm internationally was becoming increasingly ascendant as these institutions were established in Australia (see Chapter 1.7), needs for spiritual expression and the right of long-term residents to express this aspect of life were nevertheless recognised in psychiatric institutions; hospital chaplains and multidenominational chapels were common. The concrete presence of a hospital chapel and acknowledgment of the right to worship created a manifest presence for religion and spirituality in mental health care within such institutions.

In contrast, mental health practice in present-day contexts often occurs in settings where there are significant constraints on the recognition of a spiritual dimension to people's lives. Hospitals still typically have spaces set aside for worship, prayer or contemplation, whereas many community mental health care settings are well away from hospitals and typically do not. A hospital chaplain may not visit. The setting of work in publicly funded mental health services is one where there should be an underlying assumption that religious or spiritual beliefs should not affect access to health care and its benefits. Yet this can contribute to an avoidance of the issue of spirituality completely. Staff in such services will often regard each other's spiritual directions as a very personal matter, and spiritual experience may rarely be discussed, and even viewed as outside the bounds of permissible workplace-based discourse.

A complicating factor can occur when public mental health care is being delivered by institutions that have roots in a particular religious tradition, as is not uncommon in Australia. Spirituality or religion and science may be hard to reconcile, and the pressure to be scientific may hold practitioners away from the topic area. There often may be a strong social taboo against discussing religious matters, which serves to protect the workers from potentially damaging arguments about strongly held beliefs that may be at odds with each other if declared. It may not be an uncommon experience to work for many years with other practitioners and yet have little or no knowledge of their personal religious or spiritual affiliation or level of engagement. These factors may not be conducive to the potentially important task of opening out frank discussion about spiritual or religious needs and hopes of clients of the service (see Chapter 2.3; Oman, 2018).

2.2.9 INTERAGENCY WORKING AND SERVICE NETWORKS

NOEL RENOUF & FIONA SMITH

Many of the principles of effective teamwork apply to the working relationships established with individual practitioners and organisations outside the organisation. Consumers and their families require good access to a wide range of health and community services. Mental health services sit within a service network, receiving referrals from other services, referring on to them, and sometimes working together. The need for mental health workers to collaborate with other service providers has been made increasingly explicit in national and state policy as well as service standards, e.g. The Fifth National Mental Health and Suicide Prevention Plan (Department of Health, 2017). However, this endeavour has been made more complex with the recent implementation of the NDIS and the shift to personalised care (Brophy, Bruxner, Wilson, Cocks, & Stylianou, 2015).

Wherever organisational boundaries exist there is a need to address issues associated with interagency working. This applies within mental health service systems: across the boundary between a community mental health service and an inpatient unit for example; across the boundaries between child and adolescent, youth, 'adult' and aged persons mental health services; across boundaries with each of the many elements of a specialist mental health service system (forensic mental health, personality disorder services and so on). It applies to boundaries between public and private mental health service providers, and boundaries with organisations representing consumers and family carers. It also applies to relationships with a wide range of services in other sectors important to mental health, including physical health, alcohol and drugs, intellectual disability, housing, child and family welfare, employment and vocation, income security, education, and police and corrections, and potentially many others (Cooper, Evans, & Pybis, 2016; Parker et al., 2018). Furthermore, to address the mental health needs of particular groups (such as people from different cultural backgrounds, Indigenous people, people with disabilities), it will often be necessary to establish and maintain specific collaborations with groups and organisations with expertise in each of those areas.

Intersectoral linkages are not an adjunct but an integral component of mental health work which sit alongside services provided directly to consumers and their families and population-based mental health services (Gulbinat et al., 2004; Townsend et al., 2004).

ESTABLISHING AND MAINTAINING RELATIONSHIPS WITHIN A NETWORK OF SERVICES

The size and complexity of the service system might seem overwhelming, though in rural and regional areas especially, we might wish for a greater diversity and availability of services. To engage effectively mental health services need a workable strategy. Clear formal partnerships between clinical services, NDIS providers and primary health care sit at the core of the system of relationships for a mental health system (Victorian Government Department of Human Services, 2009; Department of Health, 2010; State of Victoria, 2013; Department of Health & Ageing, 2013). Beyond this, each service will need to give priority to the establishment of other key partnerships that reflect the needs of consumers and their families, while remaining open and receptive to new relationships. Some of these partnerships are likely to be well-established and ongoing: for example, adult mental health services always need a good working relationship with child and family services because there will always be a significant number of parents among mental health consumers. Some partnerships might be more fleeting and opportunistic, established to address the needs of one or two consumers at a particular time. While the principles apply more generally, the following section will focus on child and family services as an example.

The development of linkages and partnerships between services and organisations might start simply by gathering good information about the community and its services (in itself often a considerable task) and, reciprocally, making sure our own organisation is well known and its purposes and ways of working well understood in the community. For example, effective work with a consumer who is a parent may involve collaboration with a child and family welfare agency, a teacher or playgroup convenor, and others. The pioneering work of Cowling (1999, 2004) and others has developed into a very rich understanding of the ways in which effective collaborations can be established to meet the needs of parents with a mental illness and their children (Goodyear et al., 2015; see also Australian Charities and Not-for-profits Commission (ACNC), 2011 and Chapter 2.7 for further information about supports for parents with a mental illness and their children).

Further examples of collaborative models of care between sectors and collaborative ways of working to support specific populations for whom cultural, language and geographic barriers may otherwise limit access to effective mental health care can be found elsewhere (e.g., Lee, Keating, de Castella, & Kulkarni, 2010; Purdie, Dudgeon, & Walker, 2010). These demonstrate the growing body of knowledge and experience in establishing partnerships for mental health service delivery within diverse community contexts. The role of care coordinator or support facilitator has emerged as an important role in the development of partnerships and in assisting consumers to navigate the complexity of the health and welfare sector (Brophy et al., 2014). Another role to support this work is that of 'boundary spanner', someone who can mobilise resources and ensure system changes that are in the interests of consumers accessing the support and care they need (Brophy et al., 2014). The boundary spanner needs to be able to exert authority 'that enables an integrated and sustained system response focused on the needs of the client' (p. 399).

Another element in the development of partnerships involves receptiveness to approach from agencies, professionals or community services. This will sometimes involve the establishment of formal arrangements for consultation. The person providing the consultation brings expertise: specialist knowledge about mental health problems; skill in responding; knowledge and influence within their agency and service network; and willingness and ability to impart their expertise to others. More than this, effective consultation is a partnership:

> Consultation is joint exploration partly of the question at hand, partly exploring the alternatives for managing it, and partly exploring what there is in oneself, in the consultative relationship and in the work setting that helps the work advance (Steinberg 1989, cited by Luntz, 1999, p. 28).

A recovery-oriented philosophy along with the more contemporary principles of co-design and co-delivery draws on a richly textured set of definitions. Luntz, for example, distinguishes three levels of mental health consultation which, since they remain in wide use, are listed here:

1. In *primary consultation*, the consultant is first briefed and then meets the client, and then a joint decision is taken about what might happen next.
2. In *secondary consultation*, the consultant does not actually meet the client, but rather discusses the situation and offers suggestions based on information that is put together by the consultee.
3. In *tertiary consultation*, the discussions focus more on agency structure and functioning, rather than the interactions between workers and their clients (Luntz, 1999, 2000).

Child protection services, for example, require access to the specialist knowledge and skill of mental health workers to do their work effectively because parental mental health problems, along with substance misuse and domestic violence, are commonly present in the families of children in need of protection, and because many such children have mental health problems themselves. Child protection and mental health services will sometimes have clients in common, sometimes not. In any case, community mental health services (both adult and

CAMHS) must find ways to make available their specialist expertise in a way that it can be used by child protection workers (Akister, 2011).

Drawing upon research into mental health services and child protection (Cooper et al., 2016; Darlington & Feeney, 2008; Darlington, Feeney, & Rixon, 2004; Darlington, Feeney, & Rixon, 2005a; Darlington, Feeney, & Rixon, 2005b), some of the issues that need to be addressed to ensure successful interagency collaboration can be identified. Each agency needs to give explicit support and guidance to its workers to develop collaborative working, recognising that it takes time and resources. While often relying on effective interpersonal contact between individual workers, it cannot succeed in the long term unless supported by the management of each organisation (Webber, McCree, & Angeli, 2011).

Formal organisational structures that embed collaboration as part of both practice and organisational culture provide two key advantages that cannot otherwise be achieved. First, whether a client will have the advantage of interagency collaboration will not be dependent upon the worker to whom they are allocated. Second, protocols and service level agreements provide clear procedures and boundaries that can facilitate contact and provide clarity around confidentiality requirements. That is, formal structures can facilitate effective communication (Darlington & Feeney, 2008, p. 196).

Issues of confidentiality and information sharing need to be addressed explicitly, and clearly, by formalising consent processes and establishing protocols for information exchange. Different agencies may have different legal requirements and organisational practices, and all parties concerned—in particular, the client and their family—need to know the circumstances under which information of different kinds can, and cannot, be shared. Gaps in knowledge about the respective agencies need to be addressed, including basic information about services available, the roles of workers and the best contact points. Staff of each agency need to develop a realistic understanding of what they can realistically be expected to achieve, and the legislative, policy and other parameters within which each operates. Different organisational priorities and cultures within agencies (such as the differences in professional orientations within the team) can sometimes lead to misunderstanding. All of this suggests that a lot of attention needs to be paid to frequent clear communication of information at all levels and, wherever possible, joint education and projects (Darlington et al., 2004). As with the challenges of interdisciplinary teamwork, the critical issue within service networks is to keep the focus firmly on meeting the needs of the consumer, remembering the fundamental purpose of the collaboration.

CONCEPTUALISING COLLABORATION WITHIN A SERVICE NETWORK

Many partnerships of this kind will be within a health and social welfare service system, with some involving multiple organisations. For each of the elements to work effectively they must be grounded in a matrix of both formal and informal relationships involving the key stakeholders contributing to the health and wellbeing of people with mental health problems.

Interagency networking is the development and maintenance of a system of inter-organisational linkage characterised by collective decision making and a set of positive feedback relationships between the internal structure, systems and values of participating organisations and the inter-organisational network of which they are all members (Trevillion, 1999).

The vision of interagency working contained in the definition above helps workers to think about their own agencies as part of a bigger picture. It is a vision that goes beyond the preoccupations of agency-based practice with consumers. The idea of 'collective decision making' can be particularly challenging because it necessarily involves each agency and each worker giving up some degree of control about the outcome of the collaboration and moving beyond 'routinised coordination' to allow the possibility of something new and creative (Hood, 2011). Herein lies one of the main challenges of working collaboratively, because the anxiety associated with having to step outside the comfort of the familiar processes of one's own agency and the uncertainty can lead to collapse of the collaboration. Woodhouse and

Pengelly identified just such an outcome in relation to interagency collaboration.

> The more threatening the anxiety, the greater and more fraught it becomes to enter imaginatively into each other's working world for fear of losing hold of their own. Practitioners may then fall back on the 'bedrock' of a narrowly defined primary task. Boundaries tend to become defensive bulwarks instead of the definition of a secure base for commerce and negotiation (Woodhouse & Pengelly, 1991, p. 229).

Issues of this kind may affect interagency work at all levels from the simplest to the most complex. For example, a willingness and capacity to remain involved during a period of transition can make all the difference to the success of a referral from one agency to another. When interagency collaborations fail, it may be a sign that the workers have (momentarily at least) lost sight of the fact that effective work with consumers inevitably requires a capacity to collaborate outside our own workplaces.

2.2.10 COLLABORATING AND PARTNERING IN THE COMMUNITY SECTOR FOR BETTER OUTCOMES

LAURA COLLISTER

INTRODUCTION

Non-government community-managed services are one element of mental health services in Australia. The organisations are diverse, varying in scale, geographic reach and foci. Some organisations exclusively focus on mental health, while others have a wider scope incorporating, for example, primary health and disability. Specialist organisations, such as Aboriginal community-controlled organisations, provide specialist services to a defined cohort.

Notwithstanding this diversity, a common feature of all NGOs is their willingness and capacity to work collaboratively with other organisations providing treatment, support and assistance to the people they serve. This happens at an individual level where the focus is on addressing client needs at an organisational level, where services are planned and delivered in partnership, and at a systems level where organisations join together to advocate for system reform.

REASONS FOR FOSTERING COLLABORATION AND PARTNERSHIP

People with mental health issues can experience a range of needs. Some are the direct result of illness, however many are not—rather they are consequential to mental health treatment and the social and economic disadvantage experienced by people with mental health issues. The National Mental Health Commission reported:

- People with mental health issues have poorer physical health, for example people with psychotic illnesses have a rate of diabetes three times that of the general community.
- People with mental health issues experience high rates of unemployment, for example 67.3% of people with severe mental illness are employed compared to 22.3% of people without mental health issues.
- 20% of people experiencing mental health issues used alcohol excessively, or have a drug addiction (National Mental Health Commission, 2014b).

Lack of housing security is also a key issue for many people experiencing mental health issues. The Australian Bureau of Statistics (2014a) reported that approximately one-third of people between the ages of 25 and 54 years who reported having a mental health condition had experienced homelessness in their lifetime while The Survey of High Impact Psychosis (Morgan et al., 2011) found 5% of people were currently homeless at the time of the survey. Based on this data alone, it is obvious that no one agency has the capacity to provide an adequate, evidence-based response to the array of needs that may be experienced by people with mental health issues.

From a consumer and carer perspective, the mental health service 'system' is often experienced as fragmented, difficult to access and confusing. The system has been described as not well linked or integrated, and not designed to enable service coordination and integration (National Mental Health Commission, 2014b).

Partnership and collaboration underpin NGO responses to addressing the needs of people experiencing mental health issues and their families. This strategy enables:

- The expertise of each organisation to be harnessed to provide a coordinated and comprehensive response to each service user and their family's needs.
- Individuals and their families to be assisted in navigating and accessing the most appropriate support to meet their needs.
- Duplication and gaps in the existing service 'system' to be most efficiently managed.

From an evidence-based perspective there is ample evidence that coordination of services, enabled by partnership and collaboration, results in better outcomes. For example, the individual placement and support model delivers superior employment outcomes for people with severe mental illness and has, as a fundamental ingredient, integration of mental health and employment supports (Drake, Bond, & Becker, 2012). Likewise, Housing First approaches include a partnership between mental health support and housing providers (Padgett, Henwood, & Tsemberis, 2016) (See Chapter 2.6.).

PARTNERSHIP APPROACHES AND STRATEGIES IN USE

Partnerships between NGOs and other agencies range from informal agreements to collaborate on the care of individual service users, to formal contractual relationships. The key areas that partnership agreements typically encompass are:

- Mechanisms for ensuring coordinated care is provided to service users of the clinical service and the NGO in a defined geographic area. This area usually reflects the catchment area of the clinical service.
- Structured processes for joint area based planning.
- Joint staff training mechanisms to build interagency relationships and common approaches to recovery.
- Streamlining of information gathering, referral and communication.
- Processes for information sharing, including informed consent.
- Agreed processes for evaluating service effectiveness, including agreed Key Performance Indicators.
- Contractual arrangements for the provision of services.

Positive examples of partnership programs in Australia are:

- Community living support services in NSW. Psychosocial rehabilitation and support is provided by an NGO to people experiencing severe mental health issues in each Local Health District (LHD) in NSW. A Service Level Agreement between the NGO, and the respective LHD is a requirement of the program. The two organisations are mandated to develop and implement shared assessment and review, risk assessment and care planning processes. Collaboration with a housing provider is required. Information sharing protocols are required to ensure services are coordinated and duplication is minimised.
- Step Up, Step Down services (or Prevention and Recovery Care services) offer a sub-acute residential support option for people leaving acute inpatient care or experiencing a relapse of mental health issues. Typically, the residential environment and psychosocial rehabilitation elements are provided by the NGO, whereas the clinical treatment, risk management, entry and exit decisions are provided by the clinical service. The intention is for consumers and their families to experience a single integrated service response.

While most formal partnerships occur between government-funded agencies, including NGOs, there are some innovative programs that extend beyond these typical boundaries. The Doorway program based on the Housing First model, operated by Wellways Australia supports people to choose, find and sustain housing in the private rental market. An essential component of the program is the creation of an 'integrated team' comprising the service user (and their family), clinical provider, Housing and Recovery Worker, employment provider and real estate agent (Dunt et al., 2016).

CHALLENGES AND WEAKNESSES OF THE PARTNERSHIP APPROACH

While both the clinical and NGO sector recognise the benefits of partnerships, the challenges of this approach are also well acknowledged. Effective partnerships require intentional effort and time to deliver the intended outcomes. Practically speaking, effective partnerships require the support of senior staff from both agencies who are able to negotiate and agree partnership principles, roles of each respective agency, funding parameters, Key Performance Indicators and conflict resolution procedures. Typically shared roles exist that may lead to 'battles over territory', and differences in the recovery orientation of each agency emerge. Addressing these issues in a timely manner is essential for the benefits of partnerships to be realised. Governance mechanisms, such as bi-monthly partnership meetings, monitor the effectiveness of the partnership, address issues as they arise and ideally take a proactive approach to reaping the benefits of the partnership.

As described, partnerships are usually driven by the need to provide coordination across agencies for the benefit of service users and their families. Typically, however, partnerships predominate between the NGO and tertiary mental health services, and to a lesser extent NGOS and housing/homelessness agencies. There are fewer examples of partnerships between NGOs and employment agencies, NGOs and general practitioners, and NGOs and educational institutions. While the clinical and NGO sector have been encouraged to operate in partnership by government bureaucracies the same level of encouragement is not evident across these other sectors despite the potential to offer considerable benefit.

Partnerships are an effort to improve service user outcomes and experiences. They are a response to a fragmented system containing duplication and gaps. Meeting the aspirations articulated in the Fifth National Mental Health and Suicide Prevention Plan (Department of Health, 2017) of coordinated treatment and supports for people with severe and complex mental illness will require large scale redesign of the existing service system. While it is imperative we work together to achieve this end, existing service level partnerships will not be enough to achieve this outcome.

FUTURE OF PARTNERSHIPS

The non-government sector has a strong track record of working in partnership, especially with clinical mental health services. The changing landscape of mental health services across Australia will demand a broader set of partnerships and partnership skills into the future. Primary Health Networks are taking leadership in identifying needs, planning and commissioning mental health services at a regional level. This involves a range of stakeholders, including general practitioners, local councils, carers and consumers. NGOs, as a sector, have an important contribution to make to these regional based planning processes, and more broadly to influence state and Commonwealth mental health reform.

Equally, the roll-out of the NDIS has and will continue to impact on the NGO sector. Existing NGOs are challenged by the current pricing structure which provides little to no funding to support case conferencing and partnership activities. A raft of new providers are entering the sector and consumers will increasingly select providers based on their current needs and preferences. This environment challenges traditional partnership approaches which have been predicated on a relatively stable small number of area based providers.

In conclusion, the collaboration and partnership approaches used in Australia have been productive. They will continue to be important for NGOs but will be required to adapt to the new mental health service system. Partnerships will need to be broader and provide more efficiency to deliver benefit into the future.

2.2.11 COLLABORATION WITH PRIMARY CARE: ISSUES AND BEST PRACTICES

GRAHAM MEADOWS

Many people with mental health problems will receive their mental health care in the primary health system (Burgess et al., 2009; see Chapter 1.6), so often outside the structure of a team. Many others will receive care from multiple providers, whether or not these people communicate with each other. Although severe behavioural disturbance and lower levels of functioning promote contact with specialist services, many people in contact only with primary care may have concerns and problems just as complex as do those in contact with specialist services. Where significant effort from public mental health services has at times been put into general practitioner (GP) shared care, as in the case of primary mental health teams in Victoria (see Chapter 1.7), the evidence suggests that complexity and chronicity are characteristic of the clients seen in these services (Jespersen et al., 2009).

Ideally, a sophisticated system of collaborative work should be in place, based around primary care to ensure that when necessary there is access to specialist consultation, and that additional specialist needs are met. For example, a general practitioner may need to be able to work with a consulting psychiatrist and, from time to time, refer to other professionals, such as social workers, occupational therapists and psychologists. Referral back into primary care should be easy and well supported in terms of information flows, shared understandings and respectful relationships between the participating clinicians. Stepped care models (see Chapter 1.5) can assist in clarifying relationships and criteria for referral through different levels of the service system. (Kates et al., 2018)

Building such collaborations takes significant time investment (Meadows, Harvey, Joubert, Barton, & Bedi, 2007). GPs have now been systematically encouraged for over two decades to work in collaborative ways with other mental health practitioners through Medicare items and other incentives that allow remuneration for activities such as case conferencing and discussion of cases with psychiatrists on the telephone or in shared care arrangements. Innovations to funding arrangements through Better Outcomes and Better Access initiatives (see Chapter 1.7) have allowed increased access to psychological and, to a more limited extent, other professional services where the GP is the gatekeeper for the services.

In principle, there now exists a set of Medicare rebates that would be compatible with extensive shared care and other collaborative arrangements between GPs and private psychiatrists; however, it is evident that the existence of the rebates alone will not suffice to ensure that such collaboration takes place. Positive models for such collaborations do exist (see Craven & Bland, 2006; Kates et al., 2018). By way of example, in the CLIPP model (Meadows et al., 2007), psychiatrists regularly visited GP clinics; there was a pattern of formal and informal relationships through co-located care provision; and an approach to long-term management for people typically with schizophrenia was introduced (Meadows, 2003) that involved the very active involvement of a psychiatric nurse. It would now be the case that all of these activities involving complex collaborations between public and private sector providers could be resourced from Commonwealth funding (see Chapter 1.7). However, the incentives of this funding do not necessarily encourage such systematic use of the opportunities that these rebates present, and liaison is typically not this well organised. Nevertheless, the opportunities for cross-sectoral collaboration with the shifts in financial provisions for care from the Commonwealth are now very considerable. It may repay workers in the various sectors to look creatively at the possibilities that these developments offer.

2.2.12 COMMENTARY AND REFLECTION

NOEL RENOUF & GRAHAM MEADOWS

Collaboration is pivotal to effective working with consumers, families and colleagues in teams and other services to achieve positive outcomes for consumers and families. It has also become a central theme in national mental health policies and standards related to direct care and to interagency and cross-sectoral work necessary to ensure access to effective and coordinated mental health care. This is another aspect where the imperatives of development in clinical decision making (see Chapters 1.1 and 2.3) will apply. Relevant themes here include: skills and habits of reflection, the inner capacity identified as dialectical thinking to hold in mind some of the discussions, at time tensions, that teamwork may involve, and openness to the reality of communities and mental health care delivery systems as having features of complexity. So working collaboratively can be both complex and challenging, but there are some straightforward measures to take to build effective collaborations with consumers, families and agencies within and outside mental health services. Respect and recognition of differing perspectives, open communication and goodwill need to be cultivated in interpersonal interactions, at the interagency level, and in interactions with broader society and communities.

2.3

ASSESSMENT IN MENTAL HEALTH

GRAHAM MEADOWS, BANI AADAM, SALLY BUCHANAN-HAGEN, MARILYN CUGNETTO, INDIGO DAYA, JOHN FARHALL, SABIN FERNBACHER, ELLIE FOSSEY, CAROLINE JOHNSON, ROBERT KING, LYN MAHBOUB, HARRY MINAS, MELISSA PETRAKIS, CATH ROPER, NEERAJ SAREEN, JUSTIN SCANLAN & TIMOTHY WAND

2.3.1 ASSESSMENT IN MENTAL HEALTH PRACTICE: AN INTRODUCTION

GRAHAM MEADOWS & JOHN FARHALL

Depending on the context, assessment in mental health practice might focus, among other possibilities, on formulating a specific presenting problem, assigning the most useful diagnosis, understanding where a consumer is at in their personal recovery, or comprehensively clarifying needs across life domains to develop a case management plan. Best practice is to do this work alongside the person. Appropriately, this chapter opens with a consumer perspective, cogently illustrating the human impact and complexity that practitioners need to take into account in their practice.

The clinical mental health assessment approach of the psychiatry tradition (see Chapter 1.1), adopted in most clinical mental health services and used by interdisciplinary teams (see Chapter 2.2), is presented next. In general, the purpose of assessment is to provide the information that enables a practitioner to gain an understanding of the person who is requiring assistance, their presenting need or problem, and the context in which this is happening. This initial gathering of information and observations then starts the ongoing process of developing and revising a 'formulation'—a practitioner's hypothesised explanation of how these issues have arisen, why they are now a focus of attention for this person, and how the person's life context may be influencing the issues. Importantly, it is the formulation, rather than the problem itself or the diagnosis, which can typically most meaningfully prompt ways of working. A critical set of questions arise around application of diagnoses and how they might be communicated, raising issues of ethics (see Chapter 1.5) and of preventive implications (see Chapter 1.5). Incautious problematisation of distress in the form of a disorder can be disabling (see Chapter 1.5), so there are questions to be addressed not just of what the diagnosis might be but how likely it is that there is one, and so whether and how to have conversations about this with the consumer and others involved. Recognising others may have different ways of explaining what is happening, especially cross culturally is vital to consider too (see Chapter 1.3). Conceptually, clinical expertise can be viewed as one set of expertise, to be considered alongside the expertise of the person in front of you, who may or may not share the clinician's world view. In relation to diagnosis, a critical decision in this text has been to structure our diagnostic considerations around ICD-11 (World Health Organization, 2018b). An important driver of this decision is that ICD-11, unlike DSM-5 (American Psychiatric Association, 2013), is readily available on the internet. So consumers and others can access the diagnostic descriptions and openly discuss their opinions/ideas about diagnoses with the clinician while at the same time, clinicians can be curious about how the person understands what is happening for them.

Much of the interdisciplinary practice in clinical mental health services reflects some version of the clinical assessment within a biopsychosocial framework introduced in this chapter. However, the degree to which nonmedical professionals have been specifically trained in this or developed service-specific skills varies according to discipline (e.g. diagnosis is a required competency for psychologists) and role (e.g. crisis team work requires high-level assessment skills from team members regardless of discipline). In addition, a role- or discipline-specific framework–such as psychological therapy, medication prescribing–will sometimes be the most relevant aid for connecting the particular expertise of the mental health worker to the assessed needs and wishes of a consumer.

In this chapter, we consider some established and some newer frameworks that are helpful in prompting thinking about how to move from assessment to practice: that is, exploring with the consumer actions and ways of working that might be helpful. Needs Assessment and the Vulnerability-Stress-Coping model have proved useful for more than two decades, and are presented first. The present shift towards a recovery orientation in policies and services (AHMAC, 2013a, 2013b) has led to the development of practitioner frameworks and guidance for translating this into action: the PULSAR-REFOCUS approach is presented in Section 2.3.7 as an illustration. Trauma-informed assessment and care is then discussed as increasingly accepted as best practice across widely differing mental health services and supports, and strongly resonates with consumers.

Lastly, in this chapter we present discipline-oriented assessment from general practice, nursing, occupational therapy, psychology and social work perspectives. Some of these contributions address the broader context of discipline-oriented assessment, such as the philosophical stance, and models informing assessment; some focus on assessment methods and specific instruments.

At points in these presentations we will consider the issue of rights, with awareness that while a well conducted assessment can be a vehicle for guaranteeing a person's right to quality care, assessments also by process or outcome potentially infringe human rights.

2.3.2 ASSESSMENT: A CONSUMER PERSPECTIVE

LYN MAHBOUB

Generally when I think about assessment in this context, I immediately notice my resistance to the idea. In particular, I think about how clinical assessment can so often be subjective and devoid of the person's particular history and context. I reflect on how it can involve ideas about 'mental illness' where the ontology of mental distress is heavily contested and not yet settled. I also think about the history of arguments put forward for doing things 'to people' reportedly 'for their best interests' rather than with people. I too am reminded of a number of recent ideas regarding safeguarding which have had to be put forward to safeguard people's human rights, choice and control and their right to make mistakes and learn and grow. At times, assessment unless done reflexively, can fail to do this well.

Specifically, I am troubled if someone holds the uncritical assumption that assessment is 'the way to go' and often wonder what we might do if we did not do an assessment? While on one hand I agree that a 'view from the bridge' by an external party who is considering a range of things *with us,* can bring useful ideas to the table, particularly if they are offered reflexively and in a way that works to value and privilege lived experience expertise. Simultaneously, I am aware of the potential for getting assessment so wrong. I appreciate this opportunity here to unpack some of the hidden ideas within the notion of assessment.

Firstly, it is important to acknowledge that assessment implies assessment against 'a norm or standard', and that this 'norm or standard' is settled and agreed upon. I would argue that this is often not the case. For example, within the consumer/survivor movement what it means to be human or normal is heavily contested. This shows up in the contestation of psychiatric diagnosis and the dispute of the idea that mental distress (or madness) is best described as an 'illness'. Indeed, many people from within critical psychiatry seek to demonstrate how within mental health services and psychiatry, all too often emotions and 'problems in living' are re-languaged and configured as symptomatic of 'conditions' or 'disorders', located within the individual's *psyche, mind* and/or *brain.* Such individualistic renderings let politicians and governments off the hook for attending to domestic violence, abuse, discrimination, poverty and other social and structural determinants of health. This reductionist medicalisation of distress reinforces the push for putting valued dollars into beds and brain research. For example, when the 1990s were coined 'the Decade of the Brain', this diverted research dollars into brain research, instead of helping people in poverty and stopping the distress from domestic violence (see Chapters 1.2 and 2.7). Essentially, this then reinforces the idea of continually looking for answers within interiors, instead of working to uphold human rights and social justice agendas, attending to the conditions of the exterior, and all the while forgetting to return the gaze and examine the construction of 'normal'.

A specific example of contestation or disagreement about 'the norm' can be found within the Hearing Voices Movement, which questions the construction of the 'negative symptoms of schizophrenia'. Proponents of the Hearing Voices Movement ask 'how can we be so sure we are seeing the symptoms of schizophrenia and not the impact or consequences of hearing voices?' (Szasz & Szasz, 1974; Foucault & Howard, 1988; Mosher & Burti, 1989). Others crucially pointed out, people are often experiencing real 'problems in living'—these may include: poverty, exclusion, unequal access to employment and justice, discrimination, racism and abuse, interpersonal relationship difficulties and iatrogenic problems such as direct effects of medication—weight gain, lactation, incontinence, higher mortality from cancer and other treatable diseases (see Chapters 1.2, 1.3, 2.5 and 2.6). So institutional forces, intersectional and structural inequalities may affect people socially, economically, politically, mentally and physically.

Another aspect of assessment, and the notion of being measured against a norm, that is important to consider, is the context in which the assessment is being carried out. It is essential to flag here that people using mental health services are already 'marked' (at least by psychology and psychiatry) as 'abnormal', disordered, not competent and lacking in insight. Therefore, poorly practised assessments can further cement such ideas within people and lead to disempowerment and hopelessness. Not only can such practices create the conditions for consumers to see themselves as 'lacking', but they can further serve to render the consumer's strengths invisible and lead clinicians to develop a deficit-based lens.

While thinking about these norms and standards, it is important to highlight that assessments are judgements of a kind. Therefore, the uncritical, non-reflexive use of assessment has a number of associated problems, notwithstanding the normal human fears of judgement and 'not measuring up' that can add further stress and distress. So, in reflecting on assessment, it is crucial to examine the values and expectations underpinning such (often-moralistic) judgements and question whether the measuring stick being applied is reasonable and one we might all be guided by. For example, all too often consumers report the pressure to be 'more normal than normal' (Coleman, 2011). This might especially refer to people's 'living skills'. At times unrealistic standards are applied to consumers in terms of budgeting, cleaning house and cooking which, interestingly, often are markedly different to the worker's own standards and expectations of themselves. Additionally, an individualistic white, middle-class lens commonly guides many practitioners, and the real world application of this lens is not routinely questioned. What can then follow are constructions of people as 'lacking engagement', 'apathetic' and 'lacking in motivation'. Such constructions become a truth that then often informs the clinician's feelings towards the person and takes them away from more reflexive, empathic understandings that consider the losses encountered by vast numbers of people using mental health services.

To illustrate, many consumers have lost the contents of their house several times over, and the will to re-attach and care about belongings can be massively eroded, particularly as people's grief is all too often pathologised and medicated. When there is no space to grieve the multitude of losses, perhaps it is a wise coping strategy to not get attached to one's house and possessions, particularly if one feels powerless to stop mental health services pulling you out of your home into hospital for extended weeks and months and that during this time your housing and its contents can be lost again. Perhaps such so-called 'apathy' could be a clever, hidden coping strategy that keeps one from feeling the unbearable potential loss that can occur out 'of the blue' without agreement. So, I argue for the importance of questioning our assumptions and so-called failure to meet the often white Anglo-Saxon, value-laden standards, so as to reflexively consider the unequal power relations that assessment can set up.

Here I am reminded of experiences (both witnessed and personally experienced) where assessment has been done on and to people (rather than with them) effectively reinscribing dominant power relations and often re-enacting micro-aggressions. In essence, power is exercised through enactment of the 'clinical gaze' (Foucault, 1973). In addition, and perhaps more significantly, many argue that such practices function to create 'docile subjects' who are 'compliant and well-behaved' thereby further eroding people's citizenship and self-determination (Foucault, 1979, p. 171).

It could be argued that assessments can be considered one of Foucault's 'dividing practices' which function to fabricate a separation between the clinician and the consumer (Foucault & Howard, 1988). As Turner and Samson signal, this is problematic because 'the greater the social distance between client and the professional...the greater the helplessness of the client in relation to the expert' (Turner & Samson, 1995, p. 133). Additionally, such a separation can take the clinician away from remembering/recognising that they too might have feelings and needs, which are likely not all that dissimilar to those of the consumer, should they find themselves impacted by mental distress, poverty, discrimination, abuse and other social determinants and structural barriers to health and wellbeing.

In many ways this separation works to forge the in-built assumption (or is it implication) that the clinician/practitioner/professional who is in the role of 'assessor' has specialised knowledge or skills in *observation, evaluation, measurement and prediction* and that this knowledge is potentially more valuable or superior to the person's. Furthermore, the logic then follows that they additionally possess the necessary 'know how' to, firstly, spot impairment, abnormality and insufficient functioning or deviations from the norm, but secondly (as luck would have it) that they have sufficient knowledge to know 'just what to do about it', how to 'treat it' or how to respond to what they find in this assessment. Indeed, it could be argued, to use a term coined by Smail, that this is an example of 'a pretence of therapeutic potency' (Smail, 1994, p. 3). This contrived position not only contributes to feelings of inadequacy within consumers, but so too, feelings of what has been dubbed 'imposter syndrome' can be felt by clinicians as they do not often feel 'all-knowing' and fully measure up to those norms and standards themselves.

Other important questions to consider are: 'whose interests are being served by the assessment' or 'who is the assessment being done for'? In these times of increased pressures on organisations to adhere to good governance processes and to 'demonstrate outcomes' so as to earn their government funding, all too often people are subject to highly contested assessment tools. A case in point, in particular, is the *Mental Health Recovery Star* (Triangle Consulting, 2010) which is critiqued by the Facebook-based survivor group 'Recovery in the Bin' for its individualistic, prescriptive stance (Recovery in the Bin: A critical theorist and activist collective, 2020). This group remind us that tools such as this completely ignore 'problems that exist in communities and wider society, that mental health is a profoundly political issue' and an issue that requires attention to exteriors as differentiated to interiors.

In thinking about power, it is important, with Foucault in mind, to think also about resistance. From a consumer perspective, I am deeply interested in how assessments are done. A common objection from consumers is having assessments done *to* them or *on* them, rather than with them. This grievance often marks their resistance to the power inequalities that can be visited upon them in 'being assessed'. At times, the only way to work towards clawing back control and power is to perhaps stretch or fabricate responses or simply be monosyllabic. For many of us, the imposition of the assessment device into our private lives leads us to want to get out of the assessment space as quickly as possible. For many consumers, the expectation that we will just respond to questions about the innermost corners of our lives, our past experiences, our doubts, desires and dreams without any kind of relationship with the professional is at best naïve and at worst arrogant. Couple this with many people's experiences of having shared information that led to them being threatened with becoming involuntary or made involuntary, having their medication increased without discussion and other measures often experienced as punitive. As can be seen here, unreflexive, unexamined assessment done to and on people can dehumanise people, amplify their feelings of powerlessness, create resistance and erode trust. Sadly, the very things that can work towards building trust, such as sharing power and mutual disclosure (sharing something personal of oneself as a worker), are commonly constructed as unprofessional or potentially dangerous in case consumers stockpile information on them and look them up later. All in all, this works against assessments being highly useful tools.

To conclude, I argue that when thinking about assessment it is essential for budding professionals to understand 'the complex interplay between people, their environments, their occupations that support or hinder occupational performance, participation and wellbeing' as Scanlan and Fossey suggest in Section 2.3.13. I argue that to do so requires them to reflect deeply about the lived experience of being assessed. By doing so, it can work towards making it feel safer for people to 'engage'. Combine this with a nuanced understanding of the differences between what 'person first', 'system first' and 'professional first' practice would look like and once again this may aid in rendering 'assessment' more useful from the consumer's perspective.

2.3.3 CLINICAL MENTAL HEALTH ASSESSMENT: A PSYCHIATRIC BIOPSYCHOSOCIAL PERSPECTIVE

NEERAJ SAREEN & GRAHAM MEADOWS

THE PLACE OF PSYCHIATRIC BIOPSYCHOSOCIAL ASSESSMENT

The consumer perspective contribution above has identified limitations in problem-focused and diagnostically oriented assessment in mental health care (see Section 2.3.2); so by way of an introductory comment, desirable assessment practice will include a recovery and strengths focus along with other tasks and perspectives.

Psychiatric assessment is an expectation of the National Standards for Mental Health Services (see Chapter 1.7) and may be a key element of legal treatment pathways. Often some capacity to carry out an assessment of this kind is expected across many discipline groups so can be seen as a transdisciplinary skill (see Chapter 2.2). In psychiatry and associated practice, a critical, but now conventional expansion of the scope of the medical model is the proposition that practice should be *biopsychosocial* in approach. So in this section we will attempt to chart the course from medical diagnostic classification to a biopsychosocial assessment, including the practicalities of how such assessment is carried out. In practice, these processes may be modified for the setting and purpose, as well as to address any potentially harmful aspects (see Sections 1.5.5 and 2.3.2), specific discipline perspectives and other causal considerations. We aim to provide some pointers to how this may be achieved through the frame of clinical decision making.

First, while this section will primarily concentrate on a fairly conventional presentation of biopsychosocial assessment, we acknowledge that this needs to be set in wider contexts and there are alternative philosophical frameworks and practical approaches.

Alternative framework example: The Power Threat Meaning Framework

There have always been differing explanatory frameworks for understanding mental distress, which include individual problem descriptions and Indigenous forms of understanding distress, as well as diagnostic frameworks. Coproduced with consumers, the Power Threat Meaning Framework (Johnstone et al., 2018) offers a new way of approaching people's distress, which goes beyond explanations rooted in diagnostic frameworks. Whereas in traditional mental health practice, threat responses are sometimes called 'symptoms', the Power Threat Meaning Framework focuses instead on how we make sense of difficult experiences and how societal messages can increase feelings of shame, self-blame, isolation, fear and guilt. In this way, it explicitly draws links between wider social determinants of health such as poverty, discrimination and inequality, traumas such as abuse and violence, and resulting emotional distress or troubled behaviour. Thus, the Power Threat Meaning Framework offers an approach to assessment and formulation that replaces the question 'What is wrong with you?' with four questions that can apply to individuals, families or social groups:

1. What has happened to you? (i.e. How is *power* operating in your life?)
2. How did it affect you? (i.e. What kind of *threats* does this pose?)
3. What sense did you make of it? (i.e. What is the *meaning* of these situations and experiences to you?)
4. What did you have to do to survive? (i.e. What kinds of *threat response* are you using?)

The Power Threat Meaning Framework (Johnstone et al., 2018) is not intended to replace all our current ways of thinking about and working with distress. Rather it aims to support and strengthen practices that: involve a central place for experts by experience and take meaning, narrative and subjective experience seriously; acknowledge the centrality of relational, social and cultural factors in shaping the emergence, experience and expression of trauma and distress; and emphasise the importance of working with diversity.

Alternative approach example: Open Dialogue

An example of collaborative engagement with a person and their social supports as part of their assessment is the dialogic approach was first described as 'Open Dialogue,' in the 1990s (Aaltonen, Seikkula, & Lehtinen, 2011; Seikkula, Alakare, & Aaltonen, 2011). In this approach, people experiencing crisis are met within 24 hours of contact and key members of the person's social network are invited to the meeting with the multidisciplinary team. Particular emphasis is given to the practice of ensuring that everyone has the opportunity to be heard and responded to. There are two fundamental skills required to practise Open Dialogue: the skill of responding and the skill of reflecting (Rober, 2005). The skill of responding refers to how responses from therapists further the understanding of what is being said in the session and the skill of reflecting refers to how therapists talk about their own ideas with the family. In addition, people are offered other therapies as required e.g. employment support, individual therapy, occupational therapy etc. In Open Dialogue, this particular form of therapeutic conversation has evolved (Olson, Seikkula, & Ziedonis, 2014) into a community-based treatment system. This novel way of practice, according to the pioneers, can be useful not only in acute crisis but also in more longstanding repetitive, so-called 'chronic' situations and is consistent with a human rights approach (von Peter et al., 2019; see Section 2.7.6).

Where service delivery or other settings allow for approaches such as Open Dialogue, then the considerations that follow may be less relevant. But, for many practice settings, some version of the approaches highlighted in this next section are necessary components of providing a response to the needs of people with mental health problems.

CLINICAL DECISION MAKING

A substantial literature around decision making in health care commonly uses the term *clinical decision making* (CDM) (Higgs, Jensen, Loftus, & Christensen, 2018b), though conclusions from this body of work may be useful to practitioners who may not regard themselves as clinicians. Of note among the skills that can support sound CDM are those with the prefix 'meta-'. This term indicates a concept that is an abstraction from another concept. In the case of *meta-cognition*, this is the ability to observe actively and monitor one's own thinking and thought content and processes. In some psychotherapeutic traditions, experience of a personal therapeutic journey may be expected to support development of such skills. More recently introduced into practice in psychotherapies, though with a deep history in spiritual traditions, are practices that target the development of mindfulness skills (see Chapter 2.6). There is developing evidence that the cultivation of mindful awareness through techniques such as meditation can contribute to the development of positive qualities in the practitioner, making for greater effectiveness and empathy (Hick, Bien, & Segal, 2008). Neither a formal mindfulness practice, nor psychotherapy training, is a necessary prerequisite for successfully developing open-mindedness in one's approach to assessment and engagement. Nevertheless, awareness of internal mental states on the part of the clinician; an ability to monitor one's own choice of strategies for the task, their success or otherwise, and to shift course if necessary; and an ability to consider one's own reasoning processes are all features of highly effective practitioners. When combined, these abilities can assist us as practitioners in sound reasoning about the conduct and interpretation of assessment and in avoidance of critical errors of interpretation such as confirmation bias or over-interpretation.

With a consumer perspective already introduced and the introduction of the concept of Open Dialogue, we note that this chapter will include contributions from a range of conceptual and discipline perspectives. The process of balancing these perspectives and developing sophistication as a practitioner may helpfully be seen as the application of meta-skills in monitoring and constantly checking or revising choices in the awareness of the context, the location of reasoning and the task impact.

The path of a developing practitioner in CDM can be considered as a journey involving progression through various levels (Higgs et al., 2018b), with key concepts summarised as:

- *Novice*: factual, rule-driven, relies on others, cannot see the whole situation.
- *Advanced beginner*: objective facts; begins to use intuition in concrete situations; uses both analytic reasoning and pattern recognition.
- *Competent*: can devise new rules based on the situation; sees the big picture; better use of pattern recognition with common problems.
- *Proficient*: comfortable with evolving situations; intuitive behaviours replace reasoned responses; can tolerate uncertainty.
- *Expert*: can align thought, feeling and action into intuitive problem recognition; where intuition is not developed, reasoning is applied.
- *Master*: demonstrates practical wisdom; sees the big picture; reflects in, on and for action; demonstrates moral agency.

Making progress on this path involves gaining capacity to shift between different modes of cognitive processing, for instance, by increasingly making more skilful use of what has been characterised as a dual-process model of cognition (Higgs, Jensen, Loftus, & Christensen, 2018a). In this, the dual processes are rapid and intuitive thinking often with important contributions from pattern recognition; and methodical, analytic thinking that involves purposeful rule-following. Progress on this path then may be facilitated by development in four critical skill areas (Higgs et al., 2018b), again with key concepts summarised as:

- Reflective thinking: involves consideration of a situation to make better sense of it and can occur *in* the situation, in retrospect *on* the situation, and then in preparation *for* further instance of similar situations.
- Critical thinking: has a strong metacognitive emphasis and includes active preparedness to question and seek to clarify erroneous assumptions.
- Complexity thinking: involves openness to considering a situation from multiple perspectives and frameworks, and may be assisted by the perspectives of complexity science. (See Chapter 1.1.)
- Dialectical thinking: involves a quality of fluidity of reasoning process between multiple perspectives and integration of these in decision making.

DIAGNOSIS IN MENTAL HEALTH PROBLEMS

GRAHAM MEADOWS AND JOHN FARHALL

A brief description of the medical model as applied in psychiatry

Medical assessment includes history taking and examination. Interviewing of the patient–and possibly others–collects *history* which includes information on subjective experience of ill-health. The medical assessor may then classify these accounts into a recognisable pattern of experience, being a *symptom*. Conventionally, this history taking is followed by examination, during which *signs* are detected. *Signs* in medicine are particular groups of physical or other observed characteristics identified as meeting a particular pattern by the examiner. In much of medical care, the physical examination will be a particularly important aspect of this. This is important in psychiatry too, but also critical is the Mental State Examination (MSE). The very proposition of MSE implies that mental states can be examined, something that can be philosophically challenged since many aspects of the MSE are inferred rather than directly observed. Nevertheless, with training and practice, and with consideration and reflection on these complexities, reasonable reliability of reporting of MSE findings can be achieved.

Considering psychiatric assessment as a special case of the medical model, this process creates the set of observations that are then used to decide on the most likely diagnosis, which may be a disease, disorder or syndrome. The three terms of *disease*, *disorder* or *syndrome* are not used entirely consistently. However, common usage can be described as follows:

- A *disease* is most typically an entity with well-characterised structural and associated functional disturbance, very possibly with a known aetiology or specific associated cause, such as an identified infective pathogen or specific biochemical or physiological dysfunction.
- *Disorders* may also be well-characterised disturbances of body systems or mental functions, but the term carries less implication of an understanding of cause. Psychiatric diagnoses are most commonly presented as disorders.
- *Syndromes* comprise collections of signs or symptoms, which tend to be found in association and can be seen to have valid implications for treatment and prognosis.

Psychiatric classification

The International Classification of Diseases (ICD) is the formally recognised diagnostic classification system in Australian health care administrative systems. The ICD dates back to ICD-6 (1949)–lower numbered versions had designated only mortality causes and ICD-6 was the first to specifically include mental disorders. ICD-10 came into use in 1994 (World Health Organization, 1993). WHO member states agreed at the Seventy-second World Health Assembly in May 2019 to adopt ICD-11 and that it should come into effect for reporting to WHO on 1 January 2022. Also in common use in Australia is the American Diagnostic System—the Diagnostic and Statistical Manual of Mental Disorders of the American Psychiatric Association, now in its fifth edition—DSM-5 (American Psychiatric Association, 2013), which, as the name suggests, covers only mental disorders. DSM diagnoses are more operationalised and detailed, which has the advantage for learners of specificity, and for researchers and health funders of enabling greater consistency across raters; however, given the complexity of the human experiences that diagnostic systems attempt to corral, there is no guarantee that diagnoses using one system are more 'valid' than diagnoses using the other. Fundamentally, the two systems are similar: each cross-references the diagnostic codes of the other, and in their periodic revisions, both draw on much of the same worldwide research trends and findings.

Since DSM-5 has been widely used in Australia, we have for some time had a situation where many clinicians were using a diagnostic scheme that differed from the coding system used to describe their work. This introduces possible problems with translation across the coding schemes and would make one reason to prefer ICD over DSM but DSM had the advantage of recency through the period when DSM-IV, DSM-IV-TR and then DSM-5 were more recent constructions than ICD-10. As ICD-11 (World Health Organization, 2018b) is now available, that advantage no longer applies.

DSM-IV introduced *multiaxial diagnosis*, a framework that many clinicians found useful for ordering their thinking around diagnoses, and which may still be referred to. The five axes as used in DSM-IV are:

- Axis I: Clinical disorders and other conditions that may be a focus of clinical attention
- Axis II: Personality disorders and mental retardation
- Axis III: General medical conditions
- Axis IV: Psychosocial and environmental problems
- Axis V: Global assessment of functioning.

This system was dropped for DSM-5—but as many clinicians have found it useful over the years, we consider where related content may be found in ICD-11, noting that ICD-11 does allow for assignment of multiple diagnostic codes to an individual episode:

I Most of the content of ICD-11's chapter 6, 'Mental, behavioural or neurodevelopmental disorder' would be in the domain defined by Axis I.

II The disorders grouped in Axis II are found in ICD as categories for instance in the neurodevelopmental disorders or personality disorders sections.

III ICD-11 as a full diagnostic system across the whole of health care includes what in DSM-IV would be listed under Axis III.

IV ICD-11 also has a range of codes in chapter 24, 'Factors influencing health status or contact with health services' that would relate to issues previously considered in Axis IV. For instance, here we find 'Problems associated with: finances; employment or unemployment; education; social insurance or welfare; upbringing' and a good many others.

V Axis V in DSM-IV was a single scale, the Global Assessment of Functioning; in ICD-11 we find Section V, a supplementary section for assessment of functioning, a number of measures bearing on this.

While categorical descriptions of mental disorders are commonly applied, it is also argued with substantial supporting evidence (van Os, Guloksuz, Vijn, Hafkenscheid, & Delespaul, 2019), that mental disorders may often be better described using sets of symptom dimensions. ICD-11 has in places taken a more dimensional approach to classification, where for instance a broad diagnostic label may have subcodes permitting recognition of different levels of severity of particular features. This is found particularly in the approach to ICD-11 descriptions of personality disorders (see Chapter 4.9) and schizophrenia (see Chapter 4.9).

ICD-11 is designed to be easy to use and aims to make diagnostic activity in mental health care accessible to a wide range of clinicians including non-specialists. Another very important advantage of ICD-11 for the purposes of this text is that the core descriptions of the classification are available on the web for anyone who has internet access to view. This is not the case for DSM, which is copyright to the American Psychiatric Association (APA) and with a purchase cost listed at US$128 at time of writing.

Given the emphasis in this text on collaborative practice including on sharing information and openness and transparency of process, the application of a diagnostic scheme that is unavailable to consumers when a contemporary one is publicly available no longer seems defensible. So in this text, and as noted in the introduction, we weight diagnostic consideration to ICD-11. A very valuable companion to the ICD classifications is the associated Clinical Descriptors and Diagnostic Guidelines (World Health Organization, 1992)—when the version for ICD-11 is released, this will be an important additional source on use in practice of the classification. The WHO also is developing ICD-11 Primary Health Care (PHC). Similarly to the ICD-10 version (World Health Organization, 1996), this will be a more simply constructed and written version of ICD-11 that may be useful for non-specialist settings and practitioners.

Making a diagnosis and defending against common errors

The way in which doctors and others may make a diagnosis may vary depending on the problem in question and the practitioner. In line with CDM concepts introduced earlier relatively junior and less expert practitioners often generate a number of hypotheses, each of which will be tested against the available evidence. One alone may remain as credible or clearly supported, or several may remain based in the available evidence, constituting a differential diagnostic list. More senior and expert practitioners may rely more on pattern recognition and may consciously generate a smaller range of possible diagnoses. In doing so, they may be relying on balancing outputs from different cognitive systems. Whatever way the practitioner goes about it, there is a need to guard against possible errors in reasoning (Schwartz & Elstein, 2008).

Often during an interview, a clinician will formulate a small number of hypotheses regarding what the diagnosis might be, and one of these may for some reason be favoured. The clinician may then proceed with collecting information in ways biased towards collection of material that would confirm this diagnosis, avoiding collection of data that might better support an alternative hypothesis. This has been described as *confirmation bias*. Over-interpretation is another such error, wherein data which is insufficient to support a diagnostic hypothesis or to suggest another, is interpreted as confirmatory of the current train of thinking. For readers with an interest in historical or classical references, these can also be seen as related to a more traditional medical metaphor of Procrustean error (Baskerville, 2010). The metacognitive capacity of being able to monitor reasoning and practice, seeking errors and adopting remedial courses of action if indicated, will be important in avoiding these important sources of bias.

While psychiatric diagnosis is usually made by clinicians, following interviewing and synthesising the information collected in a semi-structured way, more structured instruments are used in research, and in formal psychological assessment to maximise reliability (see Chapters 1.4 and 2.3.14). Familiarity with such instruments can be valuable for the practising clinician since, for instance, they provide resources for approaches to questioning that the practitioner may find useful, either for regular use or as alternative strategies. In situations of diagnostic uncertainty, sometimes application of instrumentation originally developed for research purposes may shed light on the clinical diagnostic challenge.

The biopsychosocial model as invoked in psychiatry

The biopsychosocial grid

Australian psychiatrists training within the last two decades at least will have been encouraged to think of themselves as practising within something called the *biopsychosocial model*. A frequent tool of which trainees may make use is that of the biopsychosocial management grid. On one axis of the grid, we find the three categories of the biological, psychological and social. On the other axis of the grid, we may find the time spans of short term, intermediate term and long term. Into the cells of the management grid, the hopeful candidate may enter summaries of management strategies of the appropriate types. Undoubtedly this can be a very useful tool; however, it may be seen as something of a simplification, and possibly even a corruption, of a rather subtler construct.

The broader biopsychosocial construct

If we look back at the history of the term, it owes most in this context to the contribution of George Engel, an American psychiatrist. His exposition of the model (Engel, 1980) is somewhat different from that above. Engel uses the term biopsychosocial in contrast to the term biomedical. In using the term, Engel is setting out to emphasise the need for a broadly based systemic approach as opposed to a narrow construction of medical disorder. Engel describes this approach as drawing strongly on the contributions early in the twentieth century from the domain of biology. The key principles here of systems thinking are that each system is at the same time a component of higher systems, and that in the continuity of natural systems every unit is at the same time a whole and a part. Engel thus argues not for a model with three categories, as in the management grid cited, but for a multilevel organisational and systems hierarchy. The proposed use of the systems hierarchy is as something that is flexible, and the conceptualisation of the systems will vary from case to case. However, the continuum of natural systems may be seen as including subatomic particles, atoms, molecules, organelles, cells, tissues, organs and organ systems, a nervous system, a person, a two-person system, a family, a community, culture and subculture, society or nation, and the biosphere. An important aspect of Engel's work was his repeated assertion of the position that the biopsychosocial model was every bit as important in the approach to patients with apparently general medical problems as it was to those whose problems were evidently, or by presentation, psychiatric, and its contribution to thinking in mental health practice has been profound. This broader conceptualisation of the biopsychosocial category also resonates with, and can be complemented by, consideration of much mental health practice as set out within complex adaptive systems (see Chapter 1.1).

2.3.4 CLINICAL MENTAL HEALTH ASSESSMENT IN PRACTICE

GRAHAM MEADOWS & NEERAJ SAREEN

INTRODUCTION

Standards and expectations

The Standards for Mental Health Services (Australian Government, 2010b) make clear that the process of entry to a mental health service should include assessment, giving consideration to risk and safety, urgency, distress, dysfunction and disability; and that attention to diagnosis is expected in a comprehensive assessment. These same service standards also expect that mental health services actively support recovery and promote recovery-orientated values and principles in their policies and practices (see Chapters 1.3 and 2.6), but they do not indicate what this means for assessment practices specifically.

Recovery orientation in assessment practice

Slade (2009a) suggests that this requires undertaking assessments in a way that counterbalances the focus on problems, difficulties, dysfunction of clinical assessment, with attending more closely to the person's lived experience, views, strengths and resources. The considerations identified above in the section on CDM including application of metacognitive awareness of location of reasoning and task impact will be relevant. Some general principles derived from Slade (2009) that may be useful for clinicians in orientating their styles of questioning and conversation towards supporting recovery during assessment include:

- using assessment to explore, develop and validate meaning and making sense of what is happening

- using assessment to amplify strengths and assets of the person in his or her life context through the language and focus adopted
- using assessment to foster choice and self-determination through partnership relationships in which information and decisions are shared, rather than assuming or taking over responsibility for the person
- using assessment to support and amplify the person's development or redefining of an identity connected with personal qualities so as to differentiate himself or herself from the illness (which may at times become very prominent)
- using assessment to develop hope through focusing on the person, and possibilities for promoting wellbeing and recovery.

A guide to tasks of assessment

In Table 2.1, we have adapted and extended a list of assessment tasks from an American text (Hales, Yudofsky, & Gabbard, 2010), which may be applicable to many general mental health care settings. We qualify this with the above concern to approach this from a recovery orientation as well, a consideration to which we return in more detail. We note that specialist care settings may influence these components on basis of context or tasks (see Section 2.3.3).

GETTING STARTED

First, it is important to consider the assessment purpose and the setting in which it takes place, as both of these will influence how the assessment is conducted, and the tasks involved.

Table 2.1 Key components and tasks of clinical assessment in community mental health practice

Major task groups	Tasks of assessment
Getting started	Consider the assessment purpose and setting
	Establish goals
	Cover orientation as necessary
	If necessary deal with expectations regarding payment
	Establish rapport
	Develop a collaborative relationship
Interview techniques	Communicate empathically
	Maintain appropriate boundaries
	Communicate in a language the patient understands and avoid jargon
	Feedback and verify
	Monitor the emotional intensity and other aspects of the interview and adjust as necessary
	Manage time
Beginning a biopsychosocial assessment	Gather pertinent history data
	Perform a mental status examination
	Assess patient reliability
	Assess risks
	Assess physical health issues
Extending the range of information sources	Consider relevant laboratory investigations
	Assess patient vulnerability or other risks
	Review any advance directives, previous records and other available data
	Interview others as appropriate

Continues

Table 2.1 Key components and tasks of clinical assessment in community mental health practice (*continued*)

Major task groups	Tasks of assessment
Extending, deepening and formalising assessment	Use a structured instrument as a guide
	Further understand clients' experiences of everyday living
	Assess family context and carer needs
	Administer outcome measures
	Consider and acknowledge the person's explanatory model, paying attention to any cultural or minority context
Synthesis and sharing of information	Document accurately
	Make a narrative synthesis and formulation
	Discuss applicable diagnostic and treatment issues
	Discuss needs and priorities
	Develop a plan of action, collaboratively where possible, including for possible emergencies
	Allow time to ask questions

Purposes of assessment

Assessment serves a number of purposes in relation to the opening, continuing and closure phases of a service's contact with a client or consumer, in which differing tasks may take priority. The National Standards for Mental Health Services (Australian Government, 2010) include standards specific to assessment at entry, ongoing review and planned exit from services, and so these are also highlighted.

Opening

Within the opening phase of a clinical contact, assessment may focus on orientation, triage, risk assessment, engagement (or possibly disengagement, with advice as to another referral option), developing a provisional diagnosis and initial understanding of the issues for further action. Early tasks can also include gaining of informed consent to treatment, sharing information with the person (as about service options), and the taking of the decision as to whether to proceed to comprehensive, possibly multidisciplinary, assessment.

In this opening or entry phase of contact, the Service Standards (10.3) expect that the entry process to a mental health service meets the needs of its community and facilitates timeliness of entry and ongoing assessment (Australian Government, 2010b). In terms of conducting assessments, this includes:

- making entry processes, inclusion and exclusion criteria known in written form to consumers, carers and other service providers, including police, ambulance services and emergency departments
- having a documented system of prioritising referrals according to risk, urgency, distress, dysfunction and disability
- providing timely advice and/or response to all those referred, at the time of assessment
- keeping delays and duplication to a minimum in assessment and care planning.

Continuing

Here assessment occurs within the context of ongoing care planning, monitoring of progress and review of treatment and services being provided, including the continued vigilance for change that indicates the need for major review of the management plan and for the appropriateness of progression towards closure.

Service Standard 10.4 is specific to assessment and review during this phase. Here, comprehensive, timely and accurate assessment and regular review of progress should be provided during this phase of consumers', families' and carers' contact with mental health services (Australian Government, 2010b). This includes:

- conducting assessments and making diagnoses using evidence-based and accepted methods and tools
- assessments being conducted by appropriately qualified staff experienced and trained in assessing mental health problems, and where possible in a consumer's preferred setting with consideration for the safety for those involved
- with the consumer's informed consent, including carers, other service providers and others as nominated by the consumer
- development, documenting and regular reviewing of plans in relation to treatment, care and recovery throughout the consumer's contact with the service.

Closure

Often in a community mental health service, closure will represent a point of transfer of care to primary care settings or to another service where the person is moving to another location. The specific Service Standard (10.6) pertinent to closure and exit from a mental health service emphasises the importance of developing exit plans with consumers over time and well before exit; ensuring that consumers have accessible information about these plans, other service options and arrangements for re-entering the service if required; and the involvement of nominated family or carers in making these plans and arrangements, with the consumer's informed consent (Australian Government, 2010).

Hence, the quality of information and the accuracy of the assessment underpinning it are important at this closure phase. This may be especially so if someone has been a client with a particular service for a long period, since there is a risk that long-established views about a person's diagnosis and essential understandings of their situation may have become accepted. In this circumstance, not uncommonly, the resulting assessment is actually different from the assessment that a new observer would make, because the picture has subtly changed over time. In medicine, this may be considered a more protracted variant of the so-called 'crime of Procrustes'. Alternatively, such a difference could reflect a deeper understanding of the person and their needs that grew through working together and observing ups and downs over time.

Space as determining relationships and roles

Assessment may occur in a hospital or other health care facility; a residential or custodial institutional setting, the client's home, a primary care setting, a public place or somewhere else that is none of these. It may occur in the middle of a major city, in a country town or in an extremely remote area. The place will have an impact on: the power relationships of the situation; the extent to which privacy and safety can be assured; what actions are possible within the social, cultural or organisational boundaries of the setting; the perceived urgency of situations; the kinds of behaviour that are tolerable; and how the behaviour of the person being assessed may be interpreted. It may also influence the time available for making an assessment, and range of options available for the actions that might follow the assessment and the likely possible outcomes. As examples, in clients' homes, clinicians are generally present as guests, and the presence of family may or may not facilitate clients expressing their views; health care settings may be less familiar and potentially forbidding territory for clients, in which they have less influence; and in public places, privacy is often lacking, securing the safety of the person and others present may be uppermost, and sometimes the police may be present, in addition to clinicians.

Appropriate assessment space

Assessment activities need to be conducted in a manner that upholds the rights of the person being assessed, and is safe for consumers, carers, families, visitors, staff and members of the public (Australian Government, 2010). A safe assessment space, then, will be one in which consumers are provided with access to written and verbal explanations of their rights and responsibilities; treated with respect and dignity; their safety and wellbeing in the assessment are promoted; and they are protected in relation to potential risks of abuse, harm or exploitation.

Space should be adequate in size, and where possible sufficiently tidy and well decorated, such that all involved preserve their dignity in the space. There should be adequate attention to the issue of privacy. Furnishings should be appropriate to the task and provide reasonable comfort. Some consideration to layout of the interview space will often pay dividends. Conducting an interview across a large desk will often be seen as distancing and emphasising the clinician as dominant in the power relationship. Often arranging furniture so that the chairs are not face-to-face but angled will be more comfortable for all, so that direct eye contact is not imposed, but rather can be intermittent and modulated according to the phase and task of the interview.

Methods of recording as an influence on space

Increasingly computers are used in mental health care consultations (Higgs et al., 2018b). Many practitioners still use pen and paper to make notes during the session given difficulty in accurately recalling material especially when a significant amount of detail is collected. It is essential that the interviewer maintains nonverbal communication with the consumer in such scenarios. On occasions where the practitioner chooses (or is expected to) collect and enter information into a computerised interface during an assessment interview (using a tablet computer with pen entry), this may affect the use of space similarly to using a pen and paper, and similar rules may apply. In contrast, a fixed desktop work station may impose an unhelpful dynamic into the shared space (Rosen, Nakash, & Alegría, 2016).

Work on this issue in primary care (Greatbatch, Luff, Heath, & Campion, 1993; Pearce, Trumble, Arnold, Dwan, & Phillips, 2008; Ruusuvuori, 2001; Silverman & Kinnersley, 2010) shows that where influenced by the presence of a PC, a practitioner has the lower part of their body aligned well away from an axis that more closely matches the frame of the client, then empathy is reduced in the consultation. Focusing on the desktop screen can also make the practitioner less sensitive to nonverbal cues and less able to engage in empathic expression. A better strategy may sometimes be to make use of the computer for defined blocks of time during a consultation, making clear and negotiating this use of time with the client, perhaps then reviewing the material entered with them. While there is no simple solution, the practitioner who pays attention to this challenge can make purposive choices about how the computer is used, monitoring its impact on empathy and rapport, and responding sensitively if this occurs.

Safety

Most people with mental health problems present no risk of harm to the person doing the assessment. However, there are occasions, many of which can be reasonably anticipated, when the person being assessed may be more likely to become violent. Assault of clinicians by consumers and even murder have occurred, albeit most infrequently. Where indicated, sensible precautions should be taken to minimise the risk to the clinician, the consumer and others present in relation to possible risks of harm or aggressive or violent behaviour, albeit that these may be relatively infrequent events in many settings.

Some key points are:

- be aware of the need to anticipate violence, and do not ignore the presence of weapons, threats, cues that someone is angry or histories of prior violent behaviour
- be clear about the limits of tolerable and acceptable behaviour in the assessment context; for instance, be prepared to insist that people being assessed are not armed. Be prepared to terminate interviews, possibly abruptly, on the grounds of concern for safety
- be prepared to involve the police, for instance, in disarming armed persons. Particularly where weapons have been used, their use has been threatened, or available weapons are thought to pose a risk, such matters should be referred to the police so that weapons can be removed before assessment occurs
- in assessment spaces, potential weapons should be considered and removed, and the availability of escape routes for the interviewer noted; multiple

exit routes with outward opening doors limit the likelihood of being trapped in a room
- avoid being alone with a person when there is a known risk of violence
- listen to your intuitive and emotional responses to the situation, and be open to acting on them. Be prepared to escape a situation in which you feel threatened, or call for help
- on occasions, it may be important to acknowledge the existence of violent impulses that clients may have, and not necessarily to be frightened by them. However, this should not be confused with bravado or machismo
- avoid presenting as threatening to the person being assessed; people may become violent because they are frightened or feel disempowered about what is happening
- remember that satisfactory conduct of physical restraint of a person requires enough (often at least five) properly trained people; and that administering sedative drugs, particularly intramuscularly and intravenously, in settings without full medical support has been associated with fatalities and usually is to be avoided
- be clear about how assistance can be called for, including any availability of duress alarms, and know clearly what response can be expected if such an alarm is activated.

Orientation

Often it will be important to have a discussion and share some information about the interview from the point of view of the service provider, and also seek an understanding from the client about their expectations of the process. Understanding of the content of any referral and the associated information included in this, and expectations regarding record keeping and confidentiality, will commonly benefit from attention here. If a computer is being used for record keeping, then its place and role may need to be explained. Sometimes it will be appropriate here to share written information about the assessment process or other aspects of the service in which the work is set. It may be important to address the issue of payment. In services funded by state health departments in Australia, services will typically be free, but in other settings patient payments, availability of necessary referrals and assignment of Medicare rebates all may need discussion.

Interviewing techniques

Clinicians should have an understanding of how posture and eye contact communicate paying attention, the use of open postures and the practicalities of handling note taking. Specific conscious but nonverbal techniques, such as postural echo and the deliberate use of intention movements, can be pivotal in facilitating the effectiveness of apparently more sophisticated interventions.

Within the verbal interactions, the practitioner should be familiar with use of open and closed questions and more or less directive approaches, and aware of how to choose the most appropriate for a particular moment.

While recording in the interview is important and the space should be well set up to support this (see Section 2.3.4), there may be times in the interview when it is better to put down a pen or clearly move away from a computer to make it clear that your attention on the client is undivided and focused. Particularly in opening phases of the interview, this may be important in supporting the client in beginning to share his or her story.

The service and the individual will have positions on levels of disclosure by the interviewer and other aspects of boundary setting. Commonly, feedback and verification will be useful in interviews to assure the client that he or she is being correctly heard and understood. Monitoring the interview flow is also important from a number of perspectives. Information may emerge that leads to a need to change the goals of an interview, especially if some previously unanticipated issue of risk emerges. If the emotional tone of the interview is becoming distressing or otherwise unhelpful for the client, then there may be need for a pause for reflection and a shift in approach. An interview or questioning style that is proving ineffective in achieving the interview goals may need to be reconsidered.

LANGUAGE AND CULTURE: COMMUNICATION WITH PEOPLE FROM NON-ENGLISH-SPEAKING BACKGROUNDS

HARRY MINAS

Nonverbal communication

There is wide cultural variability in matters such as appropriate forms of address and greeting, acceptability of touch (as in shaking hands), appropriate distance, seating posture, the hand with which things are offered and accepted and the nature of eye contact or avoidance thereof. Arising from these variables, there is much room for error of interpretation and unintentional giving and taking of offence. Clinicians should inform themselves about appropriate rules of nonverbal communication, at least among consumers and families from cultural groups with which the clinician is in relatively frequent contact. When in contact with a person or family from an unfamiliar cultural background, sensitive attention to the nonverbal behaviour of the consumer and family, and an appropriate level of formality and deference in the initial contact, will usually be a sufficient guide to establishment of rapport and avoidance of cultural *faux pas*.

Verbal communication

Clarity of communication is essential for all aspects of clinical practice. Clinical assessment is an interpretive process. Clinicians ask consumers questions, receive responses and interpret those responses to indicate the presence or absence of illness and make judgements about diagnosis, disability, prognosis and treatment. They provide information, explanations and advice concerning treatment. It is vitally important for clinicians to check that they have understood the consumer correctly, and that the consumer has understood the clinician's explanations and advice correctly. Errors of interpretation, common even when the clinician and consumer come from the same cultural background and speak the same language, are more likely to occur when clinician and consumer and family do not share the same language and culture.

When communicating with a consumer who has limited English fluency:

- use simple English and avoid slang and jargon
- speak clearly and avoid speaking too quickly
- use short sentences and avoid complex sentence constructions, such as the use of double negatives
- reinforce what you say with appropriate (and not exaggerated) nonverbal communication
- be patient and unhurried
- listen carefully and attentively
- encourage the consumer to ask questions
- check that you have understood correctly, and that you have been understood.

Working with an interpreter

Communicating with consumers who speak little or no English presents significant challenges. Even when consumers appear to have a reasonable knowledge of English it is well to remember that the consumer may have limited knowledge of vocabulary, grammar, syntax and use of English idiom. A consumer with reasonably good knowledge of everyday English may not have the necessary fluency to express or understand in English complex issues such as emotional states or relationships. In the presence of delirium, dementia, anxiety, depression or thought disorder, a consumer's capacity to communicate in a second language often declines. A well-trained and skilful interpreter is essential to enable communication between clinician and non-English-speaking consumer.

If, on the basis of your own impression of the consumer's English fluency, you are not certain whether an interpreter is required, book an interpreter. Before making such a booking, and during the interpreted interview:

- ensure that you know which language (and dialect) the consumer speaks before booking an appropriate interpreter. Knowing the country of birth is not necessarily an adequate guide to which language the consumer speaks
- if possible, check whether the gender or ethnicity of the interpreter is important
- ensure, in a pre-interview briefing, that the interpreter is aware of the nature and purpose of the interview

- keep in mind the complexity of the interpreter's task, and conduct the interview in a way that will simplify this task as much as possible
- be aware of the needs of the interpreter; for example, a number of clinical situations (such as descriptions of torture or other trauma) may cause significant distress in the interpreter. Remember that many interpreters have had similar experiences to those of immigrant or refugee consumers
- carry out a debriefing after the interview when this is required, either to clarify issues in the interview or to ensure that any difficulties the interpreter may have experienced are understood and appropriately responded to.

Guidelines for working with interpreters will assist the clinician to establish effective communication with the assistance of an interpreter. Guidelines developed for use in mental health settings are readily available (Miletic et al., 2006). It is worth remembering that a properly conducted interpreted interview will require more time than other types of interview.

Cultural relativity of specific phenomena

Some types of mental state, including certain dissociative or trance states, are considerably more common in some non-Western cultural groups than in Western cultures (Minas, Klimidis, & Tuncer, 2007). It is important to keep in mind that such phenomena do not necessarily indicate psychiatric illness. There are many examples of such phenomena being a normal part of religious experience or other ritual activities.

CONDUCTING A BIOPSYCHOSOCIAL ASSESSMENT

GRAHAM MEADOWS, HARRY MINAS, NEERAJ SAREEN & JOHN FARHALL

Gather pertinent psychiatric data

Items of history

Different disciplines receive training with different sequences and emphases for the gathering of historical information. The following categories derive from standard accounts of the psychiatric history, and are presented as a useful guide to the content of history taking to enable psychiatric assessment. This kind of guide should not be regarded as inflexible, and for particular individuals the sequence of inquiry may vary in response to emergent stories. For instance, if someone has moved town, region or country many times in his or her life, taking the history may be difficult until the sequence of relocations has been clarified. The account here is a relatively brief one, and the reader is referred to comprehensive psychiatric texts for alternative detailed treatments of these items of history (see Bloch, Green, Janca, Mitchell, & Robertson, 2017; Castle, Bassett, King, & Gleason, 2013; Tasman, Kay, Lieberman, First, & Riba, 2015; Johnstone, Owens, Lawrie, McIntosh, & Sharpe, 2010; Sadock, Sadock, & Ruiz, 2014).

The taking of history needs to be tempered by considerations of the respect for privacy of the individual who is being assessed, and for his or her cultural background. For people from some cultural backgrounds, issues such as loss of libido or menstrual changes or concerns may be impossible to divulge or discuss with a stranger, particularly one of the opposite sex.

Reason for referral

The origin of the referral and any information about why the referral has occurred belongs here. It may be very important to consider who prompted the referral, and to what extent the identified consumer or client is an active party to this process. There may be a specific referral question and, if so, it should be carefully considered.

Consideration of the impact of trauma on a person's mental health, at least as a contributing factor or as the reason for a person's current problems, needs to begin during assessment as part of good mental health care. (For information about how to ask about trauma and evidence of its links to voice hearing and other experiences, see Section 2.3.9.) When the consumer is a refugee and may have experienced severe trauma or torture, the clinician must make a judgement about the extent to which these experiences will be explored, particularly in the early phase of establishing a therapeutic relationship.

Current situation

This profiles the person's situation in terms of his or her current living situation, marital situation and employment. If the person is unemployed, it may be helpful to discuss how he or she is spending his or her time during the day. Collecting this information has an important role in rapport building, by the interviewer demonstrating interest in the life of the person, and by beginning with a set of questions that can be framed in ways that are not threatening or unduly intrusive.

Presenting problem

Here information is collected on the problems that the person is having now, and what he or she would like acted on. Giving the person an opportunity to tell the story as he or she sees it is important. The line of questioning here should at least initially be of an open nature. People being assessed will vary in how much they want or need the clinician to impose some order on this exploration. Some will have a clear account well worked out for presentation, and some will have only an unclear idea as to how best to present the problem, and will appreciate structure provided by the interviewer. For cultural groups in which mental illness is particularly severely stigmatised, or in which familiarity with mental illness and treatment is low, it is less likely that clearly mental and relationship issues will be offered as the presenting problem. The interviewer must decide the approach to this part of the interview after a few minutes of listening to and attentive observation of the person as he or she starts to tell his or her story.

History of presenting problem

A decision that has to be made is from when we may date the presenting problem. This may be clear in the case of a first presentation of a discrete problem with an abrupt onset, or it may be difficult to decide where a longstanding disorder has fluctuated over time. Perhaps the important thing is to reach a clear decision from when to date the current episode, then not vary that structure for the purpose of a particular interview record. Immigrants and refugees may have a history of unexplained somatic problems and multiple primary care consultations prior to recognition of the existence of a mental disorder (Parker, Cheah, & Roy, 2001).

Family history

This will include whether parents are still alive; if not, how long ago they died; and preferably ages at death, with causes. You should also inquire about the ages of siblings. Family medical history in terms of significant disorders, including family history of psychiatric disorders and any deaths by suicide, should be included here. For assessment of genetic risk for most psychiatric disorders, the most important information is that relating to first-degree relatives.

The nature and quality of relationships with family members should be explored, while keeping in mind that family structures and relationships vary greatly across cultures, and within broad Australian culture. This helps develop an understanding of the person from the quality and nature of these relationships, as an important aspect of their formative life experience. Also informative will be the way in which the person describes these relationships, providing an important opportunity to develop understanding as to how this person thinks about and describes social relationships.

Personal history

Here we aim to capture a life story. In recounting, it may be presented as a narrative, but this may often be best gathered under a number of specific domains of inquiry, as follows, which are also a conventional way to recount this history.

Pregnancy and birth

Asking where the person was born may help orientate the history as introduced above. Problems at this early stage of life may have roles in the development of disorders of childhood and also those of adult onset.

Preschool history

The family constellation in these early years should be noted. Was this one of significant stability or instability, including significant early separation from parents or other sources of care? What kind of memories does the person have of this time? Were there any significant physical or emotional problems that may be relevant as risk factors for later life? Was there any slowness in intellectual or physical development?

Schooling and educational history

Relationships with teachers and with other students may provide more information about the development of the person, and scholastic performance gives some indication of intellectual level. What level of education did the person complete, including university and other tertiary education? Keep in mind that level of educational attainment does not necessarily indicate capacity. Opportunity for education must also be inquired about, particularly among young refugees and immigrants from very impoverished backgrounds.

Occupational history

Work roles, length of period of work, at what level and reasons for leaving particular jobs can all provide a helpful context. Level of occupation can be misleading in immigrants and refugees since many are employed in jobs that are not consistent with their qualifications, which may not be recognised in Australia. Similarly, inquiring about a person's domestic, parenting and leisure roles can be important in understanding a person's productive roles and participation in community life, particularly when he or she is not engaged in paid employment.

Marital history

Major long-term close relationships should be considered, whatever the person's sexual orientation, and whether marriage was entered into or not.

Sexual history

This may not always be a relevant item, but inquiry should at least be considered. Sexual orientation and degree of sexual experience may give important information about the person, and may be affected by some disorders. Assessment of risk of sexually transmitted diseases because of unsafe sexual behaviour may be relevant, either because disorders such as HIV-related disease or syphilis can present with psychiatric manifestations, or because anxiety about having contracted serious illness can be a cause of mental health problems. The clinician should be particularly alert to the possibility of sexual abuse in the person's history since this is very common among people, particularly but not exclusively women, with significant psychiatric disorder.

Children

Dates of birth of children, the course and experience of parenting them will be relevant here.

Forensic history

Previous encounters with the legal system may be a pointer to risk, and also stressors such as impending court cases. Past dangerousness may be assessed here.

Past psychiatric history

It is possible that earlier inquiry will have naturally led to a review of history of presenting problems. If not, then at this point there should be a review of previous history, including onset of symptoms, severity and help-seeking behaviour, such as contacts with professionals and any periods of identifiable professional care, including hospitalisations. The kinds of treatments already received and their apparent effects on symptoms, as well as side effects, will be helpful. Immigrants from low- and middle-income countries with poorly developed mental health systems may have never presented for psychiatric assessment or received treatment, even though they may have had a long history of quite severe mental disorder.

Past medical history

Information about previous medical illnesses should be gathered here, with treatments, and their effects. Any continuing or chronic health problems should be documented.

The detection and assessment of physical problems is primarily the province of medicine, and may well be best accomplished by collaborative relationships with general practitioners or other general health service providers. However, given physical health problems among people with mental illness are common and access to effective referral and treatment of physical health conditions easily missed because of a variety of barriers, clinical mental services are recommended to play an active role in assessing physical health, lifestyle and medication effects; supported referral to general practitioners; and linkage to appropriate community health and health promotion programs (Department of Health, 2011). Therefore in clinical mental health assessment by other than doctors, inquiry should be made into medical history. This should include the history of serious illness from childhood onwards, then any current physical problems, whether under treatment or not, including problems that restrict movement and difficulties with vision or hearing. Any physical symptoms that the client is concerned about, or regards as out of the ordinary, including side effects of medication, weight gain and so forth, should also be asked about. Among important considerations in contemporary mental health care are iatrogenic effects of medications including the association of antipsychotic medication with a effects on metabolism that may contribute to obesity and increased risk for a range of health problems. (See Chapter 2.5.)

Medications

Here, if not covered before, a comprehensive list of medications and any recent changes should be collected, including psychotropic medications, medications for physical conditions and any alternative medicine preparations.

Drug and alcohol history

An individual's pattern of substance use should be explored, with specific questions at least about alcohol, tobacco and caffeine consumption. Inquiry into illicit drugs may often be more general, although this will be adjusted to cultural and service contexts in which illicit drug use, sometimes specific substances, may be more normative. The regularity, frequency and amount of substance consumed should be considered, along with any evidence of dependency or withdrawal syndromes. Review of a typical day of drug use may be helpful. Informant accounts here again may need to supplement those of the consumer. The history taking required for this item will often involve finding out what drugs the consumer uses with any regularity. Then it can be helpful for each drug to document a day's usage; for example, when is the first cigarette, drink, bong or injection taken, and then at what other points in the day are these substances taken? This will give some indication of overall intake, which can be, in the case of alcohol, rendered into standard units and compared with guidelines to determine whether the level and pattern of use is likely to be harmful. It can be useful to repeat this exercise for a normal day and a heavy usage day. The presence of symptoms of dependency for specific drugs will be significant in this assessment as well. (Discussion of this is extended, including the use of the AUDIT questionnaire, in Chapter 4.4.)

Personality

Through the course of history taking, a sense of the person should emerge from the way he or she describes his or her life experience and the kind of relationships he or she has had. The person's description of him- or herself as a person may be informative, and this may also be helpfully complemented by the descriptions of other informants, all this with due respect for confidentiality.

Including the spiritual dimension in assessment

As a dimension of the lived experience of mental health problems and responses to them and one of central importance to many people, this is often neglected in assessment. Sometimes the influence of spirituality may be negative, but just as often it will represent a positive resource for the individual and/or family in bringing meaning to life and making progress. Thus in mental health care, as physicians should with people with significant physical health problems (D'Souza & George, 2006), we should consider whether it may be useful at least to broach the subject with an introduction such as:

- Has faith (religion, spirituality) been important to you at other times in your life?
- Do you have someone to talk to about religious or spiritual matters?
- Would you like to explore religious or spiritual matters with someone?

Mental state assessment

Mental state assessment should occur during the whole course of an interaction with a client, although it also involves some specific focused tasks.

Throughout, the mental posture is one of an active observer, making mental and, where appropriate, written notes, in a methodical and structured way. An important aspect of the task is of studying mental events in the client or patient, a task described as phenomenology (Jaspers, 1963; Stanghellini et al., 2019); mood, thought, delusions and hallucinations would be some examples of mental content as subject of phenomenological investigation. Careful phenomenological inquiry involves capturing, to the satisfaction of the examiner, a mental representation of the experience the person is describing. A very real and critically important challenge is of doing that in a way that is appreciated as a helpful and well-motivated curiosity by the client or patient; also being seen as helpful and supportive by any others involved. Cues provided by verbal and nonverbal communications often will need following up with specific questions including sometimes questions targeting particularly significant aspects of experiences from perspectives of diagnosis or risk assessment (see Section 2.3.3). Once the examiner considers that they have a satisfactory understanding of the phenomenon in question, there should where possible be a sharing of this with the person to seek verification. This account should, as far as possible, be in lay terms and avoid technical usage. An agreed account of the experience can then be compared to the available phenomenological descriptions, and assigned a particular technical term. A shared agreed label may then be used with the client or patient in repeated assessment, though it may from time to time be important to check that the shared understanding of what the labelled phenomenological label signifies is consistent.

Not uncommonly, inexperienced clinicians fall into the trap of seizing on jargon terms such as 'thought block' or 'loosening of associations' because they appear to dignify an account and make it seem more professional. This can contribute to errors in decision making as identified earlier. More important than being able to use jargon is the ability to describe clearly what is observed in terms that would be understandable to a lay reader, and can be checked out with the consumer. Checking out the description with the consumer will often help accuracy, and make the experience of being assessed less threatening and even helpful.

In undertaking a mental state assessment then, the assessor is applying the above position to the acquisition of information under a number of headings. These are presented slightly differently in different texts as introduced earlier (see Section 2.3.3), but the scheme set out below would be acceptable for most settings and usages. Often there may be some degree of cultural gulf between the person assessing and the person being assessed, either in terms of language or cultural background, so at a number of points in this section mention is made of cultural issues in assessment.

Appearance and behaviour

This includes general appearance and facial appearance, choice of clothing and adornment, grooming and evidence of self-care. Posture and movement, whether increased, decreased, unexpected or violent, fall into this category. Movements may be slowed in *motor retardation* (*psychomotor* if thought processes are similarly affected) or increased in rate, including pacing and restless non-purposive activity and thinking; for instance, in (*psycho-*) *motor agitation.*

The clinical significance of appearance, grooming and behaviour can be very difficult to interpret in the cross-cultural clinical setting. The clinician may be entirely unfamiliar with what is culturally appropriate dress and behaviour in the consumer's cultural group. Before attributing pathological significance to appearance or behaviour the clinician should be satisfied through appropriate additional inquiry that the appearance or behaviour would be regarded as inappropriate in the consumer's cultural group.

Speech

This is often organised under two major categories, *form* and *content.*

Form of speech includes:

- the spontaneity with which speech occurs, whether this is normal, reduced or increased
- the rate of speech, again normal, decreased or increased

- the quantity of speech; once speech has been initiated, for how long the flow of talk is maintained
- the quality of interruptibility: will the client respond to normal and polite social cues to cease flow of talk and allow the interviewer to speak?
- the flow of speech, whether it is smooth or has sudden and unexpected shifts or stops, and the comprehensibility of the flow of ideas within it.

Content of speech includes:

- the presence of any characteristic themes or overtones to the speech, including domination of the content of talk by particular preoccupations, such as the gloomy and pessimistic views that often dominate the speech of one suffering with severe depression.

In making judgements concerning the normality or abnormality of speech and language, the clinician should be very circumspect when the person is speaking a language in which he or she is not fluent. This is even more the case when the interview is being carried out with the assistance of an interpreter. It will often be necessary to seek the interpreter's assistance in making judgements concerning such things as pitch, tone, tempo and construction of the person's speech.

Mood

The term *mood* is usually employed technically here to refer to prevailing or enduring emotional set, lasting days or weeks, while *affect* refers to shorter-term changes in emotional experience and its observed expression. Mood state is inferred partly by response to questions about the way the client feels, the state of his or her spirits, while also cues from behaviour, including posture, will contribute to the formed impression of the mood state. Mood may be normal (or *euthymic*), elevated or depressed in nature, along with other more specific descriptions. Affect may vary in range or responsiveness and in how appropriate it is in relation to the circumstance and topic of discussion.

Rules governing expression of mood and affect in various situations (such as when with a person in a hierarchically superior position, an older person, a male or a female) vary a great deal in different cultures. In some cultures, it is generally undesirable to openly express strong or negative emotions. Affects such as irritability, anger and dislike may all be expressed through a neutral smile. The cultural imperative may be to control expression of affect rather than to value affective expressivity. In such circumstances, it will be difficult to judge the quality, range and appropriateness of the person's affect. This may lead to serious errors of clinical judgement in areas such as severity of depression and level of suicide risk.

Eliciting depressed mood state may require careful and progressive questioning along with helpful nonverbal communication. Beginning with questions that involve recognition of only a mildly low mood, the interviewer can gradually build towards questions that would indicate more severe states that may be less readily disclosed. *Anhedonia* (the loss of ability to enjoy usually pleasurable activities) is a core symptom of depressive disorders.

Asking about risk of self-harm may be well placed at this point if the risk (see Section 2.3.4) is related to depression, and ought not be neglected in the context of an emergent picture of evidently depressed mood. Indicators of risk for self-harm or suicide can range at the lower end from fleeting thoughts that life is not worth living, easily suppressed, through persistent ideas, towards definite plans and making of practical plans and preparations at the higher end. Some features that may be directly associated with mood disturbance in depressive disorders are described as more biological in nature (see Section 4.3.2), and at this point in the examination it can be useful also to check that items such as sleep disturbance, appetite and weight change have been noted and recorded.

Mental state assessment findings can be supplemented by informant reports, including accounts of how the client spends his or her day, changes in observed energy levels, changes in appetite, sleep and libido, reduction in normal range of interests, and any changes in habitual patterns of activities. For continued monitoring of depressed mood, many clinicians will find it helpful to familiarise themselves with a structured monitoring tool for its assessment.

Thought

Thought is not directly observable to an examiner. It may be inferred from observations regarding speech and behaviour, or from the person's observations of their thoughts through metacognitive processes (see Chapters 2.3.3 and 2.6). Some of the assessment of thought is similar in the terms used to that applying to speech, since much of what is termed thought has features of speech that is not vocalised. *Form* of thought includes the characteristic flow and pace of thinking, abnormalities of connectedness and development of ideas within thought, while disorder of *content* involves issues such as excessive preoccupations, which may relate to obsessional phenomena or delusions referred to below. *Content* of thought may be indicative of a disorder, such as preoccupation with fear of judgement by others in social anxiety disorder or the imperfection of bodily parts in body dysmorphic disorder. The *cognitive triad* of depressive thinking includes negative estimation of the past history, the current self and the future. Some of the experiences that feature commonly in diagnosis of psychotic states (see Chapter 4.2), such as *thought broadcasting* and *thought withdrawal*, are disorders of the sense of ownership of thought, and may be recorded here within a category of 'possession of thought'.

In the cross-cultural setting, there are many difficulties in making a judgement concerning the presence and type of disorder of thought form, and disorder of thought content. Among refugees and recent immigrants, particularly those who may have suffered severe trauma or torture, mistrustfulness and suspiciousness may be adaptive, and are likely to be much more prominent when in unfamiliar or threatening environments. This may also be the case for people subjected to serious racism or other forms of discrimination. Difficulties with English may also easily lead to misinterpretation of the behaviour and intent of others. In such circumstances, the clinician may make an incorrect judgement that paranoid delusions are present. Nonlinear or allusive communication styles, common particularly in Asian cultures, may be mistaken for formal thought disorder. Use of unfamiliar metaphors may be mistaken for overvalued ideas, delusions or hallucinations. Magical beliefs concerning the causes of ill-health (for example, evil eye or spiritual causes) may be mistaken for delusions. For example, in many non-Western cultures, the spirits of deceased relatives are regarded as capable of influencing or controlling the behaviour of a person. The same error may be made in relation to culturally common and acceptable beliefs concerning magic or witchcraft.

Abnormal experiences and beliefs

Depersonalisation and derealisation

These are particular experiences associated with anxiety disorders, and sometimes with schizophrenia, that may occasionally form prominent features of disordered presentation in isolation. They involve experiences of a sense that the self or the world are, in a disturbing and disorientating sense, unreal, and can be extremely distressing. Depersonalisation may be described as feeling detached from one's body as if observing oneself; derealisation may be described as experiencing the world as two dimensional, or made of cardboard cut-outs.

Obsessional phenomena

These are intrusive thoughts, recognised as part of the self, but not actively willed, that recur despite resistance, and where the attempt to resist provokes anxiety. These constitute obsessional ruminations. They may be accompanied by compulsive actions, where the performance of some repetitive act intended to neutralise the obsessional thoughts (e.g. washing or checking in response to concern about germs) is accompanied by short term relief of anxiety, and comes to take over significant amounts of the time in the day of a sufferer.

Delusions

Delusions are beliefs that are inconsistent with the individual's background, taking into account cultural and religious beliefs, and which are maintained despite evidence that would convince a reasonable-minded person that they might be incorrect. They will be defended against challenge and usually impervious to logical reasoning (see Chapter 4.2).

Illusions

These are misinterpretations of sensory stimuli. They are common in organic disorders with clouding of consciousness.

Hallucinations

A *hallucination* is an experience with the qualities of a perception, but where there is no accompanying external physical stimulus. The most commonly encountered hallucinatory experiences in most community mental health settings will be auditory hallucinations, however these do not necessarily signify a psychotic disorder, or indeed, a disorder at all. Hearing hallucinatory voices occurs across a spectrum of experience from brief and benign experiences in many people who have no disorder, to experiences that are part of depressive disorders, stress-related disorders or responses to experiences of trauma, to frequent, intrusive and distressing experiences for some people living with schizophrenia.

Systematic mental state assessment should include at least some routine screening questions, along the lines of those described in Box 2.4.

Box 2.4: Specific questions about voices, and other abnormal experiences

- Do you ever hear voices or see things that other people do not seem to hear or see? If you hear voices:
    - Is there one voice or more than one?
    - If more than one:
        - Do the various voices talk to you or about you?
        - If yes, do they talk to each other about you?
    - Do these voices sound real, as real, say, as my voice sounds now?
    - Alternatively, are they more like thoughts?
    - Are they inside or outside your head?
    - Could you identify if the voice is
        - male or female?
        - any particular person?
        - coming from any particular place?
    - Have you done anything in response to the voices, for instance, complaining to neighbours because you thought they were making the sounds?
    - Do the voices ever instruct or ask you to do things?
    - If yes, what?
    - Do you feel you have to carry out the instructions, or is it in any way difficult to resist the voices?
    - How much of the time are these voices present?
    - How much do they bother you?
    - Do you want them to go away?
- What things have you found make a difference to the experience of the voices?
- Do you ever hear your own thoughts spoken out loud?
- Do you have experiences of such voices on the radio or television referring to you in a direct manner?
- Do you ever have experiences of your will being taken over and controlled by some outside person or force?
- Do you ever have the experience of thoughts being put into your mind from outside?
- Do you ever have the experience of being taken out of your mind by someone?
- Do you ever have the experience of your thoughts being available to others and read in any way, even if you wouldn't want them to be?

These, as well as inquiry into apparently abnormal beliefs, will provide a set of initial probes for hallucinations and abnormal ideas, such as delusions, and including ideas of reference. In fact, this set of questions will collect most of the information required to establish the presence and likely impact of what are referred to as the 'first rank' symptoms of schizophrenia. The significance of these is discussed in Chapter 4.1.

Culturally normal experiences, such as hearing the voice of a deceased relative during early phases of bereavement, and describing hearing the voice of the spirits of relatives, may be misinterpreted as hallucinations with psychopathological significance. Apparently abnormal passivity experiences can also be difficult to interpret in a person from a culture in which power hierarchies are different in nature and strength from those familiar to the assessor.

Cognition

The approach to *cognitive testing* in routine practice varies with age of the client or patient. In older people, some assessment of this will often be appropriate as routine in assessment, and at an early point, if symptoms suggest delirium or dementia (see Chapter 3.3). In younger people, the place of formal cognitive testing is less clear cut. The interviewer should be assured at least that there are no salient indications of cognitive problems, and should be prepared to commence something in the way of more formal assessment if indicated. Both delirium and dementia can occur in younger age groups, and acute delirium can be a time-critical matter for response if it indicates an underlying serious medical illness. Indications of possible problems, as revealed in regular assessment interview processes, may be found under the following headings:

- *Orientation:* Is the person orientated for time (date, day, time), for place (location of the interview) and person (name, date of birth and those of others around them)?
- *Attention and concentration*: Is the person maintaining focus on your questions and responding appropriately to tasks requested? Beginnings of formal assessment of this include counting down from 100 in 7s (serial 7s) and reciting the months backwards. In each case, time the effort and record errors.
- *Memory:* Does the person register your name, and is he or she able later in the interview to recall it? Formal testing may begin with inviting the person to remember three given reasonably common words, if necessary allowing a couple of rehearsals for this. The ability to repeat them back constitutes immediate memory, and ability to repeat after 5 minutes short-term recall. Further exploration of memory problems can include inviting recall of recent news items or of what a person ate for breakfast. Longer-term accounts of events years or decades ago, either in the way of major news events or key dates as learnt facts, may assess *semantic memory*, while accounts of specific events as experienced by the person assess *episodic memory*.
- *Visuospatial ability*, if indicated, can be assessed, for instance, with the clock drawing test (see Section 3.3.3).
- *Abstract thinking*, if indicated, may in beginning a formal assessment commence by asking the person to compare two readily available objects, for instance, the desk and chair typically in the room, and list their common qualities and differences. Interpretation of culturally familiar proverbs and sayings may also be useful here.

For a brief, structured way of assessing cognitive mental state and reporting it, the reader is referred to the Mini Mental State Examination (see Chapter 3.3), a screening tool for cognitive impairment.

Assessment of cognitive function is extremely difficult in circumstances when the patient cannot speak English. Even when an interpreter is present to assist, a number of commonly used clinical cognitive tasks (for example, spell 'world' backwards) make no sense to people from some cultural backgrounds. For example, a person who speaks and writes in Mandarin will be unfamiliar with the notion of spelling. An additional problem is that of interpreting the clinical significance of various levels of functioning in response to cognitive tasks commonly used in clinical assessment. Tests of cognitive functioning (even with an interpreter) may be quite meaningless for elderly people who have never been literate (see Chapter 3.3).

Insight

Insight is a complex concept. Assessment of insight should include, at least, an account of the client's perceptions of the nature of the problem, what gave rise to it, why it continues to be a problem and what might be done to help it resolve. Commonly, this should include an assessment of the client's view of whether the problem is of the nature of an illness (or mental health problem), and what he or she thinks about the possibility of taking medication or psychotherapy or other mental health treatment to help resolve the disorder.

A particular importance of this assessment relates to the notion that successful management arises through a process of negotiations between the clinician and the client. Before introducing or suggesting any particular intervention, it would be sensible to have a clear understanding of the consumer's own explanatory model for their experiences, in order to consider the way in which this might be received. The assessment of this component of the mental state in a systematic way constitutes an important aspect of collaboration in assessment and management planning.

Physical health assessment

Psychiatric diagnosis is made primarily on the structured history taking, mental state examination and clinical judgement of the assessor. Diagnostic tests at this point typically play a limited role in establishing psychiatric disorders but very importantly some psychiatric presentations can be a manifestation of an underlying physical health problem. The psychiatrist, as a doctor, will approach this by taking a medical history and performing a physical examination designed to detect signs of the disorders that might possibly be creating a psychiatric manifestation delirium (see Section 3.3.5). This is a particular condition in which investigation for organic causes should be vigorously pursued, but it is not uncommon for other apparently psychiatric presentations actually to be secondary to a general medical condition. Successful diagnosis and treatment of the medical condition may treat, cure or ameliorate the apparent psychiatric disorder. To take one very common example, myxoedema or low thyroid function may present with symptoms of depression, but it may be evident to a physician on examination and confirmed with testing that the endocrine disturbance is the underlying problem. Other endocrine conditions have the potential to present in this way, as do, for instance, metabolic disorders, toxic effects of drugs, be they prescribed or recreational, licit or illicit, infections, central nervous system abnormalities, cancer, immune system and cardiopulmonary abnormalities. A doctor should address this in the context of a physical medical assessment with specific investigations as indicated. Texts commonly used by psychiatrists contain accounts of these problems and approaches to their treatment.

The role of physical health assessment could be three-fold:

1 Routine Physical Health assessment and establishing baseline medical status.
2 Physical Health Assessment to rule out medical causes of psychiatric manifestations including screening for illicit drug use.
3 Physical Health assessment for side effects of medication on movement, metabolic status, cardiovascular system, endocrinal system and other systems; including monitoring of plasma levels of some psychotropic medications.

The psychiatrist as doctor also has a role in advocating for good-quality physical health care to be delivered to psychiatric patients. Sometimes this involves advocating that medical needs of a patient are properly assessed by a general health care system that may not be as responsive to their needs as it would be in the case of someone without a mental health problem.

Risk assessment

Risk and risk factors

In clinical practice, risk can be defined as likelihood of an adverse event or outcome and can be categorised broadly as risks to self, to others or from others (Flewett, 2011). Level of risk can be considered as a product of the likelihood of an event, the severity of associated adverse consequences and how imminent it appears to be. Risk factors which increase likelihood of an adverse event can be considered as static and dynamic, internal and external. Risk itself is almost never a static property, but constantly shifts in response to circumstances including decisions made; not uncommonly decisions that have some properties of reducing level of risk in some way may in some other causal connection bear the possibility of increasing that level in some other way. While no field of medicine can be practised without an element of risk and uncertainty, mental health clinicians need training and ongoing support in clinical risk assessment and risk management, and for some mental health professions, risk assessment is an expected practice competency.

While there are questions around the performance of much clinical risk assessment, there are many settings in which ethical and societal accountabilities, along with organisational and medico-legal accountabilities, require that risk assessment be carried out. Risk assessment is often an implied or explicitly stated duty in mental health legislation. Mental health legislation gives particular clinicians the power to intervene and contain people in the event where a particular risk is assessed as being there, then it creates in effect a duty that clinicians perform that role. Coroners' courts, and settings involving litigation, can create other accountabilities and potentially liabilities within which clinicians or the organisations in which they work can be held at fault and potentially suffer a range of personal, organisational financial and other negative consequences. At the same time recent Mental Health Act revisions, such as in Victoria in 2014 (see Chapter 1.7), describe the concept of 'dignity of risk' which endorses a person's right to make decisions that involve a degree of risk. This reflects a direction of change in the concept of risk that acknowledges risk taking as an essential element of personal growth and development.

Approaches to clinical risk assessment can be categorised as clinical, actuarial and structured. All of these approaches have their pitfalls and in current clinical practice structured clinical risk assessment is the most commonly recommended approach (Flewett, 2011). A further layer of understanding risk can be added by incorporating psychodynamic considerations to clinical risk assessment.

In summary, risk assessment in psychiatry is a very standard practice and accompanies most clinical assessments (Holmes, 2013). It often pre-occupies clinicians and in some cases organisations and can be given a high level of prominence in staff members' performance expectations. Often focus is on risk of harm to self and others but chronic mental health disorder is a risk factor that leads to vulnerabilities, which may include many risks such as compromises to self-care, inability to manage their accommodation, finances, physical health, or hazardous substance use.

Considering risk assessment as CDM

Earlier in the text we have introduced some elements of CDM (see Section 2.3.3). Some specific concepts were those of critical thinking, reflective thinking, complexity thinking and dialectical thinking. So here we will consider how practitioners may develop their practice in this area using these concepts. We note also that risk assessment often has strongly ethical dimensions and so principles of medical ethics, including beneficence, non-maleficence, and respect for autonomy, are also involved in this process.

A critical perspective

Risk assessment has qualities of a screening process. As we have discussed elsewhere in the text (see Chapter 1.4), screening instruments perform differently in different settings, in ways that, including other influences, are strongly affected by the prevalence of the risk to be identified. For low-frequency events, a common problem is that of false positives. To give an example, suicide is a low frequency event, typically in Australia around 10 per 100,000 population per annum, in contrast to which suicide attempts and suicidality are much more highly prevalent. Seeking, then, to predict completed suicides or even recurrent attempts faces the problem that the pre-test probability of the event is quite low so a screening instrument or process would need to perform extremely well to create a selected group of people with a very-high risk (post-test probability; see Section 1.4.7).

Some structured risk assessments, for instance the Historical, Clinical and Risk-management instrument (HCR-20), have demonstrated validity in predicting future risk of violence in forensic psychiatry, but these are often demanding in terms of training and administration so may not be suitable for routine clinical use in many settings.

Reflective considerations

Reflection, as introduced earlier, involves reflection in, on, and for situations. *In* the situation, a practitioner may reflect on the nature of possible risks that might be identified, the severity of the consequences of such risks, and the range of evidence available to consider. Reflection *on* the circumstance can involve consideration after the event of risk determinations, action taken or not, consequences and the degree of foreseeability of these, then reflection *for* the situation can involve the deliberations on how subsequent situations with an individual client or others might be approached.

Complexity thinking

The extent to which risk assessment is an expected part of professional and other roles will vary according to setting. In roles with a strongly clinical orientation, then it may be given a high primacy; in other roles and services, it may be less important. There can be very considerable complexity in an individual's psychological makeup, including effects that mental health problems such as affective or psychotic states may have on the weighing of probabilities to guide decisions. Further, the individual is far from a closed system (see Chapter 1.1). For instance, it is clear that societal measures to restrict access to certain means of completion of suicide can make major differences to suicide rates. Work in different countries has demonstrated changes associated with transitions from sedative use of barbiturates to the use of much less toxic benzodiazepines, or from coal gas, which was lethal, to natural gas, which is typically not, or access to firearms; all of these can make differences to rates of suicide and in the latter case rates of homicide. As introduced above, sometimes an intervention may have risk-reduction properties but also capacity to escalate or even initiate feedback loops. Dilemmas often accompany compulsory admission, which while potentially containing and controlling some risk-behaviours, may also be demoralising and provoke resentments that may on occasions increase risk.

Dialectical thinking

One clear example of this is can be framed in one level as the balance of beneficence and autonomy (see Chapter 1.5), and in another way issues about risk containment and management versus recovery oriented practice (Hall, 2013). Respect for autonomy and recovery oriented practice might both indicate an extent to which the individuals' decisions in relation to risk taking, particularly in relation to suicide and suicidality, may be given a high priority in the reasoning system, in accordance with the proposition, for instance, that individuals have a right to choose what risks they take in life. Balanced against this might be more paternalistic notions that the individual's reasoning may be disturbed by the nature of their disorder, either for instance by distortions and information processing in schizophrenia that may lead to delusional states, or to the extent to which negative cognitive bias is associated with depression. This may mean that the person's decision making is not in alignment with the decisions that they would make either if not affected by a disorder at that time or, how they might see these same decisions in retrospect and at a different point in their recovery.

Specific practice

Risk assessment can then helpfully be considered as a process of determining presence or absence of factors that increase the risk of a particular outcome. This approach includes the framework of static and dynamic risk factors, which could impact on outcome at the end of clinical assessment e.g. a past attempt to end life by suicide is a static risk factors but presence or absence of suicidal intent is a dynamic risk factor. This also opens the dialogue with the consumer about treatments and supports that reduce the dynamic risk factors.

Much of practice, and to some degree evidence, relates to specific risks or specific diagnostic situations. Established routine assessment of suicide attempts involves, for instance, exploration of whether a note was left, whether precautions were made against discovery, whether affairs had been tidied up before an attempt such as to minimise the difficulties for others in the event that the suicide attempt was completed, and to some degree, the lethality of means. These may guide assessment of likelihood of attempts, and then protective factors may be considered such as a degree of social supports, the degrees for instance of spiritual beliefs, and access to means.

In clinical practice, the risk management practices follow the risk assessment and given the expectation on field of psychiatry to manage the risk posed to the community, these practices have historically been of restrictive nature.

There is, therefore no 'one-size-fits-all' approach to risk assessment either for individual professionals, individual clients or patients, the times or service settings. Whatever the individual setting, the application of these four considerations of clinical decision making in the context of consideration of primary, ethical principles, can help one over time, develop a considered, appropriate defensible, valued and respected approach to the task.

EXTENDING, DEEPENING AND FORMALISING ASSESSMENT

Administer outcome measures

In Australia, the National Outcomes and Casemix Collection (NOCC) is a suite of outcome measures intended to be collected at multiple time points, including assessment, so as to routinely monitor service outcomes. They include clinician rated or consumer-rated tools. Of these, the ones applying to adult practice are:

Clinician rated

- Health of the Nation Outcome Scales (HoNOS)
- Life Skills Profile (LSP-16)
- Phase of Care (PoC).

Consumer self-report (varies across states and territories)

- Mental Health Inventory (MHI)
- Kessler-10 (K-10)
- Behaviour and Symptom Identification Scale (BASIS 32)

Outside adult practice, other measures are used. These include the following:

- Health of the Nation Outcome Scales for Children and Adolescents (HoNOSCA)
- Health of the Nation Outcome Scales 65+ (HoNOS65+)
- Resource Utilisation Groups-Activities of Daily Living Scale (RUG-ADL)
- Children's Global Assessment Scale (CGAS)
- Strengths and Difficulties Questionnaire (SDQ)
- Factors Influencing Health Status (FIHS).

Established by the Australian Government to support the implementation of these outcome measures as part of routine clinical practice, the Australian Mental Health Outcomes and Classification Network (AMHOCN) processes and analyses submitted data collected using these tools. AMHOCN also supports training in the use of these tools for clinical practice, service planning and development. For this purpose, a range of information and training resources related to use of the above tools can be accessed from their website (AMHOCN, 2020). While there has been an AMHOCN review of measures of 'Recovery' (Burgess, Pirkis, Coombs, & Rosen, 2010), there is no adopted measure in the NOCC suite.

A key and continuing deficiency of the AMHOCN data collection is that country of birth and other variables relevant to immigrants and refugees are not included in the data collection. This means that we have virtually no data on outcomes for immigrant and refugee communities (Minas et al., 2013).

2.3.5 EXTENDING THE RANGE OF INFORMATION SOURCES

GRAHAM MEADOWS

INTERVIEWING FAMILIES AND OTHERS

Consumers may be willing and keen to have family members or others involved in assessment–such interviews can add important information about the course of events and their impact on others around the identified client or patient. Families may experience a range of difficulties themselves, so it is important that their support needs are also assessed and addressed (see Chapter 2.7). While a number of tools have been developed to assess families' and carers' experiences, stress and coping (sometimes referred to as carer burden) for research use, informal interviewing and maintaining regular communication with family members may be as effective for this type of assessment in routine clinical practice (see Chapter 2.7). However sometimes consumers may not wish for there to be communication with family members or others in their social sphere and practitioners need to be cognizant of the indication for agreement from the client or patient for such interaction,

Unfortunately violence or abuse occurs within families of people with mental health problems, as it does in other family settings. Family members and clients each may suffer and perpetrate violent and abusive acts. Family members or carers may wish to share concerns or accounts about actual or possible threat or violence. To receive information from a family member is not necessarily to breach confidence. If family members wish to discuss issues of concern to them, failing to accept information about their concerns may be at least inappropriate and potentially even dangerous. It may be important to create a situation in which family members or others significantly involved with a client's life can divulge material in a safe setting. This may well involve meeting with these individuals away from the presence of the identified consumer and this presents potentially challenging issues regarding confidentiality. Some services have quite specific views and policies on this. The client has a right of confidentiality and a duty of care exists, but there also may be a duty of care to the family members. Balances of rights and duties need to be considered here and an approach to this is summarised in Figure 2.2. Most jurisdictions have mandatory reporting rules for certain types of violence, particularly child abuse and readers need to be aware of policies or legal provisions that apply in their practice context.

Figure 2.2 Framework for best clinical practice when consent is not given to share information with carers (Slade et al. 2007)

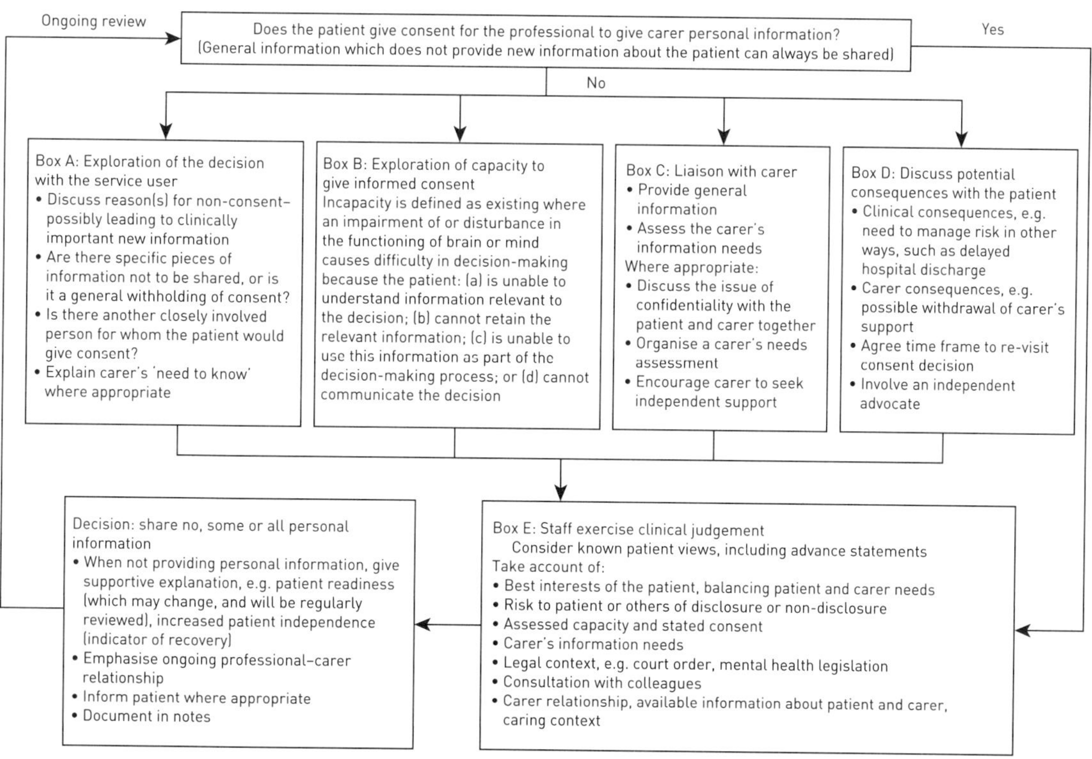

Documentation and records

Information from interviews is often usefully supplemented by material from other sources, including from client records, or case notes. If the person has extensive case notes from a particular clinical organisation, then these will be important to be aware of, and often will be helpful to review. Sometimes summaries will be available from notes, but sometimes these are not necessarily to be found at the points in the individual history that are most informative in relation to the current episode. Decisions need to be made about how much effort will go into retrieving and gaining a comprehension of the content of such sources. Consent issues may need to be negotiated for permission to seek personal information about a client from other sources, whether this be from the person's general practitioner (GP), another service or the person's family.

2.3.6 CRAFTING A SUMMARY AND FORMULATION

GRAHAM MEADOWS & JOHN FARHALL

Information collection from history taking and mental-state assessment generates a large volume of material, which is in structured formats but not synthesised. Summary and formulation are successive processes of selection and synthesis from the observational information. They help present the material in a way that is conducive to assessment of needs and care planning. Summarising may well present the information under something like the headings set out in this chapter; however, there will be a process of selection in what is presented. Negatives may well not be presented unless they are significant. The accounts may well concentrate on the aspects of the history that appear most significant and influential.

Formulation needs to be based on and typically inclusive of a summary, but goes a step further. In formulation we attempt a synthesis of the information, including some understanding of the interactions between events. A formulation may venture some judgements, such as diagnoses, or describe a particular other type of identifiable problem. It will usually be short, often a few hundred words at most, and necessarily selective. The format and content of a formulation is very dependent on the theoretical approach of the one making the formulation, since the selection of information and inferences made from it at this level are heavily theory dependent.

We will here give a useful example of one approach to development of a summary. This approach is quite biomedical in orientation and will not suit all settings, clients or problems. However, there will be services in which something like this will be expected as part of the assessment process. It can be extended to be more towards a biopsychosocial summary if the range of considerations under each heading is made significantly broader than simply medical considerations, in the way that the biopsychosocial approach recommends. Alternative approaches to summary and formulation are discussed later (see Sections 2.3.7 and 2.3.8). First, this approach is based around a mnemonic of seven Ps, which we will now discuss in order.

PERTINENT HISTORY

Commonly this will begin with statement of age, a description of gender and marital or relationship status. After this, the choice of content needs to be flexible and determined by what is important in the clinical reasoning related to this person's problems. Aspects of personal history, cultural identity, past medical and psychiatric history, including service contacts and any indicators of risk, including risk of suicidality or harm to others, are very likely to feature here. Here is an opportunity also to indicate identified strengths as evident from the personal history or other information.

PRESENTING SYMPTOMS

Here is a summary of the particular experiences, changes in behaviour or other prompts that may have led someone to be seeking help or to otherwise present problems or difficulties at a particular point in time. Some information about the onset, duration and other aspects of time course of the symptoms or problems would be expected.

PRECIPITATING FACTORS

In this section we will find information about events, often reasonably recent events or stressors that seem likely to have a role in the causation of the current episode, playing their part in determining why this person might be finding him- or herself in this particular kind of trouble or distress at this particular point in time.

PREDISPOSING FACTORS

These are aspects of the background to the life of the individual that create dispositions or vulnerabilities towards problems and perhaps towards the kind of problems currently being experienced. Sometimes this will involve a transgenerational perspective, and family history will be relevant if it indicates a biological vulnerability; otherwise the content will focus more on perhaps early life experience, acquired medical disorders or habitual patterns of behaviour, including substance misuse, for instance.

PERPETUATING FACTORS

Here we will find evident features that seem to be going against the likelihood or opportunity of recovery or remission of symptoms. These will include things that may be interfering with the functioning of innate resilience of the person that otherwise might mean they could find their own way out of or through the problem. Medical conditions, problems with engagement with services and loss of social supports—all might feature here.

PROTECTIVE FACTORS

This section cues us to attend to personal strengths of the individual that may be harnessed in treatment or that might foster optimism—for the person or the treating team—in a time where problems may appear to dominate. Similarly, paying attention to the current environmental factors that help protect and maintain the person's health and welfare, such as supportive relationships and secure housing, means a formulation can recognise their contribution in mitigating or guarding against greater impact of the problem or vulnerability.

PREVIOUS TREATMENT OR RESPONSE

This will assist planning for management, in that it will provide information on what has already been tried and what response, if any, has been achieved. Important here will be history of previous and recent contact with services, what kinds of interventions the individual has received, and what evidence there is as to whether the interventions have been of any assistance.

ADDING A DIAGNOSIS

Generally a summary such as one developed under the seven Ps structure will contain the information necessary to establish and substantiate diagnosis. Not uncommonly we may list multiple diagnostic classification labels or codes, something that may happen for various reasons:

- a diagnostic picture may be unclear at a particular point in time, so multiple differential diagnoses may be registered, sometimes with one identified as more likely
- diagnostic grouping may increasingly involve application of dimensional concepts (see Section 2.3.3) and concepts of staging (see Chapters 1.5, 3.2 and 4.2), which may be captured in use of multiple categories
- multiple entries may represent either co-occurring or comorbid conditions, where each seems to be clearly present
- the information available may be incomplete, in which case a diagnosis may be noted as provisional and assigned on a balance of probabilities; perhaps noting the need to collect more information, what that might be and where it might be found.

In practice, the development of a summary and assignment of diagnosis as set out against these axes is not a simple linear process. A first consideration or draft of the summary may be developed. Then, when the diagnostic picture is considered to be lacking critical pieces of information, the summary content may be revisited so that it becomes more inclusive as needed, and more internally consistent.

2.3.7 WORKING MODELS OF PROCEEDING FROM ASSESSMENT TO PRACTICE

GRAHAM MEADOWS & JOHN FARHALL

NEEDS ASSESSMENT AND GOAL IDENTIFICATION

Expanding the scope

Assessment in most mental health care is not an end in itself but rather a step towards some action on the part of service providers, clients, families or others. This can be described as needs assessment (what might helpfully be done or offered?) and also goal identification (what it is hoped the intended actions might achieve?). Information required to inform needs assessment and goal setting includes the various components of an appropriate, appropriately comprehensive, clinical, functional, social and environmental assessment. It also includes an understanding of the wants, requests or demands of the client, and other relevant participants in the social system. However, this information may fall short of being a source for comprehensive needs assessment and goal setting. Problem lists and diagnostic descriptions may be constrained in scope and even if they can identify that a need is present, they may not clearly identify what the need is for or what goals might best be to aim for.

Various approaches to addressing this, such as application of the Camberwell Assessment of Need Short Appraisal Schedule (CANSAS) (Trauer, Tobias, & Slade, 2008; Macpherson, Varah, Summerfield, Foy, & Slade, 2003) which includes staff and consumer-rated versions for appraising needs in 22 service categories: food; accommodation; looking after the home; self-care; daytime activities; physical health; psychotic symptoms; information on condition and treatment; psychological distress; safety to self; safety to others; alcohol; drugs; company; intimate relationships; sexual expression; childcare; basic education; telephone; transport; money and benefits. In Australian Community Surveys (Meadows & Burgess, 2009), the Perceived need for Care Questionnaire (PNCQ) has been repeatedly used to assess consumer-rated perceived needs for care (see Section 1.6.7). The PNCQ involves items of: information; medication; counselling and psychotherapies (includes: psychotherapy; cognitive behaviour therapy; counselling); social intervention (help to sort out housing or money problems); skills training (includes: help to improve your ability to work, or to use your time in other ways; help to improve your ability to look after yourself or your home; help to meet people for support or company). A brief self-report version of this designed for primary care condenses these items for self-report of needs as an element of collaborative planning (McNab & Meadows, 2005).

These approaches and instruments may be helpful in planning action based on assessment. But assessment based on the processes that we have considered so far may be lacking in scope. While a well conducted biopsychosocial assessment process can be broad in scope and for some clients adequate to the indicated task, the movement towards recovery oriented practice suggests this process can usefully be conducted somewhat differently.

REFOCUS-PULSAR: Training and resources for supporting recovery oriented practice

This framework for encouraging recovery oriented practice is one of a number available in the literature (see Chapter 2.6). It is unlikely that it is singularly effective, but at the time of writing it is unique in having high-level—and Australian—evidence that when used as a staff training resource, it can promote consumer-assessed experience of recovery (Meadows et al.,

2019). A manual setting out the key elements of the model—which represents an Australian development of a model first elaborated in the United Kingdom—is available on the web (Slade, Bird, Le Boutillier, Williams, & Leamy, 2016) and is in the public domain.

It should be noted that the evidence about its effectiveness, which several authors of this text were involved in developing (Meadows et al., 2019), was based on a specific staff training program which strongly featured consumer involvement; this sought to increase relevant knowledge and promote attitudinal changes in participating staff as well as applying the principles and processes set out in the manual. It included a strong emphasis on encouraging a relationship grounded in principles of coaching including use of an approach to interactions guided by the 'REACH' framework (reflect, explore, agree, commit, hold-to-account) and with considerations of domains of recovery guided by the scope of the CHIME framework (connectedness, hope, identity, meaning-and-purpose; and empowerment; Leamy, Bird, Le Boutillier, Williams, & Slade, 2011). In this context, the model introduced three working practices:

1 understanding values, treatment and support preferences
2 assessing strengths and
3 supporting goal striving.

An important aspect of aiming to get to agreed needs and goals in a way that extends the interactions beyond what we may see with conventional assessment (see Section 2.3.4) is the use of two particular interview guides, one guiding discussion of values, treatment and support preferences and another being a strengths worksheet. Alternative suggested approaches in the manual (Slade et al., 2016) include mapping strategies for gathering this information.

Use of these guides will prompt, by way of example, discussion of: cultural identity and its implications, gender roles and their importance, sexuality, meaning of 'mental illness' experience, previous experiences of service, and effects of stigma and discrimination; income, sources of satisfaction, spirituality and self-care actions. Once these issues have been raised—and especially if this is done in the clinical or other client-provider relationship context identified above—then the identification of personally valued goals and possible needs may be different from those identified following a more conventional assessment.

Next is to work together as partners to identify steps for pursuing those goals, which will involve:

- The person themselves prioritising the goal(s) to focus on.
- Identifying which strengths are relevant and can be built on to pursue goal(s).
- Identifying how the person's values, treatment and support preferences will impact on the action plan.
- Breaking goals down into smaller manageable steps and making plans for who will do what and when—informally or using the SMART (Specific, Meaningful, Attainable, Realistic, Timetabled) approach.
- Supporting the person to undertake independent or joint actions rather than accepting passive actions.

The resulting recovery oriented care plan will, it is to be hoped: focus on personally valued goals; reflect the person's values, treatment and support preferences; build on the person's strengths; and use a coaching approach to support the person's actions in pursuit of his or her goals (adapted from Slade et al., 2016).

The systemic importance of setting goals

Setting goals contributes to defining and planning actions or intervention, monitoring progress and evaluating outcomes. Setting goals can be an integral part of regular interactions between service providers, consumers and carers, with whom plans are negotiated and progress is reviewed; these may occur relatively informally within effective alliances. When goals are clearly defined in terms that identify the intended outcomes of a course of action, they may also be used to more systematically monitor and evaluate the effectiveness of service provision. Thus, a structured process of setting and documenting goals and defining action plans with consumers, and with carers where applicable, introduces transparency and accountability in services to those for whom the service is provided.

Stages of personal recovery as a formulation frame

Descriptions of recovery oriented principles and practice are often presented as logical steps that assume an effective working relationship between consumer and helper, and by emphasising that the principles are universal, may give the impression that recovery oriented practice is a straightforward process of hearing the consumer's goals and offering one's expertise to help the consumer proceed in their chosen direction. However, the reality of human service work is often otherwise. Professionals may assume the relevance of what appears to be a sensible pathway to better wellbeing then find that it is seen in a different light by the person, or may struggle to find a way to meaningfully apply the interventions in their skill set for the benefit of the consumer. In Chapter 2.6, we discuss many facets of the implementation of recovery oriented practices; here we present a way of formulating where a consumer is up to in their personal recovery journey that can help workers consider what services or interventions they may offer, or what may be helpful foci of conversations about meaningful assistance for the person.

The formulation framework has two key concepts: *Stages* and *Tasks* of personal recovery. The idea that people may be at very different points in their relationship with a mental health issue has become widely accepted though a framework referred to as the 'stages of change' (Prochaska, Diclemente, & Norcross, 1992), best known in the field of addiction for its application in motivational interviewing (Miller & Rollnick, 2012). The earliest stage represents the situation of those who as yet are unaware that the problem observed by others is impacting their life and those who do not accept that any change is required. The most adaptive stage describes a level where the person is managing the issue in their life and continuing to grow as a person. The processes of moving through stages of change between these is not necessarily linear—we can slip back and move forward again—and not necessarily consistent across all aspects of the journey—we can be getting on with life challenges better in some domains than others—an important consideration for formulation and collaborative treatment planning.

This phenomenon of stages of personal change has resonated with consumers' descriptions of the process of recovery from mental ill-health (Davidson, 2003; Leamy et al., 2011). Here it is summarised in five stages that equate to those of Prochaska et al. (1992)—Pre-contemplation; Contemplation; Preparation; Action; and Maintenance & Growth—however we use descriptions and language drawn partly from Spaniol, Wewiorski, Gagne, and Anthony (2002) that better relate to the focus here on recovery from mental ill-health. The Collaborative Recovery Model (Andresen, Oades, & Caputi, 2011) also usefully applies the notion of stages of change to psychological recovery from mental illness:

Stage 1. *Overwhelmed by* mental ill-health describes people who at present seem confused, disconnected from others and social roles, and with no goals.

Stage 2 *Acknowledging* an impact of mental ill-health describes those who are aware that something needs to change and have some directions of change in mind, but without yet acting.

Stage 3 Those who are *Struggling with* mental ill-health may have a beginning explanatory model and realise the need to cope better into the future, but face fears, and loss of confidence.

Stage 4 *Living with mental ill-health* means having found some personally relevant way to come to terms with it, being reasonably confident in managing it, having some meaningful place in life, but feeling constrained by disability.

Stage 5 Those who are *Living beyond* mental ill-health (Davidson, 2003) have a relatively normal and satisfying life but one where ill-health or vulnerability may be present and need attention.

The notion of recovery *'Tasks'* refers to directions of adaptive growth that many will encounter in their own personal process of recovery (Davidson, 2003; Spaniol et al., 2002). Common tasks include:

Recovery Task 1. *Understanding my mental health and what it means for me.* Essentially, this means the consumer working towards finding or creating a personally meaningful explanation for their experiences that helps them get on with life

Recovery Task 2. *Taking charge of my mental health* means finding ways to manage mental health issues

Recovery Task 3. *Living a life that I value* refers to engaging with life outside of mental illness experiences that brings meaning and satisfaction

Returning now to formulation, the Stages and Tasks can aid formulation by prompting consideration of what stage of recovery the person may be in at present in relation to the key tasks they are grappling with (or confronted with). For example, someone who describes where she is at in getting on with life (Task 3) as *'I tried to go back to my old job but it was just too stressful. I now work part-time as a peer support worker—It's really great to help others'* might be described as being at the stage of *Living with* the impact of her illness or vulnerabilities (Stage 4), and may wish to contemplate *'Living beyond'* (Stage 5). Another way in which these concepts can aid formulation, is to help match the offering of professional or peer services, with the stage of recovery, and the recovery tasks they are confronted with. For example, in relation to *understanding my mental health* (Task 1), providing 'psychoeducation' information in the form of illness concepts to someone showing typical symptoms of a psychotic disorder may appear to be good practice; however, if their current explanatory model for their difficulty is that *'it's just the weed I smoke'* (i.e. perhaps at Stage 1 or 2 in relation to this task), psychoeducation of this sort may alienate rather than educate. As an alternative, being curious about their current explanation and how well this is working for them, may open up opportunities for helpfully expanding their picture together over time.

Table 2.2 suggests examples of how one might formulate using these five stages and three recovery tasks.

Table 2.2 An aid to formulating stages and tasks in supporting personal recovery

Stage of personal recovery				
1. Feeling overwhelmed	**2.Acknowledging change is needed**	**3.Actively struggling with mental health**	**4.Living with impact of illness or vulnerability**	**5.Living beyond illness or vulnerability**
Recovery Task 1. Understanding my mental health—and what it means for me				
Confusion about what happened & what it means	Awareness that something needs to be understood or sorted out	Has a beginning explanatory model	Has come to terms with it	Comfortable with own personal understanding of experiences
Recovery Task 2. Taking charge of my mental health				
No deliberate coping	Realises need to cope or change	Is sometimes trying ways to cope or change	Generally confident in managing persisting illness or vulnerability	Mental health experiences interfere little with life
Recovery Task 3. Living a life that I value				
Disconnected from people, social roles and personal growth	Would like to be more connected to people, social roles and personal growth	Is sometimes trying ways to connect and change	Has found a place in life but still limited by disabilities	Has a 'contributing life'

Source: Adapted from Recovery Practice Guide, Senior Psychologists Group, NorthWestern Mental Health, Melbourne (unpublished).

2.3.8 VULNERABILITY: STRESS-COPING MODEL AND ASSESSMENT

JOHN FARHALL & MARILYN CUGNETTO

The *vulnerability-stress-coping model* is an extensively researched theory of psychopathology. In general psychological practice, it serves as a framework to prompt domains of assessment to aid case formulation and intervention. This section first outlines the model, then illustrates how a clinician or team may use this model to explore with a consumer how past and current factors may be interacting to explain the current mental health problems, and to suggest ideas for action.

THE MODEL

The vulnerability-stress-coping model of psychopathology (Ingram & Luxton, 2005; Zubin & Spring, 1977) proposes that everyone is potentially susceptible to any mental disorder, and that episodes of a disorder arise depending on relative levels of vulnerability, stress and coping.

- *Vulnerability*: People differ widely in their degree of vulnerability to any disorder, not only due to their genetic or biological makeup, but also to cognitive and interpersonal factors 'acquired' through developmental experiences and life events, especially those of childhood (Brown, 2011). Although conceptualised as an enduring endogenous trait, vulnerability is potentially modifiable. Vulnerability alone cannot explain the episodic nature of mental health problems: it is the interaction of vulnerability with the impact of stressors, moderated by the person's coping ability, that determines whether a breakdown in 'normal' functioning occurs, leading to observable signs and reported symptoms.
- *Stress*: Factors that disrupt a person's equilibrium are considered 'stressors'. These can be 'external' to the individual or 'internal'. Adverse (but also positive) life events, such as bereavement or job promotion, as well as daily 'hassles' (Phillips, Francey, Edwards, & McMurray, 2007), are external stressors that impact mental health (Kanner, Coyne, Schaefer, & Lazarus, 1981) dependent on how the stressors are appraised. Disruption of a person's equilibrium can also occur by the action of 'internal' stressors, including maturational changes and physical illness.
- *Coping*: The model recognises that people are not passive 'victims' of all stressors; stress can potentially be managed by coping actions. Much self-management of distress or symptoms involves some type and intensity of coping (Jorm, Griffiths, Christensen, Parslow, & Rogers, 2004). When a stressor (for example, criticism) is experienced, the typical response is to automatically attempt to readjust or 'cope' to restore equilibrium (Lazarus & Folkman, 1984), either by altering the environment (for example, leaving the stressful situation or arguing in an attempt to rebuff the criticism) or by changing in some way (for example, deciding that the critic had a point, or deciding that the critic's opinion was not important). Often a person's automatic or conscious coping responses are sufficient to restore equilibrium in their functioning. However, if there is insufficient coping effort or coping ability, functioning may decline. If the person's functioning falls below their 'threshold' for emergence of symptoms, signs of the disorder may show up.

Evidence and directions

The model's simplicity makes it a useful general framework for clinical practice, and also for working with specific problems or symptoms that are affecting consumers—coping enhancement for distressing voices is an example (Hayward, Strauss, & Kingdon, 2018). A considerable body of evidence supports each element of this model across a wide range of disorders (Ingram & Luxton, 2005), but the disorder to which it has been most extensively applied over time is schizophrenia. Research is filling out the picture of the interactive relationships between stress, vulnerability and coping. For example, in explaining the phenomenon of auditory hallucinations, it may be that specific genetic vulnerabilities (such as a marked inability to filter out irrelevant stimuli) or acquired vulnerabilities (from early childhood trauma) combine with particular stressors (interpersonal hassles) and maladaptive coping styles (experiential avoidance) in a synergistic pathway to symptom formation (Goldstone, Farhall, & Ong, 2012). In addition, the science of epigenetics has demonstrated that some environments play a mediating role, effectively activating or inhibiting the expression of a genetic characteristic, rather than simply influencing the *degree* to which it is expressed (Shorter & Miller, 2015).

Assessing vulnerability

Although vulnerabilities are relatively enduring, their assessment may not only aid understanding, but also suggest preventive or rehabilitative interventions. The following assessment themes may elicit information suggestive of vulnerability to mental disorders:

1. Genetic: Does the consumer have biological relatives diagnosed with a mental disorder? For many disorders, a family history of a similar condition increases the risk for the disorder.
2. Neurodevelopmental: Check out factors that may interfere with normal maturation and growth of the brain from gestation to adulthood (Harrison, 1997; Smucny, Olincy, Eichman, Lyons, & Tregellas, 2013). These may include maternal stresses or other adversities during gestation and birth and major physical illnesses in childhood or adolescence. Ask about head injuries, particularly involving loss of consciousness.
3. Personal and social adversity: The emotional environment during childhood and development can be sufficiently adverse as to stifle emotional development or individuation. Neglect, abuse and trauma during childhood and adolescence may render the person less resilient or more vulnerable to a range of disorders, including schizophrenia, mood and personality disorders (Hammen, 1992). (See Section 1.2.2 for a deeper treatment of social determinants of mental health issues.)

Assessing stress

Stressors can trigger symptoms, or may serve as the direct cause of symptoms. To identify the role of stress, both in the genesis of the disorder and in influencing relapses and remissions, consider the following:

1. In the period before the disorder's onset, and before later exacerbations of symptoms, has the consumer faced any major life events? Significant life events, whether welcome (for example, a new job, migration to a new country), neutral (for example, a change of case manager) or adverse (for example, a loved one's death, or becoming a refugee), involves a process of reorientation, during which old ways no longer fit and new ways need to be developed. Such changes are usually stressful to some degree.
2. Have there been daily hassles, such as relationship problems, overdue bills or an environment in which the consumer experiences criticism, hostility or blame (that is, high 'expressed emotion') from family (Miklowitz, 2004) or even mental health workers (Oliver & Kuipers, 1996)? Has the consumer experienced mental-health-related public stigma, self-stigma or discrimination (Thornicroft, Rose, Kassam, & Sartorius, 2007)? Consumers from Indigenous, migrant and other minority groups report frequent experiences of 'micro-aggressions', or brief verbal or behavioural racial insults often unintentionally communicated by majority group members (Sue et al., 2007). The stressful effect of persisting 'minor' hassles may be as great, or greater than the impact of major life events (Lazarus, 1990, 1999).
3. Is the physical, social and familial environment over- or under-stimulating? Both sensory overload (Nuechterlein et al., 1994) and social isolation (Hoffman, 2007) are stressors that may result in re-emergence of symptoms for people vulnerable to schizophrenia.
4. Is there evidence of internal stressors such as a physical illness or condition (for example, virus or diabetes), or behavioural stressors, such as overwork, drug abuse or sleep deprivation?

Assessing coping

The original formulation of this model by Zubin and Spring (1977) considered *coping* to encompass the automatic and deliberate responses of the person to specific stressors. In addition to these 'personal protectors', Nuechterlein proposed 'environmental protectors', such as supportive psychosocial interventions (a useful representation of this model is reprinted in Goldstein, 1987), thus recognising that our coping at any one point in time depends on the environment as well as our own actions. Thus, assessment should consider not only the person's coping skills but also the presence or absence of relevant supports and resources in the person's environment. In assessing coping strengths and weaknesses, include both the consumer's subjective report of coping actions and available observations from others. Note that asking the consumer how they typically cope can be empowering and enhance collaboration.

1 Coping with the stressor. Ask about problem-focused coping, directed at changing the stressor, and emotion-focused coping to manage distressing emotions (Folkman & Lazarus, 1980; Lazarus & Folkman, 1984). Consider coping style: Does the consumer look to others for help or do they tend to manage alone? Do some stressors lead to helplessness, or avoidance? It is easy to persist with responses that simply do not work, so check out how effective the consumer rates their coping strategies.
2 Coping with symptoms. Although symptoms (for example, feeling anxious or experiencing voices) may be precipitated by stressful experiences, they can also be a stressor in themselves. Consumers develop various ways of coping with symptoms, which can range from highly effective to self-defeating (Farhall, Greenwood, & Jackson, 2007).
3 Coping via treatment adherence. To what extent does the consumer cope with the disorder by taking medication or participating in psychosocial interventions as advised? How does the person's explanatory model of the disorder and their experience of past and current treatments influence how proposed treatments are now accepted? A deeper assessment of personal coping can include analysis of skill strengths and weaknesses, particularly in relation to the current problem and immediate goals.
4 Coping via supports. Assessment of coping should include assessment of support and resource strengths and deficits in the consumer's environment (DeLongis, Folkman, & Lazarus, 1988). Does the environment provide sufficient helpful personal supports (for example, family, friends, co-workers)? Can available resources address emotional and relationship problems, and stressors arising from housing needs, finances and employment (for example, via therapy, low-cost loans, advocacy)?
5 Coping via uplifts. Positive experiences or 'uplifts' (Kanner et al., 1981) may counteract the effect of stressors, by increasing feelings of wellbeing, thus being a powerful antidote to stress. In assessment, the clinician may check the nature, frequency and source of uplifts, and whether these have diminished or increased. For example, the temporary absence of a volunteer visitor may constitute the loss of a critical regular uplift that was protective against stress arising from isolation. Furthermore, how does the consumer respond to positive moods elicited by 'uplifts': do they 'savour' the good feelings, or are they 'dampened'? The consumer's typical emotion regulation strategy may be involved in the maintenance of mood disorders (Feldman, Joormann, & Johnson, 2008).

Formulation

A mental health assessment culminates in a formulation that attempts to integrate the known information about the problem with an understanding of the person in his or her life and socio-cultural context in order to guide treatment planning. Guided by a theoretical framework, the goal of a formulation is to generate hypotheses to explain why and how the person developed the mental health problem, what factors might be maintaining it, and how the consumer is currently managing it, including coping strengths and challenges.

2.3.9 TRAUMA-INFORMED CARE ASSESSMENT AND PRACTICE

INDIGO DAYA & SABIN FERNBACHER

Trauma is a major public health issue.

> Individual trauma results from an event, series of events, or set of circumstances that is experienced by an individual as physically or emotionally harmful or life threatening and has lasting adverse effects on the individual's functioning and mental, physical, social, emotional or spiritual wellbeing.
>
> *Substance Abuse and Mental Health Services Administration–USA (SAMSHSA, 2014), p. 7.*

Interpersonal trauma that occurs over longer periods of time is called 'complex trauma' (Kezelman & Stavropoulos, 2017).

A reaction to trauma can be immediate or can occur many years later.

The impact of trauma comes from more than just the traumatic experience. The context within which trauma occurs plays a role, as shown in the figure. For example, some people may have had little life opportunity to build resilience prior to trauma, which may mediate the impact. Life events after trauma also provide an important context: many trauma survivors speak about the devastating impact of not being believed, and these impacts can be a critical element of the trauma impact. What happens to a person after traumatic experiences can be restorative or may compound the traumatic impact. These factors can be helpful for clinicians to consider when working with people to understand the impact of past trauma.

People accessing mental health services experience higher rates of interpersonal violence than the general population. Overall around 66% of people admitted to inpatient mental health services have experienced child abuse (Read, Fink, Rudegeair, Felitti, & Whitfield, 2008) while around 85% have experienced child abuse and/or physical or sexual assault as an adult (Goodman et al., 2001).

Figure 2.3 Life context impacts on trauma

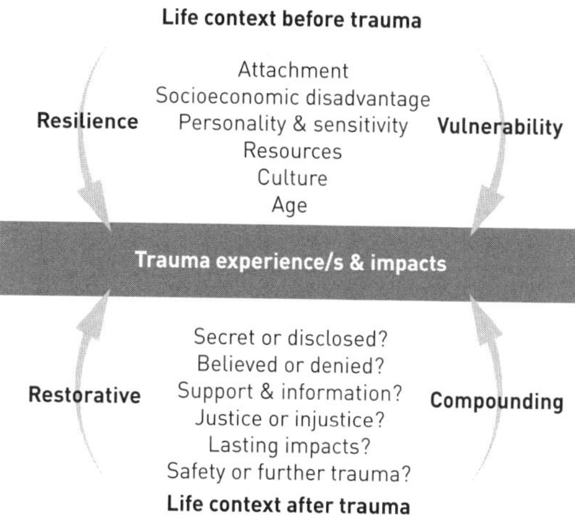

Source: Daya, 2020

Internationally, Trauma-Informed Care and Practice (TICP) has been developed to increase service provision that responds sensitively to trauma and its impacts.

MENTAL HEALTH ASSESSMENT AND TRAUMA

Trauma needs to be considered at least as a contributing factor or, as is frequently the case, the reason for a person's current mental health problems. It thus makes sense to consider the impact of trauma on a person's mental health throughout their mental health care, and this needs to start at the beginning during the assessment phase (Bloom, 2000; Harris & Fallot, 2001; Klinic Community Health Centre, 2008; Perry, Pollard, Blakley, & Vigilante, 1995; Saakvtine, Gamble, Pearlman, & Lev, 2004; van der Kolk, Roth, Pelcovitz, Sunday, & Spinazzola, 2005; Warshaw, 2007).

Taking a trauma history into account during assessment then becomes part of the approach to good mental health care.

A trauma inclusive approach to mental health assessment means that mental health workers can:

- Know that consumers are more likely than not to have experienced interpersonal trauma in their lives; just because it has not been talked about, does not mean it has not occurred.
- Understand that past events are likely to present as current concerns.

- Inquire sensitively about current or previous events in which trauma may have occurred; the inquirer (clinician) needs to be able to respond adequately.
- Understand that it is not always appropriate to ask about trauma—especially if the person is in state of heightened anxiety or in crisis; if this is the case support the person towards increasing safety and to gain control. Appropriate questions are 'How can I help you? What needs to happen to help you feel more in control now?' These questions are specifically helpful at first engagement/assessment as well as being helpful at other times.
- Know that violence and trauma can shape a person's belief system, feelings, self-perception, and relationships with others.
- Be alert to potential for retraumatisation through work-practices; if retraumatisation occurs, offer debriefing and support to the consumer where possible by an agreed third party (to avoid the potential for a staff member who may have been part of retraumatisation to then offer debriefing).
- Normalise a person's response to trauma—this needs to be combined with an understanding about how trauma manifests for the individual person.
- View adaptive behaviour and coping strategies as strengths rather than weaknesses—for example, avoidant behaviour can be a survival technique that a person has developed over a long period to manage their flashbacks to trauma in the past, whether or not it continues to be beneficial in the present.
- Inquire about current level of safety; if the person is currently experiencing violence, work on increasing safety and regaining their sense of power. Avoid strategies that aim to persuade the person to leave their current situation or make decisions that they are not ready to make (however, you must always ensure safety of children). Seek assistance from your local specialist trauma services (e.g., family violence, sexual assault or refugee services) to develop a 'safety plan'.

Is it possible to be 'trauma creating' and 'trauma-informed'?

As a survivor of child abuse, and of traumatising, compulsory mental health services, I passionately want every service to be trauma-informed. Yet, I urge clinicians to be wary of tokenistic approaches to TICP. Is it really possible for a service to be trauma-informed while compulsory treatment, seclusion or restraint are commonly practised These practices are inherently traumatising and they conflict with TICP principles. I remain unconvinced that a place which creates trauma can also be trauma-informed. Instead, I suggest that the first step before becoming trauma-informed is to work towards eliminating practices that create trauma.

Indigo Daya, giving a consumer perspective on implementing TICP

TRAUMA-INFORMED CARE AND PRACTICE

The US Government's Substance Abuse and Mental Health Services Administration (SAMHSA) provides a summary of a Trauma-Informed Care and Practice (TICP) approach, that includes the following (SAMSHSA, 2014).

Realise the widespread impact of trauma und understand potential paths for recovery

Trauma can contribute to or be the primary reason for a person's current mental health condition. People accessing mental health services have most likely experienced trauma. If trauma is not considered as part of mental health care, a large part of a person's experience is neglected.

Recognise the signs and symptoms of trauma in clients, families, staff and others involved with the system

TICP provides a way to understand the impact of trauma on a person and re-focuses sensitive inquiry from asking 'what is wrong with you?' to 'what happened to you?' It provides a way to understand behaviour as coping strategies or meaningful responses to trauma, rather than labelling it as 'problematic' or as symptoms of illness. Within a TICP approach, self-harm or problematic substance use can be understood as coping strategies to manage flashbacks. Hearing voices can be understood as a dissociative experience that holds important information about past trauma, including clues to issues that need to be understood and resolved to progress recovery.

Table 2.3 Example: A 50-year-old obese woman

Lacking TICP	TICP
Clinical assessment notes: a 50-year-old obese woman, poorly dressed, no eye contact. Presents in the context of increased distress about recurrent command hallucination with nihilistic content; currently non-compliant with medication; little insight. High risk of suicide. Hints at abusive father? Impression: Exacerbation of treatment resistant schizophrenia. Recommence medication and observe.	The woman is offered the opportunity to work with a therapist to explore her voices. She profiles her voice, which she first started hearing after leaving home at 15, and identifies that it sounds like her father. She is too distressed to talk in more detail but is comfortable to say that 'something terrible happened'. This indirect trauma disclosure is enough for the therapist to work with her. She accepts a referral for ongoing trauma counselling to make sense of how her childhood experience may contribute to this frightening voice, and to develop coping strategies for the future.

Respond by fully integrating knowledge about trauma into policies, procedures, and practices

TICP is an organisation-wide approach that seeks to review policies, procedures, practice and organisational environment. All staff need to develop an understanding of trauma according to their roles and responsibilities. TICP seeks to provide every employee with adequate support to enact the core principles. This includes

- how someone is welcomed into the organisation by the receptionist/admitting nurse
- the person cleaning understands what entering a room can mean for someone
- how people's care and treatment is discussed, and options are provided
- if people are offered assistance from a peer support worker
- how people's referral to a trauma specialist service or any other service is facilitated

This should lead to rethinking many different practices:

- the impact of bed checks in residential and inpatient services
- creating safe spaces for all genders
- clothing and dignity (for example, 'one-size-fits-all' hospital clothing can lead to feelings of vulnerability when too loose, gaping, or too tight)
- the impact of compulsory detention and treatment
- promoting choice rather than 'rules'
- greater use of counselling and therapy
- seeking behaviour explanations through a trauma lens.

A TICP organisation will ensure that people with lived experience of a variety of backgrounds and ages (including people with a history of trauma recovery) provide advice on TICP implementation

Seek to actively resist retraumatisation

TICP acknowledges that everyday events can be a trigger for someone to feel unsafe and as if they were 're-living trauma'. A TICP organisation will actively work against retraumatisation. However, mental health services work under mental health laws which can have an impact that is contrary to the intention of TICP, by enforcing detention and compulsory treatment, and allowing for seclusion and restraint. These are not the only practices that can be experienced as retraumatising, for example, nursing bed checks during the night, lack of bedroom door locks, or nursing checks during showering can all potentially be traumatising for people with a history of sexual violence or abuse.

Actively working against retraumatisation will not guarantee that someone does not feel retraumatised. At best, an organisation strives towards eliminating retraumatisation and at a minimum it would develop strategies to respond and support people when they are traumatised.

What might a trauma-informed response look like?

A young woman admitted to an inpatient unit is increasingly distressed during her admission. A nurse engages the woman in conversation and asks if anything is making her feel unsafe or distressed. She says that she is having flashbacks of past abuse, and she thinks the unit is making it worse.

The nurse explores the past few days with the woman, and they realise that the combination of locked doors, single beds, and feeling exposed in hospital pyjamas are all triggering abuse memories. The nurse apologises for the distress that has been caused and the young woman expresses gratitude for listening and believing her. They organise some clothing which provide more privacy, more frequent leave, and they make an agreement to check in more regularly to be sure that everything feels safer.

A more formal trauma-informed practice for people who experience auditory hallucinations is the international 'Hearing Voices Approach', developed collaboratively by psychiatrists and consumers, which can be helpful when working with people. It uses psychological approaches, such as the Voice Dialogue technique and Voice Profiling to support people to make sense of their voices and find ways to live well with the experience. Consumers can relate characteristics or content of their voices to past trauma, and this knowledge informs practical strategies for empowering ways of living with the experience.

KEY PRINCIPLES OF TICP

TICP frameworks provide key principles that underpin organisational and interpersonal practice. This is SAMHSA's version of TICP principles:

Safety

SAMSHA suggests 'staff and the people they serve, whether children or adults, feel physically and psychologically safe' (SAMSHSA, 2014). Additionally, interpersonal interactions must promote safety (Orygen The National Centre of Excellence in Youth Mental Health, 2018). Safety is defined by the person receiving the service and needs to be understood by those providing a service.

Table 2.4 Example: A 63-year-old fearful man

Henry is 63 years old. Since moving into his new flat, he talks about feeling unsafe at night in case someone gets in through the window. He's scared to go to bed, his sleep is disrupted, and he has difficulty focusing on work.	
Lacking TICP	**TICP**
His clinician assures him that his unit is safe, and given that it is on the third floor, how would anybody be able to get in? Given Henry had problems with sleeping before, the clinician suggests a higher dose of....	Henry's clinician acknowledges his fear and the impact on his life. The clinician inquires if something like this has happened before. While Henry had talked about childhood abuse before, he begins to recall that the noise he hears during the night reminds him of....

Safety and emotions: A consumer perspective

Trauma survivors can feel unsafe in mental health services. It is a real, but solvable problem, that the emotional impacts of psychiatric treatment can sometimes mirror the emotional impacts of past trauma.

Table 2.5 Trauma survivors can feel unsafe in mental health services

Fear	Anger	Despair/sadness	Shame
Emotions from trauma experiences			
I don't feel safe from being hurt	This is wrong, unfair	It will never get better, I can't change this	I'm a bad person, it's my fault
Unsafe impacts from mental health services			
Restraints, locked doors, side effects	Compulsory treatment, not able to get an advocate, rights are breached	Trying to speak up and not being heard, being ignored, disabling side effects	Judgemental language or attitudes by staff
Trauma-informed mental health responses			
Ask people what would help them feel physically and emotionally safe. Provide that.	Provide maximum choice, respect and fairness.	Therapeutic conversations to find hope for recovery and meaning in experience.	Validate people's struggle and strengths; convey that people are valued.

Trustworthiness and transparency

Trauma inevitably damages trust in others. TICP services adapt by going above and beyond to demonstrate trustworthiness.

Table 2.6 Example: A woman's feelings about visitors

Milly asked the contact nurse to discuss the pending visit of her relatives. The nurse promises she'll see Milly in ten minutes. Milly waits at the nurses' station and after 30 minutes goes to her room. When the nurse comes into Milly's room 1.5 hours later, Milly seems irritated.	
Lacking TICP	**TICP**
The nurse feels irritated, it wasn't her fault she had to assist a new admission. She knows the visit isn't for a few days, so she doesn't understand why Milly's so upset. She is annoyed at Milly's behaviour.	The nurse apologises for taking much longer than she promised. 'On reflection, I should not have promised that I would be back in ten minutes' she says, adding that 'I will try to be more realistic next time, I'm sorry Milly, I know how important this conversation is to you.'

Other practices that can damage trustworthiness and transparency:

- speaking to family without the person's consent
- nursing observations without engagement
- compulsory treatment
- not explaining treatment side effects
- failing to include the person when formulating diagnosis or treatment.

Peer support

Peer support is grounded in trauma-informed perspectives (Mead, n.d; Blanch, Filson, & Penney, 2012). The benefit of being supported by someone with a shared experience increases hope and promotes recovery (SAMHSA, 2014).

Table 2.7 Example: A man joins a new peer support group

Lacking TICP	TICP
Kim has been coming to the community clinic for several years, but each of his case managers has said he is 'difficult to engage' due to his paranoid ideation.	Kim joins a new peer support group at the clinic. Over time, Kim talks about being bullied at school and the spiritual being who came to protect him. He is fearful that clinical staff want to medicate him to take away his protector, and then he won't be safe. Validation from his peers gave Kim the confidence to start talking to his case manager about his recovery needs: a bit less medication, then some therapy about the bullying impacts.

Collaboration and mutuality

Disempowerment underpins many trauma-related mental health problems, so a helpful practice is to use collaboration and mutuality to create a positive experience of power in relationships. Collaboration and mutuality require the 'professional' to give up some of their power, and to acknowledge that both people have strengths and vulnerabilities.

Table 2.8 Example: A woman encounters painful feelings

Amina told her case manager that during last week she really wanted to hit a man speaking at a local community centre, but she didn't actually do it. She described feeling ashamed all week. Her voices are telling her she deserves to die.	
Lacking TICP	**TICP**
Amina's case manager said she'd make an appointment with the psychiatrist to review medication. She suggested Amina make more use of PRN medications. The case manager arranged for the mobile support team to check in over the weekend.	Amina's case manager validated the painful feelings and shared that sometimes she has scary thoughts too. The case manager asked Amina if they could work together to make sense of what happened and come up with a plan that feels supportive. They worked out that Amina had been reminded of a past trauma and brainstormed ideas for what to do next time. Amina told her voices to be quiet because she's allowed to get angry and hurt sometimes and that's nothing to be ashamed of.

Empowerment, voice and choice

It is not possible for one person to 'empower' another, but it is possible for a worker to:

- Recognise their own potential power over the client (e.g., power to detain or apply compulsory treatment)
- Acknowledge power imbalances to the client, discussing the implications together (e.g., explicitly naming power differences, inviting the client to talk about what this feels like, sharing own feelings, particularly any discomfort or ambivalence)
- Decide to avoid, or at least minimise, decisions that the person does not agree with
- Encourage and support people to make their own choices (e.g., ask about what the person wants, provide accessible information about options, ask if the person would like support or time to make decisions).

These kinds of actions create space for empowerment.

Table 2.9 Example: A woman reacts to children playing in a sandpit

Ruth has been a member of the supported playgroup for a few weeks. During springtime, the activities move outside. The children are invited to play in the sandpit. Ruth seems annoyed and stressed, saying, 'I didn't join the group for the kids to get dirty'.	
Lacking TICP	**TICP**
The playgroup leader says that these are the planned activities, and, for safety reasons, everyone must stay together. She points out that sand play is important for children.	The playgroup leader invites Ruth for a private chat. She acknowledges Ruth's concerns and asks Ruth what could be done differently to make the day fun and positive for her and her children. Ruth gets teary and starts talking about what happens when the children's clothes get the smallest speck of dirt onto them. She tries to avoid the verbal abuse, the shouting and being 'told off' that she has experienced many times from her partner. This has left both her and the children fearful. Keeping the children 'clean' is one way of trying to protect them and herself from abuse.

Cultural, historical, and gender issues

TICP applies an intersectional approach to diversity to assist in taking a person's many characteristics into account in sensitive inquiry. Cultural and historical contexts are particularly important to consider when working with Aboriginal and Torres Strait Islander people (see Chapter 1.3; Dudgeon, Milroy, & Walker, 2014), people from refugee and asylum seeker and CALD backgrounds. Issues of identity, gender and sexual orientation when working with someone from the LGBTIQ community need to be considered.

RESOURCE ORGANISATIONS

Blue Knot Foundation: (blue knot foundation, 2020)

Mental Health Coordinating Council of NSW (MHCC): (Mental Health Coordinating Council (MHCC), 2020b)

Substance Abuse and Mental Health Administration USA (SAMHSA): (Substance Abuse and Mental Health Administration (SAMHSA), 2020))

Voices Vic: (Voices Vic, 2020)

International Hearing Voices Network: (inter Voice, 2020)

Centre for Psychiatric Nursing, Recovery Library, The University of Melbourne: (The University of Melbourne, 2020).

2.3.10 DISCIPLINE-SPECIFIC ASSESSMENT IN PRACTICE

The following sections present discipline-oriented assessment from general practice, nursing, occupational therapy, psychology and social work perspectives. They address the context of discipline-oriented assessment, such as the philosophical stance and models informing assessment; some focus on assessment methods and specific instruments.

2.3.11 ASSESSMENT BY THE GENERAL PRACTITIONER

CAROLINE JOHNSON

> It is more important to know what sort of person has a disease than to know what sort of disease a person has.
>
> *Hippocrates*

HOLISTIC CARE

Doctors who become GPs are trained in the same assessment methods as doctors who later become psychiatrists. In other words, they develop skills in clinical reasoning as outlined earlier in this chapter, acquiring a language of mental disorders that focuses predominantly on the symptoms people experience and the impact these symptoms have on functioning. Alongside this 'biomedical' approach to assessing people with distress, the biopsychosocial model (see Section 2.3.3) has become a cornerstone of the discipline since it was first described as a framework by George Engel in the 1970s (Engel, 1977; Greenhalgh, 2007) encouraging assessment that looked beyond the illness the person might have towards an in-depth understanding of the person themselves (Freeman, 2005).

Therefore, the GP assessment is not simply a truncated or simplified version of what psychiatrists do, impacted by the time constraints of the environment GPs work in and their exposure to less intensive training in the discipline of psychiatry. Unlike psychiatrists, the GPs' role in assessment has a much stronger focus on holistic care, encompassing all the patient's health care needs, including integration of physical and mental health care and the 'problem list' the patient presents to the GP. For patients who have attended a GP over time, a current mental health assessment can draw on the GP's personal knowledge of the patient and records of care for previous health and mental health concerns, although episodic treatment for discrete and varied concerns over a period of time may sometimes make retrieval and integration of information challenging for the practitioner.

DETECTING MENTAL ILL-HEALTH

The GP also plays a much greater role than any other mental health professional in *detecting* people with mental ill-health who may not be explicitly seeking help. To do this, GPs are trained in advanced communication skills that include open-ended questions and a patient-centred approach, alongside either screening or case finding methods. In primary care, screening typically refers to the assessment of asymptomatic people to ascertain if they are likely or unlikely to have (or develop) a specific disease, whereas case finding refers to the assessment of people already considered to be at risk of a specific condition (RACGP 'Red Book' Taskforce et al., 2005). This is an important distinction to make in the primary care environment where allocation of time and resources to tasks that are likely to achieve the best outcome for the population need to be prioritised.

To enable GPs to detect common mental health conditions in such an environment, brief questionnaires have been developed to speed up the process of detection of common conditions such as depression and anxiety. These tools are problematic as primary prevention screening tools to be administered to all people presenting to the GP, due to the lack of specificity of the results they produce, making them inefficient for use in the primary care setting (see for example: Thombs, Ziegelstein, Roseman, Kloda, & Ioannidis, 2014). Yet they do enable the time-poor GP to at least target questions to people who are known to be at higher risk of certain mental health conditions, as long as the GP follows up with a more comprehensive assessment and ensures that those identified as needing care are actually referred to that care (RACGP 'Red Book' Taskforce et al., 2005).

TREATMENT PATHWAYS

Following on from screening or case finding, a targeted assessment as to the 'caseness' of the problem the person is experiencing is a common next step in the GP assessment process. In other words, is there a diagnosis that can be made and a treatment pathway to offer? Not paying attention to this step can lead to the problem of both under- and over-diagnosis of mental disorders in the community, both of which have important consequences for the health of the population (Plos Medicine Editors, 2013). If a diagnosis is made and treatment deemed necessary by both consumer and clinician, it is notable that many treatments that follow are delivered within the primary care setting. Other treatments require the GP to use this initial assessment to act in a so-called 'gatekeeper' role to other services, with the aim of ensuring consumers receive both evidence-based and cost-effective care.

Making decisions about best care pathways for individual patients means that assessment in general practice benefits from a strong focus on the person's context (Gunn et al., 2008) and their explanatory model for their experience. This enables a shared understanding of the types of solutions available via the health care system and outside of it (Kokanović et al., 2013). Indeed, qualitative research into how GPs conceptualise depression demonstrates that they use a different taxonomy to understand their patients' presentations than a traditional psychiatric approach, taking into account their patients' psychosocial stressors, alongside the severity and nature of their symptoms (Clarke, Cook, Smith, & Piterman, 2008).

These differences between primary and secondary/tertiary care are not surprising, given that the GP is able to see anyone and everyone seeking care via the Australian health care system. No referral system or other filter is required, other than the need (in some cases) to make an appointment or (in some cases) to afford a co-payment. When patients present to their GP, their problems are not only unfiltered but also *unrehearsed* (Klinkman & Gask, 2009), which means the assessment may require a different structure and approach in order to avoid narrowing down the focus too early in the clinical encounter. While this may account for the oft-reported concern that GPs miss cases of people with common conditions like depression (Pence, O'Donnell, & Gaynes, 2012), it also presents a powerful opportunity for people to be heard without being inappropriately labelled or judged and to feel safe in engaging with the health care system. The importance of this cannot be over-estimated in the face of the Australian National Mental Health Survey findings that showed most consumers (57%; Meadows & Burgess, 2009) who had symptoms of a mental disorder also advised they had 'no need for care'. For these reasons, the GP assessment process needs to be highly centred on the relationship between doctor and patient and benefits from good continuity of care over long periods of time (Jeffers & Baker, 2016; Lynch, Askew, Mitchell, & Hegarty, 2012).

With regard to the issue of the 'caseness' of a person presenting for care, GPs are encouraged to use the ICD-10 (and now the ICD-11) criteria, despite the fact that their psychiatric colleagues more commonly refer to DSM-5. The criteria for diagnoses in the ICD-11 are undoubtedly more user-friendly for the GP setting, because of their focus on clinical utility over reliability (Tyrer, 2014), but this can impact on the clarity of a shared clinical language when consumers, carers, primary and secondary/tertiary care clinicians communicate about the needs of individual patients.

DIAGNOSTIC AND PRACTICAL CONSIDERATIONS

Beyond the debate about which classification system is best for general practice is the crucial issue of dimensional versus categorical approaches to diagnosis in such a setting, which rightly focuses on prevention and early intervention for mental health concerns. In the primary care environment, many people will be seen who might not yet qualify for a 'categorical' diagnosis according to formal psychiatric diagnostic criteria, but who may benefit from receiving treatment earlier, at the point they are engaged and receptive to treatment, rather than waiting until symptoms progress. GPs commonly operate from a dimensional perspective, weighing up the pros and cons of using a label in a health system where certain types of treatment are only available for people with categorical diagnoses, as seen for example with the requirement of the Better Access to Mental Health Care program, which is limited to people meeting ICD-10 criteria for diagnosis (Department of Health, 2014).

Another challenge that is unique to the GP assessment process is the requirement to complete mandatory steps as part of the Mental Health

Treatment Plan (MHTP) as part of the Medicare Benefits Schedule reimbursement requirements. An assessment for a MHTP requires a much broader level of inquiry than that which would enable a diagnosis to be made, including the requirement to use an outcome measure, to conduct a formal Mental State Exam, to record some specific goals for the consumer, to assess risk, to discuss an appropriate crisis plan, to assess who the consumers will access for nonclinical supports (i.e., the carer or significant others) and to make recommendations for treatment and follow up (Johnson, 2007). While these requirements of the MHTP represent consensus opinion on what constitutes best practice in primary mental health care assessment, it remains unclear as to the benefits that completion of such a plan offers overall. Nevertheless, a MHTP should certainly be regarded as more than a simple 'referral' to another provider and is instead a document that can help clarify the goals of the person seeking care and encourage ongoing review of the progress of care. Qualitative research into the opinions of people experiencing depressive symptoms suggests that they regard the idea of a MHTP as an important mechanism to enact recovery (Palmer et al., 2013). Due to the MBS payments allocated to the MHTP, it also allows the clinician to spend more time with the patient seeking care, in an environment that otherwise rewards shorter consultations over longer ones; and spending more time with patients is a key ingredient to important outcomes when offering a holistic approach to health care (Wilson & Childs, 2002).

2.3.12 NURSING ASSESSMENT

SALLY BUCHANAN-HAGEN & TIMOTHY WAND

MENTAL HEALTH NURSING ASSESSMENT AND PRACTICE

In the field of mental health, conducting nursing assessments is considered a central activity and a high priority from a clinical to organisational level. Conventionally, mental health nursing assessments have focused on documenting presenting problems, a personal history, current symptoms, mental state, and risk factors. This typically leads to a formulation, diagnosis and plan for 'treatment' or care. Such assessments are often referred to as 'formal', 'comprehensive' or 'full'. There are numerous sources available for guidance on the format for these assessments. Indeed, health services in most states and territories across Australia provide clinicians working in the public health sector with templates or 'standardised' formats for conducting assessments.

Given this information is widely available and constitutes the basics of mental health assessment (see Section 2.3.4), this chapter concentrates on the principles, reflections and approach that mental health nurses bring to the assessment process. This is informed by contemporary thinking and practice that encompasses the principles of recovery, trauma-informed care and a strengths-based orientation written from a nursing, consumer and academic perspective.

APPROACHES TO NURSING ASSESSMENT

Nursing assessment is a continuous process integrated within the routine therapeutic interaction between the mental health nurse and the consumer. Moreover, consumers have expressed an aversion for being asked the same questions repeatedly and consider many questions about their developmental history irrelevant to their current health challenges. Instead consumers have identified a preference for therapeutic intervention 'on the spot' and emphasised the fundamental therapeutic benefits of being listened to and understood (Wand et al., 2016).

Undrill (2007) argues that the amount of information gathered during the typical nursing assessment process is often superfluous to the current presentation and has the potential to overcomplicate clinical decision making. He proposes that a stance of 'bounded rationality' is more beneficial for making decisions on less information rather than expend time and energy on accumulating and documenting excessive amounts of personal information that is of marginal utility. In addition, it is important that nursing 'assessment' is not conducted with an overly formal, mechanical or 'tick-box' style. Rigid and formalised mental health assessment can be intimidating, placing the person 'under the spotlight' with the feeling of being examined.

Mental health nurses must be aware of power imbalances between the nurse and consumer, and cognisant of how these power imbalances affect the consumer's view of mental health services, mental health workers, the assessment process, and sense of self. In every instance, power imbalances (and strategies to minimise these) must be considered and enacted. This includes recognising and redressing paternalistic attitudes. Paternalistic attitudes held by nurses can impact on mental health assessment by assuming the mental health nurse 'knows all' and thus is not receptive to recognising the expertise of the individual during the nursing assessment. The mental health nurse brings his or her knowledge and expertise as a health professional, while the consumer brings his or her knowledge and expertise through, and of, their lived experience. This enables reciprocity of learning and shifts the dynamic of the nursing mental health assessment from the consumer being a passive recipient of care to an active participant, fostering a collaborative process between the mental health nurse and consumer. When acknowledging expertise consumers bring to the nursing assessment, an approach of genuine curiosity, openness and interest is essential. People should be reassured, supported, listened to and understood. Curiosity does not mean the mental health nurse is simply curious about the person's current circumstance. It is curiosity with the intent to understand without judgement the person's experience from their perspective and to incorporate this understanding into nursing practice. This can challenge traditional understandings of mental illness and mental health based in the biomedical model, and may require some 'unlearning' on the nurse's part. However, being genuinely curious about someone's experience and understanding the situation from their perspective enables connection, contributing to the partnership between the mental health nurse and consumer. Further, adopting a non-judgemental and affirmative stance can be motivating for individuals. Normalising the situation provides an opportunity to 'de-pathologise' the person's experience by explaining to the individual that their difficulties are shared and not uncommon. Encouraging people to see their problems as shared difficulties of life is intended to humanise the nursing assessment and reassure, not minimise their situation.

Alongside adopting a curious mindset, nurses must be mindful of how their use of language impacts on nursing assessment. Using negative language to describe assessment findings leads to ongoing judgement and labelling, influencing the type of care the person receives. For example, describing someone as having impaired judgement contributes to paternalistic and restrictive practices. Likewise, labelling someone as not having insight has a myriad impacts that are beyond the realm of this chapter. However, this type of labelling during nursing assessment limits the opportunity to connect with and truly understand the person's experience from their point of view and communicate that understanding to other health care workers.

Traditional nursing assessment formats are structured to seek out problems, illness and pathology in the individual and are by no means 'comprehensive'. The end result with this approach is an impression of the person that is focused on problems and thus biased toward identifying only negative characteristics. Contemporary thinking around mental health nursing assessment, aligned with positive mental health and a strengths-based orientation, provides for a more balanced stance that includes an exploration of the person's strengths, attributes, assets, abilities, resources, coping skills, past successes, goals and future hopes. Questions that surface the positives in people's lives concentrate on: what the individual does well; what has helped in the past to surmount challenges; how the person has coped through adversity; individual interests, hobbies and activities that the person derives pleasure, purpose and meaning from; and how the person envisages their life beyond their mental health problems or their current mental distress.

BACKGROUND; CHALLENGES TO THE STATUS QUO

Major shifts in thinking and practice are occurring in mental health care and service delivery. Conducting formalised 'risk assessments' had until recently dominated mental health services. Although evidence-based practice has always been considered a cornerstone of health care, it became increasingly evident that there was no evidence that clinical risk assessment and management practices (which were often mandated by mental health services) have any impact on reducing acts of harm. For example, while suicidal thoughts are common, the act of suicide is statistically rare. Therefore, the 'numbers needed to treat' in order to circumvent one adverse outcome are enormous (Morgan, 2007).

Carter and colleagues (2017) estimated that 5.5% of patients classified as 'high risk' of suicide can be expected to suicide after long periods of follow-up. Therefore, 95% of people assessed as 'high risk' of suicide do not go on to end their lives. Moreover, most suicides occur in the low risk category as this group consist of many more members than the high-risk category and there is no evidence that a focus on risk factors has any impact on circumventing suicide (Large, Sharma, Cannon, Ryan, & Nielssen, 2011). There are also no studies demonstrating that risk categorisation (high, medium or low) has any clinical utility in reducing acts of harm (Wand, 2012). The recently published Royal Australian and New Zealand College of Psychiatrists clinical practice guidelines for the management of deliberate self-harm for example, have recommended that 'Risk assessment scales or tools or any other methods of risk stratification are not warranted for determining the need for clinical services or follow-up' (Carter et al., 2017, p. 960).

Assessing for aggression and violence risk is another preoccupation in mental health services. While mental illness is one of many risk factors for aggression and violence, people who have a mental illness are more likely to have harm perpetrated against them, rather than be the perpetrators of harm (Hiday, 2006; Peterson, Skeem, Kennealy, Bray, & Zvonkovic, 2014). A large body of research has demonstrated that the majority of people with mental illness are not violent while the majority of violent people do not have a mental illness. The far greater danger to the public is posed by people who misuse alcohol and other drugs (Wand, 2012). As with the assessment of self-harm and suicide risk there is no evidence that the routine application of risk assessment for aggression and violence risk provides any clinical benefit for reducing such acts and has the potential for unfair restrictions on freedom to be imposed on individuals (Ryan, Nielssen, Paton, & Large, 2010). Nielssen (2013) highlights the ethically questionable practice of performing risk assessments without an individual's full knowledge or consent, and points out that including the person in discussions regarding their risk of harm and future plans is likely to lead to better outcomes. With these limitations in mind, consider how many individuals are subjected to potentially harmful interventions and restrictions on personal liberty due to inherently flawed risk assessment frameworks. These pose competing risks for consumers such as being kept in hospital too long, excessive medication and side effects, loss of freedom, privacy, control, and dignity (Sykes, Brabban, & Reilly, 2015).

In addition to a lack of evidence regarding the effectiveness of risk assessment, an over-emphasis on risk within mental health nursing assessment can limit connection, negatively impacting therapeutic relationships; and depending on the resultant interventions employed, potentially traumatise or retraumatise individuals. Since risk assessment focuses on physical safety, while neglecting emotional and psychological safety, interventions based on nursing risk assessments typically involve restriction of freedom as an attempt to maintain physical safety. However, research has shown that restricting individual freedoms (for example, frequent or constant observation) decreases the person's feelings of emotional safety, thereby reducing overall feelings of safety (Berg, Rortveit, & Aase, 2017). Hence, interventions to address the outcome of nursing risk assessments generate competing risks such as the individual feeling resentful, unsafe, demoralised and less likely to seek help for fear of future coercive and restrictive practices.

MOVING TOWARDS RECOVERY ORIENTED AND TRAUMA-INFORMED NURSING ASSESSMENT

Mental health services have traditionally been influenced by biomedical models of illness and disorder and an associated emphasis on pharmacological treatments. However, with a growing emphasis on recovery, a transformation in nursing practice is indicated (Stickley et al., 2016). Recovery principles, which are enshrined in health care policy internationally, emphasise collaboration, self-determination, autonomy, hope, citizenship and the promotion of a meaningful life beyond the constraints of diagnosis (Commonwealth of Australia, 2013). Recovery principles transcend models of mental illness and disorder, and notions of separateness associated with asylum-era thinking that the causes of mental illness are primarily biological and therefore an 'all-or-nothing' phenomenon. Instead recovery embraces both a person-centred and population health perspective, recognising that regardless of aetiology or diagnosis, all mental health challenges are met at the individual level, and that mental health is relevant to all.

While genetics and biology undoubtedly play a role in mental health and wellbeing, as they do in all aspects of human experience, the degree to which they contribute to mental ill-health remains a matter of speculation. What is known without question is that mental health and wellbeing are principally determined by what happens to people after they are born, not what they are born with. Childhood abuse, adversity and instability, and numerous traumatic human experiences are all far more predictive of mental illness than heredity (World Health Organization, 2013c). Therefore, knowledge of trauma-informed practice is integral for performing empathetic and holistic nursing assessment to support consumers along their unique journey of recovery. Trauma-informed practice directs the focus from what is 'wrong' with a person to what has happened to a person and hence, where appropriate, mental health nursing assessment needs to reflect this shift in understanding of mental distress. Consumer accounts highlight that recognition of past trauma can be limited during mental health assessments, resulting in integral information being 'missed', undesired treatment being initiated, self-stigma being reinforced and a lost opportunity for the person to create meaning from their experience of mental distress, all of which limit working with a strengths-based approach.

Consistent with recovery oriented practice, nursing assessment must integrate a strengths-based approach. This includes discussions about positive risk taking. Positive risk taking weighs the potential benefits of a decision against the potential risks so strategies can be instigated to circumvent or minimise risks. Positive risk taking is an important part of individual recovery as it enables agency over decision-making processes and promotes autonomy and self-determination. Positive risk taking allows for the dignity of risk where people have the opportunity to learn by making their own decisions (Commonwealth of Australia, 2013). During the nursing assessment, the person's preferences for care should be discussed and documented verbatim. This could include preferences that carry a degree of risk and strategies to support preferences and decisions while also minimising the associated risks need to be discussed. Discussions about how to support positive risk taking should begin with asking the consumer what strategies they want to try, rather than determining the strategies for the consumer. Supported decision making is linked to positive risk taking and the dignity of risk (Gooding, 2013) and must also be included during the mental health assessment. As with positive risk taking, supported decision making promotes recovery by enabling consumers to regain control and autonomy over their treatment by identifying services and resources to support decision making.

In summary, with no evidence that lengthy nursing assessment formats make any discernible difference to the outcomes for individuals accessing mental health care, their continued dominance within the mental health system needs to be challenged. This is especially relevant as individuals are routinely (and repeatedly) required to recount personal experiences from their past that are potentially distressing and of questionable utility to addressing the current problem. A major shift in practice and an alternative way of thinking and working with people is required to truly align mental health clinicians and services with a recovery mindset. Nurses are in a position to work collaboratively with consumers by incorporating the consumer's expertise within the assessment process, moving from a problems and diagnosis focus to a strengths-based approach. By seeking to truly understand the individual's experience and adopting an open, curious and non-judgemental stance during nursing assessment, nurses are uniquely placed to collaborate with and support consumers in their recovery right from the outset.

2.3.13 OCCUPATION-FOCUSED ASSESSMENT

JUSTIN NEWTON SCANLAN & ELLIE FOSSEY

Occupational therapists' particular contribution and expertise in the area of assessment is concerned with seeking to understand the factors contributing to people's patterns of participation in daily life, including the activity disruptions and difficulties in doing daily life that may arise in the context of experiencing ill-health, disability and social and economic disadvantage (Krupa, Fossey, Anthony, Brown, & Pitts, 2009). Occupational therapists use assessments to seek to understand a person's everyday living and the interrelationships between what they do and their health, recovery, wellbeing and social inclusion.

EXPLANATORY FRAMEWORKS FOR UNDERSTANDING HUMAN OCCUPATION

Explanatory models about human occupation are typically designed to help understand the complex interplay between people, their environments and their occupations that support or hinder occupational performance, participation and wellbeing. Among the most widely known are: *Enabling Occupation* (Canadian Association of Occupational Therapists, 2002; Townsend & Polatajko, 2013), *Kielhofner's Model of Human Occupation* (Taylor, 2017), the *Person Environment Occupation Performance model* (Christiansen, Baum, & Bass, 2015) and the *Occupational Performance Model (Australia)* (Chapparo, Ranka, & Nott, 2017).

Person factors include individuals' values, beliefs and motivations, as well as their sensory, motor, biomechanical, cognitive and psychosocial capacities. Assessing these person factors allows the occupational therapist to understand what drives the individual to engage in occupations and to consider functional strengths and challenges that might support or impede performance.

Environmental or contextual factors include the built, social, cultural, political and economic environment as well as factors such as time and space. Three important implications for assessment are: that knowledge of the person's context is essential for identifying occupations that are relevant to focus on; that an understanding of social and cultural expectations about their performance is likely to be important; and that contextualised, or ecologically valid, assessment is likely to provide more accurate information about a person's strengths and difficulties in everyday living (Fossey & Harvey, 2001).

Occupation factors include the demands of activities involved in the occupation as well as how these various activities are organised and performed. Occupations are sometimes considered in terms of categories, such as self-care, productivity and leisure.

While occupational therapy assessment may focus on one or more particular person, environment or occupation factors, in an overall sense occupational therapists are interested in what individuals desire for their lives, what activities and occupations they wish to participate in and how they orchestrate their daily lives. They are also interested in how daily activities combine together to create meaning and purpose as well as how these activities support individuals to enact valued life roles. It is also important to consider the importance of occupations in creating individuals' identity and their sense of competence and mastery. Each of these aspects has an important influence on individuals' recovery (Doroud, Fossey, & Fortune, 2015).

METHODS OF ASSESSMENT

Occupational therapists' assessments include interviewing, self-report questionnaires and rating scales, and performance-based assessments. Assessments can involve consumers, family members or significant others, and other care or service providers.

Given their expertise in understanding occupational performance and participation, occupational therapists are often called on to assess consumers' strengths, difficulties and supports in various aspect of daily life. This can include basic activities of daily living (ability to care for one's self), instrumental activities of daily living (money management, food preparation/acquisition, medication management, home maintenance, community access, shopping, etc.), specific tasks required at a workplace or activities associated with caring for others.

One of the most common areas occupational therapists are called on to make an assessment is to determine the supports that might be necessary to assist an individual to live independently. This can occur if concerns have been raised about individuals' ability to manage in their current living situation or if they are wishing to (or required to) move into a different living situation.

Occupational therapists are also frequently requested to provide assessments in the context of applications for supports under the National Disability Insurance Scheme. This has added complexity to the overall assessment process, as the necessity to highlight the level of 'disability' experienced by the individual can undermine occupational therapists' focus on strengths and capabilities.

Occupational therapists also use assessments for a wide variety of other purposes, most especially to support the process of working with individuals to establish goals for the future and for determining the steps necessary to work towards these goals. Some of the assessments used by occupational therapists in mental health settings are described in the next section.

Interviews and self-report methods

Interviewing and self-report methods are typically used to identify what the person does, what she or he wants to do and is expected to do, as well as identifying occupational issues of concern from the person's own perspective. Several interview-based assessments are designed to capture individuals' perspectives about their current and desired occupational engagement. Both the *Canadian Occupational Performance Measure* (COPM) (Law et al., 2005) and the *Occupational Self Assessment* (OSA) (Baron, Kielhofner, Iyenger, Gladhammer, & Wolenski, 2006) explore individuals' perceptions of their current performance and satisfaction with performance in important or meaningful activities of daily life. The COPM and OSA are designed to support collaborative goal setting and can also be used as outcome measures. The *Occupational Performance History Interview II* (OPHI-II) (Kielhofner et al., 2004) takes a broader life-course perspective. The OPHI-II allows for the exploration of individuals' occupational choices, challenges and successes and occupational changes over time (Apte, Kielhofner, Paul-Ward, & Braveman, 2005; Kielhofner, Braveman, Fogg, & Levin, 2008). With its focus on exploring meaning, the OPHI-II can be helpful in building partnerships and supporting goal striving towards growth and recovery (Chaffey & Fossey, 2004; Ennals & Fossey, 2009).

The *Worker Role Interview* (WRI) (Braveman et al., 2005) and *Work Environment Impact Scale* (WEIS) (Moore-Corner, Kielhofner, & Olson, 1998) are two further interview-based tools of relevance respectively to explore return-to-work issues, and the impact of the workplace environment on participation and workplace adjustments (Kielhofner et al., 2008; Williams, Fossey, & Harvey, 2010).

The *time use diary and interview* can also be used to explore patterns of daily time use (Farnworth, 2003). Rather than focusing on one area, such as work or activities of daily living (ADL), daily time use information draws attention to the pattern of a person's participation across occupations and social contexts (Krupa, McLean, Eastabrook, Bonham, & Baksh,

2003). Interview-based methods are advantageous in practice for ease of completion and to adequately contextualise a person's time use (Farnworth, 2003). The *Profiles of Occupational Engagement* (POES) (Bejerholm, Hansson, & Eklund, 2006) is an example of an interview-based time use assessment.

Performance-based assessments

Performance-based assessments are used to assess how the person performs activities, preferably in life-relevant environments (for example, home, workplace and local community) wherever possible. Assessments of real activities within real contexts are referred to as 'ecologically valid' assessments. When this is not practical, performance of real-life tasks in environments that simulate naturalistic settings are used, but predictions about performance in another setting or context should be more cautious when based on such assessments (Brown, Moore, Hemman, & Yunek, 1996; Hamera & Brown, 2000).

Two examples of ecologically valid assessments used by occupational therapists in community mental health practice are the *Assessment of Motor and Process Skills* (AMPS) (Fisher & Bray Jones, 2012, 2014), and the *Perceive Recall Plan Perform* (PRPP) system of task analysis (Chapparo & Ranka, 1997). Australian examples include their uses in community rehabilitation, supported housing and outreach services (Fossey, Harvey, Plant, & Pantelis, 2006; Patterson, Goldman, McKibbin, Hughs, & Jeste, 2001). Both the AMPS and PRPP can be used to evaluate individuals' strengths and challenges in relation to everyday tasks, and to identify how the environment or activity could be modified or strategies could be applied by the individual to facilitate the ease, safety or effectiveness with which individuals can carry everyday tasks that they need and want to perform.

Two simulation-based assessments used by occupational therapists in Australia are the Performance Assessment of Self-Care Skills (PASS) (Rogers & Holm, 2016) and the University of California San Diego Performance-based Skills Assessment (UPSA) (Patterson et al., 2001). Both use simulated activities to assess individuals' skills in a range of daily living tasks. Overall results are used to identify strengths and challenges in daily activities and are used to help inform recommendations and intervention planning. These assessments can be useful to explore individuals' capabilities and capacities, especially in the context of considering moving into an environment with fewer supports (e.g., moving out of the family home or moving from a boarding house into independent accommodation). Additionally, as these are standardised assessments, they can be helpful in formally evaluating the effectiveness of interventions targeting daily life skills as well as monitoring change over time.

Performance-based assessments can also be completed for performance in other areas (such as driving, school or work) depending on individuals' needs and the practice setting (Rogers & Holm, 2016).

Finally, occupational therapists also complete assessments that focus on a specific component of occupational performance, such as functional cognition and sensory processing patterns. Two examples are the Allen's Cognitive Levels Screen (ACLS) (Allen et al., 2007) which can be used to evaluate global or functional cognition and the Adult/Adolescent Sensory Profile (AASP) (Brown & Dunn, 2002) which can be used to evaluate individuals' sensory response patterns and preferences. Results from these types of assessments are used to guide the design of interventions to enhance a person's strategies for managing aspects of occupational performance with which they are having difficulties. For example, results from the ACLS can guide the occupational therapist to make environmental adaptations or teach compensatory strategies that will support independent performance of valued activities. This could include developing skills to travel to an unfamiliar destination using public transport or using environmental cues to prompt medication-taking (Cairns, Hill, Dark, McPhail, & Gray, 2013). Results from the AASP can be used to develop individually tailored self-management strategies to assist in emotion regulation or manage anxiety related to daily activities.

2.3.14 PSYCHOLOGICAL ASSESSMENT

ROBERT KING

Psychologists bring both broad perspectives that form part of the discipline and specific skills based on training and subsequent professional development. The broad perspective is familiarity with and typically, endorsement of psychometrics as an important component of assessment. Psychometrics is the use of standardised and reliable instruments to quantify mental phenomena such as cognition and personality. Key issues in psychometrics are the reliability and validity of instruments used for measurement as well as their sensitivity to the specific mental phenomena being assessed. There is some further discussion of these issues below.

Psychologists can be expected to have at least some knowledge of the key principles of psychometrics as well as some training and experience in the selection and use of standardised instruments. However, the number and range of instruments is so extensive that it is unlikely that a psychologist will be knowledgeable about more than a small proportion of the potential instruments. However, they should have sufficient knowledge to be able to locate instruments and make some evaluation of their potential value. Specialists in clinical psychology, neuropsychology, educational and developmental psychology, organisational psychology and forensic psychology are likely to have more detailed knowledge of instruments relevant to their field of practice than will general psychologists.

It should be noted that not all psychologists make use of psychometric information. Many conduct assessments and treatments on the basis of clinical information only. Routine use of psychometric information is more common among psychologists whose practice framework is strongly informed by cognitive behaviour therapy, and those in work settings where formal assessment is part of the role, such as private practice or inpatient units.

DIAGNOSTIC ASSESSMENT

Clinical psychologists have substantial training in diagnostic assessment, which is recognised in social security legislation (see below). General psychologists can be expected to have familiarity with diagnostic systems but may have limited training in diagnostic interviewing or formulation.

Psychologists with limited training in diagnostic interviewing can achieve reliable diagnoses by using purpose specific tools such as the Composite International Diagnostic Interview (CIDI) which yields an ICD diagnosis or the Structured Clinical Interview for DSM-5 (SCID). These tools work by providing standardised questions and use algorithms that make the interview efficient by narrowing the questions once a diagnosis or group of diagnoses have been excluded because of the participant responses. Both instruments require some training, but the amount of training required to achieve satisfactory diagnostic reliability is manageable and some useful training materials are available.

COGNITIVE AND INTELLECTUAL ASSESSMENT

Cognitive and intellectual assessment makes use of standardised tests to obtain information about a person's higher brain functioning and/or capacity. It enables comparison with others of similar age and, to a lesser extent, with previous functioning. Test administration and interpretation requires specialist training and is mostly the domain of psychologists, although other mental health professionals can be trained to use simple tests such as the Mini Mental State Examination. Within psychology, more complex cognitive assessment is the domain of neuropsychologists.

There are several circumstances where cognitive and/or intellectual assessment is an important part of mental health assessment. Before looking specifically at these circumstances, it is worth distinguishing cognitive and intellectual assessment. The key distinction is that intellectual assessment aims to evaluate global intellectual capacity. It yields an intelligence quotient (IQ) and enables a person's global capacity to be situated within population norms. It is especially important in identifying people who are likely to struggle with everyday functioning and decision making and participation in mainstream activities. Cognitive assessment is more molecular and focuses on one or more specific functions such as memory, processing speed or planning. A standard intellectual assessment such as the widely used Wechsler Adult Intelligence Scale (WAIS) contains a battery of cognitive tests as well as measures that evaluate accumulated knowledge and understanding. A focal cognitive assessment is more concerned with current functioning and is interested in accumulated knowledge primarily as a means of estimating changes in current functioning. A focal cognitive assessment aims for depth of evaluation of one or more specific areas rather than an estimate of global capacity.

A common reason for intellectual assessment is behaviour problems, social problems and learning difficulties of children. Such problems and difficulties can be secondary to mental health issues such as anxiety disorders, oppositional defiant disorders, autism spectrum disorders or attention deficit disorders. However, below average intellectual functioning can be either the primary reason or a significant contributor. Understanding the role of intellectual functioning in these kinds of difficulties is important both in treatment planning and in mobilising appropriate supports.

Among adults there is less need for global intellectual assessment as scholastic and vocational achievement usually provide sufficient information. However, instruments such as the WAIS may be used to provide information about current cognitive functioning and evidence to assist with estimation of recent change. The most common reason for cognitive assessment of adults presenting with mental health difficulties is to exclude organic causes of symptoms. Brain damage, whether caused by head injury, toxic substances, infection or tumour can result in symptoms that mimic psychosis, mood disorder and/or anxiety. When there is reason to suspect such damage, cognitive testing can quantify the impact on functioning and assist with clinical decision making.

Among adults there may also be a role for cognitive testing to assist with differential diagnosis among people who present with symptoms such as delusions and hallucinations that are common features of schizophrenia but can less commonly occur in other conditions. Schizophrenia often affects cognitive functioning, especially processing speed. Evidence that cognitive functioning is intact suggests the need to give consideration to other explanations for symptoms.

Among older adults cognitive testing is most widely used to assist in identification and quantification of early dementia (which is a form of brain damage). The focus is often on memory functioning but when dementia is more advanced, global functioning may be an important consideration in care planning.

Cognitive assessment of people with mental health problems is complicated by the fact that common conditions such as anxiety and depression and less common conditions such as schizophrenia interfere with cognitive functioning (Rock, Roiser, Riedel, & Blackwell, 2014). This means that it may be difficult to determine to what extent impaired cognitive functioning is secondary to a permanent organic condition such as dementia or a potentially temporary and treatable mental health condition. The pattern of results may be relevant but sometimes a clear picture on emerges with the passage of time and, in particular, treatment response or otherwise.

PERSONALITY ASSESSMENT

Personality is generally understood to be a set of enduring traits that influence thinking, emotional experience and behaviour. Personality has a genetic component and is also shaped by early life experience. Personality is not static and can evolve over the course of life. However, the prominent features of personality continue to have an influence. A personality disorder is diagnosed when prominent personality traits have a significant effect on a person's capacity to function effectively in society and/or experience satisfaction and enjoyment in everyday life.

The aim of personality assessment is to obtain a comprehensive and reliable picture of personality functioning, especially as it is relevant to psychopathology and/or potential response to treatment. Personality testing involves the use of standardised measures. The most commonly used measures are large self-report inventories, with substantial normative data and reliable guides to interpretation of results. Some of these come with the option of computer-driven reports, reducing the role of the clinician in interpretation. One of the most widely used personality inventories is the Minnesota Multiphasic Personality Inventory (MMPI). The MMPI has undergone a number of revisions to maintain its currency. The Personality Assessment Inventory (PAI) has been more recently developed than the MMPI and has a closer alignment with current diagnostic groups, including personality disorders.

The diagnosis of personality disorders is usually made on the basis of one or more clinical interviews that include a detailed personal history. The information obtained is then cross referenced with standard diagnostic criteria. However, standardised self-report instruments, such as the PAI can be used in conjunction with a clinical interview. The Millon Clinical Multiaxial Inventory (MCMI) is an instrument with particular sensitivity to personality disorders.

Aside from identification of personality disorders, personality assessment can also be used in clarification of diagnosis and in treatment planning. It can also contribute to court reports and may be more widely used in a forensic context than in other areas of mental health practice.

Sometimes a specific dimension of personality is assessed using a more focused instrument. For example, perfectionism is a personality trait that has been found to complicate treatment of common mental health problems. Identifying the presence and strength of a trait like perfectionism can assist with treatment planning and can also assist the person seeking help to develop realistic goals.

Personality can also be assessed using projective tests. Projective tests assess personality on the basis of a person's response to a standardised task. Projective tests are more difficult to administer and score than self-report tests but can be valuable when there are problems with literacy or when there is concern that the person being tested will deliberately respond falsely on a self-report test. The best-known projective test is the Rorschach Inkblot Test. This test has several standardised interpretive systems some of which can be computer assisted. Projective tests are less widely used than self-report tests because they are more difficult to administer and require training in administration and interpretation that does not typically fall within the standard training of mental health professionals.

There are also less formal and less standardised means of assessing personality and/or temperament that are more commonly used with children. These include observation of semi-standardised play and observation of drawing and other kinds of art work, which may also be semi-standardised with set tasks such as drawing a house, tree, person or family.

STANDARDISED TREATMENT RESPONSE AND TREATMENT OUTCOME ASSESSMENT

The assessment of treatment response and treatment outcome has both potential clinical value and potential service evaluation value. Treatment response and outcome measurement may focus on symptoms or functioning or a combination of the two. A wide range of self-report and clinician rated measures can be used for these purposes but there are measures that have been specifically designed for evaluation of treatment response and measures that the Commonwealth has recommended for outcome measurement in Australia's public mental health services.

Treatment response is assessed through repeated measures during an episode of treatment. Treatment outcome is measured by comparing baseline (commencement of treatment) scores with end of treatment scores. Treatment response measures also provide information regarding treatment outcome that may be more reliable than a single outcome measure as regular measurement shows the pattern of recovery and not just recovery status at a single measurement point, when the overall recovery may be distorted by situation factors present at the end of treatment.

The Outcome Questionnaire (OQ) is an example of a widely used self-report instrument designed for routine use over the course of an episode of psychological treatment. It is typically administered prior to each session, with the results being matched to an international database that yields information about the extent to which treatment progress is in accordance with expectations and whether completion of treatment is indicated. The OQ can assist the clinician with treatment planning and implementation by providing information that assists judgements about whether the current treatment is effective or whether a change in approach might be warranted. There is a reasonable body of research suggesting that clinicians who make use of the OQ or similar instruments get better client outcomes and better client throughput than clinicians relying solely on clinical judgement. However the magnitude of the outcome difference is small suggesting that while use of routine treatment response assessment is useful it is unlikely to have a major impact on the progress or outcome of treatment.

There are many instruments designed for measurement of symptoms characteristic of specific disorders (see Section 1.2.6). The availability of such measures provides the clinician with the option of tracking treatment response via changes to one or more disorders, rather than through use of a broad-spectrum measure such as the OQ. Some measures are restricted and/or must be purchased, but many have been developed for research purposes and are freely available.

Routine outcome measurement, at intake and discharge and at three monthly intervals during an extended episode of treatment, is mandated for public mental health services in Australia. Furthermore, it is expected that the results of outcome measurement will form part of ongoing client progress reviews. The measures recommended for this purpose include both self-report measures and clinician rated measures, which, if fully implemented, can provide a broad spectrum of information regarding symptoms and functioning. Research undertaken so far suggests that implementation has been patchy but with a trend suggesting improving acceptance of and compliance with routine measurement. There is typically more clinician-rated data than client-rated data and more inpatient than outpatient data. However, there are probably still significant gaps in data, suggesting that clinicians sometimes have other priorities and, even when clients are invited to complete a self-report outcome measure, they may decline.

There is limited evidence regarding the use of the mandated outcome data in treatment planning or service evaluation in Australia's public mental health services. This makes it difficult to determine whether the implementation of a national outcome measurement program has been of direct benefit to clients or of indirect benefit through service improvement. (For a broader discussion of routine outcome measurement, feedback to clinicians and implementation in practice settings, see Bickman et al., 2016.)

ASSESSING IMPAIRMENT/ DISABILITY

Psychologists are sometimes asked to assess impairment or disability. This may be in the context of a compensation claim, a claim for a social security payment such as disability support pension, or to assist with service planning (increasingly under the National Disability Insurance Scheme) regarding support needs. In such assessments, it is important that the assessor has a good understanding of the kind of information that is relevant and important.

In the case of disability support pension, qualification is dependent on meeting the requirement of 20 or more impairment points under the mandated Impairment Tables. An impairment rating can only be assigned when a mental health condition has been diagnosed by a psychiatrist or, if the diagnosis was made by another medical practitioner, there is evidence from a clinical psychologist.

Impairment to mental health function is rated using Table 5, which specified six areas of mental health function. The number of impairment points assigned under Table 5 depends on the level of difficulty a person experiences with most of these six areas of functioning. If the assessment is to be of optimal value to the person claiming disability support pension, it needs to collect information relevant to each of these six areas. Intellectual impairment is assessed using Table 9. Under Table 9, the applicant must have been assessed as having an IQ in the range of 70-85. Once an IQ in this range is established, the number of impairment points assigned, depends on the score attained from an assessment using the Adaptive Behaviour Assessment System (or equivalent). The relevant professional can readily access the Impairment Tables online and should do so and read them carefully prior to undertaking the assessment.

The diagnosis and assessment of autism spectrum disorders is of increasing importance, as both children and adults affected by these conditions can be eligible for support at school or in the community. While the diagnosis can be (and is often) made by a paediatrician, psychiatrist, clinical psychologist or other specialist in the area on clinical information alone, standardised testing often forms a part of assessment (Loureiro, Pio-Abreu, Machado, Gonçalves, & Cerejeira, 2015). There are many standardised instruments available to a psychologist assessing a child or adult for an autism spectrum disorder. The assessment of autism spectrum disorders typically also includes a cognitive/ intellectual evaluation.

PSYCHOMETRIC ISSUES

The key psychometric issues are reliability, validity, sensitivity and specificity. Reliability is about whether or not the test consistently yields accurate information. With self-report measures, reliability is a function of the measure itself. It is usually possible to obtain information about the reliability of a measure. As a general rule, self-report measures that are commonly used in research are likely to have acceptable reliability. Clinician rated or clinician administered instruments also depend on the competence of the clinician. More complex instruments such as the WAIS require considerable training for reliable administration.

Validity is concerned not with accuracy but with whether the scores generated are good indicators of the underlying condition or state that is being measured. Validity is sometimes debatable. For example, there is room for disagreement as to whether tests of intellectual capacity have the breadth to provide a valid indication in the form of an IQ score of a person's global intellectual functioning. Instruments widely used in research tend to be valid as well as reliable. However, it is easier to evaluate reliability than validity. This means that it is fairly common for such instruments to have better quality information regarding reliability than validity.

Sensitivity and specificity refer to the extent to which a measure yields false positives and false negatives, and are important factors in validity. Sensitivity and specificity are especially important when the aim of the measurement is to assign a person into one or other category—such as having or not having a specific mental health condition. An insensitive measure yields false negatives, that is, indicating the person does not have the condition when this is not the case. Self-report measures may lack sensitivity when the person completing the measure has a motive to under-report symptoms. Poor specificity occurs when scores yield too many false positives, that is, people may be classified as having a condition they don't in fact have. Self-report depression measures tend to be nonspecific as symptoms of depression may be found in a wide range of disorders other than depression. Some measures, such as the MMPI, contain subscales designed to detect under-reporting and over-reporting so that the clinician is at least alerted to the risk. As a general rule classificatory decisions such as diagnosis, should not be made on the basis of self-report questionnaire scores alone.

RESOURCES

More information can be found for the tests on the following organisation's websites.

ABAS: (Harrison & Oakland, 2015)

DSP Impairment Tables: (Australian Government, 2011)

MCMI: (Millon, Grossman, & Millon, 2015)

MMPI: (Butcher et al., 2001)

OQ: (OQ Measures, 2020)

PAI: (Morey, 2010)

SCID-5: (American Psychiatric Association, 2018)

WAIS: (Wechsler, 2008)

WHO-CIDI: (World Health Organization (WHO), 2017b)

2.3.15 SOCIAL WORK ASSESSMENT

BANI AADAM & MELISSA PETRAKIS

SOCIAL WORK AND ASSESSMENTS

An assessment is considered an intervention tool (Day & Petrakis, 2018) and correctly takes its place in a biopsychosocial model (Australian Association of Social Workers, 2010). Assessments should be undertaken in collaboration with the person seeking assistance and address life domains such as relationships (including family where consent is given), housing, finance, employment and both physical and mental health.

The object of a social work assessment is to work with service users to identify the best and most effective plan of treatment and support to assist in building resilience and a more sustainable recovery for individuals. Undertaking an assessment that is ethically humanistic by using a mixture of trauma-informed, strengths-based and relational recovery tools is critical. This approach is applicable and should underpin all assessments along the service spectrum, including entry, ongoing and exit assessments.

HUMANISTIC ETHICS

Humanistic ethics can be thought of here as a values-based approach for social work practice and resolutely views human nature as essentially positive; as people having potential, with the ability to change and grow. This view aligns with theories of human development and self-realisation with 'latent hope' located at the core of all people (Pulla, 2017, p 104; Dolgoff, Harrington, & Loewenberg, 2012, p. 57). Social workers whose practice is guided by humanistic ethics believe that every person has the innate capacity to attribute responsibility to themselves and the ability to take ownership of their choices that are true to their values and identities. Through this, the person who is seeking support, rather than their illness and diagnosis, occupies the centre of consideration for social workers.

For the social worker who is informed by this approach though, tensions will be created, since their core interests and passion lie in inspiring and enabling individuals or groups to achieve 'self-actualisation' (Dolgoff et al., 2012, p. 57) rather than to be regulated by oppressive processes and structures that mitigate healing. As such, workers operating primarily under this approach can seemingly be at odds with colleagues who are coming from a more clinically pragmatic standardised and rationalistic approach, attempting to be efficient and effective in their practice setting. This may be because the mental health care system predominantly works towards adapting and maintaining function within its existing social order (Dolgoff et al., 2012). It is absolutely crucial then that the following three frameworks, values and philosophies—trauma-informed practice, strengths-based approach and relational recovery—are used to assist social workers become more ethically orientated.

TRAUMA-INFORMED PRACTICE

While trauma involves experiences that overwhelm a person's ability to cope (Emerging Minds, 2019), trauma-informed practice can be described as an approach to mental health service delivery that is founded on an understanding of how trauma can at times adversely affect people's wellbeing and functioning and how (social) workers can identify services that are needed for people's recovery (Fallot & Harris, 2008, pp. 6-7). In this context, practitioners should locate trauma-informed practices as central to their assessments. While there is a surplus of grey, black and peer-reviewed literature on what trauma-informed practice may look like, the specific prerequisite foundations social workers need to have when conducting an assessment, and the principles that should underpin them, follow.

When conducting an assessment, practitioners should ensure the following six principles underpin and permeate through their work. These have been adapted from SAMHSA, 2018. They are:

1 *Safety*—so that people feel psychologically and emotionally safe, making sure that the implementation of their recovery will not (re) traumatise them;
2 *Collaboration, inclusion and self-determination*—so that the relationship is on an equal footing, people are empowered and to allow people to have choice giving them ownership of their recovery;
3 *Individuality*—being responsive to the cultural, religious, historical and gender needs of people and allowing them to maintain their identity;
4 *Relationships*—to family where appropriate, peers and peer organisations for added support, linkages and connectedness;
5 *Privileging people's voices*—people are their own experts and know what and how things affect them;
6 *Accountability*—so that people are informed, and so trust and transparency can be cultivated.

Being trauma-informed and having assessments that echo the above principles will alleviate people's anxieties, particularly if they are on a community treatment order (CTO) and have been coerced. Coercion diametrically opposes trauma-informed practice because it can place an individual in a position of particular disadvantage and unique vulnerability through diminished (and deprived) autonomy, control and decision making (Maylea, 2017). And despite social work practice running on the assumption that there is a need for coercion, it is argued that 'social work as a profession should reject the notion of involuntary treatment and work towards a mental health support system which respects capacity, agency and recovery' (Maylea, 2017). Further, Maylea adds that if social workers have the opportunities to facilitate a less restrictive, less traumatic and less stigmatising route, then through the exercise of their given powers, they have an obligation to pursue that pathway.

Social workers are required to respect the inherent dignity, worth, and autonomy of every person, and minimise the use of compulsion (Australian Association of Social Workers, 2010). Assessments should generally recognise people's needs and treat them in a manner that will empower service users (SAMHSA, 2018). By reducing coercion and advocating for treatment in the least restrictive manner, social workers can formulate goals that will lead to a sustainable recovery, as well as fulfilling their role on being ethically humanistic.

FOCUSING ON STRENGTHS

A strengths-based approach is a philosophy of positive exploration of consumer strengths that may be used as stepping stones in their recovery. Strengths can be in the form of people's passions, interests, skills and assets, as it seeks to remind, reiterate and use these with people. A strengths approach has been shown to promote health, wellbeing (Xie, 2013) and self-fulfilment (Francis, 2014).

Social workers can look at both what has worked before, and what is known and familiar, to drive recovery. An additional advantage of this inclusive collaborative work is that it provides people with opportunities to take ownership of their health (Pulla, 2017, pp. 98–99). Assets can be tangible supports, like a home, which can facilitate a smoother and quicker transition back into ordinary life—rather than a person staying in the system longer than they need because they are waiting for accommodation. Assets can also be intangible, like confidence in one's ability to speak to people, which can be useful when meeting different clinical staff members or going for a job interview. Knowing that a person has this asset (confidence when talking with strangers), social workers can shape a recovery plan that incorporates elements of this asset into their plans, ultimately aiming to empower the individual in their recovery. The implication here though, is that the relationship between social workers and service users becomes more genuine and substantive, and goes beyond mere clinical inquiries, picking up on things that are not obvious or clearly stated.

Although there is an abundance of principles to guide a strengths-based approach in the literature at the moment, it may be useful for us to combine thoughts (Rapp, 1993) and training guidelines (St Vincent's Hospital, 2014) when designing a mental health strengths based assessment to include:

- focusing on the individual's strengths rather than their deficits
- creating a genuine collaborative inclusive relationship
- creating a support/transition plan that is directed by the person
- focusing on what can be done with the resources and supports available
- operating with the least restrictive interventions and in an environment that people can recover in
- believing that people have potential to grow, change and develop.

A strengths-based approach does not necessarily focus only on strengths, but it does start and work with the strengths of a person to endeavour to (re) build capacity and resilience. It further provides assistance in prompting the commitment of the person to engage with the support provided. This is because a strengths approach actively engages people in a process where their recovery plan cannot be developed without their collaborative input and engagement. It is hoped that through this process, hope, resilience, self-determination and creativity—among many other attributes—proliferate and are cultivated so that people are able to achieve greater awareness of their own abilities, skills, capacities, and potential (Xie, 2013; Francis, 2014).

CREATING CONNECTEDNESS AND RELATIONSHIPS

While personal recovery is generally thought of as a unique and personal journey that is individualistic in nature, relational recovery is understood when connections and relationships become central to the treatment and support of people's lives. The reason for relational recovery is that while the personal recovery approach in mental health is ubiquitously applied across multiple mental health settings, it is not without its detractors. Central to these critiques are that personal recovery focuses too much on the 'inner' subjective experience over and above the interpersonal connections that people find themselves in. And although many models of recovery recognise relationships or connectedness, it is argued that these 'largely obscure the interpersonal contexts of recovery' (Price-Robertson, Obradovic, & Morgan, 2017, p.1).

Relational recovery can thus be considered the 'interface' between people and the environment (Hyde, Bowles, & Pawar, 2014), the space and interaction between person and context, including 'personal relationships, physical space and other economic, social and cultural factors' (p. 10). Relationships, or the engagement in relationships, is thus where meaning and recovery can be generated. Bland and colleagues endorse this notion:

> Human existence is situated in relation to society, history, culture, the economy, the political landscape and the ecology of our constructed and natural environments. Whatever the impact of biology, there is rarely a psychiatric crisis without a wider context. Social work, with its unique focus, has always acknowledged this, recognising that recovery takes place within supportive relationships and environments (Bland, Renouf, & Tullgren, 2015, p. 21-22).

Within relational recovery then, individualism is replaced by relationships and human connection as a fundamental necessity. Relational recovery is essential for growth, as individuals are inextricably linked to their environments, working interdependently as part of an ecosystem. This interconnected system includes linkages with consent to family, friends, the workplace, social and sporting groups, and other structures, and aligns neatly with social work's mental health assessments on life domains that include employment, accommodation, finances, social supports, family engagement, etc., where psychological phenomena such as hope and empowerment are allowed to transpire' (Price-Robertson et al., 2017, p. 9).

Essentially, relational recovery is an appreciation that people's personal experiences are 'inseparable from the social and cultural milieus from which they emerge' (Price-Robertson et al., 2017). From this perspective, recovery is not only a product, but is seen as a social changeable achievable process (Price-Robertson et al., 2017; Bland et al., 2012, p. 401).

Characteristically then, mental health assessments are directed towards mitigation or management of risk, alleviation of symptoms and improvement of function. The National Standards for Mental Health Services (Australian Government, 2010) make clear that entry into a mental health service should include assessments that give due consideration to risk and safety, urgency, distress, dysfunction and disability, with due attention given to the underlying diagnosis. A counterpoint to a rationalistic, risk captive, neoliberal health system is the offering of assessments using trauma-informed, strengths-based and relational recovery tools and theories. This will ensure that social workers are applying ethically sound and evidence-based practice.

2.3.16 COMMENTARY AND REFLECTION

Graham Meadows

This chapter has taken a series of focus points on different conceptual, professional, procedural, societal, practical and interpersonal aspects of assessment. In Section 2.3.3, we introduced the CDM developmental framework involving firstly meta-cognition, then reflective, critical, complexity and dialectical thinking—there is plentiful opportunity roaming across the content of the chapter to explore these approaches to deepening understanding, practical capacities and wisdom. The reader may be interested in applying these principles in considering linkage with earlier parts of this text, for instance historical perspectives (see Section 1.1.3), social determinants (see Section 1.2.4), application to specific groups (see Chapter 1.3), issues of research including screening concepts (see Section 1.4.7), prevention and stepped care (see Sections 1.5.5 and 1.5.6), public health and community perspectives (see Chapter 1.6), roles of different disciplines (see Chapter 2.1), teamwork and cross-sectoral working issues (see Chapter 2.2). Later chapters will link assessment processes to various intervention options through the rest of Part 2, then considering lifespan issues in Part 3 and disorder-specific matters in Part 4. So considering assessment as a learning and capacity-building task, it both draws on much of the material set out earlier in the text and forms a critical capacity in making use of the learnings to be developed later in the work.

2.4 CASE MANAGEMENT

ELLIE FOSSEY, CATH ROPER, SANDY WATSON, KATH THORBURN, VRINDA EDAN, JAZ CHISHOLM, MELISSA PETRAKIS, BRIDGET HAMILTON, CAROL HARVEY, NIKOLAOS KAZANTZIS, NEIL THOMAS, HARRY MINAS & LISA BROPHY

2.4.1 INTRODUCTION

ELLIE FOSSEY & CATH ROPER

This chapter explores the concept and practice of case management in community mental health care. Case management in some form is widely practised across many sectors of health, welfare and community services in Australia as the vehicle for delivery of various kinds of assistance, support and service. Historically, since the National Mental Health Policy was introduced (Australian Health Ministers, 1992), *case management* has become a prominent feature of its community mental health service system as the vehicle for the provision of various kinds of assistance, support and services for people experiencing mental illness, their families and other support networks.

This chapter begins with consideration of the terms *case management* and *case manager*. The work of case management is then positioned from the perspective of consumer-directed recovery, and in relation to supported decision making and advance statements, practices central to supporting consumers in directing their own recovery.

A range of ways in which case management is understood and practised in mental health services are described, including: clinical case management; brokerage and care coordination approaches that have recently become more prominent within the community mental health sector and with the introduction of the National Disability Insurance Scheme (NDIS); and strengths focused and assertive approaches to case management. Some key roles of case managers, the centrality of relationships, and implications for case management practice of working with interpreters and diverse populations are discussed. Contemporary directions in policy and law and their implications for involuntary treatment in the community are then considered to provide guidance for case management practice in this context.

LANGUAGE AND CONTEXT

The terms 'case management' and 'case manager' are widely used in mental health services, but they should also trouble us. Their usage implies there are 'cases' to be 'managed', yet consumers are people not 'cases', and may seek assistance and support but do not need to be 'managed' (Davidson, Rowe, & Tondora, 2008; Rapp & Goscha, 2012). At the very least, these terms do not reflect the nature of the relationship, but their origins in business and law suggest they may more accurately refer to the managing of services or resources (Longhofer, Kubek, & Floersch, 2010). These terms also locate power and expertise with the mental health practitioner, diminishing the consumer as a person with expertise in his or her own right. Thus, sensitivity to its negative connotations is important if using the term case management; there are also alternatives such as key worker, care coordinator or service coordinator. In Australia, non-government, community-managed mental health and community support services in particular have tended to use such alternative terms. The term 'case manager' is also increasingly challenged from a recovery-orientated perspective, as discussed later in the chapter (see Section 2.4.2). Other terms, such as recovery guide or coach, may be more reflective of the roles that mental health professionals might undertake in recovery-orientated alternatives to case management practice (Davidson et al., 2008; Slade, 2009b).

People accessing mental health care are not routinely allocated a case manager or provided with any form of case management service, and are much less likely to experience case management in primary care or private sector service contexts than in publicly funded clinical mental health services. Indeed, the majority of adult Australians who consult a health service provider about a mental health issue are most likely to visit a general practitioner, whereas only 0.3% of the adult population are estimated to meet criteria for diagnosis of a psychotic disorder and to be in contact with publicly funded mental health services (Morgan et al., 2011; see Chapter 1.6). Case management services are provided by public clinical or non-government community mental services for the majority of this latter group, as well as for some youth, older adults or people with other diagnoses accessing mental health care through these service providers. So, while case management is provided to a relatively small proportion of all Australians accessing mental health care, it may be a critical feature of their service experiences.

2.4.2 CONSUMER-DIRECTED RECOVERY AND CASE MANAGEMENT

SANDY WATSON & KATH THORBURN

Putting aside, for the moment, problems of terminology and meaning, case management, from a recovery-oriented perspective, is positioned within a framework of citizenship. This involves understanding and supporting self-directed recovery by embodying the principles of self-determination; personhood; choice and decision making; rights; participation and inclusion, and personal control. Recovery is not about 'getting better', 'graduating from support', 'becoming normal' or 'fitting in' (Slade et al., 2014; Repper & Perkins, 2009). It is not about earning your place in society. Rather it is about the right to define one's own identity (Bracken, 2003) and to full social and economic participation, essentially expanding what counts as citizenship (McWade, 2016).

Traditional (clinical) approaches to case management, and mental health services more broadly, locate problems of exclusion within the individual resulting in an emphasis on individual treatment (Slade et al., 2014). A recovery-oriented approach to case management involves recognising and responding to the ways that self-determination and citizenship for people labelled 'mentally ill' are impeded by systems, social structures, and practices, and the attitudes and assumptions that drive them.

The work of case management that supports self-directed recovery not only requires an understanding of the processes and principles of recovery (see Chapters 1.1 and 2.6), and a commitment to supporting the processes of regaining a sense of identity, autonomy, meaning and life purpose. It also involves an understanding of the barriers to inclusion, and supporting individual and collective efforts to challenge these. Within this framework, the person's own understanding of his or her experience and context, and the broader lived experience knowledge base must inform all understandings of, and responses to, mental distress and recovery.

RECOVERY AND CASE MANAGEMENT: RECOGNISING THE TENSIONS

The language of case management is inherently problematic from a self-directed recovery standpoint. The terminology and underlying assumptions are antithetical to the principles of self-determination and empowerment. Continued use of the term perpetuates traditional notions of expertise and power, which are inconsistent with an overarching recovery framework. It has been assumed that it is inevitable this language will change in a way that reflects the shift towards more democratic and holistic approaches and relationships and yet it continues to persist, reflecting, perhaps, limitations in our fundamental understandings of both recovery and the significance of language and meanings conveyed in recovery-oriented practice.

Other tensions associated with case management practice and recovery, which may also be understood as the consequence of a shift in the way we understand and respond to mental distress, relate to: constructions of noncompliance, resistance and risk; the role of case management in mandated treatment; the issue of pacing (the person's own versus system imperatives); and concerns around autonomy and choice.

Tensions also arise from differing conceptualisations of the term recovery, which has a number of meanings depending on one's perspective. Table 2.10 outlines the distinction between traditional notions of recovery from a clinical perspective (*clinical recovery*) and the broader notion of *self-directed (personal) recovery*.

Table 2.10 Distinctions between clinical recovery and personal recovery

Clinical recovery	Self-directed (personal) recovery
Mental illness and disorder, pathology	Crisis of being, legitimate and valued human experience
Driven by professional expertise and knowledge	Driven by lived experience expertise and knowledge
Recovery is an outcome of treatment	Recovery is a process of personal growth
Focus is reducing deficits and symptoms	Focus is enhancing strengths and potential
Recovery is rated by professionals	Recovery is rated by the person
Crisis is interpreted as failure or relapse	Crisis is an active space that can contribute to growth

Source: Adapted from Glover, Kalyanasundaram, & Tooth, 2008; O'Hagan, 2011; Slade, 2009b

Recognising these tensions can assist us to better understand and respond to the changing nature of mental health practice, analyse possible conflicts and address potential or actual barriers to recovery-oriented practice. This shift in awareness creates many opportunities for workers to support interactions, approaches and environments that harness and encourage people's own self-directed efforts towards recovery.

RECOVERY AND THE RELATIONSHIP

Case management is about relationship, and the nature of the relationship is a key factor in recovery-oriented practice. Research confirms that it is *who* the worker is, not what he or she *does*, that is most often experienced as helpful in the recovery process (Borg & Kristiansen, 2004) and that relationships that support personal recovery are experienced as 'hope inspiring' (Repper & Perkins, 2009). Consumers identify the following characteristics of workers who support hope and recovery:

- the ability to build respectful relationships
- demonstrated genuine interest in and concern for the person
- conveying and (when needed) holding hope in/for the person
- upholding and supporting personal control and agency

- assisting access to peer support and other opportunities

(Brekke, Lien, & Biong, 2018; Sælør, Ness, & Semb, 2015; Borg & Kristiansen, 2004).

A recovery approach recognises that it is the consumer who decides the value of the relationship, and what she or he wants from it. This is in line with research findings that the consumer's rating of the alliance is the best predictor of positive outcomes (Duncan, 2012).

IMPLICATIONS FOR CASE MANAGEMENT

The idea that recovery is a self-defined, self-directed process challenges the way services are envisioned and offered, and by whom. This has implications for the mental health workforce in its entirety, and has also led to the development of the mental health peer workforce, a strong peer presence being one of the hallmarks of a recovery-oriented service.

The implications of a recovery orientation for case management are extensive. Broadly, case managers need to:

- become thoroughly informed about recovery principles and the recovery process, drawing on personal recovery narratives, lived experience research, consumer movement history and consumer-driven practices
- recognise and accommodate the diverse ways in which people make sense of their experiences relating to mental distress
- recognise the importance of citizenship and work from a human rights framework, upholding the rights of service users, as well as understanding discrimination and how to reduce it
- recognise the role of peer work, consumer-operated alternatives and self-help networks in recovery-oriented services, and demonstrate commitment to working effectively with peer providers
- work inclusively with significant others in people's lives in the person's own context, and according to her/his/their preferences
- recognise and support service users' personal resourcefulness, and their valid efforts to cope with complex and difficult experiences, respecting the importance of agency and personal control
- cultivate self-awareness, and be able to recognise and respond to the conflicting pressures (tensions) that are inevitable in recovery-oriented work (for example, risk management versus risk sharing)
- demonstrate cultural competency and an ability to respect and respond to diverse cultural perspectives on mental distress, to access relevant resources for working cross-culturally
- maintain awareness of developments in approaches to supporting people with experience of mental distress; and importantly
- convey belief in the person, and hope for the future, while validating the person's experience and demonstrating acceptance of the person as she or he is now.

Within the work of case management, specific practices central to supporting consumers in directing their recovery include supported decision making and the use of advance statements.

2.4.3 SUPPORTED DECISION MAKING

CATH ROPER

Supported decision making refers to the process of enabling a person to make and communicate decisions regarding personal or legal concerns (Office of the United Nations High Commissioner for Human Rights, 2009). In supported decision making, the individual is always the primary decision-maker, however, the person may communicate and execute their decisions in a range of ways including with the support of others such as family members, friends or the support of mental health practitioners (Pathare & Shields, 2012). 'The central principle underlying supported decision making is autonomy, that no person should have another person appointed to make a decision on their behalf, if they could make the decision themselves with assistance and support' (Chartres & Brayley, 2010, p. 1). Three levels of support that individuals may want include: support in formulating purposes and making choices, supports to engage in the decision-making process and supports to act on decisions made (Bach & Kerzner, 2010). Types of decisions might include life planning, advocacy, relationships, administrate support, informational support. Practically speaking, in the context of supported decision making, the pertinent question is: what supports are needed to ensure this person can exercise their human right to decide?

Important background to understanding supported decision making is the United Nations Convention on the Rights of Persons with Disabilities (United Nations, 2006). Globally, mental health legislation has been increasingly influenced by a human rights focus and an emphasis on consumers' rights to make their own treatment decisions. The United Nations Convention on the Rights of Persons with Disabilities (the Convention) has accelerated this tendency as the domestic laws of signatory countries are required to be in alignment with its underpinning principles of equality before the law, for all people with disabilities, including 'psychosocial disabilities' (the language used in the Convention). It was ratified in Australia in 2008.

The Convention is underpinned by respect for the inherent dignity, individual autonomy and independence of persons which includes the freedom to make one's own choices. It is founded upon respect for difference and acceptance of persons with disabilities as part of human diversity and humanity, and emphasises the principles of non-discrimination, equality of opportunity and the full and effective participation and inclusion in society of people with disabilities. Therefore, whereas a biomedical model of disability locates 'deficits' or disability within an individual, the Convention adopts a 'social model' of disability, in which disability is regarded as the interaction between an impairment and social conditions, environments and attitudes (Gooding, 2013). For example, according to the social model of disability, it is disabling when a building has no lift and can only be accessed by stairs making it inaccessible for people with wheelchairs. So, the social model identifies the problem as located in the lack of access; the problem is not the person's impairment. The person experiences inequality because of this lack of access.

Article 12 of the Convention requires that 'parties shall take appropriate measures to provide access by persons with disabilities to the support they may require in exercising their legal capacity' (United Nations, 2006), p.10). Under the United Nations Convention on the Rights of Persons with Disabilities (UNCRPD), legal capacity includes two ideas: 'legal standing' in the sense of being viewed as a person before the law, and 'legal agency' which is being able to act within the framework of the legal system (such as being able to marry, make a will, sign contracts, etc.). It also means being protected from other people making decisions for an individual (McSherry & Wilson, 2015).

This requires a shift away from substituted decision making, whereby practitioners make decisions on behalf of consumers, and towards a focus on what resources and supports the consumer wants/needs to retain legal capacity and be able to stay in control of decision making. Support can take the form of information provision in a format that the person best understands. For practitioners, adopting supported decision making alters the direction of practice to consider questions like: how can this person be assisted or supported to resume decision making as soon as possible? What resources might they need in order to retain decision making? And supported decision making means remembering that each person has the right to make decisions others don't agree with; they are entitled to change their minds; and they have the right to learn from experience and make mistakes. Supported decision making recognises that people often naturally seek the advice of trusted friends or relatives to make decisions, so that facilitating this is a valuable practice, as is providing access to independent advocacy, or encouraging self-advocacy.

A number of tools are available for building capacity to implement supported decision making in practice. For example, to guide the implementation of a human rights and recovery approach in mental health care, the World Health Organization has developed a training module on supported decision making: (WHO, 2020).

In Australia, the Independent Mental Health Advocacy service recently developed a self-help tool to support consumers' decision making in mental health units (see Independent Mental Health Advocacy, 2020). This tool has many good uses, including for peer workers to use with consumers who express concerns about their treatment; as a way for clinicians to learn about consumer rights; as it tells something about the law; and because it takes people through the practical steps that they might need to exercise their rights. It is also useful for knowing how to access supports like second opinion services.

2.4.4 ADVANCE STATEMENTS

VRINDA EDAN & CATH ROPER

In the context of physical health, advance care planning is a process whereby a patient, in consultation with health care providers, family members and important others, makes decisions about his or her future health care (Singer, Robertson, & Roy, 1996). Grounded in the ethical principle of autonomy and the legal doctrine of consent, advance care planning helps to ensure that the norm of consent is respected should the patient become incapable of participating in treatment decisions. Advance health care directives, also referred to as 'living wills' or 'Ulysses agreements' are documents that enable the person's wishes regarding health care to be known, in instances when the person cannot make those wishes known.

In the context of mental health, advance statements are documents made by consumers to indicate treatment preferences prior to becoming a compulsory patient. They often also include consumers' preferences about environments, visitors and activities (Maylea, Jorgensen, Matta, Ogilvie, & Wallin, 2018; Reilly & Atkinson, 2010). Because mental health legislation can override the individual's health care preferences and engender substitute decision making (where the psychiatrist makes treatment decisions on behalf of patients), any and all tools supporting people's autonomy are particularly significant to ensure that whenever possible consumers' treatment preferences are known and adhered to, and that they are engaged in decision making.

There is evidence that advance statements increase consumers' sense of autonomy and participation in decision making (Elbogen et al., 2007; Amering, Stastny, & Hopper, 2005), that consumers experience less coercion in crisis situations if they have one (Weller, 2013; Kim et al., 2007) and that they are important to the provision of recovery orientated services (Saraf, 2015). However, there are significant barriers to implementation of advance statements, such as poor knowledge of psychiatric advance directives by service providers (Kim et al., 2007) and processes making it difficult for psychiatrists to find and utilise them (Saraf, 2015). Consequently, all mental health practitioners have an extremely important role in: understanding the local processes in place for the development of advance statements; as well as facilitating conversations with people about their treatment preferences, assisting them to understand what advance statements are, helping them reflect on and discuss with appropriate people the decisions they wish to include in advance care planning.

2.4.5 CASE MANAGEMENT: OVERVIEW OF APPROACHES IN MENTAL HEALTH SERVICES

JAZ CHISHOLM & MELISSA PETRAKIS

Case management has become the dominant framework for delivering publicly funded community mental health services in Australia. Case management was historically designed to provide coordinated community support to people with mental illness post-deinstitutionalisation (Howgego, Yellowlees, Owen, Meldrum, & Dark, 2003). Providing a single contact person to coordinate access to services and support is a key aim of case management. This can include, but is not limited to, crisis intervention, work with families, support with daily living skills, counselling, psychoeducation, alcohol and other drug support, assessment, referral and liaison with other services (King, Meadows, & Le Bas, 2004).

Case management services in Australia are provided by clinical and nonclinical community mental health organisations, with case management considered a key mechanism for facilitating integration and continuity of care in its service standards (Australian Government, 2010b). Most Australian states and territories have adopted strategic plans that underpin case management with recovery-oriented practice (RoP) principles, each drawing to varying extents on the recovery-oriented practice framework and expectations of services and practitioners set out in national policy (Australian Government Department of Health, 2013; Australian Health Ministers' Advisory Council, 2013) (see Chapter 1.7).

No particular case management approach is specified in these policies and service standards, and individual mental health services across Australia have chosen to adopt different approaches to implementing RoP within case management. Examples include St Vincent's Hospital (Melbourne) (Chopra et al., 2009; Petrakis, Wilson, & Hamilton, 2013) and Sydney Mental Health Services, each of which uses the Strengths Model of case management (Fukui et al., 2012), described later in this chapter. Other recovery-oriented practice frameworks are increasingly shaping the ways in which case management is provided. For instance, the Collaborative Recovery Model (CRM) (Oades, Deane, & Crowe, 2017) is being implemented in mental health and community support services in several states, while the REFOCUS approach (Bird, Leamy, Le Boutillier, Williams, & Slade, 2014) has recently been adapted and trialled in community mental health services in south east Melbourne (Meadows et al., 2019; Shawyer et al., 2017). These services have all employed peer consumer and peer carer workers to provide training and support to consumers, families and staff. For further information about the Collaborative Recovery Model and the REFOCUS recovery-oriented practice framework, see Chapter 2.6.

Other case management approaches have developed over time to address the needs of particular client groups. For example, assertive community treatment (ACT) was designed to provide services for people who were unwilling or unable to attend outpatient services, to offer support with daily living, emotional and social functioning, and to help reduce hospital re-admissions (Baier, Favrod, Ferrari, Koch, & Holzer, 2013; Mueser, Bond, Drake, & Resnick, 1998). Here, the differences are first delineated between the clinical case management and brokerage approaches, the latter having become more relevant since the introduction of the National Disability Insurance Scheme (NDIS). Later in this chapter, strengths focused and assertive approaches to case management are discussed (see Sections 2.4.6 and 2.4.7).

CLINICAL CASE MANAGEMENT

Clinical case management originated with a biopsychosocial view of mental illness, underpinned by the use of clinical psychiatric practices (Kanter, 1989; Yellowlees, 1997). This aimed at coupling collaborative and therapeutic relationships between clinicians and consumers to improve social, personal and psychological aspects of a consumer's life with treating the illness (Kanter, 1989). Thus, case managers build therapeutic relationships with consumers through the use of their capabilities and proficiencies to identify needs and strengths (Simpson, Miller, & Bowers, 2003). Other types of case management have since emerged, but clinical case management remains for those people with severe and enduring mental ill-health (Brophy, Hodges, Halloran, Grigg, & Swift, 2014). The term 'case management' is also still widely used, despite concerns that it is denigrating to many people using mental health services, as discussed earlier in the chapter.

The principles of clinical case management centre on having a single point of contact in the coordination of services, and the receiver of the services experiencing improvement in their quality of life and functioning (King et al., 2004; Rapp & Goscha, 2004). It aims to provide continuity of care

(Ross, Curry, & Goodwin, 2011) and lower rates of hospitalisation (Holloway & Carson, 2001). To achieve this, clinical case managers work collaboratively with other clinicians in a multidisciplinary team providing services that include psychosocial and risk assessment (Noordsy et al., 2002). They also aim to work collaboratively with consumers on individual recovery plans and goal setting, work with families, and provide support and assistance with day-to-day concerns, as well as referrals for specialised support, recreation and rehabilitation, psychoeducation education and treatment options (King et al., 2004; Noordsy et al., 2002). In Australia, clinical case managers are typically mental health clinicians with professional qualifications in nursing, psychology, occupational therapy or social work, working in multidisciplinary teams with psychiatric registrars and consultant psychiatrists to provide treatment and monitor fluctuations in mental state and risks, so as to ensure people can function at their optimum (Sawyer, 2008; Simpson et al., 2003; Yellowlees, 1997). The provision of clinical case management services may be episodic or longer term due to the often cyclic nature of episodes of mental ill-health. For instance, following a period of case management support, people with mental health issues may remain well for long periods of time and not require case management services, whereas others may helped by more assertive or prolonged periods of case management support and treatment.

BROKERAGE APPROACHES AND CARE COORDINATION

Like clinical case management, the brokerage model was initially implemented post-deinstitutionalisation and had an emphasis on linking people with other services, monitoring needs, making assessments and planning (Holloway & Carson, 2001; Yellowlees, 1997). In the early to mid-1990s, the clinical and brokerage models of case management borrowed some components from each other (Mueser et al., 1998; Yellowlees, 1997) with both approaches emphasising a single point of contact to assess and coordinate services. However, clinical case management includes the provision of clinical services whereas in the brokerage model, the case manager is only the broker of services (King et al., 2004) and typically has a larger caseload than their clinical counterparts (Holloway & Carson, 2001).

Brokerage models emphasise service coordination, with the aim to meet the service needs in the most cost-effective way, without necessarily building strong connections and relationships with their clients (Hannigan, Simpson, Coffey, Barlow, & Jones, 2018; Holloway & Carson, 2001). The brokerage model is making a resurgence in Australia through the implementation of the National Disability Insurance Scheme (NDIS), which has introduced a personalised funding approach to support for people with disabilities, including those with psychosocial disabilities (Brophy, Bruxner, Wilson, Cocks, & Stylianou, 2015). Referred to as care coordination, it differs from traditional brokerage models in aiming to give people with mental health issues and psychosocial disabilities greater input in determining the services they want and need, and working with NDIS support coordinators to have their needs met (Brophy et al., 2015). The recovery movement led by consumers past and present has also been pivotal in bringing about this change to how services are delivered (Brophy et al., 2015).

The interaction of care coordination and brokerage models with the NDIS

Care coordination models are somewhat like brokerage models, however they are a nonclinical approach responsive to people with severe and persistent mental illness. For example, one of the most common in Australia is Partners in Recovery (PIR), the intent of which is to create partnerships and linkages between community health and social care services, so as to provide wrap-around care and support tailored to individuals with severe and persistent mental illness (Banfield & Forbes, 2018). PIR support facilitators are considered valuable in providing coordinated recovery-oriented care (Brophy et al., 2014), a source of continuity and stability for consumers, and building support networks around them, so that on the whole the care coordination model has been successful (Banfield & Forbes, 2018).

With the implementation of NDIS, some community mental health support services have ceased to provide direct support to consumers, but care coordination is proving to function in a complementary way with the NDIS by brokering other community mental health agencies to provide a specific service desired (Brophy et al., 2014; Smith-Merry, 2018).

Care coordination is a person-centred approach to coordinating services with people and assisting them to navigate the network of frequently disjointed services including housing, social, health and other supports (Brophy et al., 2014; Smith-Merry, 2018). It has its roots in person centred and recovery-oriented practices where workers are committed to connecting consumers with providers who can meet their identified needs and desires, although sometimes caseloads can create difficulties in meeting all needs successfully (Hannigan et al., 2018). What has been identified in recent years is that, for some people, a longer-term form of case management is likely to meet their needs much more effectively. Care coordination aims to take into account a person's longer term needs and to address these issues as they arise (Rapp & Goscha, 2004), so that there is no need for discharge from the care coordination service because the care coordinator will draw in relevant care and support services as required across the person's life span. This is where the NDIS approach to personalised funding and care coordination may fund the delivery of various kinds of support as a person requires them over time. In a study exploring the choices about support that people with psychosocial disabilities from mental health services might make if offered individualised funding packages, Brophy and colleagues (2015) found participants identified health; their economic situation; social connection; housing; and personal relationships as their priorities for support. These priorities indicate a role for case coordination that is distinct from the focus of clinical case management.

Next, we consider applications of the strengths model of case management and intensive case management in Australian mental health service settings.

2.4.6 STRENGTHS MODEL OF CASE MANAGEMENT

BRIDGET HAMILTON & ELLIE FOSSEY

One distinctive approach to case management, the *Strengths Model of Case Management*, was developed in Kansas beginning in the 1970s. Rapp and Goscha (2012) have articulated and refined the principles and practices of the model over 30 years and three key text editions. Broadly speaking, the model focuses on strengths, abilities, resources and potentials of people and their communities, promoting a more optimistic approach to working with individuals with mental illness, and the communities within which they live, learn, work and socialise. The strengths model was perhaps the first to offer an alternative to the clinical and rehabilitative orientation previously described.

Six key principles underpin the Strengths Model (Rapp & Goscha, 2012):

1. *People with psychiatric disabilities can recover, reclaim and transform their lives*. This principle sets expectations about people's continuing agency in their social and everyday life. It challenges ideas (based in biological psychiatry) that can highlight neurological or cognitive impairment, that are sometimes associated with expectations of psychosocial decline. This principle is aligned to more current understandings of neuroplasticity and recovery in mental health (Kays, Hurley, & Taber, 2012).
2. *Focus is on individual strengths rather than deficits,* not pathology, symptoms, weaknesses, problems or deficits. The understanding is that solving problems at best restores a person to the status quo, whereas developing her or his strengths and encouraging her or his dreams and aspirations leads to growth and accomplishments. Another benefit of focusing on strengths is that one is more likely to uncover the uniqueness of an individual than if one focuses on the person's deficits, which may be common to a large group of similarly disabled.

3 *The community is viewed as an oasis of resources*, not as posing obstacles for clients and case managers to overcome. The wider community is the source of mental health, providing a wealth of opportunities for social interacting, belonging and contributing. There are far more naturally occurring resources than those that can be provided by mental health teams and specialist programs. The emphasis is on engaging people in existing, ordinary services, as opposed to creating targeted services only for use of people within a disability group.

4 *The client is the director of the helping process.* Self-determination is described as a cornerstone of the model. No actions are taken without the client's approval. The client has the right to determine the form and direction of help received, and to make mistakes and to learn from them.

5 *The worker-client relationship is primary and essential.* This principle identifies the contrast between strengths case management and programs that ignore or even prohibit the development of a relationship. The case manager needs to be there beside the client when the going gets tough, and not just by appointment or in office hours. The client needs someone to confide in, to share in her or his struggles and achievements.

6 *The primary setting for our work is the community.* In other words, it is preferable to see the client in the park, the home or a cafe, than to see the person in the office. Case managers and clients learn a lot more about each other this way than from always being based in practitioner or home contexts.

Most widely implemented in the United States within the community support sector, strengths model case management teams are generally small and have intensive caseloads, comparable with ACT teams elsewhere (Rapp & Goscha, 2012). Centred at Kansas University, a research and development team provides training and assists in fidelity and progress evaluations, for services that take up the strengths model in a range of settings.

In Australia, strengths-focused models of practice have arisen, aligned to the national and state policy directions for recovery-orientated models of care.

AN AUSTRALIAN CASE EXAMPLE OF STRENGTHS-FOCUSED CASE MANAGEMENT

St Vincent's Mental Health in Melbourne is one clinical mental health service in Australia that has adopted the strengths model (Chopra et al., 2009; Slade, 2009b; Petrakis et al., 2013). The organisation enlisted the support of a service in Timaru in the South Island of New Zealand to mentor senior staff and provide training throughout the implementation. The key leaders in Timaru had several years of experience with the model and ties with its proponents in Kansas.

The elements of *strength assessment, goal planning and strengths-orientated* staff supervision are core to the model implemented at St Vincent's. Compared to the *individual service plans* (ISPs) implemented as part of case management practice in the 1990s (for further explanation, see *Mental Health Services: Case Managers* at www.betterhealth.vic.gov.au), the trainers and the clinicians identify several differences in practice with *goal plans* as used in this model. First, while ISPs identify client goals, these are blended with clinician-identified priorities, whereas goal plans put first the (usually nonclinical) goals of the consumer. Second, in conventional clinical documents, consumer strengths are most often identified as mitigating factors in risk assessments or relapse prevention plans, rather than as central attributes to work with.

Likewise, clinicians report that team meetings and supervision sessions take a different character from their past experience, with a greater emphasis on brainstorming ideas and rarely on probing problems.

At St Vincent's Mental Health, aspects of ongoing evaluation include: fidelity audits and evaluations of outcomes; looking at psychosocial outcomes for consumers; and economic outcomes for the organisation. In a qualitative interview study co-produced with consumer researchers (Hamilton, Bichara, Roper, & Easton, 2012), consumers of the service identified the elements that they value in strengths case management as: the friendly and positive tone of the case management relationship; accessibility of case managers; and practical assistance to achieve goals. These align with essential features identified by Rapp and Goscha (2012). Consumers also identified less satisfactory or problematic areas as: too much emphasis on medication; and the undermining impact of lack of choice, associated with legally mandated treatment such as via community treatment orders (Hamilton et al., 2012).

Beyond clinical services, St Luke's, a large health and welfare provider in Central Victoria, has embraced and implemented the strengths model since early 2000s across wide-ranging services provided to diverse populations, including children, families, youth families and people with mental health problems. St Luke's services are free and available to people regardless of their beliefs and backgrounds. It is a hub for strengths model training in the region and a source of strengths-oriented casework resources (St Luke's Innovative Resources, 2019).

There is scope for the strengths model to be widely applied in Australian settings. Rapp and Goscha (2012) offer explicit guidance to service providers addressing the deficit-oriented requirements of Medicaid, so that strengths case management can be funded under that scheme. These recommendations are potentially useful also in the Australian context, if services are to deliver case management through the National Disability Insurance Scheme.

EVIDENCE SUPPORTING THE STRENGTHS MODEL

The evidence for the strengths model has been modest but has grown steadily since the early 1990s, to include a variety of quasi-experimental evaluation studies with a pre-post design, between-group comparison, or secondary data analyses, and one RCT. The lack of comparable studies hampers the potential of meta-analysis to compare outcomes of strengths model versus other approaches to case management (Ibrahim, Michail, & Callaghan, 2014).

A critical review by Tse et al. (2016) confirmed both the feasibility and relevance of implementing a high-fidelity strength-based approach in clinical settings. All research to date has tended to focus on the social outcomes and achievement of consumer goals; that is, the model does not primarily claim or show greater improvements in psychiatric symptoms. Seven studies provided some evidence that the use of a strength-based approach improves outcomes including hospitalisation rates, employment/ educational attainment, and intrapersonal outcomes, such as self-efficacy and sense of hope. Björkman and colleagues (2002) undertook the only RCT in Sweden, confirming goal achievement and concluding that there is an economic advantage for service providers associated with the strengths model, but no clear social or symptom advantage, compared with other service models.

A recent non-randomised controlled trial of Strengths Model Case Management in Hong Kong (Tsoi et al., 2019) found that service users progressed towards recovery goals. The approach was also highly valued by workers; the model was considered by them to be protective for burnout, a finding which is important for the sustainability of this practice. However, high quality experimental studies are still needed, to robustly examine the effectiveness of strength-based approaches. A recently commenced randomised controlled trial in China (Xie, Yuan, Cui, & Yen, 2015), is further testing the outcomes of the strengths model of case management, in terms of recovery experience of the service users.

Like other approaches to case management in this text, the strengths model of case management cannot be a panacea for enabling recovery. Reflecting on 30 years of strengths approach, Rapp and Goscha identified wider social challenges that limit the impact of individualised approaches:

> A focus on strengths will never ignore that there are economic and social conditions that affect the wellbeing of those with mental illness. Poverty, unemployment, discrimination, social exclusion, disparities in health care etc can be far more disabling for people than symptoms associated with a mental illness. ... But we cannot wait for

> economic and social justice to occur before we help people use the power of their own strengths and existing strengths of the community to impact their life. This would be an equal injustice (Rapp & Goscha, 2015, p. 35).

Focusing on growth at an individual level does not negate the requirement for ongoing social change to redress inequities that will always undermine most those with the least advantage. But a strengths approach is attractive to consumers and workers alike, for its potential to avert pessimism, stem further disadvantage and enhance recovery.

2.4.7 INTENSIVE CASE MANAGEMENT: ASSERTIVE COMMUNITY TREATMENT TEAMS

CAROL HARVEY

Assertive community treatment (ACT) programs were developed in Wisconsin in the United States (Stein & Test, 1980) to work with consumers with severe mental illnesses who were at risk of frequent hospitalisations, and who were unable or unwilling to attend community mental health centres for treatment. Often such consumers are not taking medication consistently and reliably; have symptoms that are resistant to treatment; experience frequent crises; are isolated because of limited social networks; and do not engage effectively with mental health services. They may also require assistance with daily living tasks, such as shopping, paying bills and maintaining their living environment. In addition, their families may be under stress and struggling to cope with how best to offer support.

CRITICAL ELEMENTS OF ACT

ACT teams provide *intensive case management* (ICM), visiting a consumer as often as several times a day when there is a crisis, and the ratio of case managers to consumers is generally around 1:10. However, it is misleading to think of this approach as solely about intensive case management, since the ACT model seems to rely on a number of other critical elements for its effectiveness (Burns et al., 2007; Catty et al., 2002). These critical elements are:

- integrated health and social care
- extended hours of operation
- in vivo contact (or home visiting) and
- a team-based approach (Burns et al., 2007; Catty et al., 2002).

Case managers in effective ACT teams address the consumer's social as well as health care needs, providing rehabilitation focused on participating in the community, such as access to employment, assisting the consumer to negotiate the health care system, and working where necessary with other service providers, family members and landlords (integrated health and social care). ACT teams operate an extended-hours service, seven days a week. Another critical element involves reaching out proactively ('assertive outreach') to engage with consumers in their own communities (Ryan & Morgan, 2004). Therefore, the majority of the work typically involves in vivo contact in consumers' homes and localities rather than at mental health facilities. Finally, the team-based approach involves ACT clinicians meeting together daily, or even twice daily, to plan and share responsibilities for their work with consumers. This feature of the ACT model enables frequent discussion of ideas about how to engage and work effectively with consumers (Killaspy et al., 2009), as well as providing better continuity of care and mitigating the adverse impact of changes of key workers (Davidson & Campbell, 2007). ACT research continues to confirm the importance of this team-based approach to better outcomes (e.g., van Vugt et al., 2011).

IS ACT EFFECTIVE?

The Cochrane review of ACT (Marshall & Lockwood, 1998) reported that, compared with consumers receiving standard community care, those receiving

ACT were significantly more likely to remain in contact with services and significantly less likely to be admitted to hospital. They also spent less time as an inpatient. It is important to note, however, that reduction in time spent in hospital was only experienced by consumers who were high users of hospital care over the previous 12 months (Burns et al., 2007). This indicates that the ACT model is only appropriate for a subgroup of consumers, usually around one in five, or one in 10 of people living with severe mental illnesses. A corollary of this is that, although early studies suggested that consumers should receive time-unlimited services, in practice consumers are seen less regularly when they are stable, and if this continues, transfer to a community mental health program is arranged. The early randomised controlled trials conducted within the United States were soon followed by successful replications and service evaluations in Australia that also reported good outcomes for consumers, including more stable housing and better employment rates (Hambridge & Rosen, 1994; Hoult, 1986; Issakidis, Sanderson, Teeson, Johnson, & Buhrich, 1999). This has led to widespread implementation of the model in Australia. For example, ACT teams were established throughout Victoria since the mid-1990s, where they are known as mobile support and treatment (MST) teams, although some have been closed or reconfigured into 'diluted' forms more recently. The equivalent teams in Queensland are called mobile intensive treatment (MIT) teams and in Western Australia, intensive community (rehabilitation) outreach teams (ICOT). These continue to operate.

The case for the efficacy of ACT in Europe has been less clear and may be partly responsible for the closure or reconfiguration of some ACT teams in Australia and elsewhere (Rosen, Killaspy, & Harvey, 2013). Overall, the findings suggest that consumers remain in contact, and express greater satisfaction with ACT services than with comparison care, without the other beneficial outcomes reported in the United States and Australia (Killaspy et al., 2006; Sytema, Wunderink, Bloemers, Roorda, & Wiersma, 2007). Various explanations have been advanced for this failure to detect an effect of ACT in some countries. It is difficult to conduct research when the health care and social support systems of these countries are quite different. Thus, a beneficial effect would be unlikely to be detected if the comparison care in a particular country was of a higher standard than in the original trials. ACT teams that were not established for long enough or followed up for a sufficient period to obtain significant outcomes, or not operating closely enough to the original ACT model, may also provide some explanation for divergent findings. For example, there is some evidence that there are differences in implementation of critical elements of ACT (home visiting, team-based approach) between London and Melbourne (Harvey et al., 2011).

Intensive case management (caseload < or = 20) has been compared with non-intensive case management (caseload > 20) for people with severe mental illnesses in the latest Cochrane review (Dieterich et al., 2017). Most of the ICM interventions were modelled on the ACT approach. The authors reported that ICM was effective in reducing hospitalisation, improving social functioning and increasing retention in care. Like previous reviews of ACT, this review concluded that ICM is of value at least to people with severe mental illnesses who are in the subgroup of those with a high level of hospitalisation (about four days per month in the past two years). It also supported previous reports that the intervention works best when it closely resembles the original ACT model (Dieterich et al., 2017). The latest developments in assertive community treatment include adapting the model for other consumer groups; for example, most specialised early psychosis programs now include ACT principles (e.g., Nordentoft et al., 2015; Rosen et al., 2013). ACT has been trialled as an adjunct to other service models e.g. Housing First for homeless individuals with severe mental illness (Aubry et al., 2016) and is increasingly disseminated across low and middle-income countries in the Asia-Pacific region and elsewhere (e.g., Lee et al., 2015).

Assertive outreach and intensive case management may be integrated functions of the community mental health team in parts of Australia, especially in regional and rural areas. Increasingly, this approach to service delivery is being adopted in metropolitan areas. These developments may mirror the emergence of international variants of ACT such as Function ACT (FACT) in the Netherlands and UK. Research into these models is still limited although comparable outcomes to ACT for consumers living with severe mental illnesses have been reported (Drukker et al., 2011; Firn, White, Hubbeling, & Jones, 2018; Firn, Alonso-Vicente, et al., 2018; Rosen et al., 2013). Given the latest Cochrane findings, it will be important to monitor the extent to which these developments are in line with the ACT model and to evaluate whether they offer similar benefits to consumers and families and to understand their relevance to different health care and social support systems. More research into the features of ICM that may improve outcomes for consumers is certainly required (Dieterich et al., 2017; Harvey et al., 2011).

EXPERIENCE OF ACT SERVICES

The success of the ACT model in helping clinicians engage with previously marginalised consumers, many of whom have experienced inadequate help from mental health services in the past, should not be ignored (Killaspy, 2007). Interestingly, the qualitative literature suggests that ACT clinicians use more collaborative approaches than clinicians working in other community mental health teams (Angell & Mahoney, 2007). They are also more informal, flexible and responsive, and provide more help with practical issues and informal support to families (Killaspy et al., 2009; Krupa et al., 2005). These observations might partly account for the success of ACT clinicians in engaging consumers and are reinforced by available qualitative research exploring the perspectives of consumers receiving ACT services.

Box 2.5: Positive experiences of consumers receiving ACT services

'Gentle persistence' and assertiveness

'They just stuck with me.' One of the most striking aspects of the interview with Nikki related to her appreciation of the persistence of ACT staff. She noted, 'They kept showing up ... they didn't drop me or let me get off the medications ... they didn't give up ... they just stuck with me' (Chinman et al., 1999, p. 151).

Building trust and relationships, and breaking down isolation

'We've got somebody that we can rely on when we need them. And if we're not in need of them they're still there helping us' (Krupa et al., 2005, p. 20).

Jill believed that it was when her clinician and the rest of the team started to get to know her that she could then trust what they were saying and begin to give up her world of isolation and daily drinking. As a result of that trust, she then began to allow her clinician to become her 'guide to the psychiatric world' (Chinman et al., 1999, p. 151).

'I anticipate them coming to the door because I don't have many friends, you know' (Krupa et al., 2005, p. 20).

Assistance with negotiating the illness in the community

'You feel safe knowing the staff will recognise the symptoms before you do and help keep you out of hospital by giving you treatment' (Krupa et al., 2005, p. 21).

Assistance with meeting goals and promoting growth and change

Participants expressed the need for ongoing self-development ('Being sustained isn't good enough'), to get out and do 'more normal things' such as work, volunteering, recreation, saving money, getting a driver's licence and socialising (Krupa et al., 2005, p. 21).

Source: Adapted from Chinman et al., 1999; Krupa et al., 2005

Key elements of ACT that consumers associated with improvement were: the persistence demonstrated by ACT clinicians in engaging their clients; the trust that clients developed in their clinicians; and, as a result, the process by which their clinicians became 'guides' to the world of psychiatric and social services that further facilitated their clients' community adjustment (Chinman, Allende, Bailey, Maust, & Davidson, 1999). Although consumers' experiences of ACT are positive overall, some of the tensions inherent in receiving ACT services are also described by Krupa et al. (2005), including stigmatising aspects of the service and authoritative and controlling practices of individual staff. See Box 2.5 for examples of positive consumer experiences.

A number of commentators argue that the ACT model is only a vehicle for the delivery of treatment of adequate content and quality (Issakidis et al., 1999; Rosen, Mueser, & Teesson, 2007). Thus, its success is likely to depend on the extent to which clinicians are equipped to provide rehabilitation and evidence-based psychosocial interventions, such as vocational rehabilitation and family psychoeducation (see Chapters 2.6, 2.7). In this respect, clinicians in Melbourne and London have recognised that they have training needs in these areas (Harvey, Killaspy, Martino, & Johnson, 2012). A recent Dutch study (Sytema, Jörg, Nieboer, & Wunderink, 2014) concluded that delivering evidence-based interventions to consumers receiving ACT was not particularly feasible, suggesting difficulties in implementing quality care require further investigation. Many of the aforementioned approaches used by ACT clinicians to engage with consumers are also consistent with recovery-informed practice. Further, it is noteworthy that even though this work is intensive and potentially challenging for clinicians, they are mostly satisfied with the work and do not experience significant burnout (Harvey et al., 2012). The team-based approach may provide supportive and constructive containment in working with challenging clients, a finding echoed by mental health professionals working in the FACT model (Harvey et al., 2011; Killaspy, 2007; Killaspy et al., 2009; Lexén & Svensson, 2016). Further evaluation of the benefits of this team-based approach for consumers, carers and clinicians could be helpful.

Earlier in this chapter, we highlighted differing ways in which case management may be conceptualised. It should be apparent that the organisational context and client group with whom case managers are working each also shape the practice of case management.

2.4.8 BEING A CASE MANAGER

JAZ CHISHOLM & MELISSA PETRAKIS

Being a case manager in a contemporary mental health setting requires the ability to balance facets of entrenched and evolving practice, which reflect clinical and recovery oriented practices informed by evolving evidence, policy and legislative frameworks. Recovery-oriented practice (RoP) is the guiding practice framework across mental health services, and follows policy direction set nationally (Australian Government Department of Health, 2013; Australian Health Ministers' Advisory Council, 2013) and at state level around the country. All states and territories have produced reports and plans for implementing RoP that embrace recovery values and principles, albeit in slightly different ways, and guide the ways in which case managers and other mental health workers practice.

Australia's national recovery-oriented practice policy and service framework includes the following principles: using language of hope and optimism; connectedness; person first and holistic treatment, inclusive of age, race, gender, sexual orientation, and religion; dignity, respect; real choices; uniqueness of the individual; identity; meaning; challenging stigma and discrimination; rights; collaboration; communication; empowerment; and evaluating recovery (Australian Government Department of Health, 2013; Oades et al., 2017). This framework places considerable expectations on case managers, in terms of their skills, knowledge and confidence, especially given they work with people whose experiences of mental health issues vary and at differing times during their recovery journeys, as well as in mental health services that may be variable in resources and organisation. Consumers may also be grappling not only with other comorbidities, such as substance use issues or forensic issues, metabolic and other physical health concerns, but also with challenging social conditions such as poor housing, poverty, inability to find employment, and limited social support. These issues can also make case management more complex.

The overall tasks in the work of being a case manager are to find a way to connect with each individual, to create hope and opportunities for growth by supporting each person to see his or her potential, make choices and to strive towards self-directed goals. Here, the national framework for recovery-oriented mental health services (Australian Health Ministers' Advisory Council, 2013) guides practitioners, such as case managers, to follow recovery focused principles in working with people to support their recovery.

THE ROLE

Case management involves the provision of services, including engagement with consumers and their family and/or support people to work with them towards self-directed goals, using the recovery model of the service. Working with families and support people is a very prominent and important part of case management as families and support people have a wealth of knowledge about their family member and provide a substantial amount of care and encouragement to their loved one. Case managers work closely with families and support people and may not always agree but with the consumer at the centre of care, a resolution to best suit the consumer while considering risks is achieved. Applying for and liaising with support services is a part of a case manager's role. More recently, this includes supporting consumers to apply for and access personalised supports through the National Disability Insurance Scheme (NDIS) (Quinlan, 2014; Williams & Smith, 2014); and for people who are not deemed eligible for an NDIS package, finding alternative services and supports.

Case managers also complete psychosocial and risk assessments with the person to identify needs for care and support; provision of psychoeducation about factors affecting mental health issues negatively and positively, for example illicit substances and alcohol, side effects including metabolic, lifestyle behaviours, and family issues and education. A case manager works collaboratively with the person and other team members, sometimes a registrar and a consultant psychiatrist. They also undertake regular reviews, write reports and complete other documentation related to consumer wellbeing and progress, as required by the service.

Evidenced-based practices undertaken by case managers may also include family therapy using a 'systemic framework', working with dual diagnosis using 'motivational interviewing' (Petrakis, Robinson, Myers, Kroes, & O'Connor, 2018), relapse prevention programs using 'Early Warning Signs' (Birchwood, Spencer, & McGovern, 2000), psychological therapies like 'cognitive behavioural therapy' and parenting programs like 'Let's Talk About Children' (Kujala, Jokinen, Ebeling, & Pohjola, 2017; Tchernegovski, Reupert, & Maybery, 2015) (see Chapters 2.6, 2.7 for further details). Case managers may also take on a portfolio needed by the service in terms of specialisation areas in some positions around Australia. These tasks will vary between services, but examples include: leadership of change toward RoP; support for setting up specific service developments, such as peer-facilitated support group for consumers and families; and leadership of initiatives to promote better linkages with local housing or employment services.

Mental health recovery is a unique experience, and from a recovery-oriented point of view changes the ways in which case management and clinical practice are now applied. For example, a person with mental health issues may prefer to take a lower dose of medication to reduce its unpleasant side effects, even though this may mean continuing to experience a degree of symptoms. The team working in a recovery-oriented way would support this person to make this decision him or herself and respect his or her choice, including by providing information about options, such as medications that may have fewer side effects and other strategies that may assist in managing ongoing symptoms or side effects. This represents a more collaborative way of working than traditionally practised in the clinical realm, where managing symptoms was seen as predominantly the aim and expertise of clinicians.

Being a case manager is therefore a powerful place from which a recovery stance can be taken and fostered within the team. A case manager can advocate for a person's choices in managing their mental health. This may be in a case meeting where the worker is providing feedback to clinical or other staff based on what the consumer has said about their treatment preferences and recovery. An effective working alliance between a consumer and case manager goes a long way to creating possibilities for good outcomes and self-determined goal achievement. There has been a history of a 'one-size-fits-all' approach where people were placed in groups or programs without choice, perhaps because these programs were perceived as beneficial by staff. For example, a walking group may be experienced as paternalistic irrespective of the intentions behind running it. While this may be well-intentioned, recovery oriented practices are characterised by ensuring choice and assuming people are the experts in their own lives. Hence, it is important that people are informed through various means, so that they can make their own choices.

Case managers bring their own personal opinions, beliefs, cultures, experiences and professional perspectives to their practice. Therefore, self-awareness and a non-judgemental stance are important. Having a growth mindset for oneself and the consumer and family, with whom one is working, is important for hope and optimism in recovery. Having a growth mindset means believing one's most basic abilities can improve through effort and encouragement (Oades, Crowe, & Nguyen, 2009). Derived from positive psychology, Dweck (2008) coined the term 'growth mindset' to distinguish this concept from a fixed mindset. If a person has a fixed mindset, they do not believe in their capacity to cultivate their abilities, whereas a person with a growth mindset does. One can develop a growth mindset whereby one can acquire knowledge and resilience for discovering new knowledge and ways of being (Dweck, 2008).

THE LEGAL ASPECTS OF CASE MANAGEMENT

Mental health legislation underpins the rights of consumers and their families or support people, and directs the approach to decision making and judgements about capacity that can be legally made in relation to persons with mental illness. In Australia, this legislation varies between states and it is important the case managers are familiar with the mental health legislation that applies to their practice. Persons with mental illness may be subject to involuntary treatment orders by law in certain circumstances. For a case manager, it can be tricky to maintain an effective working alliance at times when a consumer is subject to involuntary treatment and in the aftermath. Managing the autonomy and rights of this person alongside risks and your legal role and professional ethical duty of care can be challenging, especially when family and support people are also involved and naturally also have their own views, suggestions and preferences about how to best support a loved one. For a more detailed discussion about working with consumers' subject to community treatment orders under mental health legislation, see Section 2.4.11.

WORKING WITH THE BROADER MENTAL HEALTH SECTOR AND OTHER SERVICES

A further aspect of being a case manager involves working with other services within and beyond the mental health system. For instance, this may include liaison with inpatient services to plan for safe and effective discharge when consumers require hospital care for a period; or working with a crisis assessment and treatment team to support a consumer to manage a relapse or crisis without an admission.

Another important role in case management involves linking consumers, families and carers with other services and supports. This may include referring consumers for ongoing follow-up by a general practitioner and linking them to other services that provide group support, one-to-one support. An individual's support plan may include study and work goals, recreational pursuits and connecting with family and friends. There also may be coordination of care when a person has several needs. For example, a person may need referrals to legal services, other health services (e.g., for psychological therapies, diabetes management), housing and/or employment assistance. A case manager may refer to and work in coordination with these services to ensure comprehensive planning and care. Services such as Partners in Recovery (PIR) (Brophy et al., 2014) and the Primary Health Networks (PHNs) also assist case managers in coordinating these services and provide extra supports like primary mental health nurses (see Chapter 1.7). Similarly, with the implementation of the National Disability Insurance Scheme (NDIS) to enhance personalised care, individual choice and access to resources for full participation in community life, case managers also need to liaise with other services and support workers involved in the provision of supports to consumers with psychosocial disability who are eligible for NDIS funding (see Chapter 1.7, where the NDIS is discussed).

2.4.9 FUNDAMENTAL THERAPEUTIC RELATIONSHIP SKILLS IN MENTAL HEALTH PRACTICE

NEIL THOMAS & NIKOLAOS KAZANTZIS

The practice of case management is underpinned by interactions and relationships between consumers, families and service providers. In the absence of a working alliance or partnership, neither recovery-oriented practice nor any case management approach will be effective. Hence, relationships are central to case management practice, requiring awareness, reflection and skills and ongoing negotiation on the part of the case manager to balance common tensions that exist to some degree in all interdependent relationships: between dependency and self-sufficiency, doing for and doing with and enabling self-determination versus management (Longhofer et al., 2010). While the nature, focus and style of these relationships may vary in terms of the frequency and location of contact, as well as the types and complexity of the work involved (King et al., 2004), it is the quality of these interactions and relationships that are thought to be more important for effective case management than the number or frequency of contacts (Rapp & Goscha, 2012). Therefore, some understanding of the potential dynamics of relationships is necessary to enable case managers to: work effectively with clients, families, colleagues within teams and across services; respond effectively to the emotional content of interactions and relationships; appreciate and establish helpful relationship boundaries; and be aware of the role of power and its impacts in these relationships.

THE EVIDENCE BASE

The provision of treatment and support pivots on the relationship that develops between the mental health practitioner and the client. This has not been studied very well at all. If we consider the advances that have been made over the past 50 years in psychotherapy process research, we have not made all that many gains. The focus is still on the 'alliance', which is generally operationalised as client-therapist agreement plus the therapeutic bond. However more nuanced relationship features have been missed, including centrally important elements of evidence-based therapies, such as cognitive behaviour therapy, including collaboration, empiricism, and Socratic dialogue (Kazantzis, Dattilio, Dobson, & Beck, 2017).

The best evidence exists for the alliance, sometimes referred to a 'working alliance' or 'therapeutic alliance'. It is notable that the features introduced by Rogers (1957), now pervade thinking about all client-therapist relationships and every major evidence-based therapy (see Kazantzis, Dattilio, & Dobson, 2017 for a CBT example). There is widespread agreement that these features are fundamental to effective helping relationships:

- *empathy*: understanding and appreciating nuances of the client's experience
- *unconditional positive regard*: warm acceptance of whatever the client experiences, without condition
- *genuineness*: being oneself rather than enacting a contrived role with the client.

This is often mistaken to refer to the entire professional (or therapeutic) relationship between practitioner and client, but it is only part of it. In fact, following Bordin's (1979) definition, the alliance is generally operationalised as 'agreement' about the goals of therapy, the tasks needed to attain those goals, and a therapeutic 'bond' comprising of mutual respect, positive regard, expressed empathy, and mutual liking. Adapted for the context of case management, these would include:

- *the relationship bond* between the practitioner and client: trust and attachment
- *agreement on goals of working together*, such as reduced anxiety, increased socialisation, return to study or work, preventing relapse
- *agreement on tasks or methods* to be used to achieve those goals, such as developing understanding of symptoms and what triggers them, developing alternate ways of coping, discussing past trauma, taking medication more regularly, investigating community supports to enable engagement in activities of interest.

In practice, goals or tasks can be difficult to navigate agreement on, or become misaligned during the course of the relationship, often without the practitioner realising. In psychotherapy research, there are robust, although small, correlations between the strength of client-rated alliance early in therapy and subsequent outcome, which is typically interpreted as evidence that the relationship contributes to the effectiveness of therapy (Cuijpers, Reijnders, & Huibers, 2019; DeRubeis, Brotman, & Gibbons, 2005; Kazantzis et al., 2018; Lorenzo-Luaces & DeRubeis, 2018). This has led to the American Psychological Association developing 'evidence-based therapy relationship' guidelines (Norcross, 2001; Norcross & Lambert, 2011) within specific therapeutic approaches or methods. These guidelines include communicating empathy and positive regard, collaboration, monitoring the alliance by requesting feedback from the client on the relationship and direction of therapy, and flexibility in implementing treatment protocols to adapt to client variability (Norcross & Wampold, 2011).

Fewer studies have been conducted on the practitioner-client relationship in mental health services, yet it appears no less relevant to routine mental health care (Howgego et al., 2003; Kirsh & Tate, 2006). Indeed, collaborative supportive relationships are commonly seen as integral to recovery-orientated service provision, as noted earlier in this chapter. There may be a number of challenges in forming collaborative relationships within these settings. Showing oneself to be reliable, empathising with the impact (rather than reality) of symptoms, focusing on shared goals and being cautious about being drawn into a persuading role in relation to treatment may be helpful in building workable therapeutic relationships. This may be particularly important with clients with poor awareness of their symptoms, who may have difficulties trusting others, or who are in receipt of treatment involuntarily (for more detail, see Section 2.4.11).

It is important to note that use of these fundamental therapeutic skills, also referred to as supportive counselling skills, do not represent a complete therapeutic intervention in their own right. Sometimes an artificial distinction is made between using these skills versus using therapy techniques. Contemporary thinking is that these skills operate more as a foundational 'layer' of practitioner behaviour on which intervention delivery (e.g., problem-solving, relapse prevention planning, suggesting new coping strategies) takes place. Consequently, these often feature as competencies in the context of the delivery of formal psychotherapies such as cognitive behavioural therapy, as well as in professional training (see Chapter 2.6).

DEVELOPING SUPPORTIVE THERAPEUTIC RELATIONSHIPS

Most case management and therapeutic practices begin with an initial 'stage' of engagement and assessment led by the practitioner. The aims of which are to lead to a preliminary formulation of the person's presenting issues and the establishment of shared goals, which are each important in guiding the course of further work together. However, due to the real-world pressures in the delivery of mental health services, practitioners often face challenges such as rapidly forming a relationship while conducting an initial intake assessment, or maintaining rapport while discussing risk management or medication adherence.

As a parallel, there may be a need to communicate an understanding of the overall structure of meetings (e.g., frequency and number; what they will generally involve), boundaries of confidentiality and commitment required. This is plainly respectful and reflects an ethical principle of 'informed consent'.

As services progress, practitioners need to pace and balance meetings appropriately to contain appropriate content while not overwhelming the person, either emotionally or with too much new information. In addition, they need to adapt their approach to the client, taking into account the broader person beyond the presenting issues. This may require judgement of the need to retain or promote the client's autonomy; addressing ambivalence about the process of change; encouragement of hope and self-efficacy, and consideration of client preferences for the degree of structure, self-expression, information, emotional support and so on during the course of meetings.

CORE COUNSELLING SKILLS

Beyond the establishment of a supportive working relationship, the counselling skills that form an important component of most helping relationships include: active listening (including use of nonverbal behaviour and simple verbal responses such as paraphrasing), questioning, reflecting and summarising. In the context of therapeutic interactions, questioning is used not merely as an information-gathering process, but also as a method for the practitioner to steer the process of talking in productive ways for the client. In particular, questioning can assist clients in elaborating upon their story, further exploring their difficulties, and at times directing their attention towards relevant issues that they might otherwise overlook. The use of a Socratic questioning style—in which the therapist guides clients in working things out for themselves, rather than providing a different perspective directly—is an embedded feature of most therapeutic approaches. Similarly, reflections can be used as interventions to guide the person in paying attention to particular themes or experiences.

If used over a course of sessions, counselling will typically progress from initial work focused on exploring clients' difficulties in order to help deepen their understanding, towards work that is more focused on developing new understandings, behaviours and experiences that result in adaptive change (see, for example, Egan & Reese, 2018). Finally, there may be a focus on maintenance of gains, managing setbacks, and on facilitating the client continuing independently following the completion of sessions.

In specialist mental health services, this work may face a few challenges. When clients are thought disordered, distractible or labile, the use of Socratic dialogue may be more challenging, although here the therapist may be serving a particularly important function in helping clients stay on track with their thinking (Kazantzis, Dattilio, & Dobson, 2017). There may be converse challenges in forming rapport and use of questioning when clients are affectively blunted or show poverty of speech, in which case more directive methods might be considered. A further challenge presented is that of ambivalence about change. This may be strong in persons with addictions or risk-related behaviour, where problems are often minimised or externalised. There may also be considerable difficulties contemplating making changes in persons with longstanding problems, where the person may be holding on to an equilibrium of just getting by, which would be threatened by change. This can easily lead to a dynamic emerging with the client expressing reluctance and the practitioner falling into a 'persuasion' role. Motivational interviewing (Miller & Rollnick, 2012) provides a detailed framework for strategic use of questions and reflections in order to sidestep this dynamic by 'rolling with the resistance' and building on the client's own consideration of change. This is increasingly becoming a core skill in working in mental health services (see, for example, Rosengren, 2017 for an accessible guide to skills).

Effective working relationships are also built on sensitivity to and respect for diversity, including in age, gender, sexuality, disability, spirituality, culture and language.

2.4.10 WORKING WITH INTERPRETERS

HARRY MINAS

When working with consumers, families and carers who do not speak fluent English, the interpreter is an essential member of the mental health team (see Sections 2.1.12 and 2.3.4). Mental health interpreting is a highly specialised skill, enabling accurate and effective communication between the consumer, family member or carer and mental health workers, such as case managers.

Interpreters translate the language used by the mental health worker and the consumer as accurately as possible, with the requirement that the interpretation conveys meaning and connotation as accurately as possible. It should be noted that many words (particularly in the mental health setting) do not have direct equivalents in different languages, so the interpreter's task is to accurately convey the meaning of what is being said. In some situations, such as when significant thought disorder is present and a person's speech is confused or incoherent, a word-for-word translation is the more accurate way of communicating the structure and content of his or her speech. Interpreters may need to be alerted that thought disorder, flight of ideas, or dysphasia may be present, and that, in such circumstances, they should translate it directly rather than attempt to impose structure or meaning to the person's speech. Here the mental health worker will be relying substantially on the interpreter's judgement, and may need to clarify certain issues with the interpreter either during or after the interview.

In mental health services the use of technical language and clinical jargon abounds. It relates to diagnosis (such as schizophrenia, bipolar disorder), symptoms (such as delusions, hallucinations) and treatment options (such as counselling, case management, electroconvulsive therapy, psychosocial rehabilitation, supported accommodation, disability support). Names and acronyms for service programs (such as Acute Care Team (ACT) in Queensland or Crisis or Community Assessment and Treatment Team (CATT) in Victoria) are frequently used by staff without explanation and are often confusing to consumers, families and carers. The use of these types of technical terms should be avoided as far as possible when communicating with consumers, families or carers, so as to promote clear communication and understanding. If the use of technical terms is unavoidable it is essential that the terms are fully explained in clear non-technical language, and that the mental health worker checks that the meaning of the terms is fully understood. Remember that, while the interpreter is a professional partner in the interpreted session, the interpreter is usually a generalist, and not specially trained or educated in mental health issues or terminology. Hence, the use of clear non-technical language is important to assist the interpreter to enable accurate and effective communication, given many technical terms will either not have a direct equivalent in the second language, or the equivalent terms may not be widely used or understood.

It is important to stress to the consumer, family or carer (and the interpreter) that all information is confidential. Interpreters are bound by a clear code of ethics to ensure that they maintain confidentiality in their work, but many consumers, families and carers are unaware of this. Concern about what happens to information divulged in the presence of an interpreter may be based on past experience; for example, where unqualified staff, or relatives, or bilingual cleaners or administrative staff have been asked to interpret. This is a particularly important issue for small immigrant and refugee communities where an interpreter and consumer may be known to each other. It may also be an issue in communities that are divided along religious, political or ethnic lines, and where there may be animosity or conflict between the groups with which the consumer and interpreter are identified. Maintenance of confidentiality is a relevant consideration for all members of staff, including mental health workers, administrative staff and interpreters.

Where there is a high degree of stigma concerning mental illness within a community, consumers may not want to be identified as having a mental illness (or having a family member with a mental illness) (see Chapters 2.3.4 and 2.7). This may result in the consumer, family or carer being reluctant to have an interpreter present in meetings with mental health workers, even if their English language skills are insufficient for effective communication.

Whenever possible the same interpreter should be called for a consumer. Where an interview has progressed well and trust has developed between the consumer, family or carer and the interpreter, working with the same interpreter is good practice. As far as is possible, the consumer, family or carer should not be presented with the challenge of re-establishing rapport with new interpreters. Feedback from consumers, families and carers about their attitudes to, or comfort with, a particular interpreter can be gained by telephoning them using the Telephone Interpreter Service in the case of spoken language interpreters, or using the National Relay Service to obtain feedback from deaf consumers.

WORKING WITH DEAF PEOPLE AND INTERPRETERS

Auslan (Australian Sign Language) is the language of choice for many deaf people, and is formally recognised in Australian federal policy as a 'community language other than English'.

There have been significant contributions to the area of mental health interpreting from Deaf interpreting services and training providers. The key national professional body representing the interests of Auslan interpreters is the Australian Sign Language Interpreters Association. Auslan interpreters will largely interpret simultaneously, with a small time lag; it is less common to interpret consecutively.

There are some specific issues to be aware of in relation to mental health interpreting with the deaf and hard-of-hearing community. It is important to consider aspects of Deaf culture, in addition to ethnic community cultures and other cultural variables, such as gender, age, social class, educational experiences, and communication preferences. Mental health workers should be aware that there is a highly articulated and unifying Deaf culture in Australia. Auslan is at the centre of Deaf culture, its single most unifying characteristic, and respect for Auslan is a core value. Another core value is that Deaf is normal–'in a room full of Deaf people, it is the hearing person who cannot sign who is disabled'. For deaf people, eye contact is extremely important, and it is acceptable to touch a person to gain his/her attention (a light touch on the arm or shoulder). Deaf people prefer to stand or sit further apart than hearing people, and facing each other, so they can see each other's 'signing' space. The mode of communication is generally more direct and may seem to hearing people to be blunt or abrupt. People who are part of Deaf culture are bilingual (fluent in Auslan and in written English) and bicultural.

Within the Deaf and the hard-of-hearing community, there are some necessary distinctions. 'Deaf community' refers to Auslan users who identify with the minority Deaf community, and use Auslan, regardless of the physiological hearing loss. Hearing-impaired people do not usually require interpreters, and do not identify with the Deaf community, but may still experience similar issues in regard to communication, comprehension, and access, particularly where technical jargon is used.

WORKING WITH REFUGEES AND SURVIVORS OF TORTURE

Interpreting when torture and trauma material is disclosed poses many challenges. The account of torture and trauma can be overwhelming and may evoke powerful emotional responses in the interpreter, particularly if the interpreter has had similar experiences. Interpreters may inadvertently alter their interpreting because they are trying to cope with the material, or because of discomfort with what the material conveys about events in their country of origin.

The pre-briefing with the interpreter should include information about the anticipated content of the interview. Interpreters will be better prepared to manage the traumatic nature of an interview if they are advised that they could find it upsetting. Interpreting in torture and trauma situations is often a new experience for interpreters. It can be helpful to establish ground rules and expectations of interpreters. On a practical level, a prior agreement should be made about how the interpreter should clarify anything that he or she does not understand, and how the interpreter should convey that he or she is becoming distressed or otherwise disturbed by the interview.

Debriefing with the interpreter regarding the emotional content of the session may also be necessary. You may need to initiate a debriefing, as many interpreters are reluctant to do so. If this is likely to be necessary, then the time needed should be thought about when making the booking for the interpreter.

Victorian Foundation for the Survivors of Torture Inc. have published *Rebuilding Shattered Lives* (Kaplan, 1998) to assist in the improvement of services to survivors of torture and trauma. The focus of the guide is on adults and the family.

For further information about trauma-informed care and working with consumers and families who have experienced trauma, see Section 2.3.9.

2.4.11 INVOLUNTARY TREATMENT IN THE COMMUNITY

LISA BROPHY & CATH ROPER

This section focuses on involuntary treatment in the community. Explanations are provided and best practice principles presented, with reference to supported decision making. Whether involuntary treatment in the community is effective and whether it should be used at all is discussed.

WHAT IS INVOLUNTARY TREATMENT IN THE COMMUNITY?

Involuntary treatment in the community (also known as outpatient commitment) is when people are given compulsory psychiatric treatment (usually medication) against their will while they are living in the community. Like most developed countries, all Australian states and territories have mental health laws that permit the provision of involuntary treatment in the community to people who meet certain criteria. These are legal orders known as community treatment orders (CTOs). Legislation varies between the states and territories in how CTOs are made, their duration, the periods between review as well as access to advocacy and external review (Brophy, Healy, & Maylea, 2018).

The issue of involuntary psychiatric treatment itself is the subject of ongoing critique and advocacy among the consumer/survivor movement, mental health law reformers and human rights activists. Cath Roper, as a person with lived experience of coercion in psychiatry, describes:

> If the state overrides my autonomy and bodily integrity, these are ethical wrongs, potentially with serious, multiple and ongoing consequences and they are a matter for regret, regardless of justification, or otherwise, for compulsory treatment (Roper, 2018, p. 85).

It is important to understand the ways in which human rights are different from consumers' rights under mental health legislation. Principally, CTOs can prevent consumers from exercising their human right to refuse treatment; they enable forced treatment; override a person's preferences and choices; and breach bodily integrity through the administration of that treatment (Roper, 2018). Whereas, under mental health legislation consumers' rights are likely to include, for example, having information, involvement in treatment decisions, access to advocacy and appeals processes,

IMPROVING PRACTICE

Awareness of human rights and acknowledgement of the ways in which CTOs violate these are essential foundations of a respectful, transparent relationship. Assisting consumers to express their views and preferences, and knowing how to access advocacy and legal services to challenge CTOs, are important skills. This is especially so in rural areas where there may be few services.

Box 2.6 outlines practice principles proposed by Brophy (cited in Fossey et al., 2012) and incorporates guidance from the UNCRPD related to supported decision making.

In line with the UNCRPD, contemporary mental health legislation is increasingly moving away from a 'right to health' foundation towards consideration of other human rights such as dignity and self-determination. Under the constraints of CTOs, this means implementing the principles of supported decision making that focus on the consumer's views and preferences. Kokanović and colleagues (2018) developed a model based on a large qualitative study to provide guidance regarding the implementation of supported decision making. The model begins with the use of legal mechanisms to support a person's decision-making authority, such as advance statements and nominated persons. Advance statements are documents written by the person capturing their treatment and other preferences (Henderson, Swanson, Szmukler, Thornicroft, & Zinkler, 2008; de Jong et al., 2016), while nominated persons are informal supporters nominated by a person to advocate for his or her preferences.

Workers and services need to have a continuous focus on how and why CTOs are being used. In these discussions, interpersonal skills such as being respectful, authentic and transparent, as well as cultural sensitivity, are important to facilitate opportunities for people to express and discuss their views and preferences (Brophy, cited in Fossey et al., 2012; Kokanović et al., 2018). The purpose of such discussions is to build genuine relationships and enable more opportunities for moving to less restrictive care. Questions to be mindful of include:

- What outcomes are important to enable the consumer to be discharged from the CTO?
- How can these best be achieved?
- How can I form relationships with consumers building on their strengths and interests?
- How can I address barriers to recovery and wellbeing, including the disempowerment that may be experienced as a result of the CTO itself?

Box 2.6: Practice principles related to supported decision making

- Acknowledge together with the person (and their family and other networks), ways in which involuntary treatment interferes with a person's autonomy and human rights.
- Regard involuntary treatment as a last resort and direct practice towards the person regaining control of their decision making.
- Ensure all consumers have access to information about their rights in a manner that is accessible and easy to understand. A brochure or written information complements a conversation and is not a substitute for this essential discussion.
- Be aware of and introduce consumers to legal mechanisms such as advance statements, nominated persons, second opinions and how to access advocacy.
- Work in respectful, authentic and transparent ways.
- Explore the meaning and impact of the CTO with the person (and their family and other supporters or networks).
- Build on strengths, hope, self-determination and empowerment.
- Reframe risk conversations to acknowledge the dignity of risk.
- Use supervision as a space to explore ethical and human rights tensions in practice.

- How will I continue to encourage hope, self-determination and empowerment?
- What is the meaning attached to the CTO and its impact on family relationships?

Empowerment can be facilitated through access to advocacy, second psychiatric opinions, peer support, and other strategies ensuring each person's expert experiential knowledge is heard and valued.

Management and leadership is required to promote culture change and support desired shifts in practice within mental health settings (Light et al., 2016). Supervision is a space to have supportive conversations about how to stay hopeful not fearful, and openly acknowledge the difficulties of practices that interfere with people's will and preferences.

Risk conversations

Good practice can involve having transparent and negotiated conversations about risk with consumers, as well as with family and other informal supporters, where the consumer wishes. For example, questions to consider include:

- How does the consumer define what's risky, for themselves?
- What are the risks to the person's autonomy, dignity, confidence and sense of future?
- What does the consumer say has worked in the past?
- What supports might the person require to mitigate risks?

Service providers should not be so overtaken by the pressure to manage risks that they avoid trying to minimise coercion. Minimising the use of coercion is important from a human rights perspective, and is likely to assist recovery (Mancini, 2007; Davidson, Brophy, & Campbell, 2016).

WHY ARE CTOS CONTENTIOUS?

There are three main reasons why CTOs are contentious. First, as already noted, they violate rights to refuse treatment, bodily integrity and other freedoms. Second, their effectiveness is in dispute (Brophy, Ryan, & Weller, 2018). Notions of what 'effectiveness' means are also hotly debated: according to whom and by what criteria? Third, there is critique about CTOs being used for the 'wrong' reasons.

Effectiveness of CTOs

Those who seek conventional and gold standard sources of evidence will find minimal support for CTOs. A recent randomised controlled study in the United Kingdom was unable to establish that CTOs were effective on a range of measures (Burns & Molodynski, 2014), and the subsequent Cochrane systematic review of the evidence found:

> no clear difference in service use, social functioning or quality of life compared with voluntary care or brief supervised discharge. People receiving CCT (compulsory community treatment) were, however, less likely to be victims of violent or non-violent crime. It is unclear whether this benefit is due to the intensity of treatment or its compulsory nature (Kisely, Campbell, & O'Reilly, 2017, p. 2).

Some Australian evidence has been used to try to support the ongoing use of CTOs, especially from cohort studies conducted in Victoria and NSW (Segal, Hayes, & Rimes, 2017a; Segal, Hayes, & Rimes, 2017b; Harris et al., 2019), but it is still not strong (Brophy, Ryan, et al., 2018; Ryan, 2019).

The most recent systematic review and meta-analysis again found that CTOs had limited impact on reducing readmission or length of inpatient stay, however, it did suggest CTOs influence people to take their medication and improved their access to community services (Barnett et al., 2018). In qualitative studies when people on CTOs are asked their views, participants often discuss the benefits of CTOs but also experiences of harm and distress, including that experiencing coercion and involuntary medication can lead to feelings of humiliation and oppression (Brophy, Ryan, et al., 2018; Corring, Apos, Reilly, & Sommerdyk, 2017; Nyttingnes, Ruud, & Rugkåsa, 2016). Hence, even if CTOs might help people stay out of hospital or improve their access to community services, there is considerable potential that CTOs may also be doing harm and impeding recovery.

Are CTOs being used for the 'right reasons'?

Shorter inpatient admissions are a common feature of contemporary mental health services which may contribute to increased use of CTOs. If inpatient beds are a precious resource, service providers may discharge consumers on CTOs, who otherwise would remain in hospital (Sawyer, 2008). Rather than strictly following legal criteria, service providers may support the use of CTOs where it is thought consumers would not otherwise engage voluntarily with services and agree to take medication (Munetz & Frese, 2001).

CTOs encourage an emphasis on compulsory medical treatment, particularly medication, and, at least in Australia, higher usage of antipsychotic medication administered by injection (Lambert, Singh, & Patel, 2009). These practices persist despite the contemporary focus on human rights and efforts to discourage forced psychiatric treatments. Achieving 'compliance' with treatment also persists as a goal in use of CTOs even though, as Thorne (1990) previously suggested, 'noncompliance' may be constructive for some consumers as they negotiate what works—and doesn't work—for them.

Current policy and law encourage 'the dignity of risk'—the idea that having a life of one's own choosing inevitably involves a degree of risk (Davidson, Brophy, & Campbell, 2016). Yet, concerns about serious harm from self-neglect or potentially dangerous behaviours often drive practice. Studies in Australia and internationally indicate that the use of CTOs can be a proxy for establishing a contract that guarantees community-based care between service providers and consumers (Brophy, Ryan, et al., 2018). For instance, consumers in a study by Brophy and Ring (2004) valued CTOs as a way to ensure help is available in a crisis; they also perceived that it would be easier to get back into hospital, if required, with less 'red tape' when on a CTO. This is a persistent theme in qualitative research about the use of CTOs (Corring et al., 2017).

Mental health service providers express frustration that economic constraints may lead to inadequate standards of care (King, Lloyd, & Holewa, 2008). So, if CTOs are being used as a substitute for service innovation or relationship building, it is people on CTOs who may be most affected. CTOs are commonly associated with a 'net widening' effect; that is, once they are introduced, their use expands beyond those groups for whom they were intended. Use of CTOs to resolve systemic deficits in skills and resources is problematic and may contribute to service cultures with a high tolerance for coercion. This would be inconsistent with contemporary directions in policy and law, especially the UNCRPD (Davidson, Brophy, Campbell, et al., 2016).

Should CTOs be used at all?

Whether CTOs should be used at all is increasingly contested, and there are calls for greater understanding of their potentially negative impacts. While CTOs have been adopted in many countries, including Australia, New Zealand, Canada, the United States and more recently the United Kingdom (Davidson, Brophy, Campbell, et al., 2016), other countries have resisted their introduction. For instance, in the Irish context (Brosnan, 2018), describes concerns about the potential for 'legislative creep' that may lead to the abuse of such powers.

Recovery principles emphasise self-determination and autonomy, as well as challenging the dominance of a biomedical approach to treatment that CTOs tend to encourage (Brosnan, 2018). Thus, the use of CTOs is seen as incompatible with the support for self-determination and respect for citizenship that is central to recovery orientated practice (Slade et al., 2014).

In conclusion, community treatment orders (CTOs) are a persistent feature of Australian mental health service delivery, despite evidence that the associated experiences of coercion and involuntary medication can lead to feelings of distress, humiliation and oppression. The use of CTOs is counter to the underpinning principles of the UNCRPD, which emphasise that people should be provided with the supports they need so they can make their own decisions. Evidence suggests that CTOs are over used, misused and their effectiveness is inconclusive. Furthermore, CTOs may not only impede recovery for consumers but also interfere with the adoption of recovery oriented practices by service providers. Systemic and individual advocacy are required to enable change. Decreased use of CTOs requires leadership of culture change.

2.4.12 COMMENTARY AND REFLECTIONS

ELLIE FOSSEY

Historically, the rise of case management was a response to the lack of coordination between mental health and other services in the community sector, as well as the complexity of the service system. These continue to present formidable barriers for consumers and families seeking care and support, as well as ongoing challenges in community mental health services to providing effective care.

Recovery-oriented perspectives and personalised and collaborative ways of working with consumers, families and carers call for the transformation of case management so that consumers are at the heart of all processes. The place of case management within the service system is also being challenged as a more diverse workforce evolves (such as with the growth of peer support roles) and differing approaches to care coordination are developed. Examples of this diversity include the implementation of Partners in Recovery (PIR) and the National Disability Insurance Scheme (NDIS). While practitioners bring many differing backgrounds to case management and care coordination, these roles involve shared areas of practice in coordination as well as developing and sustaining respectful and supportive working relationships with consumers, families and others.

2.5 PSYCHOPHARMACOLOGY

NICHOLAS KEKS, JUDY HOPE, GRAHAM MEADOWS & CARMELA SALOMON
(AUTHORSHIP BY KEKS, HOPE & MEADOWS, EXCEPT WHERE INDICATED)

2.5.1 INTRODUCTION

THE IMPORTANCE OF MEDICATION IN MENTAL HEALTH CARE

Use of medications is one of the three cornerstones of treatment for mental health disorders, together with the psychotherapies and social interventions. Use of psychotropic medication is ubiquitous in the community mental health setting. In a survey of an Australian inner urban community clinic, 77% of clients were being treated with an antipsychotic medication. One hundred per cent of ongoing clients of that service were being prescribed at least one psychotropic drug, and 72% were on two or more drugs (Keks et al., 1999).

While the importance of psychosocial factors in the aetiology and management of mental health disorders is a given, biological factors also make a contribution to the brain mechanisms underlying abnormal mental states. This is readily apparent at the most basic level from the psychological effects of substances such as stimulants or hallucinogens, which alter emotions and perceptions through action on brain neurotransmitters such as dopamine and serotonin. Physical illnesses affecting the brain range from endocrine disturbances such as thyroid disorders to tumours and infectious and immune disturbances such as HIV disease. These and brain injuries however acquired can result in emotional and behavioural changes that mimic mental illnesses such as schizophrenia and depression. (See Chapters 4.2 and 4.3.)

HISTORICAL CONSIDERATIONS

The use of substances to promote sleep, reduce anxiety, induce euphoria and alter consciousness dates back to antiquity. Medications for the specific treatment of mental disorders were mostly developed increasingly during the twentieth century. Among the first medications used to treat psychoses were opiates, stimulants like amphetamines and tranquillisers such as barbiturates. Antidepressant and antipsychotic drugs were then developed in the 1950s, followed by benzodiazepine anxiolytics and mood stabilisers (see Section 1.1.4).

All of the original psychiatric drugs were developed from serendipitous discovery, but neuroscientific research has now taken over and the development of new drugs is now a highly regulated scientific process, primarily undertaken by the pharmaceutical industry. Mechanisms of action in the brain for psychotropic drugs have gradually been elucidated, so that the development of new medications now occurs through a process of experimental development starting in the laboratory and proceeding through multiple levels of double-blind placebo-controlled trials until approval for therapeutic use from regulatory authorities is achieved (see Section 2.5.9). Subsequently there is post-marketing surveillance, as some of the adverse effects of new drugs will not become apparent until they have been used by many thousands of people for prolonged periods.

EFFECTIVE, WITH SOME QUALIFICATIONS

Psychiatric drugs have clearly demonstrated effectiveness, but in many cases, response is only partial. In psychoses, there is little doubt that many people who would previously have been institutionalised can now live in the community because drug treatment usually reduces the severity of psychotic symptoms. However, some psychotic symptoms persist despite treatment in a proportion of patients, resulting in chronic disability. This may be termed treatment-resistant illness, which affects many of the clients of mental health services. It is important to recognise another important cause of limited or non-response to a treatment. That is if the treatment is being applied in settings or for conditions where the evidence does not clearly support its use. If the diagnosis is incorrect, the treatment prescription not in line with evidence based practice or if it is being applied to a condition with milder severity that the states for which the evidence base is clear, then it is not rational to expect the prescription to bring about positive change.

Drugs are also quite imperfect with respect to side-effects, and many people experience major problems, particularly with long-term treatment. Some of the adverse effects are life threatening, such as the agranulocytosis and cardiomyopathy that may be caused by clozapine. Weight gain, diabetes and heart disease can also occur with a number of the newer antipsychotics, raising serious concern over long-term health consequences for consumers (see Section 4.2.4).

These two paragraphs make it clear that prescribing of medication should be done with awareness that to do so may for some people be a highly important and helpful intervention, but for some others there may be little or no benefit, and may cause harm. Two statistics used in evidence-based practice (see Chapter 1.4) may be helpful here. Both require specification of a specific outcome, desired or undesired (for example remission of depressive episode within eight weeks, or occurrence of disabling headache as a side effect). The Number Needed to Treat (NNT) then is the number of people on average who need to be given the treatment in order for one of them to experience the positive benefit while the Number Needed to Harm (NNH) is the number of people on average who need to be treated such that a harmful event will typically occur for one of them. The NNT and NNH are simply related to clinical trial statistics since the NNT is 1/(Absolute Risk Reduction) and the NNH is 1/(Absolute Risk Increase). In both clinical decision making and the discussions with patients that form such an important part of sound prescribing practice these can be helpful numbers to have to hand. Later on in the chapter, a worked example of application of the NNT (see Section 2.5.2) may help clarify the application of the statistic.

In the circumstances, it is reassuring to note that major epidemiological studies have found that antipsychotic medication actually has significantly improved the life expectancy of consumers, with improved outcomes for both general health as well as suicide. The benefits were strongest for clozapine. Duration of antipsychotic therapy was correlated with improving life expectancy, compared to no medication use (Tiihonen et al., 2009). A key principle in the use mental health medications is that the benefits must outweigh the risks.

This chapter will address some of the key issues surrounding use of medication (and briefly, some other physical therapies) relevant to community mental health practice. For detailed information on specific medications and treatment of particular disorders the reader is directed to standard textbooks such as the *New Oxford Textbook of Psychiatry* (Gelder, Andreasen, Lopez-Ibor, & Geddes, 2012; see also Sadock, Sadock, & Ruiz, 2017).

Table 2.12 Medications used to treat common symptoms and subsyndromes

Symptoms of mental disorder/subsyndrome	Drugs commonly used to treat
Anxiety	Anxiolytics, antidepressants
Agitation	Anxiolytics, antipsychotics
Depression	Antidepressants, anxiolytics, antipsychotics, mood stabilisers
Hostility and aggression	Antipsychotics, mood stabilisers
Positive symptoms (delusions, hallucinations, formal thought disorder, bizarre behaviour)	Antipsychotics
Negative symptoms (flat affect, poverty of speech, amotivation, impaired concentration)	Atypical antipsychotics
Mania	Mood stabilisers, antipsychotics, anxiolytics
Insomnia	Sedatives and hypnotics, some antidepressants and antipsychotics
Obsessional symptoms	Antidepressants

2.5.2 USING DRUGS FOR MENTAL HEALTH DISORDERS

GENERAL PRINCIPLES

Medications used to treat mental health disorders mostly fall into four main categories, according to predominant clinical effects:

- anxiolytic and sedative/hypnotic (mainly benzodiazepines, such as diazepam and temazepam)
- antidepressants (selective serotonin reuptake inhibitors (SSRIs), serotonin norepinephrine reuptake inhibitors (SNRIs), tricyclics (TCAs) and others)
- antipsychotic medications (typical and new generation atypical antipsychotic drugs)
- mood stabilisers (lithium, valproate, carbamazepine and lamotrigine).

However, there are a number of complications with this classification. There is poor correlation between the types of medication and the disorders for which they are used. For instance, anxiolytics may be used in anxiety disorders in addition to psychotherapy, but even more frequently, anxiolytics are used to treat anxiety and agitation in patients with acute psychoses such as schizophrenia and mania. The most commonly used medications in the treatment of anxiety disorders are actually antidepressants, which reduce anxiety over weeks of treatment.

Antidepressants are effective for depressive illnesses. However, mild reactive depressions do not tend to benefit from antidepressant medications; the treatment of choice is cognitive behaviour therapy. At the other end of the spectrum, severe psychotic depression will also not usually respond to antidepressant medication alone. Antipsychotic medications and mood stabilisers may need to be added to antidepressants to achieve a response, and the most effective treatment for psychotic depression is electroconvulsive therapy (ECT).

In fact, indications for various psychotropic medications correlate more accurately with symptoms and subsyndromes rather than overall disorders. Common symptoms and subsyndromes, and the medications that may be useful to treat those states, are listed in Table 2.12. While multiple medications are indicated for a particular clinical state, this does not mean that the medications have equivalent or even similar actions. Often the benefits of the different types of medication are complementary, so that there may be additive effects from using drugs together. However, simultaneous use of multiple drugs introduces the possibilities of increased side-effects and drug interactions, some of which can be dangerous. Use of multiple medications at one time is called *polypharmacy*, a term often applied with criticism of the prescribing practice and implied preference for simpler regimes.

Patients with schizophrenia and schizoaffective disorder may require antipsychotic, mood stabiliser, antidepressant, anxiolytic and sedative-hypnotic medications, not uncommonly all at once. Polypharmacy, as introduced above, is traditionally frowned upon; clinicians are urged to find a single effective drug. While clinicians should always try to rationalise medications to the simplest possible effective regime, the use of polypharmacy is now the rule rather than the exception in the treatment of psychotic disorders (Zink, Englisch, & Meyer-Lindenberg, 2010) as responses to monotherapy are inadequate in many patients.

When drugs from different therapeutic classes (such as antidepressants and antipsychotics) are added to each other, the strategy is called *augmentation*. When drugs from the same class are used together, treatment is termed *combination therapy*. The possibilities of problematic interactions and amplification of side-effects are in general greater for combination, rather than augmentation therapies.

There are also hierarchical rules for the use of psychotropic medications. People with psychoses are likely to be made worse if they are treated with antidepressant medications in the absence of initial stabilisation with antipsychotic medications. People in the depressive phase of bipolar disorder may become manic if given an antidepressant alone; mood stabilisation is first required.

While traditional mood stabilisers have been used for bipolar and depressive mood states for some time, recently it has become apparent that some of the atypical antipsychotics are also mood stabilisers (assisting mania, depression and mixed states), and are particularly advantageous in patients with bipolar disorder (see Section 4.3.5) who also manifest psychotic symptoms (about 60% of bipolar I patients). Antipsychotic drugs are now often used alone in mood disorders, but many patients require the simultaneous use of mood stabilisers and antipsychotic medications.

ANXIOLYTICS

Most anxiolytics are benzodiazepines, such as diazepam, oxazepam, alprazolam and clonazepam. These medications directly reduce anxiety symptoms soon after administration, and as such, often provide rapid relief from severe emotional distress. Benzodiazepines have a higher margin of physical safety than the older barbiturates, which were lethal in overdose, and have been widely abused. Clinical experience has revealed a tendency of benzodiazepines to cause dependence (the induction of tolerance and withdrawal on cessation) and addiction (excessive and usually harmful abuse of medications outside the parameters of medical advice). Clinicians try to minimise the use of benzodiazepines, and when unavoidable, use these drugs for short periods only. Side-effects include drowsiness, incoordination and impaired memory, so that using machinery and driving can be dangerous if benzodiazepines are being taken.

ANTIDEPRESSANTS

The original antidepressants were monoamine oxidase inhibitors (MAOIs), which have dangerous food and drug interactions, and subsequently, tricyclic antidepressants (TCAs). TCAs are still not infrequently used because of their possibly increased effectiveness in severe depression and in some older people, but have troublesome side-effects, such as impairment of heart conduction, dry mouth, constipation and weight gain. TCAs are also lethal in overdose.

In contrast to anxiolytics, which work immediately, antidepressants start working after weeks of continuing treatment. Antidepressants help symptoms of both depression and anxiety, and some help obsessional symptoms. Improvement may continue for up to 12 weeks of treatment. Good adherence to ongoing treatment is essential for effective use of antidepressants (as is also the case with antipsychotics and mood stabilisers).

The most commonly used antidepressants today are SSRIs, such as sertraline, escitalopram and especially in adolescents, fluoxetine. These medications are much physically safer than TCAs in most circumstances, but problems can occur in certain individuals with physical illness. Initial side-effects tend to be nausea, sleeplessness and nervousness. Paradoxically, some people can become agitated and develop suicidal thinking and self-harm impulses in the early part of treatment. This is particularly relevant for adolescents, who need to be monitored closely at treatment initiation. SSRIs tend to have a withdrawal syndrome if stopped abruptly, so it is best to withdraw the medications gradually.

SNRIS are also available, and include venlafaxine, duloxetine and desvenlafaxine. SNRIs may be more activating than SSRIs in some patients, and are commonly used in community mental health settings because of perceived better efficacy (generalisations about comparative antidepressant efficacy are unreliable due to individual and illness-type response variability). Side-effects are similar to those of SSRIs, but SNRIs can elevate blood pressure and may not be appropriate in patients with heart disease. Mirtazapine is often utilised for its sedative properties, but is prone to cause serious weight gain.

Antidepressants have been a focus of media attention lately with concern being raised about over-diagnosis and overprescribing, and with some suggestions that the effectiveness of the drugs has at best been overstated. The recent context in many countries including Australia has been of progressive increases in prescribing so that now as many as 10% of Australians may be taking these medications (Cipriani et al., 2018; Davey & Chanen, 2016). Sound clinical practice involves giving people the opportunity to benefit from psychotherapies as well as medications but this is not always done and sometimes it is not practicable. A prominent meta-analysis in *The Lancet* in 2018 presented compelling evidence that antidepressants have demonstrated effectiveness but it may be helpful to take a look at its findings through the perspective afforded by the evidence-based practice statistic of NNT introduced earlier (Cipriani et al., 2018). *The Lancet* analysis did indeed show that the 21 drugs examined typically were more effective than placebo with Odds Ratios (OR) favouring remission within eight weeks of depressive states of typically around 1.7. But let us consider in the worked example below what that OR statistic might mean from the perspective of the NNT (Centre for Evidence-Based Medicine, 2018).

Placebo response rates in psychiatry are often ~ 35%. So the odds of response to placebo are typically 0.35:0.65 = 0.53. With an OR of 1.7 this would mean the odds of response in the treatment condition would be around 0.9 (0.90/0.53=1.7). This equates to a 47% response rate. (47/53 = 0.9). So the Absolute Risk reduction for non-response is 12% (47%-35%); the Number Needed to Treat (NNT) is 100/12 = 8. The NNT statistic—usually expressed as an integer—necessarily can be heavily rounded and in this case: If eight people are treated with placebo we expect on average 3 to get remission in the time-period (~35%), while if eight people are treated with active treatment (here ADM) we expect on average 4 to get remission in the time-period (~47%). So on average one extra person out of eight has an early remission associated with ADM treatment as compared with placebo. The NNT is the group size threshold at which the ARR equates typically to an integer change in outcome, or to one additional person experiencing change compared with placebo. We usually don't treat fractions of people in medicine so it works with whole numbers with the intent that is makes for a more approachable statistic. Of course to the treating clinician this will typically look like a NNT of 2 because the ADM treatment also includes placebo effects.

This may sound like a pretty weak effect and certainly the patient receiving the medication as well as the clinician prescribing it would be unwise to rest entirely on this effect. Rather, judicious combination of a well-chosen psychotherapy with the antidepressant would be typically the better bet for a good response. But this may not correctly capture how these drugs work in different clinical settings. The antidepressants are typically more effective where the depression is more severe. A major meta-analytic study found that benefit of antidepressants over placebo increases with severity of depression symptoms, and may be minimal in mild or moderate symptoms. In very severe depression, the benefit of antidepressants over placebo is substantial (Fournier et al., 2010).

ANTIPSYCHOTIC MEDICATIONS

Antipsychotics result in the sustained reduction or elimination of positive symptoms of psychosis: delusions, hallucinations, formal thought disorder and bizarre behaviour among others (see Chapter 4.2). Antipsychotics can also be mood stabilising, antimanic, tranquillising, sedative-hypnotic and antidepressant, depending on the drug. Some have initial sedative and tranquillising effects (particularly quetiapine and olanzapine), but others (such as aripiprazole) can be activating. Antipsychotic drugs take weeks to months to exert full therapeutic effects.

Antipsychotics are classified into first generation (older drugs, also called typical) and second generation (more recently developed drugs, also called atypical) categories. Older antipsychotics, such as chlorpromazine and haloperidol, tend to cause movement disorders (extrapyramidal side-effects [EPS]) at the doses required for clinical effectiveness. Atypical drugs such as risperidone, olanzapine, quetiapine, aripiprazole, brexpiprazole, paliperidone, ziprasidone, amisulpride, lurasidone and asenapine are variably less likely to cause EPS at clinically needed doses. EPS include muscle spasms (dystonias), restless legs (akathisia), stiffness and slowing (pseudo-Parkinsonism) and abnormal movements (tardive dyskinesia). EPS can be tormenting, stigmatising and disabling. That most people with psychosis can now be treated without suffering EPS is a major therapeutic advance.

Unfortunately, new generation antipsychotics have their own major drawbacks. Most have a variable tendency to promote weight gain through an increased appetite, with a consequent increased risk of diabetes and other physical complications, including heart disease. Olanzapine and clozapine have the highest risk for weight gain while ziprasidone and lurasidone have the lowest risk. Patients taking atypical antipsychotics need to be regularly monitored physically, a responsibility usually undertaken by general practitioners. Case managers frequently need to ensure that appropriate monitoring is facilitated for their clients.

Antipsychotics have a variety of other side-effects that may come to the attention of community mental health staff. Loss of periods and sexual dysfunction occurs, particularly with risperidone, paliperidone and amisulpride. Dry mouth and dental problems can occur with a number of the drugs. Excessive sleepiness and dizziness on standing is a feature of quetiapine, olanzapine and some other antipsychotics.

Clozapine is the most effective antipsychotic. Because of its side-effects (sedation, weight gain, lowering of white cell count in the blood (agranulocytosis), dizziness on standing, and the potential for diabetes, heart problems and convulsions) clozapine is reserved for patients with treatment resistant psychoses. Despite the apparently dangerous side-effects of clozapine, this drug has been shown in a recent major epidemiological study to be the most effective antipsychotic in reducing mortality with long-term treatment far more effective than the untreated state, and proportionately more effective than any other antipsychotic (Tiihonen et al., 2009).

MOOD STABILISERS

> One of the things that baffles me ... how there can be so much lingering stigma with regards to mental illness, specifically bipolar disorder. In my opinion, living with manic depression takes a tremendous amount of balls. Not unlike a tour of Afghanistan (though the bombs and bullets, in this case, come from the inside). At times, being bipolar can be an all-consuming challenge, requiring a lot of stamina and even more courage, so if you're living with this illness and functioning at all, it's something to be

proud of ... They should issue medals along with the steady stream of medication.

Carrie Fisher

The first mood stabiliser, lithium, was developed by an Australian, John Cade. While working as the superintendent of Royal Park Hospital in Melbourne during the 1940s, Cade observed that lithium reduced manic excitement (Cade, 1949). Lithium remains one of the most effective treatments for bipolar mood disorder, but can cause serious toxicity through effects on the kidney, the function of which has to be carefully monitored with regular blood tests. The required dose of lithium is established through repeated serum levels. Lithium has a number of other challenging side-effects, including thyroid dysfunction, weight gain, thirst, excessive urination and skin disorders. It can also cause foetal abnormalities when used in the first trimester of pregnancy.

As a result, valproate (a drug developed for treatment of epilepsy) has been used more frequently, but it has its own challenges, not the least, serious and frequent foetal abnormalities, so that contraception needs to be carefully addressed in women of childbearing age. Carbamazepine (also an anticonvulsant) is another option that can cause serious effects on the blood (aplastic anaemia), albeit rarely. Lamotrigine is often useful for bipolar depression, but is not especially effective in the treatment or prevention of mania.

INITIATING DRUG THERAPY

Prior to initiating drug therapy, the issue of contraindications need to be addressed. Various medications used to treat mental health disorders can have serious physical consequences. Before initiating a number of the medications described above, relevant physical health and safety must first be established. This requires a physical history and examination, which may be obtained through a general practitioner as well as medical staff working in the mental health service. Some of the medications cannot be used in certain physical states: TCAs and SNRIs, and the antipsychotic ziprasidone, are relatively contraindicated in people with heart disease, for instance. Quetiapine and lithium can also be problematic where there is cardiac dysfunction. Liver and kidney impairment can be a barrier to the use of some drugs, and require dosage adjustment of others. Blood tests, including full blood examination, hepatic and renal function, thyroid function, blood glucose and blood lipids, can be useful as a baseline prior to initiating drug therapy.

2.5.3 OVERALL EFFECTIVENESS OF DRUG INTERVENTION

Psychiatric medications are among the most rigorously investigated treatments in modern medicine. No psychotropic would be approved for public availability by authorities such as the Therapeutic Goods Administration in Australia (the equivalent of the American Food and Drug Administration or the European Medicines Agency), without multiple, audited double-blind placebo controlled trials. Unethical practice by some in the pharmaceutical industry (such as failure to publish negative trials) is now less of a concern, since all clinical trials now need to be registered with regulatory authorities (see Section 2.5.9). The issue of possible bias in drug company-sponsored trials remains a concern, but again, such studies are rigorously audited by regulatory authorities.

The fact that a drug is statistically more effective than placebo, or equivalent to an existing treatment in a carefully supervised study with highly selected subjects usually excluding comorbid conditions such as substance use (though randomly allocated to drug and placebo groups) does not mean that full effectiveness will occur in a given patient. A way of approaching discussion of likely benefits and harms has been introduced earlier with the NNT and NNH statistics (see Section 2.5.9). Much pharmacotherapy remains an art, requiring a trial-and-error process of selecting the correct drug and finding the right dose for the particular individual, while monitoring carefully for side-effects, and providing support and psychoeducation to enhance adherence to treatment for the client and family.

Nonetheless, the scientific validity of the effectiveness of psychotropic medications for the treatment of mental health disorders is overwhelmingly established. There is a massive scientific literature reporting studies that have been undertaken investigating the efficacy of psychotropic drugs, for example. To facilitate overview of the available evidence, many meta-analytic studies (which analyse the results of many studies at the same time) have been undertaken to report summary conclusions. The Cochrane Database of Systematic Reviews, which presents the results of meta-analyses involving multiple drug trials, is a treasure trove of information. One of the first Cochrane publications concerned the effectiveness of chlorpromazine (Adams, Awad, Rathbone, & Thornley, 1998). Chlorpromazine revolutionised treatment of psychoses by improving symptomatology by an average of about 50% from the pre-antipsychotic medication era. It is still regarded by the World Health Organization as an essential medicine in the treatment of mental disorders (World Health Organization, 2009).

In the Australian setting, use of chlorpromazine is now unusual, since new generation antipsychotics have become the most frequently prescribed antipsychotics in community practice, as many clinicians have concluded these drugs are more effective and cause fewer side-effects than typical antipsychotics (Monshat, Carty, Olver, Castle, & Bosanac, 2010). However a recent authoritative publication presenting meta-analytic data concerning antipsychotics found that these impressions of clinicians concerning efficacy advantages of the newer antipsychotics can only be partially sustained, and there are important differences between atypicals with respect to effectiveness and toxicity (Huhn, Nikolakopoulou, & Schneider-Thoma, 2019). Some of the newer drugs are no more effective than older drugs such as haloperidol and chlorpromazine, although the risk of movement disorders (particularly tardive dyskinesia) are unequivocally lower with atypicals. Older antipsychotics remain appropriate for some patients.

While undoubtedly effective from a scientific viewpoint when compared to placebo, antipsychotics are only partially effective in many people with psychosis (in other words, treatment does not achieve full recovery). Treatment tends to diminish positive symptoms and to improve function, but about one-third of consumers continue to experience psychotic symptoms to some extent despite maximal drug therapy, and over half experience negative symptoms to some extent, which are only marginally improved by antipsychotic medications. Such treatment-resistant illness constitutes grounds for initiation of clozapine.

With respect to antidepressants, these are actually among the most commonly prescribed drugs of any kind in primary care settings. As the lifetime risk of major depression ranges from 7–12% in men and 20–25% in women (see Section 1.6.2), treatment of even a proportion of the overall population at risk means that the absolute numbers of people treated are high. In an initial treatment trial, 30–40% of patients with major depression can expect to achieve a remission from illness within six weeks. Many more patients will show some improvement, but up to 30% will not improve at all (Labbate, Fava, Rosenbaum, & Arana, 2010). Change in medication, alteration of the dose or introduction of other treatment measures will be necessary for patients failing to fully respond. Augmentation and combination treatments of various kinds are employed for treatment-resistant depression. The risk of side-effects increases with increasing complexity of treatment, and has to be weighed against the suffering caused by depression. Subjective quality of life is primarily determined by the severity of a client's depressed mood.

It is important to emphasise that in no way does use of pharmacotherapy exclude simultaneous provision of psychotherapeutic or other psychosocial interventions. Much evidence exists in virtually every area of mental health treatment to indicate clearly that a combination of medication with psychotherapeutic and other psychosocial measures is generally more effective than individual treatments alone. Unfortunately, the psychotherapeutic interventions that can benefit people are not uniformly available across the country (Meadows, Enitcott, Inder, Russell, & Gurr, 2015). While GP mental health care, commonly including prescribing, is available fairly evenly across much of Australia, the same cannot be said of specialist psychological care. There is at least three times higher rates of MBS-funded clinical psychological treatment in more affluent areas where the rates of mental health problem are a third of those in poorer areas, for many people in more deprived areas of the country (see Chapter 1.2); the medication may be all that they will be offered to help them through a depressive episode (Meadows, Enticott, & Rosenberg, 2018b).

2.5.4 HOW AND WHY DRUGS WORK

THE NEUROCHEMICAL BASIS OF MENTAL DISORDERS

Brain activity, expressed through chemical and electrical communication between neurons, underlies all behaviour, feeling and thinking (cognition). The most important chemicals (or neurotransmitters) of relevance to behaviour are amines:

- dopamine
- noradrenaline
- serotonin.

Dopamine is relevant for cognition and motivation. Noradrenaline is involved with fear responses and reward learning. Serotonin is relevant for impulse control, aggression and appetites.

A number of other neurotransmitters are also important for aspects of behaviour. The major nerve pathways involved in behaviour are related to the limbic system (located deep in the brain) and to the frontal lobe (the fore part of the brain, responsible for logic, reasoning and behavioural inhibition).

Neurotransmitters are released by one neurone, then affect another neurone by acting on the receptors for that particular transmitter. Most drugs that treat mental disorders exert their action through effects on receptors for particular neurotransmitters (the analogy being that the neurotransmitter is the key, and the receptor is the lock on the door to the neurone). This results in modification of the neurochemical activity in the brain.

When a mental disorder is associated with a particular kind of neurochemical dysregulation, a drug is potentially able to correct the chemical imbalance and normalise behaviour. For example, psychosis (characterised by the presence of delusions, hallucinations, formal thought disorder and disturbed behaviour) occurs because of dopaminergic overactivity in the mesolimbic pathway in the middle part of the brain. Mania appears to involve overactivity of brain dopamine in the frontal part of the brain. Some symptoms of schizophrenia may be due to underactivity of dopamine in the brain's frontal lobe.

Depression tends to be associated with underactivity of serotonergic and noradrenergic mechanisms in the part of the brain involved in mood regulation (the limbic system). Antidepressants augment brain serotonin and noradrenaline through long-term effects. Dopamine can also be involved.

It is likely that dopamine, serotonin and noradrenaline receptors exert effects through protein synthesis within neurones, as the effects of antidepressants and antipsychotics tend to be long lasting, and not merely dependent on the presence of the drug in the brain. On the other hand, removal of drugs gradually results in the recurrence of neurochemical dysregulation and relapse of the mental health disorder.

Many other neurochemicals are involved in different mental health disorders and medications. Anxiolytics and some mood stabilisers work through an inhibitory amino acid called gamma amino butyric acid (GABA). Psychosis may also involve an excitatory amino acid called glutamate, which is affected by illicit drugs such as phencyclidine (angel dust). Dementia tends to involve a neurotransmitter called acetylcholine.

The neurochemical basis of mental illness and the neurochemical effects of drugs used in mental health should not be seen as an opposing or alternative explanation to the psychosocial perspective. The approaches are complementary, and enable mental health disorders to be addressed through collaborative biopsychosocial interventions.

PHARMACOKINETICS

The way a drug is handled by the body depends on various pharmacokinetic parameters. Route of administration is a primary consideration. Most drugs are taken by mouth and absorbed in the stomach at varying rates. Rapidly absorbed drugs will generally start to work quickly. Some medications need to be absorbed through mucosa under the tongue, and may be absorbed differently, or not at all, if swallowed. Other drugs, such as long-lasting antipsychotic medications and some tranquillisers, need to be injected into the deltoid (shoulder) muscle or the gluteal (buttock) muscle. Some drugs, such as nicotine patches, can be absorbed through the skin.

Once absorbed, a drug is distributed around the body. For drugs used in mental health, the vital consideration is that the medication reaches the relevant part of the brain. To do so, that drug needs to cross the blood–brain barrier, which can be a problem for some substances. The drug is then eliminated over time, usually through the liver and/or kidney.

A useful measure of the pharmacokinetics of a drug is its half-life. Repeated dosing with medication results in increased blood levels until a steady state is reached. It takes about five half-lives for a particular drug to achieve steady state with regular dosing. A particular regular dose of drug will be associated with a steady state, which tends to vary from patient to patient, mainly because of variation in the genetics of mechanisms that eliminate the drug. People can thus be fast or slow metabolisers of particular drugs. Impairment in liver or kidney function will often slow down drug elimination and result in toxicity (a major danger with lithium).

PHARMACODYNAMICS

What a drug does to the body is called its *pharmacodynamics*. Most drugs used in mental health affect brain receptors for neurotransmitters such as dopamine. Lithium has its effects on second messenger mechanisms within certain nerve cells in the brain. Mood stabilisers, such as valproate and carbamazepine, are also anticonvulsants, and have effects on brain electrical activity.

2.5.5 HOW DRUGS ARE TAKEN

PRESCRIBING DECISIONS

Ideally, the decision to prescribe medication should be made through collaborative agreement between the client and other mental health professionals involved in treatment. Detailed information about medication options, including the varying side effects and effectiveness of different medications should be provided in non-technical language. The discussion ideally should include advice on indications, the way the medication works, the time until efficacy, the way in which medications should be taken and the likely duration of treatment. The clinician's expertise around medication is then married with the client's wishes, values and needs. Some people feel that efficacy is more important than any possible side effect, but others may feel that some side effects are unacceptable. At times side effects may be beneficial in some circumstances, such as sedation in persons suffering from insomnia.

The clinician needs to provide their informed opinion (for instance, to suggest which medication is most likely to suit the person's clinical problem, other medical conditions, value set and lifestyle), while maintaining respect for choice. Time between consultations to consider options can be useful. Even in involuntary situations, there is usually scope for choice between several medications. This can take a great deal of time and effort given the obvious complexities, but failure to do so is likely to reduce adherence to treatment.

When a decision has been reached, written information about the drug (usually the Consumer Medicine Information) should be provided. Some patients will opt to obtain this information directly from the internet.

Monitoring of medication decisions is critical in good prescribing practice. Review of efficacy and tolerability underpins safe practice. The frequency and intensity of review depends on the clinical situation, patient preference and often on available clinician resources. Ideally, medication prescription aims to find the medication with the best balance of high efficacy and no or minimal side effects.

ADMINISTRATION

Most mental health drugs are taken by mouth once or twice a day. It is easier to remember once-a-day administration, and this will assist adherence to treatment regimes. Some need to be taken with food or the amount of drug absorbed is reduced. Some of the medications need to be dissolved in the mouth. Many consumers are wary about taking several tablets at once; it is seldom a problem. Safe access and storage to medication may be an issue. Appropriate counselling for consumers about how to take their medications is a critical role for case managers, doctors and pharmacists. Information about missed doses is available in the Consumer Medicines Information.

Antipsychotic medications can also be given by injection. These preparations are designed to slowly release in the body, so are given between fortnightly and three monthly. Relapse rates of psychosis are lower on injectable or depot forms of medication, and overall outcome is often improved, especially if adherence has been problematic (Tiihonen et al., 2017).

DOSE ADJUSTMENT

For all medications used in mental health, information is supplied by the drug manufacturer about appropriate doses and dose ranges on the basis of clinical trial experience. Such recommendations will be appropriate for the majority of clients. For a minority, there will be significant variations in the dose required which may be outside the suggested dose range. The drug's effectiveness and its side-effects will also vary, depending on the particular individual. Frequent and careful monitoring of patients is an essential component of mental health drug treatment. The aim is to achieve effective treatment of the target symptoms and overall state, with minimal side-effect burden. This can only be achieved through careful monitoring of what is effectively informed trial and error in an individual treatment trial.

SIDE-EFFECTS

Unfortunately, significant side-effects are a very common occurrence during treatment with psychotropic medications. While the fortunate few patients can obtain treatment with no side-effects, many experience various problems, depending on the particular medications and individual characteristics and vulnerabilities of the consumer. Careful clinical monitoring is essential but can be difficult. Some patients will not recognise side-effects for what they are, while others will attribute them incorrectly. Intolerable side-effects are one of the key reasons for cessation of treatment; illness relapse will often follow.

2.5.6 COMPLIANCE AND ADHERENCE

Most mental health medications need to be taken regularly, and over long periods, in order to achieve therapeutic effectiveness. Mental illnesses such as schizophrenia and bipolar disorder are prone to relapse; antipsychotic medication is crucial for relapse prevention in schizophrenia. Notably, psychosocial interventions augment the benefits of antipsychotics in preventing relapse. And yet, failure to comply with treatment is probably the commonest cause of psychotic relapse.

The causes of nonadherence are various and complex. Some people will choose not to have treatment for rational reasons: many side-effects can be frankly intolerable. However, such issues can usually be addressed through modification of drug dose or change of drug. Good communication between client and mental health professionals is essential, as frequently side-effects leading to the cessation of treatment are not recognised and addressed.

The provision of a dialogue around symptom causation and the implications of both treatment, non-treatment and alternative treatments is invaluable in ensuring consumers are able to provide informed consent. Utilisation of skilled communication techniques underpins this dialogue, requiring adaptation for every clinical situation.

Some clients with psychosis may have impaired insight, and may not recognise their illness and the need for treatment. Dialogues involving psychoeducation, support and encouragement can assist patients in making decisions in their own best interests.

The cost of medication to the consumer can be a major hurdle. Strategies may be available to facilitate more affordable treatment, such as obtaining medication from a single pharmacy to facilitate benefits from safety nets.

Some clients are affected by cognitive dysfunction, and may find complex treatment regimes impractical. Once-daily administration, use of dosettes or Webster packs, phone reminders, targeted cognitive strategies, and direct support from mental health workers can assist.

At times it may be necessary to utilise long-acting injectable antipsychotic medications (*depot drugs*). In the past, depots were not a popular treatment option with consumers, as many suffered severe and unrelenting EPS. Several atypical antipsychotics are now available in depot injectable form, creating alternatives for those who chose or require depot treatment.

There are various strategies for identifying nonadherence, from good communication, to monitoring of medications and prescriptions, the use of compliance-enhancing devices and measurement of drug concentrations in the blood where possible. TCAs, lithium, valproate, carbamazepine and some antipsychotics (clozapine, risperidone and olanzapine) can be measured in the blood. Only lithium levels are highly accurate, however. In a small minority of patients, involuntary treatment through use of the *Mental Health Act* is unavoidable because of risk considerations (Andrews, 2014).

2.5.7 MEDICATION IN COMMUNITY MENTAL HEALTH, AND EXPECTATIONS OF DIFFERENT DISCIPLINES

COMMUNITY MENTAL HEALTH DISCIPLINES

As so many clients of community mental health services are taking medication to treat mental illness, medication issues are of some relevance to all disciplines. Reasons for choosing a particular drug in a given individual, the expectations of drug therapy in terms of therapeutic effects and side-effects and monitoring requirements need to be part of comprehensive team awareness in all concerned. The key parameters of drug administration (indications, contraindications, effectiveness, side-effects and the consumer's perspective) need to be reviewed at every service contact. While particular responsibility rests with the prescribers and their supervisors, all team members concerned need to contribute to the review process.

Although prescribing has been limited to doctors, administration and monitoring is a role shared by disciplines. Not only do many nonmedical practitioners hold a wealth of knowledge about psychiatric medications, but almost universally see the patient more frequently, and are well placed to respond to problem side-effects or lack of efficacy. The sharing of such information to the medical practitioner then allows timely medication adjustment.

Interestingly, it is only since the 1970s that psychiatrists have developed particular expertise in mental health prescribing. Trainees and medical officers carry out most of the prescribing in community mental health services, but will often require consultative input from psychiatrists. Several Australian states have recently passed legislation establishing mental health nurse practitioners, who are now also able to prescribe psychotropic medications. Challenges with respect to appropriate education, supervision and support have been identified.

GENERAL PRACTITIONERS

General practitioners, who have the same prescribing rights as psychiatrists, are mostly in private practice, though many are now also able to provide assistance from affiliated nurses who work with general practitioners. Over the last few years, the treatment of depression has become a core activity of general practice in Australia. General practitioners have become increasingly confident with use of antidepressant medications, largely as a result of extensive educational activities around the country. Use of antidepressants by general practitioners has often been coupled with their ability to complete mental health plans through a Federal Government funding initiative (see Section 1.7.2), and thus give their patients access to cognitive behaviour therapy from psychologists, social workers and occupational therapists.

Many consumers have thereby received relatively comprehensive treatment for anxiety and depressive disorders in general practice. However as introduced in Section 1.2.5, the benefits of this program have not been felt evenly across the country.

Pharmacologic treatment of schizophrenia and bipolar disorder remains a major educational challenge for most urban general practitioners. There is far less knowledge among general practitioners concerning antipsychotic medications and mood stabilisers in contrast to antidepressants. A small minority of general practitioners are quite skilled in the use of antipsychotic medications; these GPs often specialise in working with patients suffering from chronic psychoses. Many GPs will agree to work collaboratively with community mental health services for clients with major mental illness, but restrict their role to providing physical rather than mental health care.

General practitioners have an essential role in the monitoring of short and long term side effects of medications. There is a particular emphasis on monitoring of metabolic syndrome, weight reduction, cholesterol and diabetes treatment and smoking cessation. These interventions are aimed at reducing the long term effects of psychotropic medication, and improving life expectancy in mental health patients.

2.5.8 CLINICAL PRACTICE GUIDELINES

Use of mental health medications is extremely knowledge intensive. Additionally, pharmacotherapy has to fit into the complexities of treating particular mental disorders, given that medication use is generally indicated for subsyndromes in symptoms rather than disorders overall. Invariably, medication use will need to be combined with a comprehensive mix of psychosocial interventions for optimal outcomes. Traditionally, textbooks have been the usual source of information for clinicians. However, textbooks tend to be discipline specific. For comprehensive treatment planning, *clinical practice guidelines* (CPGs) for particular mental illnesses have emerged as useful resources. Quite frequently, CPGs provide a 'gold standard' or benchmark against which treatment plans can be evaluated.

The Royal Australian and New Zealand College of Psychiatrists has issued a number of CPGs, which are available on the college website. The mood disorder clinician guidelines were updated in 2015, and those for schizophrenia were updated in 2016. Many excellent guidelines are also available from the National Institute of Clinical Excellence in the United Kingdom and the American Psychiatric Association.

2.5.9 REGULATORY ISSUES

In Australia, virtually all medications used to treat mental illness require a prescription written by a registered medical practitioner or registered nurse practitioner. A small number of over-the-counter medications, such as antihistamines, can be useful for problems such as insomnia. Alternative therapies are also available.

All prescription drugs and over-the-counter medications are approved by the Therapeutic Goods Administration (TGA), a division of the Australian Government Department of Health and Ageing. Pharmaceutical companies that propose to market a new medication must make detailed submissions, which are subject to extensive expert scrutiny by a series of committees.

The use of certain medications, such as amphetamines and related substances, is monitored by state health departments, and requires their permission.

NEW DRUG DEVELOPMENT

It has been estimated that the cost of developing a molecule, to the point where it could be submitted to a regulatory authority for approval to be used by prescribers, is over US$800 m (in year 2000 dollars) (DiMasi, Hansen, & Grabowski, 2003). Drugs have to be taken through three testing phases:

- *Phase 1*: tests on animals and human volunteers
- *Phase 2*: double-blind placebo-controlled studies
- *Phase 3*: extensive studies, which may include placebo, but usually involve comparisons with standard treatments.

Studies are usually carried out at multiple sites around the world, with the aim of achieving approval by the Food and Drug Administration in the United States and the European Medicines Agency. Most drugs undergoing development are abandoned along the way for any number of reasons. When the drug achieves marketing approval, the reward for the pharmaceutical company is a ten-year period in which the patent is protected. At the conclusion of patent protection, other companies can market generic forms of the drug. Some countries, such as India, do not protect drug patents.

After a drug is released on the open market, *Phase 4 testing*, which involves post-marketing surveillance, is undertaken. Many drugs do not reveal drastic side-effects until many people have taken the drug for long periods. A number of psychotropic drugs have been withdrawn in the short term after initial regulatory approval because of Phase 4 testing results.

2.5.10 ACCESS ISSUES

PHARMACISTS AND PHARMACIES

While medication is prescribed by doctors and nurse practitioners, it is made available to consumers by pharmacists who are usually running pharmacies, or are a working in public hospital pharmacy departments. Pharmacists have a vital role in the logistics of drug delivery, but even more importantly, in the education and support of consumers. It is of some concern that pharmacists are not generally considered to be a part of mental health services, despite the considerable role that they may play in providing education and advice to consumers and carers, which may or may not be consistent with the community mental health service treatment plan.

Collaborative arrangement between community mental health services and pharmacists has been extremely constructive in the provision and monitoring of clozapine administration. Pharmacists can greatly assist mental health professionals with information about medications. Collaborative educational programs including pharmacists have been of great benefit to all disciplines involved, and thereafter to consumers.

PHARMACEUTICAL BENEFITS SCHEME (PBS)

In Australia, the cost of most mental health medications is supported by the Federal Government through the Pharmaceutical Benefits Scheme (PBS). Once a drug gains marketing approval through the TGA, the pharmaceutical company negotiates a price with the PBS in order for the drug to be subsidised. Most new psychotropic medications can cost hundreds of dollars a packet. If the PBS agrees to subsidise the medication, consumers pay a co-payment of $38.30 ($6.20 with a concession card), at time of writing, for a month's supply of medication. If a person is taking multiple medications, the co-payment can rapidly become prohibitive. Once the consumer has paid $1521.80 in a calendar year ($384.00 for concession card holders), further prescriptions will cost $6.20 (no charge to concession card holders).

Sometimes a pharmaceutical company cannot reach agreement with the PBS and the drug remains unsubsidised. Recently, federal cabinet has taken on the responsibility of approving PBS decisions, and decided to delay or withhold subsidy for new drugs used to treat depression and schizophrenia. After a delay of many months, approval has been gained for some, but not all of the new medications.

At least two important mental health medications in Australia are not subsidised by the PBS, as the pharmaceutical companies concerned will not negotiate with the PBS. Lamotrigine, used to treat bipolar depression (which is frequently treatment resistant), and clonazepam (which is used for panic disorder and is technically preferable to the subsidised but potentially addictive alprazolam) are not supported by the PBS. The cost of lamotrigine can be prohibitive, particularly for clients who are not able to engage in paid employment.

PUBLIC HOSPITALS

Public hospitals in Australia are funded by state governments, which in turn are funded by the Federal Government (see Chapters 1.6 and 1.7). Previously, each hospital had to pay for the medications being used at the hospital from its own budget. New medications needed to be approved at the state hospital level, as federally through the TGA and PBS. As the Federal Government has taken on funding, the importance of local hospital pharmacopoeias has diminished for drugs available on PBS. Hospitals still need to pay for drugs approved by the TGA but not subsidised by the PBS out of their own budgets, which means that non-PBS medications will often be denied to consumers.

REGIONAL AND REMOTE ISSUES

Regional and remote areas tend to have poor access to community mental health services and private psychiatrists (Meadows et al., 2015). General practitioners frequently provide the only mental health service available. Some are quite skilled in the psychopharmacological treatment of psychoses, including the requisite diagnostic assessment, but others are not. Attempts are also being made to promote telepsychiatry through funding and logistical arrangements.

CONSUMERS, CARERS AND FAMILIES

At the end of the day, apart from unusual circumstances where involuntary treatment plays a role, it is the consumers and their carers or families who decide whether they will take prescribed medication and adhere to the mental health service plan. Social and cultural factors, such as stigma, play a role in deciding whether treatment is acceptable (see Chapters 1.6 and 1.7). Decisions regarding what is in the best interest of the community mental health service client are not always made on rational grounds.

In the past, consumers and carers mostly relied upon information and education from prescribers and service staff. Today, many will immediately investigate the advice of professionals on the internet. This is often useful and empowering, but usually, it is important to provide consumers and carers or families with guidance as to what constitutes quality information. It is important that external agencies such as the patient's general practitioner (if not involved with the service) and pharmacist provide advice and information consistent with mental health service professionals.

2.5.11 DISCONTINUING PSYCHIATRIC MEDICATION

CARMELA SALOMON

Psychiatric medications may be discontinued for a number of reasons. In some cases, medication discontinuation is recommended as standard practice after a period of sustained recovery. When medication proves ineffective in treating the person's symptoms, a switch to a different medication may be needed. Sometimes people disagree with the need for psychiatric medication, or wish to manage their symptoms using non-pharmacological methods. Intolerable or life-threatening side effects or pregnancy may also trigger a need to stop or swap medications (Velligan, Sajatovic, Hatch, Kramata, & Docherty, 2017; National Institute of Health and Clinical Excellence (NICE), 2016; Bandelow et al., 2008; Salomon, Hamilton, & Elsom, 2014).

Specific switch over or discontinuation schedules vary between medications. However, clinicians should bear the following general principles in mind when supporting people who are stopping or swapping psychiatric medications:

- Decisions relating to stopping or swapping medications should occur as part of an open dialogue between the person and the treating team. Research shows that in many cases, when shared decision-making is not supported, people will attempt to stop medications unilaterally (Salomon & Hamilton, 2013). This can lead to increased risk, stress and isolation during the discontinuation period. Several tools have been developed to support open discussion about medication related decisions (Zisman-Ilani et al., 2018; Deegan, 2010).
- With the exception of life-threatening situations, medications should be stopped slowly to decrease

the risk of developing discontinuation or 'rebound' symptoms.

- The person should be made aware of the possibility of discontinuation symptoms prior to stopping. They should be offered appropriate support if symptoms do develop. Discontinuation symptoms are usually transitory and do not necessarily indicate a need to recommence treatment. Discontinuation symptoms may include: *insomnia* (particularly if the person is stopping a medication with sedating properties); *flu-like symptoms with anxiety, malaise, diarrhea and nausea* (particularly if the person is stopping a medication with a high affinity for the muscarinic M_1 receptor); and *extra-pyramidal symptoms* and *rebound psychosis* (more likely if stopping an agent that is loosely bound to the dopamine 2 receptor). It is important to consider the timing of symptom onset when seeking to distinguish between a true relapse and rebound psychosis. Rebound psychosis tends to occur much sooner after discontinuing than would be expected from a true psychotic relapse (Galletly et al., 2016; Salomon et al., 2014).
- The person should be closely monitored and supported throughout the discontinuation period, and an advanced directive rescue plan should be made in collaboration with the person prior to stopping (Galletly et al., 2016). This plan should include a list of warning signs that may indicate that a decline in the person's mental state or social functioning is occurring, and a plan to monitor and address these signs. Encouraging the person and their network to think about any changes in behaviour or thought processes that they noticed when the person was unwell in the past may be helpful when developing this list. The advanced directive plan should also support the person to consider if, when and how they would agree to restart medication or other treatments if symptoms re-emerge. In cases where the person or their treating team is concerned that a post-discontinuation decline in the person's mental state may impact on their decision-making ability, the person should be encouraged to nominate a person or persons whom they trust to be involved in decision-making if the need arises.

2.5.12 DEVELOPMENTS IN THE DRUG TREATMENT OF MENTAL HEALTH DISORDERS

PSYCHOSES

It has become increasingly apparent that the historical division of psychoses into schizophrenia and manic-depressive illness is not supported by much of the genetic and other neurobiological scientific evidence (see Chapter 1.4). This is consistent with clinical approaches to drug treatment, which are directed at subsyndromes and symptoms (see Table 2.12), rather than overall diagnoses: the medications used for schizophrenia are basically the same ones used for bipolar disorder and psychotic depression. It has therefore been strongly suggested that psychoses be treated as an overall group or spectrum, consisting of a number of treatment-relevant dimensions (such as positive symptoms, negative symptoms, cognitive dysfunction, mood symptoms (mania, depression, mixed states), anxiety and motor disturbances). While regulatory authorities still focus on treatment of illness categories (such as schizophrenia and bipolar illness) and clinicians use drugs to treat subsyndromes or illness dimensions, a major and irreconcilable disconnect is developing between the realities of clinical treatment and governing regulations.

Quite apart from illness dimensions, clinicians also need to differentiate between phase of illness. Different diagnostic and treatment considerations are apparent for young persons presenting with early psychosis, as opposed to people with an established illness (see Chapter 3.2). Psychoses tend to begin between the ages of 15 and 30, and it may take five to ten years for established illness to develop. A majority of patients achieve full or near full remission between recurrent illness episodes, but on the other hand, about one-third of patients develop chronic treatment-resistant illness with ongoing symptoms and disability despite treatment. Emphasis on intervention has been on the treatment of early psychosis, with the aim of improving longer-term outcomes.

Antipsychotic medications remain the cornerstone of drug treatment for psychotic disorders. New generation drugs have reduced the side-effect burden from movement disorders, but have introduced the challenges associated with weight gain as described above. The most important recent study in psychosis has been the CATIE study, which compared various antipsychotics over an eighteen-month period, established the effectiveness of clozapine, while casting doubt on the greater efficacy of atypicals versus typical antipsychotics. The need for physical monitoring of people on long-term antipsychotic medication was emphasised by the findings (Lieberman et al., 2005).

Most patients with psychoses will require lifelong treatment, so the consequences for physical health in terms of diabetes and heart disease are a serious concern. In this context, we note the findings of the Finnish epidemiological study (Tiihonen et al., 2009) that treatment with clozapine, and to a lesser extent other antipsychotics, substantially improves life expectancy, while lack of treatment with antipsychotics is associated with highest mortality. Further studies have verified that lack of drug treatment for schizophrenia is associated with the greatest reduction in life expectancy, but also found that depot medication is most effective in reducing mortality, lowering risk of death by 30% compared to oral antipsychotics (including clozapine) (Taipale et al., 2018).

A major trend in the therapy of treatment-resistant psychoses has been the use of combinations of antipsychotic drugs (Malhi et al., 2010). There is some supporting evidence for the addition of drugs such as aripiprazole and amisulpride to clozapine, where treatment response to clozapine alone has not been adequate. The possibility of greater toxicity from combinations is an ever present danger, however.

For clients with predominantly bipolar mood manifestations, mood stabilisers and antipsychotic medications, usually in combination, are the mainstay of treatment. Bipolar depression can be extremely treatment resistant. While most clinicians will attempt to use antidepressants (in addition to mood stabilisers), research evidence does not support the use of antidepressants to treat bipolar disorder: a proportion of patients will develop mixed states, mania and rapid cycling from one mood state to another while taking antidepressants.

Recently, the antipsychotic lurasidone has become available, and may offer some advantage in treatment of psychoses with mood disturbance. The depot antipsychotic, paliperidone palmitate, which is unique because it can reach therapeutic levels in eight days and is therefore useful in the acute setting (as well as for long-term maintenance), is now available in monthly and three-monthly injections. Long acting injectable aripiprazole, which has tolerability advantages, has also been introduced.

DEPRESSION

For the client presenting with depressed mood, there is also a complex diagnostic exercise. Many physical conditions and drugs (especially alcohol) cause depression. Physical evaluation as needed and treatable factors need to be addressed. Depression can be psychotic, bipolar or melancholic. Each poses particular treatment implications, with the need for biological therapies the common theme. Severely depressed patients are not likely to benefit from any psychotherapy until there is some improvement.

The majority of consumers with depression have reactive, situational or personality-related problems, for whom cognitive behaviour therapy and other psychotherapies are likely to be the treatment of choice. Some patients with more severe depressive symptomatology, such as anxiety, disturbance of sleep, loss of weight, low energy and suicidal ideation, may benefit from antidepressant medication, which will usually be an SSRI or SNRI. The combination of psychotherapy with medication is the most effective treatment.

Agomelatine, an antidepressant that normalises circadian rhythms (which are disrupted in depression) and has few side-effects (particularly, little sexual dysfunction or appetite increase, which can be troubling with other antidepressants) has become available. A multimodal antidepressant vortioxetine has also been introduced; it is similar to the SSRIs. Neither drug is supported by the PBS.

Infusions of ketamine, a dissociative anaesthetic, have recently been demonstrated to rapidly relieve depression and suicidality, in a matter of hours. Longer term safety and efficacy, particularly with respect to abuse potential, has not yet been demonstrated, and further research is needed (Arunogiri, Keks, & Hope, 2016).

2.5.13 OTHER PHYSICAL TREATMENTS

Electroconvulsive therapy (ECT) attracts much social controversy and condemnation. It is frequently misunderstood as 'electric shock' (in reality, it is a voltage field that induces neuronal synchronisation resulting in a convulsion which in turn, is fully modified through an anaesthetic). ECT is the most effective treatment for severe depression. Technical developments have rendered the treatment far less troublesome for consumers, particularly in relation to memory problems. ECT is most often used in patients with life-threatening illness, and saves many lives.

Transcranial magnetic stimulation (TMS), which involves application of alternating magnetic fields to the brain, has been established as an effective treatment for depressive disorders, and is now endorsed by authorities such as the American Psychiatric Association. Although not as effective as ECT, TMS causes much milder side-effects. TMS is not funded by Medicare but is available in many private hospitals.

Vagal nerve stimulation (which requires chest surgery) and *deep brain stimulation* (which requires neurosurgery) have also been endorsed as effective treatments for treatment resistant depression.

2.5.14 FUTURE DEVELOPMENTS

Apart from ketamine and related compounds, there is little prospect of major breakthroughs in new drug development over the next few years. The emphasis will be on improving the way currently available treatments are used while mechanisms underlying brain function continue to be investigated. TMS is becoming more widely available and may soon become a standard treatment.

Genetic testing, which assists with the prediction of the likely required dose of medications, is now available but often not particularly informative. Testing for whether a person will respond to any particular treatment is not yet available. At present, patients have to endure prolonged periods of trial and error to find a medication that is effective. These newer developments individualising treatment have been termed *personalised medicine*.

2.5.15 COMMENTARY AND REFLECTION

Community mental health services mostly treat clients with major mental illness. There is impeccable scientific evidence concerning the effectiveness and safety of various medications in the treatment of major mental illness. A number of different medication types are available, each with its indications and contraindications. Drugs tend to treat particular symptoms rather than overall illnesses, but there are many complexities. Most consumers attending mental health services are taking some kind of medication, often more than one. Drug treatment is an important component within the overall mix of treatments needed by people with mental illnesses. Improvement as a result of treatment can be considerable, but side-effects can be troublesome. The key principle is to ensure the benefits outweigh risk and problems.

Medications for mental health disorders usually need to be taken long term and the effects have to be closely monitored at both physical and psychosocial levels. Adherence to treatment in long-term therapy is always a serious challenge, especially as many of the drugs can cause problematic side-effects and may only be partially effective in treating illness. All disciplines involved in working with clients must be aware of medication issues and participate in the process of monitoring drug effects and the promotion of adherence to treatment.

2.6

SUPPORTING RECOVERY AND WELLNESS

ELLIE FOSSEY, CATH ROPER, PRISCILLA ENNALS, MARC MOREL, JOHN FARHALL, ROBERT KING, NEIL THOMAS, NIKOLAOS KAZANTZIS, ALEXANDRA PETRIK, FRANCES SHAWYER, SARAH FRANCIS, TARA HICKEY, ANNE WILLIAMS, ROB STANTON & BRENDA HAPPELL

2.6.1 INTRODUCTION

ELLIE FOSSEY & CATH ROPER

> For decades now, an evidence base informed by experiential and scientific research has been accumulating in support of psychosocial, recovery-oriented services and support and non-coercive alternatives to existing services.
>
> *UN General Assembly Human Rights Council, 2017, p. 8*

> The recovery approach, when implemented in conformity with human rights, has helped to break down power asymmetries, empowering individuals and making them agents of change rather than passive recipients of care. Tremendous strides have been made in this area, with evidence and recovery-based support and services in practice across the world today that restore people's hope (and trust) in services, as well as in themselves.
>
> *UN General Assembly Human Rights Council, 2017, p. 18*

These quotes from the United Nations' Special Rapporteur report (United Nations General Assembly Human Rights Council, 2017) signpost the situating of recovery and recovery oriented practices with a human rights framework. Consideration of human rights is especially important in a field of health where, in most countries, separate mental health legislation allows for treatments to be administered against people's wishes and people can be hospitalised without their consent. The United Nations' Special Rapporteur report acknowledges the role of unequal power when individuals do not have opportunities to lead their own recovery. Experiential knowledge, held by people who are engaged in journeys of recovery, is positioned as important and necessary expertise to be learned from. Further, this report emphasises that a recovery orientation involves offering care and support that promotes recovery, and upholds rights to health and citizenship on equal terms with others.

This chapter presents a broad range of approaches focused on social, occupational, psychological and physical dimensions of health and wellbeing, which can contribute to promoting personal and social recovery. Some of these approaches have long been used in mental health care, while others have developed more recently, so that they vary in the extent to which their origins explicitly align with contemporary recovery oriented frameworks and principles. Therefore this chapter begins with an overview of recovery oriented principles as the context within which these approaches need to be practised if they are to be experienced by people in recovery as supportive of wellbeing.

Approaches to addressing housing issues and enabling education and work participation are presented, and highlight the importance of attending to social determinants of health and recovery. There follows an overview of psychological therapies, including supportive counselling, educational and cognitive behavioural and mindfulness focused therapies, and an introduction to the developing area of internet-based approaches for promoting recovery, with their potential to enable access to support highlighted by challenges such as the COVID-19 outbreak (see Sections 1.2.4 and 2.6.13). Last, but by no means least important, the chapter draws attention to promoting physical health as a crucial element in promoting personal recovery and wellbeing.

As also argued in Special Rapporteur report, these psychosocial interventions and support should neither be viewed as luxuries, nor as peripheral to the right to mental health, and 'should be the first-line treatment options for the majority of people who experience mental health issues' (United Nations General Assembly Human Rights Council, 2017, p. 18).

2.6.2 RECOVERY AND RECOVERY ORIENTED SERVICES

ELLIE FOSSEY & CATH ROPER

Mental health policy and service frameworks in many countries internationally, including Australia, have embraced the term 'recovery' in describing their visions, principles, programs and practices (Amering & Schmolke, 2009; AHMAC, 2013a; AHMAC, 2013b). The term itself originates in the psychiatric survivor/consumer movement, which in turn was highly influenced by global civil rights movements. The use of this term signalled social justice concerns, such as having the freedom to make one's own choices, and be self-determining. A focus on recovery was seen as a way people could combat unhelpful ideas about the 'prognosis of doom' (Deegan, 1996, p. 92) associated with a diagnosis of mental illness and the hopelessness and low expectations flowing from this and instead, became a way for people to reclaim value in their lives. The concept of recovery embodied a paradigm shift because it said that people could experience symptoms but this in no way prevented them from living meaningful and important lives. Key to this idea of recovery was that it had to be led by the person themselves. However, the term 'recovery' has arguably been co-opted by the mental health field (Byrne, Happell, & Reid-Searl, 2015; Slade et al., 2014) and this becomes evident, for example, when we see services or practitioners, focusing solely on the management of symptoms, usually with medication (Slade, Amering, & Oades, 2008) with the person having very little say. Nevertheless, recovery has come to connote a positive, hopeful direction for reforming mental health care.

At its core, recovery is a *lived experience*, so that there cannot be one single or universal definition to describe what 'recovery' means to individuals. For instance, 'recovery' may be described as a personal journey, a process of healing or transformation; as a process of regaining hope, getting life back on track or developing a meaningful and satisfying life. There is a rich experiential evidence base on which we can draw in mental health services to understand what recovery might mean; to value and respect individuals' views and experiences; and to embrace the possibilities for recovery and wellness (Llewellyn-Beardsley et al., 2019). Recovery also occurs within the contexts of relations with family, friends, peers and communities, so that it is also contextualised by culture, experiences of discrimination, oppression and social determinants of health (AHMAC, 2013b). As a consequence, while recovery is often described as a personal or psychological process, it cannot be disconnected from the structural experiences of inequality and injustice within which emotional distress is also situated (Harper & Speed, 2012). So, as these authors argue, a framework 'more fully grounded in everyday experience' (p. 21) individually and collectively is needed to prioritise practices that address structural barriers and facilitators of recovery, such as secure and adequate income, housing, and meaningful occupation to ensure mental health.

A key distinction to make between recovery and recovery-oriented services can be put simply as: recovery is *lived* and *experienced* by individuals; what recovery-oriented services do is provide supports and interventions to *facilitate* people in recovering. In other words, recovery cannot be done *to* or *for* someone. Rather, recovery-oriented services need to offer genuine and respectful relationships and to create environments of support through which people can reclaim their lives and thrive beyond experiences of mental health issues or distress, disempowerment and discrimination (Glover, 2009).

Embracing a recovery orientation across mental health service systems requires that services do things differently: this entails significant shifts in thinking about what is done in practice, how services are orientated and how resources are used at every step and turn of service delivery (Amering & Schmolke, 2009; Davidson, Rowe, & Tondora, 2009; Slade, 2009a). This includes re-orienting services so that the lived experience and insights of people with mental health issues and their families are at their heart. A recovery lens is used to shape the language of mental health services and emphasis is placed on maximising choice and self-determination, while reducing coercion, restraint and discriminatory practices. In addition, recovery practice involves working collaboratively with people with mental health issues, families, and with lived experience workforce and peer-led organisations (AHMAC, 2013b; MHCC, 2018).

For mental health workers, this does not mean that their professional knowledge bases have no value or relevance in recovery-oriented practice, but it does necessitate recognition that the traditionally dominant professional knowledge bases in mental health services are insufficient in, and of themselves. Without enquiring into and taking the lead from people's own subjective experiences, preferences and expertise, knowledge about how to support and care for individuals also runs the risk of making assumptions and being experienced as 'power over'. Experiences of distress are valuable and contribute to the richness of contemporary mental health knowledge (Byrne et al., 2015; Slade, Oades, & Jarden, 2017). In essence, as O'Hagen described:

> A competent mental health worker understands recovery principles and experiences, supports service users' personal resourcefulness, accommodates diverse views on mental health issues, has self-awareness and respectful communication skills, protects service users' rights, understands discrimination and how to reduce it, can work with diverse cultures, understands and supports the user/survivor movement, and understands and supports family perspectives (O'Hagen, 2004, p. 2).

PRINCIPLES TO GUIDE RECOVERY-PROMOTING PRACTICES

The highly individual nature of the processes of recovery means that people may find differing approaches helpful along the way, at different points in their journey, and need different resources from different people at different times. So, there is no single recipe for recovery-orientated practice. A key point here is that elements of practice may either be helpful or harmful, but we cannot assume what will be beneficial without reference to the perspectives of those to whom services are offered, their values and preferences, and the nature of the options presented to them. This means above all, that the most important principle is to avoid assumptions, by getting to know the person with whom you are working and finding out what matters to them.

The following ten principles, summarised from Davidson and colleagues (2009) provide a useful framework within which to consider the practices described in this chapter, and their uses in support recovering and wellness. These principles include that mental health practice:

- *promotes recovery*: is grounded in an appreciation of processes of recovery and facilitating each person's efforts towards recovery (including gaining hope, power, purpose, skills and connections)
- *is person driven*: fosters choice and self-determination, self-chosen goals and directions
- *is strengths-based*: focuses on discovering interests, talents, gifts, personal resourcefulness and possibilities for who each person can be and what she or he can do
- *is community focused*: occurs in community contexts and focuses on strengthening community connections of choice
- *allows for reciprocity in relationships*: fosters involvement in roles and activities that build a sense of worth, value and having something to contribute to others
- *is culturally responsive*: is sensitive to socially and culturally diverse needs, values and preferences
- *is grounded in the person's life context*: appreciating each person's unique life story, experiences, circumstances, aspirations and sense of themselves as individuals
- *addresses the socioeconomic context of the person's life*: identifies and minimises barriers to the person's participation and engagement as a result of contexts such as poverty, housing difficulties and dislocation
- *is relationally mediated*: recovery is fundamentally a social process; relationships are central
- *optimises natural supports*: fosters connections and supports within the community.

Self-determination, choice, hope and the development of personalised strategies for dealing with illness, distress and everyday living are central in recovery. Hence, authentic recovery-based practice at its core is about inspiring hope, meaning and purpose, and supporting individuals' rights and efforts towards self-determination in their lives, recovery and treatment (Amering & Schmolke, 2009; Le Boutillier et al., 2015).

Recovery-oriented practice is operationalised as a set of practices through which mental health professionals employ skills, values, attitudes and behaviours that support individuals in their recovery (Slade, Bird, Clarke, et al., 2015). A number of guides to recovery-oriented practice have been developed over the past decade, variously informed by lived experience-based knowledge, person-centred approaches, the social model of disability, concepts from positive psychology, coaching and health promotion, and strengths-focused practices (Amering & Schmolke, 2009; Davidson, Rowe, & Tondora, 2009; Tondora, Miller, Slade, & Davidson, 2014). In Australia, the Collaborative Recovery Model (CRM), (Oades, Deane, & Crowe, 2017) and the REFOCUS approach (Slade, Bird, Le Boutillier, et al., 2015; Meadows et al., 2019) have each been implemented and evaluated in community mental health services.

The Collaborative Recovery Model (CRM) (Oades et al., 2017) is a well-established framework for applying recovery and wellbeing oriented principles that has been widely used in community mental health organisations. A strengths based, person-centred coaching approach informed by theories of change and empowerment from positive psychology, it uses strengths and values clarification, collaborative goal striving and motivation enhancement to support consumers to develop a life vision founded on their values and aspirations about recovery. CRM can support translating recovery-oriented policy and knowledge into community mental health practice, and is perceived as valuable in supporting recovery by consumers and staff (Wolstencroft, Deane, Jones, Zimmermann, & Cox, 2018).

Similarly, the REFOCUS intervention developed in UK focuses 'working relationships' and 'supporting personally defined recovery' as central to supporting personally defined recovery

(Slade, Bird, Le Boutillier, et al., 2015). As with CRM, a coaching approach to interactions with consumers is emphasised, and three key working practices are also described: understanding values and treatment preferences, assessing and enhancing strengths, and supporting goal striving. The CHIME framework, drawn from a systematic review that identified five key recovery processes as connectedness, hope and optimism, identity, meaning and purpose, and empowerment (Leamy, Bird, Le Boutillier, Williams, & Slade, 2011). It is integrated into the REFOCUS approach a means to collaborate with consumers in developing a shared understanding of personally defined recovery from their perspective. The REFOCUS approach has been adapted for use in Australian community mental health services and trialled in Victoria, indicating that recovery-focused staff training can positively impact consumer experiences of care (Meadows et al., 2019). Hence, guiding principles for recovery oriented practice are not only available to support the development of a recovery orientation in services but can be implemented within Australian community mental health practice contexts.

The knowledge that informs a recovery orientation to practice then is unique within the mental health field in the extent to which it draws on and privileges lived experience-based knowledge. Important perspectives for understanding 'recovery' have been presented in earlier chapters, including foregrounding what is meant by consumer perspective and lived experience (see Sections 1.1.6 and 2.2.1). Earlier chapters also described distinctions between conventional and recovery oriented approaches to case management (see Sections 2.4.2); consumer endorsed approaches of supported decision making and the use of advance statements (see Sections 2.4.3 and 2.4.4); peer support, peer-led approaches to promoting wellbeing and the use of co-production in mental health services (see Sections 1.1.6, 2.1.3, 2.2.3 and 2.2.4).

Here we turn to what mental health practitioners and services can do to support people in recovering and enhancing their wellness.

2.6.3 HOUSING AND SUPPORT

INTRODUCTION TO HOUSING ISSUES

PRISCILLA ENNALS

Stable, safe, affordable housing is a foundation for good mental health and wellbeing. Yet, for many people living with mental ill health, insecure tenure, precarious or poor quality housing, stress, danger and ontological insecurity (ongoing uncertainty about events in one's life) are commonly experienced in relation to housing. The housing preferences of people with a mental illness are similar to those of other Australians: home ownership is the most preferred option, followed by public housing, private rental, boarding houses, and unsupervised group homes are the least preferred option (Brackertz, Wilkinson, & Davison, 2018). Homelessness is increasingly common in Australia, with a large percentage of people experiencing homelessness, including rough sleeping. The 2016 Australian census identified that more Australians are renting (30.9%), and paying more for rent (ABS, 2016c), and that on census night 116,000 people were homeless, of whom 8200 people were sleeping rough (Pawson, Parsell, Saunders, Hill, & Liu, 2018).

Many people experiencing homelessness are also living with mental illness. A bidirectional relationship exists between mental illness and housing instability. Marginal housing or homelessness can exacerbate mental illness, while mental illness, accompanied by the accumulated social and economic adversity frequently experienced by people with mental illness, increases the risk of homelessness or living in marginal housing (Stafford & Wood, 2017). Marginal housing may include housing that lacks security of tenure (high risk of eviction), safety, amenity for social relationships, privacy (for example due to overcrowding), or does not have basic or adequate facilities. The housing careers of people with psychiatric disability vary, but some are characterised by housing instability, marginal housing, frequent moves and periods of homelessness as people try to adapt to their fluctuating mental health, periods in and out of employment, and variable access to government support payments (Beer & Faulkner, 2008). Hence, caravan parks, boarding houses, and unlicensed shared housing can present as the only access to shelter for some people with ongoing mental health issues.

Housing affordability is currently a major driver of housing instability and homelessness for Australians. Costs in the Australian private rental market have increased substantially in real terms and as a proportion of income (Thomas & Hall, 2016). The 2018 rental affordability snapshot by Anglicare (2018) found that for all household types on income support payments, only 6% of properties were affordable, and 28% were affordable to those on minimum wage. However, at the time of the survey, for people on Youth Allowance or Newstart payments, only three of the 67 000 sample of properties available for rent across Australia were affordable. Social housing–public housing managed by the states and territories in Australia, and housing managed, and often owned, by not-for-profit community housing providers–is also available to meet the needs of people on low incomes and with low economic assets. Yet, Australian census data from 2016 found that the percentage of households in social housing is at a 35-year low of 4.2%, compared with a high of 7% in 1991 (Brackertz et al., 2018) and almost 190 000 people were on the waiting list for social housing in 2017, many of whom may never be placed due to a lack of social housing stock (AIHW, 2018d). These figures illustrate the pressures on affordable housing for the Australian population as a whole, and those people with mental illness on low incomes or government support, represent a highly vulnerable group under housing stress with this population.

Some people living with mental ill health will benefit from support to obtain and sustain a tenancy. Economic and social disadvantage are the primary reasons that most people living with mental illness seek support, while others will need ongoing active support with their mental health and practical aspects of daily living. For people with complex mental health, social and housing needs, housing placement should be seen as the first of a range of resources and supports required to maintain stable housing, rather than the end goal (Padgett, Henwood, & Tsemberis, 2016).

Service systems that are not integrated can exacerbate the challenges experienced by people with mental ill health. For example, people with mental illness receiving support through state funded mental health providers can be evicted from social housing due to symptoms and behaviours resulting from their mental illness, yet mental health providers may know little about the housing needs of the people they support (Pawson et al., 2018). Home based outreach programs, for example the Housing and Accommodation Support Initiative (HASI) in NSW, are typically delivered through non-government providers, offer individualised support according to need, and linkage to foster community connection and participation. In recent years, increasing efforts have been made to understand the complex and intersecting needs of people with mental illness in relation to housing, with a range of approaches trialled to integrate and coordinate health, social and housing support. Traditional approaches of moving people through a range of levels of housing, for example crisis support to transitional housing to independent community housing, with an emphasis on 'building readiness' for permanent housing, is now understood to present many challenges (Y Foundation, 2017).

HOUSING FIRST APPROACH

The approach gaining strongest momentum and building evidence of effectiveness is the Housing First approach (Tsemberis, 2010). Housing First principles argue that the primary need for people without housing is to be permanently housed, and that supports and connections to address their additional needs should be 'wrapped around' them through assertive engagement once they are housed. Originating in the United States in the 1990s to address high rates of chronic homelessness, Housing First is now implemented in many countries including Australia. Housing First can be delivered in congregate settings (a cluster of housing) or in scattered sites (housing integrated into the community).

Housing First principles include: '(a) eliminating barriers to housing access and retention, (b) fostering a sense of home, (c) facilitating community integration and minimizing stigma, (d) utilizing a harm-reduction approach, and (e) adhering to consumer choice and providing individualised consumer-driven services that promote recovery' (Stefancic, Tsemberis, Messeri, Drake, & Goering, 2013, p.240).

Several Australian programs have invested in strong, longitudinal methodologies to understand the impact of Housing First implementation trials. In Perth, Western Australia, 50 Lives 50 Homes, a partnership led by RUAH Community Services, provided wrap-around support and housing for people who had experienced chronic homelessness. The project sustained tenancies for 88% of the 149 people who were housed and demonstrated reductions in presentations to emergency departments, hospital admissions, and criminal offences for people who were housed (Vallessi et al., 2018). In Melbourne, Sacred Heart Mission developed Journey to Social Inclusion (J2SI), which provides permanent housing and intensive relationship-based, trauma-informed support over three years for 60 people who have experienced chronic homelessness. While the program and evaluation is still in progress, first-year outcomes showed the J2SI group had higher rates of housing (60% compared to 31%), lower hospital use, decreased substance use, and decreased overall health costs in comparison to a control group (Flatau et al., 2018). A third example is Doorway, a three-year pilot integrated housing and support program delivered in Melbourne by Wellways (formerly known as MI Fellowship). In the Doorway program, participants have access to rental subsidies and brokerage support so they can source and choose properties through the open rental market, and receive individualised wrap-around supports. The pilot evaluation showed significant decreases in hospital usage, health care costs, improvements in health and social outcomes (measured through HoNOS and the Homelessness Outcomes Star), and decreased psychological distress (Dunt et al., 2017).

An internationally recognised expert in housing and homelessness, Nicholas Pleace, argues that while Housing First approaches are highly effective for people with high and complex needs, it is not in itself a complete solution to address homelessness or the housing needs of all people with mental illness (Pleace, 2018). In addition to Housing First, he recommends strong prevention, critical time intervention approaches and utilisation of the full range of existing housing and homelessness supports as part of an integrated homeless strategy. Of critical importance is matching the support needs of people, as they vary over time, with relevant resources. Adelaide is trialling a collective action project bringing housing, homelessness, health and business together to respond to rough sleeping in a coordinated fashion. The Adelaide Zero Project (Don Dunstan Foundation, 2020), based on Zero Projects in the US, is recording all rough sleepers by name and need, and allocating housing to match those who are most vulnerable.

Reviews of qualitative research focused on the experiences of people with mental illness in supported housing (Krotofil, McPherson, & Killaspy, 2018; Watson, Fossey, & Harvey, 2019) highlight how obtaining housing after homelessness affords many benefits, including control, privacy and the opportunity to rebuild identity, but also that privacy can mean loneliness for some so establishing social connections, including with service providers, is critical. Australian research shows how people with mental illness are highly active in their efforts to improve their overall housing situation, and frequently experience discrimination on account of their mental illness in relation to housing. For example, research in NSW, involving people with mental illness in receipt of housing support, explored the processes they used to actively manage their housing situations (Honey, Nugent, Hancock, & Scanlan, 2017). Participants identified personal and social resources they relied on such as organisation, clear thinking, assertiveness, emotional resilience, resourcefulness, persistence and the use of social and material resources, as they negotiated challenges related to their housing and tried to optimise their housing situations. They described how mental ill health could impede their use of these resources, sometimes leaving them homeless, couch surfing or rough sleeping. Many relied on additional supports to advocate on their behalf with housing services around tenancy issues, property maintenance, and managing conflicts with neighbours and local residents.

Many examples of good practice are developing to address the housing needs of people with mental illness in Australia, but to improve outcomes more broadly all of the following are required:

a high level, multisector, strategic policy and planning
b efforts to address structural issues including general housing affordability and lack of social housing
c greater coordination and integration of services on the ground and
d continued research and evaluation that centres the voices of people living with mental illness, to further understand the issues of precarious housing, homelessness and housing success, and the impact of service responses to these.

IS THE HOUSING SYSTEM READY FOR A PEER WORKFORCE? A REFLECTION

MARC MOREL

I am employed as a peer worker in a program supporting people who have been homeless into housing. Being a peer means that I previously lived on the street and was supported by the organisation that now employs me—Neami National in Sydney. I am reflecting here on whether the system—homelessness, housing, mental health—is ready to make the most of a peer workforce.

The peer workforce in housing and support programs is a good idea for many reasons:

- Providing meaningful employment and a route out of poverty for people who would otherwise struggle to find work after living through long periods of homelessness.
- We understand that no one becomes homeless voluntarily.
- Through our own and others' experiences we know what leads to homelessness, the realities of sleeping rough, how great and tough it can be to transition to housing, and all about the pros and cons of maintaining a tenancy while trying to manage your mental, emotional and physical health.
- Peer workers can assist other staff to navigate what is akin to operating in a foreign environment; we provide an 'ask a local' feel to outreach work.
- We can educate other workers, especially those starting in the sector fresh and students on placements, by sharing our experiences of how best to connect with people who have been marginalised, who have complex needs, given poor physical and mental health, addiction and traumatic past experiences.
- We can quickly build trusting relationships with people—they know we have been there too.
- We can support staff by taking on a range of tasks—checking in with people, organising appointments or providing support with day-to-day tasks, and providing feedback to our teams.

But negotiating these roles is tricky:

- Initially the roles were not well defined. Managers, teams, and peer workers all had to work out what the roles were about and how they would fit into the existing framework of the organisation. This takes time.
- People can resist change that takes them out of their comfort zone. We often felt that peer workers made staff feel uncomfortable. More experienced staff have embraced the peer roles more readily than those who have just completed education and placements. We are involved in some research seeking to understand more about this and how staff can be supported to make the most of peer workers.

Ways that services could support peer workers and capitalise on their benefits:

- Provide training for peer workers that match the 'gaps' in their experience e.g. information technology, delivery of service, working in teams. Ask rather than assume what people know. Our involvement in research and discussions over the first year of these roles has been vital in providing definition and direction to peer roles at Neami National.
- Help us understand the role of other staff in the team, so we get a greater appreciation of the pressure and demands of other roles.

- Support the entire team to understand how peer roles can contribute.
- Give peer workers time to develop autonomy. This will relieve some pressure on teams through the practical support that we provide to clients, and by giving support and advice to staff.
- Remember that peer support means support to all involved and is not exclusive to clients.

2.6.4 ACTIVITY PARTICIPATION, RECOVERY AND WELLBEING

ELLIE FOSSEY

What people do in daily life—all of us as consumers, family members, practitioners and everybody else—impacts our health and wellbeing in ways that are both more and less apparent. For instance, many people will be familiar with public health messages that encourage being physically active, healthy eating and limiting alcohol consumption as part of maintaining a healthy lifestyle. Yet, there are a range of other ways in which our activities and activity patterns contribute towards wellbeing (Moll et al., 2015; Gewurtz et al., 2016).

Involvement in self-chosen, personally and culturally meaningful activities is a commonly reported factor contributing to recovery (Doroud, Fossey, & Fortune, 2015). Participation in many kinds of activities have potential to contribute to processes of recovery and support wellness, but each person differs in the activities through which value and meaning are found, and recovery and wellness are experienced. Frameworks such as the Do-Live-Well framework (Moll et al., 2015) and approaches such as Action over Inertia (Krupa et al., 2010) suggest potential ways to consider and discuss the broad connections between activity patterns and wellbeing within recovery-oriented mental health practice.

Here we focus on access to education and employment in particular because, more than other activities, they are recognised rights and promote opportunities for participation, social inclusion, and access to essential resources for material wellbeing. Furthermore, lack of educational and employment opportunities increases the risks not only of lifelong social and economic exclusion but also of poorer physical and mental health (Waddell & Burton, 2006).

The next two sections (Sections 2.6.5 and 2.6.6) focus on supports for people to pursue education and to participate in the workforce. Each highlights the barriers and challenges to participation; approaches that aim to support people to participate in learning and working of their choosing; and strategies that can be implemented to create inclusive and supportive educational settings and workplaces.

2.6.5 ACCESS TO EDUCATION

PRISCILLA ENNALS

INTRODUCTION

Young people and adults with mental illness at varying phases in recovering seek to engage or re-engage with education to obtain qualifications, to enhance their employment choices and opportunities, and for personal development (Corrigan, Barr, Driscoll, & Boyle, 2008; Ennals, Fossey, Harvey, & Killackey, 2014; Killackey et al., 2017). The onset of mental illness in late adolescence and early adulthood frequently interrupts secondary or tertiary education, while its episodic nature can make return to study more challenging, with negative consequences for employability, workforce participation and career options (Waghorn, Chant, Lloyd, & Harris, 2011). Hence, re-engagement in education and successful attainment of qualifications can be an important priority to positively influence longer-term employment outcomes, earning potential and quality of life.

Prevalence rates of mental ill health in Australian students is difficult to establish for a range of reasons including students choosing not to disclose (Venville, Street, & Fossey, 2013), a lack of systematic measurement (Veness, 2016), and definitional inconsistencies. One Australian university survey identified increased psychological distress in 25% of students (Larcombe et al., 2014) a figure that is broadly consistent with international findings (Eisenberg, Hunt, & Speer, 2013; Ibrahim, Kelly, Adams, & Glazebrook, 2013). Mental ill-health is acknowledged as an issue of concern for Australian students in secondary schools, vocational training and universities (Brett, Norton, & James, 2012; Hughes, Corcoran, & Slee, 2016; Lawrence et al., 2015; Veness, 2016), with universities making recent efforts to develop frameworks and guides to support student wellbeing (see, for example, *Resources for University Educators, 2020* published by Sydney University, which is a blueprint for student mental wellbeing in universities).

Barriers and challenges in returning to learning

Participation and completion rates in postsecondary education are lower among students with mental illness than for many other students (Waghorn et al., 2011), and they experience wide-ranging barriers to entering or re-engaging with education, sustaining studies and successfully completing courses. These barriers may include financial costs, including course fees and expenses associated with studying (such as internet, computer and transport); competing responsibilities and scheduling issues or inflexible course structures; lack of or inaccessible study supports for struggling students within educational settings; managing mental health issues or fear of relapse; the need to disclose mental ill-health in seeking assistance; lack of knowledge, encouragement or support from mental health workers; and the complexity of systems to navigate to access education and financial entitlements (Ennals, Fossey, & Howie, 2015; Ringeisen et al., 2017; Shor, 2017).

Risk factors for dropping out of postsecondary educational settings include the impact on studying of thinking difficulties associated with symptoms and medication effects, lowered academic self-confidence, reluctance to disclose, and discriminatory and unhelpful responses to disclosure in academic settings (Megivern, Pellerito, & Mowbray, 2003; Shor, 2017). Previous failed attempts or prior experience of inadequate support to engage in education can compound a sense of failure and further alienate adults with mental illnesses from returning to study (Ennals et al., 2015). Hence, prolonged absence from study, previous study experiences and ill-health may combine to make re-engagement with education especially challenging without additional supports.

SUPPORTED EDUCATION INITIATIVES

A range of supported education initiatives—programs and courses designed to provide pathways and supports for re-engagement in education—have been developed internationally with the aim of enabling people with mental ill-health to access and successfully participate in mainstream postsecondary education (Waghorn, Still, Chant, & Whiteford, 2004; Mowbray et al., 2005). Supported education was initiated in the United States, but varying approaches have been described internationally, including in the United Kingdom, New Zealand, Canada, Israel and Australia (Clayton & Tse, 2003; Isenwater, Lanham, & Thornhill, 2002; Killackey et al., 2017; Sasson, Grinspoon, Lachman, & Ponizovsky, 2005).

Based on the principles of supported employment, supported education programs have developed in response to local needs and as ideas and understandings of recovery, disability rights to full participation, and of the capacity of people living with mental illness to lead full and contributing lives have become more prominent. Consequently, these programs vary in their structure and settings. Mowbray and colleagues describe four models to classify supported education programs:

- the *self-contained classroom* approach, which provides closed classes for people with mental illness delivered within mainstream educational settings
- the *on-site model*, which provides support to individuals to study within mainstream settings, such as colleges and universities
- the *mobile support approach*, usually under the auspice of a mental health service, with supporting services provided by mental health staff

- the *free-standing model*, whereby educational and personal development courses are offered within a clubhouse or at the sponsoring agency's site (for example, a rehabilitation or community mental health service) (Mowbray et al., 2005).

These models are distinguished by the nature of the curricula, and the source and types of support provided. For example, programs may include: courses designed and tailored specifically for people with mental illness returning to learning; provision of personal supports within and outside mainstream classroom settings; access to study skills support, vocational and financial counselling; support to negotiate study accommodations such as extensions or alternative assessments; peer support; and linkage between education and mental health providers (Best, Still, & Cameron, 2008; Killackey & Cotton, 2017; Robson, Waghorn, Sherring, & Morris, 2010). Programs have tended to develop to meet the needs of a particular community, so frequently combine elements of these different models. As supported education does not have a single, clearly defined structure, goal or desired outcome, it is difficult to compare between models.

Systematic reviews (Ringeisen et al., 2017; Rogers, Farkas, Anthony, & Kash-MacDonald, 2010) have concluded that supported education can assist in the identification of educational goals, establishment of supportive resources, and the management of barriers to education. They argue that further specification and operationalisation of the specific components of supported education are required, along with further specification of the skills required by staff to effectively deliver supported education, including relational skills.

Further research, using longitudinal and experimental designs, is required to build the evidence base for this relatively novel intervention. When adapted to support return to learning, the individual placement and support principles (see Section 2.6.6) may be used to guide individualised support to identify and access courses, maintain enrolment in and successfully complete individually chosen adult learning courses.

An innovative Australian trial was conducted by Killackey and colleagues (2017) at Orygen—Centre for Excellence in Youth Mental Health by employing an experienced teacher to support re-engagement with education for young people presenting for the first time with serious mental illness. Their pilot study found that this adapted approach was both feasible and potentially effective with 18/19 young people offered, taking up the opportunity for supported re-engagement with education. Eighteen young people engaged in a course of study, with 17 engaged at a higher level than previously. In concluding, Killackey and colleagues questioned whether the lack of educationally focused interventions available in Australian mental health services represents acceptance of a vocational stigma for people with mental illness from those working in the field; acceptance of low expectations for educational success and rich vocational careers. They argue that education must be a focus of interventions if people's longer term vocational trajectories are to be improved.

Demand for formal supports is not being met within university and college settings prompting the trial of other approaches. Interventions that are acceptable to students and can be scaled to meet the high need must be identified. Peer support is one such approach that appears to be having positive impacts on large numbers of students internationally. It has been suggested that when first experiencing challenges, students with mental illness speak initially to peers before seeking professional help (Reavley, McCann, & Jorm, 2012), so peer approaches may overcome barriers to support and promote low intensity help-seeking. There has been growth in groups such as Active Minds in the United States (Active Minds, 2020), Student Minds in the United Kingdom (Student Minds, 2020), and Batyr in Australia (Batyr, 2020); all peer initiated programs promoting sharing of students' lived experience to raise awareness, promote help-seeking and provide peer-to-peer support. Ben Veness completed a Churchill Fellowship to study the international approaches to address the wicked problem of student mental health and has argued for a top down approach from University leaders to drive policy and practice change in support of student mental health (Veness, 2016).

2.6.6 EMPLOYMENT: OPPORTUNITY, SUPPORT AND INCLUSION

ELLIE FOSSEY

Access to decent, productive work and just working conditions is a recognised human right, and includes the right of persons with disabilities to work on an equal basis with others, in freely chosen work and open, accessible and inclusive workplaces (United Nations, 1948; United Nations General Assembly, 2006). Only a small portion of the work carried out in communities worldwide is paid work and other forms of work contribute substantially to families, communities and the economy (including household work, caregiving, volunteering) (Gammarano, 2019). Yet, paid work or employment powerfully shapes the personal, social and material wellbeing of individuals and families, as well as the sense of productivity, dignity and identity of individuals in society (Waddell & Burton, 2006). Hence, there are rights-based, personal, social, economic and health-related reasons for being concerned about employment and mental health.

EMPLOYMENT AND MENTAL HEALTH

Mental ill-health impacts work participation in various ways. In high-income countries, many adults in the workforce experience mental ill-health. For instance, an estimated 10% of adults in the workforce experience a mental disorder, and mental ill-health is a leading cause of sickness absence from work and long-term work incapacity in these countries (Dewa & McDaid, 2011; Harvey et al., 2014). Yet, while the majority of working aged adults with common mental disorders, such as depression, are employed (around 60-70%), people with psychiatric disabilities are much less likely to be in the workforce, with studies reporting 65-90% not working in English-speaking and European countries) (Dewa & McDaid, 2011; OECD, 2012). In Australia, the proportion of the latter population in employment has remained stable at 22% between national surveys conducted in 1997 and 2010 (Waghorn et al., 2012), so that mental ill-health can be profoundly disruptive to the lives not only of affected individuals but also in their families and social networks.

Paid employment is generally considered beneficial for mental health and wellbeing (Waddell & Burton, 2006). Consistent with this, people experiencing mental ill-health often report that working is important to their recovery or wellbeing, and many of the same benefits reported by other employed people: an income, a sense of purpose, more structured time use, status and acceptance within society, feeling productive and useful to others, more positive self-appraisals, and improved opportunities for social contact (Fossey & Harvey, 2010). Nevertheless, the nature, quality and social context of work are also important, with poor psychosocial working conditions like job insecurity, high job demands and limited opportunity to exert control over working hours can be detrimental to workers' mental health (Butterworth et al., 2011; Thisted, Nielsen, & Bjerrum, 2018). Job loss and unemployment have broad adverse effects on mental wellbeing, including loss of purpose, identity and social status, reduced subjective wellbeing, psychological distress, and poorer mental health, which also worsen over time (Waddell & Burton, 2006; Munoz-Murillo et al., 2018). This relationship is more marked where people experience greater social inequalities in employment opportunities, income and access to health care (see Chapters 1.2 and 1.3). Hence, access to decent work is an important aspect of addressing social and economic inclusion.

Taken together, these issues mean there are significant personal, social, community and economic costs associated with not adequately supporting employed people to retain and return to their work following sickness absence due to mental ill-health; with neglecting the vocational issues of unemployed adults with ongoing mental illness; and with not addressing the vocational development of young people whose employability, workforce participation and career trajectories have been interrupted by the onset of mental ill-health. To attend to these issues, a vocational focus needs to be part of primary mental health care, adult and youth mental health services.

Barriers to vocational options and employment

The labour market influences the likelihood of being employed. In other words, insecure employment, job loss and unemployment are more likely to be experienced by those who are disadvantaged in the labour market due to lack of work experience or skills, long-term health conditions, older age, disability and other stigmatised attributes. In addition, current and potential workers with mental ill-health face multiple and complex employment barriers that may disrupt their work participation, many of which are not directly attributable to mental ill-health (Gmitroski et al., 2018; Kinn, Holgersen, Aas, & Davidson, 2014; Thisted et al., 2018) as illustrated in Table 2.13.

Table 2.13 Examples of barriers to work participation

Employment and welfare systems	• complexity of systems to navigate to access job-seeking assistance and welfare entitlements • unequal availability of effective vocational services, career advice and financial counselling • lack of coordination between systems to support job-seeking and return-to-work processes • potential for financial disincentives related income support and other subsidies
Workplaces	• lack of supervisor or co-worker support • prejudice and discrimination in language use, social interactions, performance expectations or performance management practices • inflexibility in work practices, particularly for workers with fluctuating or episodic conditions • lack of coaching, workplace training and/or career development opportunities
Employers	• limited knowledge of how to provide workplace adjustments for employees with mental ill-health • reluctance to hire people with mental ill-health
Mental health services	• limited knowledge about how to address employment issues and/or access relevant employment supports • underestimation of consumers' capacities to work and discouragement of their return to work • low expectations or pessimism about work prospects conveyed to consumers • vocational issues not consistently explored or systematically addressed
Job seekers and workers with poor mental health	Lack of supports related to: • managing personal information and disclosure in the workplace • planning wellness supports, and for the potential of becoming unwell, its impacts on employment and income security • concerns about impacts of medication effects or illness-related factors (e.g. fatigue, low energy, sleeping issues, anxiety) on managing work demands or work performance • limited income and resources, such as transport, clothing and equipment, to enable job-seeking and working • making connections with peers or social networks for support in sustaining employment • addressing disrupted educational and/or work history

Despite these barriers, there are effective ways to support people with mental ill-health to access and sustain employment and careers of their choosing. In addition, there is growing recognition of the need to address employment issues not only at an individual level but also by directly tackling working conditions and practices that undermine mental health and perpetuate employment disadvantage or exclusion.

SUPPORT TO ACCESS EMPLOYMENT

Originally developed in the United States, Individual Placement and Support (IPS) is a systematised approach to supporting individuals with mental ill-health to find and secure mainstream employment. The principles of IPS emphasise a goal of competitive paid employment; eligibility based a person's choice, without prior job readiness assessment or pre-vocational training; rapid job search and job placement processes personalised to match individual preferences; individualised benefits counselling and follow-along support (Drake, Bond, & Becker, 2012). A further principle thought crucial to its success is the integration of mental health and employment services (Modini et al., 2016). In Australia, IPS-based employment support services have variously developed through intersectoral partnerships between Disability Employment Services (DES) providers and community mental health services, and separate from DES within youth mental health services (Waghorn, Killackey, Dickson, Brock, & Skate, 2019). Its implementation has become more widespread in youth mental health, where there are plans for it to become a core component of headspace primary mental health services for young Australians (see Chapter 3.2). In comparison, there are policy and operational barriers and challenges to its implementation within DES programs and adult mental health services, so that IPS services are not yet routinely available to adults with mental ill-health (Stirling, Higgins, & Petrakis, 2018; Waghorn et al., 2019). Nevertheless, there are some ongoing DES employment specialists located in community mental health teams, suggesting these challenges can be overcome.

Extensive evidence from three decades of research internationally demonstrates that employment support, when provided in a manner consistent with IPS principles, is effective in assisting young people with psychoses and adults with persistent mental illness to obtain mainstream employment, including in Australia (Modini et al., 2016). While IPS based employment support is more effective than traditional rehabilitation approaches, such as pre-vocational training, it is not effective for everyone; nor does securing a job necessarily translate into ongoing employment (Dewa, Loong, Trojanowski, & Bonato, 2018b; Williams, Fossey, Corbiere, Paluch, & Harvey, 2016). Various strategies have therefore been recommended to enhance or augment employment supports based on IPS principles. These include program level strategies, such as enhanced wrap-around supports to integrate not only mental health care and employment but also housing, welfare benefits, financial and legal assistance; and improved job-matching processes to identify jobs better suited to individual interests, skills and capacities (Lockett, Waghorn, & Kydd, 2018; Modini et al., 2016). The integration of education and employment supports, based on IPS principles, may also be valuable to enhance the employment opportunities and career prospects, particularly for young people and adults with limited vocational qualifications or work experience (Killackey et al., 2019). Combining IPS based employment supports with interventions to enhance cognitive skills and problem-solving may also be useful for some individuals in developing strategies to manage cognitive challenges in the workplace (Dewa, Loong, Trojanowski, & Bonato, 2018a). In addition, useful ingredients of IPS services from a consumer viewpoint include support to develop personalised strategies for maintaining one's job and wellbeing, and to manage disclosure as an ongoing process in workplaces (Johnson et al., 2009; Williams et al., 2016). Mental health and employment services might therefore usefully create opportunities for consumers to develop personalised wellness plans, such as Wellness Recovery Action Plan (WRAP) (Copeland Centre for Wellness and Recovery, 2014) or use mobile self-management technologies such as the WorkingWell smartphone app (Nicholson et al., 2017) as well as to develop plans for managing personal information when negotiating work arrangements with employers (McGahey, Waghorn, Lloyd, Morrissey, & Williams, 2016).

CREATING EMPLOYMENT OPPORTUNITIES

An economic development approach offers a different way to tackle employment disadvantage and improve vocational choices (Roy, Donaldson, Baker, & Kerr, 2014; Stickley & Hall, 2017). Unlike vocational rehabilitation, including IPS services, that provide assistance to obtain jobs within the existing labour market, social enterprises and social businesses match local labour market gaps with the interests, talents and resources of a particular potential workforce, thereby creating new employment options within communities (Mandiberg, 2012). They create jobs for potential workers, who might otherwise struggle to access employment, by providing community employment at market wages to individuals hired into job positions, and accessible, integrated workplaces (Gilbert et al., 2013; Krupa, 2011). Thus, these workplaces are designed with more inclusive working conditions (e.g., flexible hours or job-sharing, individualised training or mentoring, schedule flexibility to accommodate medical appointments) 'built-in' to support all workers to sustain employment (Villotti et al., 2017). This approach also offers possibilities for entrepreneurship to foster self-employment and small business development that may suit some people. For instance, self-employed individuals with psychiatric disabilities in the United States report choosing to run small businesses part-time for the freedom, flexibility, work-life balance and opportunities for innovation provided (Ostrow, Smith, Penney, & Shumway, 2019).

Another area in which increased paid employment opportunities are being created is the provision of expertise as peer advocates, educators and researchers within the mental health sector. The lived experience workforce is a unique work context in which individuals' expertise grounded in 'lived experience' can be positive qualifying attributes or qualities, rather than an experience to be hidden and not disclosed. At the same time, an organisational culture and employment practices within mental health services need to be in place to ensure safe, sustainable and equitable employment for the peer workforce (Bennetts, Pinches, Paluch, & Fossey, 2013; Lived Experience Workforce Strategies Stewardship Group, 2019). (See Chapter 2.2 for further detail.)

RETURN-TO-WORK STRATEGIES

Given mental ill-health is a leading cause of sickness absence from work (Dewa & McDaid, 2011; Harvey et al., 2014), strategies that support employees with common mental health conditions on sick leave to return to work are important. Return-to-work (RTW) is complex and influenced by many factors, including: policies related to sick leave; access to financial support; the quality of occupational health care; and person related factors, such as self-efficacy beliefs about ability to return to work (Nigatu et al., 2017). Qualitative research suggests work identity matters to employees who are on sick leave due to mental health conditions, whether or not they like their jobs, so that they are both sustained by a work identity and miss the routines, activity level and social contacts of work, highlighting the need to keep in touch with work in some way during sickness absence (Cameron, Sadlo, Hart, & Walker, 2016). Often too coordination and communication is complex, but safe, sustainable, and timely RTW may be maximised with practical working alliances and collaboration among workers on sick leave, health professionals, employing organisations, direct supervisors and co-workers (Corbiere et al., 2019). RTW interventions aim to facilitate employees on sick leave getting back to work as soon as possible. The current evidence about which specific strategies are effective in supporting employees with common mental conditions to return to work remains inconclusive, so that a person-centred approach is recommended for selecting strategies, which may include interventions based on cognitive behavioural principles, problem-solving, coping and stress management strategies, as well as work accommodations to address both physical and psychosocial issues in work (Joyce et al., 2016; Bastien & Corbiere, 2019; Munoz-Murillo et al., 2018).

PROMOTING MENTALLY HEALTHY WORKPLACES

Workplace mental health promotion initiatives may be important to reduce work-related stress and the prevalence of mental disorders among workers, as well as to better support employees who experience mental illness (Dewa, Corbiere, Durand, & Hensel, 2012). While health and safety policies and initiatives have traditionally focused on physical health and safety at work, there is increasing recognition of the need to consider job requirements from psychosocial and physical safety perspectives; to educate employers and employees about the use of reasonable work adjustments for workers experiencing mental ill-health to support their return-to-work and job retention; to implement inclusive workplace policies and practices that address risks to mental health at work (e.g., discrimination, bullying, harassment); and to support workers to balance the demands of their work and personal lives (Harvey et al., 2014). Multiple individual, team and organisational level strategies are needed to prevent work-related mental health issues and to promote mental health in the workplaces (Kirsh & Gewurtz, 2012; Reavley, Ross, Martin, Lamontagne, & Jorm, 2014), including Employee Assistance Programs that explicitly address psychosocial health at work and the use of guidelines to address work-related risks to employee mental health, for example, those developed for organisations in Australia (Reavley et al., 2014; Workplace Prevention of Mental Health Problems, 2020).

The next section describes the major psychological therapies used in mental health practice.

2.6.7 PSYCHOLOGICAL THERAPIES: FOCUS AND CONTEXTS

JOHN FARHALL

DEFINING PSYCHOLOGICAL THERAPIES

Almost any mental health service or treatment has a psychological component to it. For example, prescription of medication may raise hope and expectancy that can lead to genuine improvement, regardless of whether the medication itself is effective. Similarly, the informal modelling of problem-solving that occurs as a case manager is assisting a consumer may enhance the consumer's skills. However, to be considered a psychological treatment or therapy, an intervention would usually come from a framework that:

- understands behaviour in terms of psychological processes
- has a theoretical or empirical base (usually both) that requires training and skilled delivery
- prompts change at the level of behaviour, emotion or cognition
- is a time-limited enterprise, in relation to identified issues or symptoms
- reflects an explicit agreement between therapist and client to seek understanding, and support change
- is planned and systematic.

Wampold (2001) provides a similar definition and a discussion of the nature of psychotherapy.

This section first provides an orientation to the practice of psychological therapies in the Australian mental health context, by clarifying the range of needs that might be addressed, the variation in scope across therapies, the variety of contexts in which a practitioner might be conducting the process, and briefly offering a perspective on being an effective practitioner. The section then presents several widespread and effective psychological therapies that may be applied to a range of disorders. Further psychological treatments that are limited to specific disorders are introduced in the disorder-specific chapters of Part 4 (including Interpersonal Psychotherapy (IPT) and Dialectical Behaviour Therapy (DBT; see Chapter 4.3).

What are the psychological needs that therapies address?

Psychological therapies differ in their focus and aims: some address the past, others work with the here and now; some target symptom reduction, others the provision of support. This section outlines some important needs that therapies may address:

- *providing psychological support*: many people want to engage with mental health workers or therapists in order to gain support, to foster hope for improvement in life or to help contain distress or confusion during periods of difficulty. We focus on supportive counselling first in the next section because of its fundamental role in mental health work
- *resolving or mitigating distressing and disabling symptoms*: these are the focus of most specific therapies, but there may be more to therapy than this, as the points below illustrate

- *reducing risk factors*: therapies may be prevention orientated, such as learning stress management skills, or other measures taken to reduce risk of relapse or recurrence for people with an established mental health problem
- *fostering understanding and adaptation*: people living with persisting mental health difficulties can benefit from therapies that help develop a personalised understanding of the nature of these problems, and then help them come to terms with how best to live well when their future life may include the ongoing impact of these problems. This focus of therapy can be an enabler of personal recovery
- *addressing stigma, self-stigma and low self-esteem*: societal stigma about mental health problems can not only lead to discrimination, but also self-stigma, where individuals automatically judge themselves using society's stigmatising standards. Redressing self-stigma and building an empowered self are further foci of psychological therapies
- *preventing deterioration*: some therapies are not directed at change, but in a planned and structured way they support and assist those whose difficulties with self-efficacy, disorganisation or chronically low motivation impair their ability to live well.

THE SCOPE OF SPECIFIC THERAPIES

Most therapies are time limited and focus on just one or two of the needs outlined above. Usually they are organised in one of the following ways, although longer therapies for people with complex and enduring difficulties may be more comprehensive in their scope.

- *Diagnosis-orientated therapies*: some therapies are organised around the typical set of symptoms and needs associated with a diagnosis. For example, exposure and response prevention therapy for people who have obsessive compulsive disorder (see Chapter 4.4), addresses specific ways of learning to face, rather than avoid, fears; dialectical behaviour therapy for people who have a diagnosis of borderline personality disorder (see Chapter 4.9), provides an integrated set of awareness and skills-building interventions, delivered both individually and in a group, that address key challenges, including difficulties in emotion regulation and interpersonal relationships.
- *Symptom-focused therapies*: some therapies specifically address just one troubling symptom. For people living with continuing symptoms of schizophrenia, one form of cognitive behaviour therapy for psychosis (see Section 4.2.4) focuses on coping with command hallucinations (Birchwood et al., 2014). Other specific therapies focus on anxiety, depressed mood and social anxiety.
- *Problem-focused therapies*: some therapies are orientated to a specific problem rather than a symptom. For example, couple therapy or family therapy may address maladaptive patterns of relating. However, the context for such therapies will influence how they proceed. Couple and family therapy may help people struggling with the pressures of ordinary life as well as those affected by mental health challenges such as post-traumatic stress disorder or bipolar disorder (Miklowitz & Chung, 2016). Other problem-focused therapies include specific relapse prevention therapies for psychotic disorders (Ising et al., 2015) and major depressive disorders (e.g. MBCT; Munoz, Beardslee, & Leykin, 2012; see Section 2.6.12.)
- *Universal process therapies*: some therapies address core psychological processes that are considered fundamental to better adjustment; for these therapies, the specific presentations of a problem or disorder are considered less important to directly address. Examples include supportive-expressive therapy (Luborsky, 1984), which understands most problems through the lens of interpersonal relationships, and Acceptance and Commitment Therapy (ACT; see Section 2.6.12), which addresses all problems by increasing 'psychological flexibility' in the pursuit of valued living.

VARYING CONTEXTS FOR THERAPY

The traditional view of therapies is that, following referral from a GP, mental health worker or family member, individual clients engage in confidential, face-to-face appointments with a therapist who has just that one role. In Australia, the Better Access to mental health care scheme, whereby clients may access psychological therapy services through a GP referral and private practice settings (see Chapter 1.7) come closest to this stereotype. However, it is possible that good therapy may still occur where none of these traditional elements holds true. In short, the context of therapy is usually more complex than, and sometimes lacks the formality of, the stereotype.

Involvement of stakeholders

There are likely to be several parties interested in and interacting with the client about the therapy. Family members and friends may have a big stake in its outcome, and often talk with the client following sessions (providing opportunities for extending the work of the therapy through involvement of family members). Referrers usually have a separate ongoing relationship with the client and need to know relevant issues and outcomes. Funding bodies, such as accident or compensation insurers or Medicare, may reasonably need to know about the focus and work of therapy. All of these parties should be informed and included as appropriate, with the limits of confidentiality agreed in advance with the client, and consistent with legislation.

Therapists' secondary roles with clients

Therapists may have secondary roles with the client, in addition to the psychological therapy. In public mental health services, case managers or other team members may allocate some of their time to delivery of therapy, and some to assisting with practical and social needs (see Chapter 2.4). Even private practitioners may take some case management responsibility, particularly in helping link the client with needed other services as therapy proceeds, or in arranging post-termination supports. These additional roles need thought to manage; they may be confusing for some consumers, and structuring time for each role can help both consumer and therapist keep on track and quarantine time appropriately.

Therapy as part of a team's work

Therapy is essentially about change, and the process of change is not always a smooth ride. Clients may experience periods of confusion, worsening mood or disturbed behaviour as therapy proceeds. In interdisciplinary contexts (and also in the context of keeping families or other agencies informed) a role of the therapist is to regularly liaise with family or team members, informing them in general terms (as agreed with the client) how therapy is progressing, the issues that may come up and therapy-enhancing responses they might make. Recorded therapy goals, and methods consistent with the formulation and case management plan, provide the clearest context for all parties to be on the same page.

Therapy in informal contexts

Therapeutic interventions may occur in less formal contexts than a defined number of sessions in a consulting room. Appropriately trained case managers may take opportunities for therapeutic psychoeducation (see Section 2.6.9) or for CBT focused on social anxiety when assisting a person to link with a neighbourhood centre. Crisis team clinicians may provide a brief or single session therapy; mobile intensive support team clinicians may provide CBT for psychosis or supportive therapy. Non-government mental health workers may teach mindfulness skills in a community support service, such as a Recovery College (Perkins, Meddings, Williams, & Repper, 2018). All of these examples show opportunities for choosing and tailoring what a therapy has to offer to fit the needs of a person and their current circumstances.

Therapy without therapists

Self-help books have a long history, but more recently, the accessibility of the internet has enabled widespread dissemination of online therapies. There is good evidence for the effectiveness of a range of therapies for mild to moderate mental health problems, with therapist guidance (via email or SMS) ranging from none to considerable. The accessibility and privacy of this form of therapy can make it easier for ambivalent or anxious people to try therapy. Despite the importance of the therapeutic relationship in bringing about change in face-to-face therapies, internet based therapies can be effective with little therapist guidance (see Section 2.6.13).

THERAPEUTIC ALLEGIANCE AND EFFECTIVE THERAPY

No single therapy could reasonably be expected to address the vast variety of human individual needs, yet therapists and academics often strongly identify with just one therapy, arguing its superiority. Other therapists consider themselves 'eclectic', a term used in various ways to describe the utilisation of different therapeutic models for different people or different problems (Corey, 2001). Technical eclecticism simply draws techniques from different therapy models, without necessarily adopting the models behind them. Theoretical integration is a form of eclecticism that synthesises two or more theoretical approaches to create a new conceptual framework (Norcross & Goldfried, 2019). Common factors eclecticism draws on change factors such as the therapeutic alliance, that seem to be common elements across a range of therapies. So, if no single therapy fits all, is eclecticism the answer? What is a useful perspective for mental health practitioners to take?

A large body of theory and empirical research demonstrates that the theory-based therapeutic processes ('specific factors') such as cognitive change in CBT, are not the only, or even greatest, contributor to change (Cuijpers, van Straten, Andersson, & van Oppen, 2008; Wampold et al., 1997); much of the benefit from counselling and psychotherapy arises from the presence of 'common' or 'contextual' factors (Norcross, 2011). Common factors include the presence of an emotionally charged bond between the therapist and client, a safe setting, a culturally relevant psychological explanation of the problem, and procedures that the therapist and client do that prompt behaviour change (Laska, Gurman, & Wampold, 2014). This does not mean that the specifics of a therapy, such as the cognitive and behavioural activities in CBT, are not needed–without specific explanations and rituals a therapy cannot work. However, there are relatively few mental health conditions for which one specific form of therapy is substantially more effective than another. Reflecting on this provides a useful perspective for considering the contribution of different schools or forms of therapy and decisions of a practitioner about whether to be eclectic or therapy specific in their approach.

Eclecticism has potential advantages of drawing on a wider repertoire of therapeutic models or strategies for the benefit of clients, but has risks of losing the effective elements of therapies if only parts of one are mixed with parts of another when working with one person. By contrast, focusing on providing just one type of therapy has the potential advantage of the practitioner becoming more experienced and thus able to offer greater depth or sophistication of treatment, but risks the model being inapplicable to some presenting problems. We suggest that good counselling and psychotherapy practice involves (a) minimising technical eclecticism; (b) utilising the power of common factors; and (c) holding one's therapy assumptions lightly while practising with fidelity; that is, applying each model in the way it has been validated, while keeping in mind that other models may also be an option to help the client if this way of working does not achieve the goals.

2.6.8 SUPPORTIVE COUNSELLING AND SUPPORTIVE THERAPIES

ROBERT KING

INTRODUCTION

Supportive counselling (also known as non-directive counselling) is a widely used but not extensively studied approach to helping people with mental health problems. The core technique is active listening, which makes use of:

- open questions and clarifying questions to elicit communication from the client
- feedback in the form of paraphrasing and summarising that communicates understanding and allows for correction of misunderstanding
- feedback in the form of pointing out inconsistencies or noting omissions that challenges the client to expand thinking.

Beyond technique, at the core of supportive counselling are core principles that provide the foundation for a successful therapeutic relationship:

- belief in the autonomy of the client and the capacity of the client to make decisions in her or his own best interest
- unconditional positive regard for the client (focus on strengths and attributes rather than deficits)
- willingness to engage empathically in the inner world of the client and to see things from her or his perspective.

Supportive counsellors refrain from giving advice and instead encourage the client to find solutions. Supportive counsellors provide sufficient structure to sessions so as to ensure the counsellor has the information necessary to understand the issue or problem, to appreciate client goals and priorities and to assist the client to work towards a solution and a plan of action. However the client has a central role in agenda setting and supportive counselling is sometimes termed non-directive counselling. Supportive counselling may take place within a single session or may form the primary modality of an extended therapeutic relationship.

Supportive counselling is not manualised although there are widely used texts such as Egan's *The Skilled Helper* that set out principles and practices (Egan, 2007). Manualised interventions such as motivational interviewing and problem solving therapy share some of the principles and approaches of supportive counselling but are more therapist directed and have more clearly delineated techniques and strategies.

EVIDENCE BASE

Some of the evidence base for supportive counselling derives from its history as a 'control' condition in randomised controlled trials investigating more active manualised therapies such as CBT. While the expectation in such trials was that supportive counselling would be inferior to medication or more active psychological treatments such as CBT, supportive counselling often performed surprisingly well. For example, a randomised controlled trial conducted in Edinburgh by Scott and Freeman (Scott & Freeman, 1992) found that counselling provided by social workers was as effective as CBT provided by psychologists or medication prescribed by psychiatrists for treatment of major depression. Not only was counselling successful in alleviating symptoms, it was also rated more highly by patients than the alternative treatments. Wampold and colleagues (2002) found that when supportive counselling was used in a bona fide attempt to treat depression it was as effective as more active interventions such as CBT. Cuijpers and colleagues (2012) identified 31 studies in which non-directive supportive therapy was used as a treatment for adult depression. They found that, after controlling for therapist allegiance, supportive therapy was equally as effective as other psychological interventions. In summary, while the evidence base from high quality studies is limited to treatment of depression the findings suggest that supportive counselling is effective and may not be less effective than other psychological interventions.

ADVANTAGES AND LIMITATIONS OF SUPPORTIVE COUNSELLING

Counselling is a very flexible intervention that can be adapted to a wide range of circumstances and conditions. It is equally suited to single session interventions or to extended therapy and is widely delivered by telephone as well as face-to-face. Training requirements for providers are modest and user acceptability is high. The main limitation is that the lack of clear procedures makes quality control difficult and high quality research programs tend to steer away from investigation of interventions that are not manualised and under-specified.

Application in public mental health

Counselling is well-suited to the relatively informal and sometimes irregular therapeutic engagements characteristic of case management. It is also congruent with the contemporary recovery model, which privileges client autonomy and responsibility for decision making. The supportive counselling framework is consistent with a case manager role of accompanying the consumer on a recovery journey.

2.6.9 INDIVIDUAL PSYCHOEDUCATION

NEIL THOMAS & ROBERT KING

'Psychoeducation' refers to activities that facilitate the person's knowledge about their mental health and its management as a therapeutic intervention. Psychoeducation is an empowering intervention as it assists the person affected to make informed decisions regarding the management of a mental health condition. Psychoeducation may be delivered as a stand-alone therapy, but often forms an element of routine care or a component of broader therapy approaches. Hence it may be delivered using a range of methods, including group-format courses, one-to-one discussions and the use of written or multimedia information, and may overlap with guided use of self-help materials.

Psychoeducation is a major component of talking therapies, especially cognitive behavioural and related therapies. Psychoeducation alone, without other components of psychological interventions has been found to be effective in treatment of disorders such as depression and anxiety (Donker, Griffiths, Cuijpers, & Christensen, 2009). This suggests that knowledge and understanding of these kinds of conditions may often be sufficient to enable the people affected to manage them more successfully.

A major application of psychoeducation is to facilitate effective self-management and relapse prevention, particularly in chronic and recurrent mental disorders such as schizophrenia (e.g. Hornung, Feldman, Klingberg, Buchkremer, & Reker, 1999) and bipolar disorder (Bond & Anderson, 2015). Other applications include correcting misinterpretations of physical symptoms of stress in panic and somatoform disorders (e.g. Bouman & Buwalda, 2008; Dannon, Iancu, & Grunhaus, 2002) and preventatively promoting adjustment and coping in at-risk groups (e.g. Fisher, Wynter, & Rowe, 2010; Hauser et al., 2009).

Formal psychoeducation courses often involve multiple components. One of the most empirically supported psychoeducation courses, the Barcelona Bipolar Disorders Program (Colom & Vieta, 2006), includes five sessions of information about the condition (such as symptoms, causes, triggers to episodes and course), seven sessions promoting adherence to medication, and eight sessions on self-management strategies (such as early detection of new episodes, establishing regular behavioural habits, stress management and avoiding substance use).

Educational methods are well established as efficacious in improving health outcomes in general medicine (Lagger, Pataky, & Golay, 2010), yet the evidence base within mental health is less well developed. However, there is a growing body of high quality evidence to suggest that psychoeducation can contribute to medication adherence and may have benefits that are independent of adherence to treatment. A systematic review by Bond and Anderson (2015) identified 16 studies in which a psychoeducational intervention was included in treatment for bipolar disorder, with a control group receiving treatment as usual. They found that psychoeducation increased medication adherence and reduced the risk of further manic or hypomanic episodes. There was no evidence of impact on depression.

However in psychotic disorders, where lack of insight may be a significant barrier, there have been more mixed findings. A meta-analysis by Xia and colleagues (2011) found overall positive effects on outcomes such as relapse, readmission and medication adherence. Indeed, positive effects have been observed at up to seven years follow-up (Bauml et al., 2016). On the other hand, in a meta-analysis by Lincoln and colleagues (2007), it was noted that psychoeducation including family members reduces relapse, but there was no evidence that psychoeducation focused only on patients improved symptoms, relapse or medication adherence. It is notable that in this context that medication adherence has been particularly hard to treat in this population. Gray and colleagues (2016) identified six randomised controlled trials of adherence therapy—a focused collaborative decision-making intervention targeting medication adherence. After 12 months, there were no differences between the groups with respect to treatment adherence, even though adherence therapy participants appeared to benefit from the collaborative approach in other ways such as reduced symptoms.

Overall, the boundaries of psychoeducation often blend into self-management, psychotherapeutic or family interventions, which can make conclusions about whether it is the provision of information or other elements of the intervention that are contributing to beneficial effects. Nonetheless, at the very least, provision of quality information by health providers is important in promoting greater consumer empowerment, and more collaborative discussions about treatment (e.g., Galletly et al., 2016; National Collaborating Centre for Mental Health, 2014). In many cases psychoeducation may be an effective treatment in its own right.

2.6.10 PSYCHODYNAMIC THERAPY: AN INTRODUCTION AND OVERVIEW

ROBERT KING

INTRODUCTION

The term 'psychodynamic therapies' refers to a broad spectrum of interventions, ranging from brief manualised therapies to long-term exploratory therapies. A survey of more than 2200 North American psychotherapists revealed that psychodynamic therapy was the third most widely practiced modality (after CBT and family/systems) with 36% of the sample indicating they made some use of this approach (Cook, Biyanova, Elhai, Schnurr, & Coyne, 2010).

Shedler (2010) argued that psychodynamic therapies aim to achieve changes at the level of personality and functioning rather than symptom relief. He proposed seven distinctive features:

1. focus on affect and expression of emotion
2. exploration of attempts to avoid distressing thoughts and feelings
3. identification of recurring themes and patterns
4. discussion of past experience (developmental focus)
5. focus on interpersonal relations
6. focus on the therapy relationship
7. exploration of fantasy life.

While some of these features are likely to be present in many therapies, psychodynamic therapies tend to be saturated by these features. Psychodynamic therapies may also be characterised by: a focus on unconscious wishes, impulses or fears and by the use of the client's experience of the therapeutic relationship (transference) for in vivo exploration of how these unconscious wishes, impulses or fears impact interpersonally.

Brief psychodynamic therapies are typically manualised, and work with a simplified model of mental and emotional processes. A good example is Supportive-Expressive Therapy (Luborsky, 1984; Book, 1998). This therapy focuses on analysis of relationship episodes with a view to identifying 'core conflictual relationship themes'. The premise is that most psychological problems are associated with relationship difficulties and that these difficulties arise because of:

- unconscious wishes or expectations the person has with respect to the other
- responses of the other that do not accord with these wishes or expectations and
- responses of the self when wishes or expectations are not met by the other.

THE EVIDENCE BASE FOR PSYCHODYNAMIC THERAPIES

During the past three decades, the effectiveness of psychodynamic interventions has been investigated using randomised controlled trials and the evidence base is now substantial. This evidence is summarised in six meta-analyses conducted over the past decade.

In a formal equivalence study, Steinart and colleagues (2017) found that psychodynamic therapies were as effective as other evidence-based interventions (whether psychotherapeutic or psychopharmacological) for symptom. Cristea and colleagues (2017) found that psychodynamic therapy and dialectical behaviour therapy were equivalent in effectiveness and superior to control conditions for treatment of borderline personality disorder. Driessen and colleagues (2015) found that short term psychodynamic psychotherapies were as effective for treatment of depression as other therapies and that there was some evidence of superior effectiveness with anxiety symptoms in the context of depression. A review of controlled trials of long-term psychodynamic psychotherapy found that people with complex mental disorders had superior outcomes when treated psychodynamically compared with those treated with briefer non-psychodynamic interventions (Leichsenring & Rabung, 2011). Abbass and colleagues (2011) found that short-term psychodynamic therapy was effective for treatment of depressive disorders with comorbid personality disorder and that the effect size was at least equivalent to that obtained by other therapies. Psychodynamic therapies are also reported to be effective or probably effective in treatment of psychological and physical symptoms associated with psychosomatic disorders and beneficial with respect to social adjustment (Abbass, Kisely, & Kroenke, 2009).

In summary, there is compelling evidence that psychodynamic therapy is effective and most likely as effective as other forms of psychotherapy across a broad range of mental health problems that typically respond well to psychotherapy. Notwithstanding the claims of some, such as Shedler (2010) there is little evidence that it is markedly superior to other therapies, nor even that its effectiveness derives from characteristics specific to its theories or methods. The evidence available from routine practice settings suggests that while effect size is reduced, this is no different from the reduced effectiveness found in real world applications of other therapies (Paley et al., 2008).

ADVANTAGES AND LIMITATIONS OF PSYCHODYNAMIC THERAPY

Psychodynamic therapy is not typically symptom or diagnosis focused and allows the client the central role in setting the therapy agenda. This makes it attractive to clients who seek to develop personal understanding on their own terms, rather than being told how their mind works by a newly graduated psychologist. However this comes at a cost. Even the short-term focused psychodynamic therapies require substantially longer periods of treatment than therapies such as CBT. For example, the minimum standard treatment of supportive-expressive therapy is 16 sessions. In a comparative trial, Shapiro and colleagues (1995) found that it took 16 sessions of psychodynamic therapy to achieve the sustained beneficial impact on depression that was achieved by CBT after eight sessions. The relative inefficiency of psychodynamic therapy makes it unattractive to third party funders who are more concerned about cost of symptom reduction than a client's quest for personal understanding.

Is there a role for psychodynamic therapy in public mental health?

At first glance, psychodynamic therapy might seem to be poorly suited to public mental health services because of its relative inefficiency. However, consumers of public mental health services are not equivalent to people who participate in psychotherapy efficacy trials. Their disorders are typically more severe and more complex, and they have usually failed to respond well to standard treatment. Such people are likely to need more extended and more intensive psychological treatment than a standard course of CBT or equivalent. Psychodynamic therapies may be suitable whenever a problem is sufficiently complex to require something more than a brief intervention. The fact that psychodynamic therapy is not programmatic is an advantage when a longer term involvement is required. The risk with programmatic therapies is that they become repetitive and that therapist and/or client become exasperated when the treatment has run its course but has only achieved modest gains.

Combining brief psychodynamic therapy and CBT

A long history of contention between proponents of these therapies has meant that there has been little consideration of scope for integration. This is unfortunate in my view. While psychodynamic therapy is more exploratory and CBT more psychoeducational, both promote development of insight and understanding as the means of managing symptoms of anxiety and depression. Clients with access to both frameworks have the opportunity to make use of perspectives that best promote their own understanding. The availability of high quality online CBT programs through websites such as e-couch, mental health online and on-track means that it is possible for a client to work through a CBT program at home while addressing interpersonal issues in therapy sessions. This is not recommended unless the therapist has sound understanding of CBT and is willing and able to provide some support to the online CBT during sessions, as well as addressing interpersonal issues.

2.6.11 COGNITIVE BEHAVIOUR THERAPIES

NIKOLAOS KAZANTZIS & ALEXANDRA PETRIK

INTRODUCTION

The advent of the cognitive model (Beck, 1967; Beck, 1979) emphasised the centrality of moment-to-moment conscious thoughts, assumptions, broader beliefs, and images to the development and maintenance of psychopathology. Other influential cognitive models were also being developed by Ellis (1962) and Meichenbaum (1973). However, Beck's work grew as a result of its scientific basis, and what originally began as a specific treatment of depression is now accepted as a major system of therapy that has influenced mental health care, across all professions, worldwide.

Beckian therapy has been widely researched, and is considered an empirically supported first-line treatment for acute phases of a variety of mood and anxiety disorders (e.g., National Institute for Health and Care Excellence (NICE), 2011a). The underlying theories and procedural practices of CBT have also been continuously increasing in diversity, with various applications of CBT now being recommended therapies for other disorders ranging from borderline personality disorder to psychosis. Hence, the term 'cognitive therapy', commonly referred to as 'cognitive behaviour therapy' (CBT), no longer exclusively refers to the model developed by Beck. Many therapies are part of the family of CBTs, including those that emphasise specific change processes (e.g., acceptance based approaches), those that emphasise a specific therapeutic style (e.g., motivational interviewing), and those that focus on specific techniques in CBT (e.g., mindfulness based approaches) (see Section 2.6.12).

THEORETICAL UNDERPINNINGS OF CBT

The cognitive model proposes that the ways in which individuals interpret their past and current experiences influences how they perceive their external environment. This idiosyncratic interpretation of events influences emotional reactions and future behaviour, and is termed the 'information-processing hypothesis' of CBT. Biased or unhelpful thinking patterns can act as a 'filter' through which individuals interpret internal and external events. For example, in depression, this filter can be negative or pessimistic, and involve selective memory of experience supporting negative appraisals. Applications of CBT to different disorders emphasise specific thought processes (e.g., intrusive thoughts, worry), specific beliefs (e.g., metacognitive beliefs), as well as specific content of beliefs (e.g., vulnerability across the anxiety disorders, defensiveness and abandonment in borderline personality disorder). Indeed, these themes in cognitions can be expected to be associated with specific emotions (e.g., a strong sense of entitlement is usually associated with hostility, frustration, and low empathy) and behavioural patterns (e.g., competitiveness, domineering, and critical style in entitlement), which together form a 'schema' and can be a focus of intervention from the outset of CBT.

Thought biases (often termed 'cognitive distortions') were a hallmark of the early CBT literature, including both Beck and Ellis's contributions, but have limited utility as they are not clearly defined and have been criticised for pathologising normal styles of human thought. A modern practice of CBT could, but does not necessarily, invite clients to become aware of these biases in the interests of a shared case conceptualisation.

As an integrative therapy, CBT incorporates behavioural theories and associated change processes such as operant and classical conditioning. Identification of situational triggers and antecedents and consequences to behaviour remains a cornerstone to the analysis of behaviour and comprehensive case conceptualisation. The mediational role of cognitions (such as thoughts, desires, images and beliefs) in the development of psychological problems is of course the important addition of CBTs. The essential idea is that cognitive changes are central in determining emotional, behavioural, physiological and environmental-systemic changes.

CBT involves attention to three levels of thought—the situationally specific 'surface' level thoughts, cross-situational rules and assumptions and deeper level beliefs. Thoughts that occur quickly on a moment-to-moment basis are defined as being 'surface' level, or *automatic* thoughts (for example, 'I can't cope'). Automatic thoughts are evaluations of specific moments in time or situations, and for many people are part of their current awareness. Automatic thoughts that are clinically important are generally those associated with strong emotional distress. At the intermediate level of cognition, cross-situational beliefs, rules or assumptions are beliefs often learnt in early development, either as part of a person's familial, cultural or social context (for example, 'I should think of others'). These cognitions guide behaviour and determine a client's current coping strategies (for example, 'If I avoid situations I'll feel better').

In addition to identification of automatic thoughts and cross-situational beliefs, the modern practice of Beck's therapy involves identification of 'core' level appraisals of the self, other people and the world, and the future. These rigid, overgeneralised beliefs are generally more difficult and potentially distressing to access and change. Core beliefs can either be adaptive and helpful (sometimes referred to as 'positive', such as 'I am a capable person'), or unbalanced and less helpful (sometimes referred to as 'negative', such as 'I am a useless person' or 'I'm a failure'). Core beliefs are also developed in early childhood, and often reflect social experiences (for example, an individual reared in an environment with critical parents might develop a belief about him- or herself as 'I'm not good enough' or 'Unless I excel, I won't be accepted'). It is beyond the scope of this resource, but core beliefs, assumptions, emotions, and rehearsed ways of relating are clustered in the definition of schema; according to theory, and some supportive community studies, maladaptive schemas often coexist and are triggered from moment to moment in distressing situations.

It is this attention to cognition that is pinpointed as the main reason for CBT's enduring effects and superior treatment outcomes (compared to pharmacotherapies and other talking therapies) in the treatment of anxiety and mood disorders (e.g., Hollon & DeRubeis, 2009).

Despite their conceptual similarities, CBTs differ to a great extent in their relational styles. For instance, rational-emotive behaviour therapy relies on a confrontational style of disputation, or challenging, and a high degree of directiveness, which is contrary to the humanistic (client-centred) and collaborative nature of the therapeutic relationship in CBT. Similarly, in dialectical behaviour therapy (see Section 4.9.6), the therapist will use irreverent questioning and dialogue to convey authenticity, but this is not usually part of Beckian CBT. Furthermore, the clinician practising schema therapy, a close variant of CBT, will make overt efforts to convey to the client that they disagree with the client's belief system and challenge its origins.

CBT: MOVING FROM INITIAL ASSESSMENT TO THERAPY

From the outset of treatment, the CBT therapist is to gain an understanding of the client's presenting problems using a basic problem formulation (see Sections 2.3.6 and 2.3.14). However, in order for this to be more than a basic psychosocial formulation, the therapist is required to attend to different levels of thought. Specifically, it is important for CBT therapists to develop a 'collaborative case formulation' (or 'individualised case conceptualisation') with the client surrounding (1) diagnosis; (2) current problems; (3) underlying unhelpful beliefs or thoughts that are associated with the problems; and (4) how the client copes with the beliefs through adaptive or maladaptive behavioural, cognitive or affective mechanisms (Beck, 2011).

CBT is a structured therapy, but the term 'structured' is misleading. Unless in a group therapy or technology delivered format, CBT should be flexibly delivered and responsive to the unique needs of the client. That is, session agendas should not be predetermined, and the actual session itself should not rigidly follow a time allocation or set of priorities. Like any psychotherapy, CBT's interventions exist within a (therapeutic relationship) relational context (Kazantzis, Dattilio, Dobson, & Beck, 2017).

CBT is also deceptively straightforward. Expert clinicians are adapting their case conceptualisation on a moment-to-moment basis, taking into account their personal responses to the client, reality testing their own perceptions, while adapting the component parts of the therapeutic relationship to best suit the client. For some, being asked to provide feedback (a core collaborative behaviour) is too emotionally distressing early in therapy. Similarly, being asked to share in decision making, or to offer their own perspective on the goals of therapy, is too emotionally risky, and moreover, many clients try very hard to inhibit their emotions because of familial, societal, and/or cultural beliefs and norms about the experience and display of emotion. As with all human communication, multiple schemas are being triggered to a greater or lesser extent from one second to the next, and important clinical decisions should be informed through attention to, and adaptations of the delivery style and choice of interventions during the conduct of CBT.

IN-SESSION PROCESSES THAT DEFINE CBT

A collaborative and empirical therapeutic relationship

Generic elements of the therapeutic interaction—such as genuineness, empathy, warmth, agreement on tasks and goals, and positive regard are considered 'evidence-based' relationship elements (Norcross & Wampold, 2011). However, the CBT practitioner is required to develop relationships that are characterised by a collaborative interaction, which engages the client in an empirical examination of their experiences. Put differently, clients are not passive recipients of change, but rather develop and refine strategies to help themselves. In short, a core aim of cognitive therapy is to teach the client to become his or her 'own therapist' (Beck, 2011).

In addition, there is a requirement to tailor the therapy, from assessment through relapse prevention, to the individual client's life situation. This is achieved by heralding the client's experience as the basis for selecting and evaluating the utility of interventions—and in this way, CBT takes a phenomenological emphasis and does not assume a 'correct' view of the world. It is the client's 'data' (thoughts, beliefs and subjective experiences) that are collected and 'tested' through a variety of cognitive and behavioural strategies (see Beck, 1979; Tee & Kazantzis, 2011).

Between-session activities (or therapeutic 'homework')

As well as in-session strategies, between-session work, or 'homework', has always been considered crucial to the generalisation and maintenance of adaptive skills (Beck, 1979; Kazantzis, Deane, Ronan, & L'Abate, 2005). This is the process by which clients generalise the specific skills introduced during sessions to the situations in which their problems actually exist: increasing the client's adaptive functioning. There is strong evidence for homework's causal and correlational effects in CBT (see meta-analyses by Kazantzis, Whittington, & Dattilio, 2010; Kazantzis et al., 2016).

CBT TECHNIQUES AND STRATEGIES

Because the model underpinning the therapy conceives the human experience as a cognitive one—that is, thoughts and beliefs exist in every moment—those interventions that have a behavioural focus are conceptualised as a means to achieve cognitive change (Beck, 1979; Persons, 1995; Petrik, Kazantzis, & Hofmann, 2013).

Behaviourally focused techniques

Fulfilling relationships with family and friends, productive work and study, productive communication, transitional and expected reactions to stressful life events, and absence of alcohol and other drug abuse or dependency are all central clinical considerations when evaluating a client's functioning. It makes sense that those same observable behaviours form the centre of attention in CBT. Behavioural interventions are aimed at increasing knowledge and skills, enhancing positive change and targeting unhelpful or avoidance behaviours. Operant conditioning theory states that events that are positive will increase a behaviour, those that are negative will decrease a behaviour, and those that are neither positive nor negative will extinguish a behaviour. Put simply, clients engage in behaviour (helpful or unhelpful) that works for them.

Behavioural activation for depression relies on reinforcement schedules and an individual's responses to contingencies. As depression can develop through continuous reinforcement (such as low rates of positive reinforcement, and high rates of punishment; Martell, Dimidjian, & Herman-Dunn, 2010), this part of CBT involves self-monitoring and scheduling of activities associated with pleasure and mastery. This aspect of CBT has demonstrated empirical support as a stand-alone intervention for acute phase depression (see Dimidjian et al., 2006).

Other behaviourally focused techniques in CBT include exposure and arousal reduction (also known as relaxation) strategies (designed to reduce general or situationally specific feelings of stress and anxiety) and interpersonal skills training. The latter focuses on facilitating communication between families and friends, teaching assertiveness or social skills training (Beck, 2011).

Cognitively focused techniques

Strategies that have a cognitive emphasis are generally assessed in terms of the benefit in reducing unpleasant emotions and physiology, and improving important relationships or functioning in other areas. Techniques that have a cognitive focus in CBT include identifying and evaluating cognitions and patterns in thinking, problem-solving, reattribution of responsibility and guided imagery. The broad category of identifying and evaluating thoughts can be achieved through a variety of strategies including, but not limited to, thought records, weighing up pros and cons of unhelpful thoughts and the identification of more 'balanced' thoughts. Focusing on different aspects of a client's belief system through cognitively and behaviourally focused techniques depends on the client's stage in therapy.

Therapeutic work typically begins with surface level cognitions before access to deeper level beliefs is achieved. Socratic questioning, another fundamental feature of CBT, is used throughout various processes and interventions. Despite its name, Socratic questioning (or dialogue) differs a great deal from the teaching style of Socrates, because its goal is to reach a discovery that is not predetermined (Padesky, 1993; Kazantzis & Stuckey, 2018). Socratic dialogue involves (a) gaining a mutual understanding of the client's concern; (b) exploring new information or existing information in a new way; (c) applying the explored information to the original concern; and (d) seeking feedback from the client about the value of the discovery in terms of its helpfulness, meaningfulness and importance. Examples of typical questions a therapist may use to identify or evaluate cognitions are: 'Is there any evidence against the idea that ...?', 'What if it were true that ...?' and 'What does that mean?' In the latter example, the therapist is eliciting a deeper level belief: a core belief that may be underlying many situations:

Therapist: Okay, so let's suppose that the automatic thought that you were not good enough to raise your children was true. What would that mean?

Client: I'm not sure ... If I can't even raise my children properly then I'm completely useless. I'm a failure.

If we think about previously mentioned concepts such as collaborative empiricism and the fundamental aim of enabling a client to become his or her own therapist, Socratic dialogue in CBT facilitates these central change mechanisms.

PRACTICE ILLUSTRATION: COGNITIVE BEHAVIOUR THERAPY

Jane, who was 37 years old, was receiving CBT for major depressive disorder and a comorbid panic disorder without agoraphobia. Jane had completed six sessions of therapy and was quickly able to complete a thought record assignment. Although Jane effectively completed a thought record after an event, she had difficulty making use of the skill in situations in which she experienced emotional distress. Jane had been raised in a family where she learnt to suppress her spontaneous emotional experience. In discussing her family history, Jane remembered her mother having extreme feelings of anger and suspicion, which eventually deteriorated into widespread paranoia and delusions, causing her to be hospitalised and medicated. Jane came away from these early life experiences believing that experiencing emotion was a 'bad thing', and, 'If I experience emotion, then I am out of control.' Guided discovery was helpful for Jane because it enabled her to identify these rules. In particular, Jane observed that she had a series of automatic thoughts whenever she experienced emotion, including, 'I must stop this feeling'; 'I can't let myself feel this way'. It was helpful to engage in Socratic dialogue and guided discovery within the session about the experience, as well as the suppression and acceptance of emotions, and then to extend it as the next homework assignment. In later sessions, the rationale for cognitive restructuring using thought records was discussed as a means for Jane to deal with negative emotions and be aligned with her own coping strategies.

Source: Adapted from Kazantzis et al., 2005, pp. 383–4

CONTEXTUAL FACTORS TO THE PRACTICE OF CBT

CBT is considered 'short term' in many forms of application. 'Short term' generally means a range of 16 to 20 sessions, and there is now emerging evidence for continuation phase CBT in the prevention of depressive relapse (Jarrett, Vittengl, & Clark, 2008). However, the length of treatment is dependent upon the severity or chronicity of the client's presenting problems; more longstanding and complex difficulties generally benefit from a longer-term therapy. The extent to which the client is suitable for CBT treatment (has the ability to understand the CBT model) is also important to consider.

Evidence base for CBT

CBT has been well established for depression and suicide (Beck, 1979; Wenzel, Brown, & Beck, 2009), anxiety disorders and phobias, panic disorder, substance abuse, chronic pain, personality disorders, schizophrenia, chronic fatigue syndrome and eating disorders (see Epp & Dobson, 2010 for a review). As well as working with adults, CBT has also shown to be effective in the treatment of other populations, such as adolescents, children and older adults (e.g., Creed, Reisweber, & Beck, 2011).

Self-help and internet-based delivery modes

Low-intensity interventions such as group psychoeducation, individual self-help and guided self-help may be a useful initial treatment option for some individuals before accessing more high-intensity options (such as CBT, applied relaxation or drug treatment). However, the classification of 'low' versus 'high' intensity interventions is mechanistic and not universally accepted—since any given technique can be utilised for a multitude of reasons.

Internet and smartphone delivered CBTs may also be useful (see Bakker, Kazantzis, Rickwood, & Rickard, 2016). The technology administered delivery has many benefits, including easy accessibility for individuals with restricted mobility, or who reside in rural areas.

Local training opportunities

CBT is taught in the majority of accredited postgraduate clinical psychology training programs throughout Australia; however, the availability and depth of training for other health professionals is more limited. In order to develop therapist competence, post-qualification CBT training courses are advisable. The Australian Psychological Society's Institute offers a range of training and professional development in CBT (APA, 2020d). Further interdisciplinary professional development, training and conference opportunities can also be found at organisations such as the Australian Association for Cognitive and Behaviour Therapy (AACBT, 2020), the Association for Behavioural and Cognitive Therapies (ABCT, 2020) and the European Association for Behavioural and Cognitive Therapies (EABCT, 2020). The Academy of Cognitive Therapy (Academy of Cognitive and Behavioral Therapies (ACT), 2020) provides certification in CBT.

Guides for practice can be found through the APS (APS, 2020) and the American Psychological Association (APA, 2020a). The Beck Institute of Cognitive and Behaviour Therapy is an essential resource for clinicians (BECK Cognitive Behavior Therapy, 2020). There are many resources available for clinicians wishing to gain access for treatment manuals and guidelines for practice through the above organisations.

2.6.12 THIRD-GENERATION COGNITIVE BEHAVIOURAL THERAPIES

FRANCES SHAWYER

NEW GENERATIONS

The past four decades have seen the rise of so-called 'third generation' or 'third wave' behaviour therapies (Hayes, 2016); the key examples include mindfulness-based stress reduction (MBSR; Kabat-Zinn, 1982, 1990), mindfulness-based cognitive therapy (MBCT; Segal, Williams, & Teasdale, 2002; Segal, Williams, & Teasdale, 2013), dialectical behaviour therapy (DBT; Linehan, 1993) and acceptance and commitment therapy (ACT; Hayes, Strosahl, & Wilson, 1999, 2012). Other therapies, namely mindfulness-integrated cognitive behaviour therapy (MiCBT; Cayoun, 2011; Cayoun, Francis, & Shires, 2019) and compassion focused therapy (CFT; Gilbert, 2010a) have been subject to less rigorous evaluation but show significant promise. There are numerous other third-generation therapies, such as mindful self-compassion (MSC; Neff & Germer, 2013) and MBSR/MBCT relatives such as mindfulness-based eating awareness treatment (MB-EAT; Kristeller & Wolever, 2011), which will not be considered here but which the interested reader may wish to investigate. Rather than changing the form and content of thought and emotion, these approaches focus on changing the relationship to thought and emotion, emphasising the mindful acceptance of difficult psychological experience (Chiesa & Malinowski, 2011). The regular practice of mindfulness itself is thought to reduce reactivity to thoughts and emotions and increase self-awareness, self-acceptance and the capacity to make adaptive choices (Surawy, Roberts, & Silver, 2005).

The third generation therapies have been divided into mindfulness-*based* therapies (MBIs) that centre on intensive training in mindfulness meditation (including MBSR, MBCT and MiCBT), and mindfulness-*informed* therapies that have a broader technological foundation that includes mindfulness as one process but may or may not include meditation practices (including ACT, DBT and CFT) (Baer, 2003; Crane et al., 2017). MBIs have been further divided into first-generation MBIs (e.g., MBSR, MBCT) and second-generation MBIs (e.g., MiCBT) (Van Gordon, Shonin, & Griffiths, 2015). Both generations are secular in approach but inspired by Buddhist practices with second-generation MBIs being more explicit about their spiritual roots (Van Gordon et al., 2015). First-generation MBIs tend to be narrowly focused on mindfulness practice (Van Gordon et al., 2015). Here the emphasis is on the development of attention and *non-judgemental* awareness as exemplified by Kabat-Zinn's oft-cited definition of mindfulness as 'the awareness that emerges through paying attention on purpose, in the present moment, and nonjudgmentally to the unfolding of experience moment by moment' (Kabat-Zinn, 2003, p. 145). In contrast, second-generation MBIs (e.g., MiCBT) teach mindfulness in conjunction with other Buddhist practices such as ethics and Loving Kindness meditation. In relation to mindfulness, second-generation approaches advocate a more *discriminating* awareness as exemplified in Cayoun's definition of mindfulness 'as an *informed* exploration of the present moment and a corresponding means of *holding in mind* what is beneficial from what is harmful..., with clear discernment, from moment to moment, whether one is meditating or not' (Cayoun, 2017, p. 169, italics in original).

MINDFULNESS-BASED STRESS REDUCTION (MBSR)

MBSR is an eight-week group program that uses intensive training in mindfulness meditation to teach people to live more skilful, healthier lives (Kabat-Zinn, 1996, 1999). It was founded at the University of Massachusetts in 1979. Although secular in application, MBSR is grounded in Buddhist Dharma (teachings). Indeed, the term 'stress reduction' was chosen for its universal appeal, based on the First Noble Truth that life involves suffering (or dukkha) (Kabat-Zinn, 1999). Mindfulness (as defined by Kabat-Zinn, 1999) is cultivated through both formal and informal meditation practices. The primary formal practices include body scan meditation, sitting meditation, hatha yoga and mindful walking. Informal practices include awareness of various daily life experiences, such as eating a raisin mindfully, and awareness of pleasant and unpleasant events.

Based as it is on the universality of suffering, MBSR is regarded as broadly applicable and as relevant to health professionals as to the people they treat (Segal et al., 2002). Classes have an educational orientation, are relatively large (20–40 participants) and are two-and-a-half to three-and-a-half hours long. There is an all-day silent retreat during the weekend of the sixth week. Homework is integral to the program, including a minimum of 45 minutes of meditation practice per day plus other informal exercises, six days a week (Santorelli, Meleo-Meyer, Koerbel, & Kabat-Zinn, 2017).

The minimum qualifications for a trainer in MBSR are stringent (see UMass Memorial Health Care, 2020 for details), and it is considered mandatory that MBSR instructors have a longstanding meditation practice and that they attend extended meditation retreats. A detailed curriculum guide is available (Santorelli et al., 2017), however this is not an operational manual and does not replace the formal training and personal practice required for effective teaching.

MINDFULNESS-BASED COGNITIVE THERAPY (MBCT)

MBCT is a group program that was developed to prevent depression in remitted or recovered patients with a history of recurrent major depression. Although the content is modelled closely on MBSR (Segal et al., 2002), MBCT is based on a model of depressive relapse derived from cognitive science, and specifically targets the dysfunctional patterns of thinking characteristic of depression using methods borrowed from cognitive behaviour therapy (CBT) as well as MBSR. MBCT aims to cultivate a decentred view of thoughts by teaching clients to become more aware of, and relate differently to, thoughts, feelings and bodily sensations; in particular, to view thoughts and feelings as passing events in the mind rather than as necessarily reflecting reality. The program also teaches skills in disengagement from habitual dysfunctional cognitive routines, especially depression-related ruminative thought patterns. Emphasis later in the course is on combining CBT techniques, such as activity scheduling, with meditative practices into synergistic strategies for responding to negative mood states, culminating in a written 'relapse prevention action plan'.

MBCT comprises an initial individual orientation session followed by eight weekly, two-hour group training sessions for up to ten to 12 people. The purpose of the initial individual session is to assess eligibility and foster realistic expectations about the treatment process. As the course requires significant personal investment from participants, it is important that participants are well prepared for what is involved to avoid demoralisation and early dropout in this vulnerable population. Like MBSR, the style of the group is more like an education class rather than a traditional psychotherapy group. Group sessions incorporate mindfulness practices similar to MBSR as well as CBT exercises and homework involves around an hour a day, six days a week.

Initially developed for patients as a relapse prevention intervention for those with a history of at least two episodes of depression, evidence to date suggests MBCT is effective only for those with three or more episodes of depression (Ma & Teasdale, 2004; Teasdale et al., 2000). Despite the specificity of the MBCT protocol for preventing depressive relapse, it has now also been applied as a direct treatment of depression and a range of other disorders (see Dimidjian & Segal, 2015).

For those interested in becoming an MBCT instructor, stepped training pathways have been documented from novice to advanced (Segal et al., 2016). Minimum entry criteria for the MBCT training pathway include: a personal mindfulness practice, participation in the eight-week MBCT program, and professional competencies and experience to work therapeutically with the target population including, for example, knowledge of CBT and skills to identify and manage risk. Although MBCT has a published manual (Segal et al., 2013), as for MBSR, this does not replace formal training and a 'cookbook' approach to the use of the manual is discouraged.

MBSR and MBCT courses for participants are now readily available through online formats delivered live through video conference or as a self-paced video program.

ACCEPTANCE AND COMMITMENT THERAPY (ACT)

Introduction

Acceptance and commitment therapy (ACT) is a well-described psychological treatment (Hayes et al., 1999, 2012) based on a functional contextual approach to human language and cognition known as relational frame theory (RFT; Hayes, Barnes-Holmes, & Roche, 2001). Unlike the other third-generation therapies described in this text, ACT has no direct links to Buddhism, although there are interesting parallels between them (Hayes, 2002). For example, both ACT and Buddhism are grounded in a model of universal suffering that is broadly applicable, and many of the techniques used have similar aims in building nonjudgmental observation of experience (Hayes, 2002; Hayes et al., 1999).

ACT consists of six interrelated processes that together have the general goal of building psychological flexibility, defined as 'the ability to contact the present moment more fully as a conscious human being, and to change or persist in behaviour when doing so serves valued ends' (Hayes, Luoma, Bond, Masuda, & Lillis, 2006, p.7). At its core, ACT is a behavioural treatment, grounded in producing functional change so that all ACT techniques are geared towards helping the individual live in accord with his or her values (Hayes et al., 1999, 2012). Each of the ACT processes is described below.

Acceptance

The first phase of ACT often involves a reconceptualisation of the client's presenting problem. Typically, clients will start therapy looking for relief from symptoms, such as from anxiety, depression or psychosis, so that they can think or feel differently. However, from an ACT perspective, it is neither the presence nor content of these 'symptoms' that is the problem, but the tendency of clients to take them literally and fight against them to the extent that functional living is impaired (Hayes, 2004). In the context of reviewing the client's past approaches to 'solve' his or her problem, and through the use of various exercises and metaphors, acceptance is presented as a radically alternative approach to the natural tendency to try and control private events. Acceptance is further cultivated through the interrelated areas of defusion, contact with the present moment and self-as-context.

Defusion

Techniques are taught to distinguish thoughts and images and other verbal content from literal reality and to break the connection between verbal content and behaviour. 'Workability'—whether a thought will help the client move in a valued direction—is presented as a more functional alternative to 'truth' for judging whether thoughts should be taken seriously or acted upon.

Contact with the present moment

Various exercises are used to develop the nonjudgmental acceptance of thoughts, emotions and perceptions in the here and now; for example, observing thoughts like leaves on a stream or mindfully drawing the client's attention to what is going on in the session as it unfolds.

Self-as-context

Various perspective-taking exercises and metaphors are used to assist clients to contact a transcendent aspect of self: to experience the distinction between themselves and various aspects of their experience, such as thoughts, feelings, sensations, memories and roles, in order to reduce engulfment with these phenomena.

Values

Here the aim is to help clients clarify what gives their life meaning and then develop some goals and actions to help clients live this out. Barriers to action are also identified—particularly negative thoughts and feelings—with the ultimate aim of making the connection with willingness to experience these negative states for the sake of committed action.

Commitment

Using their acceptance based skills, clients are encouraged to undertake behaviours that are consistent with their values despite the presence of symptoms. This part of therapy often involves elements of traditional behaviour therapy, such as exposure exercises, although the underlying rationale for the exercises differs.

ACT sessions

ACT sessions are typically active and experiential so that, as far as possible, learning is drawn from the client's experience rather than 'taught' didactically. The degree to which each area of ACT is addressed depends on the client's situation. There is no prescribed number of sessions, and session length is flexible.

Resources

As well as the original and updated ACT manuals (Hayes et al., 1999, 2012), there are now a substantial number of other publications, including training resources, and client and self-help workbooks. The Association for Contextual Behavioural Science (ACBS, 2020) web community is large, with several highly active ACT and RFT listservs. As an experiential therapy, professional training workshops are a particularly useful and effective way of learning and consolidating ACT skills (Richards et al., 2011). There have been a large number of randomised controlled trials published testing ACT across a range of conditions. At the time of writing, some 304 studies were listed on the ACBS website.

MINDFULNESS-INTEGRATED COGNITIVE BEHAVIOUR THERAPY (MICBT)

SARAH FRANCIS

Mindfulness-integrated cognitive behaviour therapy (MiCBT; Cayoun, 2011; Cayoun et al., 2019) is a therapy used in both group and individual therapeutic contexts (Cayoun, 2011) having been first introduced into mental health services in Tasmania, Australia, in 2001. MiCBT was developed as a transdiagnostic therapy, recognising the frequency of comorbidities in psychological illness. Therapy is typically delivered as an eight to ten-week program but may be adapted for specific circumstances. Home practice of about an hour a day is expected to develop appropriate levels of skill. MiCBT is firmly based on Theravada Burmese Vipassana Buddhist teachings specifically those of Satya Narayan Goenka (Goenka, 1987; Hart & Goenka, 1987). Utilising an information processing model, MiCBT, originally called 'Equanimity Training', integrates cognitive behaviour therapy principles with traditional mindfulness training.

The co-emergence model of reinforcement (Cayoun, 2011) underpins MiCBT and provides the rationale for engaging the various meditation practices and in particular demonstrating experientially the relationship between self-referential thinking patterns, the arising of body sensations and the subsequent reactivity. According to the co-emergence model, body sensations are the reinforcers of reactive behaviour. Sensations considered to be pleasant are positively reinforcing while those evaluated as unpleasant are negatively reinforcing. Sensations will be stronger in personally important situations creating a trigger for reactivity unless there is equanimity. Equanimity is therefore a key component and is developed through the extensive body scanning practices requiring focused attention on body sensations while remaining non-reactive. Other tools in MiCBT include the Interoceptive Signature Scale, which assists with decentering from sensations and allowing for a 'scientific' objective observational stance towards arising body sensations. This scale is also used in pain management and referred to as the MIET–mindfulness-based interoceptive exposure task (Cayoun, Simmons, & Shires, 2017).

MiCBT training has four stages that integrate psychological principles of operant conditioning, neural network theory, extinction and interoceptive awareness as well as connecting Loving Kindness practice with counter-conditioning.

Stage one, the so-called personal stage, teaches mindfulness meditations to facilitate attention regulation to promote both metacognitive and interoceptive awareness and thus acceptance of current internal aspects of experience. The meditation practices are mindfulness of breath and body scanning. Progressive Muscle Relaxation is taught as a preliminary skill to the meditation exercises and the co-emergence model is introduced. In *stage two,* the externalising stage, more advanced body scanning techniques are introduced to increase speed of neural connectivity in order that early distress cues can be readily detected before they become overwhelming. Exposure techniques are taught in which participants are asked to work on an avoided activity by engaging in imaginal exposure to both worst, and best case scenarios, while remaining equanimous to the arising sensations. This 'bipolar' exposure is used to address avoidance and increase self-confidence. *Stage three,* the interpersonal stage, continues with still more advanced scanning methods and broadens the external focus from self to others as well as teaching mindfully assertive communication to address the psychological issues associated with interpersonal difficulties. It is proposed that this builds self-confidence and assists with relapse prevention. The final stage, *stage four,* the empathic stage, introduces still deeper and faster scanning methods. This stage also includes behavioural experiments about the psychological impact of adhering to or ignoring ethical considerations while also teaching empathy skills by introducing Loving Kindness meditation.

MiCBT teachers are required to have a personal meditation practice and to have undertaken formal MiCBT training. Competencies are clearly described and assessed for certification purposes. There are three levels of training, Level 1 (foundation), Level 2 (certification level) Level 3 (maintenance of certification). Several publications describe the MiCBT method, both for clinical implementation (Cayoun, 2011; Cayoun et al., 2019) and as a manual for personal wellbeing (Cayoun, 2015).

COMPASSION FOCUSED THERAPY

TARA HICKEY

Introduction

Compassion focused therapy (CFT) is a multimodal therapy that builds on cognitive behaviour (CBT) and other therapies yet it is primarily rooted in clinical science rather than any particular approach to therapy. The origins of CFT arose from a number of observations by its founder Professor Paul Gilbert (2014a). First, when using traditional cognitive behavioural interventions clients often did not report a change in their emotions, particularly those with traumatic backgrounds. They could understand the logic behind changing their thoughts about their experience but did not find it helpful in changing how they felt. Gilbert discovered that often the emotional tone in which people would 'hear' alternative thoughts in their head was cold, logical, detached and at times even aggressive. He encouraged clients to clients to imagine a warm, friendly voice offering them the alternatives. Gilbert also noticed many clients had difficulty feeling supported and cared about by others despite intellectually knowing it. When he asked clients to generate and practise emotional tones of warmth and support many refused or found it very difficult. This led to a focus on evolutionary origins, and mechanisms of feeling reassured, content and calm, particularly through social relationships.

Theory

CTF uses a three-circle model of emotion derived from recent research by Depue (2005), into the neurophysiology of emotion. The three interacting systems are threat and protection system; drive, resource-seeking and excitement system; and contentment, soothing and social safety system. Each of these systems is explained below.

Threat and protection

The function of the threat system is to alert us to danger and to respond in a manner that will protect us. In the past, threats to human lives were predators but nowadays we are more likely to come preoccupied with detecting and responding to social threats—signs that someone is negatively judging us or may cause us harm. We can also become preoccupied with internal threats such as difficult thoughts, emotions, images or uncomfortable physical sensations (Welford, 2016). The threat system is our most dominant system and has a 'negativity bias'. When activated the most common emotions to be experienced are anxiety, anger and disgust. Most clients present with and seek help for threat emotions. CFT explores the origins and meanings linked to these emotions.

Drive, resource seeking and excitement system

The function of the drive system is to provide us with positive feelings that motivate us to source things such as food, sex and friendships (Gilbert, 2009). There is an increasing concern that the drive system is over-stimulated in modern society. However, this system can be diminished when experiencing depression, psychosis and a host of other mental health difficulties. CFT explores the functions behind a person's goals. It also focuses on whether the threat system is activated when a person fails to meet their goals. This may be in the form of self-criticism or an attack on others.

Contentment, soothing and social safety systems

Depue (2005) demonstrates there is a specific affective system, which is not based on threat or drive but is associated with feeling calm and content, which has been largely ignored by clinical psychology. Once there are no threats to deal with or a goal has been achieved the parasympathetic nervous system can be activated. Depue points out that this system is influenced by a person's attachment experience. Therefore, CFT integrates concepts and findings from attachment research. Many clients, especially clients from trauma or abuse backgrounds, will have a difficulty accessing this system. It may be unfamiliar to them and trigger aversive feelings. Working with fear of compassion and fear of safeness is a central focus of CFT (Gilbert, 2014b).

Goals and components of treatment

The three-circle system can become unbalanced and the goal of treatment is to rebalance these systems. Client-therapist formulations are organised around the system model. Central to CFT is compassionate mind training (CMT), which involves learning the attributes and skills of compassion. The standard definition of compassion used in CFT is the sensitivity to suffering in self and others with the commitment to try and alleviate and prevent it (Gilbert, 2010b). CMT helps clients change how they relate to their suffering, assisting clients to turn towards the difficult. The attributes of compassion are:

- caring for wellbeing
- sensitivity
- sympathy
- empathy
- non-judgement
- distress tolerance.

These attributes support clients to develop a motivation to reduce suffering and enhance their wellbeing. They encourage clients to pay attention (sensitivity) to suffering rather than block or turn away from it and be emotionally moved (sympathy) by these experiences. Clients are thought to compassionately tolerate uncomfortable experiences and are supported to understand the experience of the person suffering (empathy) while doing their best not to criticise or judge. The compassion skills involve creating feelings of warmth and support across a range of activities. The skills focus on compassionate:

- attention
- reasoning
- behaviour
- imagery
- feeling
- sensation.

These skills focus on the alleviation and prevention of suffering and are transformative. Compassionate attributes and skills combine to build and maintain the soothing and safety system. Many CFT interventions use standard CBT strategies such as Socrates questioning, generating alternatives, looking at the evidence, practising graded exposure and behavioural experiments. While these skills are not distinctive to CFT it is the context and manner in which they are applied that is unique (Gilbert, 2010b).

Evidence

CFT is receiving increased interest in the treatment of a range of psychological disorders including depression, anxiety, eating disorders and schizophrenia. The evidence base for CFT is growing but is currently limited. Leaviss and Uttley (2015) conducted an early systematic review. They concluded CFT might be more effective than no treatment or as effective as treatment as usual. There was insufficient evidence to show whether it is more effective when compared to standard treatments such as cognitive behavioural therapy. They highlight that this conclusion is based on a lack of large-scale high quality trials and not an indication of the existence of negative evidence. They reported a low attrition rate within a clinical context suggesting it was acceptable to clients. CFT specifically showed promise for individuals high in self-criticism. More large-scale high quality trials are currently required before it can be considered evidence based.

Australian context

A modest but growing number of practitioners are trained in CFT in Australia. Compassionate Mind Australia (Compassionate Mind Australia, 2020) is a hub for practitioners and the general public who are interested in the study and application of Compassion Focused Therapy in the Asia-Pacific Regions. It is a sister site to the Compassion Mind Foundation founded in 2006 by Professor Paul Gilbert.

2.6.13 INTERNET INTERVENTIONS FOR SUPPORTING RECOVERY

ANNE WILLIAMS

Internet interventions delivered via the web and mobile phones are increasingly being developed for and offered to people who live with persisting mental illness (Álvarez-Jiménez et al., 2012; Naslund, Marsch, McHugo, & Bartels, 2015). This growing use of internet-based interventions is supported by research demonstrating that people who experience persisting mental illness use the internet, own mobile phones and are interested in these interventions (Firth et al., 2015; Thomas, Foley, Lindblom, & Lee, 2017) and that they are acceptable and feasible (Berry, Lobban, Emsley, & Bucci, 2016; Gire et al., 2017). There is also early evidence that internet-based interventions for people living with persisting mental illnesses are effective (Álvarez-Jiménez et al., 2014; Gaebel et al., 2016).

Internet-based interventions have potential to support recovery and living well, as they can offer self-determined access, round-the-clock availability and access to a community of other users, with anonymity if preferred (Ben-Zeev et al., 2012). Many digital mental health resources are now available in Australia, New Zealand and internationally. In Australia, a website sponsored by the Australian Commonwealth government, Head to Health (Department of Health, 2019), listed over 370 digital resources for mental health in 2019, including websites, apps and forums. The website provides several links to recovery-specific information, tools and forums offered by organisations including Beyond Blue, Black Dog Institute, headspace, Sane Australia and HighRes, a website for Australian Defence Force members. New Zealand based PeerZone, a peer-led social enterprise, operates a website with a recovery-oriented toolkit designed for international use by English speakers (PeerZone, 2019). The toolkit covers challenges that people with mental distress may experience in nine life domains such as mental and physical wellbeing, self-management, work, relationships and others. Each topic includes stories from people with lived experience of mental distress, strategies to manage distress, activities to support exploring and resolving challenges, and a conversation or supporter's guide. Resources such as these are freely available online for anyone to use, either fully independently or with a supporter or mental health worker if they choose. Their focus is frequently on providing information or self-management tools, with fewer online resources providing specific therapeutic interventions.

There are also internet interventions that connect users with a community of peers and mental health providers online. An example from Australia is Horyzons, designed to support long-term recovery among people experiencing first episode psychosis and described as 'moderated online social therapy' (Álvarez-Jiménez et al., 2013, p.145). Horyzons is accessible from a computer, tablet or mobile phone and incorporates an online peer-to-peer network and interactive psychosocial interventions with moderation by clinical psychologists and vocational workers. A trial of a digital tool with similar components, known as Waka, has recently commenced in New Zealand (McBeth, 2018; Tapsell, Mathews, & Toi, 2018). Waka is designed to support self-management for people who have a diagnosis of schizophrenia and includes information, a peer support social community and online advice from a mental health coach. A third example is an international trial involving participants in Australia, Canada, the United States and the United Kingdom, which is evaluating the impact of a five week, self-paced, online program (ORBIT) on quality of life among people with late-stage bipolar disorder (Fletcher et al., 2018). The mindfulness focused intervention incorporates social support via a peer-moderated forum and asynchronous email contact with an online coach. In these examples, the online professional may have no other relationship with people who use the site or tool.

RECOVERY-ORIENTED INTERNET RESOURCES DESIGNED FOR USE BY CONSUMERS WITH MENTAL HEALTH WORKERS

Recovery-oriented internet interventions designed for users of mental health services and their workers together are beginning to emerge. The Self-Management And Recovery Technology (SMART) website was developed in Victoria, Australia and used by people experiencing persisting mental ill-health and mental health workers in clinical and community services from 2014–17 (Thomas et al., 2016). The website content was organised into topics including recovery, managing stress, health, me, relationships, empowerment and life (see Table 2.14).

Each topic incorporated videos of people sharing their lived-experience, reflective exercises and text summarising the content (See Figure 2.12). Peer workers moderated a forum that was closed to workers. The website was designed so that individuals could use it independently, or both independently and together with a worker. Interviews with 52 participants who used the website, including 15 workers, identified that the lived experience videos were highly valued by users. Service users felt less alone and gained hope for their own recovery (Williams, Fossey, Farhall, Foley, & Thomas, 2018), while workers valued the natural way that the videos opened-up discussions about the service users' lived experience. These outcomes were achieved when

Table 2.14 SMART website topic areas

Website topic	Key content
Recovery *5 sections*	• Introduced concept of recovery • Recommended starting point, included guidance on using site
Managing stress *6 sections*	• Relationship between stress and mental health symptoms • Common stressors and coping strategies
Health *9 sections*	• Relationship between physical and mental health • Self-management including diet, exercise, sleep, medication
Me *11 sections*	• Identity, including effects of stigma • Personal growth through lived experience, focusing on strengths
Relationships *7 sections*	• Interactions between relationships and mental health • Nurturing existing relationships and fostering new connections
Empowerment *8 sections*	• Empowerment in interactions with mental health service providers • Getting the most out of services; rights and advocacy
Life *9 sections*	• Developing new meaning in life • Personal values and identifying related goals

the website was used regularly, with service users appreciating being able to discuss topics that the website raised with their worker. If meetings were infrequent, or other pressing issues consumed the available meeting time, use of the website could peter out.

Figure 2.12 Sample image of lived experience video

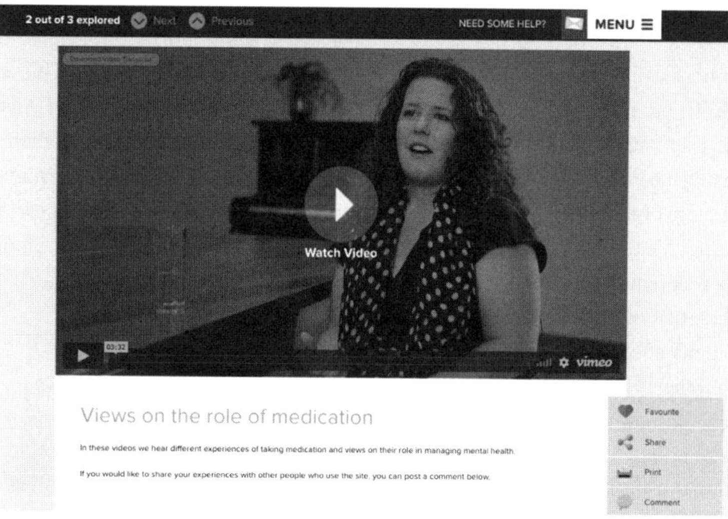

Source: SMART website

Another example of a researched recovery-oriented internet intervention, ReConnect, comes from Norway. ReConnect was an internet portal designed to be used by service users and mental health workers to support service users' recovery, and to facilitate service user involvement in their care and service user and worker collaboration (Gammon et al., 2017). The multi-dimensional website included interactive tools with access to personal content controlled by the service user, an anonymous peer-to-peer forum and messaging between service users and their workers. Service users chose how they wanted to use the website, including using the website independently, sharing work that they had done with workers through the website, or using the website tools together when they met. Twenty-nine service user and worker pairs used the website for up to six months in 2015–2016. The peer-to-peer forum was the most used component in the website, with this and service users' personal control of the website tools considered to be influential in activating personal recovery processes (Strand, Gammon, Eng, & Ruland, 2017). Workers' use of the website varied, with 30% not engaging with service users through the website. This was a source of disappointment for some service users. The researchers concluded that while the website had benefits for service users, introducing a recovery-oriented website was not likely to shift practice towards supporting personal recovery without further service commitment to recovery principles (Gammon et al., 2017).

In summary, some key points about internet interventions and their future include:

- Internet interventions will continue to develop and appear likely to be an important source of information and peer support for people who experience persisting mental illness.
- The number and range of internet interventions is large and increasing. Mental health service users and workers will need education and support to know which interventions will best suit their needs.
- Internet interventions offer a pathway to connect service users to others who share their lived experience, which can have a powerful influence on their hope for recovery.
- Internet interventions have potential beyond being a resource for people experiencing persisting mental illness to use independently.
- To realise the potential of integrating recovery-oriented internet interventions into mental health services will require workers and service users to have an active plan for how they will use the internet-based resources together, and time together to do so.

2.6.14 INTERVENTIONS TO SUPPORT THE PHYSICAL HEALTH OF MENTAL HEALTH CONSUMERS

ROB STANTON & BRENDA HAPPELL

PHYSICAL HEALTH DISPARITIES OF PEOPLE WITH MENTAL ILLNESS

It is now well-accepted that people with mental illness experience significant disparities in physical health compared to the general population. Rates of obesity and type II diabetes are up to three times that of the general population, while the prevalence of metabolic syndrome, a cluster of risk factors associated with the development of cardiovascular disease and type II diabetes is more than 60% in people with severe mental illness (Morgan et al., 2013). Furthermore, the burden of additional physical health concerns leads to early mortality of up to 30 years compared to the general population. This situation is clearly unacceptable in contemporary Australia and requires urgent attention, especially when the mortality gap is largely attributable to preventable and treatable diseases. To date, greater understanding has not led to improved outcomes and an implementation gap is clearly evident.

Physical health care in mental health services

There are a number of reasons why physical health care fails to draw the attention it demands. One factor is the competing priorities of clinicians. With mental health care the over-riding priority in many cases, time for physical health care is often perceived as insufficient. This leads to a lack of physical health data being recorded, and file audits show that even the most rudimentary physical health measures, such as waist circumference or blood pressure, are not, or not routinely, performed (Happell, Platania-Phung, Gaskin, & Stanton, 2016; Rosenbaum et al.,

2014). Similarly, inadequate staff training and lack of resources have been highlighted as contributors to the poor monitoring of physical health, despite the perceived responsibility of treating practitioners to undertake this task, and the potential medico-legal implications of failing to do so (Laugharne, Waterreus, Castle, & Dragovic, 2015).

In circumstances where physical health care data are recorded, reporting is frequently neither clear nor prominent in the consumer's case file, even when there are multiple contact points in a consumer's care team (Lawn, Zabeen, Rowlands, & Picot, 2018). Audits of electronic metabolic monitoring forms show that for more than half of consumers where data is recorded, a diagnosis of metabolic syndrome cannot be made due to missing data (Stanton, Platania Phung, Gaskin, & Happell, 2016).

Another factor contributing to the poor physical health of mental health consumers is diagnostic overshadowing, where physical health symptoms are attributed to mental health causes. This form of misdiagnosis potentially delays recognition and treatment of physical illness. Diagnostic overshadowing is well-recognised by clinicians, mental health care organisations, and consumers alike. Evidence suggests more than half of consumers believed their personal concerns regarding physical health were overlooked, describing this as a failure of the health care system to meet their needs (Happell, Ewart, Bocking, Platania-Phung, & Stanton, 2016). Consumers also reported their physical health concerns being ignored and their own strategies for promoting health and wellbeing as frequently belittled and dismissed (Ewart, Bocking, Happell, Platania-Phung, & Stanton, 2016). Lack of genuine partnerships with consumers may well lead to an unwillingness to disclose physical health concerns due to the disempowerment associated with their trivialisation by clinicians (Byrne, Schoeppe, & Bradshaw, 2018; Happell, Ewart, Bocking, et al., 2016). Similar concerns have been raised by family carers of people with mental illness, including physical health concerns being neglected, ignored and considered symptomatic of mental illness. As a result, carers often found themselves the coordinators of physical health care for their loved one (Happell, Wilson, Platania-Phung, & Stanton, 2017).

When considered in light of the fragmented health system that separates mental and physical health care and negatively impacts continuity of care, it is clear that systemic changes are needed (Cranwell, Polacsek, & McCann, 2017). Consumers and carers must be acknowledged as key stakeholders in the development, implementation and evaluation of interventions aimed at improving physical health.

In spite of these concerns, there is emerging evidence that some types of physical health care interventions show promise for mental health consumers, particularly where the consumer is engaged in the process, and the intervention delivered by dedicated specialist staff.

EQUALLY WELL

Equally Well is an organisation established to address the physical health inequities faced by people diagnosed with a mental illness, to improve outcomes and enhance quality of life. The Equally Well Consensus Statement was developed as a call to action to recognise the inadequate and unacceptable state of physical health care currently available and to improve access to high quality and better coordinated care (National Mental Health Commission, 2017). Equally Well therefore supports initiatives that move beyond identifying the problem, to the development and implementation of strategies to effect real change.

Targeted interventions appear to be beneficial

Approaches to better support the physical health care of mental health consumers have been trialled. In the United States, peer-navigators, that is persons with lived experience of mental illness who encourage self-management of physical health through psychoeducation and behavioural strategies, have been shown to be effective in improving physical health symptoms and improve health care utilisation for mental health consumers (Kelly et al., 2014). In Australia, nurse-led interventions have demonstrated considerable potential in identifying and addressing physical health problems for people diagnosed with mental illness. For example, a study of two community mental health services in Melbourne demonstrated that when case managers were supported in routine care by a mental health nurse with specialist skills in cardio-metabolic health, up to 78% of consumers received cardio-metabolic monitoring compared to just 3% when care was provided by case managers alone. The specialist nurse also referred consumers to a wider range of consumer-relevant services, including dietetic, physical activity, diabetes care and smoking cessation programs, whereas case managers referred consumers exclusively to general practitioners (GPs) (McKenna et al., 2014). This GP-only referral may not have met the unique and complex needs of mental health consumers and thus been ineffective in managing cardio-metabolic health.

Secondly, a small pilot study comparing the addition of a specialist physical health care nurse, to usual care alone, showed an increased rate of physical health-related referrals in the nurse-led group, with a very high 92% follow up rate. This group also demonstrated improvement in health behaviours, such as decreased smoking, increase in fruit and vegetable intake, and increase in physical activity (Happell, Stanton, Platania Phung, McKenna, & Scott, 2014). Although limited by a small sample, these findings offer proof of concept for the physical health nurse consultant role. Together with the findings of McKenna and colleagues (McKenna et al., 2014), a dedicated nursing role to support the physical health care of people with mental illness appears feasible and acceptable. Importantly, support for this role has been demonstrated by consumers (Happell, Ewart, Platania-Phung, et al., 2016), carers (Happell, Wilson, Platania-Phung, & Stanton, 2016) and nurses in mental health settings (Happell, Stanton, Hoey, & Scott, 2015).

A potential solution to an enduring problem

The positive findings described above led to the development of the Physical Health Nurse Consultant (PHNC) role (Happell et al., 2019). A two-year trial of the proposed role has received funding from the National Health and Medical Research Council. A dedicated mental health nurse with specialist training and expertise in physical health care will be employed in a community mental health service in the ACT. The role will adopt a shared decision-making approach to improve service navigation so as to maximise the use of available physical health services. It is hoped this novel service will address many of the barriers to accessing physical health care for mental health consumers, while at the same time, providing a service that has high acceptability, and is cost effective (Happell et al., 2018).

Important to remember in the design of physical health interventions for people with mental illness is the inclusion of the consumer perspective. Not only is this aligned with the essential elements of the Equally Well Consensus Statement (National Mental Health Commission, 2017), but it acknowledges the autonomy and 'expert by experience' approach to co-designed physical health care. Physical activity planning lends itself well to a co-designed approach. Identifying consumers' individual barriers and enablers to physical activity participation using structured checklists can assist clinicians in developing a consumer-centred and acceptable program (Wheeler, Roennfeldt, Slattery, Krinks, & Stewart, 2018). Factors to consider in such a plan include support networks, location and affordability, access to trainers with an understanding of mental illness, the consumers' short and long-term physical health goals, and their physical activity preferences and experiences. Addressing systemic barriers and facilitators to physical activity promotion are also relevant. Lack of training, resources, and organisation support are often-cited reasons limiting physical activity promotion by mental health clinicians (Stanton, Happell, & Reaburn, 2015; Way, Kannis-Dymand, Lastella, & Lovell, 2018). Education alone, however, may not be the answer since translating new knowledge into practice can be hampered by organisational culture and role delineation (Hennessy & Cocoman, 2018). These barriers may, in part, be addressed by a specialised physical health care coordination role linking mental health consumers with physical activity opportunities that are feasible and acceptable, and that meet their individual needs.

In summary, physical health and physical health care are urgent priorities for mental health consumers. Nurse-led interventions that adopt a person-centred approach where autonomy and lived experience are valued, and are cognisant of the crucial role played by carers appear to be the way forward. Such approaches are valued by to all key stakeholders and studies are underway to better understand how they can be implemented as part of usual care for this vulnerable population.

2.6.15 COMMENTARY AND REFLECTION

ELLIE FOSSEY & CATH ROPER

First, and foremost, this chapter highlights the principle that a person-led approach and rights-based practice are essential to promoting self-determination, recovery and wellbeing. The chapter provides an overview of approaches that address social, occupational, psychological and physical dimensions of health and wellbeing. Despite evidence of their usefulness, these approaches have often been viewed as adjuncts to biomedical interventions in mental health care. Internationally, there is growing recognition that psychosocial interventions and support are central in attending to social determinants of health and recovery, and fostering good mental and physical health for all. This underscores the need to make not only the approaches described in this chapter but also peer support and peer-led services (see Sections 1.1.6, 2.1.3 and 2.2.4) more widely and consistently available in community mental health care. In turn, mental health practitioners need to develop collaborative ways of working with consumers, families and carers to support facilitate their access to psychosocial interventions and support (see Sections 2.2, 2.4.3 and 2.7). Furthermore, this requires practitioners to work with and synthesise person-led, rights-based and evidence-informed practices (see Section 2.3.3). Hence, a reflective stance is necessary to working across these differing perspectives and remaining alert to the practice tensions that arise in efforts to support, rather than hinder recovery and wellness.

2.7

WORKING WITH FAMILIES

BRENDAN O'HANLON, CAROL HARVEY, ABNER POON, ROSE CUFF, PETER MCKENZIE & JEFF YOUNG

> At the end of the day, life is about being happy being who you are, and I feel like we are so blessed to have the support system and the best family to really just support each other no matter what we're going through.
>
> *Kim Kardashian*

2.7.1 INTRODUCTION

BRENDAN O'HANLON & CAROL HARVEY

This chapter addresses the experiences of families in relation to mental illness and mental health care. It explores how families are affected when a family member develops a mental illness. It considers the impacts on different family members and relationships, including as the spouses, siblings and dependent children of parents with a mental illness, and frameworks for understanding the stresses of mental illness on family carers as well as the rewards of such caring roles. Intersecting issues for families such as family violence and the impact of cultural background are briefly addressed.

To understand how mental health services can and do engage with families, the relevance of the concept of recovery for families and relationships and the policy context for service responses to families are outlined. A framework for a comprehensive response by mental health services to families, *the pyramid of family involvement*, is then described. Within this framework, a range of family inclusive practices are described that differ in duration and levels of supporting evidence. Family sensitive practice, single session family consultations, family therapy, family psychoeducation, and carer education and peer support are each described, including practices directed towards families generally, and those for families where a parent has a mental illness. The substantial evidence demonstrating the potency of family interventions for improving both consumer and family member outcomes is also summarised.

The term 'family' in this chapter includes the client and those with a significant personal relationship with the client. This includes biological relatives, partners, ex-partners, people in co-habitation, offspring, parents, siblings, friends, carers, community and others who play a significant role in the person's life. The term refers equally to same-sex partners and same-sex-parented families. The terms 'Families' and 'Family Member' are the broadest descriptors applying to anyone in a family and social network who might be impacted by the mental illness of an individual, while the term carer is usually reserved for those family members who assume an active caring role. In practice (and in this chapter), the terms 'carer' and 'family' or 'family members' are used interchangeably.

2.7.2 HOW MENTAL ILLNESS IS EXPERIENCED BY FAMILIES AND AFFECTS RELATIONSHIPS

ABNER POON, ROSE CUFF, CAROL HARVEY & BRENDAN O'HANLON

In this chapter, we focus primarily on the experiences of families where a young person or adult experiences a mental illness. Yet mental health difficulties can arise at many points in the individual and family lifecycle. While adolescence and early adulthood is a point at which most mental health difficulties emerge, children and older people develop mental health problems, each creating challenges for them and their families. Parents, partners, siblings, dependent and adult children, extended family members such as grandparents, uncles and aunts, nieces and nephews, cousins and friends may all be affected and may find themselves in uncharted and complex territory that comes with most caring or support roles.

Families can play a key role in providing practical help, accommodation and emotional support that facilitates recovery and enables a quality of life for an affected family member that might not otherwise be possible. People experiencing mental illness are also not passive recipients of care but are usually embedded in a web of reciprocal family relationships in which they may both receive and provide care. For instance, according to the 2010 Australian prevalence study of psychosis, one in seven people experiencing psychosis were providing care to others (Poon, Hayes, & Harvey, 2019). This may include carrying out household chores and providing emotional support (Chen & Greenberg, 2004), while consumers who are parents provide care to their children (Campbell et al., 2012). On the other hand, sometimes family members' attempts to assist their relative may be experienced by the consumer as making things worse. It should also be acknowledged that, as in the wider community, the family is not always a 'safe haven'. Indeed, families can be a context in which the person experiencing mental illness and their family members both cause and experience physical, sexual and verbal abuse, financial exploitation and emotional abuse and neglect.

IMPACTS OF CAREGIVING EXPERIENCED BY FAMILY MEMBERS

Family carers do not choose their caring role, but often take up this responsibility out of their love and sense of duty to their family members. Many family members who provide care do not think of themselves as carers but as spouses, children, parents or relatives of persons with mental illness (Lawn & McMahon, 2014). There is a focus in the research literature and in public policy on the impact of mental illness on those in the role of the 'primary carer'. However, it is also critical to recognise that other family members who do not necessarily provide care, for example children or siblings, will nonetheless be profoundly affected by the emergence of a mental illness in their relative.

The impact of mental illness on families is well known in Australia and elsewhere (Awad & Voruganti, 2008; Pirkis et al., 2010). Since the movement to discharge inpatients experiencing mental illness to live in the community, many studies have reported that families experience disruption of daily activities, negative emotional effects and that family life can be adversely affected (Awad & Voruganti, 2008). Living in the community for people experiencing a mental illness most often involves living with or being supported by families. The impact of mental illness beyond the person with mental illness is therefore experienced by family members. In the initial phase of the illness, families often feel distressed and confused (Addington, Coldham, Jones, Ko, & Addington, 2003; Jansen et al., 2015). Families need to learn about mental illness and how to navigate the health care system to seek out appropriate treatment of the illness (Lavis et al., 2015). Over time, families may experience grief concerning the restricted opportunities and loss of potential that is sometimes experienced by a family member with mental illness, particularly those with severe mental illness. Families can also face considerable ongoing challenges to coping with the impact of the illness, such as getting relevant information from mental health services and being involved in treatment and care of their relatives.

Marital or intimate relationships may also be affected when one partner experiences mental illness. For instance, spouses sometimes report finding it challenging to manage their caring responsibilities and navigate the impact of mental illness (Lawn & McMahon, 2014), and may experience anxiety and depressive symptoms (Idstad, Ask, & Tambs, 2010).

Siblings too can be affected when a brother or sister develops mental illness. They often take on some caregiving responsibilities to assist their parents, and have to balance their caring responsibilities with meeting their own needs (Sanders, Szymanski, & Fiori, 2014). Experiences of psychological distress, trauma, ambivalence, guilt and stigma are common in siblings (Liegghio, 2017).

An estimated 23% of Australian children live in families with a parent who experiences mental illness (Maybery, Reupert, Patrick, Goodyear, & Crase, 2009) and roughly 20% of adults attending mental health services are parents (Maybery & Reupert, 2018). Children may take up a role in caring for their parent(s) with mental illness, and these added responsibilities may not be age appropriate or their own needs may by neglected or poorly attended to (Reupert & Maybery, 2016; Tabak et al., 2016). The other parent, grandparents or other relatives may assume additional caregiving responsibilities or involvement in the children's lives (Campbell et al., 2012). Despite these important considerations, it is notable that most parents participating in the 2010 Australian prevalence study of psychosis provided adequate parenting (Campbell et al., 2018). While not all children of parents with mental illness will experience difficulties because of their parent's health status—many develop resilience and thrive—there has been growing attention to the support needs of this population. Without appropriate and flexible support available, parents with mental illness and their children may, in difficult times, struggle to cope. These families are also more likely to experience poverty, disruptions to family life and social isolation. There is a higher risk for children affected by parental mental illness of developing mental health or behavioural problems (Dean et al., 2010; Mok et al., 2016) although, encouragingly, intervention can reduce the risk of these difficulties by up to 40% (Siegenthaler, Munder, & Egger, 2012). Children and families are particularly vulnerable where high levels of parental mental illness, substance misuse and family violence coexist. For instance, very high levels of closely interrelated parental drug and alcohol abuse, mental health problems and domestic violence are found in substantiated child protection cases (Scott, 2009).

Stressors and challenges experienced by families

There are different conceptual understandings of the stressors and challenges that mental illness can create for families. One widely known conceptual framework is caregiving burden. Hoenig and Hamilton (1966) first conceptualised the impact of caregiving as caregiver burden, which they classified as objective burden and subjective burden. Objective burden refers to the negative effects of caregiving that can be measured and observed, while subjective burden refers to the subjective perception and experience of carers. Not all families perceive themselves to experience burden as they are showing care and concern to their ill family members. Nevertheless, this concept remains useful in mental health practice to understand the potential negative effects of caring for a family member with mental illness.

Objective burden includes disruption to family activities, lost opportunities in study, work and social lives, negative effects on family relationships, and health problems of carers. Families may experience disruption to their lives as they need to balance their care for their family member with mental illness with their other commitments. They may give up social activities and gatherings due to avoidance of socialisation, stigma associated with mental illness, or more urgent tasks associated with caregiving (Caqueo-Urízar et al., 2017). Being socially isolated is commonly reported by many carers (Hayes, Hawthorne, Farhall, O'Hanlon, & Harvey, 2015). Some family members may experience aggression and violence from their relatives with mental illness. Carers also experience financial problems due to restricting or sacrificing their employment opportunities, the extra finances required to support consumers, or poor budgeting skills of some consumers (Lin et al., 2018).

Experiencing poor health is commonly reported by carers globally. The National Survey of Mental Health and Wellbeing reported that many carers experienced poor mental health (Pirkis et al., 2010). A study within the 2010 Australian prevalence study of psychosis found that carers' physical health deteriorated over time (Poon, Harvey, Mackinnon, & Joubert, 2017). Some carers seem to have a higher risk for diabetes and other long-term physical health problems, are overweight, or experience bodily pains and poor sleep (Poon, Curtis, Ward, Loneragan, & Lappin, 2018; Smith, Onwumere, Craig, & Kuipers, 2018).

Subjective burden includes carers' overall subjective experience and perceived quality of life. In general, carers experience poorer quality of life than the general population (Hayes et al., 2015; Poon, Harvey, Mackinnon, et al., 2017). Worrying over their loved ones is common among carers (Stephens, Farhall, Farnan, & Ratcliff, 2011), while grieving for the loss of work and other life opportunities of consumers is also a feeling that carers may experience. Other family members who are not living with mental illness may feel that they are neglected by the family member who assumes the main caregiving responsibilities (Bowman, Álvarez-Jiménez, Wade, McGorry, & Howie, 2015).

Another approach to understanding and measuring the impact of mental illness on families is the stress-appraisal-coping framework in which the appraisal of the impact of the illness by families and their coping abilities determine its effects. This framework views illness and its disruptions to family life as stressors, and how families appraise these illness-related stressors as mediating their use of coping strategies and the outcomes experienced (Szmukler et al., 1996). Social support is also a factor acknowledged to be important in terms of coping. Based on this framework, practitioners can support families by helping them to develop appraisals of their situations that support better coping and enhanced social support, so that they can experience fewer negative effects.

Positive aspects of caregiving

While much research has focused on the negative effects of caregiving, the caring experience is also recognised to include potential benefits, such as enjoying positive relations with the person being cared for and skill development (Szmukler et al., 1996). Parents may find that they have benefited from the emotional and instrumental support provided by their child with mental illness and feel that they have fulfilled their familial duties and learnt more about themselves (Schwartz & Gidron, 2002). Similarly, spouses of people with a chronic illness, including mental illness, have reported valuing their marital relationships and providing reciprocal care, despite experiencing challenges associated with the illness (Solomi & Casiday, 2017). Siblings too may gain positive psychological growth and maturity as a result of stressful experiences with siblings' mental illness (Sanders & Szymanski, 2013).

Experiences of carers from Culturally and Linguistically Diverse (CALD) communities

Australia is highly culturally diverse, yet there are few studies examining the experiences of families of consumers from CALD communities. Families from CALD communities often assume many caregiving responsibilities for their loved ones with mental illness and experience poor wellbeing and negative effects (Endrawes, O'Brien, & Wilkes, 2007; Poon, Joubert, & Harvey, 2015). The limited studies show that such families often have restricted informal social networks, are isolated from the dominant Anglo-Celtic community, and have poor English-speaking abilities (Kokanović, Petersen, & Klimidis, 2006). Due to their unique socio-cultural circumstances, carers from CALD communities experience stigma of mental illness and barriers in help-seeking, and likely experience greater negative impacts than other families in Australia.

2.7.3 RECOVERY AND FAMILIES

ABNER POON, BRENDAN O'HANLON & CAROL HARVEY

The adoption of recovery-oriented practice is promoted in national and state mental health policy and widely espoused as informing mental health care across many settings. (See Chapters 1.1.6 and 2.7 for further information about recovery and recovery-oriented practice.) As recovery-oriented frameworks influence how treatment and care is provided by mental health services, this has ramifications for the families of persons experiencing mental illness. The importance of family relationships is recognised through the inclusion of concepts such as connectedness as a domain in the recovery process (Leamy, Bird, Le Boutillier, Williams, & Slade, 2011), yet mental health services have mainly focused on the process of recovery for people with mental illness and have not adequately addressed the recovery of family members with mental illness (Fox, Ramon, & Morant, 2015; Poon, Joubert, Mackinnon, & Harvey, 2017). In response, the concept of *family recovery* has been articulated as a nonlinear process encompassing phases of; Shock, discovery, and denial; Recognition and acceptance; Coping; and Personal and Political Advocacy (Spaniol & Nelson, 2015). In this context, family members may be seen as having their own recovery journey with similarities to, and differences from, the experiences of the person with the condition (Wyder & Bland, 2014). Like the process of recovery for people with mental illness, family recovery is supported through being connected to others, having hope and optimism about the future, having an identity outside of their caring role, developing meaning in their lives, and being empowered to take control of their own lives (Wyder & Bland, 2014).

Family recovery implies the need for greater attention by service providers to addressing the impact of mental illness on family members of persons living with mental illness (Poon, Joubert, et al., 2017). It also draws attention to key familial roles and relationships that may be important for people experiencing mental illness in their recovery, such as being a parent, which have received scant attention in the recovery literature (Ende, Busschbach, Nicholson, Korevaar, & Weeghel, 2016). An alternative to family recovery is the concept of *relational recovery*. This concept emphasises that recovery is an inherently relational process and that relationships cannot be 'sectioned off' as one domain in the recovery process. The concept of relational recovery also highlights the impact of mental illness on relationships and identifies relationships between family members as a focus for intervention (Price-Robertson, Obradovic, & Morgan, 2017). This concept links well with Rolland's Family Systems Illness model, within which health conditions are seen as presenting challenges for family relationships (such as loss of intimacy or the need to move between periods of stability and acuity) and where families can be supported to meet these challenges in a way that enables them to remain connected (Rolland, 2017).

The application of a recovery-oriented framework with the families of persons experiencing mental illness has surfaced new insights about how to support the recovery of families. Further, recent Australian research concerning family carers of people living with psychosis suggests that effective psychosocial rehabilitation for people with psychosis has the potential to improve carers' own health and wellbeing (Poon, Harvey, Mackinnon, et al., 2017). Equally, the inclusion of parenting support in the delivery of mental health services has potential to promote recovery for parents and benefits for all family members (Maybery et al., 2017). This provides additional support for emphasising the relational nature of recovery. Therefore, mental health services need to address the recovery of people with mental illness and their families concurrently.

2.7.4 SERVICE RESPONSES TO FAMILIES

BRENDAN O'HANLON, CAROL HARVEY, PETER MCKENZIE, ROSE CUFF, JEFF YOUNG & ABNER POON

CONTEXT AND OVERVIEW

Here we briefly consider the policy context affecting families and carers in relation to mental health care and the extent to which the diverse needs of families are currently addressed by services. A pyramid of family involvement will be presented as a way of describing and grouping practice models and services for families. At the different levels of the pyramid, practice models facilitated by practitioners and by peer family members will be described along with those that specifically target families where a parent has a mental illness.

Policy in relation to families and carers

In the Australian context, the role of carers and families is recognised at a national and state level. The Fourth National Mental Health Plan made reference to the need to respond to families including families where a parent has a mental illness as a priority for prevention and early intervention (Australian Health Ministers, 2009). The National Mental Health Service Standards too include a standard that specifically addresses the role of mental health services in responding to carers (Australian Government, 2010b). Carer Recognition Acts exist nationally (*Carer Recognition Act 2010* (Cth)) and in most state jurisdictions, which aim to increase awareness of carers and the value of their contribution to society. State Mental Health Acts include specific provisions relating to carers and families. These typically acknowledge the role of families and the terms under which they receive information about their relative when under treatment and care. These policies and legislative frameworks create a favourable context for the constructive inclusion of families in mental health care, but neither ensures that families are included in family members' care nor that their own needs are addressed.

NEEDS OF FAMILIES AND CARERS FOR INFORMATION AND SUPPORT

Families and carers may have multiple unmet caregiving needs and they need adequate and timely information and resources to care for their loved ones (Diminic et al., 2018). Some carers may also need access to alternate caregiving arrangements, and support with family and social relationships. Their needs and the negative effects of caregiving continue to be poorly addressed within mental health services (Coker, Williams, Hayes, Hamann, & Harvey, 2016; Poon, Joubert, & Harvey, 2018). There is also considerable variability in the needs of families. The point at which mental health difficulties arise in the family lifecycle, the nature of the mental health conditions confronting families, the differing needs of families (and different members within the one family) and the changing needs of families over time create challenges for mental health services in responding well to families. This is further complicated by consumers and family members sometimes having conflicting preferences in relation to the participation of families in treatment and care. Rather than offering a single intervention to address one specific need, multiple interventions should be provided to address the needs and wellbeing of carers and their evolving needs should be revisited over time (Poon, Joubert, et al., 2018). As a starting point, actively including families in ongoing treatment discussions should be a key priority of mental health workers. Failing to include family members in care plans results in poor mental health care and perpetuates caregiving burden.

The pyramid of family involvement

Early attempts to promote family involvement in mental health services were driven primarily by the potential of family interventions to deliver improved outcomes for the identified consumer. Less attention was paid to the needs of other family members. A greater recognition of the impact on family members of supporting a person experiencing mental illness has been reflected in carer specific policy and funding across health and disability services, including in mental health services. Similarly, mental health services are increasingly expected to respond to the needs of families in their own right, rather than solely as a means of supporting the consumer. This includes specific initiatives focused on families where a parent has a mental illness, such as the Victorian Statewide FaPMI program and in New South Wales, the Support Program for Carers from Culturally and Linguistically Diverse (CALD) background. Over time this has led to the development of a range of different services and practice models for including and responding to families. Unfortunately, these developments have often been restricted to particular settings or sub-groups of families and there has been a lack of an overall vision for a comprehensive response to the needs of families and their role in caring for people experiencing a mental illness.

Building on the work of Mottaghipour and Bickerton (2005), the Bouverie Centre (a specialist publicly funded family mental health service in Victoria) has proposed a multi-tiered approach to family involvement for mental health services called the *pyramid of family involvement* (Bouverie Centre, 2016). This recognises that not all families want or need the same level of involvement in their relative's treatment and care and may benefit from different service options.

As Figure 2.13 shows, the provision of different levels of service to families (the pyramid) is seen as operating within an organisational culture (the circle) whereby inclusion and respect for family members is embedded in the organisational culture—'just part of how we work around here.' The different tiers of involvement articulate an anticipated need from families and a corresponding service response capacity, with fewer families requiring the higher levels of service response, as follows:

- **Level 1:** All families need to be offered routine inclusion and respect, as reflected in family

Figure 2.13 The pyramid of family involvement

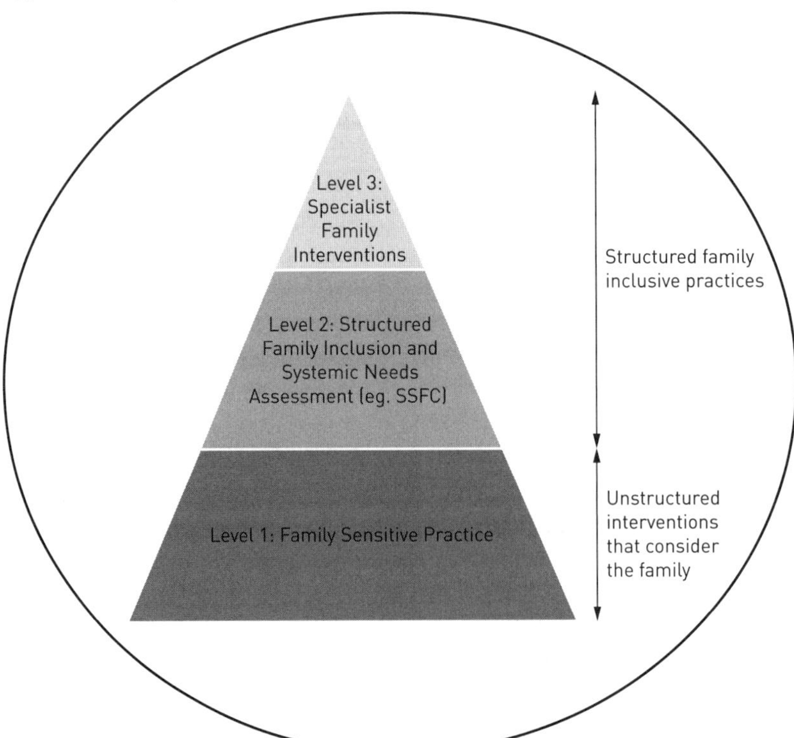

sensitive practice, and all staff within a service need to be able to practise in this way.

- **Level 2:** A significant but smaller group of families will want the opportunity to meet with their relative's treating practitioners in a more formal family meeting process, such as Single Session Family Consultation (SSFC), that allows for a more structured assessment of, and response to, their needs. Many, but not all practitioners in the service will need to be able to facilitate these needs-oriented meetings at this second level.
- **Level 3:** More intensive interventions will be offered to a relatively small group of families who are seeking and may benefit from more intensive evidence-based family interventions. At this third level, a smaller group of practitioners in the service need to be trained in these modalities or, in some instances, these interventions might be provided by external family specialists.

There are multiple advantages of such a tiered framework of response to families. Firstly, it can bring together the varied existing service responses in a coherent whole for families. Secondly, the framework articulates a pathway for families between the various service options as their needs change or become apparent over time. For example, a meeting with a family might be sufficient to address a family's needs or it might identify the potential for the family to benefit from a more intensive intervention. Thirdly, the framework provides clarity for practitioners by providing a scope of practice at each level. For example, a nurse on an inpatient unit knows their role is to practise in a family sensitive manner rather than to attempt to address longstanding family relationship issues. Finally, from a service efficiency and resource allocation perspective, the framework provides guidance to managers about the level and type of training that needs to be provided to different staff working in different roles and service settings. In the following sections, the pyramid of family involvement will be used to describe a range of practice models and services for families in a mental health context.

2.7.5 PRACTICE MODELS

FAMILY SENSITIVE PRACTICE

BRENDAN O'HANLON, CAROL HARVEY, PETER MCKENZIE, ROSE CUFF, JEFF YOUNG & ABNER POON

Family sensitive practice has been defined as 'any work role that is performed in a way that is inclusive, understanding and respectful to families and other carers, including their social and cultural contexts' (Bouverie Centre, 2016). It encompasses and places value on practices that include the ways in which practitioners work with individual clients and their incidental and less formal contacts with family members. When working with individuals, practitioners can ask consumers questions that create awareness of the importance of family and other relationships for both the consumer and the practitioner. Unplanned and informal contact with families can be an opportunity for practitioners not just to gather information, but also to acknowledge the role of family members and communicate messages of inclusion and respect.

In circumstances where family members are children, active inquiry with the parent experiencing mental illness about their children and about their parenting role is important. Such discussions need to be handled sensitively given that some parents are reluctant to involve their children and other family members in treatment because of fears regarding being judged inadequate as parents and the potential involvement of child protection (Maybery & Reupert, 2006). Creating opportunities for contact with a consumer's children (for example, scheduling a home visit when children are present) is also critical for ensuring contact happens with those family members whose needs might otherwise remain invisible.

The increasing role of carer peer workers in mental health services creates another dimension of family sensitive practice. Peer workers provide an option for practitioners to link family members who understand the experience of the family. Peer workers can also help families navigate the often complex and daunting processes of mental health care.

The value of family sensitive practice is that it can be undertaken flexibly and in a range of circumstances as the practitioner undertakes their usual work role. While it may require practitioners to change their attitudes towards families it does not require advanced training or major restructuring of existing work roles. It has the advantage that it is relevant to all staff and can 'reach' most family members including those who might be reluctant to be involved in more formal meetings or in specialist family interventions. Family sensitive practice also promotes mutual respect and trust between practitioners and families. This creates a context for the engagement of families in more structured and purposeful processes offered at Level 2 and 3 of the pyramid. As such it provides the foundation on which other services to families can be built.

PRACTICE ILLUSTRATION: FAMILY SENSITIVE PRACTICE

The receptionist at a mental health service acknowledges the sister who regularly accompanies her brother to attend the service by saying 'It's good to see you again Leila, how are you?'

A nurse in the emergency department when meeting with a person who is acutely unwell and accompanied by their parents, acknowledges the impact of the illness on all members by saying 'It sounds like you have all had a pretty tough time over the last few days.'

A service has an intake protocol with questions about who comprises 'family' for the consumer, including who they live with and those who might be particularly vulnerable such as dependent children or elderly parents.

A practitioner rings a mother to say that her son has arrived safely at the inpatient unit.

A practitioner may respectfully ask about the cultural identity of the client and their family as a starting point for talking about how to offer culturally sensitive family visits.

STRUCTURED INCLUSION AND NEEDS ASSESSMENT

At Level 2 of the pyramid of family involvement, the focus is on bringing family members together in a formally convened meeting. This typically occurs when families or members of a client's social network are invited to attend and participate in a relatively formal or structured session–usually with the client also present. This is a 'step up' from family sensitive practice that involves families by welcoming them, keeping them informed of events and discussing family issues with consumers, as described above.

Single Session Family Consultation (SSFC) is an example of a practice model developed in Australia to engage families, assess and address their needs. The SSFC is a time limited and structured process for meeting with the consumer and the family and is focused on achieving realistic and negotiated goals. SSFC was developed by the Bouverie Centre by combining Family Consultation, a brief model for responding to the needs of families affected by mental illness, with single session therapy that focuses on maximising the value of one or more counselling sessions (Jewell et al., 2012; Talmon, 2012; Wynne, 1994). A recent evaluation of SSFC showed promising results of applying SSFC in youth mental health services (Poon, Harvey, Fuzzard, & O'Hanlon, 2017).

In practice, SSFC involves processes for convening and conducting the session and following up with the family. In the convening process, particular attention is given to preparing all potential participants to make the most of the time when family members are together. There is a strong focus on negotiating the involvement of family or other social network members with the client. This aims to increase the likelihood that the session delivers a useful outcome for the consumer and does not threaten the relationship between the practitioner and consumer. The SSFC session itself includes stages of welcoming, scoping the issues, deciding on a focus, addressing the identified issues and agreeing to clarify how family members will be involved and their needs addressed. A follow-up telephone call is made to families following the session to gauge their experience of the session, to check on progress in relation to issues identified during the SSFC and to clarify the next steps.

An advantage of the SSFC approach is that sessions do not commit the client or family members to ongoing involvement, but they can set the scene for longer-term work if this is mutually agreed upon. Alternatively, SSFC can be offered on an as-needed basis, a format that suits many families. SSFC enables practitioners to match family need to available services, including more specialised options, available in Level 3.

When meeting with families where a parent has a mental illness, attention needs to be paid to consulting the parents about the participation of young children and if they are to be directly involved what will be discussed. In circumstances where children do participate in meetings, access to toys and drawing materials can help make the environment more child-friendly. The focus of these meetings can include helping children develop an empathetic understanding of their parent's illness, developing plans for what will happen in the event of a relapse (including arrangements for care of the children) and considering what other supports, both formal and informal, are available to the family.

PRACTICE ILLUSTRATION: A SINGLE SESSION FAMILY CONSULTATION

Angelo, a 58-year-old married Italian man, lives with his wife, Nella (57) and Bianca (24), the youngest of their three children. He works as a tiler in a construction business. Angelo is on sick leave following a recent episode of bipolar affective disorder, during which he became disinhibited and aggressive towards his work mates.

At the next appointment with his key clinician, Liam, Angelo talks about his work and his family. Liam identifies the opportunity to bring the family together in a SSFC session. He reflects that given they have all been through a lot, it might be good to meet with the family. Liam suggests that a meeting might help family members to know how to best support Angelo.

In the convening stage of SSFC, Liam talks with Angelo about who should attend the meeting and what might be discussed. Angelo says his wife and Bianca could attend. Angelo feels Nella doesn't understand how hard it is for him to go back to work. He knows Bianca is worried about him but doesn't know what she has been told.

With Angelo's consent, Liam invites Nella and Bianca to the meeting. Nella says she is concerned about Angelo getting back to work. She wants to support him but feels like she just upsets him. Bianca says she doesn't understand what's happening with her dad.

Liam meets with the family using the SSFC meeting structure. He summarises what each family member wants from the meeting and checks that he has understood their views. Liam suggests that he wants to make the most of the time they have together by having a focus for the session. The family agree that it would be good to be 'all on the same page' regarding Angelo's condition. Liam facilitates a discussion where Angelo shares his experience of being unwell, while Liam provides relevant information about bipolar disorder, its treatment and what helps with recovery. In appreciating how embarrassed Angelo feels about his behaviour towards his workmates, Nella agrees that she will stop asking Angelo about work. Angelo in turn offers to do a few small jobs around the house to help out. Bianca says she has found the information helpful but would like to find out more. Liam suggests websites for Bianca to find out more about bipolar disorder. While the family are grateful for the session, they opt to 'see how things go'. The family agree to Liam making a follow up phone call in two weeks' time to check-in about progress regarding the issues raised in the meeting and to clarify whether they need further assistance.

Let's Talk about Children (Let's Talk) is another practice model that could be seen as fitting at the second level of the pyramid. Let's Talk is a brief, two-to-three session recovery-oriented intervention for parents with a mental illness and their children developed in Finland (Solantaus, Paavonen, Toikka, & Punamäki, 2010). Let's Talk involves the parent identifying their children's strengths and vulnerabilities across a range of domains and deciding what might need to occur to address any identified concerns. Let's Talk adopts a stance of 'parent as expert' and focuses on the parent-child relationship with just the parent and other parent/carer in the room. This model has been adapted and trialled for use in Australia (Maybery et al., 2017).

SPECIALISED FAMILY INTERVENTIONS

The forms of family inclusive services offered at Level Three of the pyramid are more interventive, often (although not always) longer term and more intensive in nature. Interventions at this level are more likely to include models that have an established evidence base in improving client and family outcomes. Given the historical emphasis on these models in mental health care and their established effectiveness, they are considered in greater detail.

Professionals have worked with families as part of the treatment of schizophrenia and other mental health conditions since the mid-1950s. Different models for working with families have developed from differing theoretical orientations, including psychoanalysis, systems theory, behavioural and cognitive behavioural psychology. The carer movement has also strongly influenced the development of models for working with families in mental health. While each model or approach articulates distinctive features and emphases, there are many shared elements, and there has been considerable cross-fertilisation between approaches over time.

Beyond theoretical orientations, the range of approaches differ according to whether the person experiencing the mental illness participates (consumer and family or family alone); the goals of the intervention (relapse prevention, educating family members or improving family members' coping); the format of the intervention (single family or multiple family groups) and who provides the intervention (professionals or family members). Family approaches can be grouped into three main categories: family therapy; family psychoeducation; and carer education and peer support.

2.7.6 FAMILY THERAPY

BRENDAN O'HANLON, JEFF YOUNG & PETER MCKENZIE

The aim of family therapeutic models is to work with members of the whole family to change their response to the mental disorder, and to each other, by exploring beliefs, patterns of interaction and behaviour within the family to avoid unhelpful (vicious) cycles of interaction and to promote helpful (virtuous) cycles. Historically these models attracted criticism from the carer movement for inadvertently blaming parents, but contemporary family therapeutic approaches have addressed this, and promote collaboration between the person with a mental illness and his or her family. An example is the use of narrative therapy with persons diagnosed with schizophrenia, where the disorder or any of its effects are seen as separate from the person (externalised) and all family members are encouraged to join forces against the externalised disorder or its effects (White, 1987).

Family therapy has been used to address a wide range of adult, child and adolescent mental health problems (Carr, 2018a, 2018b). Family therapy and hybrid approaches that include family therapy components are in common use in child and adolescent mental health services, for example, in the successful treatment of adolescent eating disorders (Jewell, Blessitt, Stewart, Simic, & Eisler, 2016). In adult mental health services, their use has waned over the last 20 years. Their psychological and relationship focus means they can be potentially at odds with more diagnostically, biologically and individually orientated mental health services.

More recently, Open Dialogue has attracted considerable interest in Australia. Open Dialogue is an innovative therapeutic model drawing together family therapy, systemic, network and needs-adapted approaches. Originally developed in Finland, Western Lapland, where it provides a complete mental health service delivery framework, there is evidence that Open Dialogue in mental health settings delivers significant benefits for people who experience mental health crises, their families and social networks (Seikkula et al., 2006; Seikkula & Olson, 2003). There is also emerging evidence for the value of Open Dialogue in other parts of Scandinavia, the United States, the United Kingdom and Europe (Razzaque & Wood, 2015). Key features include:

- immediate help with an emphasis on being able to bring people together and sharing experiences and understandings with 'crisis' seen as an opportunity
- social network perspective and systemic collaboration
- flexibility and mobility in responding to specific needs and circumstances of all participants
- responsibility and proactive facilitation in proposing and conducting a network meeting
- psychological continuity provided in the treating team
- tolerance of uncertainty and valuing of reflective and curiosity
- dialogue and polyphony which involves a therapeutic stance creatively expressed in its dialogic and reflective practices of listening and responding and invites transparency for the therapy planning and decision making process.

In Australia, Open Dialogue's principles and accompanying practices have resonated strongly with mental health consumers and carers/supporters; there is considerable enthusiasm for its adoption in services; and emerging interest among practitioners, the lived experienced peer workforce and service leaders. Training in Open Dialogue is now being provided in Australia and adaptions of the model are being used in a small number of mental health services.

2.7.7 FAMILY PSYCHOEDUCATION

CAROL HARVEY & BRENDAN O'HANLON

Family psychoeducational approaches emerged in the early 1980s in response to research demonstrating a link between the emotional climate and the likelihood of relapse in families where a member had been diagnosed with schizophrenia. This research found that there was a greater likelihood of relapse in families where there was a high level of critical, hostile or overinvolved responses by family members towards the person living with schizophrenia (high expressed emotion), than in families where there was a low level of expressed emotion (Brown, Birley, & Wing, 1972; Vaughn & Leff, 1976). Although the concept of expressed emotion (EE) has been critiqued as family blaming, family responses associated with high EE are best viewed as an understandable and common response to the experience of living with someone with a severe and relapsing condition.

Early family psychoeducational interventions aimed to reduce relapse by reducing critical and hostile responses and helping family members cope more effectively with the illness through education, stress reduction techniques and skills training. The concept of EE provided a guide to which families might benefit most from family psychoeducation. However, family EE status is less likely to be included as a criterion for offering family psychoeducation in recent clinical practice guidelines (Galletly et al., 2016), reflecting recognition that the needs of low EE families should also be considered and addressed.

Behavioural family therapy is an example of a single family psychoeducational intervention that includes elements of education, including relapse prevention, communication skills training and problem-solving (Harvey, 2018; Lucksted, McFarlane, Downing, & Dixon, 2012). Multiple family groups bring together small groups of families to work together (including the person experiencing the disorder), which adds mutual support to the education, skills and problem-solving components (Lucksted et al., 2012). While family psychoeducational approaches were originally developed for people living with schizophrenia, there is growing evidence that they are effective for people with other enduring and relapsing conditions, such as bipolar disorder and recurrent depression (Lucksted et al., 2012).

There is uncertainty about how family psychoeducation works (Lobban et al., 2013), although various factors which may lead to change have been proposed, including improved coping by family members and enhanced social support (Kuipers, 2006; McFarlane, Dixon, Lukens, & Lucksted, 2003). Despite this, family psychoeducational interventions have generally been supported by the carer movement. This reflects that family psychoeducation responds directly to families' needs for support and information and provides ways of dealing with the common day-to-day difficulties involved in supporting a person with a mental health condition. The following practice illustration illustrates how behavioural family therapy may assist the consumer and their family.

PRACTICE ILLUSTRATION: A FAMILY'S INVOLVEMENT IN BEHAVIOURAL FAMILY THERAPY

Marley is a 22-year-old woman living with her mother, stepfather and primary school-aged siblings. Marley and her family were offered behavioural family therapy by Marley's case manager after Marley had her second inpatient admission following the re-emergence of auditory hallucinations and paranoid ideas involving her mother. This relapse of schizophrenia occurred in the context of Marley's increased intake of alcohol and escalating conflict between Marley and her mother. Initial work with the family revealed that although there was considerable conflict in the household, Marley's mother and her whole family were very worried about her. Despite the family's longstanding support for Marley, it was also apparent that their understanding of Marley's condition was limited, and that at least some of the tension in the household was a result of misunderstanding and misinterpreting Marley's behaviour. For example, Marley often managed her voices, which were more intrusive during the family's evening meal, by leaving the table abruptly and going to her room. The family interpreted Marley's behaviour as angry protest and changed their understanding and response markedly when, with the help of the case manager, Marley was able to describe her experience of the voices and her coping strategy. Members of the family were also able to understand the link between Marley's alcohol use and her high levels of anxiety.

Following this work, Marley and her family were able to develop a staying well plan that included agreed action if Marley started showing early signs of becoming unwell. As trust between the case manager and the family grew, they agreed to work on their communication skills. These were introduced in a playful manner, and the younger siblings responded enthusiastically, even holding their parents to task around completion of 'homework' in practising the skills. The first session that encouraged family members to express positive feelings towards each other yielded a noticeable improvement in the family's morale. When a crisis arose following further conflict between Marley and her mother, they were introduced to structured problem-solving by Marley's case manager. This allowed them to resolve the conflict and to see the value of learning this approach to help deal with future problems.

PSYCHOEDUCATIONAL INTERVENTIONS WITH FAMILIES WHERE A PARENT HAS A MENTAL ILLNESS

Family Talk is an evidence-based family psychoeducational intervention developed by Beardslee, Gladstone, Wright, and Cooper (2003) in the US. Family Talk aims to promote parenting and child development and prevent children's mental health problems in families with parental depression. It is designed to enhance family communication and understanding concerning depression and to support interpersonal relationships in the family and children's social life outside the family. In Australia, The Family Model (Falkov, 2012) provides practitioners and managers with an accessible, and practical approach that supports collaborative ways of working with individuals and their families in which one or more members experience mental illness. It can be used as a tool to foster engagement and facilitate thought about connections between symptoms and relationships, while highlighting a family's strengths and difficulties.

The Think Family–Whole Family Programme intervention in the United Kingdom is based on principles from behavioural family therapy, Beardslee's psychoeducational approach, and Falkov's principles of joint collaborative working. It focuses on encouraging information-sharing and family meetings, promoting shared understanding of the parent's illness and whole-family goal setting (Yates & Gatsou, 2017).

Emerging Minds is leading a federally funded consortium to establish a National Workforce Centre for Child Mental Health which is developing a comprehensive suite of resources for families and professionals including online training. (See Emerging Minds, 2020.)

RESEARCH SUPPORTING THE VALUE OF FAMILY PSYCHOEDUCATION

Family interventions are one of the most researched psychosocial interventions in mental health. Evidence indicates family interventions are effective with a range of adult mental health conditions, including schizophrenia, mood disorders, anxiety disorders and substance-use disorders. The research evidence supporting the value of family interventions is strongest in relation to schizophrenia, and particularly in relation to family psychoeducation of which there are over 50 randomised controlled studies since the 1970s (Pharoah, Mari, Rathbone, & Wong, 2010). Recent reviews and meta-analyses have concluded that family psychoeducation has positive effects in terms of preventing relapse and rehospitalisation (Pharoah et al., 2010; Pilling et al., 2002). In reviewing family psychoeducation studies, Bustillo and colleagues (Bustillo, Lauriello, Horan, & Keith, 2001) found average relapse rates of 24% compared with 64% for those receiving standard treatment. A meta-analysis by Pilling et al. (2002) found that the number needed to treat (NNT) was eight (that is, one consumer out of every eight will avoid a relapse in a 12-month period, when treated with family psychoeducation compared with standard care) and the reduction in the likelihood of relapse was 12.8%. The findings in relation to readmission were more striking for single family interventions compared with other treatments, with a NNT of three and a 48.8% reduction in the risk of being readmitted in the first 12 months.

These findings have been endorsed by the most methodologically stringent of these reviews: the updated Cochrane review by Pharoah et al. (2010), which also concluded that family interventions significantly reduce relapse and readmission rates. Pharoah and colleagues (2010) estimated the NNT to prevent relapse was 7; further, relapse events were reduced at 12, 18 and 24 months into treatment. This Cochrane review also concluded that consumer adherence with medication may be encouraged by family intervention, and hence provide another mechanism for reducing relapse (Pharoah et al., 2010). While the major focus of research has been consumer relapse and readmission, positive findings have also been reported in areas such as symptom reduction, improved social functioning and employment (McFarlane et al., 2003; Pharoah et al., 2010). In addition to the importance of better outcomes for consumers, family members are frequently adversely affected by the impact of their relative's mental health condition, as noted earlier, so that family outcomes are also important. While family outcomes from family psychoeducation are less commonly studied (Barbato & D'avanzo, 2000), the only meta-analysis of 16 studies found that family interventions can have considerable positive effects on relatives' burden and psychological distress, and on the relationship between relatives and consumer and family functioning more generally (Cuijpers, 1999). It has also been suggested that effective outcomes for consumers are more likely when family knowledge, beliefs and functioning are assessed (Lobban et al., 2013).

IMPLEMENTATION OF FAMILY PSYCHOEDUCATION IN MENTAL HEALTH SERVICES

Despite there being substantial evidence for the effectiveness of family psychoeducation in mental health, these approaches are typically not offered as part of routine care in adult mental health services in Australia or overseas. A number of studies report low rates of uptake of specialised family interventions in services, despite concerted efforts to support their implementation (Magliano et al., 2005). Common barriers to implementation include factors related to the consumer and their family (for example, consumer estrangement from family), the practitioner (for example, clinicians' fears of working with multiple family members in the same room) and the organisation (for example, workloads and the low priority afforded family work by managers) (Harvey & O'Hanlon, 2013; Lucksted et al., 2012). The growing field of implementation science in health care is identifying new strategies for achieving practice change, including post-training support, organisational consultation and monitoring of uptake as part of effective comprehensive implementation strategies (Damschroder et al., 2009; Eassom, Giacco, Dirik, & Priebe, 2014; Harvey & O'Hanlon, 2013). These strategies are particularly relevant to the implementation of family interventions, given that they have been identified as more difficult to implement than interventions involving individual consumers (Brooker, Saul, Robinson, King, & Dudley, 2003).

2.7.8 CARER EDUCATION AND MUTUAL SUPPORT

PETER MCKENZIE

Carer support and education approaches encompass a range of services and approaches to support families and carers in their caring role. This includes self-help and mutual support groups to carer group support and education programs in partnership with service providers, as well as the development of a professional lived experience carer peer workforce (Visa & Harvey, 2019). An important driver for these approaches has been the growing recognition of the impact on families of caring for a relative with a mental illness as described earlier. The most effective approaches include direct peer support, education about mental health conditions and their treatment, and teaching of practical coping strategies.

Since carer support and education are typically provided in a group context of carers supporting each other, the development of self-help and mutual support has been a key feature of these approaches. Carers coming together to share their experiences and support each other, along with education around mental illness, has become an important means to sustain their caring role. According to a UK study: 'at the core of the processes... is the sharing of personal knowledge of one's own experience' (Munn-Giddings & McVicar, 2007, p. 27). While these programs share many common elements with family psychoeducation, they are differentiated by their focus on lived experience and family coping rather than consumer outcome, and by the fact that consumers do not usually participate in these groups. Yet, positive outcomes for consumers can also be an indirect effect of carers participating in mutual support groups. In a literature review of the effectiveness of mutual support for family caregivers, the authors suggested that there is consistent evidence for the immediate positive effects of such groups on the physical and psychosocial health of both consumers and their families (Chien & Norman, 2009).

PEER SUPPORT AND EDUCATION PROGRAMS FOR FAMILIES

Family carer support and education may be facilitated by trained family members, mental health professionals or usually a combination of the two. Similarly, these programs may be delivered or auspiced by carer organisations or within the context of clinical treatment, rehabilitation and recovery services. Family support and education programs based on self-help and mutual support models are often underutilised in mainstream mental health services (Leggatt, 2005), despite evidence that they can help reduce some of the psychological burdens of caregiving for a sustained period (Stephens et al., 2011).

Several examples of carer peer support and education programs have been evaluated for their effectiveness. A peer-taught family-to-family education program in the United States (Dixon et al., 2011) reported that participants had significantly greater improvement on a range of outcomes compared to a control group who had access to existing community supports. These included problem and emotion-focused coping, reduction in distress and problem solving. Further, drawing from previous evidence (mainly from America), a study exploring the value for carers of their involvement in self-help and mutual support groups identified a range of benefits for carers including: improved self-esteem and self-confidence; mutual support; sharing coping strategies; and an expanded worldview (Munn-Giddings & McVicar, 2007). Peer support programs for children and youth whose parents have a mental illness have also been demonstrated to be useful. For example, in one study, improvements were seen in the young people's self-esteem, coping and connectedness, and reductions in relationship problems were observed post-intervention (Goodyear, Cuff, Maybery, & Reupert, 2009).

AUSTRALIAN INITIATIVES

The Carer Life Course Framework (Pagnini, 2005) is a partnership project between Carers NSW and NSW Health based on the experiences of carers and developed a theoretical and empirically based framework for understanding aspects of caring over a continuum of needs, external factors and time. It provides practical information and support interventions for carers over the course of their journeys of caring.

Mind Australia is a national community mental health support service (CMHSS) that draws on the Carer Life Course Framework in providing direct support and education for carers through a range of services, including support groups, facilitated by professionals and carers. These range from a focus on carers, families and partners, to particular diagnoses, counselling and peer support, carer education, respite and a mental health carer and family specific helpline (Mind Australia, 2020).

Wellways is another CMHSS that provides peer support and education programs designed for families, friends and carers in most/all Australian states. This includes an eight-session program supporting families/carers to maintain their own wellness and promote the recovery of family members with mental illness, along with a program specifically relating to dual diagnosis (see further Wellways, 2020).

A recent large-scale study examining the impact of the Wellways program revealed significantly decreased levels of psychological distress, self-blame and stigmatising attitudes and improved communication and relationship quality/feelings for carer participants on completion of the program and at follow-up (Farhall et al., 2019).

The Fostering Realistic Hope Workshop Series is an example of a diagnosis-specific therapeutic and collaborative psychoeducational support group for carer families living with complex Post Traumatic Stress Disorder/borderline personality disorder; it has been developed and delivered by the Bouverie Centre and is currently being evaluated.

In NSW, the Support Program for Carers from Culturally and Linguistically Diverse (CALD) Communities provides support and information to CALD carers who look after a family member or friend with a mental health problem. Twenty language-specific carer support groups have been run across the Sydney metropolitan and Wollongong areas. Large numbers of carers have participated in this support program, which has also trained a pool of bilingual group leaders to provide language-specific support for groups (Transcultural Mental Health Centre, 2020).

Carer Connect is a Queensland-based initiative that provides a mutual support and mentoring group model for mental health carers by linking more experienced carers with carers who are less experienced in the caring role.

Online carer peer support

Online technologies are also offering an increasing range of platforms for carer peer support. For example, in Australia, Mind Australia provides a direct online carer discussion forum, while Sane Australia offers a number of social media platforms for mental health carer involvement: ranging from Twitter, Facebook connections through to online forums for carers, family friends and other people caring for someone with a mental health condition.

There are also high quality international family peer support resources accessible online. For example: Rethink in the United Kingdom have created Caring for Yourself, which features a self-help workbook for family and friends supporting people with mental illness (Fadden, James, & Pinfold; Rethink Mental Illness, 2020b).

The Sibling Toolkit, developed by Rethink's Siblings Network promotes sibling wellbeing, and features personal stories and videos of siblings sharing their experiences, the challenges and what they have learned (Rethink Mental Illness, 2020a).

2.7.9 COMMENTARY AND REFLECTION

BRENDAN O'HANLON & CAROL HARVEY

The demonstrable impact of mental illness on families, evidence for the effectiveness of family interventions in supporting recovery for consumers and family members alike, and a supportive policy context are all powerful rationales for involving families in mental health care. The key challenge for individual practitioners and for mental health services is to find ways of routinely engaging families in a supportive, respectful and non-blaming manner. This provides a foundation for helping families to identify and address their needs and for offering supports and interventions that have been shown to improve outcomes for consumers and their families. Ultimately, this means that families are assisted to support consumers in their recovery, while at the same time reducing the impacts of mental illness on family members and promoting their wellbeing.

PART 03

MENTAL HEALTH PROBLEMS CONSIDERED IN THE CONTEXT OF THE LIFESPAN

The context for illness or disorder is affected by when in life it occurs. For example, phobic anxiety may be experienced by children, youth, adults or the elderly, with those phases of life shaping the presentation of the disorder, and the person's journey of recovery. In addition, some disorders typically emerge or have their greatest impact during one phase of life, such as autism in childhood and mood and psychotic disorders in early adulthood. This cues us to include a developmental context in our understanding of their origins and to consider treatments and services in relation to the current life stage.

It is no accident that mental health service systems have tended to organise around infant and child, youth, adult and elderly life contexts. Specialist assessment and treatment expertise has emerged to meet the needs of these groups, as well as links with other age-appropriate social and health services. In Part 3, we introduce mental health problems and disorders that are typically identified and treated in their lifespan context. We seek to bring together not only an overview of presenting conditions at each life stage, but also to relate these to the life context and the relevant service system. In Part 3, we have included a first-person account from a young person in Chapter 3.2, and practice illustrations in each chapter to assist the reader in contextualising the information and to link the information from Parts 1 and 2 to clinical practice, as discussed in these later chapters.

Chapter 3.1, on childhood mental health, focuses on developmental and family perspectives, as well as the conceptual underpinnings of assessment and diagnosis in this age group.

Chapter 3.2 provides a rationale for considering youth as a key developmental context for major disorders and the unique opportunities for prevention at this stage, then provides an overview of the main presenting mental health issues and an exploration of the extent to which existing service systems address these in an age-appropriate response.

Chapter 3.3, on the later years of life, presents the mental health problems experienced in the lives of the increasing number of elderly people in the population, and the treatments and services that can assist.

3.1

CHILDHOOD MENTAL HEALTH

BARBARA KEEBLE-DEVLIN

3.1.1 CHILDHOOD

Children have rights that are protected by policies, laws, program and practice principles that guide the health and welfare of children in our society. But this has not always been the case. Children have not always been valued; in fact, there is a mournful history of child abuse from the earliest of times, a history that depicts the cruellest of human behaviour, and includes periods when children were in fact on the bottom of the social scale.

We will open our examination of this topic with some historical notes on childhood as it has been seen in society, and the current legal position of children.

THE FAMILY INFLUENCE ON CHILD DEVELOPMENT

Studies of social and emotional wellbeing in childhood focus largely on the strengths of the individual child and the family, and consider the influence of the school and other social environments (Hamilton & Redmond, 2010). The most powerful influence on children's lives is the experience of their own parenting, which can exert enduring influence in the way children grow and develop (Rutter, 2006). The family constellation and education level of parents/carer, household income and area of residence are significant socio-demographic characteristics that impact on the prevalence of mental disorders in children and adolescence (Lawrence et al., 2015).

The years we spend at home living with parents who do things in a particular way, exposing their values, beliefs, ideologies and everyday opinions—from making a bed to the clothes a child wears—inevitably affect the way a child grows up. While many of the parents' opinions and ideas may be rejected, they have all had their influence by the way they have been communicated or the outcome of parents' decision making.

Early attachment between the baby and a primary caregiver is likely to be affected if there is maternal depression; marital discord, parental unemployment and the quality of child-care arrangements all have significant influence on the child (Highet, Gemmill, & Milgrom, 2011; Olesen, Macdonald, Raphael, & Butterworth, 2010; Schofield & Beek, 2014). The family, then, is a critically important context in which to seek to understand the child, and accordingly the family is also a significant focus in this chapter.

THE DEVELOPMENTAL PERSPECTIVE

There are differences across cultures and gender and universality cannot be claimed, but a pluralistic notion of development is useful in understanding prevention opportunities, and is key to successful interventions in child and youth mental health. It requires asking what a child needs at any particular age to minimise risk and foster protective factors crucial for promoting normal growth and development (Beardslee, Chien, & Bell, 2011). To understand any deviation from normal development, it is important to consider and describe the stage of life the individual has reached. We need to appreciate the patterns of continuity and discontinuity from birth to death in order to grasp the variations and differences between normal and abnormal development. Human continuity and change, lifelong growth and developmental diversity and key life transitions and events all interplay to influence an individual's development (Hoffnung et al., 2010). The age boundaries are not an exact science but they do provide correspondence with stage theories and typical developmental pathways. The third section of this chapter will therefore deal with some important views of human development.

DISORDERS OF CHILDHOOD

Historically, child development research has focused on narrowly defined concepts of individual development. More recently, the research lens has broadened to include multiple constructs that examine the dimensions of social and emotional wellbeing, the nature of resilience and coping skills, and how it is that children adapt, thrive and prosper (Humphrey et al., 2010; Lawrence et al., 2015). Children who are 'well-adjusted' are emotionally resilient in stressful circumstances and can achieve at school, demonstrating confidence in reaching their potential to develop to become healthy adults (Blandon, Calkins, & Keane, 2010; Denham, Wyatt, Bassett, Echeverria, & Knox, 2009; Pahl & Barrett, 2007). A small proportion of children, however, do not successfully negotiate developmental milestones, and are at risk of developing a range of social, emotional and behavioural or mental health problems.

The disorders presenting in this age group are commonly considered according to the age of presentation and the dominant symptoms that are usually expressed through behaviour. In the following section of this chapter, we will lay out the common disorders in the particular age ranges. The rather particular position of somatisation in childhood is given some emphasis here.

CLINICAL ASSESSMENT IN CHILDHOOD, INCLUDING FORMULATION

The last major section of this chapter will link the three perspectives above with the clinical approach to assessment of problems in childhood. While this section is focused on this particular phase of life, we believe it is also a useful complementary perspective to the earlier material on assessment in Chapter 2.3.

CLINICAL MANAGEMENT

Management of problems in childhood is not covered in depth in this chapter, as a comprehensive account of this would be beyond the scope of this work. However, there are some commonalities with case management in adult mental health practice, as set out in earlier chapters, particularly Chapter 2.3. Pointers to management also appear in the consideration of multidisciplinary team assessment, which again can be read as complementary to the material presented in Chapter 2.2.

3.1.2 CHILDHOOD IN SOCIETY

THE HISTORICAL PERSPECTIVE

In medieval times, childhood was a state to be endured rather than enjoyed. Children in Western society were often considered a burden and encumbrance because adults had little to no acknowledgment of their human needs. Very often, their gender was the only focus for individual value. If the child was of noble birth, the central focus was gender, as the social expectation was for a male heir. Children from the poor classes were included in the labour force, while their richer peers learnt 'good manners', to be employed as maids and pages in aristocratic households.

Exploitation of children as a cheap form of labour continued with the Industrial Revolution. Their value was determined by their strength, and the fact that they could be offered small wages 'and their ability to fit into small spaces beneath machinery which was generally unguarded' (Connell, 1985, p. 2). Children were regarded as small adults in both the home and society, were held responsible for their behaviour and were thus punishable by law. We can learn much about how children were seen over the centuries through paintings that portrayed children as 'miniature adults'; both in their facial and body features and the clothes they wore (Hoffnung et al., 2010, p. 13).

Interest in child development gathered some momentum in the nineteenth century with the concept of childhood developing as a distinct stage or period in a person's life. Charles Darwin (Darwin, 1877) published a detailed account of his own sons' development, later followed by Gesell (1926) who observed children at precise ages to understand their general and specific developmental achievements, and further developed the growing body of knowledge by providing generalised standards that were typical of normal development and age related (Hoffnung et al., 2010). Child behaviour studies began to explore whether heredity or environmental factors determined personality, characteristics and mental capacity. Studies by Stanley Hall in the 1880s formed the basis for interest about how children felt and behaved, rather than how adults thought they should behave. The emergence in the nineteenth century of compulsory elementary education and legislation to restrict child labour reflected a growing awareness of the needs and rights of children and how this period influences later development. Knowledge of child and adolescent psychiatry during the twentieth century was shaped by specific research in neurophysiology, neuropathology and psychology. Cognitive assessment, introduced by Binet and Simon in the early 1900s, revolutionised thinking on retardation, and promoted the introduction of remedial and psychological education. This led to the introduction of school medical services and child-focused clinics.

Early child guidance services focused on the adjustment of growing children to their environment rather than treating abnormal behaviour. Two of the more notable early child-focused clinics opened in London: the Tavistock Clinic (1920) and the Maudsley Hospital (1930). The impetus of psychoanalytic theory and behaviourism during the 1950s and 1960s paralleled the emerging specialty of child psychiatry.

Through the twentieth century, the evolution of ideas concerning the rights of children progressed considerably, with emphasis on their general and mental health. However, the World Health Organization (WHO, 1978) found that, while there had been rapid development in child health care, the mental health needs of children still required greater emphasis and inclusion in health policy and planning. The Convention on the Rights of the Child (UNICEF, 2020) states that children are entitled to the same human rights as all other people. It also creates special rights for children, recognising their particular vulnerability, such as the right to express their views freely, and that decisions affecting children must consider the best interests of the child. Securing these rights of the child in Australia still requires further development of child-sensitive laws, policies and initiatives that span vulnerable and disadvantaged groups. A major longitudinal study following the development of 10 000 children and families from across Australia will yield some exciting discoveries that will no doubt contribute to the formation of public policy for the twenty-first century (Australian Bureau of Statistics, 2018).

LEGAL STATUS OF CHILDREN

The Rights of the Child

Australia is a signatory to the United Nations *Convention on the Rights of the Child* (the Convention), whose values are encapsulated in the Australian *Human Rights and Equal Opportunity Commission Act 1986* (Cth), which in principle endorses the following:

> All children to be protected from neglect, cruelty and exploitation; to enjoy all rights without any form of discrimination; to enjoy special protection and to be given opportunities and facilities to enable them to develop in a normal and healthy manner and in freedom and dignity; to have a name and nationality from birth; to enjoy the benefits of social security, including adequate nutrition, housing, recreation and medical services; to receive special treatment, education and care if handicapped physically, mentally or socially; to education; and to grow up in an atmosphere of affection and security and, whenever possible, in the care and under the responsibility of their parents.

The convention, which has become the world's most widely ratified human rights treaty, puts responsibility on the governments of the world to promote and protect the rights of children and young people. Despite Australia's ratification of the convention, there remains a lack of a comprehensive national policy framework for children, although many states and territories have developed Acts and frameworks that promote children's safety and wellbeing, and many of the principles within the convention are embedded within child protection legislation; for example, in Victoria there is *The Children, Youth and Families Act 2005*, *The Child Wellbeing and Safety Act 2005* and *Children and Justice Legislation Amendment (Youth Justice Reform) Act 2017*; in the Northern Territory there is the *Care and Protection of Children Act 2007* and *Children's Commissioner Act 2013*; the ACT has the *Children and Young People Act 2008*; NSW has the *Children and Young Persons (Care and Protection) Act 1998* and *Advocate for Children and Young Persons Act 2014*; Tasmania has *Children, Young Persons and Their Families Act 1997* (with an amendment made to the Act in 2009) and the *Commissioner for Children and Young Persons Act 2016*. Currently, all the principles of the convention are not consistently fully integrated into Australian law and there remains a lack of enforceable remedies for many child rights violations in Australia (The Australian Child Rights Taskforce, 2011). Australian Government (2009) is a cooperative overarching document that provides a national agenda to address how Australia manages child protection matters. This will assist in reducing discrepancies across states and territories.

The age of majority

The age of majority, or full status of adulthood, in Australia is 18 years, having been reduced from 21 in the mid-1970s. Each state has its own minimum age requirements for young people to buy alcohol or cigarettes, be held responsible for criminal behaviour, obtain a driving licence or leave secondary school or the family home. Throughout Australia the legal age for consensual sex is either 16 or 17 years, acknowledging at least in law that under this age a young person does not have the psychological capacity to give informed consent. There are some grey areas in which the legal position of a young person is unclear: termination of pregnancy; access to contraception in the absence of parental consent; and the right of adolescents to consent to intrusive medical treatment or mental health treatment.

3.1.3 FAMILY DEVELOPMENT

In considering the family of the twenty-first century, we cannot assume that the dynamic processes that have shaped family development over the past decades will remain the same or continue to do so in the future. Family structure, cultural-ethnic diversity, children's rights, health-related issues and economic and social change concerns will no doubt play a role in shaping family life. It is, however, likely that in the future variations in family structures will continue to increase, as many people are cohabitating, either as a prelude or an alternative to marriage. There is also an emerging trend for young people to remain single for longer.

Family development theory focuses on common elements of diverse experiences of the life cycle or life course of a social group (predominantly for child rearing) bound together by hereditary factors and psychosocial ties and organised by environmental and social needs and expectations. The traditional concept of predictable stages that families pass through reflects the ages of parents and children but may not explain some irregularities and diversity in family groups. However, it is useful to describe a family by its own unique developmental cycle, the characteristics of which reflect individual development and the phase or stage of its members' growth together as a subsystem in society.

The family life career stage is described in Table 3.1.

While a framework for understanding family development can be useful, it is important to remember that the characteristic events of any family may fluctuate according to individual development, family constellation and sociocultural expectations and adjustments. Other considerations are necessary to applying the above framework to differing family compositions and Aboriginal and Torres Strait Islanders, for whom influences of concepts such as peoplehood and different notions of kinship and family identity may be more relevant.

DIVERSITY OF AUSTRALIAN FAMILIES

Since the 1970s, a variety of different family models has emerged, embracing blended stepfamilies, extended, same-gender (made legal by the *Marriage Amendment Act 2017* (Cth)) and single-parent families. The stereotypical nuclear family of the 1950s and 1960s (two parents with children), while remaining a powerful normative ideal in Western society, continues to decrease as family and household structures change along with changes in fertility patterns, longevity, work and family interface, and social customs, attitudes and choices. The broadening economic and cultural diversity process provides a new landscape for choices and decisions for individuals to create their own 'family' identity. Australia is a multicultural society that promotes tolerance of diversity and acceptance of optional forms of adult intimate partnership and parenting styles. This increasing cultural diversity and cultural duality has expanded the range of family lifestyle patterns, religious affiliations and labour force participation of the parents. Tracking these changes is essential if contemporary policy is to reflect and be informed by current statistical profiles (de Vaus, 2004).

Developing an ethnic identity in Australia today is supported by Australia's Multicultural Policy (launched February 2011), which recognises the importance of a culturally diverse and socially inclusive nation. This policy promotes population integration rather than the cultural assimilation models of the 1950s and 1960s, and sets out a new paradigm for inclusion and belonging with the benefit of families and children at the centrepiece. All states and territories have active policies and programs to respond to the growing issues of contemporary diversity.

As Indigenous and migrant households from diverse regions continue to expand, we can expect the defining influences of family diversity to challenge 'acceptable' family boundaries. With many women now needing to work outside the home, an increase in the number of children being cared for by people other than the parents, in both formal and informal arrangements, is occurring. The proportion of children using formal care has increased progressively since the 1980s, while the proportion of children using informal care has remained largely unchanged.

The most frequently acknowledged difference between cultures is that of family structure, and this amazing diversity provides us with a wider lens from which to view and understand childhood development. Growing ethnic diversity has forced the institutions that have an impact on children's lives (educational and recreational settings, supported in home and out-of-home family care, and the justice

Table 3.1 Family life career stages

Stage 1: newly established couple	An adjustment period, during which each partner learns his or her role and makes adjustments necessary to establish a life together. Sometimes referred to as the honeymoon period, characterised by romanticism, idealism and exclusivity. The couple may be blinded by novelty, and initially experience themselves as sharing the same values, attitudes and expectations. Individual differences are overlooked or not recognised in an effort to have agreement and sameness. Some of the challenges include building a life together and establishing or continuing with extended kinship, family and social networks. Some cultural groups may have extended family living arrangements.
Stage 2: childbearing or young family	A time of high stress for the couple as their lives change dramatically with the addition of a baby. Parenthood produces financial, emotional and time-management adjustments. Individual differences may emerge as the struggle for balance between individual and 'couple needs' becomes overt. This may be intensified at crisis points relevant to individual or family life cycles, e.g. birth of a baby; lifestyle changes for one or both partners.
Stage 3: preschool-age child family	Parents need to adjust to the needs and interests of preschool children. Parenting responsibilities take up most of their 'couple' relationship. Parents need to adjust both to the growing demands of a preschool child and the lack of privacy and time as a couple.
Stage 4: school-age child family	The challenge to the family now is to become part of a school community with other families and their children. This involves balancing the varied schedules of all family members, while encouraging children's school accomplishments, and helping children to acquire a work ethic as they master the basic skills to function effectively in society.
Stage 5: secondary school-age child family	The focus of the family now is on the adolescent's attempts to become more autonomous while remaining connected to the family and maintaining family responsibilities. The parents now have more time, and start to develop post-parental interests as the adolescents mature and prepare to leave home.
Stage 6: family with young adults	The focus for the family now is on helping young adult children prepare their lives for the external environment of work, further studies or their own partnerships or marriage. There may also be adjustments to the family home to assist the young person to remain or return to the family home.
Stage 7: middle-age family	The parents now face the empty nest, and become interested in rebuilding their 'couple' relationship in terms of extra time, activities, external interests, and preparation and planning for retirement. Some parents assume the grandparent role and continue their interest in their children through their grandchildren. Some conflicts or adjustments may involve adult children continuing or returning to the family home after completing education, or in times of difficulty: financial or relationship breakdown. This can lead to tension or be satisfying in roles and responsibilities, resources are negotiated and shared. Difficulties may arise as they prepare for retirement and face new adjustments to their status as retirees. An additional challenge for many is the care of their own elderly parents, even as they are ageing themselves (Goodfellow & Laverty, 2003).
Stage 8: ageing family	The original parents now become elderly, and their children become the members of the 'sandwich' generation. The family experiences its last days of existence as one spouse dies, and then the other. The 'original' family ceases to exist. Older adults often look back on their lives with happiness and are content, feeling fulfilled with a deep sense that life has meaning. Erikson calls this stage integrity. Some older adults look back over their lives and despair at their experiences and perceived failures. They may fear death as they struggle to find a purpose to their lives. Social inclusion, family connectedness and healthy living are all positive factors for ageing well.

Source: Adapted from Bigner, 1994; Hoffnung et al., 2010

and health care systems) to respond and adapt to the changing needs of children and families. Montazer and Wheaton, in their 2011 study of generational differences in adjustment of children of immigrants, argue that the country of origin and the migration experience play a significant role in shaping the emotional adaption process in the host country. High levels of somatisation, seen as an expression of distress, have been reported in newly arrived adult refugees, with post-traumatic stress disorder (PTSD) and other forms of psychological distress a common feature displayed by many refugees (Schweitzer, Brough, Vromans, & Asic-Kobe, 2011). Children rarely escape the influence of parental distress, with adverse life events connected to a child's poorer overall development, health and wellbeing (Olesen et al., 2010). Increasing cultural understanding and competency within our educational system, mental health and welfare sector is an imperative for working effectively with children and families in Australia. We need to understand the sources of family diversity, and the impact of diversity on family members and individual development, if we are to be effective in promoting healthy childhood development.

CHARACTERISTICS OF A HEALTHY FAMILY

> Time spent together and good communications are key strengths of functional families but this is being increasingly harmed by work pressures.
>
> *Families Australia, 2011*

Understanding how parenting or the family experience influences and shapes human development has been the subject of study for many years. It is largely understood that there are individual differences in susceptibility to parenting and other environmental influences, both on physical and emotional development. Recent literature includes work by Belsky and de Haan (2010), Olesen and colleagues (2010) and Price-Robertson, Smart and Bromfield (2010). Lawrence and colleagues indicate a growing body of knowledge relating to the detrimental effects on childhood development and later life wellbeing from negative and adverse family and parental experiences (Lawrence et al., 2015). They also report that young people in step-, blended and one parent/carer families had higher rates, especially for males, of mental illness than those living in original families (Lawrence et al., 2015). Defining healthy family functioning across such a diverse nation becomes problematic, as it requires more than the absence of adverse experience. The active investment of love, affection and encouragement, along with strengthening other protective factors, such as enabling cognitive development, are characteristics of healthy families (Hoffnung et al., 2010; Price-Robertson et al., 2010).

We can think about a healthy family as one whose members operate as a system, in the ways in which they make decisions and take actions to govern behaviour, help each other meet goals and enable the family unit to develop its unique identity and maintain individual healthy development while adapting to life changes. Hoffnung and colleagues describe the 'family life cycle as a series of predictable stages families pass through, based on the ages of children and the mother' (Hoffnung et al., 2010, p. 568). Curran describes the traits and characteristics of a healthy family as:

- Family members listen to one another; when one member has a problem, he or she is heard without being criticised or having his or her problem solved for him or her.
- All members of the family feel free to express their opinions and feelings without being discounted, judged or made fun of.
- Everyone in the family feels respected and valued.
- Everyone's privacy is respected; for example, members can lock the doors to their rooms and can feel that their mail will not be opened and read by others.
- Traditions and rituals are followed; for example, the Tooth Fairy visits a child when a tooth is lost, and certain foods are eaten on holidays.
- Arguments are not avoided: children are allowed to see their parents disagree as well as resolve differences; parents as well as children are careful to admit when they are wrong, apologise and make amends.

- Everyone has some responsibility for running the household; chores are seen as contributions to family wellbeing.
- The family does some things together as a group, such as skiing, camping, sports events, games and visiting other families.
- Members are able to laugh at themselves as well as at one another; there is a sense of support and companionship—an 'all-for-one, one-for-all' attitude.
- The family supports a strong sense of what is right and wrong, good and bad.
- The family has spiritual beliefs.
- There is a willingness to seek help from outside the family in times of crises.
- The family values service to others.
- Sharing meals as a family is done on a regular basis; conversation among members is seen as an important part of family mealtime (Curran, 1983, cited in Bigner, 1994).

Supportive childhood experiences within the family can positively define later relationships and wellbeing (Price-Robertson et al., 2010). A healthy family can be described as one that adapts to stress in a way that maintains family continuity and allows challenges to enrich the individual and family experience.

CHILDHOOD DEVELOPMENT

Individual and pathological development

The study of developmental stages and changes in behaviour over time is referred to as 'developmental psychology'. The study of changes that result in abnormal behaviour is often referred to as 'developmental psychopathology' or 'developmental psychiatry'.

Developmental psychiatry considers the interaction of biological and environmental factors, the effects of nature and nurture and the interconnections between brain and mind. The goal of developmental psychopathology is to elucidate the complex interplay between biological, psychological and social-contextual aspects of normal and abnormal development (Cicchetti & Toth, 2009). Most developmental theorists seek to address whether development is a continuous or a discontinuous process; that is, whether growth and development consist of small incremental changes or distinct stages; follow one or many pathways of change; and are influenced more or less by nature or genetic predetermination and the role of nurture or the environmental context (Hoffnung et al., 2010). To understand a child and his or her view of the world is to see the world through a child's eyes. It requires piecing together children's experiences, understanding the context in which they have grown, identifying their genetic precursors temperament, and appreciating the uniqueness of each and every child.

Trauma-informed care

Trauma-informed care is an integral component of recovery oriented practice and involves a fundamental shift in thinking, as it uses a different explanatory framework to understand mental distress and illness. Trauma-informed care emphasises the 'lived experience knowledge' and places the child and family at the centre of care.

The impact of trauma in childhood and young people can interrupt emotional regulation and may lead to a heightened stress response and maladaptive development. Young people who have experienced trauma often have severe and persistent mental health and drug use problems and can be high users of mental health and drug services. It is well known that chronic stress will affect all domains of development and neurobiological functioning, and recovery from the impact of trauma experiences will be the goal of early intervention.

For this reason it is important to take a 'holistic' (whole person) perspective when taking a developmental history and recognise that past experiences and current problems interact in a complex way. Rather than asking 'What is wrong with this child?' the question is better framed as 'What has happened to this child?' This then requires a shift from 'How do I treat this child?' to 'What does this child need to continue to develop and live a satisfying life?' How we perceive the relationship of current behaviour to early trauma is critical in formulating an understanding of what the child has experienced and the impact on growth and development.

COGNITIVE DEVELOPMENT (JEAN PIAGET 1896–1980)

Piaget's theory of cognitive development refers to the way in which people learn to think, reason and use language. He describes development as discontinuous stages, an orderly and sequential process relying on particular stimuli before specific intellectual abilities can be developed. Each successive stage is described as qualitatively different from other stages. Piaget hypothesised that children's experiences and perceptions are challenged by the external environment and that, through resolving discrepancies between their environment and their sense of reality, a more mature understanding develops. Piaget describes five major stages of cognitive development, and suggests that a child moves through each stage dependent on biological, intrapersonal and interpersonal factors.

Piaget's theory suggests that the path of cognitive development is the same for all people, and that, at each new level of development, previous achievements are incorporated and integrated. For Piaget, his cognitive development theory is the biological adaptation to the environment, which begins at birth through adaptation with the exercise of sensorimotor reflexes. Adaptations occur as the need presents, and are either automatic or inevitable. According to Piaget, an infant interprets and responds to new experiences through the process of assimilation, and through the interplay of adaptation and assimilation, new learning is broadened and deepened or modified. While Piaget does not refer to the role of nature and nurture, he does stress that the interaction of maturation, equilibration, experience and social interaction and transmission are essential for cognitive development. Piaget's theory has utility for conceptualising cognitive development in an organised, coherent, empirically supported way to understand the child at different ages (Hoffnung et al., 2010; Lewis & Volkmar, 1990). Piaget's theory and more recent neo-Piagetian approaches provide a useful framework to understand cognitive development, thinking and information processing. A criticism of Piaget's theory is that it fails to recognise continuing cognitive development across the lifespan and that emotional and multicultural factors are largely ignored.

MORAL DEVELOPMENT (LAWRENCE KOHLBERG 1927–1987)

Kohlberg's theory of moral development builds on Piaget's initial formulations, and addresses moral decision making in children and adults by focusing on the reasons why an individual makes a decision. His theory relates to moral thinking rather than action, and he related his moral stages to forms of cognition. Kohlberg proposed that moral development progresses sequentially through three levels and six stages (or types), not necessarily linked to particular developmental stages, because some individuals progress to higher levels of moral development than others. However, Kohlberg proposed that moral development was a continuous process throughout the lifespan. Kohlberg's theory has provoked criticism that it is culturally and gender (male) biased, and that there are problems with the research methods. As research methods and technology become more sophisticated and our understanding of the brain and biology broadens, we may discover if there is a biological basis or what parts of the brain are activated when a person solves a moral dilemma (Killen & Smetana, 2007).

PSYCHOSOCIAL DEVELOPMENT (ERIK ERIKSON 1902–1994)

Infant development

According to Erik Erikson, the central task from birth to 18 months is the development of trust versus mistrust. Therefore the fundamental role of the parents or primary caregiver is the fulfilment of physiological and psychological needs. Trust is enhanced when parents respond consistently to their baby's needs, and provide a safe and predictable environment in which routines are established to meet the baby's needs in a sensitive and prompt manner.

John Bowlby developed attachment theory during the 1960s as part of a theory of personality development. Attachment is defined as an enduring emotional bond uniting one person with another developed during the infant's first year of life and commonly manifested by seeking proximity and

Table 3.2 Kohlberg's stages of moral development

Stage	Nature of stage
Preconventional level *4–10 years (emphasis on avoiding punishments and getting awards)*	
Stage 1 Punishment and obedience orientation	Good is what follows externally imposed rules and rewards and is whatever avoids punishment
Stage 2 Instrumental purpose; ethics of exchange	Good is whatever is agreeable to the individual and to anyone who gives or receives favours
Conventional level *10 years and older (emphasis on social rules)*	
Stage 3 Interpersonal normative morality; ethics of peer opinion	Good is whatever pleases or helps others and brings approval from friends or peer group
Stage 4 Social system orientation: conformity to social system; ethics of law and order	Good is whatever conforms to existing laws, customs and authorities; contributions for the good of society as a whole
Postconventional level *Adolescence and older (emphasis on moral principles)*	
Stage 5 Social contract orientation: conformity to social system; ethics of law and order	Good depends on consensus principles in the face of various individual values; common principles should be upheld for the ultimate welfare of society
Stage 6 Ethics of self-chosen universal principles	Good is whatever is consistent with personal, general moral principles relating to universal justice and human rights that may be at odds with society's laws

Source: Adapted from Hoffnung et al., 2010, p. 366

contact with the attachment figure, particularly when under stress. It is a lasting psychological connectedness between human beings (Ainsworth & Bowlby, 1991; Zeanah, Berlin, & Boris, 2011). While most infants become attached to their primary caregiver in the first year, the pattern of attachment varies around the world (Hoffnung et al., 2010), with some studies suggesting that neonatal perceptions may initially influence how the parents interact with their child (Hernandez-Martinez, Canals Sans, & Fernandez-Ballart, 2011).

Attachment theory proposes that children will take initiative and interest in exploring their environment, providing they have a secure base to which they can return. Bowlby (1969) argued that, initially, exploration occurred with an attachment figure (primary caregiver or mother), with the attachment experience gradually internalised and carried forward into adulthood as mental schemata. Infant attachment status is related to many areas of childhood adaptation and development of psychopathology.

Bowlby believed that early family processes influence a child's development, and he sought to understand the nature of the relationship between a baby and the primary caregiver (usually the mother) by examining the effects of major separation.

Mary Ainsworth extended Bowlby's earlier studies during the 1970s. She developed a twenty-minute laboratory assessment of the parent–infant attachment, referred to as the 'strange situation'. Based upon the responses the researchers observed, Ainsworth described three major styles of attachment: secure attachment, ambivalent–insecure attachment and avoidant–insecure attachment.

Later, researchers (Main & Solomon, 1993) described a fourth attachment style called 'disorganised-insecure attachment', based upon their own research. A number of studies since that time have supported Ainsworth's attachment styles later in life. Secure attachment provides the basis for self-reliance, curiosity and successful relationships. As adults, those who are securely attached as infants tend to have trusting, long-term relationships. Other key characteristics of securely attached individuals include having high self-esteem, enjoying intimate relationships, seeking out social support and an ability to share feelings with other people.

Secure attachments have been shown to predict social competencies, resiliency, self-esteem and internalised self-control (Hoffnung et al., 2010; Sroufe & Fleeson, 1986). The necessary conditions for the development of secure attachment are quality of infant–mother relationship and responsiveness of the mother to infant's cues, and the ability of the infant to discriminate his or her mother or attachment figure from other persons (Hoffnung et al., 2010; Schofield & Beek, 2014).

Ambivalent-insecure attachment is characterised by extreme feelings of ambivalence towards the primary caregiver and timid, inhibited interactions with the environment. Infants who are ambivalently attached tend to be extremely suspicious of strangers. These infants display considerable distress when separated from the primary parent or caregiver, but do not seem reassured or comforted by the return of the parent. In some cases, the infant might passively reject the parent by refusing comfort, or may openly display direct aggression towards the parent.

Infants are perceptive, and are affected by responses from their caregivers. They are sensitive to maternal communications, including speech, movement, gestures and expressions, and generally react to feelings of separation from the mother or primary caregiver.

Infants with avoidant attachment pattern tend to avoid parents and caregivers. This avoidance often becomes especially pronounced after a period of separation. These infants might not reject attention from a parent, but they do not seek out comfort or contact. Infants with an avoidant attachment show no preference between a parent and a complete stranger.

Infants with a disorganised-insecure attachment style (generally found in seriously disturbed care arrangements) show a lack of consistency and clear attachment behaviour. The parent or primary caregiver is usually 'out of tune' with the infant's needs and may have unrealistic, withdrawing or rejecting ways. Their actions and responses to caregivers are often a mix of behaviours, including avoidance or resistance. These infants are described as displaying dazed behaviour, sometimes seeming either confused or apprehensive in the presence of a caregiver (Hoffnung et al., 2010).

It is now well established that parent–child attachment is a central aspect of resilience and social and emotional development (Zeanah et al., 2011; Schofield & Beek, 2014) and during times of separation, they need patience, comfort, consistency and continuation of regular routines to continue feeling secure. This has significance for children of parents who suffer a mental illness, who are emotionally unavailable at times to meet the emotional needs of their children. These children are more likely to develop emotional and psychosocial disorders than children of well parents. The symptoms of mental illness affect the ability to care and nurture a child, either through changes or disruptions to care giving (hospitalisation), or by the interruption to infant–mother relationship because of the impact of symptoms on the mother's mental status. Depressed mothers, who interact differently with their infants from well mothers, may negatively affect the infant's interpersonal relationship and developmental needs. Mothers with severe and persistent mental illness face many challenges as caregivers, both in sustaining consistent care and managing the demands of caring and raising a child (Ostler, 2010). In recent studies, Mills-Koonce et al. (2011), found that mothers with consistently insecure-avoidant attachment styles related to psychological distress are more likely to avoid or disengage emotionally from their adult partner relationships, which in turn is reflected in the less sensitive mother–child relationship.

Early childhood: preschool years

The preschool child is emerging as a social being and able to play with other children (reciprocal play) rather than beside another child (parallel play). Erikson acknowledged that play was a significant contribution to a child's development of physical, social, emotional and cognitive skills. Children's play occurs in all cultures, and although the nature and style of play may be influenced by the cultural and socioeconomic context, it allows a child to use fantasy and imagination to progressively learn new skills through imitation and advance motor skills through physical play. The composition of a child's play is influenced by the parents' or caregivers' encouragement, range of play opportunities and appropriate materials suitable for the level of the child's development (Hoffnung et al., 2010).

During the preschool years, the adaptive mechanisms that are learnt are identification, introjection, imagination and repression.

The preschool child will identify with the parent (or another significant adult) of the same sex and begin to mimic his or her behaviour and internalise the attitudes of that parent. The child assimilates (introjects) attributes of others that have an impact on his or her life. The preschooler has an active imagination, and will fantasise in play activities, often using objects in a symbolic manner; for example, a block of wood or a peg is used as a car while the child makes the noises to match his or her actions. The preschooler represses unwanted thoughts, experiences and impulses from his or her awareness. (Freud would say this is when the Oedipus or Electra complex is active). The following is the range of emotions experienced by the preschooler:

- *anger:* conflict over playthings, unfulfilled wishes, temper tantrums and crying
- *fear:* memories of unpleasant experiences, stories, pictures, TV, radio, expressed through panic, running away, hiding, crying and/or avoidance
- *jealousy:* loss of parental interest and attention expressed through reverting or regression to infantile behaviours, pretending to be ill or being naughty (attention seeking)
- *curiosity:* anything new, their own bodies, expressed through sensorimotor exploration and asking questions; a typical word for a preschooler is 'Why?'
- *joy:* sense of wellbeing expressed through smiling, laughing, clapping hands, jumping up and down, hugging objects and facial grimacing
- *envy* of other children's possessions expressed through stealing, wanting, asking and crying when denied
- *grief:* loss of anything loved or important, expressed through losing interest in normal activities; being 'preoccupied with loss'
- *affection:* bond or attachment to parents, siblings, other significant people, pets, objects that give pleasure, expressed verbally and physically.

The preschooler uses the same coping mechanisms in response to stress as the toddler, but his or her behaviour is regulated largely in response to environmental and social controls (social conditioning). Children expand their range of mental and behavioural coping strategies to regulate their emotional responses as they get older, often in an attempt to reduce fear (Sayfan & Lagattuta, 2009).

According to Erikson, developing a sense of initiative is the challenge for the preschooler or early childhood years.

Preschoolers must learn what they can do by imitating behaviour, and by using their imagination and creativity and testing the boundaries of their behaviour. This is a critical period for the development of self-concept, which is shaped largely by parental approval. The process leading to the development of self-concept begins in infancy, and is extended through early childhood, as the preschooler constructs elementary notions about his or her personal identity through physical characteristics, possessions and abilities. The preschooler learns to evaluate his or her inner self according to what others tell him or her. Children of this age see their parents as all-knowing and all-powerful, perhaps even omnipotent! The messages parents give to the preschooler about themselves and the world affect the development of their self-concept, and may have a lasting impact on their personality development. Family patterns are internalised, and the preschooler develops sets of information from which to judge the external environment. Erikson suggests that the major development crisis of preschoolers is initiative versus guilt, learning how to use assertiveness to influence the environment and feel good about themselves without fear of reprisal.

Middle childhood: Primary-school years

The ability to differentiate between fantasy and reality becomes established during this period. The school-age child consolidates earlier reactions and, according to Erikson, focuses on resolving psychosocial conflicts by acquiring a sense of industry versus inferiority. Erikson describes this as the central task of the school-age child in developing a positive, healthy attitude towards work and the desire to master certain basic skills. Industry is an extension of initiative acquired in the preschool years, with the expectation that the task or activity started will be achieved or completed satisfactorily, thus prompting a sense of mastery in the child. The school-age child learns the association between performance and rewards or acknowledgment from significant adults in their world (parents or teachers). If a child concludes that he or she cannot do anything well, he or she will adopt an attitude of inferiority, which leads to a sense of worthlessness.

School-age children are responsive to and need approval to confirm their self-worth. Children in this age bracket are heavily influenced by the significant adults in their lives and become more skilled at inferring others' mental states and traits (McKown & Strambler, 2009). The school environment provides the opportunity to work with children in achieving tasks and mastering social, emotional and cognitive skills. It is often a second chance for children who come from impoverished family environments to accomplish tasks and belong to a social group, and is an important component of children's socialisation. This age group is interested in making things and using toy equipment to act out themes dominant in their lives. The complex dynamics of human interaction are acted out in the playground and classroom as the school-age child vastly increases his or her knowledge and awareness of social communication. Children of this age group begin to compare themselves socially, and are increasingly influenced by their peer group. Changes in school-age children's perception of friendship are indicative of their psychosocial development. The school-age child learns what he or she is able and good at, perhaps in spelling, maths or sport, and what he or she is not so good at. While school-age children acknowledge positive and negative aspects of themselves, they often attribute the cause of their negative achievement to an external source (*projection*). As children develop critical self-assessment, by comparing themselves with other children of the same age group, they may internalise their problems by blaming themselves. Building a positive self-concept requires balancing self-awareness of positive and negative traits. Parents and significant adults in a child's life have a responsibility during middle childhood to interpret reality, counteract negative self or peer reviews and be aware of their own stereotypical or discriminatory judgements.

PRACTICE ILLUSTRATION: INCREASING CONCERN

Mark is eight years old, and lives with his mother and baby sister Zoë, who is two years old. Mark's parents recently separated, and his mother moved out of the family home in a metropolitan area to live in a caravan on her sister's property in the country. Mark changed schools suddenly, and is attending the small local country school with his younger cousin. His new schoolteacher asked to see Mark's mother because she was worried about Mark wetting himself during school hours, and concerned that he seemed distracted and irritable. Mark's mother did not attend the meeting with the teacher. Instead, she phoned saying that Mark would settle in soon because he was a bright outgoing lad, but he was upset over the recent changes in his life. His mother also said there were no real problems at home, except the occasional night bedwetting, and he was quieter than usual, but she understood this was to be expected given the recent upheaval. Over the next two months, the teacher phoned trying to arrange a meeting with Mark's mother, to no avail.

3.1.4 DISORDERS OF CHILDHOOD

SOMATISATION, NERVOUS HABITS, FEAR AND WORRY: NORMAL AND ABNORMAL CHARACTERISTICS

The notion that children express their distress through physical symptoms is well established (Garralda, 1996; Meltzer et al., 2009), with anecdotal evidence from many parents describing their child exhibiting pretend aches and pains to gain attention and achieve their needs, especially when frightened or fearful. Age is a significant correlate of childhood fear, and it is not unusual for younger children to have fears of the dark, the environment or loud noises and supernatural beings (Meltzer et al., 2009). Fears are only labelled as phobias when they impair or delay functioning and development, and culture may play a role in the traditions and values in the expression of fear (Meltzer et al., 2009). Small children may not be able to verbalise their distress or needs, and will often resort to using physical symptoms—for example, tummy aches and generalised pains or a sore finger—to get a response from a parent or caregiver. Many parents feel able to distinguish between the pretend or imagined pain and real pain. The use of physical symptoms as an expression of psychological needs is common in small children, and is normal when it is transient, and responsive to parental reaction and encouragement to cease the symptoms and find 'healthy' ways to communicate their needs. Stressful events and family adversity can contribute to the onset and/or maintenance of somatisation in children, especially in psychologically vulnerable children and when there are high levels of physical symptomatology in their parents (Olesen et al., 2010). Distinguishing between pathology and learnt behaviour is difficult initially, but the cues are in the child's ability or inability to verbalise distress. Where the child's only means of communicating distress is through somatic symptoms, and this tendency leads to an exaggeration of physical impairment or handicap and recurrent medical intervention, it is more likely to become pathological. The mechanisms underlining somatisation in children are still not fully understood, but somatisation in small children is common and, if transient, is understood as normal, given the child's limited vocabulary for emotional expression (Garralda, 1996). There is some suggestive evidence that childhood somatisation is linked to the emotional wellbeing in families, family functioning and to anomalies in children's social relationships (Ford & Ramchandani, 2009; Olesen et al., 2010).

Further common behaviours and phenomena in children are nervous habits and worry. Sadness is an affective expression, often difficult to differentiate from frustration and anger in small children. Children's methods for handling their feelings, anxieties and frustrations range from angry impulses, evasion, avoidance and withdrawal to the point of appearing obstinate. These behaviours can all be observed in normal children, but are transient, with the child responding to external controls and gradually internalising a 'locus of control'.

DISORDERS USUALLY DIAGNOSED FIRST IN INFANCY

This period (birth to two years) is a time of repeated contact with health services for mothers and their infants with reliable identification of health problems (Royal Australian & New Zealand College of Psychiatrists, 2010) and implementing early intervention strategies can promote long-term benefits for ongoing development. Defining a disorder in a small child is not an easy task, as children's behaviour generally shows wide variations, with difficulty discerning what is contextually normal or abnormal for any given age. While it is now recognised that infants and very young children can develop significant psychopathology, differentiation between normal episodic problem behaviours and psychopathology is often difficult to assess because of rapid developmental changes (Visser et al., 2010). Parental tolerance or intolerance of certain types of behaviour may vary considerably, and have an impact on the child's or parent's help-seeking behaviour. The quality of the parent–child attachment is fundamental in understanding the origins of behaviour, and can often be assessed in naturalistic observations with attention to 'presence or absence of child parent behaviours that reflect proximity-seeking, avoidance, resistance or disorganisation in response to distress or separation' (Zeanah et al., 2011). We use classification schemes to organise patterns of psychological disturbance, personality characteristics, levels of adaptive functioning, types of psychosocial situations and general health or illness. There are few disorders that are first diagnosed in infancy, but there are a number of indicators for subsequent psychopathology. General practitioners usually refer to a paediatrician in the first instance for assessment of development and often treat most infant ailments before referring onto mental health services. The most common disorders in infancy that may be referred on include:

- *Sleep, feeding and eating disorders*: Sleep disorders are common, affecting 30-40% of infants with parent advice and support usually resolving problems. Maternal mental health is important in managing sleep problems (Waters, Suresh, & Nixon, 2013).
- *Pervasive developmental disorders*: see Chapter 4.1.
- *Relationship problems or attachment disorders:* Reactive attachment disorder is serious and can prevent a baby from forming healthy bonds with parent/carer and impact on later life relationships.
- *Anxiety disorders or separation anxiety*: Separation anxiety disorder can be a serious emotional disorder where insecure attachment impacts on the infant who feels unsafe and can be clingy to parent/carer. Differs from normal separation anxiety in intensity of anxiousness and fear. Usually a treatable condition with effective parenting education.
- *Motor skills disorder*: Developmental coordination disorder symptoms vary with age and performance of tasks. In infants the delays in motor skills may be noticed with difficulty achieving normal motor milestones like hand control and walking. Usually diagnosed in preschoolers or school-age children when they are expected to become proficient at motor skills activities.

Infant psychiatry has been described as a subspecialty of child and adolescence psychiatry (Luby, 1994), requiring alternative methods of assessment and intervention. The central importance is the relationship between the child and the primary caregiver and the developmental context; therefore intervention approaches should target the dyad and the environment in which the infant is being raised. Symptom identification is more ambiguous than with older children. A multiaxial diagnostic system for infants, which includes assessment of the environment, interpersonal relatedness, infant–parent relationship and caregiver characteristics, would assist the diagnosis of infant psychopathology.

As a mental health clinician, you can make some useful observations from the waiting room to the first interview, including: how the infant or toddler and parent shows affection, how the infant or toddler gets the parent's attention and what sort of response is elicited, how the parent and infant or toddler communicate, how attached or close the parent and infant or toddler appear, and what is their reaction to you. While these are your first set of observations, they will provide you with data that you can corroborate further or with other sources. The assessment interview is your chance to develop rapport or a treatment alliance, while observing the interactions and communication patterns between the parent(s) and the infant or toddler.

DISORDERS USUALLY FIRST DIAGNOSED IN CHILDHOOD

Childhood (2-11 years) is a period of rapid development across all domains (emotional, social, physical and intellectual). While symptoms differ from child to child it is generally understood that the impact of mental disorders on children can affect school functioning, social and family relationships and self-esteem and early intervention is critical in improving outcomes for healthy development.

Around one in seven children and adolescents (aged from 4-17) experience a mental disorder. Attention deficit hyperactivity disorder (ADHD) is the most common disorder for males into their teen years. Sadly children and adolescents living in rural/regional areas i.e. outside of the greater capital cities, have higher rates of mental disorders particularly for males (Lawrence et al., 2015). Classification of disorders in childhood fall into two approaches: the first reflects a categorical approach and assumes that mental disorders, like physical disorders, have relatively clear boundaries that assist in distinguishing abnormal behaviour from normal behaviour; the second, dimensional approach, assumes that most forms of psychopathology are not categorically different from normal behaviour. In this approach, psychopathology is therefore described on a continuous dimension that reflects the degree to which a child demonstrates abnormal or maladaptive behaviour, and very often the behaviour can be grouped under broader dimensions of externalising or internalising problems (Tackett, 2010; von Stumm et al., 2011).

The ICD-11 is a tool for recording, reporting and grouping conditions and factors that influence health and provides clinicians with a diagnostic tool to begin the process of understanding what symptoms mean with hypotheses about the disorder categories that are most relevant to the child's main problem. Clinicians favouring the dimensional approach would begin the diagnostic process by using behaviour checklists that rate the extent to which a child shows particular maladaptive or problem behaviour. The child, parents and teacher may be asked to complete questionnaires or checklists. The results provide an opportunity for grouping of like behaviours with severity indicators in different settings. A commonly used dimensional method is the child behaviour checklist (CBCL) (Achenbach, 1997). Two broad dimensions that are useful to apply in understanding a child's pattern of behaviour are externalisation and internalisation.

Externalising behaviour (disruptive behaviour or social disorders) probably causes more concern initially, as it primarily involves disruptive behaviour that is persistent and causes a nuisance and a bother to others. Generally these externalising behaviours can be grouped into aggressive and delinquent. These behaviours violate the basic rights of others and indicate a loss of failure to develop internal controls, and are often referred to as under controlled behaviours.

Attention deficit disorder (ADD) and ADHD, oppositional defiant disorder (ODD) and conduct disorder (CD) are examples of externalising behaviours. These disorders are diagnosed more often in boys than girls, show high levels of comorbidity and indicate a risk for continuing antisocial behaviour or problems in adulthood. ADD and ADHD subtypes are not necessarily discrete and stable categories, as there is wide variation with some children 'shifting from inattentive to hyperactive-impulsive and vice versa' (Larsson, Dilshad, Lichtenstein, & Barker, 2011). Children do not seek treatment on their own. Referrals to mental health services usually come from any concerned adult (e.g., GP, teacher, parent or family member) who is worried about the child. Some research has found low levels of agreement among informants' reports of child problem behaviour, and the clinician may need to prioritise concerns with the parents in relation to what they see as the problem.

Internalising behaviour (anxiety or fear-related disorders) includes: panic disorder, agoraphobia, specific phobia and social anxiety disorder. Symptoms of excessive fear and anxiety and related behavioural disturbances must persist for at least 6 months and be severe enough to cause impairment and significant distress across areas of development and functioning.

Generally, you will find that parents and others will provide more reliable information about externalising behaviour (because it affects others), and the child will often be able to tell you more about internalising behaviour (mood, sleep and thoughts and fears) and the things they worry about that distract them from being and feeling happy. Parents will often report that 'something is not quite right', but may be surprised about what their child knows and is worrying about, and the depth of feeling.

PRACTICE ILLUSTRATION: OUTCOME

Nine weeks later, a nurse from the mental health service made contact with Mark's mother, and said that Mark had been referred to the child and adolescent mental health service by the school. The nurse reported that the school had grave concerns for Mark, as he was not settling in, either socially or academically. He was withdrawn and sullen, and did not play with other pupils during the recess times. The teachers had noticed he had lost weight, and always looked tired. He was often tearful, but would not talk about anything with other pupils or with the teachers. Mark's mother agreed to one appointment with the nurse, saying that Mark was just adjusting to a different life and was 'no trouble at home'.

The initial interview was attended by Mark, his mother and his baby sister, Zoë. The interviewers were a social worker and a nurse. From the outset, it was clear that most of Mark's mother's attention was devoted to the very active Zoë, who was clingy, fidgety and sought her mother's attention continuously. Mark was solemn, but responsive to his sister, and made numerous attempts to occupy her and keep her quiet when their mother became distressed at his sister's constant demands.

The nurse took Mark to the playroom while the social worker continued to talk with Mark's mother about her recent life changes. Mark, although quiet, engaged quickly in drawing. The nurse asked Mark to draw his family, himself and a free drawing of his choice. Mark drew three figures, his mother holding his sister, and himself quite separate. He also drew a black sky with a shape that he described as his 'lost dad'. He drew himself as quite small against a very large bare tree. His free drawing was a family group of four all smiling with a yellow sun in a blue sky. He described the drawing as 'My family when we were all happy'. By the end of the session he was chatting freely to the nurse about how he missed his dad, and that he wished he had been good. He described dreaming 'all the time' of everyone living together so he could play with his old friends. He talked about all the things he missed, and how he worried that his mother might leave him alone with his auntie. He said he cried every night, but would not tell his mother, because she would think he was naughty.

Meanwhile, it was apparent that Mark's mother was not coping well, and in fact described being quite depressed. She had lost weight, was not sleeping and spoke of feeling guilty for leaving her husband. She could not understand why she left, other than to say she needed to be on her own, but described symptoms of depression prior to leaving. Mark's mother was seen by the treating psychiatrist, and commenced antidepressants.

Mark was seen for six sessions to assist him to express his feelings. His mother was seen at the same time by the social worker, who provided her with assistance to access financial support, and introduced her to a support group for newly separated mothers. This group helped introduce her to new friends in the area, and assisted her to discuss her feelings with women who had a similar experience.

3.1.5 THE PSYCHIATRIC EVALUATION OF THE INFANT AND CHILD

INTRODUCTION

A comprehensive approach to assessment in childhood and adolescence differs in emphasis from assessment in adulthood. It views the child or young person in the context, which includes multiple lines of development, family history and functioning or development, and the social environmental structure. The clinical interview will here be considered as a viable technique for data gathering, clinical observation and engagement of family cooperation in the assessment and treatment process. The mental status examination (MSE) will be discussed as a component of the psychiatric evaluation.

PARTNERSHIP AS A CONTEXT FOR WORKING WITH CHILDREN AND FAMILIES

The characteristics of families presenting to mental health services varies widely, with some families experiencing various levels of disadvantage by a range of socioeconomic impacts and other factors, which may include poverty, family disharmony and violence, substance abuse, parental ill-health or mental health issues and diverse forms of disability. This rising complexity, combined with the number of families seeking services, presents numerous challenges for the way in which services adapt and operate to meet the needs of families who are sometimes in crisis. Finding ways to make best use of the resources and maximise outcomes for children and families requires services to work together to enhance positive outcomes for children and families. Joint assessment and treatment processes and recognition of the roles of other services in the broader system of care will provide a greater capacity to meet the needs of children and families experiencing mental health problems. We know that there are many agencies outside public mental health services that work with families and children, and that effective interagency work is more likely to improve the experience and outcomes for families and children. National and state government policies articulate the need for effective intersectoral partnerships, and linkages between services are seen as integral to the provision of seamless care. There are a range of services that a mental health worker may need to liaise and work with to support families and children, including: schools and other educational settings; housing; family counselling and health services; child protection; police and emergency services; drug and alcohol services; intellectual disability; and recreation and employment support services. Health privacy legislation and other legislation that covers confidentiality, while being a genuine concern, should not be the reason to avoid interagency working and partnerships. When working with families who require multiple services, gaining agreement on what can and cannot be shared at the outset and under what circumstances is an important step to begin working effectively with the family. Partnerships in service delivery are the current context for working with children and families.

THE CONTEXT OF REFERRAL

Referral for a psychiatric assessment is often influenced by a number of factors, and usually instigated by a concerned adult who may be a professional mediating between the family and mental health service. The child instigates very few referrals. Understanding the context of referral is therefore a key component of the assessment process. Useful questions to ask are:

- Why is the referral being made now?
- Who is most worried or concerned about the child?
- What is it they are concerned about, and why?
- What will happen if the child is not seen?
- Who else has seen or assessed the child?
- What has been tried before?

These questions assist in focusing on the social context and manner of referral as well as the child. The assessment process begins with understanding the context of the referral.

THE ASSESSMENT PROCESS

Principles underlying assessment

This developmental perspective is critical, as children behave differently at various ages and often in different settings, and the clinician needs to know the range of behaviours and abilities expected at each age to be able to discern what is normal and abnormal. Developmental theories provide a framework of principles and concepts for normal development and psychopathology, and have direct application to assessment, because they point to the type of information required and provide benchmarks for interpretation of data. Assessment instruments that are comprehensive and developmentally sensitive, along with parent reports and questionnaires, assist in gathering initial information that will help build a profile of the child's functioning. There are a number of useful principles and concepts underlying assessment (see Cox, 1994; Hamrin, Gray Deering, & Scahill, 2008).

- The psychiatric evaluation of a child needs to be based on what is known about child development and child psychiatric disorders.
- Humans are social beings, and social development is related to interactions and transactions with the social environment.
- The timing of experiences influences impact because of the stage of neurodevelopment, the individual's emerging psychological capacities and the relevance of happenings that are felt in their specific context, including the response of others.
- Intrinsic and extrinsic factors interweave, and both are crucial.
- There are continuities and discontinuities in outward behaviour, and particular behaviours may reflect different psychological processes at different ages.
- Conversely, behaviours may change their form, but nevertheless still be manifestations of the same basic process.
- Major life events and transitions occur in a social context that requires negotiation and experience, and reflects individual difference and responses.
- Attention must be given to evaluating protective factors as well as risk factors.
- It is necessary to disentangle direct and indirect effects and the chaining of events, capacities and behaviours.

Mode of assessment

While the ideal is for the first contact to be with the 'whole family', various restrictions often prevent the whole family attending, and the clinician has to employ a flexible approach, not only to engage the family but also to match the assessment mode to the referral information. Certain assessments are indicated for particular problems; for example, an individual assessment is indicated in the first instance for a referral of a young person with psychosis or depression). If a particular therapy is indicated from the referral information, assessment in that mode is preferable. For example, from a referral that indicates family distress and parent-child relationship problems, a family assessment facilitates a smooth transition to family counselling or therapy. While centre-based assessments maximise economy of time for clinicians, it is not always expedient for families who have difficulties with transport and/or distance or other problems that make attending a clinic appropriate. To sustain cooperation and provide the most efficient and effective mode of assessment, home-based and school-based assessments have their value. In rural areas, outreach clinics may be provided from various venues to promote accessibility and responsiveness.

In most cases, assessment information is required from various sources. If the trust of family members is to be gained and to observe confidentiality, information must not be sought or given without their permission. The limits of confidentiality must be established at the outset, as the parents may wish to disclose information that they believe is not known to their child or children, and the young person may wish to discuss with the clinician issues that are not related back to the parents. The clinician has an ethical obligation to keep in confidence the information discussed with a client, but also must let him or her know of possible pathways for information reporting should issues of risk emerge. It is wise to set the boundaries at the outset, about what can and cannot be kept in confidence. This provides an opportunity to discuss with the family that information related to risk or safety is excluded from the bind of confidentiality. It is important to recognise that there may be disagreement or conflict between the interests of the child and those of his or her parents, and while providing opportunities for all members to 'tell their story', the clinician needs to decide the most useful and constructive manner to use the information in the best interest of the family.

The clinical interview with the family

If we view a child's role in society through a 'family lens' (which fosters the principles of the Rights of the Child), the family, as a critical structure in a child's life, needs to be included or considered in all forms of assessment and treatment for the child. This inclusion should be extended to service planning and evaluation and imperatives for change. Service planning and development will therefore need to embody a mechanism that captures family-sensitive practice.

There are numerous approaches to family interviewing, with most clinicians agreeing that the assessment process should benefit the family (at the very least, do no harm) and result in some kind of healing process. How the clinician begins with or engages the family is likely to have an impact on family cooperation and course of contact. The literature on engaging the family in assessment and treatment is quite clear about the core components of effective and sensitive family work as being willing to be respectful and able to work collaboratively with all members of the family in seeking a shared understanding of the treatment for the presenting problems. The early work of Minuchin, which remains valid for today, describes the process of engagement with families as 'joining and accommodating', which referred to the clinician's acceptance of the family's organisation and style initially to 'blend' with the family (Minuchin, 1974). Framo, Hayley, Friedman and Crosby extended the concept of engaging and joining, with particular reference to conducting the first interview (Framo, 1980; Hayley, 1987; Friedman, 1985; Crosby, 1992). Several core components of engaging families in the assessment process, which ultimately have an impact on family cooperation for ongoing treatment, are described in essence as leadership; establishing a holding environment; empowerment; and establishing a working alliance. Essentially, these components should foster trust where emotions can be expressed, explored and contained.

There are differing schools of thought within the family therapy domain as to particular approaches, but the goals of effective family interviewing remain similar. Moore and Seu explain that correlating with social and policy trends to observe the rights of children is the concept of accepting that children can 'construct therapy within powerful and prevalent discourses' (Moore & Seu, 2011, p. 298), if the therapist can respect the ability of the child to understand by explaining the context of the family meeting.

The clinical interview with the child

The mode of communication with a child will depend on the child's age, level of development and communication preference, but it is always useful when talking to use simple, unambiguous and clear vocabulary and phrase your questions so that the child can answer in his or her own way. The child's cognitive ability and moral judgement are in a state of constant development. The child's understanding or insights into problems are contingent upon his or her own level of development and the influence of parents' or carers' opinions. Interviewing the child is only one aspect of assessment, but it is a valuable component of the assessment process. It is not unusual for a child to 'know' more about the family functioning and business than the parents realise, and it can be very useful to interview the child and parents separately. Begin the initial interview with the child by establishing an accepting and neutral attitude and an interest in the child's opinion. Depending on the age and interests of the child, games or toys can be a useful method to encourage children to express themselves. The mental health assessment of a child differs from an adult, as you are specifically addressing the developmental level of the child in relation to the child's use of language, social, emotional and cognitive skills, and commenting on family and child resilience, protective and inhibiting factors.

The MSE

Much of the data for the MSE emerges spontaneously throughout the interview process, while structured questioning, tasks and activities gather other data. An outline for the MSE is detailed in Table 3.3.

It is useful to summarise the MSE with some comments on the child's overall temperament, and the compatibility between the child's capacities, demands and expectations of family environment. You can summarise the temperament of a child as easy, difficult or slow to warm up temperament (Hamrin et al., 2008). The concept of 'goodness of fit'—that is, compatibility or match between people who have to relate together in the interests of optimal development of each individual—is applicable here in determining suggestions for adaptive behaviour.

An assessment of a child may include referral for specific assessments, such as language or speech and occupational therapy, along with a comprehensive general health assessment from a GP or paediatrician, and may include a range of pathology tests. As noted

Table 3.3 Mental status examination (MSE) for children

Appearance	Description of the child's size, manner of dress, mannerisms, tics, physical attributes and identification should be recorded. It is not informative to state that a child is dressed 'appropriately' unless there is a description of what this means. Social groups and subcultures may have very different 'appropriate dress'. It is important here to comment on nutritional state, any bruising or distinguishing marks, neurological signs and level of self or parent care.
Sensorimotor development	Comment on gross and fine motor coordination. Observe whether the child is clumsy or awkward with movement, and note his or her eye or hand coordination. Drawing, manipulating small objects, throwing and catching a ball are useful activities to assess sensorimotor development, along with clinical observation of the child walking and moving. A referral to an occupational therapist may be indicated if the clinician observes any delays or difficulties.
Manner of relating to clinician and family	Does the child exhibit extreme anxiety when separating from parents or too much ease? Observe how the child relates to family members. Is the child indiscriminate and overfriendly, or shy and withdrawn? With whom in the family does the child feel safe or ambivalent?
Mood or affect	What are the predominant feelings displayed by the child during the interview? Does his or her mood fluctuate or change? How does the child appear: relaxed, flat, withdrawn or sad? Does the child display the full range of affect in response to the content of conversation? Is the child's self-concept positive or negative?
Capacity and level of play	Does the child engage in age-appropriate activities? Is the child spontaneous or inhibited or disinhibited? Does the child integrate skills during activities? Does the child exhibit curiosity, imagination and fantasy?
Thought processes and content	A child's thought process and content can be assessed during play or activity. Observe themes that emerge during the play or activity; children often 'tell' the interviewer about their world through activities or drawings. It is useful to encourage the child to talk about his or her drawings and write such comments on the drawing. Fantasy is an integral part of the thinking process for children, as well as a major coping mechanism. Healthy children exhibit fantasy material through play and storytelling, but it does not dominate their time. The extremes are where a highly anxious, inhibited child presents little fantasy and is difficult to engage in play, and the acutely psychotic child, in whom fantasy dominates his or her waking hours. Many healthy children 'work out' their real-life problems through the use of fantasy, and some anxious children use fantasy as an escape or coping mechanism. Fantasies may be revealed through free play, drawings, wishes, and dreams or nightmares. It is important for the clinician to assess the child's ability to distinguish fantasy or make believe from reality.
Perceptual abilities	Does the child have a grasp on reality commensurate with his or her age in relation to general orientation? What kinds of impressions does the child offer in relation to differentiating fact from fantasy? Does the child use all of his or her senses (sight, hearing, touch, taste and smell)?
Cognitive abilities and intelligence	The clinician will gain a general understanding of the child's cognitive abilities during the interview. The best source of cognitive ability is from the school the child attends. If the school has had concerns about a child's intelligence, there may already be psychological tests completed. If not, the clinician will need to refer for an educational assessment or discuss appropriate testing with the child psychologist.
Attention level or concentration	Is the child able to 'pay attention' to requests by the clinician? Can the child attend to activities to complete tasks? Do external stimuli easily distract the child? What level of activity does the child display, ranging from lethargic and preoccupied to hyper-alert, easily distracted and constantly moving around? The clinician needs to differentiate between disorganised activity and hyperactivity. Hyperactivity is often more noticeable at school or in groups of children than in one-to-one situations.

Continued

Table 3.3 Mental status examination (MSE) for children (*continued*)

Language and speech	Extent of vocabulary for age; use of expressive language or gestures in place of words. Are there any abnormalities of expressive language (echolalia, neologisms, misuse of pronouns and gender)? If any speech or language delay is detected, the child should be referred to a speech pathologist for a comprehensive assessment.
Concept of self	This area includes object relations and self-concept and identification, as they are intimately related. A child's concept of him- or herself is linked to his or her identification and the quality of relationships established with family, peers and others. How does the child see him- or herself (strong, weak, good or bad, attractive or unattractive)? With whom does the child identify and compare him- or herself? How does the child interact with others, including the clinician? How does the child characterise others in the world (starting with family, teachers, peers and others)?
Positive attributes or adaptive capacities	Can the child problem solve? What are the strengths of the child that may also serve as protective factors? What interests does the child have? How does the child defend him- or herself against stress? What is the child's defence organisation? Judgement and insight can be included here in determining what the child thinks the problem is, and what caused the problem, how upset the child is about the problem, and what the child thinks might help solve or minimise the problem. How does the child think the clinician can help solve the problem?
Temperament	Based on nine behavioural dimensions: • Activity level: the amount of physical motion exhibited during the day • Distractibility: the ease of being interrupted by sound, light, and unrelated behaviour • Rhythmicity: regularity of patterns of eating, sleeping and elimination • Approach: initial reaction to novel situations • Attention span: the extent of continuation of behaviour with or without interruption • Adaptability: the ease of changing behaviour in a socially desirable manner • Quality of mood: emotional expression, positive or negative • Intensity: the amount of energy exhibited in emotional expression • Responsiveness to stimulation: the degree to which the person reacts to light and sound.

Source: Adapted from Chess & Thomas, 2002

previously, the psychiatric assessment may vary in the number of sessions and time required. It is important to use yourself therapeutically in establishing trust with the child and parents. Presenting for a psychiatric assessment may mean many different things to children, parents and families. It is often the 'last straw' for many parents, who may feel guilty, blamed, frustrated and angry, and a sense of loss of the perfect child idealised in their desires. These feelings should be recognised, acknowledged and responded to realistically and in an empathetic manner. Every child has strengths, and it is important that the child is seen as a whole, and that positive aspects are recognised. It may be useful for the parents to be reminded of such qualities to balance their view of the problem, and help with alleviating their distress.

The multidisciplinary team

As you can see, evaluating children's functioning requires a range of specialist skills across a diverse area. Many clinicians in child and adolescent psychiatry have developed their knowledge beyond their generic discipline area, including systems theory, family therapy, specific psychological treatment and counselling modalities for children, lifespan development, educational, speech and language assessments and abnormal psychology.

For most if not all assessments of children, a multidisciplinary approach facilitates the sharing of differing perspectives in order to arrive at an evaluation that best represents the nature, cause and treatment of the problem. Understanding the child and family in their social context is part of the evaluation process. Specific tests or further assessments may be required to complete the clinical assessment of the child. This responsibility falls to the multidisciplinary team, which may consist of medical, psychological, psychiatry, speech pathology, occupational therapy, nursing, special education and social work domains. The combined generic training of these discipline areas, along with extended knowledge, provides the matrix of skills required in child and adolescent psychiatry. Child and adolescent services in metropolitan areas are usually resourced with a range of disciplines. In rural or remote areas, services may not be able to recruit or retain the full complement of resources for a multidisciplinary team, and may need to work with other services or liaise with specialists in metropolitan areas.

DIAGNOSIS AND FORMULATION IN CHILD PSYCHIATRY

The diagnostic process

As a clinician working with children and families, it is imperative to know the usefulness and limitations of a diagnosis. Arriving at a diagnostic label for the condition or symptoms presented by the child is the outcome of a comprehensive evaluation, which leads to treatment planning. There are a range of questions that are useful in conceptualising and preparing for the diagnostic process:

- Does the child have any type of 'diagnosable' psychiatric disorder?
- If yes, does the clinical picture fit that of a recognised clinical syndrome?
- What are the various roots of that disorder in terms of intrapsychic, family, sociocultural and biological factors?
- What are the relative strengths of each of these root causes for this child?
- What forces or conditions are maintaining or predisposing the problem?
- What forces are facilitating the child's normal development (protective factors)?
- What are the strengths and competencies of the child and family?
- Untreated, what is the likely outcome of the child's disorder?
- Is intervention necessary to assist the child in his or her growth and development and prevent further difficulties?
- What types of intervention are most likely to be effective and acceptable to the family?

The diagnostic appraisal is ideally a joint activity shared by the multidisciplinary team. Many clinicians believe that the process itself is therapeutic, and cannot be separated functionally from treatment. It is, however, useful to distinguish conceptually between the assessment and diagnostic process and targeted treatment interventions, keeping in mind the impact and effect of the assessment process on the child and family. Quite often the assessment experience for the child and family will bring about change through altered perceptions, attitudes, feelings and behaviours. It is often helpful for families to talk through their concerns and worries, and find their own solutions from this experience.

As discussed earlier, there are two principal schemas used to describe psychopathology: the diagnostic system ICD-11 and the dimensional approach, which relies on standardised instruments and procedures, designed to assess the psychological characteristics of a child. Both approaches are used to complement the understanding of a child's symptoms. In child psychiatry, the term 'symptom' may refer to almost any behavioural manifestation that comes to the attention of the parents, teachers or others. It is therefore necessary to establish the frequency, intensity, circumstances or place and antecedent behaviour of the symptoms described. There are a range of symptom checklists that can be used to assist parents and teachers in understanding frequency and severity of symptom manifestation. When certain behaviours or traits are occurring frequently, causing concern and interrupting normal development, this is accepted as symptoms that may or may not define a condition or syndrome. The validity of describing symptom behaviour depends on the accuracy of the informant or observer.

Difficulties may arise during the diagnostic process because some maladaptive behaviour may not 'fit' into a particular category, and may arise out of different factors, intrinsic defects or immaturities that make the child vulnerable to normal demands. In clinical practice, you will find children presenting with some features of a given syndrome but lacking others. Most of the descriptions of syndromes depict typical or prototypical clinical presentations.

Summary

It is wise to question constructs of psychopathology and consider dimensional qualities of assigning a diagnosis to presenting symptoms. There is currently no best way to understand or describe adequately a child's experience and expression. The current health care system requires a common approach to communicate the scope and nature of disorders in children. While we work amid dichotomies of practice, where individual ideology sometimes assumes that some behaviours are normal and others are not, and some behaviours indicate differences in brain structure to problems in family adaptation, what is clear is that a standardised approach to communication about disorders is only as effective as the informant's ability to describe the signs and symptoms accurately. Current nosological systems of psychopathology rely on the clinician's appreciation of the process whereby children develop impairments in emotional, behavioural and mental functions.

3.1.6 COMMENTARY AND REFLECTION

This chapter has confined itself to a limited set of aims, being an overview of the thinking and particular approaches used in assessing disorder in this phase of the lifespan. Readers who will be active as clinicians in this area of practice are encouraged to consult more specific textbooks to take their skills and knowledge beyond the overview provided here. However, for the non-specialist reader, this chapter should have served to lay out some of the guiding principles of clinical mental health practice in childhood, and to define some of the distinguishing features of work in these areas.

PRACTICE ILLUSTRATION: THE THREE-MONTH FOLLOW UP

At the three-month follow up, Mark's mother was feeling much better, and had contacted her husband to arrange visits with the children. The school reported that Mark was now settling in well and had made new friends. The joint interview with Mark, his mother and Zoë was quite different from the initial interview. Mark and Zoë sat either side of their mother, and enjoyed poking fun at each other while she spoke about their progress. They presented as a united family who were discussing issues openly while still feeling saddened by the changes. It remained unclear as to why their mother had initially left her husband and the family home, but both parents had agreed to go to counselling to discuss reconciliation. Despite a lengthy period before accepting or seeking help, this family have overcome the impact of significant life changes, and they are adapting to a new phase in their lives.

While it is unknown whether the family unit would have progressed or worsened without professional mental health support, it is clear that Mark benefited from the intervention by his general demeanour and school performance.

3.2

YOUTH MENTAL HEALTH

CRISTINA MEI, FAYE SCANLAN, ROXXANNE MACDONALD & PATRICK MCGORRY
[WE SINCERELY THANK ASSOCIATE PROFESSOR ROSEMARY PURCELL, PROFESSOR ALEXANDRA PARKER AND DR SHERILYN GOLDSTONE FOR THEIR CONTRIBUTION TO THE PREVIOUS EDITION OF THIS CHAPTER. WE ALSO THANK ALL OF OUR COLLEAGUES AT ORYGEN AND HEADSPACE AROUND AUSTRALIA, AND COUNTLESS YOUNG PEOPLE WHO HAVE SHAPED THE REFORM AGENDA IN YOUTH MENTAL HEALTH.]

> Mental disorders are the chronic diseases of the young.
>
> *Insel and Fenton, 2005*

As mental health services struggle to evolve in the era following deinstitutionalisation, Australian policy makers have come to understand that it is critical that such services be re-engineered to match the pattern of mental ill-health across the lifespan. In particular, the epidemiological variable of the age of onset of mental disorders (McGorry, Purcell, Goldstone, & Amminger, 2011) must become the key influence on service design and investment if the impact of emerging mental disorders is to be reduced. An equally important influence on service culture and structure is the changing face of developmental psychiatry in the twenty-first century. The most significant change is the evolution and expansion of the transition from childhood to adulthood. Adolescence has been transformed and extended into emerging adulthood (Arnett, Žukauskienė, & Sugimura, 2014), creating the expanded transitional life stage of youth. This has had a range of implications for society and the provision of preventively orientated mental health care. Australia is at the forefront of these changes in theory and practice, and has a unique opportunity to contribute to reducing the impact of mental disorders, not only at this life stage, but across many decades. In this chapter, an overview of the life stage of youth is provided, followed by an outline of the management of youth mental disorders, with a particular focus on the epidemiology, assessment and treatment of anxiety, depression and psychosis.

3.2.1 YOUTH AND ITS DEMOGRAPHY

The life stage of youth, beginning around puberty and covering the transitional stage of early adolescence and young adulthood, is among the most important developmental periods to maximise personal growth and potential (Patton et al., 2016). While it is widely acknowledged that the commencement of adulthood at the arbitrary age of 18 years is discordant with recent trends of a protracted adolescent phase owing to shifting biological, maturational and societal trends (Arnett et al., 2014), the precise age definition of 'youth' remains debated. An age range of 10–24 years has been proposed (Sawyer, Azzopardi, Wickremarathne, & Patton, 2018) although some authors have suggested a more prolonged transition to mature adulthood that concludes at 29 years of age (Arnett et al., 2014). Across Australia, the age range of 12–25 years has guided the re-design of mental health services for young people (McGorry, Goldstone, Parker, Rickwood, & Hickie, 2014), aligning with the peak age of onset of mental disorders (McGorry et al., 2011).

Within Australia, young people aged 12–25 years account for nearly 20% of all Australian residents (Australian Bureau of Statistics, 2017). As a percentage of total population, the youth population in Australia (aged 10–24 years) has been relatively stable between 2013 and 2017 (Australian Bureau of Statistics, 2017). However, the population of culturally and linguistically diverse (CALD) young people (12–24 years) has demonstrated a faster rate of growth than their Australian-born counterparts, reflecting immigration to Australia from CALD countries.

3.2.2 CHALLENGES AND TRANSITIONS OF YOUTH

Young people are uniquely vulnerable to, and often heavily impacted by, the onset of a mental illness for complex biological and sociological reasons (Paus, Keshavan, & Giedd, 2008). Adolescence and early adulthood is a time of dynamic structural and functional change in the brain, driven by a complex series of maturational processes that result in the refinement of the neuronal circuitry and a recalibration of the inhibitory/excitatory balance, particularly in the frontal cortex (Paus et al., 2008). The transition from childhood to independent adulthood presents new developmental challenges that must be met against the background of these highly dynamic changes in brain architecture. Young people are in the process of defining their individuality and autonomy, which includes establishing and negotiating their own social networks, beginning sexual relationships, completing their education and entering the workforce. This transitional process has changed qualitatively and quantitatively in recent decades, particularly in Western societies, now extending from prior to puberty into the late twenties, before fully independent adulthood is securely achieved (Arnett et al., 2014). Pubertal timing has accelerated, which can increase the risk for mental illness via underlying neurobiological and hormonal changes that intensify susceptibility to environmental stressors (Whittle et al., 2012). This heightened vulnerability to mental ill-health extends to the emerging adult years where brain maturation continues (Lebel & Beaulieu, 2011), increasing susceptibility to stressors, risky behaviour and psychopathology (Paus et al., 2008). Trauma, which is commonly experienced by young people, can adversely impact brain and cognitive maturation processes (Teicher & Samson, 2016), increasing the risk of mental disorder onset.

As lifespans have increased, the transition to adulthood has been stretched and made less secure, largely due to the rapid pace of change in our social, economic and technological environments. Within Australia and other developed countries, many young people now face an extended period of education, unstable job prospects, financial insecurity, and prolonged parental dependency (VicHealth & CSIRO, 2015). It is hardly surprising that mental illness, even when brief and relatively mild to moderate, can seriously disrupt this developmental trajectory and limit a young person's potential.

3.2.3 INFLUENCES OF YOUTH ON DISORDERS AND SERVICE PRESENTATION

PREVALENCE OF MENTAL DISORDERS

Mental ill-health is a key health issue facing young people globally, and if it persists and develops into forms of serious mental disorder, the distress and disability caused can last for decades. The incidence and prevalence of mental illness in young people is well documented, and is the highest of any age group. In Australia, the 12-month prevalence of diagnosable mental disorders is estimated at 14.4% between 12-17 years of age (Lawrence et al., 2015a) and 26.4% between 16-24 years (Slade, Teesson, & Burgess, 2009). In the United States, the National Comorbidity Survey Replication indicated that 75% of people suffering from a psychiatric disorder experienced its onset by 24 years of age, with the onset of most of the adult forms of mental illness falling within a relatively discrete time band from the early teens to the mid-twenties, and peaking in the early twenties (Kessler et al., 2005). This pattern of onset has led to the proposal that the mental disorders be considered the 'chronic diseases of the young' (Insel & Fenton, 2005). While many of the risks factors for later disorders are present in childhood, and certain disorders such as autism and attention deficit hyperactivity disorder (ADHD) have their onset prior to puberty, most major disorders do not declare themselves until adolescence or early adulthood (McGorry et al., 2011).

HELP-SEEKING BEHAVIOURS AND MENTAL HEALTH SERVICE DESIGN

Although young people with early signs of mental illness present with a genuine need for care, 75% of those aged 16-24 years with a 12-month diagnosis of a common mental disorder do not seek professional help for their symptoms (Burgess et al., 2009). This rises to as high as 87% in young men. The minority of young people who do access professional help often fail to engage with services or have insufficient contact to allow the provision of minimally adequate treatment (Sawyer, Reece, Sawyer, Hiscock, & Lawrence, 2019), resulting in little or no benefit for clinical or functional outcomes (Cosgrove et al., 2008). Service-level factors can create critical barriers to accessing and engaging with services due to their design, appropriateness for young people, confidentiality, cost, availability, location, décor, and safety (Ambresin, Bennett, Patton, Sanci, & Sawyer, 2013). Young people themselves are often reluctant to seek help, which can stem from a range of beliefs such as wanting to solve their own problems, perceived stigma of mental illness, and negative attitudes towards services (Rickwood, Deane, & Wilson, 2007).

The traditional and existing design of specialist mental health services follows the paediatric-adult medical model: child and adolescent mental health services, and adult mental health services. Child and adolescent services focus on the needs of younger children and are better equipped to manage disorders that typically emerge pre-puberty (e.g., ADHD, CD, and developmental disorders) than adult-type disorders that begin to emerge during adolescence (e.g., mood, psychotic, substance use and borderline personality disorders). Child and adolescent services are typically provided until around 18 years of age, after which the young person is transferred to the adult service stream for continuing care. This service split takes no account of the pattern of age of onset of mental disorders nor of sensitive developmental and cultural issues for young people (McGorry et al., 2011). It creates massive service discontinuity from child and adolescent mental health services at a time when developmentally appropriate and expert mental health care is most needed. The system is 'weakest where it needs to be strongest' (McGorry, 2007). The need for mental health care very often continues or emerges for the first time beyond this point; however, transition to adult mental health services is often suboptimal and adult services are simply not designed to cater for the developmental and cultural needs of youth with emerging mental illness and their families (Singh et al., 2010). With a predominant focus on older patients with severe and persistent psychotic disorders, adult services neglect a significant proportion of young adults with less severe non-psychotic disorders who require care (McGorry, 2007) as well as young people with emerging mental illness more broadly who typically lack sufficient symptom specificity and severity to meet adult-type diagnostic criteria.

EARLY INTERVENTION IN YOUTH MENTAL HEALTH

How then can mental health services be designed to better fit the needs of young people? A new 'youth mental health' approach, that incorporates adolescents and young adults (12-25 years of age), is required that builds on, but is qualitatively and quantitatively different from, the existing child-adolescent and adult services. Specialist mental health services for young people are appropriate because this population is heterogeneous, with varying and clinically uncertain illness trajectories, and tends to present blends of multiple comorbidities of variable intensity, particularly substance abuse and challenging personality traits, that require an integrated model of care. Youth-specific services are needed that employ developmentally and culturally appropriate approaches to the management of emerging mental and substance abuse disorders, and acknowledge the complex and evolving pattern of morbidity and symptom fluctuation seen in this age group. Young people's unique life stage issues are not all resolved by the arbitrary age of 18. Their individual and group identity and their help-seeking needs and behaviours need to be central to any service model. Ideally, youth-specific services should be provided in an accessible, community-based, nonjudgmental and non-stigmatising setting, where young people feel comfortable and can feel a sense of trust.

The sheer scale of the incidence and prevalence of mental ill-health among young people and the high stakes in terms of outcome calls for a layered approach to service provision that has both the capacity to deal with the high volumes involved, as well as the depth necessary to manage the diversity of need. Different service levels that cover the entire spectrum of need among young people are required: from services that could benefit the entire community, through to primary care services for those with mild to moderate mental ill-health, then specialised services for those with complex or severe presentations. These could include:

- services that improve community capacity to deal with mental health difficulties in young people by providing education, mental health first aid training, e-health and self-care initiatives
- primary care services, provided by frontline service providers such as general practitioners, teachers, school counsellors and other school-based programs, community health workers and other youth workers
- youth-specific mental health enhanced primary care services providing comprehensive and holistic assessment, treatment, and social and vocational recovery services, with general practitioners co-located or integrated with mental health and multidisciplinary specialists.

Australia's innovative response to youth mental health reform, informed by an evidence-based approach, has been modelled around the world. This began in the 1990s through the establishment of an early psychosis paradigm that has been influential in not only establishing evidence for the effectiveness of early intervention (Correll et al., 2018), but also in promoting national and international efforts for reform in services and treatment approaches for those with a psychotic illness (McGorry, 2015). The success of this model of reform and its 'proof of concept' has encouraged the wider application of early diagnosis and specialised treatment for the full range of emerging disorders in young people, including the mood and anxiety disorders, substance use disorders, eating disorders and personality disorders (McGorry et al., 2014; McGorry, Hickie, Yung, Pantelis, & Jackson, 2006).

Over the last decade, the Australian government has increasingly recognised the need for reform in the provision of mental health services, particularly for young people, and a series of policy frameworks and new programs have been put into place to address this major public health issue. The National Youth Mental Health Foundation, headspace, was established in 2006 with the mission to promote and support early intervention for young people with a range of mental disorders, including substance use disorders (McGorry et al., 2014). Since its inception, headspace has expanded from 10 services in 2007 to 110 in 2018, with an additional 30 centres or satellite centres committed in the 2019 Federal Budget. A major part of the headspace mandate is to establish youth-friendly, highly accessible centres that target young people's core health needs by providing a multidisciplinary enhanced primary care structure with close links to locally available specialist services and community organisations. The significant focus on ensuring that headspace centres provide a 'youth-friendly' environment is vital, as this is rarely available in the primary care or the specialist mental health systems, and provides a 'soft entry' point that is more appealing and effective in attracting young people into the service. This is achieved by the co-location of primary care (e.g., general and sexual health concerns) and vocational/educational services along with mental health care. Further in this chapter, we detail the outcomes of headspace.

3.2.4 SPECIFIC MENTAL DISORDERS COMMONLY ASSOCIATED WITH YOUTH

The broad focus of headspace aligns with the range of mental disorders that commonly emerge during adolescence or young adulthood, including anxiety, depression, psychotic disorders, substance use disorder, eating disorders, bipolar disorder, and personality disorders (Kessler et al., 2005; McGorry et al., 2011). These disorders may continue across the lifespan and, in some instances, may emerge during other phases of life; the onset of certain anxiety disorders can occur during childhood, while some adults may present with late-onset psychosis or mood disorders (Kessler et al., 2005; McGorry et al., 2011). While a small proportion of ADHD cases may present as late-onset, its peak onset is during childhood (Sibley et al., 2018). Youth mental disorders that form the focus of this chapter are anxiety, depression and psychosis.

PHENOMENOLOGY

A recent review of the phenomenology of major depression found that commonly reported clinical symptoms were lowered mood, impaired cognitive functioning, psychomotor changes, and altered volition/motivation (Kendler, 2016). Other reported symptoms were anxiety, slowing of speech, somatic complaints, and changes in sleep and appetite. For psychosis, delusions and hallucinations are common in addition to other symptoms such as depression, subjective thought disorder, disorganised communication, and lack of motivation (Morgan et al., 2011). As can be seen, symptoms can be shared across diagnostic entities. When symptoms of major mental disorders do emerge, they typically present as a fluctuating mixture of clinical features that can include depression, anxiety and other nonspecific symptoms such as sleep disturbance, withdrawal and apathy (Hartmann, Nelson, Ratheesh, Treen, & McGorry, 2019). These early symptoms can follow different pathways, either diminishing or progressing into several possible directions (Kim-Cohen et al., 2003) and often crossing traditional diagnostic boundaries, before meeting criteria for a specific (though typically comorbid) psychiatric diagnosis.

FORMAL DIAGNOSIS

Prior to meeting formal diagnostic criteria (see Table 3.4 for ICD-11 descriptors), young people typically present with subthreshold symptoms that are characteristically mild, undifferentiated and frequently changing. This means that traditional diagnostic systems, which reflect cross-sectional symptoms of well-established mental disorders, are often inappropriate for young people experiencing the early stages of mental disorders. In response, a transdiagnostic staging approach to guide early diagnosis and treatment has been advocated (McGorry et al., 2006). In brief, this approach places an individual on a continuum of illness ranging from asymptomatic (stage 0), nonspecific (stage 1a) and attenuated mental syndromes (stage 1b), full-threshold disorder (stage 2), recurrence and persistence (stage 3), and severe, chronic mental illness (stage 4). Compared to traditional diagnostic systems, the model differentiates early and mild clinical presentations (stages 1a/b) from those that are more severe and established (stages 2+), with progression to later stages not considered evitable. This differentiation acknowledges the need for care prior to a first episode and enables the selection of treatments that are more effective, simpler and safer for earlier stages. Importantly, treatment provided is proportional to both the presenting clinical need and the risk of progression to later stages that are associated with greater severity and impairment. In this sense it offers pre-emptive intervention rather than stepped care and is more proactive and ambitious in seeking better outcomes.

Table 3.4 ICD-11 descriptors for anxiety, depressive disorder and psychosis disorders

ICD-11 category	Descriptor
Anxiety or fear-related disorders	Excessive fear and anxiety and related behavioural disturbances, with symptoms that are severe enough to cause significant distress or significant impairment in personal, family, social, educational, occupational, or other key areas of functioning.
Depressive disorder (single episode)	Almost daily depressed mood or diminished interest in activities lasting at least two weeks accompanied by other symptoms such as difficulty concentrating, feelings of worthlessness or excessive or inappropriate guilt, hopelessness, recurrent thoughts of death or suicide, changes in appetite or sleep, psychomotor agitation or retardation, and reduced energy or fatigue.
Schizophrenia or other primary psychotic disorders	Significant impairments in reality testing and alterations in behaviour manifest in positive symptoms such as persistent delusions, persistent hallucinations, disorganised thinking, disorganised behaviour, and experiences of passivity and control, and negative symptoms such as blunted or flat affect and avolition, and psychomotor disturbances. Symptoms occur with sufficient frequency and intensity to deviate from expected cultural/subcultural norms.

Source: International Classification of Diseases (ICD-11). Geneva, World Health Organization, 2018c.

PREVALENCE

Anxiety disorders and depressive disorders are the leading contributors to the total burden of disease in young Australians aged 15-24 years (Australian Institute of Health and Welfare, 2016). Although psychotic disorders are less common, they also represent a significant burden (Access Economics, 2009). In Australia, the 12-month prevalence of common mental disorders among 12-17-year-olds is 5% for major depressive disorder and 7% for anxiety disorders (Lawrence et al., 2015b). For 16-24-year-olds, the prevalence rates are 3% and 15%, respectively (Australian Institute of Health and Welfare, 2011b). The 12-month treated prevalence of psychotic disorders is 4.0 cases per 1000 population aged 18-24 years (Morgan et al., 2011). Although findings are conflicting, there is some evidence to suggest that the prevalence of major depression has increased over time (Sawyer, Reece, Sawyer, Johnson, & Lawrence, 2018c).

HOW CAN WE UNDERSTAND THE ORIGINS?

The origins of youth mental disorders are typically multifactorial and include a range of biological, psychological and social risk factors. Genetic factors commonly contribute to the causation of mental disorders, with heritability estimates ranging from 31-

42% for major depression and 64% for schizophrenia (Lichtenstein et al., 2009; Sullivan, Neale, & Kendler, 2000). While mental disorders have been traditionally conceptualised as discrete entities, there is increasing evidence to support the sharing of genetic risk factors across diagnostic categories, including depression and schizophrenia (Caspi & Moffitt, 2018).

Environmental factors are an equally important contributor to the causation of mental disorders (Polderman et al., 2015) and are also commonly shared across disorders (Uher & Zwicker, 2017). However, not all individuals exposed to the same adverse event will experience a mental disorder, suggesting an important role of gene-environment interactions. Environmental factors associated with mental disorders include parental history of mental illness, parental discord, social disadvantage, urbanicity, child abuse or trauma, substance abuse, discrimination, marginalisation, and bullying (Lereya, Copeland, Costello, & Wolke, 2015; Uher & Zwicker, 2017). Early experiences of socioeconomic disadvantage (including low-income households, low levels of parental education and higher levels of parental unemployment) are strongly associated with higher rates of mental disorders in Australian young people (Lawrence et al., 2015b). The onset of mental illness may represent a cumulative effect of risk factors whereby exposure to multiple forms of adversity increases the risk of depression and psychotic symptoms (Bentall, Wickham, Shevlin, & Varese, 2012). Specific risk factors may also suggest a poorer prognosis; for example, childhood maltreatment is predictive of recurrent and persistent depressive episodes as well as poor long-term functioning in young people at ultra-high risk for psychosis (Nanni, Uher, & Danese, 2012; Yung et al., 2015).

Up to 75% of Australians have experienced a traumatic event (Mills et al., 2011), placing them at risk of a range of mental disorders. Trauma is particularly common in young people with a history of out-of-home care, involvement in the youth justice system, or certain occupations (e.g., armed forces), and among those who are refugees, homeless, or identify as lesbian, gay, bisexual, transgender, intersex or queer (LGBTIQ) or Aboriginal and Torres Strait Islander people (Bendall et al., 2018). For Australian Indigenous populations, a connection to their traditional land and community is a key determiner of mental health status in addition to experiences of intergenerational trauma and loss, racism, environmental adversity, and social disadvantage (Dudgeon, Milroy, & Walker, 2014). Early experiences of trauma, including abuse, neglect or adversity, can detrimentally influence brain and cognitive development, which can play a complex role in the emergence of psychopathology (Teicher & Samson, 2016). Negative or disrupted attachment relationships, which are common among children and adolescents who have experienced trauma or statutory care, can lead to psycho- and neurobiological alterations of the developing brain, increasing the risk of a range of emotional, behavioural and mental health problems (Schore, 2001).

In some cases, the mental health effects of bullying can exceed child maltreatment (Lereya et al., 2015). Peer victimisation is an independent contributor to poor mental health outcomes, including emotional problems and suicidality, with its effects long-lasting (Copeland, Wolke, Angold, & Costello, 2013). Possible mechanisms underlying this association include changes in the physiological response to stress (e.g., hypothalamic-pituitary-adrenal axis dysregulation) and distorted cognitive responses to negative events (Arseneault, Bowes, & Shakoor, 2010).

As society evolves, new trends that may potentially impact the mental wellbeing of young people have emerged. Within Australia and beyond, this includes educational pressures and a more competitive and insecure labour market, increased cost of living, changes in globalisation and technology, increased time spent online and poorer physical health, increased diversity and potential discrimination, and environmental factors such as climate change (VicHealth & CSIRO, 2015).

COURSE AND IMPACT

Mental ill-health in young people is often associated with ongoing disability, including impaired social functioning, poor educational achievement, un- or under-employment, substance abuse, violence and victimisation (Dean et al., 2018; Gibb, Fergusson, & Horwood, 2010). This can lead to a cycle of dysfunction and disadvantage that can be difficult to break, as emphasised by the over-representation of individuals with a mental disorder in prisons (Fazel, Hayes, Bartellas, Clerici, & Trestman, 2016) and the high percentage of Australian adults (71%) and youths (53%) who are homeless and report a diagnosed mental disorder (MacKenzie, Flatau, Steen, & Thielking, 2016; Spicer, Smith, Conroy, Flatau, & Burns, 2015). The physical health of individuals with a mental disorder is also commonly compromised due to a variety of reasons such as lifestyle and medication side effects (De Hert et al., 2011), and contributes to the excess and premature mortality in this population (Olfson, Gerhard, Huang, Crystal, & Stroup, 2015). The impact of mental ill-health extends more broadly to family members and carers who may experience caregiver burden, distress, stress, grief, stigma and reduced quality of life (Bowman, Alvarez-Jimenez, Wade, Howie, & McGorry, 2017).

At an economic level, the annual financial cost of mental illness in Australia has been estimated to be $12.8 billion for high prevalence disorders (Lee et al., 2017) and $56.7 billion for the cost of the burden of serious mental illness in adults (Royal Australian and New Zealand College of Psychiatrists, 2016). In young people, the cost of mental illness in Australia per annum is estimated between $6.29 and $10.6 billion (Access Economics, 2009; Hosie, Vogl, Carden, Hoddinott, & Lim, 2015) with much of this attributed to lost productivity due to lower employment, as well as work absenteeism and premature death. This equates to $10 544 per annum per young person with a mental health disorder in Australia (Access Economics, 2009). However, these figures are likely to under-estimate the true cost of emerging mental ill-health in young people as they do not account for school absenteeism and compromised education achievement, which can have ramifications for future tertiary education and vocational pursuits.

An influential World Health Organization (WHO) report on the global burden of disease estimated the peak age for the maximum negative social and economic impact of a disabling illness to be 22 years (Murray & Lopez, 1996). This is because our society invests heavily in its young people to enable them to reach adulthood and become socially and economically productive in their turn, and therefore any disabling illness that prevents a young person from fulfilling their potential, is a social and economic calamity (McGorry & Purcell, 2009).

3.2.5 ASSESSMENT

Given the potential lifelong impact of mental disorders, comprehensively assessing a young person's mental health is essential for accurate diagnosis and to develop effective and appropriate treatment plans. The assessment phase presents a critical opportunity towards preventing the escalation of symptoms, deterioration in functioning and exacerbation of risks that young people are likely to face if they do not receive appropriate treatment (Burns & Birrell, 2014). In practice, the processes of engagement, assessment and treatment are inextricably intertwined; conducting a comprehensive assessment in which the young person feels heard, understood and validated is likely to engage them and can be therapeutic in itself (Power & McGorry, 1999). Moreover, neither assessment nor engagement ceases after the initial clinical contact with a young person, both are ongoing and dynamic processes. While recognising that engagement, assessment and intervention are inextricably connected, for clarity, it can be helpful to consider best practice within each area separately.

ENGAGEMENT

Engagement is used here as a broad term that includes the extent that a young person is engaged with the help-seeking process, interventions, a health service, and with individual clinicians. Engaging a young person and building trust and rapport are essential components of any intervention (McGorry, 2012) and should be considered important goals of assessment in youth mental health settings (Orygen, 2016a). Youth participation (e.g., involvement in decision making and the design and delivery of services) and peer support programs (described further below) are valued components of early intervention services that can facilitate youth engagement (Health Workforce Australia, 2014; Hetrick et al., 2017). While engagement is a critical consideration within mental health care at any point in the lifespan, it is particularly important for clinicians working with young people to consider how to engage this population in every step of their journey from help-seeking through to recovery, given the specific and unique engagement challenges associated with developmental and phase of life factors.

Young people's desire to build or enhance their autonomy (a core developmental task) may manifest in a preference for solving problems independently, mistrust of authority figures and/or a reluctance to confide in others, all of which may hinder the process of engagement and assessment. Furthermore, young people's help-seeking is often initiated by others (e.g., parents, teachers), therefore, the assessment process may be perceived as coercive (Stallard, 2002a). In this situation, the young person may be ambivalent or entirely averse to seeking support. They may perceive that the clinician is there to serve the needs of others rather than their own needs. Young people are also likely to have more reservations about talking to health professionals about their mental health and personal lives than other age groups, particularly due to concerns about maintaining confidentiality (Rickwood et al., 2007). So it is perhaps not unexpected that they are also less likely than adults to disclose mental health concerns to a GP (Highet, Hickie, & Davenport, 2002). Young people are particularly disconnected from medical professionals (Hickie, Fogarty, Davenport, Luscombe, & Burns, 2007) and for many, their point of engagement with health services may represent their first encounter seeking support from a health professional independently (McGorry, 2012). There is also increased potential for clinicians to misinterpret certain aspects of young people's presentation as 'resistance' or ambivalence about engaging in care than there is with adults. For example, adolescents presenting with depressive symptoms are more likely than adults to experience irritability as their primary mood disturbance (Katz, Fotti, & Postl, 2009). Additionally, young men often present with non-traditional symptoms of depression, for example externalising behaviours such as anger and aggression (Martin, Neighbors, & Griffith, 2013), and may be reluctant to openly discuss their mental health. For a young person who is feeling very irritable, sitting through an assessment in which they are asked to answer numerous questions may be particularly challenging, while the clinician may also struggle to 'sit with' their irritability and hostility and may interpret it as 'resistance'. It is important to see beyond the surface emotion and behaviour. A standard mental health assessment can also be taxing on young people in terms of their cognitive, emotional and social skills. Depending on a young person's stage of development in these domains, they may struggle to respond to open-ended questions and articulate their experiences, which may manifest in limited responses to questions or disengagement in the assessment process. Disclosing self-harm can be difficult for young people, especially for those who may have previously experienced stigma from health care professionals, necessitating the need for compassionate and useful responses to self-harm, including building trusting relationships and leading helpful conversations (Robinson, McCutcheon, Browne, & Witt, 2016).

Due to the challenges that both a young person and clinician may encounter in the engagement process, it is recommended that clinicians spend more time building engagement with young people than they might with other age groups. For many young people and their families/carers, the time of help-seeking represents a crisis (Power & McGorry, 1999). Every effort should be made to focus on starting out 'on the right foot', building rapport and establishing continuity of care for the young person and their family/carers (Power & McGorry, 1999). It is important not to rush the assessment and time should be taken to 'set the scene' by explaining the assessment process, providing opportunities to ask questions and raise concerns. Clearly explaining confidentiality and its limitations within the assessment, and the service more broadly, from the outset is a critical part of creating a safe space for young people to discuss sensitive issues. Clinicians should maintain a non-judgemental stance and communicate respectfully with young people at all times (Patton et al., 2016) in addition to demonstrating a genuine interest in the young person's perspectives on their current situation and social environment, and identifying and empathising with their main source of distress (Power & McGorry, 1999). Remaining present in the room with a young person, actively listening to them and exploring their motivation for treatment have all been shown to enhance engagement (Jungbluth & Shirk, 2009). Providing practical assistance regarding any immediate needs the young person may have (e.g., letters of support or referrals for housing, financial issues) can also help build rapport and demonstrate a willingness to support the young person's needs, with the aim of enhancing recovery and reducing potential sources of stress and distress (Macneil et al., 2014). It is also good practice to ask a young person about their previous experiences of help-seeking. This can provide key information and allows the clinician to understand and address any particular challenges related to previous experiences. Exploring young people's perceptions of mental illness, previous exposure to individuals with mental illness and any concerns they may have related to the assessment process can also be helpful (Chisholm, Patterson, Greenfield, Turner, & Birchwood, 2016) in addition to conducting the assessment interview outside of the typical clinical setting.

It is important to remember that engagement is an ongoing process and to remain vigilant for potential barriers to engagement and address these when they arise. Rather than making assumptions about why a young person may not be engaging, clinicians may explore barriers to engagement (including their own communication style and systemic factors such as appointment times, fees) and actively attempt to address these.

GOOD PRACTICE IN ASSESSMENT WITH YOUNG PEOPLE

Trauma-informed assessment

All help-seeking young people should be routinely screened for trauma (Bendall et al., 2018). The screening and assessment process should be conducted in a manner that considers the needs of young people who have experienced trauma, ensuring that any distress occurring during disclosure is managed to prevent retraumatisation. Trauma experiences often involve impaired attachment relationships, which can contribute to a lack of trust in health professionals. Establishing a trusting therapeutic relationship is an essential step in helping young people feel comfortable to discuss trauma experiences. Developing this relationship may require multiple sessions.

Establishing a shared understanding of the goal of assessment

It is important to ensure that the clinician and young person have a shared understanding of the purpose of the assessment and its process. Beyond engagement, the goal(s) of assessment will depend on the clinician's role and ongoing involvement in a young person's care. For GPs, the goal may simply be to establish if there is a need for clinical care and/or further specialised assessment. For mental health clinicians, the goal typically involves clarifying the presenting issues, establishing differential diagnoses and working towards collaborative development of a treatment plan. Wherever possible, a psychosocial assessment should be conducted (Parker, Hetrick, & Purcell, 2010). The decision as to whether or not clinical care or further assessment is indicated should be based on the intensity of the young person's distress, the severity of symptoms, the degree of impairment in functioning (including on relationships, health), the effectiveness of the young person's current coping mechanisms, the level of social support available to them, their level of risk and the persistence of distress, risk and impairment (McGorry, 2012).

Use of language

It is best to avoid introducing medicalised or psychiatric language when working with young people, at least initially (Macneil et al., 2014). Using normalising questions and reflecting the young person's own terminology is recommended (e.g., 'stress' rather than 'anxiety', 'not travelling so well' rather than 'being unwell'). It can also be helpful to initially focus on conversation topics that young people may find less challenging (e.g., their interests) (Parker et al., 2010). As discussed later in this section the choice of language is especially relevant to young people from CALD backgrounds or Aboriginal and Torres Strait Islander communities.

Considering a young person's developmental level

A one-size-fits-all approach to assessment is inappropriate in any age group, but particularly so in adolescence (Sauter, Heyne, & Westenberg, 2009) and early adulthood given the amount of developmental variance. A developmentally sensitive assessment can be defined as one which takes into account 'the critical developmental tasks and milestones relevant to a particular adolescent's [or young person's] presenting problems (e.g., pubertal development, cognitive development, the development of behavioural autonomy and social perspective taking during adolescence)' (Holmbeck, Devine, Wasserman, Schellinger, & Tuminello, 2012, p. 430).

There are important reasons to ensure that assessment is conducted in a developmentally sensitive way with young people. Firstly, adolescence and early adulthood represent a critical period in the lifespan when the developmental trajectory can be dramatically altered for better or worse (Patton et al., 2016). Opportunities for early intervention are likely to be missed if developmental factors are not taken into account during the assessment of adolescents (Holmbeck et al., 2012) and young adults. Secondly, age is not a precise indicator of cognitive and neural development (Holmbeck et al., 2012). This means that an assessment needs to be tailored to the young person's emotional, social and cognitive stage of development versus their age or physical development (Sauter et al., 2009). Thirdly, poor alignment between a young person's developmental level and the level at which assessment is 'pitched' is likely to hamper engagement and the establishment of a strong therapeutic alliance (Briere & Lanktree, 2013). For example, while metacognition (i.e., the ability to 'think about thinking') typically develops in early adolescence, many adolescents are still developing metacognitive skills and may struggle to reflect on their thoughts and identify connections between their thoughts, feelings and behaviours (Garber, Frankel, & Herrington, 2016). This may manifest in difficulty responding to open-ended or reflective questions, and providing limited responses to questions (Garber et al., 2016). Similarly, young people who have limited ability to engage in perspective taking would struggle to consider or respond to questions about how their difficulties may be impacting others, while young people who have less developed emotional awareness and literacy skills may struggle to articulate their difficulties, and respond to questions about their emotions (Casey, 1996).

There are several strategies that can be helpful in 'matching' assessment style to a young person's stage of development. First, language should be 'pitched' at the right level and the possible impact of developmental factors should be considered if the young person provides limited responses or seems to be struggling to respond (Sauter et al., 2009). Second, consider whether a young person can use the specific cognitive skill in the specific context that they are being asked of during an assessment (Garber et al., 2016). Some young people may struggle to see things from others' perspective due to their stage of development. Lastly, clinicians should try to clarify and understand the views of young people rather than challenging them (Stallard, 2002a).

Involving family/carers in the assessment process

It is considered best practice to involve young people's family members/carers in the assessment process if possible (Beyondblue, 2011; Orygen, 2016a). The concept of 'family' can be considered broadly to reflect that for many young people, and particularly those from non-Western cultural backgrounds, this extends beyond their immediate biological family (Dudgeon et al., 2014).

While some young people may have poor relationships with their family that may negatively impact on their mental health, for many young people, family members can act as 'scaffolding' or key 'treatment allies' (Masten et al., 2004). When a young person engages with mental health services, they are often in crisis, and experiencing a range of intense emotions (e.g., shame, fear, guilt). Often, family members are similarly concerned about the wellbeing of their young person and are looking for answers about what is going on (both from the young person and professionals) (Oldershaw, Richards, Simic, & Schmidt, 2008). Involving family members in the assessment process can be helpful in providing some containment for the young person and family alike. It also provides a valuable opportunity to seek collateral information about a young person's mental state and functioning, the circumstances surrounding their current episode of mental health difficulties, their family history, and current risk and protective factors (Macneil et al., 2014). Moreover, it provides an opportunity for clinicians to assess how a family is coping and if they may benefit from being offered further support (e.g., engaging with a family peer support worker, referral for individual support) (Crisp, Creek, Fraser, Stavely, & Woodhead, 2014). Parental mental illness is often associated with depression in adolescents and needs to be treated for the adolescent to fully benefit from treatment (NICE, 2005).

Family involvement in a young person's care can range from no involvement, to family members actively participating in assessment and intervention. The degree of involvement should take into account the young person's wishes and circumstances, their age and stage of development (Beyondblue, 2011). Clinicians should talk with a young person early in the engagement process to establish their preferences. Regardless of the young person's preferences, the clinician should always be clear that confidentiality will be breached in the event that it is deemed necessary to fulfil duty of care (Beyondblue, 2011). Clinicians should also be clear with the young person and their family about the young person's ability to consent to treatment independently. This will be influenced by their age (typically ≥14–15 years), cognitive capacity, and local laws and policies. It can be helpful to discuss with a young person the benefits of a family inclusive approach and the potential pitfalls of not including them, as well as addressing any reluctance from the young person (Beyondblue, 2011). Alongside managing the young person's mental health, strong and sustained support should be provided to their family members who nearly always experience distress and need guidance during the management process (Jansen, Gleeson, & Cotton, 2015).

Inclusive practice in assessment

Young Australians are a diverse population that includes a range of minority groups, such as young people from CALD backgrounds, Aboriginal and Torres Strait Islander young people, and young people identifying as sexuality or gender diverse, who often face additional barriers to accessing and engaging with services compared to their peers (Brown, Rice, Rickwood, & Parker, 2016). The reasons for this are that services are often not easily available, are not close enough, and/or they are not culturally sensitive or culturally safe (Brown et al., 2016). This means that services need to actively implement strategies to facilitate engagement (e.g., providing outreach and a culturally sensitive service, increased opening hours); and clinicians need to be sensitive to their experiences. This may include asking young people about previous help-seeking experiences, validating any negative experiences such as discrimination, and ensuring that they feel supported in addressing barriers to care that may arise.

Increased vulnerability to mental health problems among minority groups is related to young people's increased exposure to multiple adversities including discrimination, harassment and trauma. Therefore, it is particularly important to assess exposure to economic and psychosocial adversity among young people from marginalised groups and consider how these factors may be contributing to their presentation. Even if the young person's symptoms meet diagnostic criteria for a mental disorder, it is important to validate that their experiences may be occurring in the context of multiple adversities (Dudgeon et al., 2014).

Culturally and linguistically diverse young people

Clinicians should talk with young people and their families from CALD backgrounds about their understanding of mental health and illness as it may differ significantly from Westernised perceptions. Rather than making assumptions based on a young person's ethnicity or race, it is important to ask the young person and their family about their perspective. Demonstrating a willingness to try to work with them from their perspective can be helpful in facilitating a relationship in which a young person and their family can feel they are trusting someone who understands and respects their perspective (Dudgeon et al., 2014). Instead of introducing a Western language around 'mental illness' or specific disorders, it can be helpful to explore the young person's (and their family's) understanding of their symptoms and use their language. This approach ensures that the care of the young person is tailored to their and their family's values and beliefs, and that treatment goals are shared. These considerations also apply when working with young people who are refugees in addition to understanding the potential added complexities of working with this population (e.g., trauma, violence, loss, forced migration, resettlement stress) (Mental Health in Multicultural Australia, 2014).

Aboriginal and Torres Strait Islander young people

Similarly to when working with CALD populations, perceptions of mental health and illness should be explored with Aboriginal and Torres Strait Islander young people, and the use of Westernised language around 'mental illness' should be avoided. It is generally agreed that traditional concepts of mental health and mental illness are unhelpful and inappropriate with this population. Instead, adoption of the young person's terminology is advocated (e.g., 'feeling not quite right', Dudgeon et al., 2014) as well as the awareness that the concept of 'family' is much broader than within Western cultures. (See Section 1.3.2.)

When assessing Aboriginal and Torres Strait Islander young people, clinicians should follow a less-structured and formal approach as the use of formal assessment protocols and screening tools can damage rapport and engagement, and most have not been validated with this population (Dudgeon et al., 2014). Health is conceptualised holistically by Aboriginal and Torres Strait Islander people, incorporating both the health of an individual and the community. Given this strong connection, engaging with the young person's community and broader family is an important aspect of care. Aboriginal and Torres Strait Islander communities have unique protective factors, including the sense of kinship, connection to land, culture, community and ancestry, and a history of extraordinary resilience (Dudgeon et al., 2014). A strengths-based approach, described below, is advocated.

LGBTIQ young people

All mental health services for young people should be inclusive for those who identify as sexuality or gender diverse. Although a young person's sexual or gender identity may not be related to their reason for seeking support, it is important that clinicians adopt an approach to engagement and assessment that enables all young people to feel safe to discuss sexuality, sex and relationships of all kinds. Such an approach provides a space to affirm the young person's sexual and gender identity and address the unique challenges that LGBTIQ young people are more likely to experience than their heterosexual and cis-gender peers. Distinct barriers to accessing mental health care that LGBTIQ young people may experience include fear of harassment and being misunderstood, heterosexual assumption, lack of accurate information about sexuality diversity, and being outed (Brown et al., 2016). To ensure that services are safe and inclusive for LGBTIQ young people, a number of service- and clinician-level factors can be addressed. These include incorporating inclusive practices into organisational policies and procedures, promoting the service as a safe and supportive environment, engaging with LGBTIQ young people in service planning processes, and using language and terms that are respectful and consistent with the young person's self-understanding (Orygen, 2019).

While we have focused on the three population groups above, inclusive practice should extend to other groups including young people experiencing homelessness, those with comorbid substance use issues, and those in the forensic system or out-of-home care. For the latter, engagement with young people should continue after they leave out-of-home care and during their transition to independence, with a holistic approach to address arising challenges, including housing and employment where indicated (Herrman et al., 2016).

Assessing and monitoring suicidality

Assessing and managing suicidality among young people is a challenging task. Clinicians need to balance the need to assess suicidality and implement safety planning and intervention (as indicated) with the tasks of engagement and maintaining/building rapport. This can be particularly challenging if there is a need to disclose risk to crisis or emergency services and/or caregivers (Rice et al., 2014). Using a structured approach to assessing suicidality may be containing for clinicians' anxieties (Rice et al., 2014). However, while certain structured suicide risk assessment tools were recommended in the past, evidence suggests that they have little clinical utility in predicting risk and they may interfere with therapeutic rapport (Large et al., 2016). Both within Australia and internationally, clinical guidelines related to the management of self-harm (in both young people and adults) clearly state that risk assessment scales, tools and other risk stratification methods should not be used to determine the need for clinical care (Carter et al., 2016) or to predict future risk of self-harm or suicide (NICE, 2011b). Rather, a comprehensive psychosocial assessment of a young person's needs and risks should be undertaken (NICE, 2011b).

Risk assessment should work towards collaboratively identifying with the young person the specific risks of suicidality they face, taking into account their personal circumstance, risk and protective factors, significant relationships that may be protective or represent increased risk (e.g. abusive relationships), their coping methods and both acute and longer-term risks (NICE, 2011b). When working with young people who self-harm, a strong risk factor for suicide, a psychosocial assessment focusing on needs, strengths and personal circumstances should be performed to inform a management plan (NICE, 2011b). This response should be provided with compassion, understanding and positivity (Robinson et al., 2016).

It is important that professionals encountering young people who are experiencing suicidality, or who have a history of doing so, are knowledgeable about suicidality among young people, and are able to respond empathically (Orygen, 2017a). Discussions concerning suicidality should be conducted in a sensitive nature, using normalising questions (e.g., 'when young people are feeling distressed, stuck or not travelling so well, they might hurt themselves intentionally or think about, plan or attempt suicide. Have any of these things been going on for you?'). Outside of the clinical setting, evidence-informed guidelines are available to help young people communicate safely about suicide on social media (Robinson et al., 2018).

Assessing and monitoring other risk factors

It is important to assess risk more broadly, rather than focusing solely on assessing risk of harm to self. Other risk factors to consider include risk of deterioration in the young person's mental health and/or functioning, risk of causing harm to others, and risk of harm from others/exploitation.

Maintaining a strengths-based perspective

It is important to assess a young person's strengths and supports rather than focusing solely on their vulnerabilities and difficulties (Dunne, Bishop, Avery, & Darcy, 2017). Asking a young person about times in their lives when things have been feeling better, their interests, how they cope, and what is currently getting them through can provide helpful information. Instilling a sense of hope in a young person about their prognosis is an integral part of the assessment process (Jansen, Pedersen, Hastrup, Haahr, & Simonsen, 2018).

Youth peer support

Youth peer support, where young people with a lived experience of mental illness assist others in their recovery, is a key component of youth mental health services that is both acceptable to young people and potentially economical (Hamilton et al., 2017a). This approach promotes care that is holistic, strengths-based, patient-centred and recovery oriented. In addition to the patient benefits (e.g., reducing hospital admissions and stigma), peer support is also beneficial to the workers themselves in enhancing their mental health and wellbeing (Health Workforce Australia, 2014). When combined with shared decision making, peer support can assist young people in feeling more involved in the assessment and treatment decisions process (Simmons, Batchelor, Dimopoulos-Bick, & Howe, 2017).

Shared decision making

Shared decision making is a consultation process that enables a clinician and a young person to jointly participate in making a health decision having taken into consideration the options, the benefits and harms of each, and the young person's values, preferences and circumstances (Hoffmann et al., 2014). Shared decision making is considered to be a particularly important process in supporting a person to make decisions about their treatment when the evidence does not clearly support one clear option (Hoffmann et al., 2014). As such, it is ideally positioned for use within youth mental health care. Moreover, it is patient-centred and is likely to appeal to young people as it encourages their active participation in their care, autonomy, and self-efficacy in a supported manner. Implementing shared decision making with young people experiencing mental illness can be complex given that a young person's age and their clinical condition can impact on their capacity to participate in decision making (Simmons, Rice, Hetrick, Bailey, & Parker, 2012). Involvement of another adult during the decision-making process should be considered on an individual basis depending on the young person's presentation, local laws and policy related to consent (Simmons et al., 2012).

Moving from assessment towards treatment planning

Treatment planning should be based on the clinician, the young person, and their family/carers (if involved) having a shared formulation of the young person's presenting issues. The clinician should take care to normalise their distress in the context of stressors, and provide a rationale for further support rather than simply suggesting the young person has 'something wrong with them' or 'needs help' (Macneil et al., 2014, p. 32).

Treatment planning needs to be developmentally appropriate, tailored to the individual's clinical needs, including consideration of their family and social circumstances and their cultural background (NICE, 2005a). If a young person is experiencing significant psychosocial problems, the initial focus should be on establishing how they can be supported to ensure that their basic needs are met (e.g., housing, safety, referral to support agencies). This discussion should always be conducted in a way that is empowering to the young person, using a collaborative approach and acknowledging their preferences about how best to support them. Adolescents often adopt a short-term problem-solving perspective rather than wanting to engage in longer-term work (Stallard, 2002b). Focusing on some short-term goals and trying not to get the young person to commit to too much too soon is likely to be more helpful than longer-term treatment planning.

COMMON ISSUES AND DILEMMAS IN ASSESSMENT

Reluctance to diagnose

Concerns within the medical field about pathologising young people's distress can contribute to a reluctance in health professionals to diagnose mental health problems in young people in addition to concerns that young people will be prescribed medication unnecessarily or 'medicated' (McGorry, 2012). Although premature and excessive prescription of medication can occur, reliance on pharmacological or combined therapies over nonpharmacological interventions to manage young people's mental health in primary care does not seem to be excessive (Hickie et al., 2007). Moreover, as the vast majority of young people with diagnosable mental disorders in Australia still face challenges in access to health care, overdiagnosis and overtreatment are unlikely (McGorry & Goldstone, 2011).

Clinicians may also struggle with diagnosing young people as current diagnostic systems in mental health do not adequately address the complex and fluctuating nature of emerging mental illness (McGorry & Goldstone, 2011). The need for care typically precedes the capacity to apply current major diagnoses from the traditional systems. The latter also fail to adequately acknowledge the role of stressors in contributing to young people's mental health difficulties (Watt, 2017). Using a staging model to conceptualise young people's presentation (as discussed earlier) and adopting a trauma-informed approach to assessment and treatment is recommended.

Identifying when to intervene

Across the lifespan, but particularly among adolescents, it can be difficult to differentiate between transient and normative emotional distress and/or behavioural changes and what may represent early signs or the onset of mental illness (McGorry & Goldstone, 2011). Among young people, emerging mental health problems may reflect an exacerbation, or change in course of childhood-onset mental disorders (e.g., CD, ADHD). More commonly, they reflect the onset of a mental disorder in the absence of any history of childhood mental illness (McGorry, 2012). As described earlier, the emergence of mental illness is usually preceded by a period of nonspecific, but increasingly severe symptoms, such as depression, anxiety, self-harming behaviours, cognitive changes, sleep and appetite disruption, accompanied by increasing distress and disability. Young people, their parents/carers and professionals may ask 'is this 'normal' or something more serious?' (McGorry, 2012). While no one wishes to mislabel normal developmental stress, there can be a real tendency to accept, minimise or dismiss signs of mental distress in young people as 'normal', 'the troubled teens' or simply as reflecting 'the worried well' (McGorry, 2012).

When working with young people, it is good practice to set the 'threshold' for intervention lower rather than higher (Hamilton et al., 2017b). Waiting for a young person to clearly exhibit symptoms of a full-threshold disorder sets the bar inappropriately high and may encourage an over-reliance on 'watchful waiting' approaches which can cost lives (Hamilton et al., 2017b). While subthreshold mental health symptoms may indeed resolve, this does not mean that they do not warrant intervention given that they are often associated with significant distress, functional impairment, risk of self-harm, suicidal thoughts and behaviours, and substance abuse (Rickwood, Telford, Parker, Tanti, & McGorry, 2014). Such thresholds are simply not applied in physical health, where the consumer voice is better respected in defining need for care.

HELPFUL ASSESSMENT INSTRUMENTS AND GUIDES

A range of evidence-based resources are available to assist in the engagement and assessment of young people, as summarised in Table 3.5. These cover diverse populations, including young people from CALD backgrounds and young people presenting with early psychosis, challenging behaviours, self-harm or suicidal ideation.

Table 3.5 Engagement and assessment resources

Author	Population	Topic	Resource type
Engagement			
Orygen (2017b)	Young people (12–25 years) with challenging behaviour (e.g., resistance, self-harm, aggression, disorganised, intoxication)	Responding to challenging behaviours and engagement considerations	Clinical practice point
Orygen (2016b)	Young people with early psychosis	Factors influencing engagement How to promote engagement What to do when young people do not engage	Clinical practice point
Assessment			
headspace (2013)	Young help-seeking people (12–25 years)	headspace Psychosocial Assessment that assists with engaging and building rapport while assessing a range of mental health disorders	Assessment tool
Orygen (2016a)	Young people with early psychosis	Access to care, assessment and treatment	Clinical practice guideline

Orygen (2015a)	Young people with early psychosis	Assessment, management and service models for risk of violence	Clinical practice point
Orygen (2016c)	Young people with early psychosis from CALD communities	Importance of working with CALD young people and their families Management strategies Cultural explanatory models of illness Working with interpreters	Clinical practice point
Simmons et al. (2012)	Young people accessing mental health care	Shared decision making and its components	Evidence summary
Dudgeon et al. (2014)	Children and young people	Identification of emotional problems Culturally appropriate assessment measures	Book (particularly chapter 22)
Assessing and managing suicidality			
Carter et al. (2016)	Management of deliberate self-harm (hospital and community-based)	Epidemiology Organisation of services Assessment and intervention Working with special populations (e.g., children and adolescents)	Clinical practice guideline
NICE (2011b)	Individuals aged 8+ years who self-harm	General principles of care Primary care Psychosocial assessment in community mental health and other specialist settings Longer-term treatment and management Treating comorbid conditions	Clinical practice guideline
Rice et al. (2014)	Young people (15–25 years) experiencing ongoing suicidal ideation	Engagement and consistency of care Risk assessment Crisis planning Engaging systems of support Engendering hopefulness Development of adaptive coping Management of acute risk Consultation and supervision	Practice principles

3.2.6 EVIDENCE-BASED AND OTHER TREATMENTS (BIO/PSYCHO/SOCIAL) AND SERVICES

KEY PRINCIPLES OF CARE ACROSS ALL DISORDERS IN YOUNG PEOPLE

A staged care approach

A staged rather than stepped care approach is recommended when working with young people experiencing mental health difficulties. Generally, initial intervention focuses on monitoring, psychoeducation, support and low-intensity psychological interventions, with more intensive psychological interventions being offered to young people with moderate to severe symptoms. Although the stage at which medication should be considered differs across disorders, it is not routinely offered as an initial intervention for earlier stages. 'Staged care' is conceptually distinct from the more common term 'stepped care' in that it aims to be proactive rather than reactive. Staged care does not wait for treatment to fail before intensifying the effort. The health system generally needs to adopt this approach for all potentially persistent and recurring illness.

A focus on functional recovery

When working with young people, equal emphasis should be given to functional and symptomatic recovery (Orygen, 2016a). Getting a young person engaged in age-appropriate activities (e.g. education, work) is a key component of their recovery process (Killackey et al., 2019).

Family/carer involvement in treatment

It is considered best practice to involve the family/carers of young people in the treatment process when possible. It is also important to consider and respond to the needs of family/carers across a young person's episode of care. The extent in which family/carers are involved during treatment may vary from case to case, ranging from no involvement to active participation. Family/carer interventions aim to educate families, provide support, and develop problem-solving skills and coping strategies. (See Chapter 2.7.)

Below, guideline recommendations and research findings that are considered current best practice are drawn upon to summarise treatment considerations for anxiety, depression and psychosis during adolescence and young adulthood.

ANXIETY

In the absence of recent Australian guidelines on the treatment of anxiety disorders in young people, clinicians can refer to the NICE guidelines for international best practice. The NICE guidelines on social phobia provide specific recommendations for adolescents and adults (NICE, 2013). In contrast, those on generalised anxiety disorder (GAD) and panic disorder solely cover treatment for adults aged 18 years and over (NICE, 2011a). As no adolescent specific guidelines for GAD or panic disorder are available, clinicians can refer to the adult guidelines. However, special considerations should be applied when adapting adult guidelines for use with young adults, including considering the impact of systemic factors (e.g., school, peers, family) when planning treatment; involving family/carers treatment where appropriate, and having a lower threshold for onward referral. Specifically, when engaging in treatment planning with adolescents presenting with anxiety disorders, it is important to consider the possible impact of parenting behaviours in maintaining symptoms and to consider whether peer victimisation, or victimisation of the adolescent in any other setting is contributing to their presentation (NICE, 2013). Furthermore, regardless of which anxiety disorder(s) a young person may be presenting with, a young person's age should be taken into account when considering prescribing medication. Prior to prescribing selective serotonin reuptake inhibitors (SSRIs) to a young person, clinicians should always explain their potential risks, including an increased risk of suicidal thinking and self-harm in a minority of people under 30. They should also consult best practice guidelines for further recommendations on considerations in prescribing, monitoring and ceasing medication with young people. Prompt follow up should occur if SSRIs are prescribed with regular monitoring.

Current therapies for anxiety are limited, with relapse occurring in 52% of young people (Ginsburg et al., 2014), necessitating the need for new evidence-based treatments. Virtual reality has emerged as a treatment method that can potentially exceed the benefits of standard treatments although further research is required (Freeman et al., 2017). Potentially safer and more efficacious pharmaceutical treatments for anxiety, such as cannabidiol, are currently being trialled (Amminger, 2017).

Staged care for anxiety disorders in young people

A staged care approach is recommended for the treatment of all anxiety disorders in young people with care proceeding from lower to higher intensity interventions depending on the severity of a young person's symptoms, associated risks, degree of impairment in functioning and responsiveness to treatment (NICE, 2011a, 2013). Psychoeducation about anxiety disorders and treatment options should be offered to all young people presenting with suspected anxiety disorders alongside psychoeducation about the benefits of exercise, a healthy diet and sleep routine in managing anxiety disorders (NICE, 2011a, 2013). Individual cognitive behavioural therapy (CBT) is often the recommended treatment of choice although this may depend on the young person's clinical symptoms and stage of illness (NICE, 2011a, 2013). SSRIs may be offered where a young person declines CBT or as a combined treatment (alongside CBT) or if a young person's symptoms only partially respond to treatment (NICE, 2011a, 2013). For anxiety co-occurring with moderate to severe depression in young people (15–25 years), evidence suggests that CBT combined with fluoxetine is significantly more effective in reducing anxiety symptoms than CBT alone (Davey et al., submitted).

DEPRESSION

As there are no current, youth-specific Australian guidelines for treating depressive disorders, this section considers treatment for depressive disorders based on current best evidence. As noted in the Beyondblue clinical practice guidelines (now rescinded), 'health professionals, young people and parents/carers must be aware of the dangers of not treating episodes of moderate to severe depression. Depression is the major risk factor for suicide' (Beyondblue, 2011, p. 28).

Staged care for depressive disorders in young people

Although a number of approaches may be effective for adolescents presenting with mild depression (in the absence of significant signs of comorbidity or suicidal ideation), behavioural therapies, including CBT, show the most robust evidence for effectiveness. Antidepressants should not be prescribed for adolescents with mild depression although they may be considered in those who are unresponsive to psychotherapy and whose condition persists or worsens. Medication should also be considered (in combination with psychotherapy and healthy lifestyle strategies) in young people with moderate to severe depression and when psychotherapy is refused (Davey & Chanen, 2016). If no improvement is observed, an increased dose should be considered (after 4–6 weeks) and an alternative medication may be prescribed (after a further 6 weeks) (Davey & Chanen, 2016). Given that treatment-resistant depression is prevalent, further approaches may be considered where clinically indicated, including intensive psychosocial interventions, augmented pharmacotherapy, and neurostimulation (Davey & Chanen, 2016). For young people experiencing depression with psychotic features, augmenting treatment with the addition of an atypical antipsychotic may be considered.

Some young people may present with complex and severe depression including risk to life and severe self-neglect. Complex depression includes 'depression that shows an inadequate response to multiple treatments, is complicated by psychotic symptoms, and/or is associated with significant psychiatric comorbidity or psychosocial factors' (NICE, 2009a, p. 17). In these instances, a specialist mental health assessment should always be conducted and medications managed under supervision of a consultant psychiatrist. If the young person is at significant risk of suicide, self-harm or self-neglect, inpatient care including developing a multidisciplinary care plan is indicated.

Clinical considerations in using antidepressant medications with adolescents

Although fluoxetine is the recommended first-line antidepressant for adolescents, it is not an effective treatment for all cases, particularly those aged <18 years (Davey et al., 2019), and other antidepressants must often be considered. However, fluoxetine can offer benefits to those with moderate to severe depression who are >18 years of age (Davey et al., 2019). All adolescents prescribed antidepressant medications must be closely monitored for adverse reactions, general progress and review of mental state. All professionals and others involved in care should monitor for the appearance of suicidal behaviour, self-harm and hostility. This is particularly important within the first four weeks of the adolescent commencing an antidepressant treatment but also with continuing vigilance and monitoring throughout the episode of care. The frequency of monitoring should be determined on a case-by-case basis (e.g., weekly contact for the first four weeks and fortnightly thereafter).

Clinical considerations in prescribing medications to young adults (aged 18–25 years)

The choice of antidepressant should be discussed with the young adult adults (aged 18–25 years) and their parents/carers as appropriate. An SSRI is usually the first choice of antidepressant type. Both the young adult and their family/carers should be advised of an increased risk of developing suicidal behaviour because of the potential increased prevalence of suicidal thoughts in the early stages of antidepressant treatment for this group. Similar to adolescents, any young adult commenced on antidepressants should receive close monitoring of their mental state, progress, and adverse side effects.

PSYCHOSIS

Clinicians should follow the most current version of the Australian Clinical Guidelines for Early Psychosis when working with young people in the ultra-high risk phase (indicated by subthreshold psychotic symptoms accompanied by functional decline), or in the acute or recovery phases of first episode psychosis (FEP) (Orygen, 2016a). A staged approach is recommended, with the intensity of care matched to stage of illness. At any phase of illness, a thorough assessment of mental state, risks and functioning is an ongoing process throughout the intervention. If a young person presents with unexplained functional decline, the possibility of psychotic disorder should be considered. As a first step in the assessment and intervention process, developmentally and culturally appropriate psychoeducation about the ultra-high risk mental state or FEP (as appropriate) should be offered to all young people and their families including information about treatment options. The following Practice illustration provides an example of the management and outcomes (from engagement to treatment) of a young person with psychosis.

PRACTICE ILLUSTRATION: ENGAGEMENT AND ASSESSMENT

Jake presented as a young man who experienced an involuntary inpatient admission due to hallucinations and persecutory delusions. A conversation about Jake's diagnosis of psychosis was had between him and his treating clinician. Jake mentioned that he felt psychosis referred to 'when you think things are not real and stuff... and when you see stuff.' Jake was asked if he thought this reflected what was happening to him. This ensured a shared understanding of Jake's experience.

Jake agreed that he was experiencing these symptoms. The clinician explained what psychosis meant, ensuring that Jake understood the explanation and that any misconceptions were clarified (e.g., permanence of symptoms). It was stressed that the label of psychosis was not important and that recovery was more crucial. Jake's strengths were highlighted, which included his determination and signs of recovery. To validate Jake's experiences, the clinician acknowledged the fears previously expressed by Jake (e.g., not knowing who to trust, feeling scared) and how he was able to talk about his experiences despite these fears.

Initially, Jake's family worried about what people would think if they knew of his diagnosis and had reservations about treatment. They benefited from the support of a family peer worker and being involved in Jake's care.

Following this diagnosis, a shared decision-making approach to treatment was utilised. This included asking Jake about his treatment goals (see section 3.2.5 discussing the various treatment options, and providing Jake with the opportunity to voice his values and preferences.

Jake mentioned that he was reluctant to commence antipsychotics as he didn't want to turn into 'a zombie'. After discussing why Jake felt like this and what information he knew about antipsychotics, the clinician described their potential benefits and side effects, and compared them against other treatment options. This discussion took into consideration how the different options and their side effects may specifically impact Jake.

Jake decided to commence an antipsychotic and was discharged to outpatient care in the early intervention service.

Source: Adapted from EPPIC National Support Program Writing Group, 2014; Macneil et al., 2014

The ultra-high risk phase

Intervention in young people at ultra-high risk for psychosis has the potential to delay or even prevent a first episode (van der Gaag et al., 2013). The treatment of choice for young people in the ultra-high risk phase is frequent assessment of the young person and their families (every 2-4 weeks) in addition to ongoing psychosocial support (preferably including CBT). Assessment should focus on monitoring the young person's mental state and safety. Antipsychotic treatments should not typically be prescribed for young people in the ultra-high risk phase, however they may be considered in certain circumstances following multidisciplinary assessment. The largest study to date examining the efficacy of omega-3 fatty acids in preventing transition to psychosis failed to replicate earlier findings, with further research needed to delineate its role in reduction of psychosis risk (McGorry et al., 2017).

Acute phase of FEP

The interventions of choice in the acute phase of FEP are frequent assessment and monitoring combined with antipsychotic medication and psychological therapy. Intensive assessment and intervention is recommended for all young people at this phase.

Antipsychotic medication should not normally be used during the first 24–48 hours of treatment in order to facilitate assessment. Benzodiazepines, even in high dose, are a practical alternative in most cases. Second generation antipsychotics (SGAs) are the antipsychotic of choice, with the side effect profile guiding the choice of which SGA to prescribe. A shared decision-making approach should be implemented when discussing treatment choices, including discussion of potential side effects (including metabolic, weight gain, extrapyramidal motor symptoms, and sexual side effects). Ongoing monitoring for, and early intervention in the case of, adverse side effects should then be implemented with a preventive focus if possible (e.g., weight management strategies implemented prior to treatment initiation). It is important to distinguish affective and non-affective psychosis to enable appropriate treatment (i.e., mood stabiliser). Polypharmacy should generally be avoided (except if indicated by specific situations (Orygen, 2016a), particularly the prescription of multiple antipsychotics. Conversely, if manic features are prominent, it is crucial that lithium is utilised promptly. Adherence should be monitored and explicitly addressed where necessary. When comorbidity is present, treatment of the primary psychotic disorder should be prioritised unless comorbidity leads to high levels of risk to self or others, or clinical judgement indicates that the comorbidity has a major impact on the primary psychotic disorder (e.g., cannabis dependence).

CBT is the psychological therapy of choice in FEP, demonstrating the most immediate benefit. Supportive therapy and befriending may also be considered.

PRACTICE ILLUSTRATION: TREATMENT

The following dialogue demonstrates how Jake and his case manager (CM) went on to develop some shared treatment goals around his experience of psychosis.

CM: Jake, now that we have spent some time understanding some of what has been happening for you, I was wondering what you think would be helpful for us to work on together?

Jake: I just want to be able to see my friends and go to work and be normal. Just to be able to leave the house and see people without getting into fights all the time.

CM: It's been really challenging for you to continue with work and seeing friends recently. What do you think would need to change for you to reach that goal?

Jake: To be able to get out of the house I would need to be less worried about the cops. That they are setting me up.

CM: Sure, you've said that you spend a lot of time thinking about that at the moment. What else would look different?

Jake: I overreact pretty quickly, especially when I hear the voices. To be a bit calmer and not get so angry or scared would help.

CM: Fantastic. We can definitely work on those things. It sounds like there are a number of smaller steps there. Let's write them down:

- To be less preoccupied with my worry that the cops are trying to set me up.
- To be able to calm myself down and relax when I hear voices.

There are a number of indicated cognitive behavioural strategies to support Jake to meet his goals. These include developing a shared formulation, identifying 'thinking errors', gathering evidence for beliefs, coping strategies and behavioural strategies for responding to feelings of fear or anger.

Source: Adapted from Orygen, 2015b

Early recovery phase FEP

Young people should be closely monitored in the early recovery phase to assess treatment response and adherence. This should include: seeing a case manager (CM) weekly, a doctor at least fortnightly, and seeing or contacting families at least fortnightly. A young person's early response to antipsychotic medication should be considered as an indication of prognosis. CBT interventions may be indicated to enhance recovery and outcomes (Orygen, 2016a). As relapse is common, this should be discussed with family and carers in the context of developing a 'relapse action plan.' Addressing vocational recovery is a key component of the recovery stage. This can be achieved through an individual placement and support (IPS) model, which aims to assist individuals as they enter employment. This model has shown promising results, with high employment rates of young people with FEP (Killackey et al., 2019).

Relapse of FEP

Relapse of FEP should be treated promptly. Psychosocial factors and illicit drug use must be assessed as likely contributors alongside adherence issues. Medication should be recommenced or increased at early signs of relapse. When considering whether to maintain antipsychotic therapy in relapse prevention, the potential benefits need to be weighed against potential risks, including the impact of side effects on functioning. It is particularly important to implement relapse prevention strategies (including more regular review and provision of information about rapid access to care) if the dosage of medication is decreased or medication is ceased. All young people experiencing relapse of FEP should be offered specialised FEP interventions alongside combined family and individual CBT specifically focusing on preventing relapse.

FEP incomplete recovery, medication discontinuation and discharge

Regular contact with the treating team is key for all young people in the late recovery phase. It is important to try to identify young people experiencing persisting positive or negative symptoms early. Clozapine should be considered for young people who have not responded to adequate trials of two antipsychotic medications (including one SGA). Antipsychotic medication may be continued for 12 months or more beyond resolution of positive psychotic symptoms. A shared decision-making approach based on a comprehensive evaluation of the risks and benefits of ongoing medication should inform treatment decisions.

CBT should be considered as an adjunctive therapy during late/problematic recovery. More intensive and structured interventions should also be considered for families, emphasising problem solving and communication skills.

Ongoing regular monitoring of risk is particularly important for young people during transitions from acute care and at discharge from the service.

Planning for discharge should be done in a timely and comprehensive manner with clinicians clearly communicating and documenting a discharge plan at least three months prior to discharge. This plan should be shared with the young person, their family, their GP and the new service provider at this early stage. Wherever possible, clinicians should assist young people in their care with the transition process by providing orientation and engagement with future treatment providers (e.g., a joint visit and clinical handover to the designated clinician).

PRACTICE ILLUSTRATION: OUTCOMES

Jake engaged well in psychological treatment and mostly adhered to taking his medication. He recovered from his initial episode of psychosis while living with his family. Once his symptoms stabilised, Jake's goals changed, with the main one being to recover his independence. Jake engaged with a vocational recovery program at the early intervention service. He reengaged with university on a part-time basis and moved into share accommodation. This initially worked well. However, as Jake was socialising more, partying and using alcohol and other drugs, he became increasingly erratic in his adherence to his oral medication. He often missed doses and forgot to collect his scripts.

As a result of this period of non-adherence and other contributing factors (including drug use, sleep interference), Jake began to experience a return of psychotic symptoms of disorganised thinking and hallucinations. Using a shared decision-making model, further treatment options were discussed and compared with Jake, including a long-acting injectable and resuming oral medication combined with psychoeducation and support strategies. After considering the positive and negative aspects of each option, Jake decided to continue with the oral medication. Jake's CM worked through additional psychoeducation with him, as well as trying to implement prompts to remind Jake to take his medication (e.g., linking it with a daily activity). The CM also worked with Jake's family to ensure he had a strong support network and positive relationships. These strategies were successful with only occasional relapses. After several months, Jake noticed a significant reduction in his symptoms and an overall improvement in his thinking, motivation, social interactions and sleep. In combination with psychosocial strategies, Jake's misuse of substances was also managed.

Source: Adapted from EPPIC National Support Program Writing Group, 2014

TREATMENT CHALLENGES FOR MENTAL HEALTH CLINICIANS

Youth engagement

Young people experiencing mental health difficulties are at high risk of dropping out of treatment prematurely. The risk of non-adherence to treatment and disengagement from services is substantially higher among individuals with FEP than those with more chronic illness (Robinson et al., 2002). Particular risk factors for non-adherence and treatment disengagement among young people with FEP include a previous forensic history, less severe illness at baseline, living without family at discharge, and persistence of substance use throughout treatment (Conus et al., 2010; Schimmelmann, Conus, Schacht, McGorry, & Lambert, 2006).

Treatment engagement can also be challenging when working with young people with depression (Goodyer et al., 2017). Given this, there is an increasing interest in evaluating the effectiveness of brief interventions, with promising evidence emerging for anxiety and/or depressive symptoms (Parker et al., 2016; Weersing, Gonzalez, Campo, & Lucas, 2008). In Australia, this approach is also being reflected in youth mental health care settings, with some headspace centres offering 'brief intervention clinics' to those with mild to moderate symptoms in the absence of clinical complexity or safety concerns (Schley et al., 2019).

When using modular treatment approaches, clinicians should carefully consider which treatment components should be prioritised earlier in the course of treatment, as these may be the only ones that get delivered. It is also important for clinicians to regularly check in with young people and their families/carers to obtain their feedback (positive and negative) on the sessions. Finally, clinicians should revisit treatment goals intermittently to ensure they are working towards the young person's goals as they currently see them.

Adherence to medication

Young people may also struggle to adhere to medication as prescribed. Young people may discontinue their medication completely even in the absence of any medical supervision. This can be dangerous in the short-term and is associated with an increased risk of relapse and suicidality (Orygen, 2016a).

When working with young people prescribed psychiatric medications, clinicians should monitor and affectively address adherence issues. A shared decision-making approach should be used when discussing options for recommencing/switching or ceasing medication taking into account the potential risks and benefits of each option (Orygen, 2016a). For young people with FEP, long-acting injectable (depot) medications may be considered to address known or suspected adherence issues (Orygen, 2016a).

Recovery and relapse

In addition to causing marked human suffering, mental illnesses that tend to emerge early in life, and are often recurrent, place a particularly large burden on the community (Gore et al., 2011), partly due to reduced economic and social participation. Young people with mental disorders often have difficulty completing education, gaining employment and securing housing. As mental health services for young people are often not fully integrated with other service systems (e.g. employment, housing), young people can experience difficulties in accessing these services to aid their recovery.

It is important to be vigilant for symptoms of relapse in young people and to refer promptly for further assessment and intervention as indicated (NICE, 2005). Clinicians should talk to young people and their families/carers about the risk of relapse during their treatment and collaboratively develop 'relapse action' or 'wellness plans', including noting any previously successful strategies, early warning signs of relapse, potential triggers, and where to seek further support if needed (Orygen, 2016a).

Complex presentations

Young people often present with complex presentations. In fact, working with severe and complex presentations has been identified as the biggest challenges facing clinicians working with depressed adolescents (Hetrick, Simmons, Thompson, & Parker, 2011). Depression with onset prior to 18 years of age is more severe and complex (poorer functioning, increased comorbidity, and increased suicidality) than late-onset depression (Zisook et al., 2007). The complexity and severity of adolescent depression may detract from engagement and treatment outcomes (Hetrick et al., 2015). It may also make treatment planning more challenging, particularly if treatment is restricted to a certain number of sessions. When deciding which symptoms to prioritise targeting, clinicians should take into account symptom severity, risk issues, the extent to which each symptom is developmentally atypical, and its impact on functioning (Holmbeck et al., 2012; NICE, 2005).

TREATMENT CHALLENGES FOR YOUNG PEOPLE

Access to care

In Australia, prior to the establishment of headspace, it was estimated that only 13% and 31% of young men and women, respectively, seek professional support for mental health problems (Slade et al., 2009). Factors that contribute to young people's reluctance to seek help include: poor mental health literacy, lack of awareness of how to access mental health support, confidentiality concerns, a preference for solving problems independently, stigma, and previous negative experiences (Dunne et al., 2017). Young people living in rural and remote areas are particularly disadvantaged when trying to access mental health care (Brown et al., 2016). Lack of knowledge among parents and young people alike about where and how to get support for mental health problems can be a significant barrier to accessing mental health services (Brown et al., 2016). Unfortunately, even when young people do seek professional support for mental health problems, accurate detection and evidence-based or minimally adequate treatment remains the exception rather than the norm (Sawyer et al., 2019). It has been argued, that within primary care, this reflects 'a lack of a systemic approach to identifying and providing appropriate and evidence-based interventions rather than any individual doctor-based failure' (Burns & Birrell, 2014). Other challenges faced by young people include the limit of therapy sessions under the Medicare Benefits Schedule, as reflected in Roxxanne's experience (see Box 3.1). It is essential to address these systemic problems to improve outcomes for young Australians experiencing mental illness.

Several initiatives have been launched in Australia to increase young people's access to mental health care. These include headspace (targeting young people experiencing high prevalence disorders) (McGorry et al., 2014), a series of Early Psychosis Prevention and Intervention Centres for young people experiencing psychotic disorders (McGorry, 2015), and more recently the GPs in schools program in Victoria (Department of Education and Training, 2018). The Royal Australian College of General Practitioners offers specialised training for GPs on youth mental health. A series of online services are also available for young people nationwide, including ReachOut.com by Inspire Foundation, eheadspace, lifeline, and evidence-based online intervention such as Mood Gym (Burns & Birrell, 2014).

Over the last five years, increasing numbers of young people have accessed headspace services. While it is a positive outcome that young people are seeking help, responding effectively to this demand has been challenging. The 2018 national survey of headspace centres revealed that resource constraints due to underlying systemic issues have negatively impacted the wait times for young people (headspace, 2019). Key factors limiting the ability of headspace centres to meet service demands include workforce availability, difficulty recruiting and retaining staff, and the physical constraints of centres (e.g., number of consultation rooms). The majority of headspace services are bulk billed, making them easily accessible and more likely to attract young people, leading to increased wait times.

In 2018, a number of state and federal announcements were made to strengthen mental health services. The Federal Government pledged an additional $51.8 million in funding to strengthen existing headspace services and improve access to care. The 2019 Federal Budget included $461 million for youth mental health services and suicide prevention. In response to a dedicated advocacy campaign and increasing recognition of the need for transformational change, a Victorian Royal Commission into mental health care was announced as well as a Federal Productivity Commission inquiry into mental health care across Australia. Outcomes of these processes have the potential to bring major reform and much needed investment in mental care to strengthen the health system and provide better access to and quality of care for people with mental illness.

'Missing middle'

Despite the above progress, there still remains a gap in the system between primary care initiatives such as headspace and specialist mental health services. Due to the pressure on the specialist system, many young people experiencing mental health problems are unable to access services within this system. They may, however, present with needs that are too complex or symptoms that are too severe to be managed within primary care. As a result, many young people 'fall through the gaps'. This can potentially contribute to a range of detrimental outcomes including housing insecurity, criminality, increased reliance on welfare, and premature death. Alarmingly, nearly three-quarters of young people who do not qualify for community-based mental health services (despite significant morbidity and functional impairment) have attempted suicide in the last 12 months (Orygen, unpublished data). The absence of appropriate services for this group can result in young people and their families seeking assistance via hospital emergency departments during times of crisis. However, when care is provided in these settings, it can be traumatic or harmful (e.g., restraint, sedation). Enhancing service provision for this group of young people should be prioritised in service planning and policy development. This requires increased investment for, and strengthening and integration of youth mental health systems to adequately treat the full spectrum of presentations. A focus would be ensuring seamless transitions from primary to tertiary care and coordination with social systems through a vertically integrated system with state and federal funding streams.

Treatment delays

Despite the fact that mental disorders are highly prevalent among young people, delays in accessing treatment can span 15 years (Burns & Birrell, 2014). This poses a major threat to their prognosis, with a longer duration of untreated illness associated with poorer treatment outcomes (de Diego-Adeliño et al., 2010). The peak onset of mental disorders during adolescence and early adulthood coincides with a developmental period where an individual's knowledge and experience of mental health disorders may be underdeveloped, which may contribute to delayed access to treatments (Jorm, 2012). GPs may in turn be less likely to detect mental health problems when a young person does not conceptualise them as such (Jorm, 2012). However, in Australia, research suggests that even when young people have a reasonable knowledge of high prevalence mental disorders, and are able to identify symptoms, this does not transfer to a willingness to engage with professional services (Burns & Birrell, 2014). Some of this hesitance likely reflects a broader lack of confidence across the community about the potential benefits of seeking professional mental health support, however, compared to other age groups, young people are particularly disconnected from medical professionals which exacerbates this problem. While ongoing efforts are needed to address systemic barriers to young people accessing mental health care (Brown et al., 2016), evidence-based strategies, such as intensive community education and mobile detection teams, can reduce treatment delays even for more serious illnesses such as psychosis to a median of only 5 weeks (Melle et al., 2004).

KEY RISKS OF HARM IN TREATMENT ATTEMPTS

Side effects of medication

Medication should always be used cautiously with young people experiencing mental health problems and only be offered in the context of a thorough assessment, ongoing monitoring and shared decision making. Careful consideration must be given to the relative benefits and risks, including the risks associated with not using medication if it is clinically indicated. Generally, a 'start low and go slow' approach is recommended when considering commencing medication and dosage (Orygen, 2016a). The risk of toxicity should always be considered prior to prescribing any medication to young people who are assessed to be at risk of suicide (NICE, 2005, 2009a). Whenever antipsychotic medication is prescribed, frequent monitoring of adherence and adverse side effects is critical (including metabolic monitoring) (Orygen, 2016a).

Adverse effects of seclusion and restraint

Seclusion and restraint are traumatising practices currently used in emergency or inpatient settings to manage patient behaviour. This may involve seclusion, bodily restraint or mechanical restraint, and forced sedation. From a trauma-informed care framework, seclusion and restraint should be avoided and phased out of frontline care due to their harmful effects including injury, retraumatisation and, in extreme cases, death (Bryson et al., 2017). Staff safety is also a priority and the management of violent and aggressive patients is a real challenge with which an

BOX 3.1: ROXXANNE'S EXPERIENCE

It wasn't until I made strides in treatment for my anxiety with a psychologist at headspace that my depression became noticeable to me. It worsened after moving out of home. I was working full-time, studying full-time, and caring for my sister who was in Year 12. For me, it felt like I couldn't tell what was true and what was my depression clouding how I saw reality.

I continued to see a psychologist and called any helpline that would talk to me in between. My appointments were just enough to keep me afloat. Even though I was experiencing suicidal thoughts and profound emotional pain, it seemed like the professionals I saw didn't think it was that bad because I looked so high functioning. I felt like no one would take me seriously unless they could see something physical. Eventually I began medication, and that was the first thing that actually improved my health.

I still take medication and have depression. Recently my new psychologist told me that maybe when I was earning enough, I could afford the care that I need, that is, care not bound by the 10 session maximum of a Mental Health Treatment Plan. I left headspace after that and found a state-funded counselling service that is not capped at 10 sessions. Unfortunately the service is in such high demand that the difficulty is in actually getting an appointment.

I understand myself and the health system better now, and I've learned how to advocate for myself. But I learned through bad experiences, and I'm not okay with that. At the moment I'm working with a number of youth mental health organisations to advocate for a better mental health system, and am working towards a career in health.

underfunded and demoralised mental health system is struggling to cope. However, the situation can be hugely enhanced with reform and investment plus new skills and approaches.

GOOD PRACTICE EXAMPLES

Best practice management, as described above, should be delivered within models of care that are developmentally and culturally appropriate for young people. The headspace model is a key example of best practice in youth mental health within Australia that has guided youth mental health reform worldwide. This was created following the success of specialised early intervention services for psychotic disorders, which is regarded as the gold standard model of care compared to treatment as usual (Correll et al., 2018). A key principle of the headspace model is providing early intervention within an integrated and preventive framework that offers evidence-informed stepped care guided by risk-benefit considerations and shared decision making, with social and vocational outcomes as the key targets (McGorry et al., 2014). These services are guided by the principles of integrated care, whereby clinical and non-clinical multidisciplinary care is provided within one location and is tailored to the needs of young people and their families (Porter & Lee, 2013). This allows primary mental health care to be delivered within the context of physical health care, substance abuse management, educational and vocational support, and social care. This service approach has been shown to improve access to care and yield favourable recovery outcomes (Hetrick et al., 2017).

The headspace model is comprised of 16 core components that currently represent best practice to deliver and reform youth mental health care (Rickwood et al., 2019). These core elements consist of 10 service components (youth participation, family and friends participation, community awareness, enhanced access, early intervention, appropriate care, evidence-informed practice, four core streams, service integration, supported transitions), and six enabling components (national network, Lead Agency governance, Consortia, multidisciplinary workforce, blended funding, monitoring and evaluation).

The organisation headspace, including its online service (eheadspace), addresses early intervention, particularly for the high prevalence mental health problems, but a back-up system is necessary for young people with complex presentations or more severe conditions, who typically require intensive, specialised treatment and a longer tenure of care. Orygen Youth Health (OYH), established in 2002, is Australia's largest youth-specific mental health organisation, and comprises an integrated research and clinical program. OYH provides a range of community-based clinical services for young people aged 15–25 years living within a catchment area of approximately one million people in north-western metropolitan Melbourne, including:

- triage and assessment services
- extended-hours mobile multidisciplinary teams providing intensive community-based crisis response and home treatment
- mobile youth-intensive case management services for young people with complex needs who are difficult to engage in office-based care
- psychosocial case management and therapeutic individual and family services
- specialist services for young people with severe personality disorders (Helping Young People Early, HYPE), mood disorders (Youth Mood Clinic), psychosis (Early Psychosis Prevention and Intervention Centre, EPPIC), and those at ultra-high risk of developing a psychotic disorder (Personal Assessment and Crisis Evaluation clinic, PACE)
- consumer and carer peer support programs
- comprehensive group-based personal, social and vocational recovery programs
- a specialist youth inpatient unit.

The primary goal of OYH is to focus on the onset phase and early course of these potentially serious mental disorders. The model acknowledges the complexities of service provision in an age group where comorbidity is the norm, and therefore linkages with other mental health and general support agencies are essential in ensuring quality service provision (McGorry, Edwards, Mihalopoulos, Harrigan, & Jackson, 1996). Given the complex and multifaceted needs of young people experiencing mental illness, and their families, client services at OYH have been designed to be comprehensive, flexible and responsive to the phase and severity of illness. Orygen now needs to extend to cover the full age range and later stages of illness and to vertically integrate with local headspace centres also operated by Orygen. This is a current project which requires major investment and restructuring.

Similar approaches to headspace that operate within an integrated model have appeared worldwide (Hetrick et al., 2017). Across New Zealand, Youth One Stop Shops provide a range of holistic and accessible youth-friendly health, social and employment services to young people aged 10–25 years, which have delivered positive outcomes (Bailey, Torrie, & Osborne, 2013). Other services across the globe include Jigsaw in Ireland, which is an accessible and effective community-based mental health service for young people aged 12–25 years (O'Keeffe, O'Reilly, O'Brien, Buckley, & Illback, 2015). Further international youth mental health services include: Youthspace in Birmingham, headspace in Demark, the Netherlands, and Israel, and soon California, Access Canada and the Foundry in British Columbia, and @ease in the Netherlands.

3.2.7 WHERE AND HOW DO YOUNG PEOPLE GET HELP?

Despite increased provision of youth-specific models of care, seeking help for a mental disorder can be a challenging and complex process for young people that is influenced by multiple factors (Rickwood et al., 2007). Initially, young people are likely to seek informal help through family or friends. How young people seek formal professional care can vary depending on their developmental phase. During adolescence, family are the key influence to seeking face-to-face services, whereas from late adolescence, this influence reduces. In contrast, accessing online services is more likely to be self-initiated by both adolescents and young adults (Rickwood, Mazzer, & Telford, 2015).

Based on the most recent Young Minds Matter survey (2013-14), the most common health service providers for emotional or behavioural problems between 12-17 years of age were GPs (41.6%), psychologists (29.1%), and counsellors or family therapists (29.0%). This reflects that GPs are a common initial contact and source of referrals to other health professionals or services such as Medicare-funded specialised mental health care. This age group was also found to access a range of services, including school-based services (48.7%), online services (10.9%, including those provided by headspace, ReachOut and Youth Beyondblue), hospital-based care (8.1%, including emergency, outpatient or inpatient services), and specialist mental health services (5.7%). Trends in mental health-related emergency department visits have shown a rising increase in presentations, reflecting inadequate investment in specialist community mental health care for children and youth (McGorry, Chanen, & Robinson, 2018).

As reflected in the following section, headspace has played an integral role in enhancing access to mental health care, particularly for minority groups. In the 2016/2017 financial year, a total of 80 237 young people accessed a headspace centre and almost 32 000 accessed eheadspace (headspace, 2017).

3.2.8 THE IMPLICATIONS OF THE DIVERSITY OF AUSTRALIA

While Australia boasts a unique and varied geographical and cultural environment, this diversity also highlights the disparities in youth mental health across Indigenous, remote and other minority populations. Aboriginal and Torres Strait Islander people are a longstanding marginalised group within Australia who have endured inequalities across a range of outcomes that includes mental health. Despite a lack of epidemiological data on the mental health outcomes of Australian Indigenous populations (Black et al., 2015), mental and substance use disorders are common in Indigenous adolescents (Azzopardi et al., 2018). Compared to their non-Indigenous counterparts, young Indigenous Australians are more likely to report depression and significant psychological distress (Azzopardi et al., 2018), and are five times more likely to die by suicide (Australian Institute of Health and Welfare, 2015). Yet access to mental health care by Aboriginal and Torres Strait Islander young people can be hindered by the cultural appropriateness of services, confidentiality concerns, stigma and shame, language or literacy difficulties, and poor service knowledge (Brown et al., 2016).

Aboriginal and Torres Strait Islander people often reside in remote or rural areas where access to health care can be restricted due to increased wait times, shortages in trained health professionals and limited infrastructure (Australian Institute of Health and Welfare, 2018e). Across the general population of young people living in remote areas of Australia, access to mental health services is poor due to factors such as lack of anonymity in smaller towns, perceived lack of services and qualified mental health professionals, accessibility of services, transportation, stigma, and self-reliance (Brown et al., 2016). This is despite the higher incidence of youth mental illness and rate of suicide in rural regions of Australia compared to urban areas (Bowman, McKinstry, & McGorry, 2017; see Section 1.3.2).

Similarly, access to mental health services is low among CALD backgrounds despite demonstrating a higher rate of psychosis than Australian-born individuals (Stolk, Minas, & Klimidis, 2008). A number of adverse circumstances can increase the risk of mental health problems in young people who are refugees from CALD countries, including exposure to violence and trauma, detainment in immigration detention centres, and resettlement stress (de Anstiss, Ziaian, Procter, Warland, & Baghurst, 2009). Accessing mental health care can be challenging for this population due to language barriers, distrust of services, stigma, as well as service systems inadequately responding to the mental health needs of CALD populations (de Anstiss et al., 2009).

Although challenges remain in adequately responding to the mental health needs of young people within marginalised groups, promising gains have been made. A key finding from the most recent independent review of headspace was the enhanced access to care for a number of marginalised and at-risk groups (Hilferty et al., 2015). In particular, headspace was shown to be accessed by a significant proportion of young people who reside in regional areas (39%), have an Indigenous background (7.4%), identify as LGBTIQ (20.2%), or experience homelessness or insecure housing (16.7% of 18–25-year-olds). This reflects the majority of headspace centres being strategically located in regions with relatively poor access to standard mental health services, particularly in regional and rural parts of Australia and metropolitan regions with high need. While access to headspace by young people from CALD backgrounds remains a challenge, strategies to improving access and engagement have been proposed, including engagement with local CALD communities and ensuring a culturally inclusive environment (Rickwood, Telford, et al., 2015).

3.2.9 COMMENTARY AND REFLECTION

The emergence of 75% of mental disorders prior to 24 years of age makes the life stage of youth critical for the prevention and early intervention of mental disorders. Mental health care for young people has significantly strengthened over the last two decades through the development of early intervention models of care and youth-specific mental health services that are informed by best practice across the areas of engagement, assessment and intervention. The construction of a youth mental health stream, that bridges the gap between existing child and older adult psychiatry, has been shown to enhance access to care and provide age-appropriate, acceptable and effective mental health assessment and intervention. Services for the developmental period of 0-25 years should be culturally and developmentally appropriate, with a flexible boundary between child and youth services.

Initiatives such as headspace and Orygen Youth Health (OYH), as well as similar models that have emerged internationally, provide examples of how to address the need for reform in service provision for this age group, who experience the highest prevalence of mental illness among any Australians, yet the lowest use of mental health services. As these reforms challenge existing (often longstanding) practice, they have provoked resistance in some quarters, despite the undeniable unmet need in this age group. Nonetheless, these initial ground-breaking approaches, designed to deliver better health, social and economic outcomes, provide an encouraging example for youth mental health care worldwide that many countries are examining with growing interest.

A new wave of reform is now needed. There remains enormous and urgent need and scope for further improvement in order to sufficiently meet the mental health needs of young Australians. Firstly, the headspace model is currently being expanded to increase its provision to young people with severe and complex presentations. To adequately care for this 'missing middle', who are too complex for primary and care and yet locked out of specialist mental health services, substantial and ongoing investment is needed (McGorry & Hamilton, 2017). The target is to establish a vertically integrated system of care across primary to tertiary services that provides seamless patient management. Secondly, valid and clinically useful diagnostic methods for young people with emerging mental disorders are needed, such as transdiagnostic clinical staging, to improve not only the utility of diagnosis, but also facilitate the selection of more effective, simpler and safer interventions for earlier stages. Lastly, clinical staging would allow treatment planning and selection to be guided by a staged-based stepped care approach, enabling a more pre-emptive and personalised approach to care. This could generate significant benefits to young people, their families as well as the broader community, including the potential prevention of mental illness, enhanced social and workforce participation, and increased economic productivity at an individual and societal level.

3.3

MENTAL HEALTH OF OLDER ADULTS

CHRISTOS PLAKIOTIS, SAGARIKA DE FONSEKA, RHODA LAI & DANIEL O'CONNOR

3.3.1 INTRODUCTION

Old age psychiatry concerns itself with the entire spectrum of mental illness affecting older adults. This includes the majority of psychiatric conditions seen in younger adults but, in addition, disorders manifesting primarily via their effects on cognition. Cognitive impairment represents a key focus of an old age psychiatrist's work, as in addition to being a primary source of attention itself, it may also influence the manifestation of other psychiatric conditions in older people, such as depressive and psychotic disorders.

THE DEMOGRAPHY OF AGEING

Australia's population is ageing as a result of two factors—with good documentation of these mainly from the Australian Bureau of Statistics. The first is that Australian families have been having fewer babies since the late 1960s, with the birth rate falling below the replacement rate. The second is that people are living longer. For example, life expectancy was 68 years for males born in 1960, for females 74 years; it is 81 years for males born in 2015 and 85 years for females. With a declining birth rate, and more people living longer, progressive ageing of our population is the natural tendency. While inward migration of typically younger people counteracts the natural trend to a degree, the number of people aged 65 years and over is projected to double in the early twenty-first century from 13% (2.5 million) of the population in 2001–02 to around 25% (6.2 million) by 2042. Population growth will be even more rapid among Australians aged 85 and over, from around 300 000 in 2002 to 1.1 million in 2042.

The ageing of Australia's population will naturally entail an increase in the number of older adults with mental health problems. This is clearly illustrated by projected figures for dementia prevalence over coming decades. In 2020, it is estimated there are 459 000 Australians living with dementia, projected on trend to increase to 590 000 by 2028 and 1 076 000 by 2058 (Dementia Australia, 2020). Against this background, the demand for old age psychiatry and related multidisciplinary services will rise dramatically, making knowledge of the field essential for all mental health care providers

3.3.2 MENTAL HEALTH CARE PROVISION FOR OLDER ADULTS

MEMORY CLINICS

In Australia, memory clinics usually operate parallel to but separate from aged psychiatry services. Memory clinics undertake multidisciplinary diagnostic assessment and treatment planning–involving geriatricians, social workers, neuropsychologists and psychiatrists–for people presenting with concerns regarding cognitive impairment. Such clinics do not generally have the age-based entry criteria of public psychiatric services. Furthermore, while psychiatric comorbidity (such as a depressive disorder) or behavioural or psychological disturbances in dementia (BPDD) may be identified as part of the assessment process, management of these conditions is not a primary focus. Most memory clinics operate within the public health care sector, although equivalent privately run clinics exist in some metropolitan areas.

PUBLIC PSYCHIATRIC SERVICES

Specialised aged persons mental health services (APMHS) for adults aged 65 years and over operate within the public health sector in most parts of Australia, especially in large metropolitan sectors. These services provide multidisciplinary mental health care to older adults suffering from the entire spectrum of mental illness. APMHS also occasionally treat younger adults who present with early-onset dementia. Unlike memory clinics, public aged psychiatry services do not usually become involved in diagnosing and treating patients with dementia in the absence of related behavioural or psychological symptoms warranting mental health service involvement. APMHS vary widely across Australia in configuration and available resources. An 'ideal' service consisting of a community team, inpatient unit and specialist residential units is described below, but this mix is not uniformly found across the country.

Where they exist, APMHS are generally operated by mainstream health care services (Local Health Networks or LHNs) and divided according to geographical regions or catchment areas. Within each region, there is usually a centralised telephone triage service through which all referrals to the service are channelled. Each service operates acute aged psychiatry inpatient wards, which are sometimes referred to as assessment units. Some services also operate psychogeriatric hostels (low-level care) and nursing homes (high-level care) for patients with mental illness requiring specialised longer-term psychiatric treatment that cannot be provided in mainstream aged care facilities.

Each area also operates a community team for the assessment and management of people living in the community, either in their own homes or within mainstream residential care facilities. These teams are usually standalone, but may be integrated with adult community teams in some regional and rural areas. Community teams often see patients in their own environment, rather than as outpatients at a clinic, thereby overcoming the difficulties frail older adults may experience in transporting themselves to appointments. At the centre of the multidisciplinary model of care provided is case management (see Chapter 2.4), whereby each patient is allocated a case manager (CM; usually a psychiatric nurse, social worker or occupational therapist) who is responsible for coordinating all aspects of a patient's care, and serves as the primary contact person for patients and carers in their interaction with the service. CMs are able to access input from other disciplines as required, such as consultant psychiatrists, psychiatry registrars, clinical psychologists and neuropsychologists as well as social workers and occupational therapists (outside the case management role).

Apart from providing case management to patients with continuing care needs, some teams operate sub-teams focused on providing specialised interventions to particular patient groups. Examples of such teams are those that provide intensive community treatment as an alternative to hospitalisation; those providing support to aged care facilities in caring for residents with emotional and/or behavioural difficulties; and those providing home-based psychosocial support.

PRIVATE PSYCHIATRIC SERVICES

Some of the larger metropolitan private psychiatric hospitals also have acute aged psychiatry inpatient units that are able to provide multidisciplinary care to voluntary inpatients. Private old age psychiatrists are concentrated in metropolitan areas (see Chapter 1.5), and often have to engage in shared care arrangements with public sector community teams in order to meet the complex, multidisciplinary care needs of their patient population.

THE CONTRIBUTION OF INFORMAL CAREGIVERS

Carers are significant stakeholders in the mental health care of older adults, providing emotional and practical assistance to relatives with a range of mental disorders residing at home (see Chapters 1.1, 2.1 and 2.7). In 2015, 11.6% of the Australian adult population—almost 2.7 million people—acted as carers. Primary carers (those who act as the main source of informal assistance to a person needing care) are most likely to be relatively older females, being aged 55 years on average. As a result of their role, carers may experience significant mental health problems of their own (in the form of worry, anxiety and depression) as well as increased physical impairment and financial pressure. A lack of social support and intrafamilial conflict, coupled with greater responsibility for household chores, may further compound their distress. Provision of interventions to support carers and alleviate carer burden is therefore crucial and should be a guiding principle of all aged mental health clinical work. Aged mental health services sometimes have designated carer consultants (see Chapter 2.1) who can work directly with families to provide counselling or arrange linkage with support services to ease carer burden. It is imperative, however, that all clinicians working in the field familiarise themselves with community resources available to assist carers in fulfilling their role (Butterworth, Pymont, Rodgers, Windsor, & Anstey, 2010; Australian Bureau of Statistics, 2015b).

Perceptions of inadequate support from health services have been found to be greatest among carers of older people with profound mental (rather than physical) disability. Greater availability of formal services for patients with physical disabilities and/or a need for more or different types of resources by carers of people with mental disabilities are possible explanations. Rising levels of dementia (Australian Institute of Health and Welfare, 2012) coupled with demographic changes (see Section 3.3.1), such as declining fertility rates and greater workforce participation by women, will place increased pressure on a shrinking pool of informal carers in future with which support services will need to keep pace. At the same time, however, existing services may be underutilised by carers because of a perceived lack of need or lack of knowledge. Reducing the stigma of dementia, improving public awareness of services and encouraging referrals from health practitioners may help address barriers to service use (Brodaty, Thomson, Thompson, & Fine, 2005; Vecchio, Stevens, & Cybinski, 2008).

3.3.3 MENTAL HEALTH ASSESSMENT AND MANAGEMENT OF OLDER ADULTS

HISTORY TAKING

Direct patient interview is always the centrepiece of any psychiatric assessment (see Chapter 2.3). However, collateral history has a particularly important role in old age psychiatry, more so than in general adult psychiatry, because of the possible presence of cognitive impairment in older adults, which may have an impact upon the reliability of the history provided. As in other areas of psychiatry the history taken in old age psychiatry comprises the following key elements: (a) basic demographic information; (b) presenting complaint; (c) history of presenting illness and systems review; (d) past psychiatric history; (e) alcohol and drug history; (f) forensic history; (g) family history; (h) personal history; and (i) premorbid personality.

In adapting this schema to older adults, inquiring about possible cognitive decline and the ability to carry out activities of daily living is particularly important, as both physical frailty and cognitive deficits may give rise to functional impairments. Patients and their caretakers should be asked whether they have noted any difficulties with the person's orientation and memory for recent events and, if present, the nature and time course of such difficulties. It is particularly important to inquire about behaviours that may place a patient or others at risk (see Chapter 2.3), such as wandering away from home and getting lost, or forgetting to turn off the stove. Determining the extent to which short- and/or long-term memory are affected may be helpful in characterising dementia severity and subtypes. The ability to attend to personal care activities (such as washing and dressing), prepare and eat meals, go shopping and manage finances should be inquired about, and the degree of any required assistance determined. Extensive assistance by family members or sticking with familiar routines may sometimes obscure the true extent of a patient's cognitive and functional impairments. For example, a patient who reports regularly driving a great distance to visit relatives may admit on closer questioning that he would be entirely unable to find his way if required to make a detour from a highly familiar route that has been travelled for many years. Sometimes cognitive impairment may become more apparent when a patient leaves a familiar environment, as may occur following a move from home into residential care. Clinicians should also inquire about the presence of other behavioural difficulties that may stem from a dementing illness, such as agitation and verbal or physical aggression.

The extent to which the above elements of history (relating to cognitive decline) are emphasised, and their location in the order of history taking, will depend on the nature of the presenting complaint and the patient's overall presentation at interview. Where dementia is the presenting problem, this questioning will be integral to obtaining the history of the presenting complaint. In the case of a seemingly cognitively intact and highly functioning individual, questioning regarding cognition may be considered an important extension of the psychiatric systems review.

MENTAL STATE EXAMINATION AND BEDSIDE COGNITIVE TESTING

Mental state examination in older adults

Aspects of the mental state examination (MSE) (see Chapter 2.3) that are of particular relevance to older adults are outlined in Table 3.6.

Cognitive screening: The Mini Mental State Examination

In addition to the standard MSE performed in younger adults, cognitive examination is required in assessing older adults. At a very basic level, this may involve testing orientation to time, place and person, and short- and long-term recall, in an unstructured way. In practice, the Mini Mental State Examination (MMSE; Folstein, Folstein, & McHugh, 1975) is frequently administered by aged mental health services as a cognitive screening tool, as its wide familiarity among clinicians will assist in this aspect of the assessment being conveyed to colleagues.

The MMSE has its limitations, particularly in appraising frontal lobe functions such as complex planning skills, leading to a variety of newer cognitive screening tools being proposed as more complete alternatives. Examples include the Montréal Cognitive Assessment (MOCA) (Nasreddine et al., 2005); the Addenbrooke's Cognitive Examination-Revised (ACE-R) (Mioshi, Dawson, Mitchell, Arnold, & Hodges, 2006); and the Neuropsychiatry Unit Cognitive Assessment Tool (NUCOG), which was developed in Australia (Walterfang, Siu, & Velakoulis, 2006). These tools are more sensitive than the MMSE to mild cognitive impairment.

Table 3.6 Aspects of mental state examination (MSE) in older adults

Appearance and behaviour
Poor hygiene and grooming in older adults may arise due to poor physical health and frailty as well as cognitive impairment, in addition to the range of psychiatric illnesses (such as depressive or psychotic disorders) affecting younger individuals. It is important to identify sensory impairments, as these may impede effective patient assessment (cognitive testing especially) and management. Psychomotor agitation or retardation is particularly common in depression in older adults. In this age group, however, psychomotor retardation may be confused (or coexist) with the bradykinesia of Parkinson's disease, or be a feature of apathy, rather than depression. Apathy is common even in mild dementia and, compared to depression, is characterised by lack of interest rather than withdrawal, and a lack of drive to engage in activities rather than an inability to passively enjoy them (anhedonia).
Speech
Paucity of speech is a feature of both depression and dementia in older adults. Impairment in language ability, known as dysphasia, is a feature of dementia but not of depression. Word-finding difficulties may be an early sign of emerging cognitive problems in dementia. Conditions resulting in neurological damage, such as stroke or Parkinson's disease, may also give rise to motor difficulties in articulating speech, known as dysarthria.
Mood and affect
Anxiety may be a more prominent accompaniment of depression in older than younger people. Mood elevation, in addition to occurring in manic illness, is seen in frontal lobe dementias. Cerebrovascular disease may give rise to mood lability. Clinicians should be aware of a tendency among some older adults to minimise mood-related symptoms.
Thought
Complex delusional beliefs occur in both early and late-onset psychoses, but are unusual in dementia. More common in patients with dementia are delusions regarding theft or misidentification. Patients with dementia may believe they share their home with nonexistent people or may converse with their own image in the mirror, which they fail to recognise. The onset of cognitive decline may alter the clinical presentation of pre-existing psychotic illness. For example, a patient with schizoaffective disorder may present with predominant irritability and agitation during acute illness episodes and no longer convey florid delusional beliefs with his or her previous clarity.
Perception
The presence of hallucinations in modalities other than the auditory (and olfactory) should prompt a search for an underlying medical or neurodegenerative cause. Patients with delirium often experience visual and tactile hallucinations. Formication—the sensation of insects crawling on or under the skin—is particularly characteristic of alcohol withdrawal delirium. Complex visual hallucinations are a hallmark of dementia as a result of Lewy body disease. Charles Bonnet syndrome (CBS) is a condition in which mentally healthy older adults with impaired vision experience complex visual hallucinations. These are often 'Lilliputian' in nature, involving people, animals or objects that are smaller than usual. An auditory variant also exists, typically involving the experience of protracted musical hallucinations.
Cognition
Older adults with preserved social graces may appear cognitively intact, but clues to emerging cognitive deficits are often present even before formal cognitive screening. Inquiring about age and date of birth at the outset of an interview, while gathering demographic data, is non-threatening and may immediately reveal significant cognitive problems. A further clue to underlying cognitive difficulties is a sense of 'vagueness' in the patient's history. This may be accompanied by confabulation, whereby a patient describes fictitious events in an effort to bridge gaps (arising from memory deficits) in the history he or she can provide. Formal cognitive screening tests are discussed elsewhere in this chapter.
Insight and judgement
Patients with mild dementia may retain considerable insight into their emerging cognitive deficits, but vary in the degree to which these are acknowledged. With progression of dementia, insight is usually very limited. Even where some awareness of cognitive deficits is present, insight into their functional impact is often absent, and may contribute to patients displaying poor judgement in making important decisions. For example, a patient may insist on living independently or driving even when clearly unable to continue doing so.

Source: Adapted from Ames, Chiu, Lindesay, & Shulman, 2010; Thomas, 2013

Another locally developed cognitive screening instrument, the Rowland Universal Dementia Assessment Scale (RUDAS), may be more suitable than the MMSE among people from culturally and linguistically diverse (CALD) backgrounds (Storey, Rowland, Conforti, & Dickson, 2004). However, none has attained the widespread acceptance and familiarity of the MMSE, and the significance of their scoring may not be readily apparent to clinicians who are unfamiliar with their use. For this reason, the MMSE supplemented by a clock drawing task, and frontal, parietal or temporal lobe screening tests if required, may yield more readily interpretable results. Testing should be conducted via an interpreter in patients whose primary language is not English.

Supplementing the MMSE

The clock drawing test taps into a wider range of cognitive domains than the MMSE, including verbal understanding, memory, concentration, abstract thinking, spatial knowledge, planning and visuo-constructive abilities. It is easy to administer and has the characteristics of a good screening procedure for moderate and severe dementia (Park, Jeong, & Seomun, 2018). Although a variety of administration methods and scoring systems have been proposed, the standard instructions (using a pre-drawn circle of approximately 10 cm diameter) are: 'This is a clock face. Please fill in all the numbers and set the time to ten minutes after 11.' Difficulties with conceptualisation and planning, and the presence of perseveration, may be evident on qualitative evaluation of the result. Where a scoring system is preferred, it may be best to use a simple one such as the following four-point scale: 0 = intact clock; 1 = mild impairment; 2 = moderate impairment; 3 = severe impairment (Borson et al., 1999). In either case, the clock drawing test provides a basic visual record of patients' cognitive abilities, and is well suited to serial testing and comparison over time.

Where impaired frontal lobe function is suspected, consideration should be given to supplementing the MMSE with additional frontal lobe screening tests. The Frontal Assessment Battery (FAB) represents a structured option for screening frontal lobe functioning (Dubois, Slachevsky, Litvan, & Pillon, 2000). Although perhaps undertaken less frequently in clinical practice, bedside cognitive testing of parietal and temporal lobe functioning (beyond that afforded by the basic MMSE) is also possible, and may be particularly indicated in assessing patients who have had a stroke or other acquired brain injury.

3.3.4 MEDICAL INVESTIGATIONS IN OLDER MENTAL HEALTH PATIENTS

INTRODUCTION

Older mental health patients may have undetected medical conditions that very occasionally cause their mental disorder and, more usually, reduce their level of functioning. People with severe, chronic mental illness are especially likely to have poor medical care and poor compliance with medical treatments. Medical investigations therefore play an important role in the psychiatric assessment (see Chapter 2.3) of this group of patients. For example, new onset psychiatric symptoms in an older adult may point to delirium, in which case accurate identification of the underlying cause is important for guiding treatment. Some investigations, such as brain imaging, will be important in clarifying dementia-related diagnoses, whereas others, such as thyroid function tests, will be important in the case of depressive disorders. Serum drug levels should be performed where patients are already established on medications, psychiatric or otherwise, that require such monitoring, to rule out toxicity and guide further treatment. In addition, baseline testing of fasting glucose and lipids (cholesterol and triglycerides) is recommended in all cases where antipsychotic medication is to be commenced, because of the metabolic syndrome these agents may give rise to (see Chapters 2.3 and 2.5).

Medical investigations that may be of benefit in the work-up of older mental health patients are listed in Table 3.7. It is recommended that community mental health clinicians liaise with a consultant psychiatrist or psychiatry registrar regarding the selection of appropriate investigations in any particular case. It is often possible to liaise with a patient's GP to organise such testing on an outpatient basis. Lack of a well-established psychiatric history and/or a recent thorough medical assessment may be indicators for a particularly thorough level of testing.

Table 3.7 Medical investigations in older mental health patients

Blood tests:

- full blood examination
- electrolytes, urea and creatinine
- liver function tests
- eosinophil sedimentation rate
- C-reactive protein
- calcium
- magnesium
- phosphate
- B12
- folate
- thyroid function tests
- hepatitis serology
- syphilis serology
- serum drug levels where indicated (e.g. for mood stabilisers or digoxin)

Midstream urine (microscopy, culture and antibiotic sensitivity)

Chest x-ray

Electrocardiogram

Neuroimaging

- computerised tomography (CT) brain imaging
- magnetic resonance imaging (MRI)
- Nuclear imaging:
    - single photon emission tomography (SPECT)
    - positron emission tomography (PET)

THE ROLE OF NEUROIMAGING IN AGED MENTAL HEALTH PRACTICE

Neuroimaging modalities in aged mental health practice can be broadly classified according to whether they are used to characterise brain structure or function. Structural imaging has a recognised role in characterising brain size, architecture and condition in general in clinical practice. While both classes of neuroimaging have potential applications across the entire spectrum of disorders seen in old age psychiatry, they are particularly relevant in investigating patients exhibiting symptoms of dementia. The two structural imaging modalities used in clinical practice are computed tomography (CT) and standard structural magnetic resonance imaging (MRI), whereas single photon emission computed tomography (SPECT) and positron emission tomography (PET) are the key functional imaging. modalities. Further techniques used to study dementia in research settings include functional magnetic resonance imaging (fMRI) and the emerging field of molecular imaging based on the use of radioactive tracers to bind to particular molecules of interest

In conditions such as late-life depression, schizophrenia and bipolar affective disorder, the role of neuroimaging in clinical practice to date has tended to be limited to excluding coexisting intracranial pathology, such as mass occupying lesions or strokes, and to aid diagnostic clarification in cases where comorbid dementia is suspected. Traditionally, CT scanning has been the main structural imaging modality used in aged mental health services, but the increasing availability of MRI has seen more MRI studies being ordered in recent years. Given its superior spatial resolution, structural MRI has advantages over CT scanning in demonstrating greater anatomical detail (e.g. of atrophic areas), identifying smaller lesions (e.g. lacunae and microbleeds), avoiding the confounding effects of CT-related bone artefacts, and allowing for radiation-free imaging where repeated investigation is required. These advantages notwithstanding, CT scanning may be warranted where imaging is urgently required (e.g. trauma or suspected haemorrhagic stroke), in evaluating calcification or lesions of bone, where cost and/or waiting time is an issue, where MRI is contraindicated due to metallic implants or medical devices, or if patients are particularly claustrophobic or prone to moving in the scanner.

The issue of whether patients have access to the imaging type most appropriate for their clinical condition (now primarily MRI and functional neuroimaging in the investigation of cognitive disorders), or whether financial or resource limitations are associated with less informative CT scanning being the only modality offered, is an ethical dilemma within the aged mental health field. Such concerns are not unique to Australia. To make use of its full potential in assessing aged mental health patients, brain imaging should be utilised judiciously and with a clear clinical question in mind. This question should be posed concisely in ordering neuroimaging, and relevant clinical data succinctly summarised, to facilitate correct test selection and image interpretation by radiologists and nuclear medicine physicians.

THE EMERGING ROLE OF FLUID BIOMARKERS IN ALZHEIMER'S DISEASE

A range of fluid biomarkers, that can be measured in blood or cerebrospinal fluid, are currently the subject of investigation as potential aides in the diagnosis and management of Alzheimer's disease, when performed alongside cutting edge neuroimaging techniques such as PET scanning. As in the case of some of the advanced neuroimaging modalities, it is important to appreciate that, despite the availability of commercial testing kits for fluid biomarkers in some countries, they are not yet widely used in routine clinical practice but are more likely to be encountered in research settings. It is nevertheless useful for mental health clinicians to be broadly aware of their existence as their further refinement and subsequent widespread utilisation may impact profoundly on the field of Alzheimer's disease in coming years, e.g. by allowing the prediction of the future onset of dementia well ahead of clinical symptoms and, thereby, earlier intervention to halt or even reverse disease progression (Molinuevo et al., 2018).

NEUROPSYCHOLOGICAL ASSESSMENT AND MANAGEMENT

Clinical neuropsychologists have undergone advanced, postgraduate level training in the assessment and management of patients with known or suspected brain disorders. They study changes in cognition and behaviour stemming from conditions including developmental disorders, psychoactive substance use disorders and neurological disorders such as acquired brain injury, epilepsy and stroke. In general psychiatry, they may be called upon to provide advice regarding cognitive impairment associated with long-term mental illnesses such as schizophrenia and bipolar affective disorder (see Chapters 2.1 and 2.3). Additionally, in aged mental health practice, neuropsychologists play a key role in the diagnostic assessment and treatment of patients with cognitive impairment due to dementia. In general health care settings, neuropsychology referrals are made by general or specialist medical practitioners or allied health professionals. In aged mental health settings, referrals can usually be made by any member of the multidisciplinary treating team.

Neuropsychologists employ interviewing, observation and psychological testing to assess patients' cognitive and behavioural functioning. Assessment may occur on an outpatient basis, at a patient's place of residence or in a hospital inpatient setting, and involves answering questions and performing paper-based tasks. Neuropsychological tests may be selected depending on the presenting problem and reason for the referral, and may require several hours (over one or more sessions) for their administration. Language, memory and new learning, problem-solving skills and spatial abilities are measured and evaluated with reference to a patient's age, gender and background.

Neuropsychologists are often asked to provide diagnostic clarification where cognitive impairment is suspected or apparent. However, they may also be asked to undertake medicolegal assessments to determine whether patients have decision-making capacity with regard to managing finances, making a will (testamentary capacity) or making health or lifestyle-related decisions. Furthermore, neuropsychologists may provide education and counselling for cognitive, emotional or behavioural problems related to brain disorders and assist in patient treatment, rehabilitation and discharge planning. Given these different aspects of neuropsychological assessment and management, referrers should clearly convey their specific questions to neuropsychologists. Of equal importance, the purpose and possible implications of neuropsychology referral should be explained to patients and carers from the outset, particularly where capacity-related assessment is being requested.

3.3.5 COGNITION AND COGNITIVE DISORDERS

DEFINING COGNITION AND ITS DISORDERS

What does cognition refer to?

'Cognition' refers to the higher-level brain functions whereby information is processed and knowledge acquired and applied (see Chapter 2.3). The term encompasses a range of mental processes, including attention and concentration, memory (immediate, short and long term), orientation, language and numeracy skills (verbal and written), problem solving, decision making and abstract reasoning and planning. In psychiatry, cognitive processes are usually considered distinctly from those of emotion (mood) and perception, although disturbances in both the latter may have an impact upon cognitive abilities. Cognition is an important concept in old age psychiatry because of the increased likelihood of deterioration in its functioning with increasing age.

Problems with cognition

The terms 'cognitive impairment' and 'cognitive decline' are often used where deterioration in any of the above cognitive functions is apparent. Such impairment may be acute and reversible, or chronic and irreversible. The most common cause of acute, reversible cognitive impairment is delirium. In old age psychiatry, the term 'dementia' is used to denote a range of conditions contributing to chronic, irreversible cognitive impairment. In other medical disciplines, the term 'acquired brain injury' is sometimes used to denote clinical presentations arising from traumatic brain injury that essentially overlap with the concept of dementia. In clinical practice, however, distinguishing between these two broad categories of cognitive impairment is not always straightforward, as patients may be unable to provide a coherent account of the chronicity of their symptoms. Collateral history from a close relative or acquaintance may thus assume a central role in patient assessment, with its unavailability giving rise to diagnostic dilemmas (Dyer, Nabeel, Briggs, O'Neill, & Kennelly, 2016).

DELIRIUM

Significance and characteristics

Delirium is the most common cause of acute-onset, reversible cognitive impairment among general hospital inpatients, affecting 10–18% of older adults who are admitted to hospital, 30% or more who have cardiac or hip surgery, and 50% or more of patients requiring intensive care admission. Essentially a form of cerebral organ failure, it poses a significant public health problem, being linked to prolonged hospitalisation, higher death rates, more rapid functional and cognitive decline and inflated health care costs. Despite its potentially devastating ramifications, it frequently goes unrecognised in medical treatment settings (Australian Commission on Safety and Quality in Health Care, 2016; Inouye, Westendorp, & Saczynski, 2014).

Altered consciousness or awareness, with difficulty focusing, sustaining or shifting attention, is a key feature of delirium. Cognitive impairment (such as disorientation, memory loss or language problem) or perceptual disturbances, that are not better explained by dementia, may also be present. Delirium usually develops acutely over hours to days and has a fluctuating course over the day. Evidence of an underlying medical cause is required from history, physical examination or laboratory investigations. Supportive features that are often present in delirium, but not diagnostic in themselves, include disturbances in sleep-wake cycle, psychomotor activity, perception or emotion, delusions, affective lability, impaired speech articulation (dysarthria) and EEG abnormalities (see Chapter 2.3). Accompanying symptoms such as these may contribute to misdiagnosis of delirium as anxiety, depression, psychosis or mania. However, the presence of new onset visual hallucinations in particular should raise suspicions of an underlying medical cause, rather than a primary psychotic illness, in the first instance (Inouye et al., 2014; Flaherty, 2011).

Subtypes of delirium

Delirium can be classified into hyperactive, hypoactive and mixed subtypes, based on motor activity. Hyperactive delirium presents with restlessness, agitation and hypervigilance as well as delusions and hallucinations. Hypoactive delirium, the most common subtype in the elderly, presents with sedation, lethargy and slowed motor activity. Mixed delirium entails fluctuation between the hyperactive and hypoactive forms within the same illness episode. Hyperactive delirium is more apparent clinically, whereas hypoactive delirium may be overlooked or misattributed to causes such as depression or fatigue because of its potentially ambiguous presentation. Subtle cases of hypoactive delirium among older general hospital inpatients may be detected by actively exploring their understanding of their medical care and its broader consequences on a regular basis. Delirium subtypes may reflect different pathophysiological mechanisms and carry different prognoses. For example, alcohol withdrawal and metabolic imbalance are more likely to cause hyperactive and hypoactive subtypes respectively (Han, Wilson, & Ely, 2010; Mittal et al., 2011).

Causes and pathophysiologic mechanisms

A broad array of medical and surgical illness can give rise to delirium. Delirium is more likely to manifest when the impact of any physiological insult outweighs the 'cognitive reserve' available to deal with this, thus placing older adults at particular risk. A practical mnemonic for remembering some of the most common risk factors and causes of delirium is as follows:

- D: drugs (prescribed, over the counter or illicit, including recent changes)
- E: eyes, ears (vision or hearing impairment)
- L: low oxygen states or insults (myocardial infarction, stroke, pulmonary embolus)
- I: infection (commonly urinary tract infections or pneumonia)
- R: retention (of urine or stool)
- I: ictal (postictal states)
- U: uncontrolled pain
- M: metabolic abnormalities
- (S): subdural haematoma (Flaherty, 2011).

Causes of delirium identified as particularly likely to be life threatening include Wernicke's encephalopathy, hypoxia, hypoglycaemia, hypertensive encephalopathy, hyperthermia or hypothermia, intracerebral haemorrhage, meningitis or encephalitis, poisoning (exogenous or iatrogenic) and status epilepticus (Han et al., 2010). Pathophysiologic mechanisms suggested to underlie the development of delirium include neurotransmitter dysregulation, inflammation, hypoxia and hypoxaemic injury, electrolyte abnormalities, and genetic determinants (Flaherty, 2011).

Delirium awareness, screening and evaluation

Delirium should be part of the medical vocabulary for all aged care providers, as awareness of its possible presence is the first step towards not missing it. Delirium awareness entails a good understanding of the circumstances under which this condition may arise, its variable clinical presentation (including fluctuating course, overlap with dementia and potential for being overlooked or misdiagnosed) and consequences (Flaherty, 2011; Mittal et al., 2011).

Delirium is diagnosed on the basis of clinical information, behavioural observations, and mental state and cognitive assessment. Thorough history taking where possible (see Chapter 2.3) clarifies the acuity of observed changes in cognition and behaviour and helps confirm or exclude underlying medical illnesses, medication use or substance abuse as causative factors. Physical examination and investigations (the latter drawing from the previously outlined schema for medical investigation in older adults) complement and extend the findings obtained on history. Mental state examination (MSE) and cognitive screening (see below) detect cognitive impairments and accompanying psychiatric symptoms such as affective lability or hallucinations (Mittal et al., 2011).

Delirium screening may be superior to one-off clinical psychiatric assessment in detecting and diagnosing delirium in older adults. One approach to screening is to use a validated screening tool at multiple observation points in all older adults who make contact with health care services. The frequency of screening will depend on the acuity of the treatment setting. Several scales are available for bedside delirium screening by nursing staff, with the Confusion Assessment Method (CAM) having the best supportive data (Inouye et al., 2014; Flaherty, 2011; Mittal et al., 2011).

Electroencephalography (EEG) may assist in the diagnostic investigation of equivocal cases of delirium. The classic EEG finding in delirium, irrespective of underlying cause, is generalised slowing to the theta-delta range, which resolves with treatment. The EEG sometimes displays a pattern characteristic of the underlying condition, such as rapid beta activity in sedative-hypnotic toxicity or triphasic waves in hepatic encephalopathy. EEG is also indicated in cases of delirium caused by epilepsy (Inouye et al., 2014).

Prevention and management of delirium

Nonpharmacological approaches to risk factor reduction are the first line of delirium prevention and management. The Hospital Elder Life Program (HELP) represents a formalised approach to preventing delirium and loss of functioning among older hospitalised adults through nonpharmacological means, and is the most widespread programs of its kind worldwide. Emphasising reorientation, sleep hygiene, adequate food and fluid intake, attendance to visual and hearing deficits, therapeutic activities, and minimisation of psychotropic medication use, it is cost-effective in preventing delirium by targeting the risk factor contributing to it (Inouye et al., 2014).

Where delirium does occur, treatment should be provided in a quiet environment with adequate soft lighting. Staff and room changes should be minimised, and a clearly visible clock and calendar provided. Frequent reorientation, eye contact and use of clear verbal instructions are recommended when talking to patients. Reading glasses and hearing aids should be available to address sensory impairments. Family or carer involvement in patient treatment should be encouraged. As in other practice, physical restraint should be avoided (see Chapters 1.1, 1.7 and 2.3), and evidence supporting its use as a falls prevention strategy in the context of delirium is generally lacking. Furthermore, restraint may actually increase the risk of developing delirium and its severity (Flaherty, 2011; Mittal et al., 2011; Tropea, Slee, Brand, Gray, & Snell, 2008).

Identification and treatment of the underlying cause is the single most effective treatment of delirium. Evidence regarding pharmacological approaches to preventing and managing delirium is limited, but key recommendations can nevertheless be made. Medication review undertaken when delirium is initially diagnosed may identify recent contributory medication changes. Psychoactive medications and other treatments that increase patients' risk of developing delirium should be used with care. Judicious prescription of opiate analgesia and benzodiazepine anxiolytics, so that patients benefit from their therapeutic properties while being spared from potential adverse effects, is an example of this. Evidence for the prophylactic use of risperidone and haloperidol for preventing perioperative delirium has also been promising, but mixed (Inouye et al., 2014; Ford & Almeida, 2015; Han et al., 2010).

The role of antipsychotics (see Chapter 2.5) in delirium has been suggested to be limited to a subgroup of patients experiencing severe agitation or secondary delusions or hallucinations. If an antipsychotic is used, the goal should be a patient who is awake and manageable, not sedated, and the medication should be reduced and ceased as soon as practicable since research is increasingly suggesting that antipsychotics may contribute to prolonged delirium and worse clinical outcomes. Traditionally, haloperidol has been the most commonly used antipsychotic for delirium. Haloperidol's strong dopamine antagonism (and negligible cholinergic activity) limits psychotic symptoms without further impairing alertness and attention. Haloperidol has been used in both oral and intravenous formulations, the latter having the advantage of minimising extrapyramidal side effects but requiring cautious use because of the possibility of inducing cardiac arrhythmia (QT_C prolongation and Torsades de Pointes). Newer atypical agents, (see Chapter 2.5) such as risperidone, olanzapine and quetiapine, have also been used in treating delirium, but evidence supporting their use is also limited (Inouye et al., 2014; Flaherty, 2011; Han et al., 2010).

PROGNOSIS OF DELIRIUM

The common conceptualisation of delirium as a short-lived cognitive disorder from which most patients fully recover is not in keeping with longitudinal reports of poorer outcomes among older adults. It has been proposed that the majority of older adults can recover completely and have good outcomes, but that full or partial persistence of delirium in a substantial minority of patients at the time of discharge from hospital may explain the poor outcomes seen in this population. Recognising that persistence of delirium after discharge may impede patient self-management of chronic medical illnesses and monitoring the course of delirium at discharge and beyond to ensure its full resolution have been suggested to redress this problem (Cole, 2010).

DEMENTIA

Significance and characteristics

Dementia is a syndrome the predominant feature of which is memory impairment and/or deficits in other major cognitive domains, including dysphasia (impaired language ability), apraxia (inability to perform learnt motor skills), agnosia (inability to recognise objects or people) and impaired executive function (difficulty planning, reasoning and problem solving). These deficits should not be limited to an episode of delirium or better explained by any other medical, neurological or psychiatric illness. New onset mood, psychotic or behavioural features may accompany the condition. Specific subtypes of dementia in older adults are those due to Alzheimer's disease; Lewy body disease and Parkinson's disease; vascular disease; and frontotemporal lobar degeneration (see Table 3.8). Additional causes include substance use (such as alcohol); normal pressure hydrocephalus; Huntington's disease; traumatic brain injury; HIV infection; and prion disease.

Dementia is of growing interest as a public health care problem (see section 3.3.1). Most (but not all) cases are characterised by progressive social or occupational functional decline, leading to inability to carry out activities of daily living and limiting independence. The resulting burden on patients, carers and society as a whole (for example, because of the cost of nursing home care) is enormous, and will rise further with increasing life expectancy. Presently, the average patient with dementia will survive only three to ten years, but the promise of approaching disease-modifying treatments makes early diagnosis and better understanding of disease pathophysiology increasingly important (Australian Institute of Health and Welfare, 2012).

Distinguishing between delirium and dementia

Although distinct clinical entities, both delirium and dementia involve cognitive impairment, and are often confused by health care providers. Delirium, in particular, is often missed when superimposed on dementia. However, the two conditions can usually be differentiated on the basis that cognitive decline is acute in delirium but slow to develop and chronic in dementia; a clear sensorium is typical in early dementia; and difficulty sustaining or shifting attention is more suggestive of delirium. Distinguishing delirium from severe or end-stage

Table 3.8 Dementia subtypes seen in older adults

Alzheimer's disease		
Clinical presentation	**Pathology and imaging**	**Management**
Clinical diagnosis of Alzheimer's disease (the most common dementia subtype) requires impairment in two or more cognitive domains that impedes activities of daily living and causes functional decline. The amnesia observed in AD mainly affects declarative episodic memory, namely autobiographical memories related to particular events, places, times, and emotions. When the condition is at an early stage, this is usually most apparent for recent memories. This type of memory impairment points to mesial temporal lobe dysfunction and can become evident in a number of ways. Patients may misplace items, repeat questions or discussions, or struggle to remember dates and appointments. To evaluate memory in a formal manner, clinicians can ask patients to recall and recognise a list of words or objects or to repeat a brief story that they are told. Other types of memory (e.g., procedural memory), that are dependent on structures outside the hippocampus and parahippocampus, usually remain intact in Alzheimer's disease (Erkkinen et al., 2018). Initial short-term memory impairment is followed by disturbances in language, praxis, visuospatial and executive functions, as well as longer-term memory with disease progression. Behavioural and psychological symptoms are common in more advanced cases, including agitation, wandering, aggression, anxiety, depression, delusions and visual hallucinations. Sleep disturbances include insomnia, excessive daytime sleepiness and complete diurnal sleep-wake cycle reversal.	Grossly, Alzheimer's disease is characterised by diffuse cerebral cortical atrophy and ventricular enlargement, reflecting neuronal loss and shrinkage. Loss of cholinergic neurons is particularly implicated in memory deficits. Extracellular Aβ peptide amyloid plaques and intraneuronal tau-positive neurofibrillary tangles and neuropil threads are demonstrable at post mortem. The 'amyloid cascade hypothesis' has been the dominant model of AD pathogenesis since it was first proposed in 1992. The gradual formation of diffuse plaques through fibrillar Aβ accumulation gives rise to an inflammatory reaction, oxidative stress, changes in ion homeostasis and kinase/ phosphatase activity, resulting in neurofibrillary tangles and generalised synaptic dysfunction and neuronal loss (Molinuevo et al., 2018). In patients with established Alzheimer's disease, structural MRI shows excessive bilateral atrophy of the hippocampi and mesial temporal, lateral temporoparietal, and posterior cingulate/precuneus cortices, with mesial temporal atrophy being the most typical finding in ordinary AD (Erkkinen et al., 2018). Medial temporal lobe atrophy (with hippocampal volume loss) on brain imaging points strongly towards Alzheimer's disease, but is not specific, also occurring in vascular and Lewy body dementia and frontotemporal lobar degeneration. Prominent posterior or biparietal cortical atrophy also occurs in some patients with Alzheimer's disease.	There are presently no confirmed disease-modifying pharmacologic treatments for Alzheimer's disease. However, new treatments aimed at elements of both amyloid and/or tau are a focus of active research (Erkkinen et al., 2018). Cognitive enhancing medications, which may slow progression of cognitive and functional decline, are the cholinesterase inhibitors (donepezil, rivastigmine and galantamine) and the N-methyl-D-aspartate antagonist, memantine. Other classes of psychotropic medications may play an adjunctive role to psychosocial approaches in treating behavioural and psychological symptoms of dementia.

(*Continues*)

Table 3.8 Dementia subtypes seen in older adults (Continued)

Lewy body disease (LBD) and Parkinson's disease		
Clinical presentation	**Pathology and imaging**	**Management**
Dementia due to LBD may be the second most common dementia subtype. Fluctuating cognitive impairment and spontaneous parkinsonism (which is usually less marked than in Parkinson's disease) are typically present. Supportive features include a range of sleep disturbances (especially REM sleep behaviour disorder associated with dream enacting) that may occur before dementia manifests. Psychiatric symptoms include depression and vivid visual hallucinations in particular. The clinical features of Lewy body dementia resemble those of dementia in Parkinson's disease, and the two conditions may be closely related. Parkinson's disease dementia is diagnosed when cognitive deficits emerge more than one year after the onset of parkinsonism.	Both LBD and Parkinson's disease are characterised by the presence of Lewy bodies, abnormal intraneuronal protein deposits. In Parkinson's disease, Lewy bodies are concentrated subcortically in the deeper brain structures mediating movement disorders. In Lewy body dementia, they are found throughout the brain and may affect structures involved in emotion, behaviour and cognition. Structural brain imaging can assist in diagnosing Lewy body dementia by ruling out other causes of cognitive decline. Cerebral atrophy, varying in severity with dementia stage, may also be seen on brain imaging but is not unique to LBD. When compared with healthy controls and patients with Alzheimer's disease, individuals with dementia with Lewy bodies and Parkinson's disease dementia show greater occipital hypometabolism on FDG-PET. Using tracers that bind specifically to dopamine and other monoamine transporters, PET and SPECT imaging can be used to investigate how intact the nigrostriatal dopaminergic pathways are. Reduced striatal tracer uptake can be seen in dementia with Lewy bodies and Parkinson's disease dementia and points to dysfunction within nigrostriatal dopaminergic pathways. Functional DaT imaging (a type of SPECT imaging that uses radioactive tracers that bind to the presynaptic striatal dopamine transporter—DaT) can help distinguish dementia with Lewy bodies and Parkinson's disease dementia from Alzheimer's disease, as the nigrostriatal system is better preserved in the latter (McKeith et al., 2007; Erkkinen et al., 2018).	Great caution is required in prescribing antipsychotic medication to patients with suspected LBD, as a subset has severe dopamine agonist sensitivity. Acute reactions include altered conscious state, exacerbation of psychotic symptoms and irreversible parkinsonism, sometimes together with other features of neuroleptic malignant syndrome. Other psychotropic agents, such as sodium valproate, may be preferable to antipsychotics in treating behavioural and psychological symptoms of dementia. Cholinesterase inhibitors may be particularly helpful in attenuating the vivid visual hallucinations associated with this condition.

Vascular disease		
Clinical presentation	**Pathology and imaging**	**Management**
Patients in this category exhibit cognitive deficits as a result of a diverse range of vascular pathology, established by clinical history and examination or diagnostic imaging. The clinical picture depends on the location and extent of the vascular damage, e.g. parietal lobe involvement may present with visuospatial problems. Vascular dementia is likely if vascular risk factors are present (hypertension, smoking, diabetes mellitus and atrial fibrillation) and cognitive deficits arise abruptly after a stroke, are patchy in nature or have a stepwise course. Common noncognitive symptoms include abnormal gait or frequent falls, urinary incontinence and focal neurological deficits.	The vascular changes seen pathologically and reflected on brain imaging are variable. Lesions highly correlated with dementia are large vessel ischaemic stroke or dominant hemisphere boundary zone infarcts; bilateral anterior infarcts; extensive or bilateral thalamic infarcts; inferior medial temporal lobe infarcts; and association area infarcts (parieto-temporal and temporo-occipital). Severe white matter disease may be associated with dementia, but imaging findings should be interpreted cautiously, as white matter changes are present in many older adults without clinical cognitive impairment.	While vascular dementia is not reversible, identification and treatment of vascular risk factors may reduce further cerebrovascular damage. Cognitive enhancing medications may benefit some patients with mixed vascular dementia and Alzheimer's pathology. Behavioural and psychological symptoms of dementia associated with vascular disease are managed similarly as in Alzheimer's disease.
Frontotemporal lobar degeneration or Pick's disease		
Clinical presentation	**Pathology and imaging**	**Management**
Three distinct clinical syndromes are recognised, each characterised by a predominant feature, but all involving an overlap of behavioural and personality changes and/or aphasia: **Behavioural variant frontotemporal dementia** presents with personality changes, apathy, emotional blunting, social disinhibition, hyperorality, repetitive behaviour and poor insight. **Semantic dementia** presents with lack of word comprehension and naming in the setting of fluent speech. Generic or broad terms tend to be used in place of words with a precise meaning. **Progressive non-fluent aphasia** involves effortful, grammatically inaccurate speech, with word-finding difficulties and later problems naming objects.	Inclusions that are positive for ubiquitin or tau (the latter sometimes forming spherical aggregates known as Pick bodies) are found at post mortem and have been linked to genetic mutations. Frontal and temporal lobe atrophy are often seen on brain imaging in the behavioural variant of this condition, but are not essential for diagnosis. Left-sided anterior temporal lobe atrophy is characteristic of semantic dementia, whereas left-sided perisylvian atrophy is common in progressive non-fluent aphasia.	Management is focused on relieving symptoms and supporting patients, families and carers. Psychoeducation to increase carers' knowledge of the condition and impart coping strategies (such as avoidance of confrontation and tolerance of obsessions) may improve patients' quality of life and relieve carer burden. Speech therapy may help alleviate language problems. Psychotropic medication may be cautiously prescribed for behavioural or mood disturbances. Cholinesterase inhibitors, as used in Alzheimer's disease, are not indicated in the treatment of frontotemporal dementia.

Source: Adapted from Kester & Scheltens, 2009

dementia may still be difficult, as patients with the latter can display disorganised thinking, perceptual disturbance, altered consciousness and inattention even in the absence of delirium. An acute change in mental state and worsening of baseline dementia symptoms provide clues to the diagnosis of delirium in this patient group (Han et al., 2010).

Management of medical comorbidity

Cases of reversible dementia are rarely encountered clinically, but identifying and correcting any potentially reversible medical causes is nevertheless important. The gradual cognitive decline seen in reversible dementia helps distinguish this condition from delirium, with its rapid cognitive decline (Han et al., 2010). Normal pressure hydrocephalus is a potentially treatable cause of reversible cognitive impairment that is worth looking for, but is uncommon. In other cases, identifying and correcting unrecognised medical conditions, such as anaemia, hypothyroidism, or B12 deficiency is intended primarily to maximise patients' overall level of functioning, but direct benefits on cognitive performance may occasionally ensue.

MANAGEMENT OF DEMENTIA

Management of cognitive symptoms

There are currently two classes of cognitive enhancing medication that can help to slow the progression of the cognitive and functional decline associated with Alzheimer's disease, but which cannot ultimately reverse the condition. These medications are the cholinesterase inhibitors (donepezil, rivastigmine and galantamine) and the N-methyl-D-aspartate (NMDA) receptor antagonist, memantine.

Cholinesterase inhibitors (donepezil, rivastigmine and galantamine), which are most frequently used in mild to moderate cases of Alzheimer's disease, inhibit the cholinesterase enzyme in the synaptic cleft (see Chapter 2.5), thereby enhancing the reduced cholinergic neurotransmission seen in this condition. Prior to prescription, patient and carer expectations in relation to these agents should be ascertained; potential side effects (such as exacerbation of bradycardia) discussed; and their limitations (symptomatic relief of cognitive impairment that may diminish with advancing illness) explained. NMDA receptor antagonists (memantine) offer a novel approach to Alzheimer's disease treatment by acting on the glutamatergic system, dysfunction of which results in neuronal excitotoxicity. Memantine is most frequently used for moderate to severe Alzheimer's disease, sometimes in combination with a cholinesterase inhibitor. There is little evidence supporting a switch between cholinesterase inhibitors, and decisions regarding discontinuation of any of these treatments require clinical judgement.

For many years, Alzheimer's disease research has been focused on developing a disease-modifying therapy to reduce the accumulation or promote the removal of the β-amyloid plaques central disease neuropathology. Strategies for achieving this have included trying to prevent plaque formation by impeding secretase enzyme activity on amyloid precursor protein and using antibodies to remove β-amyloid monomers, oligomers, or plaques. However, hopes of a disease-modifying therapy have been tempered by the failure of over a dozen anti-amyloid drugs, most recently aducanumab after a futility analysis indicated it had no significant prospect of clinical efficacy despite earlier data showing promise in dose-dependent plaque removal and slower disease progression. The incomplete understanding of Alzheimer's disease pathogenesis offered by the amyloid cascade hypothesis has been postulated to account for failure to progress this line of research (Forester, Patrick, & Harper, 2019).

While future research should seek to optimise anti-amyloid drug trials, diversification into non-amyloid-related research (e.g. inflammation and mitochondrial functioning) has been suggested to be important along with increased emphasis on prevention-related research (e.g. physical inactivity and other modifiable risk factors). Government sponsoring to facilitate data sharing between academia, health care providers and the pharmaceutical industry has also been proposed to propel the field forward (e.g. extensive genetic, transcriptomic and proteomic data repositories are now available which would have been unheard of when dementia clinical drug trials first commenced)

(Forester et al., 2019). Despite the setbacks identified above, Alzheimer's disease drug development has remained strong, with 132 compounds in the drug development pipeline in 2019, including 96 in disease modification trials (Cummings, Lee, Ritter, Sabbagh, & Zhong, 2019). While the ischaemic damage underlying the various types of vascular dementia is not reversible, it is reasonable to optimise cardiovascular health, such as treating hypertension and elevated cholesterol, and to consider anticoagulation with aspirin as a means of reducing future stroke risk.

Psychiatric complications and their management

A key focus of dementia care is in the management of behavioural and psychological symptoms of dementia (BPSD). This term encompasses a range of behavioural and psychological symptoms that some, but not all, patients may experience secondary to their dementia. Examples of behavioural symptoms include agitation (increased physical movement, such as pacing, that does not serve a clear functional purpose); wandering; and verbal and physical aggression. Examples of psychological symptoms include the emergence of anxiety, depression or psychosis. The term 'BPSD' covers a broad spectrum of psychopathology, and it is insufficient to simply state that a patient has BPSD without elaborating on the nature of problematic symptoms. BPSD are being increasingly recognised as a major factor in the clinical diversity seen in Alzheimer's disease, as well as being implicated in disease severity and rate of decline.

To work effectively with people with dementia, it is important to adopt an approach that is respectful of people's individuality, accommodating of their cognitive and functional deficits and mindful of their basic need for human contact. Thus familiarisation with a patient's background and preferences, as well as current symptom profile, may allow implementation of individually tailored psychosocial interventions (see Chapters 2.3 and 2.4). Taking time to talk a patient clearly through personal care interventions as they occur may help avert resistive or aggressive reactions. Similarly, withdrawing temporarily from a patient who is becoming distressed during care-related activities and revisiting the same tasks later (when the patient is more relaxed) may prevent needless activation of aggression. Positive interactions between patients with dementia on the one hand and clinicians and carers on the other are key to successful care delivery (including implementation of psychosocial treatments for BPSD), and should be aimed for at all times.

In the first instance, any reversible causes of BPSD should be identified and addressed. Loneliness and boredom, whether in residential care settings or the home environment, can be relieved by involvement in structured activities programs. Such programs are often delivered in residential facilities by specially trained activities workers. Patients residing at home with their family may benefit from an activities schedule devised by an occupational therapist (see Chapters 2.1, 2.3 and 2.6), which may include involvement in day programs outside the home. There is evidence that adequate management of pain—which may be overlooked because of patients' limited ability to communicate its presence—can help attenuate BPSD symptoms (Pieper et al., 2013; Dyer, Harrison, Laver, Whitehead, & Crotty, 2018). Close liaison with a patient's general practitioner (see Chapters 2.1 and 2.3) or physician is recommended in selecting appropriate analgesia.

Psychosocial approaches to reducing BPSD include aromatherapy, massage therapy, reminiscence therapy, validation therapy, and simulated presence therapy, though only music therapy and functional analysis-based interventions (interpreting behaviours as indicators of unmet needs) have convincing evidence (see Chapter 1.4) to support their effectiveness. Music therapy has also been found to reduce anxiety. There is also evidence that carer education, staff training in communication skills, and person-centred care are effective in reducing agitation (Abraha et al., 2017; Dyer et al., 2018). Depending on the setting in which they work, mental health clinicians may be involved in directly delivering psychosocial treatments to patients, teaching carers how to implement them or providing referral advice for accessing other treatment providers. It is worth noting that the effect sizes (see Chapter 1.4) found in studies of nonpharmacological interventions are comparable to those found in nonpharmacological interventions, and do not carry the same risks of side effects (Dyer et al., 2018).

Evidence supporting psychopharmacological approaches to managing BPSD is not robust, possibly because of difficulty undertaking well-designed medication trials in this impaired patient population. Despite this, antidepressants, benzodiazepines, antipsychotics and mood stabilisers (see Chapter 2.5) are frequently utilised and found to be clinically beneficial. Antidepressants are indicated in cases with objective evidence of depression. A short-acting benzodiazepine (such as oxazepam) may be particularly effective in relieving dementia-related anxiety and agitation. For more severe behavioural problems, such as repeated physical aggression, antipsychotic medication may be considered. The atypical antipsychotic risperidone (see Chapter 2.5) is licensed in Australia for severe BPSD. Other atypical antipsychotics, including aripiprazole, olanzapine and quetiapine, are not approved in Australia (or Canada, New Zealand, the UK and the US) for BPSD, so their use for this purpose is regarded as 'off-label'. Mood-stabilising medication, such as sodium valproate, can also be prescribed for severe cases of agitation, restlessness, aggression or disinhibition. Caution is required in prescribing psychotropic medication to patients with dementia, with low starting doses and incremental dose adjustment.

Medication use in dementia is not without risk. To compare the effectiveness and safety of atypical antipsychotics (aripiprazole, olanzapine, quetiapine and risperidone) in the management of BPSD, Yunusa and colleagues (Yunusa, Alsumali, Garba, Regestein, & Eguale, 2019) undertook a network meta-analysis. This technique, which represents a further development of traditional pairwise meta-analysis, allows inferences to be made about all possible comparisons between intervention pairs within a network of trials, even where such comparisons were never directly evaluated in the original trials. The authors concluded that a compromise between effectiveness and safety is inevitable in using atypical antipsychotics to treat BPSD and that there is no single agent with an optimal risk-benefit profile. The use of all atypical antipsychotics for BPSD was thus regarded as controversial given their advantages over placebo were modest, in contrast to their substantial risks. Specific findings from this network meta-analysis are summarised in Table 3.9.

The decision to introduce medication for BPSD should therefore be carefully considered, and medication only commenced as part of a comprehensive treatment program also involving psychosocial strategies. Once medication has been commenced, symptom monitoring is essential and treatments should be discontinued if unsuccessful. Symptoms will reduce with time, so successful treatments can be reduced or withdrawn at regular intervals (every six months, for instance) to check if they are still needed.

The correct identification of Lewy body disease (LBD) is particularly important in relation to managing BPSD. The reason for this is that antipsychotic medications, including newer atypical agents, can sometimes exacerbate rather than minimise psychotic symptoms due to LBD. While prescribing antipsychotics may inadvertently prove diagnostic, their use is best avoided if possible. Alternatively, recognition of vivid visual hallucinations as potentially LBD-related may allow their marked attenuated through cholinesterase inhibitor prescription. Where antipsychotic medication use is deemed unavoidable in this context, quetiapine is often preferred to minimise the chance of psychosis being paradoxically exacerbated.

Sundowning and its management

Sundowning (also known as 'sundowning syndrome' or 'nocturnal delirium') is the condition whereby behavioural disturbances in patients with cognitive impairment worsen in the late afternoon or evening. Sundowning is most commonly seen in dementia—but may also occur in delirium—and is associated with carer burnout and patient institutionalisation. Circadian rhythm irregularities and sleep fragmentation that progressively worsen with cognitive and functional decline are postulated aetiological factors. Measures that can be implemented to prevent the emergence of

Table 3.9 Atypical antipsychotics for BPSD: Meta-analytic findings

Measures of efficacy
• No atypical antipsychotic (aripiprazole, olanzapine, quetiapine, risperidone) demonstrated consistent superiority over others across all measures of effectiveness and safety. • Aripiprazole was more likely than placebo to be associated with an improvement across three behavioural measures (small effect size): Neuropsychiatric Inventory, Brief Psychiatric Rating Scale and Cohen-Mansfield Agitation Inventory. • Quetiapine was more likely than placebo to be associated with an improvement on the Brief Psychiatric Rating Scale only (small effect size). • Risperidone was more likely than placebo to be associated with an improvement on the Cohen-Mansfield Agitation Inventory only (small effect size). • Olanzapine did not demonstrate superiority over placebo on any efficacy measure.
Cerebrovascular accidents and risk of death
• Risperidone and olanzapine were more likely than placebo to be associated with cerebrovascular accidents. • No atypical antipsychotic agent was safer than others in relation to the risk of death.
Sedation or somnolence
• All atypical antipsychotics were more likely than placebo to be associated with sedation or somnolence. • Risperidone was less likely than olanzapine or quetiapine to be associated with sedation or somnolence.
Extrapyramidal side effects and falls
• Risperidone was more likely than placebo to be associated with extrapyramidal side effects. • Risperidone was less likely than olanzapine to be associated with injuries, fractures or falls. • Risperidone should be avoided for BPSD in the presence of Lewy body dementia or Parkinson's disease to prevent worsening of extrapyramidal side effects. • Quetiapine was less likely than olanzapine and risperidone to be associated with extrapyramidal side effects. • Quetiapine and aripiprazole were ranked most favourably for averting extrapyramidal side effects.
Other atypical antipsychotics
• Evidence to recommend or validate the use of asenapine, clozapine, lurasidone, paliperidone, and ziprasidone is lacking.

Source: Yunusa et al., 2019

sundowning or limit its severity include minimising environmental changes; reducing excessive noise; ensuring adequate light exposure; promoting participation in daytime activities; avoiding night-time disruptions; discontinuing medications that can impair cognition (for example, anticholinergics); and ensuring optimal management of medical comorbidities (Mittal et al., 2011).

MILD NEUROCOGNITIVE DISORDER/MILD COGNITIVE IMPAIRMENT

Definition and subtypes

Mild Cognitive Impairment (MCI; ICD-10 and DSM-IV) is now referred to as Mild Neurocognitive Disorder (MCD; ICD-11, DSM-5—here noting that 'MND' also has common usage for motor neurone disease). MCD is distinguished by a decline in cognitive function above that seen with normal ageing, and often apparent to patients themselves and occasionally others close to them. The shift in nomenclature from MCI to MCD can be seen as marking a transition from a syndrome to a disorder, however one that still includes multiple diseases since the diagnosis does not imply known aetiology (see Chapter 2.3). A particular significance of MCD/MCI relates to the increased risk of developing Alzheimer's disease or other types of dementia compared to similarly aged individuals in the general population, with a 40–80% five-year conversion rate in most clinic-based studies. (The rate is considerably lower in community-based cohorts; see Chapter 1.4.) In the absence of serious accompanying behavioural or psychological difficulties, patients with MCD/MCI are more likely to present for initial cognitive assessment to a memory clinic than a public mental health service. Nevertheless, many older adults seen by mental health workers for other reasons have minor coexisting cognitive deficits consistent with this condition. According to ICD-11 (World Health Organization, 2018e), MCD/MCI is:

- characterised by the subjective experience of cognitive decline from a prior level of functioning
- accompanied by objective evidence of cognitive impairment in one or more domains relative to what would be expected for the person's age and general intellectual functioning
- not of sufficient severity to significantly impede the independent performance of activities of daily living (Abraha et al., 2017).

Furthermore, according to ICD-11 (World Health Organization, 2018), the cognitive impairment of MCD/MCI is:

- not entirely due to normal ageing
- attributable to an underlying nervous system disease, trauma, infection or other condition affecting specific parts of the brain or to the long-term use of particular substances or medications
- of undeterminable aetiology in some cases (World Health Organization, 2018).

Amnestic and non-amnestic MCD/MCI subtypes are recognised by some authors. Amnestic MCD/MCI is characterised primarily by clinically significant memory impairment, with or without some minor inadequacies in other cognitive domains. While falling short of criteria for dementia, the amnestic deficits may eventually progress to Alzheimer's disease. The less common non-amnestic MCD/MCI may be characterised by minor deficits in single or multiple non-memory domains (Chertkow et al., 2008; Petersen, 2011).

Predictors of progression from MCD/MCI to dementia

Patients with MCD/MCI who have greater baseline cognitive impairment are more likely to progress to dementia, probably because they are closer to the diagnostic threshold for dementia. A variety of biomarkers has been suggested in research settings to be predictive of progression from amnestic MCD/MCI to Alzheimer's disease. However, evidence supporting their routine clinical use is insufficient, with further research required to determine their role, optimal cut-off points and reliability (Petersen, 2011; Petersen et al., 2018).

Clinical identification and management

The same general approach to diagnosing dementia—encompassing history taking, physical examination, brief cognitive testing and investigations for reversible causes of cognitive impairment—is also relevant to diagnosing MCD/MCI. In this schema, the role of brain imaging is properly limited to ruling out conditions such as vascular disease or hydrocephalus that might explain cognitive decline, rather than determining a prognosis. Detailed neuropsychological testing is warranted in many cases to differentiate subtle deficits from normal ageing. Patients should not be falsely reassured that they are normal but, rather, offered a diagnosis of MCD/MCI where appropriate and counselled about its possible implications (progression to dementia) and prognostic limitations (inability to definitively predict progression based on current knowledge). Given the unclear prognosis, clinical reassessment every six to 12 months is recommended.

In updating its 2001 guideline on MCD/MCI, the American Academy of Neurology made eight recommendations for assessing this condition (Petersen et al., 2018, see also Table 3.10). Recommendations were made by a panel of experts not only on the basis of evidence from a systematic review of the topic, but also strong associated evidence, standard management principles, and judgements. For each recommendation, a level of obligation (A—Must, B—Should, C—May and U—No recommendation supported) was determined based on the strength of these postulates and the risk-benefit ratio of following it. Importance of outcomes, differences in patient preference, financial burden and availability of intervention were factors considered in adjusting assigned levels

Table 3.10 Recommendations for assessing MCD/MCI (American Academy of Neurology)

	Recommendation	Level of obligation*
A1	Concerns about impaired memory or cognition raised by a patient or close acquaintance should prompt assessment for MCD/MCI and not assumed to be due to normal aging.	B
A2	Assessment of cognitive impairment should not be based exclusively on historic accounts of subjective memory problems (in undertaking a Medical Annual Wellness Visit in the United States).	B
A3	Validated assessment tools should be used to assess for MCD/MCI where assessment or screening is indicated. Formal clinical assessment for MCD/MCI should follow where testing is positive for the condition.	B
A4	The presence of cognition-related functional impairment should be established before a diagnosis of dementia is given to a patient with MCD/MCI.	B
A5	Clinicians lacking experience in cognitive assessment should refer patients with suspected MCD/MCI for specialist evaluation.	B
A6	Patients diagnosed with MCD/MCI should be medically evaluated for potentially modifiable MCD/MCI risk factors.	B
A7a	Patients and families enquiring about MCD/MCI biomarkers should be advised that no such biomarkers are currently accepted.	B
A7b	The option of biomarker research should be discussed with interested patients and referral to centres or organisations that may link them into this research considered.	C
A8	Serial cognitive assessments should be performed in patients with diagnosed MCD/MCI to detect changes in cognition over time.	B

*Level of Obligation: A—Must, B—Should, C—May and U—No recommendation supported

Source: Petersen et al., 2018

A range of interventions are available in managing patients with MCD/MCI, which may help minimise existing cognitive impairment and possibly delay its progression (although strong supporting evidence from randomised controlled trials is limited). Thus comorbid conditions that may exacerbate and amplify cognitive decline should be identified and treated. These include sleep disorders such as sleep apnoea and depression. Social interactions can be promoted to counter isolation. Optimal treatment of vascular risk factors, particularly hypertension, is also recommended. Both healthy older adults and those with MCI can be encouraged to set aside adequate leisure time and participate in aerobic exercise and intellectually stimulating activities as part of a healthy lifestyle. Evidence supporting the use of pharmacological interventions for MCD/MCI is currently insufficient to support regular clinical use (Chertkow et al., 2008; Petersen, 2011; Petersen et al., 2018).

In updating its 2001 guideline on MCD/MCI, the American Academy of Neurology also made eight recommendations regarding its management (Petersen et al., 2018, see Table 3.11). Recommendations were developed and a level of obligation assigned to each in the same manner as for assessment-related recommendations.

MEDICOLEGAL ISSUES STEMMING FROM COGNITIVE DECLINE

Substitute decision making

'Enduring power of attorney' is the legal process in most Australian states and territories whereby a person (the 'donor') assigns certain functions (that he or she would normally undertake) to another individual (the 'attorney'), in a manner allowing the attorney to continue exercising these functions after the donor loses capacity to do so. The term is often

Table 3.11 Recommendations for managing MCD/MCI (American Academy of Neurology)

	Recommendation	Level of obligation*
B1	Patients with diagnosed MCD/MCI should be weaned from medications that may give rise to cognitive decline and have potentially modifiable risk factors treated.	B
B2	Patients with MCD/MCI and their families should be counselled that no medications or dietary factors are known to symptomatically benefit cognition and no medications are approved by the FDA for this condition.	B
B3a	Clinicians may elect to not offer cholinesterase inhibitors to patients with a diagnosis of MCD/MCI.	B
B3b	If clinicians decide to suggest cholinesterase inhibitors, they must inform patients that such prescriptions are off-label and not evidence-based.	A
B4	Referral of patients interested in pharmacological treatment for MCD/MCI to centres or organisations that may link into clinical trials should be considered.	C
B5	Patients diagnosed with MCD/MCI should be advised to exercise twice weekly as part of their overall care.	B
B6	Diagnosis and prognostic uncertainties should be discussed with patients with MCD/MCI and patients and families encouraged to plan ahead in the areas of advance care directives, finances, estate planning and safe driving.	B
B7	Behavioural and neuropsychiatric symptoms in MCD/MCI should be examined for and treated with non-pharmacologic and pharmacologic means when appropriate.	B
B8	Cognitive treatments may be recommended in patients with MCD/MCI.	C

*Level of Obligation: A—Must, B—Should, C—May and U—No recommendation supported

Source: Petersen et al., 2018

used to denote a financial enduring power of attorney, in which authority is given to the donor to manage financial, property-related and legal matters on behalf of the donor. Appointment of a medical enduring power of attorney or substitute decision maker for health care matters follows the same principles, but involves the authority to make medical care decisions on the donor's behalf being assigned to the attorney or decision maker. Provisions also generally exist across Australia for the appointment of an enduring attorney or guardian or a substitute decision maker to make lifestyle-related decisions, such as where a person lives or who they live with. The advantage of assigning powers of attorney or appointing a substitute decision maker is that the donor is able to determine actively who can make financial, medical or lifestyle decisions on his or her behalf once he or she is no longer able to do so. A key limitation is that these powers cannot readily be reversed once activated.

The terminology used in relation to powers of attorney or substitute decision making varies between states and territories. Provisions for appointing others to make future financial, health care or lifestyle decisions vary in different parts of Australia. Planning tools available on the Dementia Australia website (Dementia Australia, 2020) provide information on these variations.Despite the increased legal attention afforded to this concept in recent years, it is the authors' experience that few older adults with mental illness or dementia avail themselves of the opportunity to formally document their future care preferences (in the event of losing decision-making capacity).

In the event of a power of attorney or substitute decision maker not having been assigned by a person prior to losing decision-making capacity, applications can be made to relevant legal bodies in some states and territories for the formal appointment of another individual to make financial decisions (referred to as an 'administrator' in some jurisdictions) or medical or lifestyle decisions (referred to as a 'guardian' in some jurisdictions). Such a process may also be applicable in the event that abuse of a previously appointed power of attorney or substitute decision maker is suspected. A key difference between substitute decision makers appointed by an individual compared to those appointed by a tribunal or similar body is that periodic reporting of how assigned authorities are being executed is usually required in the case of the latter (thereby affording individuals with dementia an additional layer of protection against potential exploitation).

Psychiatrists or neuropsychologists may be asked to determine whether a person has the capacity to assign an enduring power of attorney. In order to do so, a person should be able to explain:

- why he or she might make a power of attorney
- what the attorney will be able to do, particularly with the person's money and property
- whom he or she would choose as the attorney and why
- that if the person's medical condition deteriorates and he or she is no longer able to manage his or her own affairs, the attorney can continue doing so and this arrangement cannot be cancelled.

Testamentary capacity

Testamentary capacity is a related issue that old age psychiatrists and neuropsychologists may be called to give an opinion on. Testamentary capacity refers to an individual's ability to make a valid will. Cognitive deficits and other symptoms of mental illness, such as floridly delusional beliefs with schizophrenia or a markedly pessimistic outlook with severe depression, may impair a patient's ability in this regard. As in the case of capacity to appoint an enduring power of attorney, individuals exhibiting cognitive impairment of an equivocal nature may require detailed neuropsychological testing as part of the assessment process.

The key features required for testamentary capacity are:

- knowledge of the extent and value of one's property
- awareness of who the natural beneficiaries of the will are
- awareness of the disposition one is making
- ability to relate these elements to formulate an orderly property distribution plan.

Driving assessment

Requirements relating to the reporting of older drivers with impaired ability to drive (either established or suspected) to licensing authorities may vary between jurisdictions. Consultation with an occupational therapist driving assessor is recommended. Psychiatrists or other medical practitioners may be required to prepare relevant psychiatric and medical reports about a person's ability to drive with reference to local legislative requirements. A driving assessor may then follow up with written and on-road driving assessments (the latter using a specially modified vehicle). Together, the medical reports and the results of driving assessment allow licensing authorities to decide whether to allow an individual to continue driving.

Elder abuse

Elder abuse can occur in various forms. Financial abuse, sometimes involving misappropriation of a person's money under a previously appointed enduring power of attorney, is perhaps the most commonly recognised form. Neglect in the provision of personal care to frail older adults, with or without cognitive impairment, may also occur. Again, this may sometimes be partially driven by financial considerations, as in the case of family members who fail to access appropriate personal care services for elders—either home-based or at a residential care facility—to avoid associated costs. In more extreme cases, overt physical or even sexual abuse may occur. These latter two forms of abuse are sometimes particularly difficult to address, as the perpetrators may be aged care facility co-residents experiencing a degree of cognitive impairment themselves. However, elder abuse has received increasing attention in recent years and, in some jurisdictions, may be the subject of mandatory reporting requirements for mental health and other professionals. Parallel to this, legal services focused on assisting older adults to defend their rights have also been established. Applications for administration and guardianship sometimes need to be initiated by mental health clinicians and other health workers for cases of elder abuse which cannot be redressed less formally.

3.3.6 MOOD DISORDERS

CLINICAL FEATURES OF DEPRESSION IN OLDER ADULTS

Older people are at risk of developing depression for a range of reasons, including a past history of depression, social isolation, an anxious personality, bereavement, physical illness, pain and loss of independence (Park & Unutzer, 2011). The risk of developing depression among aged care facility residents, who may have several of these risk factors, is particularly high. Although depression is common among older adults, the diagnosis is sometimes missed as the presentation may be different to that seen in younger adults (see Chapter 4.2). Older adults are more likely to present with hypochondriacal symptoms that can sometimes reach delusional intensity. An example of this is older adults who become preoccupied with the notion that their bowel functioning is abnormal. Coexisting features of depression–such as lowered mood, disturbed sleep and poor appetite and energy–are usually apparent on careful assessment, but may be overlooked initially in the quest to find a medical explanation for the bowel complaints. The eventual identification of a depressive cause for the patient's complaints allows the introduction of appropriate antidepressant treatment. If the underlying depression proves to be medication resistant, electroconvulsive therapy may be warranted and give rise to satisfactory resolution of a patient's physical complaints and lowered mood.

DEPRESSION OR DEMENTIA?

The presence of depression in older adults can often result in secondary cognitive deficits, which may be significant enough to arouse suspicions of a dementing illness. Distinguishing between true dementia and so-called 'pseudo-dementia' secondary to depression is not always straightforward. Depressive illness may also emerge in the setting of established dementia, and secondary cognitive deficits can remain even after depressive symptoms are treated, further complicating the clinical picture. In such clinical scenarios, it is important to look for evidence of both depressive symptoms and cognitive impairment on history and examination and, if both are present, to determine the temporal sequence in which they have arisen relative to each other. Collateral history from an informant who is well acquainted with the patient may be critical in ensuring the accuracy of this assessment. Other clues may be afforded by a patient's presentation at interview. For example, a patient's approach to cognitive testing may be particularly informative. Patients with true cognitive decline may reluctantly persist with cognitive examination and assume a defensive approach in trying to minimise or rationalise any cognitive difficulties exposed by such testing. Alternatively, patients with 'pseudo-dementia' are more likely to display attention difficulties that impair memory retrieval or give up entirely on difficult test items and convey depressive, self-derogatory cognitions in trying to explain their reasons for doing so (Leyhe et al., 2017).

MANAGEMENT OF DEPRESSIVE DISORDER

A range of psychosocial, behavioural and pharmacological approaches are often required for the successful treatment of depressive disorder in older adults (Andreescu & Reynolds, 2011). While the broad principles of managing depression are the same in older and younger adults, treatment modifications are sometimes required to account for psychological, physical and social changes that occur with advancing age. There is no reason why older adults cannot participate in a range of psychological therapies for depression. Evidence suggests, however, that they are less likely to be offered such therapy in comparison to medication (Draper & Koschera, 2001). Patient preference may be one explanation for this trend, with some older people being unaccustomed to the notion of a talking therapy as a means of relieving emotional distress. The perceived stigma attached to mental illness by past generations may lead older adults to minimise psychological symptoms or attribute them to physical illness. Patient awareness of emerging cognitive decline may also discourage participation in psychotherapy. In turn, an exaggeration of such concerns by treating clinicians may limit the range of treatments they are prepared to offer patients.

Psychological treatments

Engaging older patients in a relaxed, safe environment through psychoeducation may serve as a base from which more advanced psychotherapy can proceed. CBT, interpersonal therapy and problem-solving therapy (see Chapters 2.6 and 4.3) have been shown to yield comparable improvements in depressive symptoms to pharmacological interventions, but may require adaptation to account for cognitive and sensory deficits in older adults. Conducting sessions at a rate that older adults can process, alteration of session lengths, taking a supportive rather than neutral therapeutic stance, and rehearsing important takeaway messages can help to engage patients with limited cognitive resources and increase their comprehension and uptake of the therapy (Leyhe et al., 2017).

Significant problems with effectiveness and equity of the Better Access scheme—as the major innovation in psychological care delivery in recent times in Australia—have been discussed elsewhere in this text (see Chapters 1.5 and 1.7). One very obvious gap of the scheme for much of its existence has been the exclusion of older adults living in residential care with poor access to psychologists and psychology services within the residential aged care sector (van Gaans & Dent, 2018). A detailed description of how aged care sector psychology services can be further improved is contained in a detailed submission by the Australian Psychological Society to the Royal Commission into Aged Care Quality and Safety (Australian Psychological Society (APS), 2020e).

From a psychiatry of old age perspective, it would be useful to know how effectively the Better Access scheme is accessed by older Australians, given that past data is suggestive of older adults being offered primarily biological treatments (such as medications and ECT) rather than psychotherapy for their mental health conditions. An evaluation of the suitability of psychological services delivered to those older adults who do manage to access them (either within or outside this scheme) would also be helpful. Both questions are worthy of further research.

Antidepressant medication

It is important to avoid undertreating depression in older adults. Thus while caution in initiating and adjusting antidepressants is warranted in this patient population, medications can be increased to standard adult doses if well tolerated. A selective serotonin reuptake inhibitor (SSRI), such as escitalopram, is an appropriate first-line antidepressant, given the good tolerability of this class of medications. A serotonin and noradrenaline reuptake inhibitor (SNRI), such as venlafaxine, can be considered where a first-line agent has proven ineffective (see Chapter 2.5). Mirtazapine is also frequently used in older patients, and offers the added benefit of promoting sleep with its nightly dosing schedule. Older classes of medications, such as tricyclic antidepressants (TCAs) and irreversible monoamine oxidase inhibitors (MAOIs), are also available, but infrequently used because of their greater potential for adverse effects. The anticholinergic side effects (including blurred vision and confusion) of TCAs may be particularly difficult for older patients to tolerate, and their propensity for cardiotoxicity warrants particular attention in this population. The dietary restrictions required for safe MAOI use tends to limit their use to the most extreme cases of treatment-resistant illness.

While newer antidepressants are thought of as safer overall for older patients, their use in this age group is entirely without risk. For example, newly initiated SSRIs or venlafaxine are strongly associated with hospitalisation due to hyponatraemia among older adults whereas mirtazapine and tricyclic antidepressants are associated with a small to moderate risk. To mitigate this risk, weekly sodium level checks are recommended upon initiating and up-titrating antidepressant medication in older patients. By contrast, ongoing antidepressant pharmacotherapy has not been found to increase the risk of hyponatraemia-related hospitalisation (Farmand et al., 2018).

A further risk of antidepressant use in older adults is the development of QTc interval prolongation on the ECG. A normal QTc interval is less than 450 ms for men and 460 ms for women with prolonged intervals of 500 ms or over engendering a high risk of Torsades de Pointes, an uncommon but potentially fatal polymorphic ventricular tachycardia. TCAs and citalopram are most likely to cause QTc prolongation in older adults whereas SSRIs and SNRIs on their own do not appear to increase the risk significantly (Rochester, Kane, Linnebur, & Fixen, 2018). As with sodium level checks for the detection of hyponatraemia, weekly ECGs are recommended in older adults upon initiating and up-titrating antidepressant medication to detect this potentially dangerous complication.

Electroconvulsive therapy

Older adults are particularly vulnerable to developing severe depression (Sorrell, 2016) with psychiatric hospital discharges for psychotic depression peaking in men in their early seventies and women in their late seventies (Draper & Low, 2009). Psychotic symptoms and psychomotor retardation (a physical sign of melancholia) are independent predictors of a good response to electroconvulsive therapy (ECT) (van der Wurff, Stek, Hoogendijk, & Beekman, 2003). For this reason, ECT may be an appropriate antidepressant treatment in this patient group, often (but not always) giving rise to a very satisfactory therapeutic response where medication has previously failed. Increased medical comorbidity among older adults may be a relative limiting factor from an anaesthetic perspective. However, such concerns must be counterbalanced against the risk of untreated depression giving rise to medical instability—because of inadequate intake of oral fluid, food and medication—in deciding whether ECT is a suitable treatment option on a case-by-case basis.

On the negative side, ECT may be more likely to result in immediate post-ECT confusion and short-term cognitive impairment (including problems with attention and new learning) in older than younger individuals. Enduring ECT-related cognitive deficits are uncommon, mostly involving deterioration in memory for personal and autobiographic events (autobiographical memory) (Gardner & O'Connor, 2008; O'Connor, Gardner, Eppingstall, & Tofler, 2010). Strategies used to minimise adverse cognitive effects of conventional, brief pulse width ECT include use of right unilateral electrode placement (switching to bitemporal treatment only if therapeutic response is suboptimal) and spacing treatments out from thrice to twice weekly. Apart from the traditional bitemporal approach to administering bilateral treatment, a bifrontal electrode placement may be utilised in which the electrodes are placed 3–5 cm above the outer angle of both orbits. In avoiding direct stimulation over the temporal lobes, it is hoped that bifrontal ECT will confer comparable therapeutic effects to conventional bitemporal treatment but with fewer side effects.

An additional approach in administering ECT, that is also motivated by a desire to minimise cognitive side effects, is the adoption of a 0.3 ms ultrabrief pulse width in place of the usual 0.5–2 ms pulse width. The object of this is to allow neurons to depolarise and stimulate seizures at lower electrical doses. Unilateral ultrabrief pulse ECT is effective and associated with significantly fewer cognitive sequelae than standard brief pulse unilateral treatment but response is a little slower and more treatments are required. Counterintuitively, bitemporal ultrabrief stimuli are strikingly less effective than unilateral ultrabrief stimuli. Ultrabrief pulse treatment is recommended for older people with pre-existing cognitive impairment, those who became confused after previous courses or who fear post-treatment memory loss. Despite the great emphasis placed on optimising ECT treatment technique to minimise adverse cognitive sequelae, it should be borne in mind that ECT may actually result in improved cognitive functioning in many older adults experiencing temporary cognitive impairment secondary to their depression (Verwijk et al., 2014).

Repetitive transcranial stimulation

A newer biological treatment option for depression is repetitive transcranial stimulation (rTMS), which relies on a magnetic field to stimulate parts of the brain implicated in depressive illness. A significant advantage of rTMS over ECT is that its non-convulsive stimuli do not require a general anaesthetic and muscle relaxant, thereby allowing the treatment to be administered to conscious patients on a minimally disruptive, outpatient basis. While most research in rTMS has been undertaken in younger adults, there is some evidence supporting its use in older adults (Iriarte & George, 2018). But a constraint in its use to treat depressed older adults to date in Australia has been the lack of a Medicare subsidy for the procedure. This has seen rTMS being offered almost exclusively in the private sector, where it may be out of the reach of older individuals with mental illness who do not have the means to afford private health insurance.

BIPOLAR AFFECTIVE DISORDER IN LATER LIFE

Older patients with bipolar affective disorder (see Chapter 4.3) can be considered in two broad categories (Dols et al., 2014). The first includes those with an onset of bipolar illness in young adulthood and continued illness episodes later in life. The second includes patients who develop bipolar illness for the first illness time as older adults. Late-onset manic episodes may sometimes be triggered by coexisting physical illness, such as infection or cancer, or its treatment. Identifying and treating acute physical precipitants of mania is therefore clearly important. In other cases, however, manic symptoms may be a manifestation of underlying neurodegenerative changes (relating to vascular disease, for example) that are otherwise clinically unapparent but which may progress to dementia over time. For this reason, a first episode of mania in an older adult without a past history of significant mental illness requires particularly careful assessment, management and follow up. Investigative work-up of an older adult with manic symptoms should be thorough, with applicable tests selected from the list of medical investigations outlined earlier in this chapter. Following the resolution of acute mania, there may be a role for baseline neuropsychological assessment to allow for future comparison.

Lithium (see Chapter 2.5) remains a standard bipolar disorder treatment among older people, in both acute mania and the maintenance phase. However, concerns relating to renal disease, endocrine effects, lithium toxicity and medication interactions are very pertinent in this population. Rather than abandoning lithium use in older patients, increased vigilance in monitoring serum lithium levels, renal and thyroid function and medication interactions is recommended. Older adults have also been found to need lower dose regimens to experience effectiveness (De Fazio et al., 2017). Where lithium is inappropriate, the mood stabiliser sodium valproate may be easier to use as a result of less stringent monitoring requirements. Newer antipsychotic medications with antimanic and mood-stabilising properties, such as olanzapine and quetiapine, offer an additional option for acute mania and maintenance bipolar treatment, but their use is not without complication (see Chapter 2.5.) Antidepressant prescription for patients with severe bipolar depression or recurrent depressive relapses may be unavoidable, but caution is required because of the potential for inducing mania. Optimal concurrent use of mood-stabilising medication may reduce the likelihood of a manic switch. Electroconvulsive therapy should not be overlooked in bipolar disorder, as it can treat severe depression and mania safely and effectively, including in patients who have difficulty tolerating medication side effects.

Pharmacotherapy should occur in the context of broad psychosocial support for patients and carers, including individual or family-focused psychotherapeutic approaches and psychoeducation about early warning signs of relapse, appropriate activity levels and good sleep hygiene. Multidisciplinary team members are well positioned to provide such support in public mental health care settings.

PRACTICE ILLUSTRATION: SEVERE DEPRESSION REQUIRING ELECTROCONVULSIVE THERAPY

Vicky is a 67-year-old woman of Greek origin who migrated to Australia with her older sister at 19 years of age and immediately set to work in a textile factory. She married at 21 years of age and went on to have two sons and a daughter, all of whom have remained close to their parents and continue to provide ongoing support. She experienced her first episode of serious mental illness when aged 29, being hospitalised at the time and treated with electroconvulsive therapy (ECT). Review of her clinical record indicated a complex past psychiatric history, with several further admissions in her thirties during which she did not require ECT but was variously diagnosed as suffering from schizophrenia, depression or 'manic depression'. These episodes were associated with progressive functional decline, with Vicky struggling to maintain employment in a number of factory jobs over the years because of feeling increasingly victimised by and isolated from work colleagues. Her most recent psychiatric admission had taken place ten years previously when she was aged 57. Detailed medical notes available from this admission were clearly indicative of a severe depressive episode with psychotic features. Vicky was again treated with ECT for this episode, requiring 14 treatments in total. Although her mental state remained stable on nortriptyline in the ensuing decade, the severity of this last illness episode had seriously shaken her self-confidence and prompted early retirement.

On this occasion, Vicky was referred to the public aged mental health service for multidisciplinary management by her private psychiatrist after experiencing a relapse of her depression while remaining adherent to nortriptyline. Although it was initially planned to provide her with intensive community treatment, she was admitted to hospital after experiencing prominent thoughts of ending her life by strangulation. On admission, she was cooperative in manner, appeared and reported feeling low in mood, and described a range of depressive symptoms, including prominent nihilistic beliefs that she was dying. She scored 22/30 on the MMSE. In the absence of any account from her family of cognitive decline, and no remarkable findings on initial physical investigation, it was difficult to know for certain to what extent this score was reflective of her cultural and educational background or her current depressive state.

Vicky's family reported her current presentation to be consistent with that seen at the time of her last hospitalisation. After initial unsuccessful attempts to treat Vicky's depression pharmacologically (with addition of antipsychotic medication, olanzapine, optimisation of nortriptyline dose and subsequently switching to mirtazapine), a decision was reached with her and her family to embark on a further course of acute ECT. She was initially treated thrice weekly with a right unilateral electrode placement (as had been the case ten years previously) in an effort to minimise cognitive side effects. There was no discernible response after three treatments, however, so she was switched to more effective bilateral treatment (given twice weekly to minimise cognitive side effects). Vicky responded slowly to a course of ten acute bilateral treatments, with resolution of her depressed mood, nihilistic ideation and suicidal thoughts. The approach of spacing out treatments to minimise cognitive side effects proved successful, her MMSE score reaching 27/30 by the end of her hospital stay.

Vicky agreed to a further four continuation ECT treatments, to be administered at fortnightly intervals on an outpatient basis, in order to consolidate existing gains in treating her depression and minimise the risk of early relapse while newly prescribed medications were taking effect. Attendance for these four treatments, which were completed uneventfully, was coordinated by her case manager (CM) from the community mental health team. In addition to being maintained on olanzapine, she was commenced on desvenlafaxine and established on low-dose lithium just before discharge from hospital. It was hoped that this antidepressant–lithium combination would be more effective than an antidepressant alone in reducing the risk of longer-term relapse. Following discharge from hospital, medication was adjusted in consultation with her private psychiatrist as part of a shared care arrangement. Vicky remained in remission six months after discharge and her olanzapine was withdrawn. Throughout this period of community care, Vicky's CM worked closely with her and her family to provide support, access community services (such as home cleaning), and link Vicky into a psychosocial support program for older people with mental illness. There were no depressive symptoms at the twelve-month review, and Vicky was discharged to the care of her general practitioner and private psychiatrist.

3.3.7 ANXIETY DISORDERS

ANXIETY IN OLDER ADULTS

Older adults experience the same range of anxiety disorders as younger individuals (see Chapter 4.4), but the circumstances contributing to their emergence may differ. Physical frailty, financial pressures, social isolation and caregiving duties are ageing-related factors that may give rise to generalised anxiety disorder or, less commonly, acute anxiety episodes consistent with panic disorder. Agoraphobia is more likely to develop independently of panic disorder in older adults. Alternatively, panic disorder, social phobia and obsessive-compulsive disorder—which are all relatively uncommon in old age—may be longstanding conditions that come to psychiatric attention when physical illnesses bring patients into increased contact with health care providers. Along with generalised anxiety disorder (GAD), specific phobias are relatively common among older adults. Aside from longstanding phobias, such as fears of heights or injections, age-related events such as falling may give rise to new phobias in later life. Fear of falling is the most common specific fear among older adults, especially those with a history of falls (Ramos & Stanley, 2018). Post-traumatic stress disorder (PTSD) due to events earlier in life, such as traumatic combat experiences, generally decreases in severity, perhaps due to older adults' tendency to increase avoidance. More recent events, such as being an assault victim, can also lead to PTSD later in life, though symptoms tend to be less severe than those of younger adults (Bottche, Kuwert, & Knaevelsrud, 2012).

Clinical features of anxiety disorders in older adults include affective and mood symptoms (such as apprehension, rumination and irritability) and cognitive symptoms (such as difficulty concentrating, distractibility and fear of death or illness affecting relatives). However, older individuals may also manifest anxiety via somatic symptoms of psychomotor tension (such as fidgeting, restlessness and tremulousness) and physiological arousal (such as sleep disturbance, diarrhoea and dizziness). A focus on such somatic complaints, which are attributed to physical health problems, coupled with patient reluctance to acknowledge anxious mood, may contribute to the infrequent identification and correct diagnosis of anxiety disorders in older adults. The relationship between medical illness and anxiety in this patient population is indeed an important one, and is considered more fully below (Ramos & Stanley, 2018; Bower, Wetherell, Mon, & Lenze, 2015).

The increased prevalence of medical illness in this population is particularly likely to give rise to anxiety. A common example of this is chronic pain, which can be associated with conditions such as osteoarthritis or peripheral vascular disease. Medical conditions may also trigger anxiety by challenging older adults' sense of security and independence. Repeated falls, which place patients at risk of injury, or motor strokes that render patients incapable of basic personal care activities are examples of this. Complicating this area further, certain medical illnesses manifest physical symptoms that may be misattributed to anxiety (see Chapter 4.7). Examples include the palpitations and tremor seen in hyperthyroidism and the tachypnoea of chronic obstructive pulmonary disease (COPD).

Anxiety in older adults may also arise due to a range of psychiatric conditions, such as major affective or psychotic illness, delirium, dementia, alcohol abuse and dependence or personality disorder. Comorbidity of generalised anxiety disorder and major depression is particularly common, even more so than for younger adults (Altunoz, Kokurcan, Kirici, Bastug, & Ozel-Kizil, 2018). Given the wide range of medical and psychiatric comorbidity in anxious older individuals, thorough assessment encompassing direct and collateral history taking, physical examination and investigation is essential. The previously outlined guidelines for dementia screening (see Chapter 3.3) again serve as a useful template for investigation selection.

PSYCHOTHERAPEUTIC APPROACHES TO MANAGEMENT

Nonpharmacological management of anxiety disorders is similar in both younger and older individuals (see Chapters 2.6 and 4.3). CBT, supportive therapy and relaxation techniques all have demonstrated efficacy in decreasing anxiety in older people with GAD, panic disorder, and other conditions with anxiety symptoms. CBT yields effects in older adults that are comparable to those in younger adults when used to treat panic symptoms. Though CBT tends to have smaller effects for GAD in older adults, evidence for supportive therapy has yielded greater effect sizes (Ramos & Stanley, 2018). Psychology referral is recommended to determine the most appropriate psychotherapeutic modality on a case-by-case basis, and psychotherapy procedures should be adapted to address issues relevant to older adults and to account for any cognitive and sensory deficits, as described in our earlier discussion on depression management.

PHARMACOTHERAPY FOR ANXIETY IN OLDER ADULTS

Preliminary evidence suggests that SSRI (citalopram, sertraline) and SNRI (venlafaxine) antidepressants are effective in treating GAD in older people. There is also some evidence supporting the use of these medications in panic disorder and other anxiety disorders. Tolerability of these medications in older adults is generally good, though consideration of possible adverse effects requires more attention in this population than for younger adults (Ramos & Stanley, 2018).

Use of benzodiazepines for anxiety disorders in the elderly should generally be limited to providing initial, short-term symptomatic relief while awaiting antidepressant medication to take effect. Where a benzodiazepine is considered necessary, preference should be given to a low dose of a short-acting medication (Ramos & Stanley, 2018). Agents with long half-lives should preferably be avoided because of their greater potential to accumulate in the plasma and give rise to oversedation and associated giddiness, ataxia, confusion, memory loss and other cognitive impairments. Delirium can also be precipitated. These factors increase the risk of falls in older adults, whose ability to excrete benzodiazepines may be reduced. Thus oxazepam (elimination half-life of four to 15 hours) is preferable to diazepam (elimination half-life of 20–48 hours, and up to 90 hours at age 80) in prescribing to older adults.

Occasionally, a patient referred to aged psychiatry services is already taking long-term benzodiazepines. In such cases, it is important to re-examine the need for long-term use every six to 12 months and consider whether the medication can be weaned. Abrupt benzodiazepine cessation under these circumstances is likely to give rise to rebound anxiety and be unsuccessful. Very gradual dose reduction over many months, coupled with increased emphasis on psychological interventions, is far more likely to succeed.

3.3.8 PSYCHOTIC DISORDERS

Old age psychiatrists treat two groups of older adults with primary psychotic illness that are unrelated to an underlying dementing process (Iglewicz, Meeks, & Jeste, 2011). The first of these developed a psychotic illness as younger adults and their care has been transferred to aged psychiatry services after turning 65. These patients are sometimes referred to as 'graduates'. The second group of patients includes those who first develop psychosis as older adults.

EARLY-ONSET SCHIZOPHRENIA IN LATER LIFE

Medical comorbidity and metabolic syndrome

Patients with early-onset schizophrenia (see Chapters 3.2 and 4.2) have increased medical morbidity and a decreased life expectancy. Patients with longstanding schizophrenia who survive to the age of 65 may exhibit a range of psychological and physical impairments and pose a particular treatment challenge for aged psychiatry services that take over their care. Older age in general is more likely to be associated with a range of medical illnesses, the assessment and treatment of which patients with chronic psychosis may sometimes neglect. Failure to keep medical appointments because of disorganisation or residual persecutory beliefs is an example of this. Mental health service providers who become aware of these illnesses often have to liaise with general practitioners and other health care providers in an advocatory capacity to ensure that patients access appropriate and timely medical treatment.

Some of the medical conditions requiring attention may be related to long-term use of antipsychotic medication in this population. Both older typical and newer atypical antipsychotic medications may give rise to cardiovascular morbidity with prolonged use. While newer atypical medications are less likely to give rise to movement-related problems (parkinsonism and tardive dyskinesia), this advantage is offset by their increased propensity to induce a metabolic syndrome comprising weight gain and impaired glucose tolerance and lipid metabolism. As in the case of younger patients taking antipsychotic medication, it is important to monitor vigilantly for the emergence of any features of metabolic syndrome and take preventive or therapeutic action to address these, by means of preventing future complications of diabetes or cardiovascular disease. Close liaison with a patient's general practitioner is recommended to ensure the adequate management of metabolic syndrome and its consequences, as part of the patient's overall health care plan.

Cognitive deficits in schizophrenia

Patients with early-onset schizophrenia may also eventually exhibit cognitive deficits that give rise to functional impairment, which, in extreme cases, may resemble that seen in dementia. Aged residential care placement may be necessary in such cases. The emergence of severe cognitive impairment may also alter the manner in which pre-existing psychotic symptoms are manifested. Whereas a patient may have been able to describe floridly delusional beliefs or auditory hallucinations earlier in the course of their schizophrenia, acute illness relapses may come to be characterised predominantly by irritability.

Therapeutic relationships and transitions in care

Formation of a sound therapeutic relationship is a cornerstone for providing effective, responsive and patient-centred management for individuals with enduring psychotic illness, and this includes patients who have reached old age. The progression from middle to old age may be experienced as disruptive by patients from a mental health care perspective, as this often entails a transfer of care from adult to aged mental health services. Strong links forged with a case manager (CM) and medical staff of an adult mental health service over many years may sometimes be severed rather abruptly, ahead of new trusting relationships having to be built with other aged mental health providers. Patients may be at increased risk of relapse during this period. It is therefore important that the changeover process between services and CMs be sensitively handled to ensure there is merely a transition—rather than breakdown—of continuity of care from one service provider to another. An overlapping period of shared care between the discharging and receiving services is one approach towards easing this transition, allowing patients ample time to familiarise themselves with new staff and say goodbye to trusted clinical workers.

Accommodation options for patients with schizophrenia

Individuals with schizophrenia sometimes have lifelong difficulty securing stable accommodation. While some may be fortunate enough to live with supportive family members or other carers in private or public housing, others may find themselves living in boarding houses. Boarding house quality is variable and facilities may struggle to meet the increasing care needs of ageing residents. Aged mental health clinicians are generally familiar with available residential care options in their region and are well positioned to consider whether a patient's existing accommodation is adequately meeting his or her needs or whether a formal level of care re-evaluation via an aged care assessment service (ACAS) is warranted. ACAS assessment is mandatory for accessing aged residential care placement.

Antipsychotic pharmacotherapy for schizophrenia

Psychotropic medication management in patients with early-onset schizophrenia follows the same principles as in younger adults (see Chapters 3.2 and 4.2). However, additional caution is required in medication prescribing to account for patients' increased age. As older adults metabolise drugs more slowly, lower doses of antipsychotic medications than younger adults require may be sufficient for symptom control. If an older adult with schizophrenia is having antipsychotic medication commenced or switched, medication should be initiated at a lower starting dose than in younger adults and increased very cautiously. Antipsychotic medications may prolong the QTc interval of the electrocardiogram, something that may place patients at risk of potentially fatal cardiac arrhythmias. Some antipsychotics are more likely than others to cause QTc prolongation. Ziprasidone, for example, is particularly associated with QTc prolongation, whereas olanzapine is much safer in this regard. These differences between agents should be accounted for in medication selection for older adults, who are more likely to have heart disease than younger people. These principles are equally applicable where antipsychotics are being used for other diagnoses in older adults, such as late-onset psychosis and dementia.

LATE-ONSET PSYCHOSIS

Clinical features of late-onset psychosis

Psychotic illness in older adults, whether labelled as schizophrenia or otherwise, often tends to be qualitatively different from early-onset psychotic illness (Howard & Jeste, 2011). Many older patients with psychosis tend to not have symptoms of disorganisation, and to have well-preserved personality features. Late-onset psychosis is often characterised by the presence of 'partition delusions', the belief that intruders can enter one's home not only through open doors and windows, but also by penetrating closed doors and walls as well as air vents. Patients may come to believe that intruders are stealing their belongings or moving items such as furniture around the home. Olfactory hallucinations may accompany these beliefs, sometimes in the form of toxic gases that are believed to be circulated via ventilation ducts. Patients may take various precautions to protect themselves from these intrusions, such as sealing and obscuring windows and vents, placing locks on manholes and cupboards or installing security cameras. In extreme cases, patients may become highly isolative and virtually barricade themselves inside their homes to protect themselves from perceived intruders.

Obstacles to engagement

Among the greatest difficulties encountered in managing patients with late-onset psychosis are the establishment of initial contact and subsequent therapeutic rapport. Patients may be mistrusting of others whom they feel have misunderstood and not validated their experiences. This may include police officers who have questioned any complaints made by patients themselves about perceived persecution and assessing mental health clinicians. Attempts to interview patients in relation to a mental illness they do not believe they have may be met with outright avoidance of mental health providers. The assistance of family members and occasionally police may therefore be required in order to obtain access to patients' homes for this purpose (see Chapter 2.1). Involuntary psychiatric treatment may need to be initiated where there is evidence that persecutory beliefs and behaviours stemming from these are placing patients at risk. Examples of risky behaviours include failure to seek medical treatment for serious physical illness because of a fear of a mental health referral being triggered, or hiding large sums of money on one's person to prevent its theft by perceived persecutors.

Pharmacotherapy for late-onset psychosis

The principles regarding antipsychotic pharmacotherapy for early-onset schizophrenia are equally applicable here. As patients with late-onset psychosis are likely to be medication naïve, particular care in initiating antipsychotic medication is required, with low-dose atypical agents preferred. Very occasionally, use of depot antipsychotic preparations may need to be considered under involuntary treatment provisions. Interestingly, some patients' symptoms that fail to respond adequately to antipsychotic medication may settle entirely following a move to new accommodation, only to recur many months or several years later.

It is worth noting that neither the visual 'Lilliputian' hallucinations of Charles Bonnet syndrome (CBS) not their musical auditory variant respond well to antipsychotic medication (see Chapter 3.3).

Adverse social consequences and their alleviation

Although many patients with late-onset psychosis would otherwise be highly functioning, their illness may bring about a range of behaviours and actions that lead to adverse social consequences. Patients living in private rental housing may find their accommodation jeopardised following repeated unfounded complaints to real estate agents and landlords about alleged property violations. Alternatively, efforts to escape from perceived tormentors, such as moving houses, may place patients at risk of great financial losses. Estrangement from family members, who may unwittingly find themselves incorporated into delusional belief systems, may further deprive vulnerable patients of vital support when they need it most. Substantial case management (see Chapter 2.4) and social work input may be necessary to assist patients negotiate their way through these problems. Occasionally, mental health workers may need to apply for the appointment of an administrator or guardian to protect patients from high-risk financial, social or medical decisions motivated by psychotic experiences.

Late-onset psychosis or dementia with psychotic symptoms?

Many patients with late-onset psychosis are not cognitively impaired. However, psychotic symptoms can also arise for the first time in later life secondary to dementia. Psychotic phenomena that are relatively rudimentary in nature and accompanied by cognitive impairment may help distinguish dementia-related psychosis from primary psychotic illness. In some cases, patients with probable dementia may exhibit uncharacteristically complex delusional beliefs. In others, patients with likely primary psychosis may also show evidence of mild cognitive impairment (MCI) that may progress to dementia over time. Both scenarios can give rise to diagnostic uncertainty. Occasionally, separate diagnoses of late-onset psychosis and dementia may be justified. Careful history is required, often from collateral sources, to achieve diagnostic clarity along with comprehensive physical investigation (following the previously outlined schema for medical investigation of older mental health patients). Where emerging dementia is suspected, baseline neuropsychological testing performed once acute psychosis has resolved may facilitate future monitoring of any progressive cognitive changes.

3.3.9 OTHER PSYCHIATRIC DISORDERS IN LATER LIFE

SUBSTANCE ABUSE AND DEPENDENCE

Among older adults, the frequently atypical presentation of substance abuse and dependence may result in the overlooking and underreporting of this potentially serious health problem (see Chapter 4.5). Older people may deny the presence of substance misuse and not exhibit classic symptoms of dependence, such as craving. Instead, substance misuse in this population may present with psychomotor changes (such as incoordination or falls); affective disturbance (such as irritability or depression); cognitive impairment (such as amnesia or confusion); or physical symptoms mimicking other illnesses (such as vomiting or urinary incontinence). This variable clinical picture may lead to substance misuse being mistaken for a range of other psychiatric or medical conditions unless clinicians remain aware of the possibility of its existence. Older adults at particular risk of developing substance misuse, such as those with bereavement and chronic pain, should be carefully assessed and followed up (Flood & Buckwater, 2009; McGrath, Crome, & Crome, 2005).

Older patients seen by aged psychiatry services are more likely to misuse alcohol and prescription or over-the-counter medications rather than illicit drugs. In addition to providing treatment for the primary drinking behaviour itself, management of some older adults who have been long-term drinkers may focus on physical and cognitive complications. Examples include Wernicke-Korsakoff syndrome (due to thiamine deficiency, and manifesting with ataxia, visual disturbances and memory impairment) and dementia. Vigilance in prescribing and dispensing medications that are prone to being abused, such as anxiolytics and analgesics, may help avert the emergence of (or attenuate existing) misuse. Medication review by a geriatrician to identify and reduce unnecessary polypharmacy may contribute to this overall aim, and patients and their families should be counselled to not share medications (McGrath et al., 2005; Scott & Jayathissa, 2010; Blow & Barry, 2014).

Once identified, older people with substance misuse problems appear to respond to treatment as well as, or even better than, younger adults, especially when programs are age-specific (Kuerbis, Sacco, Blazer, & Moore, 2014; Blow & Barry, 2014). Clinicians should therefore be aware of local procedures for obtaining specialised drug and alcohol support for older adults. Barriers to accessing such support include misuse of medications rather than illicit drugs, which may not be a primary focus of some drug and alcohol services; medical illness and reduced physical mobility that may render clinic attendance difficult; and a perception among some older patients that drug and alcohol treatment programs targeted predominantly at younger adults are unsuitable for them. Aged mental health workers are well positioned to deliver interventions for substance misuse to patients who might otherwise be unable to access them, so familiarity with this area is important.

PERSONALITY DISORDERS

People with personality disorders may experience attenuation in their symptoms with advancing age. For this reason, old age psychiatrists are less likely to encounter some of the more severe manifestations of personality disorder seen in younger adults (see Chapter 4.9), such as the repeated self-harming behaviours of some patients with borderline personality disorder. This does not mean, however, that personality disorders are absent among older adults. To the contrary, many older patients display difficulties in interpersonal relationships that appear to be underpinned by personality related variables. Interestingly, such difficulties sometimes only come to psychiatric attention later in life when individuals may find previously relied upon coping strategies insufficient for dealing with significant life changes. One commonly seen example is individuals who exhibit marked behavioural difficulties following admission into nursing home care. While difficulty adjusting to one's new environment is often an obvious contributor to such behaviours, careful collateral history in particular is sometimes indicative of longer-standing, maladaptive personality features that may previously have been apparent only to close family members and associates. Such patients do not always meet criteria for a personality disorder diagnosis, but recognition of behavioural difficulties as being personality related is an important first step in implementing a successful management plan. Rather than a reliance on psychotropic medication, education of residential care staff is often an important component in the successful implementation of a behavioural management strategy.

PRACTICE ILLUSTRATION: SELF-MEDICATION WITH ALCOHOL FOR ANXIETY AND PERSONALITY RELATED DIFFICULTIES

Joan was a 66-year-old separated lady with a past history of anxiety, depression and alcohol dependence who was referred to the public aged mental health service by her private psychiatrist after missing several appointments. The psychiatrist was concerned that she might be significantly depressed as she apparently lacked the motivation to get out of bed to attend appointments at his rooms.

A home visit by assessing clinicians revealed Joan to be living alone in a large, untidy and poorly maintained house. Joan was dishevelled and tremulous but cooperative with the assessment process, speaking at length with clinicians about her present circumstance and background history. Joan had been treated in the private sector for low mood and alcohol dependence since her mid-forties. She had tried multiple antidepressants and mood stabilisers with limited effect, but had never received ECT. She had also participated in inpatient alcohol rehabilitation programs, but with only partial success in preventing long-term abstinence from drinking. On a positive note, there was no history of suicide attempts or self-harming behaviours.

Joan felt her longstanding drinking problem had contributed to separation from her husband several years previously. She and her husband jointly owned the home in which she now lived, her husband allowing her to continue living there following the breakup of their marriage. The couple only had indirect contact through their two sons, who visited Joan occasionally. Although Joan did not feel directly pressured by her husband to leave the home, she found the task of property maintenance unmanageable and acknowledged that her inevitable divorce would see her requiring alternative accommodation. Overwhelmed by the prospect of having to finalise these matters, she was presently experiencing severe anxiety that culminated in intermittent panic attacks. In an attempt to relieve her emotional distress, she had taken to the comfort of her bed and increasingly resorted to drinking over previous weeks, now consuming two bottles of wine daily. She only left her home on a fortnightly basis to stock up on the frozen pizzas on which she survived. Embarrassed about the possibility of others seeing her in this state, she had increasingly isolated herself from her sons and the few friends she had over preceding weeks. Although reporting some features of lowered mood, anxiety rather than depression appeared to be the main problem currently, and she was not feeling suicidal.

Joan agreed to initial daily home visits by the aged mental health service's assertive home treatment program to supervise detoxification from alcohol. A reducing diazepam regimen was prescribed for this purpose which, fortunately, proved to be an uncomplicated process, with few symptoms of physical withdrawal. Joan subsequently indicated a preference to attend the clinic for ongoing outpatient treatment. She was initially seen weekly and subsequently fortnightly for psychotherapy and medication management. Joan attended sessions reliably over a period of several months. The sessions were informative in providing insight into childhood difficulties relating to her perception of emotionally unavailable and distant parents who she believed favoured her more outgoing older sister. These experiences had given rise to a mix of dependent and avoidant personality traits and prominent anxiety for which she had self-medicated with alcohol for many years. Early retirement and separation from her husband in the face of these ongoing mental health problems reinforced her sense of inadequacy. The perceived isolation that the finality of a divorce would entail exacerbated her anxiety further and led to renewed drinking in the lead-up to referral.

Joan appeared to derive some comfort from talking about these difficulties at considerable length, but any insight gained did not translate into significant action to change her situation for many months. Given this observation, a predominantly supportive modality of psychotherapy was adopted. Concurrent attempts to relieve her anxiety through trials of SSRI and SNRI antidepressants were met with limited success, with Joan intermittently hyperventilating during sessions. Despite her clinic attendance becoming increasingly irregular, she eventually took definitive steps to finalise her divorce and negotiate a favourable division of the proceeds from the sale of her home. She engaged in heavy drinking in the aftermath of this stressful event, however, and was almost constantly intoxicated. She also risked homelessness because of her inability to secure viable alternative accommodation.

Joan was therefore admitted to an acute aged psychiatry inpatient unit for alcohol detoxication and was discharged after a relatively brief stay to a supported residential service (SRS) with intensive multidisciplinary support to ensure the success of this placement. Joan thrived in this environment, with her severe anxiety diminishing substantially and her drinking ceasing entirely even in the absence of regular psychotropic medication or conventional psychotherapy. With the combined support of aged mental health and SRS staff, Joan was able to maintain good personal hygiene and dietary intake, establish new friendships with co-residents, and re-engage in a range of previously enjoyed solo and group activities outside the facility. She also commenced regular outings with her sons. Joan achieved such a high level of functioning and independence that active aged psychiatry involvement was no longer required and she was discharged to the care of her general practitioner.

SQUALOR SYNDROME AND HOARDING DISORDER

Squalor syndrome is a relatively uncommon but particularly intriguing condition encountered in old age psychiatry. It refers to the condition whereby usually isolated older adults are found residing in a state of abject squalor, from which they may have to be 'rescued' for their own health and wellbeing and sometimes that of neighbours also. The appalling, dirty living conditions that characterise this syndrome are often accompanied by self-neglect, whereby a minimal acceptable standard of personal hygiene and health status are not maintained. Squalor syndrome may occur as an isolated phenomenon, but sometimes there are one or more comorbid psychiatric conditions, such as schizophrenia, dementia, borderline intelligence, alcohol dependence or personality disorder.

Hoarding overlaps with squalor syndrome and may be a prominent feature of the condition. Not all hoarders, however, live in squalor. Some individuals who display hoarding behaviour may do so in an 'organised' manner; for example, many years' worth of newspapers and magazines may fill up much of the house in neat piles extending from floor to ceiling.

In 2018, hoarding disorder was added by the World Health Organization to the ICD-11. According to ICD-11, possessions are accumulated in hoarding disorder due to their unnecessary acquisition (recurring wishes or activities related to collecting or purchasing items) or non-disposal (perceived necessity to retain items and distress related to disposing them) irrespective of their real worth. The clutter resulting from accumulated possessions risks living areas becoming unusable and unsafe. The condition gives rise to considerable distress or functional impairment in key personal, familial, social, educational, occupational or other domains (World Health Organization, 2018e).

Two qualifier levels for hoarding disorder are defined in the ICD-11:

- *Hoarding disorder with fair to good insight* satisfies all classificatory provisions of hoarding disorder. The person is aware that hoarding-related attitudes and activities (relating to unnecessary acquisition, non-disposal, or clutter) are abnormal. This qualifier level is still applicable if, on demarcated occasions, the person exhibits no insight (e.g., when required to dispose of possessions).
- *Hoarding disorder with poor to absent insight* also satisfies all classificatory provisions of hoarding disorder. Despite contradictory evidence, the person believes the majority or all of the time that hoarding-related attitudes and activities (relating to unnecessary acquisition, non-disposal, or clutter) are not abnormal. The person's poor to absent insight does not obviously fluctuate in parallel to their anxiety level (World Health Organization, 2018).

It may be hoped that including hoarding in ICD-11 will draw attention to the disorder, challenge policy makers to develop better service responses, promote sympathetic depictions of hoarding in the media, and foster respect for those burdened by the condition (Burki, 2018).

Management of this diverse range of presentations is complex. Patients may have already come to local council attention ahead of referral to aged care or psychiatric services because of the public health risk posed by their properties. Psychiatric or medical hospitalisation–voluntarily or otherwise–may sometimes be warranted, particularly where there is a coexisting psychiatric condition or if a person's physical health is acutely compromised. Multiple service providers may come to be involved in these people's care. Recidivism is common following attempts to remedy the situation (by industrial cleaning of the home, for example) and provide ongoing community support. Guardianship and administration, as well as residential care placement, are sometimes necessary (Lee & LoGiudice, 2012).

3.3.10 COMMENTARY AND REFLECTIONS

As this text is being prepared, two Royal Commissions (see Chapter 1.7), one nationally into Aged Care Quality and Safety, and one into Victoria's mental health services, are ongoing. They have a potentially significant bearing on the future of aged mental health services in Australia. The fact that these Royal Commissions have been established at this time is an indicator of the level of concern in the wider Australian community regarding the quality and adequacy of existing mental health and aged care services. Between them, the two Royal Commissions offer the promise of improved models of service delivery for the twenty-first century and the establishment of sustainable funding models to support their implementation well into the future. At the same time, the different levels of government involved in their establishment and the different focus of each Royal Commission on mental health specifically versus aged care more broadly underscores the longstanding division between the state and federal sectors (see Chapters 1.5 and 1.7) in health care provision as well as the division between psychiatric and physical health or aged care services.

In parallel, the introduction of the National Disability Insurance Scheme (NDIS; see Chapter 1.7) offers opportunities for older adults with mental illness to access care packages beyond those available via clinical aged persons mental health services (APMHS) or the traditional community and residential aged care sector. At the same time, it adds another layer of complexity to service funding and provision in this domain. While generally seen as a positive development by disability advocates, the NDIS has also been criticised as being complex and expensive to administer, with providers sometimes struggling to remain financially viable and clients often requiring assertive advocacy to have their funding needs met. In the authors' experience, the interface of the NDIS with existing care systems for older adults with mental illness, and its potential to provide them with better care, is still being tested on a case-by-case basis and only time will tell how well it serves this sector of the population. From an aged psychiatry perspective, perhaps the most enduring outcomes that one might hope for from the Royal Commissions are the seamless delivery of physical and mental health care to older adults with mental illness and better integration between federal and state governments in achieving this aim.

On a positive note, rapid advances in neuroscience over the last few decades have advanced our understanding of the neurobiological mechanisms of mental illness. The promise of disease-modifying therapies may revolutionise the field of dementia care in particular and old age psychiatry with it. Fortunately, existing multidisciplinary treatment approaches in aged mental health provide a solid foundation for meeting the challenges posed by an ageing Australian population and delivering an increasing array of symptomatic and preventive interventions well into the future.

PART 04

MENTAL HEALTH PROBLEMS CONSIDERED IN TERMS OF DISORDERS

Part 4 includes a series of chapters covering some major groups of mental disorders, largely following the order in which they are presented in ICD-11. As a text oriented towards the needs of practitioners in community mental health services we have not sought to cover some disorders which we consider less likely to be main focuses of assessment and intervention in such contexts. So for instance we have not brought into scope sleep-wake disorders nor have we ventured any distance into forensic mental health. Paraphilic disorders and impulse control disorders, for instance, are not covered in the text. For consideration of these problems the reader is referred to both comprehensive psychiatry texts and specialist texts, to which reference can be found in related chapters.

The bulk of each chapter presents knowledge from professional disciplines about phenomenology and diagnosis, what is known about origins, course and impact, then assessment, treatments and services. To help readers tune into the unique ways in which mental health issues manifest in each person's experience of a disorder, we have included throughout Part 4 first-person accounts from people who have experienced many of the disorders. To deepen learning, a series of Practice illustrations support consideration of practice issues that emerge in the discussion of specific disorders.

Chapter 4.1 introduces neurodevelopmental and associated psychiatric disorders where, arguably, the mental health needs of consumers are not well understood in mainstream mental health provision.

Chapter 4.2 considers schizophrenia and other psychotic disorders, which, although occurring much less commonly in the population than many other conditions, often impact heavily on the lives of those affected, leading them be a particular priority for services in some parts of the mental health system.

Chapters 4.3 and 4.4 cover some of what are sometimes grouped in the high prevalence disorders—mood disorders and the large group of disorders where anxiety is the most disabling feature.

Chapters 4.5 and 4.6 cover less common, but often disabling or even life-threatening problems, eating disorders and disorders of bodily experience.

Chapters 4.7 and 4.8 are centred on addictive behaviours—substance use disorders—also often grouped in the high prevalence disorders—then gambling and gaming disorders.

Chapter 4.9 concludes the part with coverage of personality disorders.

4.1

NEURODEVELOPMENTAL DISORDERS AND ASSOCIATED PSYCHIATRIC DISORDERS

CHAD BENNETT, TAREQ ABUELROOS & HAMILTON KENNEDY
(CONTENT HAS BEEN CONTRIBUTED BY CHAD BENNET AND TAREQ ABUELROOS, EXCEPT WHERE HAMILTON KENNEDY'S AUTHORSHIP IS NOTED FOR A SECTION.)

4.1.1 LIVED EXPERIENCE

HAMILTON KENNEDY

There is a very particular experience that comes from navigating the world as a neurodivergent person. The difficulties that can arise as a result of experiencing the world as different to others increases when within the mental health system. It is here that so much of my behaviour and experiences could be easily attributed to either ASD or a mental illness.

For mental health services, when I bang my head due to feeling overwhelmed my personality is considered disordered. My inability to make eye contact in certain situations means I am considered to have social anxiety. When I make strong claims regarding the goodness or badness of people I am considered to be delusional or to again have a disordered personality. I have meltdowns which means I can be considered to have behavioural problems. Of course, these things could also easily be attributed to my experience of being on the autism spectrum.

For myself, there is no clear distinction between my experiences which can be labelled mental illness and experiences that could be explained by being on the autism spectrum. There is only me and my experience. The sort of person I am is highly sensitive to others and stimulus; this makes some aspects of the world challenging. I am often unable to discern other people's faces, emotions and intentions which can leave me paranoid; or worried which would be, I imagine, any rational person's response to this situation. Often this means I can get agitated or aggressive, but these experiences are not the norm and most often result from my confusion.

When you work with me, or someone like me, who is considered to both be on the autism spectrum and also having a mental illness it is important to consider a few things. Ultimately you will be treating an individual, not an illness or a predetermined set of behaviours, so problems and difficulties they may share with you are valid and need to be addressed independent of their aetiology. Where a problem comes from may be less relevant to us than having supportive and helpful responses to them. If someone is very concerned with something, it should be taken seriously and prioritised in the work, independent of whether it is caused by neurodivergency or mental illness.

I hope that those who work with people like me will also consider that when we come into contact with mental health services, either voluntarily or involuntarily this does not necessarily mean that we have a mental illness. We may have ended up here because of our neurodivergency being inappropriately pathologised. Mental health services are intimidating and full of new often overwhelming sensory stimuli (or lack thereof); this will influence how people interact with you. Accordingly, it is important to consult with friends, family, and the person to learn more about how they normally interact with others and things that will make their experience of these environments workable.

I may not be 'normal', nor do I want to be. I want to be me and I want to be treated with dignity, compassion and acceptance of my difference.

4.1.2 INTRODUCTION

The developmental disorders are a heterogeneous group of conditions shared by the onset of occurrence in the development period. There are two major developmental disabilities that are deserving of extra attention in relation to the study of mental health: intellectual disability and autism. People with both disorders are at high risk for suffering additional mental disorders and subject to a range of disadvantages in all spheres of life. The diagnosis and management of these comorbidities is hindered by the communication deficits inherent in the developmental disorders, and by other factors that may modify the presentation of psychiatric illness. Service delivery is complicated by bureaucratic boundaries and difficulties in the detection and treatment of illness.

4.1.3 INTELLECTUAL DISABILITY

WHAT IS INTELLECTUAL DISABILITY?

Intellectual disability (ID) refers to the existence of concurrent deficits, in cognitive and adaptive functioning, that have been present during the development period, which is usually taken as being before the age of 18. They are persistent and lifelong though their manifestation may change in relation to the person's personal experience, environment and developmental phase. Intellectual disability is a descriptive term and is not a diagnosis which can explain symptoms and signs, determine treatment or prognosis. It is best understood as the consequence or symptoms of an underlying disorder; for example, cognitive impairment as a symptom of Down's syndrome. As described below there are many causes for the cognitive impairment and the main purpose of a diagnosis of intellectual disability is a bureaucratic category (Greenspan, 1999) to determine access to services. However, intellectual disability is frequently associated with altered function in other psychological and biological domains, which can often be classified as other comorbid mental disorders. The presence of intellectual disability may make individuals vulnerable to environmental disruptions, and it complicates evaluation, management and treatment planning, whatever the acute current condition.

DSM-5 AND ICD-11 CLASSIFICATION SYSTEMS.

DSM-5 uses the terms intellectual disability while ICD-11 uses disorder of intellectual development, the former term is shared among different disciplines however the latter can be considered more accurate. Both systems emphasise the presence of significant intellectual deficits of two or more standard deviations below the population mean, which generally translates into performance in the lowest 2.75% of a person's age, gender and cultural group, or an IQ of 70 or below. This should be measured with an individualised, standardised, culturally appropriate, psychometrically sound measure. DSM-5 requires both clinical assessment and cognitive testing to confirm the cognitive deficits, while ICD-11 allows the use of clinical judgement only when cognitive testing is not available. DSM-5 classifies the severity based on the level of functioning while ICD-11 severity is based on the cognitive impairment as assessed by formal cognitive testing or behavioural indicators when such tests are unavailable. However, the ICD system does emphasise the importance of using clinical judgement in interpreting the results of cognitive testing and to use it as a guide.

Diagnosis

The diagnosis of intellectual disability is unusual in that it is the only psychiatric diagnosis that is statistically defined and established by the administration of standardised tests. Unfortunately, this can lead to people being excluded from services on the basis of a rigid interpretation of the test score even if they have obvious needs. Usually three specific criteria are required for a diagnosis of intellectual disability. These are:

1. intelligence quotient (IQ, a measure of cognitive function based on verbal and performance measures) of 70 or below
2. deficits in adaptive functioning
3. onset of the disability before age 18.

Usually the deficits in cognitive functioning are measured by an IQ test, such as the Wechsler scales (Wechsler, 1997), although this may not be possible in those with severe and profound disabilities when the

Table 4.1 Main features of the different degrees of intellectual disability

Level of disability	IQ	Percentage of people with intellectual disability	Percentage of total population	Characteristics	Pathology
Mild	IQ 50–70	75% of cases	1.5% of population	Can use immature language with limited academic skills. Most master basic self-care and practical activities. Needs some support to achieve independent living and employment as adults.	Brain pathology uncommon
Moderate	IQ 40–50	20% of cases	0.5% of population	Achieve only basic language and academic skills. Some may master basic self-care and practical activities. Most require considerable support to achieve independent living and employment as adults.	Brain pathology commoner the lower the IQ
Severe	IQ <40	5% of cases		Limited language skills. May have motor impairments and typically require a supervised environment with daily support.	
Profound	IQ <40	<1% of cases	0.05% of population	Very limited communication abilities and basic concrete skills. May have co-occurring motor and sensory impairments and typically require daily support in a supervised environment.	

Source: Adapted from ICD-11, 2018

diagnosis is made on the basis of adaptive behaviour. Adaptive functioning is also assessed using standardised measures, such as the Vineland (Sparrow & Cicchetti, 1985), unless deficits are obvious. Deficits must be evident in such spheres as interpersonal relationships, daily living skills (grooming, hygiene, dressing, self-care, safety and self-preservation) and managing vocational and/or recreational aspects of life across multiple environments.

Severity is no longer judged by the degree of cognitive dysfunction but by the degree of functional impairment and consists of the following categories.

Epidemiology

Prevalence

The prevalence of ID in Australia is estimated (Wen, 1997) to be 1.8%, and is the most commonly reported type of disability for disability service users, with 68.4% of disability service users across Australia having an intellectual disability. However, not all of these individuals with an ID will have access to or seek services from specialist agencies, and many will lead independent lives. ID is approximately 1.5 times more common in males than in females, possibly the result of X-linked genetic conditions, and most individuals are in the mild range of ID. The introduction of interventions to prevent people developing intellectual disability have not had a major impact on the overall prevalence, partly because they prevent conditions that are relatively uncommon, such as vaccination as a prevention for congenital rubella, and also because of the increasing life expectancy of people with intellectual disability.

AETIOLOGY

Establishing the cause of the intellectual disability can be important for the individual and the family both as an explanation but also for understanding the risks of having more children affected by the same cause. It may help explain aspects of the persons presentation such the overeating in Prader-Willi syndrome as well as identify specific medical risks and complications that can be associated with certain disorders (i.e. the cardiac problems seen in Down's syndrome). Understanding the causes of intellectual disability can inform public health measures to reduce the risks of having children with intellectual disability such as ensuring women are vaccinated against rubella as infection in pregnancy can lead to significant intellectual disability and a range of other physical problems. There has been significant improvement in yield from testing over the last two decades due to newer diagnostic techniques in dysmorphology, cytogenetics and molecular genetics neuroimaging and molecular genetics, neuroimaging and clinical neurophysiology. Advanced genetic tests such as array comparative genomic hybridisation, single nucleotide polymorphism microarray, whole exome sequencing and whole genome sequencing have allowed the detection of very small chromosomal abnormalities which used to be missed by studying the gross structure of the chromosome through karyotyping. This has resulted in at least doubling the detection of a causative genetic abnormality ranging from 7.8% up to 60%, compared to 4% using karyotyping (Hochstenbach, Buizer-Voskamp, Vorstman, & Ophoff, 2011). The superior results of advanced genetic testing has been reflected in several clinical guidelines replacing the karyotype testing with the chromosomal microarray (CMA) as first-line investigation for patients with ID and ASD (Manning & Hudgins, 2010).

Although in clinical practice the cause of the intellectual disability is commonly not known, Bower and colleagues found that with investigation it was possible to find an identifiable cause for the ID in about half of a sample of children with intellectual disability in Western Australia (Bower, Leonard, & Petterson, 2000). In this population, genetic and chromosomal conditions formed the largest proportion of known causes. Although most of the 500 or so known genetic causes are individually rare, Down's syndrome accounted for approximately 14–15% of all cases, and Fragile X was found to account for about 0.5% of intellectual disability in males.

There are many nongenetic conditions that are associated with ID, and these do so by interfering with neurological development. The increasing survival rate for very premature babies is associated with both intellectual disability and cerebral palsy (Allen, 2008), and may be associated with intrauterine infections as well as trauma and hypoxia. Preventable infections are still a major cause of ID in the developing world, and include congenital syphilis, rubella and measles, among others.

Toxins have long been recognised as a cause of intellectual disability, and now the commonest toxin in Australia is probably alcohol. The intellectual impairment associated with foetal alcohol syndrome (FAS) is permanent, and FAS is now regarded as the leading preventable cause of nongenetic intellectual handicap. It is now recorded as 0.02 per 1000 for non-Aboriginal children and 2.76 per 1000 for Aboriginal children in Western Australia (Commonwealth of Australia: National Expert Advisory Committee on Alcohol, 2002). Prenatal and postnatal infections with agents such as cytomegalovirus (CMV), toxoplasma and herpes were found to account for about 3% of intellectual disability.

Although the causes in many cases of intellectual disability are unknown, risk factors have been documented in the 'unknown cause' category. These include maternal exposures, such as smoking and alcohol ingestion during pregnancy, pre-term birth, low birth weight and multiple births (Bower et al., 2000). As yet unidentified genetic causes are also suspected, as family clustering of intellectual disability has been found in about one-quarter of cases of mild mental retardation of unknown aetiology in two European studies (Hagberg & Kyllerman, 1983; Matilainen, Airaksinen, Mononen, Launiala, & Kääriäinen, 1995).

Assessment

Individuals with more severe disability are usually diagnosed in the postnatal period, either because of obvious physical abnormalities or known risk factors, such as hypoxia. Other children may be identified as having an intellectual disability by not achieving age-appropriate milestones, providing other explanations such as deafness, visual impairments, chronic illness and deprivation are excluded. Sometimes it is at school that problems become apparent; for instance, the inability to keep up with peers which may present as depression or aggression. At this age it is important to exclude specific learning disorders (such as dyslexia), autistic spectrum disorders and sensory impairments. In adulthood, decompensation during periods of stress may result in ID being identified. At any age, the diagnosis should only be made after careful,

PRACTICE ILLUSTRATION: DEVELOPMENTAL HISTORY

Tim is a 23-year-old man living at home with his parents. He has a mild intellectual disability that is attributed to him being born prematurely at a gestation of 31 weeks and suffering from hypoxia. He has a dysarthria, making it difficult to understand him, and has longstanding epilepsy, which is well controlled on medication, although he has a fit every three to four months. He was slow to achieve his milestones, did not crawl until 18 months, and began to walk between the ages of two and three. His language was also delayed, and he was not using sentences until the age of four. He attended the local kindergarten, and remained there for two years, as it was thought he was too immature to commence primary school. He attended the local school, where allowances were made for his inability to keep up with schoolwork. He was older and bigger than the other children; if he thought he was being teased, he would hit them. As a consequence, he was often left alone. At the age of 10, he had a teacher's aide to assist with his academic skills. At secondary school, he was getting into repeated fights, and eventually attended a special school, where he was one of the more able students, and he responded well to being given extra responsibility. He has two brothers who are 10 years older, and have established relationships and employment. After leaving school at the age of 16, he attended a TAFE course for three years. He then went to an adult training centre run by disability services, but did not like to be identified with other disabled people, and stopped attending. Since this time he has spent most of his time undertaking small tasks at his father's fish-and-chip shop, but has no other activities or social outlets. His mother is an extremely anxious woman, who sees it as her role to look after him.

longitudinal, multidisciplinary assessment, and should go beyond a simple IQ test to include an analysis of adaptive skills to identify what supports may be needed.

COMMON GENETIC CAUSES OF INTELLECTUAL DISABILITY

Down's syndrome

Down's syndrome is the commonest recognised genetic cause of intellectual disability, and there are approximately 60 babies born with Down's syndrome per year in Victoria (Collins, Muggli, Riley, Palma, & Halliday, 2008). It is not typically hereditary in nature and does not run in families, but is secondary to faulty production of germ cells (sperm or egg) before fertilisation. Maternal age is the major risk factor, and the incidence of Down's pregnancies for women aged 45 and over is one in 50; for those aged 20, it is one in 2000 (Ratcliffe, Stewart, Melville, Jacobs, & Keay, 1970). Paternal age and radiation have also been implicated. Patients usually have three copies of chromosome 21 in every cell instead of the usual two, which is why it is also known as Trisomy 21. The parents have a normal chromosomal pattern, and these cases account for 95% of people with Down's syndrome. In 4% of cases, the abnormality is a translocation of genetic material to chromosome 21 (of which there are only two in affected individuals), and carriers may be found in the family.

Numerous physical stigmata characterise the disorder, including up-slanting of the opening between the two eye lids, palpebral fissures, small flattened skull with small ears and a squint, high cheekbones, tongue too big for the mouth, broad hands with stubby fingers, a single transverse palmar crease and incurved fingers. Cardiovascular pathology is common, and often led to death in childhood before advances in treatment. Most people with Down's syndrome have an IQ in the moderate or severe range. Antenatal screening is no longer limited to high-risk groups, and the syndrome is increasingly identified in the early stages of pregnancy, with up to 92% of parents then choosing to terminate the pregnancy (Mansfield, Hopfer, & Marteau, 1999). The proportion of babies born with Down's syndrome has stayed constant in many Western countries because of the rising proportion of mothers aged more than 35 years, and the prevalence has increased because of the better life expectancy (Binkert, Mutter, & Schinzel, 2002).

Fragile X syndrome

This is the commonest hereditary cause of ID, and one in 3600 males have the Fragile X gene and syndrome. It is assumed that the proportion of females heterozygous for the full mutation is the same as the proportion of males with the full mutation (Beckett, Yu, & Ngoc Long, 2005). ID is present in most Fragile X males and 60% of females (women have two X-chromosomes and are therefore less severely affected). The syndrome is so named because an arm on the X chromosome looks as if it is about to break off. Physical features, not as specific as in Down's syndrome, include large ears, long face, prominent forehead, abnormally large testes and connective tissue abnormalities (such as high arch palate, hyperextensible joints, flat feet, scoliosis, hypotonia and mitral valve prolapse; Turk, 1992).

INTELLECTUAL DISABILITY AND PHYSICAL ILLNESS

Medical problems often occur in this group, and similar problems are experienced in their diagnosis and treatment. Certain illnesses, such as GI tract problems, dental problems, epilepsy and sensory deficits, are particularly common (Beange, McElduff, & Baker, 1995). Hypothyroidism is more common in Down's syndrome, as is obesity in Prader-Willi syndrome. Untreated illness can present with behavioural problems, and some disorders, such as epilepsy, are associated with psychiatric morbidity in the normal population and, by implication, the ID population.

MANAGEMENT

Only broad management principles are discussed below, as the intellectually disabled population is extremely diverse and heterogeneous. Their needs will vary in relation to the severity of the disability and life stage. The term 'normalisation' is often cited as the guiding principle, which loosely means assisting the person to live as normal a life as possible (Wolfensberger, 1972). An educational and disability management model is used, and individually tailored based on an assessment of needs. The majority of the ID population live at home, and most services are now community-based. The range of services include long-term and short-term accommodation options, educational programs, assistance with activities of daily living (ADLs) and family supports. The medical role has been de-emphasised, and limited to the treatment of associated physical or psychiatric conditions. Under the concept of normalisation, the ID population, like the rest of the population, should be able to access generic services. However, a small but significant group require hospital-like care because of their level of disability, and there remains a large proportion of people with an intellectual disability for whom access to generic services does not occur, or remains problematic. Reasons for this are usually related to problems with communication, challenging behaviour or additional disabilities, such as mental illness or high physical support needs, in addition to an inability or unwillingness of generic service providers to meet the complex needs of this group. Conditions are often unrecognised, and, when recognised, are inadequately treated (Beange et al., 1995; Ryan & Sunada, 1997).

4.1.4 INTELLECTUAL DISABILITY AND PSYCHIATRIC DISORDERS

For many years, it was thought that people with an intellectual disability had a low prevalence of mental illness. Reasons given were that they were well cared for in institutions and they did not have to worry about the past, future or current needs. It was also thought that perhaps they did not have the same range of emotions as other people, and that their simpler thought processes might be less prone to disorder. In many ways they are less valued members of the community, and the belief that prevalence of mental health problems is lower has been perpetuated by the lack of contrary evidence. There has been a paucity of research of illness in this group, which has traditionally been regarded with a low political and professional priority. However, it is now accepted that people with intellectual disability can experience the full range of psychiatric disorders, and that the rate is considerably higher than that found in the general population. The combined point prevalence for all psychiatric disorders is probably between 30 and 50% (Smiley, 2005). In addition, there are a number of factors that result in mental illness being poorly identified and treated in this group. Unfortunately, little research has been done on treatment outcomes. Much of the content below could also be applied to people with autism, although it is presented in relation to people with intellectual disability.

CONCEPTUAL ISSUES

Frame of reference

Psychiatry treats mental illness, but unfortunately there is no good definition of what constitutes mental illness (see Chapter 1.1). Modern definitions include the concept of causing distress to oneself or others, and generally disorders of the higher functions of thought, emotion and behaviour are the focus of treatment (as opposed to neurology, which treats sensory and motor abnormalities). Traditionally, these were seen as disorders of the mind, as opposed to disorders of the brain, though the complex interplay between biological and psychosocial variables has always been recognised. The diagnostic process consists of analysing why a behaviour is presenting problems, and to whom. The communication and cognitive impairments in people with intellectual disability complicate this process, which is often additionally compromised by their dependency on others. For example, a young autistic man who lives in an extremely impoverished environment and who repeatedly self-injures by banging his head could be considered to have depression, but is it more appropriate to diagnose the patient or to attribute the problems to the environment? Another patient may present because she continually wanders off and gets lost. This is clearly a behaviour caused by a mental disorder that requires a management strategy, but does not neatly fit in to a medical model, and requires a different type of explanation to inform an appropriate management strategy. The framework to conceptualise the problems is broadened, with increased emphasis on social and psychological explanations as well as biological causes of problem behaviour. Precipitating factors for problem behaviours may include social factors (that is, changes in staff at the residential units), physical factors (that is, dental pain) or psychiatric problems (that is, depression). The expression of such a behaviour may be modified by a range of factors, including the degree and cause of disability, communication skills, past experience, pain threshold and behaviour repertoire. The psychiatrist is more than ever the detective trying to establish the cause of the troublesome behaviour in a wider frame of reference.

Diagnostic criteria

Modern diagnostic criteria, such as in DSM-5 or ICD-11 (p. 171), have been operationalised on a syndromal basis (see Chapter 2.3) in an attempt to improve reliability. The symptoms criteria are largely language based, and derived from research on the normal population. Because of various considerations, outlined below, it is unclear to what extent they are applicable to the ID population (Sturmey, 1993):

- *Communication deficits*: people with an ID may lack the verbal skills to describe their internal experiences, and thus may not reach the required threshold for a particular diagnosis. For example, the DSM-5 criteria for major depressive disorder require the ability to report depressed mood, diminished interest and pleasure. A person with an ID may not be able to describe these experiences
- *Cognitive deficits*: people with an ID may lack the conceptual skills to understand their internal experiences, and thus may not reach the required threshold for a particular diagnosis. For example, the DSM-5 criteria for major depressive disorder require the ability to report guilt. A person with an ID may not be able to understand a concept such as guilt, which involves being able to integrate a relatively complicated set of mental constructs
- *ID excluding a diagnosis*: it remains unclear to what degree the integrity of the psychological systems involved in mental operations is required to develop psychiatric illnesses. For example, the failure of the theory of the mind (that is, the inability to conceptualise another person's mental state) is put forward as a central deficit in autism (Folstein, 1999). If this is the case, to what extent are they are able to experience symptoms such as thought insertion, thought withdrawal or thought broadcast?
- *ID modifying the presentation of a diagnosis*: a psychiatric disorder may present in an altered form, and behavioural presentations of psychiatric illness are relatively common in this population. For example regressive behaviour, loss of skills and aggression may all indicate an underlying psychosis
- *The psychiatric disorder may only be present in the ID population*: self-harming behaviour, such as head banging, is generally only evident in the more severely intellectually disabled. Other types of self-harming behaviour, such as finger biting or lip biting, may be specific to certain syndromes, such as Lesch–Nyhan syndrome
- *The relationship between behaviour and genetics in relation to aetiology is not indicated*: for example, should the overeating evident in Prader-Willi syndrome be classified as a separate psychiatric disorder or be seen as part of the phenotype?

DSM-5 and the ICD-11 manuals provide detailed subcategories and related categories within diagnostic groups: given the limitations in eliciting psychopathology (both with regards to the communication skills of the adult with learning disabilities, and difficulties with informant histories), it seems inappropriate to subdivide diagnostic categories to the same extent as for the general population. Greater subdivision is likely to introduce inaccuracy and lessen validity, for example, with regards to types of dementia or nonaffective psychotic disorders.

CONCEPTUAL SOLUTIONS

Frame of reference

Various terms used to describe the behaviours that may be a focus of attention in people with an ID are as follows:

- *problem behaviour:* a problem behaviour exists if it meets one of the following criteria: it is inappropriate to a person's level of development; dangerous; constitutes a handicap for the person; causes stress; or is contrary to accepted social norms (Zarkowska & Clements, 1994).

- *challenging behaviour:* a term introduced to signify the available services that were not meeting needs appropriately; the issue is a challenge to provide appropriate services, not just a problem carried by the individual. The challenge is to find effective ways of helping people to behave and express themselves in an acceptable manner (Bluden & Allen, 1987).
- *dual diagnosis*: the use of this term has also been advocated, as it encourages us to think of alternative explanations for a person's behaviour rather than attributing behavioural problems to learning disabilities per se. Unfortunately, it is not a specific term, and has also been applied to other comorbidities. In practice, many people with these problems are managed using interventions derived from a range of different disciplines and professional backgrounds, including psychotropic medication and behaviour management programs.

CLASSIFICATION

It is generally accepted that ICD-11 and DSM-5 classifications can be applied to a person's condition until a person's IQ is less than about 50 (providing that he or she has adequate verbal skills), and that the full range of syndromes can be experienced. Below this level of IQ, it is difficult to apply standard classification criteria.

One alternative approach in the United Kingdom is the UK Royal College of Psychiatrists Diagnostic Criteria for psychiatric disorders for use with adults with learning disabilities or mental retardation, a multiaxial diagnostic classification (see Chapter 2.3) system (DC-LD; Royal College of Psychiatrists, 2001), in which a hierarchical approach is adopted through and within each axis, as follows:

- Axis I: Severity of learning disabilities
- Axis II: Cause of learning disabilities
- Axis III: Psychiatric disorders
    - DC-LD Level A: Developmental disorders
    - DC-LD Level B: Psychiatric illness
    - DC-LD Level C: Personality disorders
    - DC-LD Level D: Problem behaviours
    - DC-LD Level E: Other disorders.

Examples of how this system might be used are given below:

- Ms Susan Smith is a 37-year-old woman with severe learning disabilities (Axis I) because of Down's syndrome (Axis II), who has a six-month history of obsessive-compulsive disorder (Axis III, Level B) and longstanding self-injurious behaviour (through head banging: Axis III, Level D)
- Mr John Brown is a 62-year-old man with moderate learning disabilities (Axis I) of unknown cause (Axis II), who has a twenty-year history of schizophrenia (Axis III, Level B) and a two-year history of dementia (Axis III, Level B)
- Mr Peter Jones is a 25-year-old man with severe learning disabilities (Axis I) and autism (Axis III, Level A), who has a three-month history of depressive episode (Axis III, Level B), longstanding pica (Axis III, Level B) and longstanding self-injurious behaviour (Axis III, Level D).

EPIDEMIOLOGY

Generally, studies have shown high rates of mental illness in the ID population. The point prevalence rates vary from 20–60%, depending on the population studied, how cases were identified and the classification system used. In a recent review Smiley (Smiley, 2005) concludes that most of the research shows that the total point prevalence of mental health problems (including problem behaviour) in adults with learning disability is higher than in the general population, with a rate that lies somewhere between 30 and 50%. A figure of 3% prevalence for schizophrenia has been found repeatedly (Clarke, 1999–2001). The results from a more recent methodologically sound study using a case register are shown in Table 4.2 (Cooper, 1997).

Table 4.2 Estimated point prevalence rates of comorbid mental disorder in adults with learning disability

Disorder	Rate
Schizophrenia	3%
Bipolar affective disorder	1.5%
Depression	4%
Generalised anxiety disorder	5.5%
Specific phobia	7%
Agoraphobia	1.5%
Obsessive-compulsive disorder	2.5%
Autism	7%
Severe problem behaviour	10–15%

PRACTICE ILLUSTRATION: INCREASING PROBLEMS

For the past year, Tim has been more unwilling to go to work with his father, and instead prefers to spend most of his time sitting in his room smoking. He has now moved into a bungalow at the back of the house. He has little interaction with his parents, and he prefers for them not to come in to his room, which smells of urine, and his mother places his meals on the doorstep along with a supply of cigarettes. He has also started to drink alcohol, and has become erratic with his medication, resulting in more frequent epileptic fits. He wears the same clothes most of the time, and is unkempt and dirty in his appearance. He is irritable, and accuses his mother of trying to poison him. Recently he has started to wear ear muffs 'to stop the birds making so much noise'. He has refused to see his local doctor, but recently assaulted his mother, breaking her arm, resulting in the police being called, and, although no charges were laid, assessment by psychiatric services was requested.

RISK FACTORS FOR MENTAL ILLNESS IN MENTAL RETARDATION

Biological risk factors

- *Genetic*: some genetic abnormalities are linked with both intellectual disability and psychiatric illness. For example, Down's syndrome is particularly associated with the later onset of dementia (Collacott, Cooper, & McGrother, 1992) and Fragile X with ADHD (Turk, 1992), and there are rare genetic syndromes related to chromosome 22, in which schizophrenia and ID are associated, such as velocardiofacial syndrome (Murphy, Jones, & Owen, 1999).
- *Neurodevelopmental*: brain damage may give rise to specific personality disorders, problems of arousal and difficulties in emotion regulation. Schizophrenia is thought to be a consequence of a number of nonspecific insults on neurodevelopment; for example, obstetric complications. These may also result in intellectual disability.
- *Behavioural phenotypes*: it is becoming increasingly accepted that genes contribute to behaviour. Certain genotypes are associated with specific behavioural manifestations, including distinctive social, linguistic, cognitive and motor profiles (O'Brien, 2006).
- *Sensory disabilities*: people with an intellectual disability often have problems with hearing and vision, leading to an increased risk in the normal population for psychotic illnesses.
- *Epilepsy*: associated with both the development of depression and psychotic illnesses, and occurs in up to 20% of people with an intellectual disability.

- *Medication*: the use of psychotropic medication among people with intellectual disability is widespread, and psychotropic medication is often prescribed for people with an intellectual disability without a clear diagnosis, even following deinstitutionalisation (30% in some surveys received antipsychotics; Nøttestad & Linaker, 2003). Side effects, such as akathisia, are more likely to be blamed on the intellectual disability. Anti-epileptic medication can have a number of behavioural and cognitive side effects.

Psychological risk factors

- *Coping skills*: the presence of ID means that people are less able to develop strategies with which they can deal with the problems of everyday life, and face increased stress as a result of this.
- *Primitive defence mechanisms*: there is some suggestion that patients with an ID tend to use more primitive defence mechanisms (such as denial and projection), and can respond to stress with regressive, childlike behaviour.
- *Personality development*: may be impaired as a consequence of ID and its consequences.
- *Loss and life events*: patients with an ID are more likely to face separations from family when they are placed in respite care. Significant events, particularly bereavement, are less likely to be explained to them.
- *Labelling and stigma*: often people with an ID have been teased and insulted from an early age. Self-image may be affected by the presence of ID.
- *Communication*: lack of verbal skills may mean an inability to tell carers about problems and make use of advice concerning the resolution of any problems.
- *Altered symptomatology*: both psychiatric and physical symptoms may be modified by the presence of an ID (for example, toothache may be evident as increased aggression), making their recognition and treatment less likely.

Social risk factors

- *Supports:* likely to have fewer meaningful supports.
- *Family reaction:* the family may experience a burden of care, and may also have unresolved grief issues.
- *High levels of expressed emotion*: may be seen in families and residential units, and are associated with the exacerbation of mental illness.
- *Accommodation*: often placed in units with other people with significant problems, including aggression. Sexual abuse may occur, and is often unrecognised.
- *Access to health, education and training*: people with an ID are reliant on carers to gain access to services, cannot refer themselves and are therefore disempowered. Few choices may be given to them, and their lifestyle is often one of bureaucratic convenience.
- *Professional and carer skills*: carers often fail to recognise symptoms, so illness is often undetected for prolonged periods of time. When patients are referred, staff and services often lack the skills, resources and structure to assess and manage this group of patients appropriately.
- *Sexuality:* many people with an ID are infantilised and never receive sexual education. Consequently, when they behave in a sexual manner it is often clumsy and inappropriate. This behaviour is then labelled and treated as deviant and troublesome.

ASSESSMENT ISSUES

Several processes can influence the making of a diagnosis in a person with an ID (Sovner, 1986):

- *Diagnostic overshadowing*: refers to the common mistake to attribute psychiatric symptoms purely to an intellectual disability. It should be remembered that the only symptom attributable to ID is the deficit in intelligence, as measured by IQ testing. Psychiatric illness commonly presents with aggressive behaviour, but is treated as a behavioural problem.
- *Intellectual distortion*: refers to the concrete thinking and poor communication that can lead to difficulties in understanding the person's internal experiences. During the assessment, special care has to be taken in eliciting the psychopathology. This is because some adults have limited communication skills, and may have difficulty explaining their symptoms. They may also have difficulty understanding questions. Questions must

be asked in simple language, using short sentences appropriate to the adult's developmental level.

- *Psychosocial masking*: refers to the improvised social and life experiences that can lead to the unsophisticated presentation of symptoms that are then not recognised (that is, the manner in which clients report hearing voices is often matter of fact, and thus not recognised as being part of an illness).
- *Cognitive disintegration*: refers to the stress-induced disruption of information processing that can present as bizarre behaviour and thought disorder.
- *Baseline exaggeration*: refers to an increase in pre-existing cognitive deficits and behavioural problems that reflect the limited range of responses a patient may have. It may be difficult to recognise this as a psychiatric illness.
- *Cloak of normality*: for many people with an ID, it is very important to appear normal to avoid the stigma of having an ID (that is, denial). Thus all questions are answered in a way that will continue the image of normality, and any unusual symptoms may be denied in a similar manner. The assessor must be aware of the possibility of the adult being suggestible and giving compliant answers; for example, the person answering 'yes' or repeating the last word or phrase when given a choice of alternatives.
- *Autistic spectrum of disorders*: this can lead to particular problems, with improper use of pronouns, delayed echolalia, and other catatonic-like symptoms.
- *Developmental*: even the most able adult with learning disabilities is likely to have difficulty with some parts of the assessment process, such as remembering and describing the sequence of events and time scales. Patients may talk to themselves or have intense fantasy lives that may resemble psychotic symptoms, although they can be appropriate for the person's stage of development.

To overcome these problems, good interview technique and collateral histories are highly important in assessing a patient with an ID. It is important to look for meaning, changes and patterns of any behaviour that may be a form of communication, psychiatric illness or a response to environmental stimuli. Using frequency charts may often provide useful information. A family history of psychiatric illness often has increased weight, given the lack of other information. Assessments often take longer with patients who have an ID, and may need to occur over several visits (Levitas & Silka, 2001).

PSYCHIATRIC ASPECTS OF SPECIFIC SYNDROMES

There are a number of psychiatric syndromes associated with specific genetic syndromes. This can be useful in adding weight to a specific diagnosis and can also be used to develop specific screening programs. A selection of these is discussed below.

Fragile X syndrome

People with this condition often avoid social situations that cause anxiety (avoidant behaviours). They exhibit outburst behaviours (crying, screaming, vomiting, aggression and tantrum-like behaviours) because of being overwhelmed or overstimulated, or because of a desire to stop a perceived unpleasant situation. They may engage in repetitive behaviours that appear to be pleasurable, such as tactile or olfactory events. Diagnosable attention deficit disorder is very common, and autistic features are frequent (hand flapping, biting, gaze aversion, preoccupation with objects and difficulty adjusting to change; Turk, 1992).

Trisomy 21 and Down's syndrome

Senile plaques develop early, apparently related to genetic programming. Cognitive deterioration is usual from middle age onwards, and hypothyroidism quite commonly develops. Nowadays many live to late middle age, and may show evidence of dementia. Depression is an important differential diagnosis, and occurs at a higher rate in people with Down's syndrome as compared to other people with intellectual disability (Collacott et al., 1992).

Lesch–Nyhan syndrome

This disorder is associated with severe self-harming behaviour, including lip, cheek and finger biting.

MANAGEMENT ISSUES

Despite difficulties in making a diagnosis, it is important to generate diagnostic hypotheses whose accuracy can be evaluated against the success of any subsequent interventions (see Chapter 2.3). In general management it is the same as for the normal population for specific diagnosis such as schizophrenia. It is important to adopt a bio-psycho-social approach.

Biological interventions

Often the most important step is to exclude physical illness. Undiagnosed pain may result in aggressive behaviour. Sometimes knowing the cause of the ID can lead to specific management strategies, as in Fragile X. Medication is commonly used to control behaviours when no diagnosis has been made, and in institutions up to 50% of patients are on psychotropic medication. A Cochrane Collaborative Review (Brylewski & Duggan, 2004) found no evidence that antipsychotics change behaviour in the absence of a diagnosis. Medication should be used as in the normal population, and based on diagnostic hypotheses, but needs to be continually reviewed because of the danger of side effects that may not be reported by a person with an intellectual disability. Guidelines based on consensus have been established for the prescription of psychotropic medication in people with an intellectual disability (Reiss & Aman, 1997). It is useful to chart target responses to evaluate efficacy. Paradoxical effects are not uncommon, and this may relate to an impairment of cognition or delirium. An overreliance on medication may prevent other strategies from being used.

Psychological interventions

A careful behavioural analysis can sometimes identify patterns that can then lead to appropriate interventions. This is a highly skilled and time-intensive process, and is based on trying to understand the functions of the behaviour in an operant framework. Interventions require a high degree of motivation and cohesion among staff. Cognitive and dynamic psychotherapy techniques can be employed, but may have to be modified to allow for any communication difficulties and issues related to complexity of concepts (that is, using pictures or drama; Hollins & Sinason, 2000). Bereavement counselling can be important, as often intellectually disabled people are excluded from funerals and other processes whereby grief may normally be expressed (Bonell-Pascual et al., 1999). Anger management and anxiety-reduction techniques can also be used.

Social interventions

Most people with intellectual disability live at home with families and support is provided to maximise opportunities to lead as normal a life as possible. These include assistance with activities of daily living as well as respite care, long-term accommodation, training, education and assistance in the development of relationships and other skills. Education for patients, carers and families to increase understanding and help develop caring strategies that permit personal growth are also important.

SPECIFIC PSYCHIATRIC ILLNESS IN THE ID POPULATION

The ID population is not homogeneous, and the rates and presentation of psychiatric illness will vary with such factors as IQ and aetiology of disability. In general, diagnostic criteria can be used in the normal manner until the IQ is around 50 or lower. Below this level, modified criteria may be required, and patients may present with disorders not seen in the higher IQ ranges.

Neurotic, personality and behaviour disorders (mild ID)

These disorders can be difficult to distinguish from one another. Many patients have a background of abuse, neglect, poor parenting, inadequate education and poor social and coping skills, coupled with a low tolerance of frustration and impaired impulse control. They can often present with a range of unacceptable behaviours, such as aggression or inappropriate sexual activity (Alexander et al., 2010). They can respond to psychologically based interventions adapted to their level of understanding, such as anxiety management, anger management, behaviour therapy and CBT. Assisting them in meeting their

PRACTICE ILLUSTRATION: INTERVENTION

Although Tim refused to see a crisis team, it was thought that he was at risk because of his epilepsy, and that he presented a risk to his parents. This was considered in conjunction with the possibility that his social withdrawal and unusual behaviour represented the onset of psychotic illness, so he was certified and admitted to hospital for further assessment. On the ward he was virtually mute, and refused to answer any questions. He attempted to leave on several occasions, and was placed on the high dependency unit. Attempts to help him wash met fierce resistance, and, when he was forced to have a shower, he smeared faeces over himself. Over a period of a week, he became increasingly slow in his movements, and eventually stayed in bed staring at the ceiling, and even stopped eating and drinking. As his condition had become more urgent, a course of bilateral ECT was given over a period of four weeks. He responded very well to this treatment, becoming more alert and responsive, and able to engage in social interaction and ward activities. He was unable to explain how he was feeling prior to admission or whether he was experiencing any hallucinations. He was diagnosed as having a psychotic depression, and commenced on antidepressants and antipsychotics. Prior to discharge, he was referred to disability services, with the request that his family should be provided with additional supports to assist with day-to-day management and activities at home.

basic needs, such as accommodation, is a prerequisite before embarking on therapy.

Affective disorders

Depression has a high prevalence, and can present with expected features, such as tearfulness, lack of interest, social withdrawal and psychomotor retardation. However, cognitive symptoms such as worthlessness, guilt, recurrent thoughts of death and suicide attempts are less common in those with intellectual disability. Aggression and acting-out or self-harming behaviour may be the main presenting features, and may be the only manifestation in the more severely disabled, who are unable to communicate their feelings (Ross & Oliver, 2003). In some cases, it may present as a 'pseudodementia', with loss of skills and withdrawal. These differences in presentation indicate that modified criteria may be needed (Smiley & Cooper, 2003). Mania presents with an increase in activity, intrusive behaviour, destructiveness, irritability and sometimes self-abusive behaviour. Bipolar affective disorder is estimated to have a prevalence of 1–2%. Treatment is as for the normal population.

Schizophrenia

ID has a long history associated with schizophrenia, and seems to occur at higher rates (2–3% for ID, as opposed to 1% for schizophrenia). ID appears to be a risk factor for schizophrenia, and heralds a poorer prognosis. The symptom profile is similar, and can present with aggression, disturbed behaviour or lack of self-care. Negative symptoms can exacerbate skill loss, and cognitive changes can impair the ability to learn new skills. People with an ID may be more debilitated by a psychotic illness than the normal population (Bouras et al., 2004). It cannot be reliably diagnosed in people with an IQ lower than about 50 (Meadows, Turner, Campbell, Lewis, & et al., 1991). Treatment is the same as for the normal population, and should include psychoeducation, pharmacology and reducing expressed emotion. Some syndromes, in particular, have an increased incidence of schizophrenia (e.g., velocardiofacial syndrome: 10%; Murphy et al., 1999).

Dementia and delirium

People with an ID are more likely to develop delirium in response to events affecting brain function (that is, infection, trauma or medication). People with Down's syndrome are at very high risk of developing Alzheimer's dementia, and from the age of 40 onwards, all will have pathological changes, but only one-third will have clinical signs (but multi-infarct dementia is not seen, and they seem to be protected from this). The rest of the ID population seems to dement in the same way as everyone else, but there is some evidence it presents at a younger age because of pre-existing cognitive deficits, which can also confound establishing the diagnosis (Cooper, 1997).

Psychiatric disorder in the severely disabled

This group often has multiple handicaps, including epilepsy, sensory deficits, limited mobility and communication. They have limited responses, and the bulk of pathology consists of behaviour disorders with an unclear relationship to other forms of psychiatric illness. Impulsive, explosive and sexually inappropriate behaviours are common. Repetitive stereotyped movements often occur, and relationships with OCD or schizophrenia have been suggested.

4.1.5 AUTISM AND ASSOCIATED DISORDERS

NEURODIVERGENCE: A CONSUMER PERSPECTIVE

Autism has long been theorised as a medical disorder. However there has been increasing amounts of activism which conceptualises people on the autistic spectrum as experiencing some of the normal diversity of human existence. It frames people who have been diagnosed with as being on the autism spectrum as being 'neurodiverse' and the rest of the population as 'neurotypical'.

As this movement disagrees with the idea that autism is a disorder, it is concerned with supporting the rights and autonomy of people of autistic people. It sees the notion of 'curing' autism as offensive as they believe that there is nothing intrinsically wrong with the experience and instead proposes changing of environments, educating others and better supports for people. Similar to the ideas of the critical disability movement, it views society as a disabling factor rather than the experience of autism itself.

There has been a lack of involvement of people with autism in discussion about the nature of autism, research of the experience and policy that affects them. This has meant that often professionals and families, who have a particular perspective and not the lived experience, speak on others' behalf. There is also opposition to some of what is considered 'autism therapies' as the movement argues that these are primarily targeted at eliminating behaviours which are not harmful but are considered unpalatable for neurotypical people.

There has also been criticism of this movement as it has been suggested that its advocates are 'high-functioning' or only experience what used to be known as Asperger's. However, many autistic rights activists actually are considered 'low-functioning' and 'non-verbal' yet through assistive technologies contribute strongly to the debate.

The neurodivergent movement does not discount the very real difficulties that can be faced by people on the autism spectrum. This can range from practical issues such as housing and support staff to potential involvement in the psychiatric system. When working with autistic people it is important to remember that it is a very individual experience. It is a very particular way of being. Whether embraced or shunned by the individual it is most important to adopt a non-judgemental stance underscored by acceptance of difference. It is important for clinicians to be curious about what parts of the autism experience are celebrated or valuable parts of themself.

BACKGROUND

Autistic spectrum disorders have lifelong effects, and are based on a 'triad of impairments' in social interaction, communication and imagination (narrow and repetitive patterns of behaviour). It is a disorder of neurodevelopment and associated developmental psychology, and has a strong but complex genetic basis (Berney, 2000). Autism does not appear to be a unitary disorder, but is instead a complex disorder, or perhaps disorders, whose core aspects often co-occur but have distinct causes. As the presentation can vary with markedly different levels of severity on each of the three main dimensions, reference is often made to the 'autistic spectrum' of disorders, and DSM-IV used the term 'pervasive developmental disorders' and recognises three: autism, Asperger's syndrome and pervasive developmental disorder not otherwise specified (PDD NOS). However, DSM-5 subsumed all three disorders under the term autistic spectrum disorder, as it has not been possible to find the evidence to support the division into three separate disorders. They can be easily mistaken for schizophrenia by the unwary (Konstantareas & Hewitt, 2001; Perlman, 2000). DSM-5 also combined the impairments in social interaction and communication into one criterion because of the practical difficulty in separating the two types of deficits, which are so interdependent. This will mean that autism will have two and not three dimensions of impairment. ICD-11 adopted the same views as DSM-5 with similar criteria including:

- persistent deficits in social communication and interaction
- restricted and stereotyped patterns of behaviour, interests and activities
- onset in the early developmental period
- symptoms associated with a significant functional impairment.

Both ICD-11 and DSM-5 recognise that individuals along the spectrum exhibit a full range of intellectual functioning and language abilities.

The term is used both as a diagnosis and as an adjective; for example, some behaviours in people with schizophrenia are described as autistic and some people may be described as having autistic traits when they show some features that are not severe enough to warrant a diagnosis.

Autism can be seen as a group of deficits in social intelligence, in contrast to academic intelligence as measured by an IQ test. The percentage of people with autism who also meet criteria for mental retardation has been reported as anywhere from 25–70%, and this variation is thought to be secondary to the language problems inherent in autism that make valid IQ testing difficult. The usual assertion that many people with autism commonly have intellectual disability has been challenged and probably requires further investigation (Goldberg Edelson, 2006). However, there is agreement that it can be found, together with any level of ability, from profound general learning disability to average or even superior cognitive skill, in areas not directly affected by the basic impairments. It can also occur with any other physical, psychological or psychiatric condition.

Based on the diagnostic criteria of DSM-IV and ICD-10 classifications, boys and men are affected perhaps three or four times more often than girls and women (Loomes, Hull, & Mandy, 2017). A review of the research suggests that the best estimate for the population prevalence of all autistic spectrum disorders is close to 0.6%. Although autism is often seen as a childhood disorder, it is clearly one that persists throughout the lifespan.

CLINICAL PICTURE

The clinical picture is extremely varied, and can change with increasing age or psychiatric or medical problems and in different environments. Here a simple system of subgrouping, developed by Wing (1997), based solely on a description of the type of social impairment, will be used, as it is useful to demonstrate the range of clinical presentations.

Aloof group

These are people who appear aloof and indifferent to peers, though they may accept physical affection from familiar people. Few have cognitive ability in the normal range, and their abilities may be limited to gross motor function only. They may have motor stereotypes (odd movements of limbs and body) and odd postures, gait and movement (such as tiptoe walking, and hand and arm flapping or twisting). Speech is delayed, and has characteristic abnormalities, including immediate or delayed echolalia (copying of other people's talk). This type of speech may be meaningless, or may be used as a request, sometimes with reversal of pronouns—for example, 'You want juice' may mean 'I want juice'—because they echo the words they hear when juice is offered. Eye contact is inappropriate, play is absent and activities consist of repetitive routines, such as putting objects in patterns or insisting on following the same routes for journeys. Temper tantrums can occur if any change is introduced. Other features include oversensitivity to sensory stimuli, and fascination with simple sensory stimuli, such as bright lights, sounds, textures or smells. In some, self-injury is a major problem, along with disturbance of sleep and food fads.

Passive group

These are children who passively accept approaches from others with no spontaneous interaction. The other impairments are present in a less florid form, and this group tends to be more amenable in behaviour than the aloof group. Some have ability in the average or high range, and may manage in mainstream primary school. The diagnosis may be missed until problems with learning and social interaction begin to emerge in secondary school.

Active but odd group

This group makes active social approaches that are odd, inappropriate and one-sided. Their speech is often fluent, but repetitive and not used for reciprocal conversation. The repetitive routines take the form of fascination with and talking about particular topics, such as trains, train timetables or cars. A small proportion tends to have intense fantasies, and seems to have difficulty distinguishing these inventions from reality. Poor gross motor coordination is common. Behaviour difficulties arise from the egocentricity and resistance to doing anything other than their own preferred activities. The range of cognitive ability in this group is wide, but levels tend to be higher than for the aloof children, and a larger proportion have average or superior intelligence, as measured on standardised tests. People with Asperger's syndrome often fit this profile.

Loners

A subtle form is found in people of average, high or outstanding ability, who tend to prefer to be alone, lack empathy and are concerned with their own interests. Their schooldays are often stressful and difficult, because they will not conform to the demands of teachers or of fellow pupils. Most are happier as adults, and may follow successful careers. Some learn the rules of social interaction by rote, while others remain solitary by choice. Some marry, but partners may feel the lack of emotional rapport. A minority develops psychiatric illnesses.

DIAGNOSIS

Diagnosis is made by obtaining a detailed developmental history (from infancy) from parents or other informants, with particular emphasis on the elements of the autism triad that are present early in development. Differential diagnosis includes generalised learning disabilities, and specific disorders affecting language, reading, motor coordination, hearing or vision.

Autism can be misdiagnosed as any kind of psychiatric condition, or can be missed if a psychiatric condition is superimposed on the developmental disorder. A history and detailed assessment of the pattern of skills, disabilities and behaviour are required for correct diagnosis.

Associated features supporting a diagnosis in the autistic spectrum include a scattered profile of abilities on cognitive testing; tests showing absence or impairment of a theory of mind (difficulties in working out what people may be thinking or feeling); and poor ability to comprehend emotional expressions. Autistic spectrum disorders merge into eccentric normality. When making a diagnosis, it is also necessary to consider whether there are any physical abnormalities, including epilepsy and other specific syndromes. Examinations for possible causes should be undertaken if there are clinical indications, such as a clear history of regression in development. EEG and chromosomal investigations, including investigations for Fragile X, may be useful. The American College of Medical Genetics and Genomics recommends offering genetic evaluation and considers chromosomal microarray analysis as a first-tier test over karyotyping.

EDUCATION, MANAGEMENT, TREATMENT AND PROGNOSIS

The most effective way of helping children with autism is to maximise their abilities and minimise behaviour disturbance through structured education designed to take account of their impairments and special skills.

Disturbed behaviour may be a result of physical (such as epilepsy or pain) or psychological factors. Disturbed behaviour that is not a result of physical causes often responds to appropriate environmental and behavioural management, which is the treatment of choice. Superimposed psychiatric conditions may respond to removal of adverse factors in the environment, but may also require appropriate drug treatment. Disturbed behaviour is often evident from ages two to five years, tends to improve from six to 10 years, but may reappear in adolescents and young adults, eventually calming down in middle and later life. Depression is particularly common in response to awareness of problems in social interaction, and there is a risk of suicide. The outcome for independence in adult life is linked to level of ability. Individuals with severe learning disabilities will remain dependent all their lives. Those with mild learning disabilities may achieve some degree of independence. Most of those with average or high ability will become independent as adults, although most remained very dependent on their families or other support services. Few lived alone, had close friends or permanent employment (Howlin, Goode, Hutton, & Rutter, 2004).

4.1.6 COMMENTARY AND REFLECTIONS

The UN Convention on the Rights of People with Disability (see Chapter 1.5) emphasises that independence for persons with disabilities encompasses:

- individual autonomy
- the opportunity to be actively involved in decision making processes, and
- the opportunity to access the physical, social, economic and cultural environment (Nations, 2006).

The key strategies that promote independence are:

- assisting people to develop their identities
- supporting people to make decisions and
- strengthening families to build positive visions that guide towards independence (Stokes, 2013).

Mental health and disability services have different philosophies, organisational structures and staff. Services require careful coordination to be effective and avoid negative interactions. Staff in either organisation have particular skills in one area, but lack the confidence and training to deal with both disabilities when they occur together. This is likely to be further complicated by the roll-out of the new insurance scheme, the National Disability Insurance Scheme (NDIS) that is replacing disability services across Australia. While the NDIS was created under the premise of providing clients with more autonomy and control over the services they receive, the lack of choices in the private sector at this stage is likely to limit such capacity. Several complex cases remain under the care of the Disability Services for the foreseeable future and could not be transitioned to the NDIS. The transitioning period from the Disability Service to NDIS seemed to be the most critical period, and the Disability Service has created a new state-wide team, the Intensive Support Team, to facilitate a smooth transition for such complex cases.

In the United Kingdom, psychiatrists have remained involved in the care of this population, and it is a recognised subspecialty. In Australia the expectation is that this population should access the same services as everyone else and specialist services are limited to consultation-based service models in some states. Medicare funds an annual health assessment, but there are no other specific items relating to the care of people with intellectual disability. This contributes to the lack of political pressure groups and consumer involvement in service developments.

PRACTICE ILLUSTRATION: OUTCOME

For the first two weeks of discharge, Tim was seen on a daily basis by the CAT team. Although he would only say that everything was okay, they were able to monitor his progress through his parents' reports, which informed them that he became less irritable and more engaging in social interaction. An outreach worker was funded through disability services, which initially helped Tim attend to his personal hygiene and daily needs. As he improved, he was seen on a monthly basis at the outpatient clinic. A job was found for him at a supported work environment, and his outreach worker trained him to use public transport to get there and supported him in his first few weeks of employment. He reported that this gave him a sense of satisfaction as well as spare cash. He made friends there, and with the support of the disability case manager was able to arrange to go on holiday with them. He began to talk about moving out of home, and periods of respite care were arranged in anticipation of this.

4.2

SCHIZOPHRENIA OR OTHER PRIMARY PSYCHOTIC DISORDERS

CHERRIE GALLETLY, MARGARET GRIGG, BERNIE MCCORMICK & DAVID CASTLE
(CONTENT HAS BEEN CONTRIBUTED BY CHERRIE GALLETLY AND DAVID CASTLE, EXCEPT WHERE THE AUTHORSHIP OF ANOTHER CONTRIBUTOR IS NOTED FOR A SECTION.)

4.2.1 WHAT IS THIS GROUP OF MENTAL HEALTH EXPERIENCES LIKE?

HISTORICAL DEVELOPMENT OF THE CONCEPT

Schizophrenia remains an enigma, despite advances in understanding of the disorder over the 120 years since it was first described as a distinct condition. One of the underpinning problems is the way the concept of schizophrenia developed. In the 1890s, a German psychiatrist, Emil Kraepelin, separated this disorder, which he called 'dementia praecox', from manic depressive psychosis on the basis of differences in their longitudinal course (Jablensky, 2010). Dementia praecox was by definition a poor-outcome disorder, although later Kraepelin himself acknowledged some cases did reach full recovery. Kraepelin believed that the biological causes of dementia praecox would one day be discovered. While there has been substantial progress, Kraepelin's expectations have not been realised and the causes of the disorder and the pathological changes responsible for the various symptoms and variations in course are still not fully understood.

In 1910, Swiss psychiatrist Eugene Bleuler introduced the term 'schizophrenia', meaning 'split mind' (Jablensky, 2010). He was referring to a loss of the connections between thought processes, emotion and behaviour. He proposed that symptoms such as hallucinations and delusions were caused by this fundamental splitting of different psychological components of the mind. Bleuler understood that schizophrenia was not a single disorder, referring to a 'group of schizophrenias' with varying manifestations and varying outcomes. Unfortunately the concept of 'split mind' has led to confusion between schizophrenia and multiple personality (now known as dissociative identity disorder), although these are completely unrelated conditions with very different causes and clinical presentations.

In modern mental health research and clinical services, schizophrenia is often referred to as if it is a single, easily defined disorder. While we generally accept the current DSM-5 (American Psychiatric Association, 2013) and ICD-11 (World Health Organization, 2018d) constructs of schizophrenia as having reasonable reliability, the existence of a distinct biologically based disorder is not established. The diagnosis is made on the history and clinical assessment, and there is no diagnostic test that establishes that a person has schizophrenia.

In this chapter, we will refer to 'schizophrenia' as though it is a single disorder, in line with current practice and with the understanding that most research into schizophrenia has treated it as such (Jablensky, 2010). But readers should remind themselves that the label in all likelihood includes a group of different illnesses, with some generalisable parameters regarding aetiology, presentation, course, and treatment response.

Owen and colleagues (Owen, Sawa, & Mortensen, 2016) write that 'arguably the greatest challenge facing future research into aetiology, pathogenesis and treatment is the failure of current syndromic definitions to delineate a valid disease entity'. Recently, there has been interest in the concept of a continuum, or spectrum, of psychosis, extending from mild subclinical psychotic symptoms to severe, chronic psychotic disorders. Van Os, a researcher in the Netherlands, has been influential in developing these concepts. Guloksuz and van Os (2018) write of the slow death of the concept of schizophrenia, and the painful birth of the psychosis spectrum. Schizophrenia, as currently understood, would describe those at the severe end of a continuous range of psychotic symptoms (van Os, Linscott, Myin-Germeys, Delespaul, & Krabbendam, 2009).

PHENOMENOLOGY

The schizophrenia construct

There is ongoing debate about the validity of the concept of schizophrenia, although there is general acceptance that there are a number of symptom domains that are found to greater or lesser degrees in people considered to have schizophrenia. These groups of symptoms are:

- *Positive symptoms*: sometimes referred to as 'reality distortion', namely delusions and hallucinations. Delusions are false beliefs held with tenacity, unamenable to reason and not in keeping with person's sociocultural belief systems. In schizophrenia there has been particular emphasis on bizarre delusions, but the most common delusions in people with schizophrenia are persecutory (the belief one is being picked on, followed, spied on with malicious intent), grandiose (elevated sense of power, being chosen for some special purpose, messianic) and referential (things having special personal meaning for the individual, such as radio or TV content, sequences of number plates and so forth). These are not particular or specific to schizophrenia, and can be seen in some organic disorders and mood disorders (notably mania). More 'schizophrenia-specific' delusions are those that are very bizarre (e.g. one's hair growing on the inside of one's skull, one's internal organs being rotated, being influenced by intergalactic machines, and so forth). Passivity experiences (feeling one's mind, emotions and body are being controlled by an external force) are often attributed by the person to being a victim of an external influence such as telepathy or hypnosis. In 1959 Schneider, a German psychiatrist, introduced the concept of 'first rank' symptoms, which were seen as particularly characteristic of schizophrenia (Jablensky, 2010). While these are useful as descriptions of the range of symptoms seen in schizophrenia, a Cochrane review has shown that the presence or absence of first rank symptoms is not a reliable indication of diagnosis (Soares-Weiser et al., 2015).

- *Hallucinations*: false perceptions that can occur in any sensory modality (auditory, visual, smell, taste, somatic) but auditory hallucinations ('voices') are both the most common and the most particular to schizophrenia. Schneider (Jablensky, 2010) included a number of specific auditory hallucinatory experiences among his first rank symptoms (see Box 4.1). Command hallucinations, where the voice 'tells' the individual to enact some behaviour (e.g. 'stab the person sitting next to you in the eye with your pen') are rare but clinically important. They are highly distressing and potentially associated with dangerous behaviour. Visual hallucinations are not uncommon in people with schizophrenia but are usually fleeting and ill-formed: clear persistent visual hallucinations usually indicate underlying organic brain pathology such as drug intoxication and withdrawal states. Tactile hallucinations can be very distressing, especially if of a sexual nature, for example associated with beliefs the individual is being raped. Hallucinations involving taste and smell are more likely to be due to organic (e.g. the epigastric feeling that occurs before a temporal lobe seizure) or depressive (e.g. the smell of oneself rotting away) conditions.

Box 4.1: Schneiderian first-rank symptoms for schizophrenia

Delusions

Passivity phenomena, where the individual believes their actions, emotions or feelings have been 'taken over' by some other force: likened to being a robot or a puppet on a string.

Ego boundary permeability, encompassing thought insertion (thoughts being put into the person's mind from some external source), thought withdrawal (the reverse of thought insertion) and thought broadcast (thoughts being passively 'shared' with others).

Delusional perception where a normal percept leads to an instantaneous—often fully formed and elaborate—delusional belief system.

Hallucinations

Third person voices discussing the individual, often as a derogatory 'conversation' between the voices.

Running commentary (third person hallucinations commenting on the actions of the individual).

Thought echo (hearing own thoughts out loud).

Source: Adapted from Soares-Weiser et al., 2015

- *Negative symptoms*: Bleuler (Jablensky, 2010) considered the negative symptoms to be the primary symptoms of schizophrenia, and in many ways they can be considered as the core of the disorder: certainly they are more persistent and generally more disabling than the positive symptoms. These symptoms are characterised by *apathetic social withdrawal, restriction of affect* (a bland unresponsive facial expression that in its severest form can be labelled 'blunted') and *paucity of thought* (leading to short unembellished answers to questions and a lack of general ability to engage in social banter). The social withdrawal is distinct from that associated with social anxiety, in that there is no real desire to socialise, and there is an associated difficultly in reading social cues or understanding the minds of others (referred to as lacking 'theory of mind'); the latter has parallels with autism (see Section 4.1.5), and indeed it was described in this way by Bleuler. A crucial clinical point is to distinguish 'primary' from 'secondary' negative symptoms (Kirschner, Aleman, & Kaiser, 2017): the latter are symptoms and behaviours that manifest like negative symptoms but are caused by some other primary process (e.g. depression, or as a reaction to positive symptoms) or by some medications (notably dopamine system antagonists such as haloperidol). The importance of distinguishing secondary from primary negative symptoms lies in the former being responsive to treatment of the underlying problem (or removal of the offending agent in the case of antipsychotic-induced negative symptoms).

- Many people with schizophrenia have *cognitive dysfunction* which manifests across a number of domains and usually occurs along with negative symptoms. The components of cognitive function which have shown most impairment are executive function (high level planning and concepts) and verbal fluency (finding the right words). Such difficulties usually begin before the positive symptoms develop and tend to be enduring or even show some worsening over time.
- *Disorganisation symptoms*: The dimension of 'disorganisation' was first separated from the original positive/negative dichotomy by Liddle (1987). This dimension encompasses disorganisation of thoughts (so-called 'formal thought disorder') and of actions; as well as *inappropriate affect*, where the expressed affect is not congruent to the topic (e.g. laughing while talking about a sad event). *Formal thought disorder* ranges from mild, with vagueness and circumstantiality, to so severe that little sense can be made of the conversation (sometimes referred to as 'word salad'). Particular—but again not exclusive—to schizophrenia are tangentiality, where the flow of speech diverts from its original course and wanders away; and derailment, where there is a sudden and (to the listener at least) inexplicable jump from one topic line of speech to another: this is also referred to as 'knight's move' thinking, after the way the knight can move in a chess game. Other disorders of thought include thought withdrawal (where thoughts seem to be removed from the brain by an external agency), thought insertion (where thoughts that the person does not own, often with disturbing content, are inserted into their head), thought broadcast (hearing one's thoughts spoken aloud so everyone around can hear them) and thought blocking (where the train of thought abruptly ceases).
- *Arousal*: The three symptom dimensions described above are generally accepted as the main ones characterising schizophrenia, but other symptom dimensions can be seen when interviewing or interacting with a person with schizophrenia. Arousal tends to be more changeable than the other dimensions and is more commonly reported in acute relapse when the individual is autonomically and behaviourally agitated. It is, of course, very important clinically as agitation can lead on to aggression. It requires careful evaluation and treatment, usually including medication.
- *Mood and anxiety symptoms*: Depression and anxiety are very common accompaniments of schizophrenia, and require evaluation and focused treatment. The lifetime rate for depressive disorder in schizophrenia has been estimated at 25%, while rates of depression not meeting diagnostic criteria are very much higher (Siris, 2000). Overall, lifetime rates of 10–12% for generalised anxiety disorder, 4–20% for panic disorder, 5–20% for agoraphobia, and 30% for social anxiety disorder have been reported in people with schizophrenia (Pokos & Castle, 2006). Obsessive-compulsive disorder appears to become more common as schizophrenia progresses, such that around 11–15% of people with early onset schizophrenia might manifest the disorder, growing to 22–30% later in the course of the illness (Pokos & Castle, 2006).
- *Depressive disorder*: needs to be distinguished from negative symptoms. Key considerations in the clinical interview are eliciting the core depression items of depressed mood and loss of pleasure, as well as associated features such as fatigue, poor concentration, sleep disturbance and appetite disturbance, notably loss of appetite and weight loss. It is important to recognise that some medications used for the treatment of schizophrenia, including many antipsychotics, can impact on sleep and appetite and this needs to be borne in mind in the clinical appraisal. Exploring negative thoughts, including guilt, pessimism about the future and hopelessness, is critical. The latter is also often associated with suicidality and full assessment of suicide risk is required as suicidal acts and completed suicide are tragically common in people with schizophrenia (Hor & Taylor, 2010).

All of the anxiety or fear-related disorders are more common in people with schizophrenia, compared to the general population (Braga, Reynolds, & Siris, 2013). Again, specific questioning is required to elicit the features of each disorder and to avoid missing a treatable anxiety disorder. Social anxiety disorder, for example, can masquerade as social avoidance, part of the negative symptom dimension. The key difference is the desire to socialise in social anxiety disorder, compared to apathetic social withdrawal in the negative symptom dimension. Given the fact that people with schizophrenia have often suffered substantial adversity and trauma—including sometimes as a consequence of coercive treatments—it is hardly surprising that disorders associated with stress, particularly post-traumatic stress disorder are common in people with schizophrenia. Obsessive-compulsive disorder is of particular interest in schizophrenia, in part because some people seem to have a vulnerability to both psychotic and obsessive-compulsive symptoms and also because some antipsychotics—notably clozapine—can cause or exacerbate obsessive-compulsive symptoms.

FORMAL DIAGNOSIS (ICD-11)

ICD-11 describes three main categories of psychotic disorder, termed (1) schizophrenia, (2) schizoaffective disorder and (3) acute and transient psychotic disorder.

1. Schizophrenia and other primary psychotic disorders are characterised by disturbances across multiple aspects of mental function. Symptoms can include delusions, hallucinations, thought disorder, experiences of being influenced and control, and cognitive impairment. There may be grossly disorganised behaviour, and negative symptoms such as blunted or flat affect and lack of motivation. The symptoms occur with sufficient frequency and intensity to deviate from expected cultural or subcultural norms. The symptoms need to have been present for at least a month to make a diagnosis of schizophrenia.
2. If these symptoms are due to another mental and behavioural disorder (e.g., a mood disorder, delirium, or a disorder due to substance use), then this disorder rather than schizophrenia is the correct diagnosis.
3. The categories in this grouping should not be used to classify the expression of ideas, beliefs, or behaviours that are culturally sanctioned.
4. Schizoaffective disorder is diagnosed when criteria for schizophrenia and a manic or depressive episode (whether mixed, moderate, or severe) are met at the same time or within a few days, in a single illness-episode lasting at least a month. Catatonia (described later in this section) or other psychomotor disturbances may be seen. Symptoms must not be caused by another health condition, a substance or a medication.
5. Acute and transient psychotic disorder has an abrupt onset. The symptoms are similar to schizophrenia, but can change quickly, from day to day. The symptoms build to their maximum severity within two weeks, and do not persist for more than three months. Again, symptoms must not be due to another medical or psychiatric condition, such as a delirium or substance use.
6. Schizophrenia, schizoaffective disorder and acute and transient psychotic disorder are further divided into subtypes according to longitudinal course, including:
   - first episode
   - multiple episodes
   - continuous.

   Each of these subtypes (first episode, multiple episode or continuous) is further described according to the current presentation as:
   - currently symptomatic
   - in partial remission
   - in full remission
   - unspecified.

   So, for example, a person might be described as suffering from schizophrenia, continuous course, currently symptomatic.

Two further disorders, schizotypal disorder and delusional disorder, are included in the broad category of schizophrenia and related disorders in ICD-11.

1 Schizotypal disorder is characterised by an enduring pattern of odd behaviour, appearance and speech, along with cognitive and perceptual distortions, and unusual beliefs. These symptoms cause distress, or impaired functioning, but are not sufficiently severe to meet criteria for schizophrenia. The term 'negative schizotypy' includes constricted or inappropriate affect and anhedonia, while 'positive schizotypy' includes paranoid ideas, ideas of reference, and hallucinations. The classification of schizotypal disorder has varied over time. It is classified with both the personality disorders and schizophrenia spectrum disorders in DSM-5, and as part of the grouping of schizophrenia and related disorders in ICD-11. Conceptually, it fits with van Os's model of a continuum of psychosis (van Os et al., 2009), with a pattern of symptoms that is similar to, but less severe than, the symptoms meeting criteria for schizophrenia.

2 Delusional disorder is, as the name suggests, characterised by delusions that persist for at least 3 months, in the absence of a depressive, manic, or mixed mood episode. Other characteristic symptoms of schizophrenia such as persistent auditory hallucinations, disorganised thinking, and negative symptoms are not present, but there may be perceptual disturbances including transient hallucinations and illusions that are thematically related to the delusions. The person's affect, speech, and behaviour are typically unaffected, apart from abnormalities related to the delusional beliefs. As with other disorders in this category, delusional disorder is not diagnosed if the symptoms result from another medical or psychiatric condition.

Delusional disorder can be categorised as currently symptomatic, in partial remission or in full remission.

ICD-11 also includes a description of catatonia:

> Catatonia is a disorder of behaviour and voluntary control of movements. People with catatonia may have extreme slowing of motor activity, or simply stop moving at all and freeze in rigid, unusual or bizarre postures. Mutism and purposeless motor activity can also be observed. Catatonia is not always due to schizophrenia, but may occur in a number of different disorders including depressive episode. Catatonia was more commonly described among people living in the asylums many years ago, before the widespread use of antipsychotic drugs.

4.2.2 LIVED EXPERIENCE

BERNIE

THE EXPERIENCE OF SCHIZOAFFECTIVE DISORDER

My illness comes in the form of specific delusional thoughts and fears based in reality; depression; some mania; and ideas of reference. Suicidality is an ongoing and fluctuating symptom. These greatly inhibit my functioning and ability to live a life free from major symptoms. Some people regard paranoia as a general suspiciousness: for me it means a debilitating constant delusional fear which means I cannot function at most levels for significant periods of time. It manifests in actions like taking two different trains and a taxi home from university to avoid 'pursuers'. My illness was precipitated by a string of significant personal crises and the experience of sexual assault. Imperceptible changes in mental state over time can occur gradually without detection until it is too late, especially in first episode psychosis. I see my mental health now as a continuum on which I constantly move back and forth: it fluctuates daily at times, and sometimes substantially over months at a time.

I have been hospitalised about half a dozen times and it is important to understand what hospital (and medication) does and doesn't do, can and can't do. There have been times where hospitalisation was the only option and times where it was the worst option. On several occasions my mental health was worse after being discharged from hospital than it was prior to admission.

My illness follows recognisable patterns but the particular way it presents can be different each time therefore objective medical opinion can be required to anticipate relapse, and this is the reason I present issues as I experience them to my GP without diagnostic speculation. It's like 'this is what is happening, what do you think?' As a patient—I experience; as a doctor—he diagnoses. Sometimes increased medication in crisis is called for; sometimes the situation is assessed as 'you need a beer'. My treatment consists of flexible, experienced, timely, strategic, early intervention, and I can talk in mental health shorthand with my GP who I have known for many years. I can say things like 'this is as bad as 1991' and he will understand: we are partners in insight and hindsight. Words of encouragement mean more from someone you trust and can sometimes briefly override or negate symptomatic beliefs. We have successfully intervened over a dozen times in the last 30 years preventing relapses from occurring and mitigating those that do. There is a tacit recognition between us that I am one of the experts in my own mental health.

As much as I try I cannot 'think my way' out of psychotic experiences; they do not readily respond to reason or logical argument and tend to be circular and nebulous in nature. My experience is that it is best to 'park' particular issues/symptoms/scenarios and work in practical, immediate terms and activity, especially in crisis. The next phase is the space to analyse, reconcile and understand feelings and symptoms at a gentle pace. You can't 'create' recovery but it will happen in time, all you can do is put in place the best conditions to facilitate it when it happens. Recovery can be a slow gradual process of awakening; it's like realising that you are drunk is part of the way to becoming sober!

My mental illness fluctuates and is episodic; I therefore need a treatment and a lifestyle that is responsive and can accommodate these issues over time. Idiosyncratic responses to illnesses and situations are best determined and validated by the individual and their treating team together.

4.2.3 WHAT DO WE KNOW ABOUT THESE DISORDERS?

PREVALENCE

As described above the term schizophrenia most likely includes a number of different disorders, with a range of causes. This makes determining the prevalence, course and outcome difficult. A large review in 2008 found that the median incidence of schizophrenia is 15.2/100 000 persons. The incidence of schizophrenia is higher in men with a male to female ratio of about 1.4:1.0 (McGrath, Saha, Chant, & Welham, 2008). There is wide variation between different regions, and finding out the reasons for these variations would help in identifying the factors that can cause schizophrenia. Overall, women tend to have a later age of onset, and a less severe course of illness.

In 2010 the Survey of High Impact Psychosis (SHIP; see Section 1.6.4) surveyed 1825 people with psychotic disorders, living in eight different regions of Australia, and in contact with public mental health services in the previous 12 months. In the SHIP survey, about two-thirds (65%) of people experienced their first episode before the age of 25 years. The mean age of onset was 23 years for men and 24 years for women.

There are a number of factors even before birth, such as exposure to famine or influenza during the second trimester of intrauterine life, that are associated with an increased risk of developing schizophrenia later in life. Being born in late winter or early spring may be associated with greater risk of schizophrenia. These risk factors indicate that damage to the developing brain can confer an increased liability to schizophrenia as an adult (van Os & Kapur, 2009).

Migration is associated with an increased risk, especially in the second generation (the children of those who migrated). This observation led to the concept of 'social defeat'. Social factors such as bullying, stigma and discrimination are thought to act as stressors that can precipitate schizophrenia in those who are predisposed to develop the disorder (van Os, Kenis, & Rutten, 2010).

The 'two-hit hypothesis' is a model to help us understand the development of schizophrenia. The first 'hit' is the underlying genetic risk and factors that occur in utero and in early life, which result in vulnerability to the disorder. The second 'hit' occurs later, and includes social adversity and substance abuse (Murray, Bhavsar, Tripoli, & Howes, 2017).

Box 4.2: Environmental factors associated with an increased risk of schizophrenia

In utero and birth:

- influenza type exposure
- toxoplasmosis
- maternal anaemia
- hypovitaminosis D
- maternal stress
- late winter/early spring birth (northern hemisphere only)
- obstetric complications/foetal distress
- advanced paternal age
- urban birth.

Post-birth exposures:

- migration (notably ethnic minorities)
- tobacco exposure in teenage years
- cannabis exposure in teenage years.

People with schizophrenia die about 15 years earlier than the general population, and this premature mortality is discussed in more detail when we discuss physical health in Section 4.2.3. While this earlier mortality is most pronounced in schizophrenia, most other mental disorders including the more common disorders such as depression are also associated with poorer health and earlier death, compared to the general population (Firth et al., 2019). Contributing factors include lifestyle challenges (inadequate diet, lack of exercise, obesity, smoking, alcohol), and the metabolic effects of some medications.

HOW CAN WE UNDERSTAND THE ORIGINS?

The causes of schizophrenia are not well understood, despite considerable research effort, partly because of the challenges in defining the disorder described above.

The interaction of genetics, environment and developmental stage

The well-established fact that monozygotic (identical) twins have only around a 50% concordance for schizophrenia is often cited as compelling evidence for 'environmental' parameters being pertinent in the aetiology of the disorder (Owen et al., 2016). None of these effects are particularly powerful, most being associated with an increased risk ratio of around two. More recently the gene-environment discussion has been nuanced by a deeper understanding of epigenetic effects and gene-environment interaction effects. Thus, environmental factors interact with underlying genetic predisposition to act as potential cumulative causal factors in schizophrenia. Also of importance is the timing of specific environmental impacts, as the brain is differentially vulnerable at different developmental stages, to certain 'insults'. It is hardly surprising that periods of greatest brain growth, notably in utero, are the highest risk periods, but some factors seem to operate later, including cannabis (Hamilton, 2017) and (perhaps) tobacco consumption in teenage years.

Genetics

The strong genetic component to schizophrenia has been known and accepted for decades. The genetics is highly complex, and most likely there are many genes of small effect. Various approaches including genome-wide studies, and research focusing in specific genes, have identified over 100 genetic loci associated with schizophrenia, some related to neurodevelopment and some linked to neurotransmitters relevant to psychosis (notably dopamine; Foley, Corvin, & Nakagome, 2017). An interesting association has been found with loci on chromosome 6, which has been conjectured to have impact on neuronal pruning in adolescence (Sekar et al., 2016). A reduction in neuronal connections is recognised as a normal part of brain development and maturation during adolescence, and it is thought that this process is disrupted in people who develop schizophrenia—possibly explaining why symptoms develop at this time of life.

Intriguing as this may be, it is important to appreciate that none of the identified loci carry a very strong signal (i.e., no single gene has a major effect) and also that there is little specificity for schizophrenia. For example, a large-scale genome-wide association study of 33 332 people showed similar loci being associated with bipolar disorder, autism spectrum disorder, attention deficit disorder and major depressive disorder (Cross-Disorder Group of the Psychiatric Genomics Consortium et al., 2013). Somewhat more specific to schizophrenia are so-called 'copy number variants' (extra copies of sections of a gene), but again these are sometimes found in people with bipolar disorder and autism spectrum disorder. Sporadic *de novo* (new) genetic mutations may also sometimes cause people to develop schizophrenia.

The brain in schizophrenia

That schizophrenia is a disease affecting the brain seems obvious, but for many years there was scant attention paid to brain abnormalities in people presenting with what was considered a 'functional' (as opposed to 'organic') psychosis. This was squarely challenged by researchers at London's Northwick Park Hospital in the late 1970s (Johnstone, Crow, Frith, Husband, & Kreel, 1976). Using what was then cutting-edge computed tomography (CT) scanning, it was shown that people with schizophrenia, as a group, had larger cerebral ventricular volumes (a marker of reduced grey matter) than healthy controls. This finding has been replicated countless times, and with more sophisticated neuroimaging, yielding fairly consistent findings of reduced volumes of overall grey matter as well as smaller volumes in specific brain areas including the hippocampus and amygdala. It is important to note that these are group effects and that that there is considerable overlap in these parameters between people with schizophrenia and those without: there is no specific brain structural abnormality that can be used to tell us if someone has schizophrenia and not everyone with a diagnosis of schizophrenia is outside the normal range of grey matter volume.

One of the major questions for the field remains what causes these abnormalities. Longitudinally, it seems that these brain changes may to some extent antedate illness onset, being found in prodromal and 'high risk' individuals. They may possibly be a marker of neurodevelopmental insult, probably largely genetically mediated. Indeed, as described earlier, the neurodevelopmental hypothesis has dominated the schizophrenia field for the last 30 years (Murray et al., 2017). Put simply, it is postulated that there is an inherent early (foetal, or early childhood) developmental brain 'lesion' but the brain is not 'able' to manifest positive symptoms of psychosis until later in life (late teens and early adulthood). There are many factors supporting this model, including that longitudinal birth cohort studies have shown early childhood abnormalities (very nonspecific) of milestone acquisition (notably verbal) and socialisation among individuals who later develop schizophrenia. There are also associations of schizophrenia with minor physical abnormalities that are thought to be markers of early neurodevelopmental deviance. More recently, it has been shown that the structural brain abnormalities show an escalation at the time of the transition to psychosis (Chung & Cannon, 2015); and also that there is sometimes progression of the structural abnormalities over time (Schnack et al., 2016). Thus, the neurodevelopmental model has been modified to include a neurodegenerative element, which resonates with Kraepelin's thinking 120 years earlier.

Neurotransmitters and schizophrenia

The advent of pharmacological treatments for schizophrenia in the 1950s opened the door to attempts to understand the underlying neurochemical abnormalities associated with psychotic symptoms, and a number of different hypothesis have been proposed over the years. The dopamine hypothesis remains the most enduring of these, resting on observations that dopaminergic (dopamine releasing) medications and illicit drugs can produce delusions and hallucinations; and that all effective antipsychotic medications block dopamine D2 receptors post-synaptically. Actually the 'problem' with the dopamine system in schizophrenia is rather more complex than a simple excess, as different brain areas have differential variations in dopaminergic tone. Thus, an excess of dopamine in the mesolimbic tract could explain positive symptoms of delusions and hallucinations, while a relative shortage of dopamine in mesocortical tracts might be responsible for negative symptoms (Howes, McCutcheon, Owen, & Murray, 2017). This raises difficulties for antipsychotic medications that block all D2 receptors, as they may be effective in ameliorating positive symptoms but actually worsen negative symptoms. There is also some support for the idea that some people have a 'form' of schizophrenia associated with an overall lack of dopamine: the so-called deficit syndrome, for which early initiation of clozapine could be advocated (Howes & Kapur, 2014).

Given the many complex inhibitory and excitatory connections within and between neural networks in the brain, it is not surprising that many other neurotransmitter systems are also implicated in schizophrenia. Again, it is important to be aware that there may be a number of disorders included in the diagnostic category of schizophrenia, and these can have different patterns of neurotransmitter abnormalities. The serotonin system has an important role to play (note that serotonergic agonists such as lysergic acid diethylamide—LSD—produce hallucinations); and glutamatergic, muscarinic, nicotinic and endocannabinoid systems are all targets for drug development in schizophrenia.

Inflammation and auto-immunity

Autoimmune disorders, most notably N-methyl-D-aspartate Receptor (NMDA-R) encephalitis, can present with a clinical picture similar to schizophrenia. In this condition, the body generates antibodies to specific receptors in the brain. The NMDA receptors are activated by glutamate, an excitatory neurotransmitter, and the resulting autoimmune disorder can present with an acute psychosis. This condition was described very vividly in a book, *My Brain on Fire*, by Susan Callahan, a journalist who developed NMDA-R encephalitis. Autoimmune brain disorders can be diagnosed via blood tests and lumbar puncture, and respond to immunological treatments. There is considerable interest in the concept that there may be other auto-antibody disorders that present with symptoms typical of schizophrenia. It can be difficult to know who should be screened for NMDA-R encephalitis, so Scott and colleagues have developed guidelines to assist screening of people who present with possible early psychosis (Scott, Gillis, Swayne, & Blum, 2018).

As in other areas in psychiatry, recent research has also focused on oxidative stress and inflammation, as possibly contributing to the development of schizophrenia. These processes may affect specific brain regions and impact on neurones involved in brain development and maturation (Barron, Hafizi, Andreazza, & Mizrahi, 2017). There has also been interest in the role of the microbiome, and gut health, in schizophrenia, as in other mental disorders. The exciting aspect to these lines of research is that they may lead to new treatments, beyond the dopamine-blocking drugs currently available.

Substance use

Substance use is very common among people with schizophrenia. There are two ways of looking at this—first, does drug use increase the risk of developing schizophrenia? Second, what is the impact of substance abuse in people who have established schizophrenia?

Numerous studies have shown that use of cannabis in adolescence confers a higher risk for psychosis outcomes in later life and the risk is dose-related (Hamilton, 2017). Individuals with polymorphisms of COMT and AKT1 genes may be at increased risk for psychotic disorders in association with cannabis, as are individuals with a family history of psychotic disorders or a history of childhood trauma. Beginning cannabis use at a younger age is associated with a higher risk of developing schizophrenia (Di Forti et al., 2014).

Tobacco use has also been implicated as a possible factor contributing to the development of schizophrenia, although unlike cannabis, there is no association between smoking and earlier age of onset of psychosis (Myles et al., 2012). There are high rates of smoking among people with schizophrenia; for example in the SHIP study 70% of participants were current smokers, compared to a general population rate of around 15–20%.

The rates of other substance use in people in the SHIP survey are shown in Table 4.3. The SHIP participants were attending public mental health services, so these rates are most likely higher than for all people with schizophrenia living in the community (some of whom will only see GPs and/ or private psychiatrists). Sometimes the use of drugs or alcohol is driven by a short-term benefit in achieving reduction in anxiety and psychotic symptoms. Unfortunately, with excessive, long-term use, alcohol and illicit substances are strongly associated with a number of adverse outcomes for people with schizophrenia, including a poorer longitudinal illness course with high relapse and rehospitalisation rates, family dysfunction, physical health morbidities, violence and crime. Cannabis and stimulants are especially important. In individuals with an established psychotic disorder, cannabis can exacerbate symptoms and have negative consequences on the course of the illness. Cannabis can precipitate relapse in people with schizophrenia, despite the person taking on antipsychotic medications; and stimulants, notably crystal methamphetamine, can cause florid psychotic relapses that can be associated with violence. These addictions require a concerted therapeutic effort (De Witte, Crunelle, Sabbe, Moggi, & Dom, 2014).

Table 4.3 Rates of substance use in schizophrenia/schizoaffective patients in the SHIP study (n=1150)

Substance	Lifetime prevalence	Last year prevalence	Last year frequency of use
Alcohol	92.4%	80.7%	Monthly/weekly 33.7% Daily/almost daily 12.6%
Cannabis	98.0%	48.7%	Monthly/weekly 17.4% Daily/almost daily 17.6%
Stimulants	72.8%	39.2%	Monthly/weekly 10.8% Daily/almost daily 3.0%
Other illicit drugs	75.6%	29.5%	Monthly/weekly 5.5% Daily/almost daily 3.5%

Source: Adapted from Morgan et al., 2011

Trauma

Trauma can include distressing emotional, physical, sexual and social experiences and has recently been recognised as an important factor that increases the risk of schizophrenia. Exposure to adversity in childhood, including physical, sexual and emotional abuse, neglect, parental death, and bullying, is associated with almost a three-fold risk of developing a psychotic illness (Varese et al., 2012). In addition, disorders more common in those who have been subject to childhood adversity and trauma, such as post-traumatic stress disorder, depression, anxiety and substance use disorders are also common comorbid conditions in people with schizophrenia. It has been suggested that childhood trauma has a negative impact on recovery from psychosis (Alameda et al., 2015). Researchers are now developing models to show how genetic vulnerability, and the effects of trauma on the development of brain networks, might interact to lead to later psychosis (Popovic et al., 2019). Now that we have recognised the importance of trauma, both as a causative factor and as a cause of ongoing emotional distress, there is an urgent need to develop trauma-informed interventions for people with schizophrenia (see Section 2.3.9).

IMPORTANT INFLUENCES ON PROGNOSIS

There are many factors that can impact on prognosis, including individual strengths, family and social factors, and the quality of services provided. There is often a surprisingly long period between when the first psychotic symptoms develop, and when the person begins treatment. This period is called the duration of untreated psychosis (DUP) and a longer duration of untreated psychosis tends to be associated with poorer outcome.

Poor premorbid function and early age of onset of illness can indicate a poorer prognosis (Lauronen et al., 2007). Male gender, comorbid substance abuse, more severe and persistent negative symptoms, and greater cognitive impairment, have also been found to be more common in those with less positive outcomes.

It has been suggested that the occurrence of relapse has an adverse impact on prognosis. In a Hong Kong study of people with FEP, half of the participants stopped maintenance medication while half continued. After a period of time in the study, all participants received treatment as usual. Ten years after the study had ended, 39% of people who had experienced a period off medication had a poor outcome, compared to 21% of people who had never stopped medication (Hui et al., 2018). The argument that relapse has a toxic effect on long-term outcome has been used to advocate for wider use of long-acting injectable (LAI) antipsychotic medications, as well as continuity of community supports.

Psychosocial interventions, including several types of family interventions (see Chapter 2.7), have been shown to reduce, delay or minimise the impact of relapse (McFarlane, 2016). Community-based programs that emphasise ongoing support and treatment for consumers can also reduce relapse rates, as would be expected as such programs encourage medication adherence, ensure stability of living arrangements, help manage stressors and encourage social inclusion. Specialist community programs, known as 'intensive case management' or 'assertive' community treatment, that provide outreach to people who are unable or unwilling to access outpatient services, can reduce hospitalisation rates (Schottle et al., 2014) and be cost-effective in improving quality of life (Karow et al., 2012). In addition, many psychosocial interventions stress the identification of early warning signs and the preparation of a plan of action if these early warning signs become apparent. This process of working together to develop a relapse prevention plan can be empowering and helps with developing illness self-management skills (Morriss, Vinjamuri, Faizal, Bolton, & McCarthy, 2013).

COURSE AND IMPACT

Guloksuz and van Os (2018) point out that over time, some people recover from first episode psychosis, or from schizophrenia, and these people exit from treatment services. So, clinicians are left with a selected sample of people with poorer outcome, and this becomes regarded as the normal course for people diagnosed with schizophrenia. Sometimes when people make a good recovery, it is thought that the diagnosis may have been wrong, rather than that the diagnostic category encompasses a range of disorders with variable capacity for recovery.

As described above the onset of schizophrenia tends to occur in late adolescence or early adulthood, and often disrupts the developmental tasks of this life stage. These tasks include living independently, establishing adult relationships, and moving into the workforce. There is sometimes a prodromal period where the person gradually disengages with education, work and social relationships, and may develop nonspecific symptoms, before psychotic symptoms develop. People with schizophrenia often have fewer years of education, compared to their siblings (Tempelaar, Termorshuizen, MacCabe, Boks, & Kahn, 2017), and lower educational achievement in turn tends to be associated with unemployment and social disadvantage. There has been a push for better vocational services for people with schizophrenia, to overcome these disadvantages.

Measures to improve early recognition of psychosis can reduce the burden on the individual and their family, who may experience a distressing period during which psychotic symptoms and disturbed behaviour gradually escalate. There is also a risk of violence and suicide during this period of undiagnosed and untreated psychosis (Nielssen, Malhi, McGorry, & Large, 2012). Early intervention can improve engagement with services and treatment response, reduce illicit substance abuse, and prevent relapses (Fusar-Poli, McGorry, & Kane, 2017). There is less disruption to family, friends, and participation in work or education. Psychosocial interventions are likely to be more helpful during the early stages of a psychotic episode.

There is considerable variation in the course of schizophrenia. This is important in instilling hope—even if the symptoms are severe and the outlook appears discouraging, there may well be symptomatic recovery over the long-term. Often the earlier years are the most troublesome, and gradually the individual settles on the best medication for them, psychosocial interventions and durable social supports are put in place, and the person develops better skills in managing the symptoms. A 2001 study found that 16% of people who had unremitting symptoms in the early stages of schizophrenia achieved a later recovery (Harrison et al., 2001). Further, van Os and Kapur (2009) write that relatively good outcomes are seen in 20–50% of cases. Two large studies undertaken by WHO (Hopper, Harrison, Janca, & Sartorius, 2007; Jablensky et al., 1992) found that more than 30% of people with schizophrenia had relatively good clinical outcomes after 15 and 25 years of follow-up. A more recent study demonstrated that after initial deterioration, the trajectory of illness, on average, ameliorates by the age of 23 (Levine, Lurie, Kohn, & Levav, 2011).

Loneliness and social isolation are recurring themes among many people with psychosis (Barut, Dietrich, Zanoni, & Ridner, 2016). Social support is a key factor in facilitating recovery, but people with psychosis sometimes have difficulties with the social skills necessary for forming supportive social networks. Added to this, stigma and continuing symptoms of illness may impact on the capacity to develop and maintain social relationships. While social stigma in the broader community is the most obvious, health professionals may also express stigmatising attitudes. The SANE website (SANE, 2020) contains useful information about combating stigma, and resources and support to help with social inclusion and recovery.

Many people with schizophrenia live with social disadvantage. The majority (85%) of people taking part in the SHIP survey lived on government pensions. Lack of sufficient disposable income limits healthy lifestyle choices such as choosing good food, joining a gym, and buying walking shoes. In addition, as described above, people with schizophrenia tend to have higher rates of alcohol and illicit drug use, compared to the general population, resulting in adverse social, economic and health consequences.

While community attitudes can include fear that people with a diagnosis of schizophrenia might be dangerous, in fact people with schizophrenia are at greater risk of being victims of crime (Morgan et al., 2016). This might be due to vulnerability and lack of awareness of risks to personal safety, and to living in areas with cheap rent, but higher rates of crime. These traumatic events increase the risk of other comorbid mental disorders such as anxiety and PTSD.

As many as a third of the homeless people in our cities have schizophrenia (Teesson, Hodder, & Buhrich, 2004). Common reasons for homelessness include the use of money for substance use, as well as the presence of persecutory beliefs involving services and institutions. There is a need for stable, secure housing along with social supports to enable people to move from homelessness to appropriate accommodation.

In Australia, about 5% of prisoners have a diagnosis of schizophrenia (Nielssen & Misrachi, 2005). This can be due to crimes related to poverty and substance abuse, or to acting on delusional beliefs and command hallucinations (Yee, Large, Kemp, & Nielssen, 2011). On release, good follow-up by community mental health services is essential.

There is enormous variation, between individuals and over time, in the course of schizophrenia. The earlier years of the illness tend to be more troublesome. Many people are able to make a good recovery, with a stable living situation, meaningful social connections and regular engagement in satisfying daily activities.

Some are able to continue in demanding professions, with good supports and effective measures to reduce or manage daily stresses.

Physical health

Most people in Western countries can anticipate living into their late 70s or early 80s, but people with schizophrenia frequently die much earlier. On average, people with schizophrenia die 14.5 years earlier than expected; the years of potential life lost is greater for men (15.9 years) than women (13.6 years; Hjorthoj, Sturup, McGrath, & Nordentoft, 2017). There has been an increase in diabetes paralleling the increased use of second generation antipsychotics. However, it appears that in schizophrenia, mortality is actually highest in those who do not take antipsychotic drugs (Vermeulen et al., 2017). Antipsychotic drugs differ in their metabolic profiles, and it is obviously desirable to prescribe drugs which are less likely to cause weight gain. For example, olanzapine is associated with substantial weight gain, while ziprasidone and lurasidone tend to be weight-neutral.

People with psychotic disorders living in Australia have higher rates of virtually all common physical disorders including chronic pain, headaches, asthma and arthritis (Morgan et al., 2011). They also tend to have poor dental health. In addition, obstructive sleep apnoea (OSA) may also be more common, and less recognised, among people with schizophrenia. Sleep disturbance, tiredness and cognitive impairment may be mistaken for negative symptoms or medication side effects (Myles et al., 2016).

Table 4.4 shows rates of major cardiovascular disease risk factors among participants in the SHIP study.

Table 4.4 Cardiovascular disease risk factors in people with a psychotic disorder in the SHIP study (n = 1825)

	Male %	Female %	Total %
Tobacco			
- current	71.7	59.1	66.6
- lifetime	85.9	73.7	80.9
Physical activity			
- low	63.5	62.5	63.1
- very low	32.4	35.3	33.6
BMI			
- overweight	33.0	23.2	29.1
- obese > 30 kg	42.4	52.5	46.4
Blood pressure			
- diastolic ≥ 85 monthly	42.9	41.5	42.3
- systolic ≥ 130 monthly	35.2	21.9	29.9
Diabetes/hyperglycemia	19.8	22.4	20.8
High cholesterol	29.0	34.2	31.0

Source: Adapted from Morgan et al., 2011

People with schizophrenia have less health screening, less surgical intervention, poorer outcomes for medical treatment, and shorter survival compared to the general population with the same illness. Good quality coordination, delivery and monitoring of physical health care are essential for optimal management of this multimorbidity (Firth et al., 2019).

There has been disappointingly little decline in tobacco use among people with schizophrenia despite comprehensive public health campaigns in many countries that have resulted in substantial reductions in smoking among the general population. Reasons for such high rates of smoking in people with schizophrenia include cognitive enhancement, negative symptom amelioration, and social affiliation.

PRACTICE ILLUSTRATION: INITIAL ASSESSMENT

MARGARET GRIGG

Mary is 19 years old, living with her parents, and in her second year of university, studying Fine Arts. You first meet her when you go to her parents' home to carry out an assessment provided by an acute community treatment service following a request from her general practitioner, who is concerned about social withdrawal and possible psychotic symptoms. Her mother expresses concern that over the last six months Mary has become more isolated and afraid to leave the house, and has recently stopped attending classes or study groups. When you arrive, you note that she appears dishevelled, and is rather incongruously wearing a couple of frayed woollen jumpers despite warm weather. She is initially suspicious and reluctant to talk, but after some reassurances agrees to an interview, with reasonable confidentiality achieved by this being conducted in the kitchen while her mother does some gardening outside. During the interview, Mary is fidgety, and frequently stands up as if she is about to walk out of the room, but sits down again when you ask her to. Her speech rambles, and she loses the thread of conversation easily. She describes hearing the voice of God, as a stern, clearly heard male voice that seems to be coming from a point a few feet above her head; the voice generally speaks directly to her and tells her that something terrible will happen if she leaves the house, but sometimes also provides a steady flow of sentences talking about what she is doing, generally critically. These messages are reinforced by the radio that regularly transmits messages to her from God. She admits that she has recently been smoking up to six joints of marijuana daily, but asks that you not tell her parents. She has not used any other drugs, and does not drink alcohol. Mary is feeling frightened, but is not sure she can trust you. She would like the voices to stop and wants to return to university. Your assessment indicates that Mary has a psychotic illness, and requires intensive treatment.

4.2.4 ASSESSMENT

GOOD PRACTICE IN DISORDER-SPECIFIC ASSESSMENT

People with schizophrenia may be experiencing troubling psychotic symptoms, even while they are participating in the clinical interview. The interviewer needs to speak clearly, offer simple explanations, and maintain a respectful manner. It is important not to be intrusive, and to back off topics the person does not wish to discuss—if necessary, coming back to them later. Long silences can provoke anxiety so a gentle flow of conversation is more comfortable. During psychotic episodes, thinking tends to be quite concrete. Inappropriate affect can be confusing to inexperienced interviewers, and an interested but consistent stance on the part of the interviewer generally works best. The skills used to interview people with thought disorder are described by Galletly and Crichton (2011). Clinicians often avoid asking people with schizophrenia about exposure to trauma and abuse (Lommen & Restifo, 2009; Read, van Os, Morrison, & Ross, 2005) despite the elevated prevalence, and its importance for engagement, formulation, risk assessment and treatment planning (Hassan, Stuart, & De Luca, 2016). Some guidance for inclusion of this in assessment is provided in Section 2.3.9. The overall aim is to utilise a recovery-oriented approach, developing a collaborative and trusting relationship.

Clinical staging—conceptualising the course of a disorder, and choice of treatments, in stages—is routine for many medical conditions. Staging does not imply that the person will pass through all stages, but can be helpful in locating an individual person along the trajectory of possible illness. Over the last decade, a clinical staging model for mental illnesses has been developed (McGorry, Hickie, Yung,

Pantelis, & Jackson, 2006), which proposes that the course of illness can be described on a continuum of outcomes (see Table 4.5), where only a minority will have the poorest outcomes. Clinical staging models assume that treatments offered earlier in the course of an illness have the potential to be safer, more acceptable, more effective and more affordable than those offered later.

Table 4.5 Clinical stages of psychosis

Clinical stage	Definition
0	Increased risk of psychosis No symptoms currently
1a 1b	Nonspecific changes Mild or nonspecific symptoms of psychosis, including neurocognitive deficits Mild functional change or decline Ultra-high risk of psychosis Moderate but subthreshold symptoms, with moderate neurocognitive changes and functional decline to caseness or chronic poor function (30% drop in SOFAS in previous 12 months or < 50 for previous 12 months)
2	First episode of psychotic disorder Full-threshold disorder with moderate-to-severe symptoms, neurocognitive deficits and functional decline (GAF 30–50) Includes acute and early recovery periods
3a 3b 3c	Incomplete remission from first episode of care Recurrence or relapse of psychotic disorder that stabilises with treatment At a level of functioning, residual symptoms, or neurocognition below the best level achieved following remission from the first episode Multiple relapses with objective worsening in clinical extent and impact of illness
4	Severe, persistent or unremitting illness, as judged by symptoms, neurocognition and disability criteria

Source: Adapted from McGorry et al., 2006

Assessment should include all the usual components of mental health evaluation, as described in Chapter 2.3. For people with schizophrenia, it is usual to pay specific attention to the following.

- Symptoms and strengths:
  - detailed account of the person's experience of their symptoms, including hallucinations, delusions, thought disorder, thought insertion, withdrawal and blocking, ideas of reference, passivity experiences, and an understanding of how these symptoms impact on day-to-day life
  - current risks—detailed assessment of risk of self-harm, suicide, or harm to others
  - the person's own understanding of their symptoms, and their cause
  - their own coping strategies to manage symptoms, and daily stresses
  - strengths, resilience—how have they dealt with previous challenges?
  - collateral history from family, friends and medical records.
- Psychosocial history:
  - recent stresses—especially if there has been an exacerbation of symptoms, as generally there is a reason why the symptoms are worse just now
  - current living arrangements, income, financial situation, any legal issues
  - social supports, family relationships, friends, social activities.
- Physical health:
  - evaluation of the possibility of an autoimmune disease such as NMDA-R encephalitis (see Section 4.2.3)

   - tobacco use, as this can affect metabolism of antipsychotic drugs, and has health and financial consequences
   - physical health. BMI, fasting blood sugar and lipids, and blood pressure should be assessed.
- Comorbid conditions:
   - detailed history of drug and alcohol use, as substance abuse is a common comorbidity; urine drug screens, hepatitis screening and other specific tests such as liver function tests may be indicated
   - comorbid depression, anxiety and PTSD. Detailed assessment will guide treatment of these conditions—which can be psychological (such as cognitive behaviour therapy), medication (such as antidepressants) or a combination of psychological therapy and medication.
- Engagement with treatment:
   - engagement with services, psychosocial interventions and medications, currently and in the past; which interventions have been helpful? Which have been unhelpful or made things worse?
   - adherence to medication. Relapse, or poor symptom control, is often due to lack of adherence so this should be carefully assessed, using non-judgemental questions.

An occupational therapy assessment, to establish an individual's capacity for independent living and support requirements, should be undertaken where indicated. In addition, neuropsychological assessment can be helpful in delineating cognitive impairment and identifying cognitive strengths.

COMMON ISSUES AND DILEMMAS IN ASSESSMENT

Suicide accounts for 28% of the excess mortality in people with schizophrenia (Saha, Chant, & McGrath, 2007). Risk assessment should include factors that increase the risk of suicide including the combination of young age and male sex, high level of education, family history of suicide, the presence of insight, substance use, depressive symptoms, hallucinations and delusions (Hor & Taylor, 2010). In an Australian study, the highest suicide risk was found in the first 7 days after discharge from inpatient care (Lawrence, Jablensky, Holman, & Pinder, 2000). Standard risk assessment tools for suicide have not been shown to be effective (Large, Ryan, Carter, & Kapur, 2017), and careful assessment of the individual, and the psychosocial context, is essential. Past history of violence, use of amphetamines, and presence of command hallucinations, are important in assessing risk of harm to others.

People with schizophrenia may sometimes lack recognition of the origin of symptoms and the need for treatment. The main purpose of mental health laws is to allow for the involuntary treatment of people who do not recognise the need for treatment, while safeguarding the rights of those with mental disorders.

Although community treatment orders (CTO; see Section 2.4.13) have been associated with controversy regarding both ethics and efficacy, Australia has one of the highest rates of CTOs in the world, with as many as 10% of people with schizophrenia on a CTO (Light, Kerridge, Ryan, & Robertson, 2012). There is some evidence that involuntary community treatment may be helpful when voluntary engagement with services has been poor or sporadic and there has been a pattern of harmful behaviour or serious functional impairment associated with exacerbations of illness after refusing treatment. Involuntary community treatment is not a substitute for effective engagement by clinical staff.

Improving the person's capacity to make informed treatment decisions is an objective of recovery-oriented practice. Enabling treatment may restore the capacity to appreciate the likely consequences of their own decisions in people who have temporarily lost that capacity, and is an important function of mental health laws.

HELPFUL ASSESSMENT INSTRUMENTS AND GUIDES

Rating scales for comorbid conditions such as depression or anxiety can be useful. It has been difficult to develop brief rating scales for schizophrenia that can be used by clinicians during their routine work. Self-rating scales tend not to be very helpful, due to the complex nature of the symptoms. Most rating scales are therefore clinician rated, require training to use accurately, and are quite time consuming.

The Clinical Global Impression–Severity scale (CGI-S) is a 7-point scale that requires the clinician to rate the severity of the patient's illness at the time of assessment, relative to the clinician's past experience with patients who have the same diagnosis (Guy, 2000). It can be useful in giving a snapshot of the person's current situation, and the CGI-Improvement can also be used to record change after introducing a specific intervention (usually a new medication). One of the most commonly used scales is the Brief Psychiatric Rating Scale (Overall & Gorham, 1962), which can give more detailed objective evidence of change over time. The shortest version has 18 items. The Positive and Negative Syndrome Scale (PANSS; Kay, Fiszbein, & Opler, 1987) is longer, with 30 items, but can give scores on positive, negative, cognitive, excitement, and depression factors.

The RANZCP Guidelines (Galletly et al., 2016) note that there is no universal cognition scale that would be reliable and valid in any routine clinical assessment. The Repeatable Battery for Assessment of Neuropsychological Status (Randolph, Tierney, Mohr, & Chase, 1998) can be useful, but non-psychologists require brief supervised training with a neuropsychologist in order to use this. Other options, not yet widely adopted, are the Brief Cognitive Assessment Tool for Schizophrenia (B-CATS; Hurford, Marder, Keefe, Reise, & Bilder, 2011) and the Brief Cognitive assessment (BCA; Velligan et al., 2004).

Physical health monitoring is essential, starting from the very first contact with mental health services, as metabolic disturbances can begin early in the course of illness and treatment (Foley & Morley, 2011). The NSW Guidelines for the physical health care of people with severe mental illness (Curtis, Newall, & Samaras, 2012) provide a good template for this. The RANZCP Physical Health Expert Consensus Statement (Lambert, Reavley, Jorm, & Oakley Browne, 2017) is also helpful.

4.2.5 EVIDENCE-BASED AND OTHER TREATMENTS AND SERVICES

A collaborative therapeutic relationship is the foundation of treatment. Trust, respect, and empowerment are all important elements. It can take time and patience to build rapport with someone who is paranoid and afraid to talk about their symptoms and the challenges in their life, or who does not see any need for treatment and is an unwilling participant. The mental health clinician can often build trust while helping with immediate matters, at the same time keeping the long-term recovery goals in mind.

MEDICAL TREATMENTS AND STRENGTH OF EVIDENCE

Medications

Antipsychotic medicines treat the symptoms of schizophrenia but not the underlying causes. In the absence of new discoveries, these medicines remain the cornerstone of both acute and maintenance therapy for schizophrenia. These medications are sometimes classified into two groups, the older, or 'first generation' antipsychotics and the 'novel', or 'second generation' drugs. However, in practice it is more helpful to consider the individual properties of each medication, and its suitability for the individual, taking into account both control of current symptoms, and potential side effects.

Antipsychotic medications each have a specific side effect profile. It is essential to use the lowest effective dose and, in collaboration with the person who will be taking the drug, select a drug with the least troublesome side effect profile. There are a number of drugs available and it is essential that the most suitable is chosen for the individual patient, and that the medication is changed if it proves to have problematic side effects or lack of efficacy. Some of the drugs are available in a range for formulations; e.g. olanzapine can be given as a wafer, a tablet, a short acting injection (for acute agitation) and a long-acting injection (for maintenance treatment).

Oral antipsychotics

The RANZCP Clinical Practice Guidelines for Schizophrenia and Related Conditions (Galletly et al., 2016) give details of the various antipsychotics available in Australia; since publication, brexpiprazole has become available.

These guidelines are available on open access (Galletly et al., 2016). While clozapine is the only antipsychotic demonstrated to have superior efficacy, there can be considerable difference in how well each drug controls symptoms in the individual. There is no means to predict which person will respond to which medication. Therefore, there is often a period of trials of various medications, to identify the most effective and well tolerated drug.

Where possible, medicines with the least risk of weight gain should be selected (Bak, Fransen, Janssen, van Os, & Drukker, 2014). In general, antipsychotic medications which assist with sleep and reduce anxiety also tend to put on weight. Weight gain, metabolic syndrome and sedation are most problematic with clozapine, olanzapine and quetiapine. Clozapine is the only drug available for medication-resistant schizophrenia, so at this point there is little choice if other drugs have been ineffective. Fortunately, there are less obesogenic alternatives to olanzapine and quetiapine. In practice, olanzapine and quetiapine are very effective in the acute setting, with a calming action, improving sleep, and good symptom control. However, if the person continues on these drugs in the long-term, instead of switching to a weight-neutral drug, then there is considerable risk of weight gain and metabolic complications including type 2 diabetes. Metformin is sometimes prescribed to reduce this risk, if clozapine, olanzapine or quetiapine are prescribed long-term (Smith, Myles, & Galletly, 2017).

The less sedating drugs tend to have a greater risk of causing extrapyramidal side effects (including tremor and rigidity, which can resemble Parkinson's disease), akathisia (restlessness and pacing), and tardive dyskinesia (abnormal involuntary movements, usually of the mouth and tongue). Extrapyramidal side effects can sometimes be managed by adding an anticholinergic drug such as benztropine, but more commonly the dose is reduced or there is a switch to another antipsychotic.

Some of the antipsychotic drugs (such as risperidone) cause prolactin elevation, which can result in loss of menstrual periods in young women taking these medications. There is also a risk of an effect on cardiac condition (QT prolongation) with some drugs (such as amisulpride), so regular ECGs may be needed. The RANZCP Guidelines (Galletly et al., 2016) contain detailed information about monitoring requirements and the management of side effects of antipsychotic drugs. Only one antipsychotic at a time should be prescribed, unless the person's symptoms are do not respond to monotherapy.

Long-acting injectable antipsychotics (LAI)

The LAI are also known as 'depot drugs'. They can be given at intervals ranging from 2 weeks to 3 months, depending on the choice of drug and formulation. Treatment is usually started with the oral drug (e.g. paliperidone tablets) then switched according to a stepwise protocol to the LAI.

LAI have the advantage that medication adherence is assured, and some people find this more convenient than taking oral medications every day. The daily medication routine can be a reminder of the illness in someone who is otherwise well, and they may prefer an injection every 3 months. Consider the use of long-acting injectable (LAI) antipsychotic medicines if:

- the individual prefers a long-acting injectable medicine
- adherence has been poor or uncertain
- there has been a poor response to oral medication.

The LAI have the same range of side effects as the oral antipsychotics, and there are again individual differences in response and tolerance to the various drugs available.

Switching between antipsychotic drugs can be challenging given the different neurotransmitter affinities. Keks and Hope (2019) have developed a switching guide to assist with ceasing one antipsychotic medication and replacing it with another, minimising the risk of relapse or adverse effects during the switch.

Clozapine monitoring

Clozapine is the most effective antipsychotic drug available, and can result in improvement even after many years of illness. It is the only antipsychotic shown to reduce suicidal behaviour in people with schizophrenia (Meltzer et al., 2003). However, there are risks of agranulocytosis (a decline in the numbers of white blood cells), and myocarditis, so regular blood monitoring (weekly for the first 18 weeks, every 4 weeks thereafter) and cardiac monitoring is needed.

People taking clozapine often gain weight, and dietician advice and exercise is essential from the start. There is some evidence to support the use of metformin to minimise weight gain and insulin resistance for people taking clozapine (Chen et al., 2013).

Interestingly, a Scandinavian study found that people taking clozapine lived longer than people taking other antipsychotics—perhaps due to the close monitoring (Tiihonen et al., 2009). Clozapine can have a delayed response, so it is worth persisting for a full year if there is no initial response, and there tends to be ongoing gradual improvement, the longer the person stays on clozapine. Substance abuse is not a contraindication to clozapine, and sometimes people find it easier to reduce and cease substance use when they are taking clozapine, compared to other antipsychotics.

Lack of response to clozapine

Even with clozapine treatment, there may be persisting distressing positive symptoms, and disabling negative symptoms. Adjunctive medications (such as adding amisulpride) and electroconvulsive therapy (ECT) are sometimes used in this situation (Siskind et al., 2018).

Acute behavioural disturbance

Management of acute behavioural disturbance requires skill and care, to avoid further trauma to a person who may be agitated, paranoid and frightened. Mental health services and emergency departments generally have a protocol for these situations, and an example is contained in the RANZCP Guidelines (Galletly et al., 2016). The first step is de-escalation, listening calmly and respectfully and building a cooperative relationship which hopefully will lead to negotiation of a good outcome. If medication is needed, this is generally a combination of antipsychotics and benzodiazepines. Being subject to a coercive intervention can be traumatic and the person should have an opportunity to debrief later, to understand why the intervention took place, and to develop a plan so future treatment proceeds more smoothly.

Maintenance medication and adherence

Continuous long-term treatment is generally necessary to keep symptoms under control and prevent relapse (Emsley, Chiliza, Asmal, & Harvey, 2013). A controversial long-term study by Wunderink and colleagues (2013) suggested that in people with first episode psychosis, functional outcomes are better in those who are taking lower doses of antipsychotic medication, or no medication. There is no comparable evidence in chronic schizophrenia to suggest that functional outcomes may be improved by ceasing medication. On the other hand, there are studies suggesting that relapses may be damaging (Emsley et al., 2013; Hui et al., 2018).

The Clinical Antipsychotic Trials of Intervention Effectiveness (CATIE) study found that 74% of patients had discontinued their medication within 18 months, attributed to adverse effects and lack of effectiveness (Lieberman et al., 2005). Relapse rates are estimated to be five times higher in patients who discontinue antipsychotic medication compared to those who remain adherent (Emsley et al., 2013).

Peer workers can sometimes be more effective than clinicians in helping people work through barriers to adherence. There are a number of strategies to improve adherence including:

- behavioural tailoring strategies: incorporating medication taking into the daily routine using environmental supports
- dose administration aids

- missed-dose alarms
- pharmacy-based reminders
- reminder telephone calls.

Additional treatments

Benzodiazepines, mood stabilisers and antidepressants can be prescribed for comorbid agitation, anxiety or depression. There may be additive side effects, for example if a mood stabiliser that causes weight gain and sedation (sodium valproate) is combined with olanzapine, which also causes weight gain and sedation. Benzodiazepines can be helpful in managing sporadic symptom exacerbations, such as brief but intense periods of paranoia or auditory hallucinations, which are often accompanied by anxiety and panic. Tolerance and dependence can occur with benzodiazepines if they are taken regularly and for longer periods. Severe treatment resistant psychosis, and severe depression, occasionally require treatment with electroconvulsive therapy (ECT).

Pilot research suggests that repetitive transcranial magnetic stimulation (rTMS), a treatment that uses a magnetic field to increase or decrease activity in a specific area of the brain, might help with auditory hallucinations, positive symptoms in general, and negative symptoms. However, a Cochrane review in 2015 found insufficient evidence to support or refute the use of rTMS in schizophrenia (Dougall, Maayan, Soares-Weiser, McDermott, & McIntosh, 2015).

N-acetyl cysteine (Berk et al., 2008) and ethyl eicosapentaoic acid (fish oil; Porcelli, Balzarro, & Serretti, 2012) are supplements that are sometimes used to augment antipsychotic medications.

PRACTICE ILLUSTRATION: FIRST EPISODE TREATMENT

MARGARET GRIGG

Initially Mary agrees to treatment and is commenced on risperidone. She is visited by the acute community team who, in addition to supervising her medication, provide support and some psychoeducation to Mary and her family. However, after a few days, Mary is becoming increasingly distressed, evidently still using substantial amounts of marijuana. Her parents are anxious, and find the situation very hard to cope with. An admission to hospital for further assessment and initiation of treatment seems indicated. You discuss this option with Mary and her mother, and while her mother is very supportive of an admission to hospital, Mary refuses to go, and refuses to accept the medication or visits from the community team.

A decision is made to admit Mary to hospital involuntarily as there are concerns that she is refusing treatment because it will interfere with her special powers, her family are finding it difficult to care for her, and she poses a risk to herself in that she is neglecting herself. There are also some concerns that she may harm herself in response to the voices, although Mary has become very guarded when talking about them.

During the first couple of weeks in hospital Mary is very distressed, and will not agree to take tablets, so the medication is provided through injection. While she is in hospital she meets the peer worker, who has also personally experienced having a mental illness. The peer work provides information and support, but most importantly provides hope that she will get better. Over time she begins to feel comfortable and forms a good relationship with some of the nurses. Towards the end of her time in hospital, she becomes more open about her experiences and expresses her fears that she will not recover. Her involuntary admission is ceased after four weeks, although Mary voluntarily decides to remain in hospital as she does not yet feel ready to return home.

Six weeks later, Mary has returned home. Information from staff in hospital indicates that Mary has been taking risperidone, and that she has tolerated it reasonably well. During the interview, Mary indicates that she is no longer hearing the voice of God, but remains fearful that something bad will happen, and is anxious about being out of hospital. Her concentration also remains poor, and she has deferred her studies because she is unable to attend class. While Mary's parents agree that she is much better than before she went into hospital, they feel that she is still too unwell to study, and that she may harm herself. You also note that she seems to have gained weight during her admission to hospital. With Mary and her family you develop a plan that involves Mary continuing to take her medication, not using marijuana, providing information and support to Mary and her family, monitoring her weight regularly, organising an appointment with a dietician at the local community health centre, and attending a psychologist for cognitive behavioural therapy. A local non-government organisation will provide practical assistance to Mary and her family, assisting her to attend appointments and re-establish some recreational activities. They will also coordinate the treatment plan.

PHYSICAL HEALTH MONITORING AND INTERVENTION

Physical health monitoring and intervention should begin early in the course of illness rather than waiting until problems develop. The question of who is responsible for medical treatment and care in those taking antipsychotics is unresolved (Lambert et al., 2017). Certainly, there can be a lack of effective treatment even when the diagnosis of hypertension, high cholesterol etc. has been made (Galletly et al., 2012).

Ideally the GP should undertake monitoring and treatment, but many people with schizophrenia do not have a GP. Mental health services tend to undertake monitoring but often do not provide comprehensive treatment for these physical health conditions. Multifaceted interventions, including healthy lifestyle advice (exercise, diet) and targeted pharmacological therapies can be effective in reducing overall cardiovascular risk. *The Lancet* Commission (Firth et al., 2019) describes interventions at individual, health services and system levels that could improve the physical health of people with mental disorders.

Obstructive sleep apnoea (OSA) is most likely quite common but underdiagnosed, so if OSA is suspected, the person should be referred to a respiratory physician or sleep specialist. Effective treatment of OSA can produce considerable improvement in wellbeing and day-to-day functioning.

More information about the diagnosis and management of metabolic syndrome, and other health conditions, in people with mental illness can be found in the NSW Metabolic Guidelines (Curtis et al., 2012) or the RANZCP Clinical Practice Guidelines for Schizophrenia and Related Disorders (Galletly et al., 2016).

Group weight loss and fitness interventions can be helpful, and there are numerous studies showing promising results. The RANZCP Guidelines (Galletly et al., 2016) recommend that all mental health services should provide evidence-based programs to address obesity and lack of exercise, and there is an urgent need for these programs to be more widely available in the community. Lack of motivation, most likely related to negative symptoms, can be a barrier and more work is needed to find strategies at overcome this.

Smoking may increase the metabolism of some antipsychotic agents, such as clozapine and olanzapine, by increasing the activity of enzymes in the liver. Nicotine replacement therapy has no effect on these enzymes. If people taking these drugs cease smoking abruptly, the plasma levels of antipsychotic drugs can increase substantially, so the doses need to be reduced when people succeed in quitting smoking.

Smoking is the single most potentially modifiable risk factor for early death among people with schizophrenia and is a pressing health issue (Firth et al., 2019). Although there are high rates of smoking among people with serious mental disorders, many are keen to quit, for the same reasons as other smokers—to improve their health and save money (Ashton, Rigby, & Galletly, 2013). Measures that have helped the general population such as scary images on cigarette packets and Quit lines are generally not effective. However, there is good evidence for the success of group programs run by peer workers who have successfully quit smoking, along with a mental health worker (Ashton, Rigby, & Galletly, 2015). Again, these programs need to be widely available.

The RANZCP Guidelines (Galletly et al., 2016) recommend that all mental health services should provide evidence-based programs to address smoking, obesity and lack of exercise. The person with schizophrenia, and their carers, should be involved in strategies to ensure healthy living (diet, exercise).

PSYCHOLOGICAL AND PSYCHOSOCIAL THERAPIES

The RANZCP Guidelines (Galletly et al., 2016) state that 'comprehensive care of people living with schizophrenia requires an integration of biological and psychosocial interventions. Psychopharmacology with standard case management does not address all the domains of the illness, especially cognitive deficits, social complications and functional impairment.'

Some psychosocial interventions/therapies address illness management, while others have a greater emphasis on personal recovery. New initiatives include advance directives, supported housing, and recovery colleges (Slade et al., 2014), and web-based resources (Naslund, Marsch, McHugo, & Bartels, 2015). Individual and group family programs (both clinical and peer-led), several variants of CBT for psychosis (Wykes, Huddy, Cellard, McGurk, & Czobor, 2011) and supported employment have the most established evidence bases (Farhall & Thomas, 2013). The RANZCP Guidelines recommend psychoeducation, cognitive remediation therapy, and social cognitive therapies as first-line therapies. Both biological and psychosocial interventions are best implemented within the framework for recovery-oriented practice (Australian Health Ministers' Advisory Council (AHMAC), 2013) that seeks to guide mental health workers in how to prioritise supporting all consumers of mental health services to engage as fully as possible in a personally meaningful and contributing life.

Psychoeducation and self-management training

Psychoeducation programs for people with schizophrenia can improve adherence to treatment, with better outcomes and lower readmission rates (Xia, Merinder, & Belgamwar, 2011). Psychoeducation needs to be tailored to the individual's needs and goals. It is also important to provide psychoeducation and ongoing support for families. Some NGOs have recovery-oriented programs providing education and support groups for carers, which can be invaluable.

Illness self-management training, and Illness Management and Recovery (IMR) are more comprehensive. In addition to psychoeducation, these programs include interventions to improve adherence, social skills training to strengthen social support, strategies to manage residual symptoms and a relapse prevention plan. However, recent trials of IMR have failed to demonstrate benefit (Jensen et al., 2019). There is some evidence for the effectiveness of WRAP, a self-designed prevention and wellness process used in a range of mental disorders (WRAP, 2020; Duckworth & Halpern, 2014). However, most of the research on WRAP involves disorders other than schizophrenia. There has been considerable interest in a peer-developed and led program called Building Recovery of Individual Dreams & Goals through Education & Support (BRIDGES). BRIDGES aims to increase empowerment, self-esteem, self-advocacy, and assertiveness through peer support and the acquisition of knowledge, and has been shown to improve participants' self-perceived recovery and hopefulness (Cook et al., 2012). Web-based interventions that support self-management and specifically utilise a recovery framework are also being developed (e.g., Thomas et al., 2016; Gumley et al., 2020).

Cognitive Remediation

Cognitive remediation therapy (CRT) aims to improve cognitive impairment, with a long-term goal of improving overall functioning. The RANZCP Guidelines, along with recent reviews (Best & Bowie, 2017; Galletly et al., 2016) recommend that CRT should be available to anyone with schizophrenia who has cognitive impairment. A number of cognitive remediation programs are available online and this treatment can be quite efficient as a number of people can work through the online programs at the same time, in a computer lab setting. The programs often use a strategy called scaffolding, where new skills are mastered, then used as the foundation for the next level. A combination of CRT and vocational rehabilitation can be effective in increasing hours worked and job retention (McGurk, Mueser, DeRosa, & Wolfe, 2009). There is ongoing research to match the type of cognitive remediation to the individual.

Where CRT is not available, or the person prefers a different approach, 'cognitive adaptation therapy', should be considered. This involves the use of diaries, calendars, mobile phone apps and other practical strategies to improve day-to-day organisation (Velligan et al., 2008).

Cognitive behaviour therapy for psychosis

Cognitive behaviour therapy for psychosis (CBTp) is designed to reduce distress due to persisting symptoms, and to promote recovery. Symptoms such as delusions, hallucinations, and lack of motivation, are addressed using a CBT framework to understand the links between thoughts, emotions and behaviours. Female gender, older age, higher clinical insight at baseline, shorter duration of the illness, and higher educational attainment are predictors of good outcome for CBTp (O'Keeffe, Conway, & McGuire, 2017). CBTp was developed as an individual treatment but is now sometimes delivered in group formats. An extension of CBTp, meta-cognitive therapy (MCT), specifically helps delusions, using CBT techniques to reduce the intensity of the delusional beliefs (Balzan, Mattiske, Delfabbro, Liu, & Galletly, 2019). For example, people can learn not to jump to conclusions on the basis of inadequate evidence. MCT can be delivered as an individual therapy, or in small groups. Emerging directions include use of smartphone technology to assess experiences and coping in real time, and to provide CBT-based help when needed in daily life, rather than waiting for appointments (Bell et al., 2018; Bucci et al., 2018).

Other psychological therapies

People with schizophrenia sometimes have difficulties with social cognition, which involves the understanding of relationships between the self and others. 'Theory of mind' is the ability to infer how others would be feeling in particular situations; people with schizophrenia often have limited recognition of how the people around them would most likely feel in a given situation. Several different types of therapy have been designed to teach the skills needed to recognise and understand how others feel, and to interact successfully in social situations. Overall, social skills training does seem to be beneficial, especially for negative symptoms (Turner et al., 2018).

Integrated Psychological Therapy (IPT) and the newer, expanded version Integrated Neurocognitive Therapy (INT) aim to address neurocognitive deficits, helping people to encode, remember, interpret and respond to subtle social cues. Cognitive Enhancement Therapy (CET) similarly starts with addressing cognitive deficits, then moves on to applying these improved skills in social interactions. New strategies to improve social cognition include using virtual reality to practise social interactions, and giving oxytocin (a hormone that reduces paranoia and encourages social bonding) before starting each social cognition therapy session (Tan, Lee, & Lee, 2018).

There is interest in group acceptance and commitment therapy (ACT) for people living with psychosis (Johns et al., 2016). Mindfulness-based training (with or without cognitive therapy elements) has been used to address distressing auditory hallucinations (Chadwick et al., 2016).

AVATAR therapy is an innovative approach in which people who hear voices have a dialogue with a digital representation (avatar) of their presumed persecutor, voiced by the therapist. The avatar responds over the course of therapy by becoming less hostile and conceding power to the person who hears the voices (Craig et al., 2018). There is evidence of a reduction in auditory hallucinations using this approach, compared to supportive counselling.

While psychological therapies are well supported by research evidence, and recommended in Clinical

Practice Guidelines, they are often not available for the people who could benefit (Harvey, Lewis, & Farhall, 2018). Psychological therapies are more likely to be provided in Early Intervention and First Episode Psychosis services.

Vocational rehabilitation

Vocational rehabilitation is crucial to successful functional recovery. The RANZCP Guidelines (Galletly et al., 2016) recommend that people with schizophrenia should be encouraged to find a meaningful occupation, either paid or voluntary. This should be actively facilitated by the clinician and specific programs to deliver vocational services need to be widely established.

Unfortunately job networks and mental health services tend to be separate organisations, and it has been proposed (Galletly et al., 2016) that in planning new services, or developing existing services, vocational recovery specialists should be included in the treating team.

A Cochrane review (Kinoshita et al., 2013) found that supported employment, where the person is placed in a job then supported to perform the job successfully, was more effective than other strategies (including prevocational training) for improving vocational outcomes in people with severe mental illness. Employment can have many benefits besides the obvious economic advantages, including improved socialisation, better self-esteem, higher disposable income and reduced substance abuse.

PEER SUPPORT

Most public mental health services now employ trained peer workers, also known as lived experience workers (Nestor & Galletly, 2008). In addition, carer consultants (people with lived experience as a carer) can assist families and other carers. Peer work in Australia is growing (see Fong, Stratford, Meagher, Jackson, & Jayakody, 2018) and peer workers are often involved in programs such as smoking cessation groups, psychoeducation, enhancing adherence, and Wellness Recovery Action Planning (WRAP; Cook et al., 2012) and the BRIDGES program described above. They can also have a role in post discharge support. Some programs are predominantly delivered by peer workers, while others have clinicians and peer workers working together. Hearing Voices groups are typically peer-led, have an emerging evidence base and utilise expertise from both lived experience and research. Peer recovery programs such as the Peer Zone Workshops and online tool kit (Peer Zone, 2016) have been developed independently by those with lived experience of severe mental illness. A recent study showed that about half of a group of people with schizophrenia living in the community had access to the internet at home (Wong, King, Balzan, Liu, & Galletly, 2018). A study of the use of online peer videos in the Self-Management and Recovery Technology (SMART) research program, showed that viewing the videos typically evoked a strong sense of connection and inspired viewers in their own recovery journey (Williams, Fossey, Farhall, Foley, & Thomas, 2018), suggesting significant potential for online access to peer experience.

FAMILY INTERVENTIONS AND FAMILY SUPPORT

Interventions with the families of people with schizophrenia began more than 40 years ago. There was initial concern that these therapies blamed the parents for the occurrence of schizophrenia in their child, but subsequently a collaborative, recovery-oriented approach has evolved. A recent review (McFarlane, 2016) found that family intervention was associated with a 50–60% reduction in the rate of relapse, compared to treatment as usual. Family psychoeducation aims to work with family members to develop coping skills that counter the specific difficulties that are found in schizophrenia. Family to Family, which is a peer-led family psychoeducation course offered by the National Alliance of Mental Illness (NAMI) in the United States, has been shown to reduce carer burden and enhance family empowerment (Mercado et al., 2016). Closer to home, a large-scale evaluation of the Australian version of the program offered by Wellways Australia (Farhall et al., 2019), has shown that both the education and peer support ingredients independently contribute to reductions in distress and self-blame, and improvements in communication, relationship quality and attitudes towards mental illness.

TREATMENT CHALLENGES FOR MENTAL HEALTH WORKERS

Working with people with schizophrenia can be very rewarding. Psychosis is often an intense and troubling experience, and a sense that someone understands and wants to help is in itself beneficial. Mental health workers require patience, as the pace of change can be slow. The negative symptoms, including blunted affect, lack of energy and initiative, and social withdrawal, impact on engagement in recovery-oriented activities, and limit social activities.

People sometimes lack awareness of the need for recovery, so might not cooperate with services they do not think they need. Poor insight also contributes to high rates of medication non-adherence and subsequent relapse. Achieving lifestyle change to address physical health problems can be challenging, as indeed it is for most members of the community who are overweight and not very fit.

Addressing drug and alcohol abuse and addiction is sometimes part of the picture of comprehensive care. Community agencies are often organised into separate mental health, and drug and alcohol services. A 'no wrong door' approach where people are accepted wherever they first present would likely be more successful with better trust and engagement (Liu et al., 2016).

Finally, the gap between consumer needs and the available services means that many people with schizophrenia do not receive ongoing specialist management (Nielssen, McGorry, Castle, & Galletly, 2017). Community mental health services can be forced to focus on discharge, in order to take on new referrals, with the consequence that care of people who are still very unwell can be passed on to the GP. Case management, psychological treatments, and social and family support, may be lacking. The situation can sometimes be improved by finding NGO services that provide ongoing support and psychosocial therapies in the community.

TREATMENT CHALLENGES FOR CONSUMERS

Discrimination and stigma can be problematic, as many people in the general community do not have a good understanding of schizophrenia. It can be difficult for the person to know whether to disclose their diagnosis when filling in official forms for rental, applying for jobs etc.

Private psychiatrists can provide consistent, ongoing care, with the same doctor, but there often are gap payments. Allied health workers such as private psychologists, social workers and exercise physiologists can be very helpful, and Medicare will pay for a set number of sessions in a calendar year, under the Better Access scheme. For example, an exercise physiologist can set up a program to combat obesity and deconditioning, and psychologists can use CBTp and other methods to aid recovery. However, many practitioners charge gaps in addition to the Medicare funding.

A small proportion of people with schizophrenia may face challenges related to substance abuse and dependence, insecure accommodation or homelessness, and problems with the law. However, many are able to achieve a good recovery and live satisfying lives.

KEY RISKS OF HARM IN TREATMENT ATTEMPTS

It is essential that relapses are recognised early and treated effectively, to achieve the best possible recovery. Weighing up the risks and benefits of compulsory treatment is a dilemma for clinicians working with people with schizophrenia. Mental health clinicians need to balance the need to maintain a cooperative relationship and negotiate treatment, with concern that there may be harm to the person or those around them. Compulsory admission to hospital, using the state Mental Health Act, will ensure immediate assessment and initiation of treatment. However, admission can be traumatic, especially if the person is in a closed ward and subject to coercive treatments such as injections of

PRACTICE ILLUSTRATION: OUTCOMES

MARGARET GRIGG

Three years later, after working closely with Mary and her family through much of that time, you are preparing to discharge her from the mental health service to her local general practitioner. Mary has returned to study, and has almost finished her degree. She has moved from her parents' home to a flat with friends, and has a new boyfriend, who is aware of her illness and is very supportive. Mary has had two relapses, with admissions to hospital both associated with her reducing her medication. She has developed a good understanding of the impact of marijuana on her mental health and is committed to continuing the medication. She plans to continue to see her local doctor and a counsellor at the community health centre.

medication. Sometimes it is possible to undertake treatment entirely in the community, using a 'hospital at home' approach (Singh, Rowan, Burton, & Galletly, 2010), which is generally a better experience for the person and their family.

Similar conflicts arise between the person with schizophrenia's rights to make their own decisions, and the risks of untreated psychosis, when deciding whether to apply for a community treatment order. These orders are usually used to administer long-acting injectable antipsychotic drugs. There are also legal mechanisms for assuming control of a person's finances, and requiring them to live in a particular accommodation. Again, civil liberties and the person's own wishes are weighed up against the harms that would occur without these orders.

4.2.6 WHERE AND HOW DO PEOPLE GET HELP?

There are numerous pathways to obtaining mental health services for people with schizophrenia. In many parts of Australia, young people can access headspace. GPs are often the first clinician involved, and can liaise with mental health services to arrange a home visit, or an urgent consultation.

Sometimes people go directly to general hospital emergency services. Emergency Departments generally have mental health nurses onsite, with access to psychiatrists as needed. Some regions have hospital at home services for people with acute psychiatric disorders, which can be an effective alternative to hospitalisation.

Community services vary across Australia but typically consist of a mixture of government services with case management, specialised services such as depot (LAI) and clozapine clinics, and non-government organisations (NGOs). The NGOs can often provide longer-term community support.

Some GPs are very interested in mental health and have the advantage of treating physical health comorbidities as well as the mental disorder. Especially in rural areas, GPs can be responsible for all aspects of care including LAI medications and clozapine prescribing and monitoring. The first person account given by Bernie in Section 4.2.2 is a good example of effective collaborative practice between a consumer and his GP.

4.2.7 THE IMPLICATIONS OF THE DIVERSITY OF AUSTRALIA

RURALITY

In rural and remote regions of Australia the GP usually provides treatment, and coordinates community services if these are available. Some rural towns have visiting psychiatrists who can provide reviews when needed. Telepsychiatry consultations with a psychiatrist in a metropolitan centre can be very useful in providing a specialist assessment and management plan. Options for vocational rehabilitation programs are usually limited, but on the other hand there may be scope for voluntary work and other forms of community engagement.

AREAS OF DISADVANTAGE

Many people with schizophrenia live in disadvantaged areas, due to limited income. Socially disadvantaged regions typically have greater unemployment, more crime, and higher rates of smoking, drug use and alcohol abuse. Overall, physical health tends to be worse compared with more socioeconomically advantaged regions, with higher rates of chronic diseases, and earlier mortality (Marmot, 2017). People with schizophrenia therefore often live with these effects of social disadvantage, along with more specific social difficulties related to the illness.

ABORIGINAL AND TORRES STRAIT ISLANDER PEOPLES

In Australia, the prevalence of schizophrenia among Indigenous people has not been reliably assessed. A systematic review (Black et al., 2015) identified studies reporting prevalence rates of psychosis (including schizophrenia) from 1.68–25%. In the Indigenous population of Cape York and the Torres Strait, the prevalence of schizophrenia was 1.68%, and was higher in men than women, and in Aboriginal people compared to Torres Strait Islander people. There were high rates of cannabis and alcohol use, and comorbid intellectual disability was more frequent among Aboriginal people.

Ernest Hunter, a psychiatrist with extensive experience working with Indigenous people, has observed an increase in psychotic disorders in Indigenous Australians, attributed to cannabis, alcohol, and social adversity (Hunter, 2016). Indigenous people have higher rates of incarceration than the rest of the Australian population, and people with psychotic disorders are overrepresented. In Queensland, 23% of Indigenous women and 8% of Indigenous men in prison had psychotic disorders.

There has been very little published on treatment of schizophrenia in Indigenous Australians, but Hunter et al. (2013) have described the growth of a regionally based mental health service working with a remote Aboriginal community in Far North Queensland. In commenting on the Australian Clinical Practice Guidelines for schizophrenia, Hunter makes three cogent observations: The high levels of mental health issues, including psychotic disorders, in many Aboriginal communities 'manifestly... reflect social context' and require social change as well as clinical mental health service provision; the nature of clinical interventions should reflect best practice in wider society, but be 'informed by a nuanced appreciation of application, given local circumstances and practices', and that it is 'critical... to support the families and communities in which those people live' (Hunter, 2016, p. 1106). Chapter 1.3 presents background, issues and approaches for working with Aboriginal and Torres Strait Islander people.

CULTURAL AND LINGUISTIC DIVERSITY

Refugees and migrants have higher rates of schizophrenia compared to the resident population (Hollander et al., 2016). There are cultural differences between migrant groups, and these need to be taken into account in assessment, and in reaching a shared understanding of the nature of the disorder between mental health clinicians, the person with the disorder, and the family. An interpreter may be needed, which adds further complexity. It can be difficult to determine whether the experiences a person describes are culturally acceptable (such as hearing the voices of ancestors), or indicate mental disorder, and the advice of a person familiar with the culture may be required. In some cultures, mental illness is shameful. Refugees in particular may not trust anyone from 'the government' or seen as being in authority. Effective management requires a good understanding of the social, cultural and religious context and development of a cultural explanatory model that integrates these domains.

There are differences in tolerance of antipsychotic medication between ethnic groups. For example, East Asian people may require lower doses and be more sensitive to extrapyramidal side effects (Ormerod, McDowell, Coleman, & Ferner, 2008). The chapters in Part 2 of this book give further guidance on working with people from diverse cultural backgrounds.

LGBTIQ COMMUNITIES

There is a scarcity of literature on clinical care for LGBTIQ people with serious mental illness, as illustrated by the scoping review of Kidd and colleagues (Kidd, Howison, Pilling, Ross, & McKenzie, 2016), which found no evidence base for specific treatments for psychosis in these groups. However, clinician awareness of the increased risk of any mental health challenge experienced by these populations, and of the risks of societal misunderstanding and service discrimination that are outlined in Chapter 1.3 can be helpful in engagement and formulation; these are consistent with the recommendations of Kidd et al. (2016) for promotion of service cultures that enable inclusion and awareness. It can be challenging to distinguish gender dysphoria from delusions in a person with schizophrenia, particularly if their sexual or gender identity was unclear or apparently different prior to onset. Nonetheless, all forms of support and treatment for the gender dysphoria, consistent with the person's wishes, can be considered. Meijer and colleagues report four cases of specialist Gender Affirmative treatment in people with schizophrenia-related disorders in which psychotic symptoms stabilised and satisfaction was high at three-year follow-up (Meijer, Eeckhout, van Vlerken, & de Vries, 2017).

4.2.8 COMMENTARY AND REFLECTION

The concept of schizophrenia has proven remarkably resilient, despite a lack of evidence that it is in fact a single disorder, and the absence of a specific diagnostic test or symptom. It is most likely a collection of disorders, with different but perhaps overlapping causes, which present with some similarities and are grouped together. One positive consequence of this is that it is not possible to be accurate about prognosis, and a person with very severe symptoms can still make a good recovery over time.

DIFFERENT PERSPECTIVES

There is considerable debate about the benefits and harms of maintenance antipsychotic medication in people with First Episode Psychosis (FEP). One perspective is that these medications can be harmful in the long-term and should be gradually reduced and ceased. Another point of view prioritises prevention of relapse, and advocates for long-term medication, preferably delivered as a long-acting injection. While the evidence generally relates to FEP, the debate spills over into the care of people with established schizophrenia.

EMERGING DIRECTIONS

There is active research from both biological and psychosocial perspectives. There is ongoing genetic research, looking both at the genes themselves, and gene expression. Researchers are investigating the possibility that inflammation, and an autoimmune process taking place in the brain, might be responsible for some instances of schizophrenia. The impact of trauma on the developing brain, and the mechanisms by which trauma, and other stresses during childhood and adolescence, increase the risk of schizophrenia is not entirely understood. There is an urgent need to develop trauma-informed therapies specifically tailored to people with schizophrenia.

There is considerable interest in the question of when, and how, maintenance antipsychotic medication can be reduced and sometimes ceased. Several large randomised controlled trials are under way. This is a crucial question, and to some extent the answer may depend on our ability to separate out the different disorders currently thought to be included in the category of schizophrenia.

In addition, there is ongoing research into cognitive remediation strategies to improve cognitive function, and therefore hopefully improve outcomes. Addressing unemployment via specialised vocational programs continues. There are a number of new psychological approaches, many of them peer-led, and these require further refinement and evaluation. Effective psychosocial interventions need to be much more widely adopted.

Finally, the reduction in lifespan is a crucial issue that needs to be tackled from multiple perspectives. These include encouraging doctors to prescribe optimal medications, widespread adoption of successful interventions (such as metformin and lipid-lowering drugs) to address metabolic syndrome, and lifestyle programs to reduce weight and increase exercise.

4.3

MOOD DISORDERS

KAY WILHELM & MARLIES ALVARENGA

4.3.1 WHAT IS THIS GROUP OF MENTAL HEALTH EXPERIENCES LIKE?

LIVED EXPERIENCE

AS TOLD TO KAY WILHELM

How did it start?

My name is Jennifer, and I am 28. When I got depressed, I was under a lot of stress at work and I was suffering migraines. I felt physically and mentally exhausted, feeling blame and guilt, ganging up on myself. I was finding it difficult to do things I would normally do, like seeing friends, also getting out of bed, having a shower, just taking care of myself. I was still managing to go to work but that was about it.

So how did it develop?

I think over two weeks. I'd had depression and anxiety before, even as a teenager, but nothing quite like what happened this year. This was really dark and I was thinking a lot about suicide as the best way out. That was really scary.

How long has it taken?

The week before I had really felt like it was transient, so I had hope that it wouldn't feel like that forever but over the last few weeks, it's been every day. Before I always felt nauseous, but with this episode, I lost hope and thought it would be forever.

So what did you do about it first?

A long time ago I went to my GP and I felt better. I had counselling. This year, when I felt really bad, I knew that wouldn't be enough and I went to hospital.

What has been helpful?

I find medication can be helpful. It just creates a bit of a break and lifts a weight off. The other thing that helped is having consistency in care, seeing my GP and psychiatrist regularly, a psychologist helps to build strategies to deal with sort of acute conditions. I find that exercise has helped a lot. And the peer support worker has really helped, they've been through it and have come out the other side.

How has the experience changed you or your life?
I think I find it sometimes difficult to separate myself from my mental illness, it starts to become scary, and you start to feel like it becomes your life and it is dominating everything, all aspects of your life. I think it affected my friendships and relationships, and definitely affected my career, with lack of confidence or worry. I realise I've been battling this a little while. Yeah, I think, in terms of growth, it has made me a more empathetic and more creative person. It has made me appreciate when I am feeling 'normal' or happy that much better, yeah.

How would you know if it were to happen again?
I think catastrophising and feelings of regret. Once you start that, every decision that you make you beat yourself up, more or less defeating. I think once you start doing that, it will form into a depression.

4.3.2 HISTORICAL DEVELOPMENT OF THE CONCEPT

KAY WILHELM

FROM MELANCHOLIA AND TO MAJOR DEPRESSION

Hippocrates' Aphorisms described 'melancholia' as a distinct disease characterised by 'fears and despondencies, if they last a long time' (Hippocrates, n.d.). He attributed this to the presence of black bile (associated with coldness, blackness and dryness), and thought that melancholic individuals possessed a temperament that was essentially depressive. In the second century BC, Soranus of Ephesus (Toohey, 1990) characterised those with melancholia by 'mental anguish and distress, dejection, silence, animosity towards members of their household, sometimes a desire to live, and at other times a longing for death; suspicion that a plot is being hatched against him, weeping without reason, meaningless muttering, and occasional joviality.' This description is still recognisable today.

Berrios' review (Berrios, 1988) of historical underpinnings of melancholia and depression noted the contributions of Burton in *Anatomy of Melancholy* (Burton, 1630) who differentiated grief from melancholy and recognised suicide as an integral part of melancholy and Kraepelin, who described manic depressive psychosis (which became bipolar disorder) as distinct from dementia praecox (which became schizophrenia). In describing depression, Kraepelin, a German psychiatrist, also used endogenous (to convey a more severe depression with a biological origin), in contrast to reactive depression (to convey a reactivity to external events, more usually seen in outpatients). Burton (Burton, 1630) drew on his own experience and a number of contemporary theories to suggest that possible treatments for melancholy included a healthy diet, sufficient sleep, music, and 'meaningful work', along with talking about the problem with a friend.

The term 'depression' is more recent. While it covers a broader range of experience than 'melancholia', in the process, it has become less meaningful and harder to define. The concept of 'major depressive disorder' was first used in the 3rd edition of the *Diagnostic and Statistical Manual* (American Psychiatric Association, 1994; Wilson, 1993) to describe a depressive episode of clinical significance, meaning that it does not resolve spontaneously, has an impact on daily function, with the implication being that some intervention is required. The diagnostic category of 'major depression' was intended to increase the reliability and validity of the construct by relying more on observable symptoms and signs and less on the patient's inner life. What the early physicians described as melancholia, we would now call major depressive disorder with melancholic features, some also with psychotic features.

While the construct of major depression was intended to address the difficulties inherent in the constructs of reactive and endogenous depression, the diagnostic threshold for depression is much lower than for melancholia. In this context, a diagnosis of reactive depression implies that the depression will resolve when the triggering event is resolved and endogenous implies that the depression comes out of some bodily process and that only biological interventions will assist. The more recent thinking is that there are a host of biological and psychosocial factors that can kick-start a depressive episode and the features of the episode (symptoms, type, duration, relapse potential) are also driven by a combination of biological and psychosocial factors.

The concept of bipolar disorder, previously known as 'manic depression', dates back to 1850, when Falret's presentation to the Academy of the Paris Psychiatric Society noted *'la folie circulaire'* ('a circular insanity'; Falret, 2019; Pichot, 1995). Then, in 1854, Baillarger described 'a biphasic mental illness causing recurrent oscillations between mania and melancholia', which he termed *'folie à double forme'* ('madness in double form'; Baillarger, 1854). These concepts were developed by Kraepelin, who coined the term 'manic depressive psychosis', and noted that between the periods of mania and depression, patients returned to normal function.

Subtyping into unipolar and bipolar disorders was first proposed by German psychiatrists Kleist and Leonhard in the 1950s and they were first regarded as separate conditions in the first DSM in 1952, then taken up by ICD-8, in 1985. In 1980, DSM-III replaced the term 'manic depression' with bipolar disorder. The subtypes bipolar II and Rapid Cycling have been included since the DSM-IV in 1994 (American Psychiatric Association, 1994).

PHENOMENOLOGY

According to ICD-11, mood disorders are characterised by a 'fundamental disturbance which is a change in affect or mood to depression (with or without associated anxiety) or to elation. The mood change is usually accompanied by a change in the overall level of activity; most of the other symptoms are either secondary to, or easily understood in the context of, the change in mood and activity. Most of these disorders tend to be recurrent and the onset of individual episodes can often be related to stressful events or situations'.

Again, in ICD-11 (ICD-11 for Mortality and Morbidity Statistics, 2019), 'In typical mild, moderate, or severe depressive episodes, the patient suffers from lowering of mood, reduction of energy, and decrease in activity. Capacity for enjoyment, interest, and concentration is reduced, and marked tiredness after even minimum effort is common. Sleep is usually disturbed and appetite diminished. Self-esteem and self-confidence are almost always reduced and, even in the mild form, some ideas of guilt or worthlessness are often present (which differentiates depression from grief). The lowered mood varies little from day to day, is unresponsive to circumstances and may be accompanied by so-called 'somatic' symptoms, such as loss of interest and pleasurable feelings, waking in the morning several hours before the usual time, depression worst in the morning, marked psychomotor retardation, agitation, loss of appetite, weight loss, and loss of libido. Depending upon the number and severity of the symptoms, a depressive episode may be specified as mild, moderate or severe'.

Depression types have been conceptualised in a number of ways:

1 *Endogenous and reactive (neurotic)*: Schneider was concerned with improving the method of diagnosis in psychiatry. In 1920, he coined the terms 'endogenous depression', meaning biological in origin, and 'reactive depression', more usually seen in outpatients. This implies that endogenous depression comes 'out of the blue', whereas most depression of either type has a precipitant.
2 *Melancholic/non-melancholic*: Melancholic depression is a particular subtype, even in those who see depression on a continuum. It is associated with significant morbidity, possibility of psychosis and high suicide risk. It often constitutes a psychiatric emergency and always requires *at least* an antidepressant (often requiring an antipsychotic agent and sometimes, ECT). The signs are related to psychomotor change (see Figure 4.1). People with melancholic depression may also develop psychotic features: this is particularly likely if they are agitated and ruminating about negative thoughts—and if their family are concerned that they are 'different'. Parker and others have argued about the importance of identifying melancholic and psychotic depression types. The non-melancholic depressions are 'fuzzier' constructs (Parker, 2008) that reflect how individuals with varying temperaments respond to

stress (and are more likely to be categorised as mild/moderate depressions).

3 *Mild/moderate/severe*: Here, depressive symptoms are seen as a continuum, with severe major depression (MD) on one pole, with/without superadded melancholic and psychotic features and mild depression, with or without anxiety symptoms, at the other. However, this is problematic as it is possible to have 'mild' melancholic depression (evolving or partially treated) and 'severe' non-melancholic depression.
4 *Unipolar/bipolar*: Bipolar depression implies the presence of manic/hypomanic episodes: Depressions in bipolar disorder are likely to be melancholic in nature and the presence of bipolar disorder has treatment implications.
5 *Early/late onset*: Here earlier onset depressions are more related to genetic vulnerability, temperament/neuroticism, early childhood environment and trauma, with an onset peaking in early 20s and onset usually before age 30. These episodes are more likely to be non-melancholic, but a small but very significant group present with an early onset melancholic depression. It is important to identify early melancholic episodes because this may signal risk of developing bipolar disorder and have a genetic vulnerability to bipolar disorder. This is confounded in young people by undeclared substance use (usually stimulants) or severe trauma. Stimulant use (see Chapter 4.7) may precipitate bipolar episodes in biologically vulnerable people and substance use (including alcohol, tobacco and cannabis) complicates the diagnosis and management. Late onset depressions are more likely to be melancholic and/or psychotic, often related to microvascular disease, other neurodegenerative and illness-related factors, and often with an onset of cognitive problems apparent within the following few years.

FORMAL DIAGNOSIS

Depressive episodes are characterised by depressed mood described as sadness (or feeling down, empty or black) and/or loss of interest or pleasure. This is accompanied by feelings of guilt or low self-worth, disturbed sleep or appetite, feelings of tiredness, motor disturbance, poor concentration and feelings that life is not worth living. Self-esteem is depleted, with a tendency to ruminate over past mistakes and a pessimistic view of future goals. The person may be withdrawn, more prickly or complaining and be seen as having a 'personality disorder' if only viewed cross-sectionally. But, to complicate matters, depression does tend to amplify personality vulnerabilities and the trick is to find whether the behaviour is uncharacteristic: relatives and friends are often the best judge. In more severe, melancholic episodes, the person may be significantly mentally and physically slowed, with significant agitation and 'importuning' manner in some. This can make it difficult to be in their company if one is not aware of what is going on.

Depression can be long lasting or recurrent, substantially impairing an individual's ability to function at work or school or cope with daily life. Onset may be relatively quick (over days to weeks) or slower (gradual over months), whereby family and friends accommodate to changes without realising how depressed the person has become. These personality attributes should be reviewed after recovery, as they may be exaggerated by the presence of depression and often subside or disappear when the person is back to normal. One potentially problematic area is in postpartum depression, as some women with post-partum depression develop a melancholic and even a psychotic episode. In these cases, this may be the index episode for bipolar disorder, or some other psychotic disorder.

Manic episodes are characterised by an abnormally elevated or euphoric mood, frequently associated with an increased tendency to irritability, increased energy and activity, reduced need for sleep (as distinct from insomnia), an inflated sense of one's own abilities (grandiosity), disinhibited behaviour; increased sexual drive; increased spending or excessive generosity; tendency to make overly frank comments about others, increased subjective speed of thoughts ('my thoughts are too quick for my tongue to keep up with'); more talkative; speaking more loudly; increased distractibility; reduced ability to focus and complete tasks (despite having many plans or projects), enhanced perceptual experiences (e.g., colours seem richer than usual).

In mania, mood that is elevated is out of keeping with the person's circumstances and may vary from joviality to almost uncontrollable excitement and elation, accompanied by increased energy, overactivity, pressure of speech and decreased need for sleep. Attention cannot be sustained, often with marked distractibility. Self-esteem is often inflated with grandiose ideas and overconfidence. This plus loss of normal social inhibitions may result in behaviour that is reckless, foolhardy, or inappropriate to the circumstances, and out of character and damaging to both the person and their reputation.

Manic episodes usually have a fairly rapid onset (over days to weeks) and tend to recur. They may follow a cycle (from several times a year to annually or even every few years). Episodes may be precipitated by such events as disrupted sleep rhythms from shift work and long-haul flights, medications (notably corticosteroids, stimulants; see Chapter 2.5). These episodes can cause serious errors of judgement, including unwise sexual behaviour, spending large amounts of money, driving faster than usual, making disinhibited remarks. They may occur with psychotic symptoms that are mood congruent (i.e., matching the elevated mood so that the manic person thinks they have great intellectual gifts, can do anything, including the ability to fly off buildings).

Table 4.6 ICD-11 criteria for mood disorders

Disorders involving depression only		
Depressive episodes are characterised by depressed mood described sadness (or 'down, 'empty', black) and/or loss of interest or pleasure	Symptoms of depression: depressed mood and/or loss of interest. Depressive symptoms include: • feelings of guilt or low self-worth • disturbed sleep (too much or too little) • disturbed appetite (too much or too little) • fatigue, tiredness • motor • poor concentration • feeling life is not worth living. In more severe, melancholic episodes, the person may be significantly mentally and physically slowed, with significant agitation and querulous, 'importuning' manner in some.	
Category	**Category threshold**	**Impact**
Mild depressive episode	Persistent mild mood elevation; 2 or 3 of above depressive symptoms are usually present.	Patient is usually distressed by these but not to the extent that they lead to severe disruption of work or result in social rejection; probably able to continue with most activities.
Moderate depressive episode	4 or more of above symptoms.	The patient likely to have great difficulty in continuing with ordinary activities.
Severe depressive episode without psychotic symptoms	Several of above symptoms are marked and distressing, typically loss of self-esteem and ideas of worthlessness or guilt. Suicidal thoughts and acts are common and some 'somatic' symptoms are usually present.	The patient is likely to have great difficulty in continuing with ordinary activities. To reach criteria for melancholia.
Severe depressive episode with psychotic symptoms (psychotic depression)	A depressive episode as above but with the presence of hallucinations, delusions, psychomotor retardation, or stupor.	Symptoms so severe that ordinary social activities are impossible; may be danger to life from suicide, dehydration, or starvation.

Dysthymia	A persistent or chronic form of mild depression; the symptoms of dysthymia are similar to depressive episode, but tend to be less intense and last longer.	
Disorders involving elation and depression		
Manic episodes are characterised by an abnormally elevated or euphoric mood, frequently with an increased tendency to irritability	Manic symptoms include: • increased energy and activity (more 'wired') • reduced need for sleep (as distinct from insomnia) • an inflated sense of one's own abilities (grandiosity) • disinhibited behaviour: increased sexual drive; increased spending or excessive generosity; tendency to make overly frank comments about others • increased subjective speed of thoughts ('my thoughts are too quick for my tongue to keep up with'); more talkative; speaking more loudly • increased distractibility: reduced ability to focus and complete tasks (despite having many plans or projects) • enhanced perceptual experiences: e.g. sounds are more harmonious, colours richer than usual	
Category	**Category threshold**	**Impact**
Manic episodes	Symptoms present for at least 7 days, may be characterised by the presence of delusions and/or hallucinations or need for hospitalisation	Characterised by impairment in function. Also may have significant impact on person's safety and reputation because of manic behaviours.
Hypomanic episode	Symptoms need to be present for at least 4 days	Mood is distinctly different to normal but person is no significant impairment. Person may feel better than they ever have before. No evidence of psychosis, hospitalisation
Bipolar affective disorder Bipolar 1 and 2 disorders	Typically both manic and depressive episodes separated by periods of normal mood	Presence of manic episodes indicates diagnosis of bipolar 1, if only hypomanic episodes, called bipolar 2 disorder
Cyclothymia	Persistent instability of mood involving numerous periods of depression and mild elation, none sufficiently severe or prolonged to justify a diagnosis of bipolar affective disorder or recurrent depressive disorder. This disorder is frequently found in the relatives of patients with bipolar affective disorder. Some patients with cyclothymia eventually develop bipolar affective disorder.	

In bipolar 2, hypomanic episodes are characterised by persistent mild mood elevation, increased energy and activity, and usually, marked feelings of wellbeing and increased physical and mental efficiency. Increased sociability, talkativeness, overfamiliarity, increased sexual energy, and decreased need for sleep are often present but not to the extent that they cause severe disruption of work or social rejection. Irritability, conceit, and boorish behaviour may be more evident in more euphoric behaviour and this is not accompanied by hallucinations or delusions.

There can be difficulties with the bipolar 2 diagnosis. In some the course may remain 'true to type' with each episode, in others, manic episodes may emerge later, causing a change to bipolar 1. In some, the bipolar 2 diagnosis may be seen as more acceptable diagnosis than borderline personality disorder or stimulant misuse. This is especially an issue in young people who have more volatile mood swings overall. Here, the diagnosis can require re-examination over time.

Of note, the depressive episodes that are part of bipolar disorder are more likely to be melancholic in nature (with psychomotor change), but the 'atypical' features (increased appetite, somnolence, interpersonal sensitivity) are more likely to be accompanied by psychotic features.

Table 4.7 Differentiates unipolar and bipolar depression

Features	Bipolar	Unipolar^
Family history	Bipolar disorder (more likely) Alcohol and/or substance use (more likely)	Bipolar disorder (less likely) Alcohol and/or substance use (less likely)
Illness onset	Early onset (approx. 20–25 years)	Later onset (approx. 25–30 years)
Onset/offset	More often abrupt	More often gradual
Comorbidity	ADHD more often	ADHD less often
Duration of episodes	<6 months	>6 months
Number of prior episodes	Multiple prior depressive episodes	Fewer prior episodes
Mood symptoms	Lability of mood/manic symptoms	Depressed mood and low energy
Psychomotor symptoms	Psychomotor retardation	Psychomotor retardation less likely
Sleep disturbances	Hypersomnia and/or increased daytime napping	Initial insomnia/reduced sleep
Appetite changes	Hyperphagia and/or increased weight	Appetite and/or weight loss
Other symptoms	Other 'atypical' depressive symptoms such as hypersomnia, hyperphagia, 'leaden paralysis' Psychotic features and/or pathological quilt	Somatic complaints

Note: Depressive symptoms common in bipolar disorder are akin to atypical features. A history of hypomania may be easily missed and collateral information from family, health professionals and others is invaluable. If a person presents with this group of depressive features, clinicians should carefully assess for past (hypo)mania. Closely monitor for emergence of such should antidepressant monotherapy be utilised.
^**Unipolar** depression refers to non-bipolar depression.
References: Angst et al., 2005; Moreno et al., 2012; Perroud et al., 2014.

Source: Adapted from *Australian and New Zealand Journal of Psychiatry*, 2015, vol. 49 (12), 1–185; CPG Mahli et al, 2017, p. 14, table 7

For comparison with ICD, the Royal Australian and New Zealand College of Psychiatry guidelines (Malhi et al., 2015) provide information about DSM categories for mood disorders (see Tables 4.6, 4.7 and 4.8). Both ICD and DSM systems use much the same language and base their classification of mental disorders on observable psychopathology in the clinical evaluation for classification purposes. This was done to improve reliability of diagnosis and for this reason, both have a lack of emphasis on cognitions and internal experience. The duration criteria were harmonised and dimensional assessments were introduced in both systems.

A major difference is the role of functional impairments, as a threshold for 'disorder' is mandatory in DSM-5, but not ICD-11 (Gaebel,

2015). This means that ICD-11 rates may be higher but threshold for disorder is more applicable in research studies than in clinical situations where someone is either presenting for help or thought by others to need help, so that caseness is less of an issue. Neither DSM-5 nor ICD-11 have introduced neurobiological or genetic factors into their classification systems.

Both systems take steps towards dimensional symptom assessments, but there is no emphasis on internal meaning for the individual or on their strengths. These issues are becoming more important with increased use of bio-imaging and linking to cognitive processes. There is also more work to be done in the realm of subclinical disorders and whether minor depression and dysthymia are entities in their own right or prodromes for other disorders.

4.3.3 WHAT DO WE KNOW ABOUT THESE DISORDERS?

KAY WILHELM

More recently, there has been discussion about whether 'mood' is the prime concern, as depressive episodes affect sleep, other body rhythms, cognition and movement. These issues reflect the 'increasing recognition that current diagnostic approaches, while retaining their utility in the clinic, do not map onto underlying biology and are at odds with the continuous nature of psychiatric phenotypes' (Owen, 2014). It seems clear that we cannot continue to rely on them as the basis for understanding the pathophysiology of these disorders or for developing and testing new treatments.

Table 4.8 Facts and figures about mood disorders

	Major depression	Bipolar 1	Bipolar 2
Epidemiology			
Prevalence	Lifetime 15% 12-month 4.1%	Lifetime 0.6%	Lifetime 0.4%
Gender	Up to 2x rate in women	None	More common in women
Illness characteristics			
Mean age of onset	Mean age of diagnosis is 27 years (40% have first episode by age 20)	Mean age of diagnosis is late 20s; mean age of onset is late teens	Mean age of diagnosis is later, 29 years
Recurrence	80% have two or more episodes	Manic: depressive episode ratio is 1:3 Nearly 50% have recurrence within 2 years	Less clear
Treatment responsiveness	54% recover in 6 months, 70% within one year 12–15% develop a chronic condition	Age of onset and depressive burden predicts prognosis	
Risk of suicide	Greater with longer episodes, more severe/melancholic in nature	30–60x general population	As high as BP1

Source: Adapted from RANZCP Guidelines, tables 4–6; Malhi et al., 2015, p. 1095

HOW CAN WE UNDERSTAND THE ORIGINS?

Genetics and mood disorders

Over 20 genes have been associated with depression onset and confirmed by meta-analyses. For some families where members that have experienced multiple depression events, severe course of the disorder, or an early age at its clinical onset or in bipolar disorder, there may be single genes involved. Generally, the role of genetic factors in depression onset and progression, suggests that multiple genes are involved, with no one gene having a pronounced effect (Shadrina, Bondarenko, & Slominsky, 2018).

Many genes have been identified as having relevance to depression, some because they increase the risk of bipolar disorder (where a genetic predisposition is much clearer) and some because they are thought to increase risk of depression. The most clearly understood gene x environment interaction concerns the serotonin transporter gene (HTTLPR polymorphism; Wankerl, Wüst, & Otte, 2010), where it has been found that people with short alleles of the gene have less efficient mechanisms for handling stress and are more prone to onset of depression when challenged with a series of stressful life events. While there are detractors of this (Fergusson & Horwood, 2001), it is also possible that the larger studies have too heterogeneous a group of subjects. But not all people with the same genetic endowment behave in the same way due to the role of epigenetics (Starr, Hammen, Conway, Raposa, & Brennan, 2014) and the role of early environment, especially trauma is important here (see Section 2.3.9).

Epidemiological studies indicate that exposure to early adverse experiences can increase risk of development of depression and/or anxiety disorders, most likely through persistent sensitisation of the central nervous system (CNS; Heim & Nemeroff, 2001).

There have been some genes identified in families, but generally not replicated in others. In summary, the triggers for episodes of bipolar disorder in vulnerable people include:

1 periods of high stress, such as death, interpersonal trauma
2 traumatic head injury, especially concussion or other types of brain injury may cause symptom onset
3 substance misuse is common among those with bipolar disorder, and the conditions may trigger each other in some cases; drinking alcohol and using drugs can worsen symptoms of both mania and depression
4 disruption of diurnal rhythms, such as shift work, international travel
5 childbirth.

Social determinants of mood disorders

Allen and colleagues (2014) have stated that 'A person's mental health and many common mental disorders are shaped by various social, economic, and physical environments operating at different stages of life. Risk factors for many common mental disorders are heavily associated with social inequalities, whereby the greater the inequality the higher the inequality in risk.' As there are many types of mood disorders, there is also a wide range of social determinants but in common with other health conditions it is 'our behaviours and our habits (such as excessive and poor eating, excessive drinking and drug use, smoking, physical inactivity, and high intake of salt and processed food) that drive the lion's share (40%) of our ill health and early demise' (Allen et al., 2014; see also Chapter 1.2 for a full discussion of the social determinants of health). We know that regular cigarette smoking increases suicidal ideation and nicotine dependence increases the incidence and prevalence of depression (Flensborg-Madsen et al., 2011) and bipolar disorder (ter Meulen, van Zaane, Draisma, Beekman, & Kupka, 2017).

We also know that exercise has been shown to have preventative and modulating effects on mood disorders (Phillips, 2017) while sedentary activity has the opposite effect. There is now evidence about the effect of diet (Jacka & Berk, 2013) and reduced physical activity, which is likely to be a bidirectional relationship. There are also effects from social exclusion, loneliness and bullying. All of these behaviours are important in their own right but also can be related to low income and access to resources.

To quote an example which shows the complexity of the issues from WHO:

> Patients with type II diabetes mellitus, for example, are twice as likely to experience depression as the general population and those patients with diabetes who are depressed have greater difficulty with self-care. Patients suffering from mental illness are twice as likely to smoke cigarettes as other people, and in patients with chronic obstructive pulmonary disease mental illness is linked to poorer clinical outcomes. Up to 50% of cancer patients suffer from a mental illness, especially depression and anxiety and treating symptoms of depression in cancer patients may improve survival time. Similarly, in patients who are depressed, the risk of having a heart attack is more than twice as high as in the general population; further, depression increases the risk of death in patients with cardiac disease. Moreover, treating the symptoms of depression after a heart attack has been shown to lower both mortality and rehospitalisation rates. In light of this evidence, how can we possibly address the burgeoning epidemic of noncommunicable diseases without tackling comorbid mental illnesses? (Kolappa, Henderson, & Kishore, 2013)

Stress and diathesis conceptualisations (including the role of trauma)

The social determinants of mental health (see Chapter 1.2) principally have their affect through the body's response to stress, by epigenetic modification, altering cognitions, behaviours but also neurophysiology and even brain structure. Examples of social determinants of mood disorders include adverse childhood experience, gender, poverty and discrimination and limited access to education, food, housing and employment, health care. The impact of early trauma has also been under the spotlight. While Freud had pointed out the psychological effects, it is now clear that there are also effects on brain structures. The impact of early trauma is discussed in more depth in Chapter 3.

These issues are of particular relevance to minority groups such as Indigenous people, refugees, LGBTIQ groups, and people who are otherwise socially excluded. (See Chapter 1.3 for a full discussion of these issues in relation to the social conditions and experiences of minority and vulnerable groups.) Social rank theory (SRT) suggests depression stems from feelings of defeat and entrapment that ensue from experiencing oneself to be of lower rank than others. A recent study reported that perceived lower social rank may provide a psychosocial mechanism to explain the link between social factors (especially socioeconomic status) and depressive symptoms and that psychological variables, such as rumination or self-esteem, may mediate or moderate the relationship between social rank and depressive and/or suicidal symptoms (Wetherall, Robb, & O'Connor, 2019). These factors lend themselves to a public health approach as well as improving the lot of individuals and their families.

Important influences on prognosis

Many factors that can influence prognosis are dealt with in the next section. It is however important to consider resilience. Such movements as positive psychology, strengths-based and recovery-based care have been part of a shift away from considering deficits to considering strengths. (See Chapter 2.6 for a discussion of various psychological interventions.)

GOOD PRACTICE IN DISORDER-SPECIFIC ASSESSMENT

Assessment and management

Tables 4.9, 4.10 and 4.11 provide a pragmatic approach to some important factors for consideration.

The management of mood disorders is related to depression type and severity, presence of manic episodes, and temperament and personality factors and social context. The Biopsychosocial and Lifestyle Model (BPSL) is a good starting point for exploring these factors (Malhi et al., 2015).

Figure 4.1 Biopsychosocial and lifestyle model (BPSL)

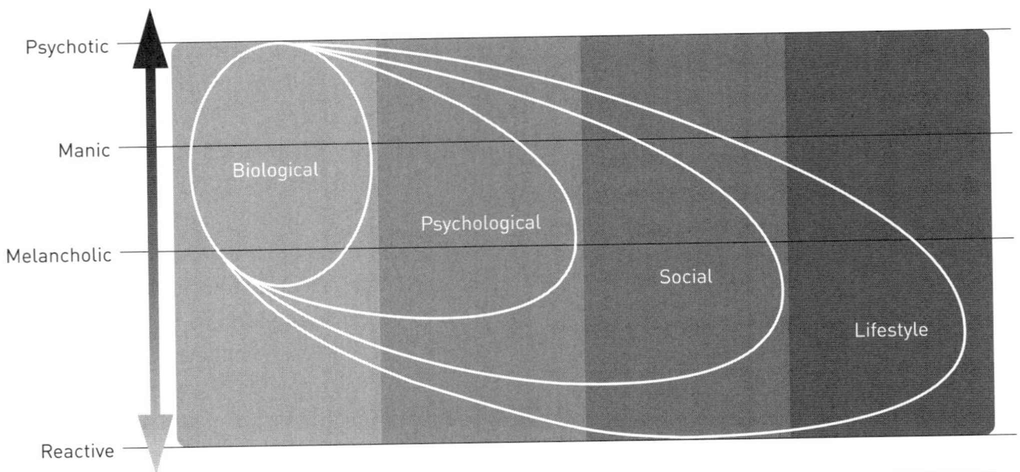

Biological Treatments	Psychological Treatments	Social Treatments	Lifestyle Treatments
• Antidepressants • Antipsychotics • Mood stabilisers • Electroconvulsive therapy • Transcranial magnetic stimulation	• Brief cognitive behavioural therapy • Formal cognitive behavioural therapy • Interpersonal therapy • Mindfulness • Acceptance and commitment therapy • Schema therapy	• Family psychoeducation • Family/friends • Formal support groups • Community groups • Caregivers • Employment • Housing	• Exercise • Diet • Smoking cessation • Alcohol cessation • Ceasing drugs • Managing substance misuse • Sleep

COMMON ISSUES AND DILEMMAS IN ASSESSMENT

Table 4.9 provides a pragmatic approach to guide clinicians through the assessment process.

Many medical conditions can precipitate mood disorders or complicate progress and recovery.

Table 4.10 outlines the physical examination needs of people with depression.

Following the assessment process, Table 4.11 provides a pragmatic approach for managing people with mood disorders. Again, the intention is to provide a series of steps and questions that may be useful in prompting discussion, with some suggested ways forward. This list of interventions is not exhaustive but does provide some useful resources that are all freely available.

Table 4.12 provides a summary of antidepressants in current usage, and indications for their use.

Table 4.9 An approach for assessing people with mood disorders

Assessment issues suggested questions for patient	
Does s/he have a depressive episode?	Are you depressed (sad, feeling low, empty)? Have you lost interest in things you usually enjoy? Has there been a change in self-esteem and/or self-worth? Are you being more self-critical or tough on yourself than usual? This is followed by questions related to depression (appetite loss, sleep loss, loss of interest and motivation, loss of concentration, guilt, suicidal ideation and plans)
Does s/he have a melancholic depression?	How are you spending your day? How different is this from normal? Are you able to look forward to things you normally enjoy, such as....? Can you be cheered up? ...enjoy activities as much as usual when you get started? What lifts your mood? How are you sleeping? What time are you waking? Is this your normal time? Is there a change in your mood and energy over the day? Has this a specific pattern? Have you found it difficult to get going, especially in the mornings? Had difficulty getting out of bed/showering? Felt apathetic? Have you felt empty inside? Are you preoccupied with any thoughts or ideas? Have you any worries that seem to be getting you down? Things you wouldn't normally worry about? Have you thought life was hopeless? Not worth living? You would be better off dead? Have you any plans to hurt yourself?
Is a self-report measure useful?	The PHQ-9 ('Patient Health Questionnaire-9 (PHQ-9)', 2019), the Gwen Adshead (2015) and the CES-D (Chisholm, Quinlivan, Petersen, & Coall, 2005) are all depression measures available online, the DMI-10 (Black Dog Institute) is useful in presence of medical illness, the GDS (The Royal Australian College of General Practitioners, 2019) is available for older people (RANZCP, 2006), p. 70.
Have there been any manic episodes? Personal or family history of bipolar disorder?	Have you ever had any mood swings where you are more energetic/ wired? Has anyone ever said you were manic? (Ormerod, McDowell, Coleman, & Ferner, 2008; Black Dog Institute, 2018)
Is there evidence of psychotic depression?	Have you been worrying a lot? Stewing over things? Could you tell me about these? Have you been blaming yourself/ guilty about past events? Have you been worried you have a serious illness even when told you are OK?
What is the age of first onset?	Have you had episodes like this before? How old were you the first time?
Precipitating factors (stress, environmental, medical)	Why now? Have there been any changes in your life? Your routine? Any recent stressors? Health issues?
Is there past history of depression? Is this episode similar to previous?	Have you had any previous episodes? Were they similar in nature? What was the first time? Worst time? What helped? How were you between episodes?
Is there a history of past manic/ hypomanic episodes? (See Table 4.6.)	Have you had episodes when you had increased energy and activity (more 'wired') and reduced need for sleep? Would you like to do a self-rating test? (Black Dog Institute, 2018).

(Continues)

Table 4.9 An approach for assessing people with mood disorders (*Continued*)

Assessment issues suggested questions for patient	
Is there evidence of cognitive change, neurodegenerative disease?	Can you tell me time, date? Can I do a short test of your memory and concentration? (Murphy, Laird, Monson, Sobol, & Leighton, 2000; Berry, Barrowclough, & Wearden, 2007.) MOCA is better test of frontal lobe problems than MMSE. If short on time, check orientation and ability to draw clock face, with numbers and time (20 to 4).
Is the person expressing suicidal ideas? Plans?	A good opening question is: Have you ever felt that life was not worth living? A review is available below (Anderson, Mitchell, & Brodaty, 2017).
Is there a history of use of nicotine, alcohol and other drugs?	Do you smoke tobacco? Do you drink alcohol? Are you using any other substances to alter your mood (prescribed or not)? Are you aware these all increase your risk of depression and suicidality?
Have there been medication changes leading to drug interactions, side effects?	Have you started any new medications (including CAM)? Check drug interactions: can consult pharmacist, clinical pharmacologist, treat as appropriate.
What about other lifestyle factors?	Do you eat balanced meals? How much time do you spend in exercise? What do you usually enjoy doing (hobbies, interests)? Do you have a problem with gambling? Any worries about eating behaviours? Are your family/friends concerned about you and your lifestyle?
What factors are likely to slow/impede recovery?	Have you any problems with family? Social network? Work? Personal finance? Health? Have you any legal problems?
What factors are likely to improve recovery?	What has helped in your recovery from previous episodes? What strengths have you applied in past life crises?

Table 4.10 Physical examination and investigation of patients presenting with mood disorders

Examination*	
	Rationale
Vital sign	Blood pressure may be altered by certain psychotrople medications and anxiety, bradycardia may occur in hypothyroid states Sinus tachycardia may reflect anxiety
Body mass index and waist circumference	To assess current general health status and gauge subsequent psychotropic associated weight gain
Signs of possible self-harm	Old scars (Including tracheostomy scars)
Endocrine disorders	Goitre, hyper/hypothyroid features, Cushingold features
Respiratory disorders	Observed sleep apnoea/snoring, restless leg syndrome, COPD features, wheeze/asthma, lung malignancy
Neurological disorders	Parkinsonism, motor/sensory deficits, cerebrovascular disease features, motor tics
Organ insufficiency	Jaundice, AV fistula for dialysis, dyspnea, peripheral oedema

Investigation*	Rationale
Full blood examination (FBE)	Some psychotropics are associated with neutropenia and agranulocytosis[a] Neutropenia has been particularly associated with clozapine and carbamazepine, and reported with olanzapine[b] Macrocytosis is seen in heavy drinkers (20–30% in the community and 50–70% in hospital patients)
Urea and electrolytes (U&Es) and liver function tests (LFTs)	Psychotropics may alter LFTs and U&Es Psychotropic pharmacokinetics may be influenced by otherwise clinically silent renal or hepatic impairments Possibility of hyponatremia especially in elderly patients on multiple medications Isolated escalation of gamma-glutamyltransferase (GGT) suggests alcohol misuse[c] GGT is elevated in 30–50% heavy drinkers in the community and 50–80% in hospital patients
Electrocardiogram (ECG)	Some psychotropics are associated with a prolonged QTc Interva[d] QTc prolongation has been particularly associated with TCAs, citalopram at high doses, ziprasidone, paliperidone, and lurasidone[efgh]
Thyroid function tests (TFTs) and thyroid auto-antibodies	Thyroid dysfunction can cause changes in mood Thyroid dysfunction can be induced by treatments such as lithium[i]
Inflammatory markers and microbial serology	Needs assessment on a case-by-case basis
Vitamin levels	There is an association between vitamin deficiencies and mood disorders Vitamin B12, folate and vitamin D, studies are relevant in some cases[j,k]
Sexually transmitted disease (STD) testing	If history suggests impulsive unprotected behaviour with sexual activity
Pregnancy testing (beta HCG)	If history suggests impulsive unprotected sexual activity Necessary prior to starting psychotropics in any woman who is potentially pregnant
Urine and blood drug screening	Screen for benzodiazepines, opioids, psychostimulants cannabis, hallucinogens.

*Dodd et al., 2011.

Note: Clinically appropriate examination and investigation needs to be conducted on an individual basis and ideally baseline investigations should be performed prior to commencing psychotropic agents. Often the person's general practitioner will be best placed to conduct an examination and consider investigations at the point of referral for specialist care. In unusual or particularly refractory mood disorders, more detailed investigation, including brain imaging, may be appropriate. Features on history should guide optimal investigation, for example history of severe insomnia and snoring may require specialist referral and sleep studies and neurological signs and symptoms may require a neurology opinion and specialised investigations such as an EEG and lumbar puncture. On occasion more extensive investigation may be required such as MRI scans of the brain. An emerging area is that of genotyping; it has been suggested that HLA-B*1502 testing should be considered in Asian patients prior to commencing carbamazepine treatment because of a potential risk of Stevens Johnson Syndrome[l], and pharmacogenetic testing may prove useful in the future in patients with a history of medication intolerance or resistance.*

References: [a] Nazer et al., (2012), [b] Flanagan and Dunk (2008), [c] Franzini et al., (2013), [d] Beach et al., (2013), [e] Ellingrod (2012), [f] Citrome (2011), [g] Camm et al., (2012), [h] Suzuki et al., (2012), [i] Hage and Azar (2011), [j] Anglin et al., (2013), [k] Matharoo et al., (2000), [l] Barbarino et al., (2015), US Food and Drug Administration (2012), [m] Hicks et al., (2013, 2015), Singh (2015).

Source: Adapted from Malhi et al., 2015

Table 4.11 A pragmatic approach to managing mood disorders

Patient feature	Intervention
What is the person's understanding of their condition?	Education: use *Understanding Your Episode* sheet (Black Dog Institute, 2019)
What is the pattern?	Use mood chart, work out best part of the day if diurnal variation, use this to structure day
Is there evidence of a physical cause of the mood disorder?	See Table 4.10 for information on how to address this
What are general principles for dealing with depression?	Educate about the need to be as active as possible, exposure to early morning light and physical activity, good diet (e.g., Mediterranean diet), good sleep, safe alcohol levels, regular exercise (e.g., weights, walking), enquire about substance use, gambling. Maintain hope: 'remember that this will pass'...
Is there an unresolved loss? History of trauma?	Consider grief counselling or psychotherapy, IPT useful here. Unresolved trauma need specific referral.
Are there current stressors precipitating depression or impeding recovery?	Offer stress management skills, relaxation skills, problem solving, cognitive behaviour therapy approaches, family support.
Is there anxiety/panic due to breathlessness?	Specific techniques to improve posture and breathing control, sleep quality, overcome panic
Is there decreased mobility?	Techniques to improve mobility using a rehabilitation framework (behavioural activation) can be useful.
Use of antidepressants	**Intervention**
Which antidepressant to use? *A more detailed overview of medication for depression (Tables 13-15) and bipolar disorders (Tables 19–20) is available in the RANZCP Guidelines.* Table 4.12 gives an overview of antidepressant medications (ADMs)	Consider target symptoms, past history, risk of overdose, medical history, current medications, sensitivities and interactions. Consider using an SSRI, generally sertraline, citalopram, escitalopram the least interactions with other medications and best tolerated (Cipriani et al., 2018) or SNRI, particularly venlafaxine; start low, increase slowly to avoid side effects, which may be more prominent in the older people, medically ill and those with genetic polymorphisms. Where tricyclic ADMs useful, nortriptyline is best tolerated.
Is there worrying, ruminations, obsessional thinking or rituals?	Consider using an SSRI (as above) have the least interactions with other medications and are the best tolerated (Cipriani et al., 2018). Clomipramine is also used as first-line treatment (Fineberg, Brown, Reghunandanan, & Pampaloni, 2012).
Are there melancholic features?	Use broad-spectrum antidepressant (e.g. venlafaxine; mirtazapine, start 7-5–15 mg (lower doses better for sleep); nortriptyline starting 10–20 mg); an antipsychotic may also be required. Patients with little or partial response may require augmentation with mood stabilisers and other medications or ECT, in consultation with psychiatrist (see Table 4.9)*
Is there significant anxiety or insomnia?	Valdoxon and melatonin helpful for resetting sleep cycle, also lithium carbonate. Use a more sedating antidepressant: mirtazapine 7.5–5 mg can help anxiety and insomnia; bupropion (available for smoking cessation) is ADM, can be used off label; some TCAs (e.g. small doses of imipramine, nortriptyline, doxepin) may assist substance withdrawal as well.* Check for manic symptoms.
Do they have bipolar disorder?	Depression in bipolar disorder is generally melancholic in nature, but be aware of possible emergence of manic symptoms. They are likely to require a mood stabiliser and psychiatric review.

Is there significant pain?	Consider treating pain with CBT, mindfulness, physical measures (such as massage and stretching). Some antidepressants (e.g. TCAs) potentiate analgesics; amitriptyline is particularly useful for pain and depression, some TCAs (e.g., nortriptyline have less anticholinergic side effects), mirtazapine can be useful*.
Is there fatigue?	Consider using a more stimulating antidepressant (e.g. reboxetine, an SSRI or moclobemide)* Encourage exercise, record on daily mood chart.
Is the patient on other medications for medical illnesses?	Consider using an SSRI (sertraline, citalopram or escitalopram or mirtazapine, which have the least interactions with other medications); consider on a case-by-case basis.*
Are they taking any OTC and/or complementary medicines?	Enquire about treatment goals for these. Consider potential interactions.
Are there issues with nicotine dependence?	Bupropion, nortriptyline both have specific anti-craving effects. Smoking changes blood levels of some psychotropics.
Is there a need to change antidepressants?	The paper listed below gives good information about making changes (Keks, Hope, & Keogh, 2016).
Is the person expressing suicidality?	Need to consider this in choice of medication, best to consider referral to psychiatrist/mental health service.
Are there issues related to culture and ethnicity?	Some of the issues related to cultural competence may related to acceptance of medication and other treatment, including psychotherapy. Ethnicity can affect metabolism of some psychotropic agents and is important in selection of ADMs.
Is the person part of a minority group with special needs?	RANZCP Guidelines: (RANZCP, 2020a).
What is best psychotherapy to use? (For more details, see Section 4.3.5.)	Best evidence is for CBT and IPT for acute and maintenance phases, supportive therapy and short-term psychodynamic therapy can be effective in acute phases and mindfulness-based cognitive therapy (MBCT) for prevention.
Are there dysfunctional cognitions and related behaviours?	CBT will be useful for mild/moderate non-melancholic depression, panic, social/other phobias and GA (see Section 4.3.5).
Are there long-term interpersonal difficulties?	Identify problems, offer interpersonal (IPT), relationship therapy, family therapy where needed, longer-term psychotherapy, including DBT may be useful.
Is there ongoing evidence of emotional dysregulation?	If present before and after the episode, consider DBT and/or MBCT.
Are there issues of self-blame about the patient's illness?	Clarify misunderstandings, guilt issues, 'unfinished psychological business', CBT can be useful here.
Are there ongoing undue concerns with health? Is there somatising behaviour? Is there a long history of health anxiety or is it recent?	Use reattribution techniques to illustrate relationship between psychological issues and body function (Knott, 2014). Consider CBT for longstanding health concerns? Anxiety about health?
Is the person expressing suicidal ideas? plans?	A good opening question is: Have you ever felt that life was not worth living? A review is available in Anderson et al., 2017.
Are there indications for inpatient admission?	Table 4.14 lists criteria to provide guidance.
What factors are likely to slow/impede recovery?	Have you any problems with family, work, personal finance bothering you? Have you had any legal problems?
What factors are likely to improve recovery?	What has helped in your recovery from previous episodes? What strengths have you applied in past life crises?

Table 4.12 Summary of antidepressants in current usage

Typical recommendation[a]	Antidepressant class	Generic name of medication	Principal mechanism of action	Features of depression for which antidepressant is most likely to be useful
1st line	SSRI	Citalopram, Escitalopram, Fluvoxamine, Fluoxetine, Paroxetine, Sertraline	Selective 5-HT reuptake blockade	Anxiety
	NARI	Reboxetine[b]	Reuptake inhibitor for noradrenaline and adrenaline	Activation (e.g., motivation & withdrawal)
	NaSSA	Mirtazapine	Blocks the reuptake of serotonin via 5-HT_{2A} & 5-HT_{2C} receptors. Also blocks $5HT_3$ & Alpha-2 receptors	Insomnia, circadian disruption, weight loss, reduced appetite
	Melatonergic agoinst	Agomelatine	Melatonin agoinst (M1 and 2 receptors) and 5-HT_{2C} antagonist	Sleep problem, sexual dysfunction, poor hedonic drive
	NDRI	Bupropion[c]	Blocks the action of the noradrenaline transporter and dopamine transporter	Fatigue
2nd line	SNRI[d]	Desvenlafaxine, Venlafaxine[e], Duloxetine, Milnacipran	Block both serotonergic and noradrenergic reuptake. Latter leads to an increase in prefrontal dopamine	Melancholia; severe depression. *Velafaxine*: treatment resistant depression. *Duloxetine*: Pain
	TCA	Amitriptyline, Clomipramine, Dothiepin, Imipramine, Nortryptiline Trimipramine	Block NA reuptake. Some also block 5-HT reuptake. All TCAs inhibit H_1, αl, & M_1, receptors. Some also block 5-HT receptors. Board spectrum of actions, including blockade of voltage-sensitive sodium channels	Pain Melancholla
	Serotonin Modulator[e]	Vortioxetine	5HTla agonist,5HTlb partial agonist, 5HT3a and seven antagonist 5HT transporter inhibitor	Melancholia Severe *depression* Enhance *cognition*

Typical recommendation[a]	Antidepressant class	Generic name of medication	Principal mechanism of action	Features of depression for which antidepressant is most likely to be useful
3rd line	MAOI	Phenelzine, Tranylcypromine	Irreversibly inhibit the mitochondrial enzymes MAO-A (metabolises 5-HT, NA & DA) and MAO-B (preferentially metabolises DA)	Melancholia Atypical symptoms[f] Treatment resistant depression Mild to moderate depression with anxiety
Adjunctive	Reversible MAOI SARI	Moclobemide Trazodone	Reversible inhibitor of MAO-A (RIMA) Serotonin 2A/2C antagonist and reuptake inhibitor (at high dosage). At low doses blocks 5-HT2A, α l, & H, receptors, (hypnotic action)	Melancholia Atypical symptoms[f] Treatment resistant depression Mild to moderate depression with anxiety Used when patients do not respond well to 1st line

Notes: (1) SSRI, selective serotonin reuptake inhibitor, NARI, noradrenaline reuptake inhibitor; NaSSA, noradrenaline and specific serotonergic antidepressant; NDRI, noradrenaline-dopamine reuptake inhibitor; SNRI, serotonic and noradrenaline reuptake inhibitor, TCA, tricyclic antidepressant; SM, serotonin modulator, MAOI, monoamino oxidase inhibitor; SARI, serotonin antagonist and reuptake inhibitor. (2) In New Zealand, certain antidepressants are not funded unless suitable alternatives have been trialled first.

***References**: Boulenger et al., 2012; Citrome, 2015; Katona and Katona 2014; Mahableshwarkar et al., 2015; Sanchez et al., 2015; Schatzberg et al., 2014.

[a] There is some flexibility in terms of 1st, 2nd, and 3rd treatment based on patient's symptoms (e.g., MAOIs would be prescribed 1st line for atypical depression); [b] Atomoxetine is prescribed for ADHD and is therefore not recommended 1st line for depression; [c] Only indicated in Australia for smoking cessations; [d] SNRIs have been positioned as 2nd line only because of greater toxicity in overdose; [e] Low dose; [f] Evidence is equivocal Trimipramine: refractory insomnia.

Source: Adapted from Mahli et al., 2015, p. 34

Table 4.13 Considerations in use of antidepressants

Antidepressant class*	Clinical considerations
SSRI	SSRIs are suitable first-line and are generally better tolerated than other classes of antidepressants but can cause emotional blunting. Sexual dysfunction and gastrointestinal symptoms are common. Many SSRIs (especially fluoxetine and paroxetine) cause significant CYP450 inhibition and care is needed when co-prescribed with other medications. Paroxetine can cause withdrawal agitation.
NARI (reboxetine)	Reboxetine is suitable first-line. Common side effects include insomnia, fatigue, nausea, dry mouth and constipation.
NaSSA (mirtazapine and mianserin)	Mirtazapine is a suitable first-line option, but is associated with increased appetite, weight gain, somnolence, dry mouth and constipation. The last three side effects are also common with mianserin.

(Continues)

Table 4.13 Considerations in use of antidepressants (*Continued*)

Antidepressant class*	Clinical considerations
Melatonergic against (agomelatine)	Common side effects include sedation and dizziness. Risk of hepatotoxicity.
NDRI (bupropion)	Common side effects include dry mouth, nausea and insomnia.
SNRI (venlafaxine, desveniafaxine, duloxetine)	SNRIs appear to be more effective than SSRIs in treating severe depressive symptoms (HAM-D>25) and melancholia. In some cases, adverse effects may limit SNRIs to second-line treatment. However, if depression is severe (i.e. HAM-D>25), then SNRIs are a suitable first-line option. Headache, sexual dysfunction, sweating and gastrointestinal symptoms are common with venlafaxine. Can also cause withdrawal agitation.
SM (vortioxetine)	Vortioxetine appears to have a particularly significant beneficial effect upon cognitive function in the treatment of depression. However the evidence requires further replication. Nausea, vomiting and diarrhoea are the major adverse effects.
TCA	In comparison to SSRIs, TCAs have a greater side effect burden (anticholinergic and CNS) and toxicity in overdose and therefore, are considered second-line. However, TCAs (especially those that have both noradrenergic and serotonergic activity such as amitriptyline and clomipramine) may be more effective compared to other antidepressants in treating severe depressive symptoms (HAM-D>25), in particular patients with melancholia and those hospitalised due to severe depression.
MAOI	Efficacious antidepressants but not recommended first-line due to risk of hypertensive crisis if necessary dietary and drug interaction restrictions are not adhered to.

Table 4.14 Recommended indications for psychiatric admission

Category of indication	Specific indication
Clinical Presentation	Severe depression with significant disability. 1a. Suicidal ideation with seemingly imminent risk 1b. Medical risk (i.e.., inadequate fluid intake)^ Mania 2a. Likelihood of escalating manic symptoms/early warning signs of imminent manic episode 2b. Significant impulsivity or reckless disinhibition in context of mania Insight is severely limited to the extent that outpatient treatment is not possible Significant psychotic symptoms
Comorbidities	Medical illness that influences course and treatment of mood disorder. Alcohol and other substance misuse (particularly psychostimulants, cannabis, hallucinogens, benzodiazepines)
Psychosocial Variables	Lack of significant social supports (especially recent loss of supports). Stressful home environment
Treatment Variables	Inability of engage in community-based care Failure to respond to community-based care Initiation of complex treatments (e.g. Electroconvulsive therapy [ECT])

*In such instances, admission to a medical setting may be more appropriate.

Note: Decisions about admission involve weighing a number of the above clinical and psychosocial factors, together with the perspectives of cares and others involved in the community treatment setting.

In RANZCP Guidelines (Malhi et al., 2015), first-line indications for ECT include (1) severe melancholic depression, especially when the patient is refusing to eat/drink (2) high risk of suicide (3) high levels of distress (4) psychotic depression or catatonia (5) previous response, (6) patient choice. Second-line indications are for patients who have not responded to several trials of medication, including for example TCAs, MAOIs.

Complementary therapies are common and some have potential interactions with prescribed medications: it is always worth enquiring about what people are using. As with prescribed medications, most complementary medications are metabolised in the liver using the same cytochrome p450 system, so that the potential for drug interactions should always be considered (see Chapter 2.5).

4.3.4 EVIDENCE-BASED AND OTHER TREATMENTS AND SERVICES

KAY WILHELM

The following discussion of evidence-based treatments is based on the NHMRC guidelines listed here.

The NHMRC levels of evidence are available to assist with evaluating psychotherapies (NHMRC, 2016; Australian Government, 2016).

- Level I — Meta-analysis or systematic review of level II studies including a quantitative analysis.
- Level II — Study of test accuracy with: an independent, blinded comparison with a valid reference standard, among consecutive persons with a defined clinical presentation.
- Level III-1 — Pseudo-randomised controlled trial (i.e. alternate allocation or some other method).
- Level III-2 — Comparative study with concurrent controls: non-randomised, experimental trial or cohort study or case-control study or interrupted time series with a control group.
- Level III-3 — Comparative study without concurrent controls: historical control study or two or more single arm study or interrupted time series without a parallel control group.
- Level IV — Case series with either post-test or pre-test/post-test outcomes.

MAIN TREATMENTS AND STRENGTH OF EVIDENCE

Antidepressants (ADMs)

There is Level 1 evidence for ADMs for the treatment of major depression following multiple RCTs, but 'the decision to treat an individual with an antidepressant remains very much a matter of clinical judgement' (Malhi et al., 2015). The main medications for mood disorders used are outlined in Tables 4.12 and 4.13 and the management section in Table 4.11 gives some ways of approaching ADM selection.

The clinical decision making in bipolar disorder is more straightforward as the clinical picture is more stable (i.e., there are fewer types and depression is more likely to be melancholic in nature). Here there is also Level 1 evidence for the use of mood stabilisers, as outlined in Table 4.12.

Comments on evidence for ADMs

There has been considerable confusion about the efficacy of antidepressant medications (ADMs). A number of psychotherapies have been found to be efficacious for the acute treatment of depression and most therapies (antidepressants and psychotherapies) seem to work over 50% of the time. In this chapter, the case is being made for tailoring treatments for depression to different individuals based on type (rather than relying on severity (Parker, 2005), duration of depression and medical, psychological and personality comorbidities). Much has been made of the lag between onset of disorder and diagnosis for bipolar disorder, often because melancholic depression is overlooked. The situation in young people may further be confounded by emotional upheavals of adolescence and substance use.

The other issue is that studies comparing ADMs and psychotherapies have used both for a discrete period of time (generally the time to provide a manualised treatment). In reality, ADMs provide symptomatic improvement of mood, may assist with emotional regulation and have been thought to even improve brain plasticity for some. The main issues are knowing when it is essential to use antidepressants prior to considering psychological therapies, when they can be used together, how long to use different modalities and when and how patients can exercise choice.

Brain stimulation

The RANZCP Guidelines (Malhi et al., 2015) note that electroconvulsive treatment (ECT) is a highly effective treatment with a strong evidence base (Level 1 evidence) particularly for the treatment of severe depressive disorders. The principal side effect is memory impairment and this has to be weighed against clinical indications. This needs to be done with psychiatrists and anaesthetists with appropriate training in properly equipped settings, all of which increases efficacy and decreases any side effects. There are handouts that can be helpful for patients and families where it is being considered at SANE (SANE Australia, 2019), Black Dog Institute (Black Dog Institute, 2019b) and Beyondblue websites (Beyond Blue, 2019b). Transmagnetic stimulation (TMS) is a more recent and less intrusive treatment, with much less burden for patients. This treatment is still being evaluated, and said to have a 50% success rate. However, ECT is still the treatment of choice for life-threatening, serious depression fitting the guidelines. (Recommendations for ECT and rTMS are listed in Table 4.11.) The RANZCP Guidelines (Mahli et al., 2015, p. 44) and the RANZCP (2020b, 2020c) both have position statements about use of ECT and TMS, which give comprehensive overviews of these two treatments.

Vagus nerve stimulation (VNS) is another interesting intervention that is being investigated but has yet to be fully proven. A recent review (Johnson & Wilson, 2018; Cimpianu, Strube, Falkai, Palm, & Hasan, 2017) concludes with the statement: 'There is an overwhelming evidence to suggest that vagus nerve is an important component of the immune response and manipulating vagal tone is a way to modulate the immune system. Using VNS to manipulate vagal tone provides an exciting new opportunity for minimally invasive therapeutic intervention in adult and paediatric patients. Most of the studies thus far have related to depression but VNS is now being explored for other psychiatric disorders and a range of medical conditions where inflammation plays a significant role.' This is noted as there is growing interest in a possible relationship between inflammation in depression, discussed later in this chapter.

4.3.5 PSYCHOSOCIAL TREATMENTS FOR DEPRESSION

MARLIES ALVARENGA & KAY WILHELM

Psychosocial treatments (or talking therapies) can assist an individual with having a better appreciation of the self and the patterns of thoughts and behaviours which can lead to the experience of distressing feelings. These therapies focus on thoughts, beliefs, values and moral perspectives responsible for how individuals view the world and deal with life's challenges and conflicts. There is also evidence that exercise, diet (Jacka & Berk, 2013) and lifestyle changes (such as ceasing smoking tobacco and substance misuse (Taylor et al., 2014), and gambling (see Chapter 4.6) can also improve mood. However, the effects are likely to vary dependent on depression type, stage and duration. These behaviours should be revisited after recovery from an episode and consideration as to need for longer-term medication and psychotherapeutic approaches to improve wellbeing, decrease relapse and address vulnerability to further episodes can be considered.

In this sense, the therapeutic relationship between a clinician and a patient is of primary importance. In addition, the formation of a therapeutic alliance has the potential to increase adherence with other forms of treatment, such as medication, and it provides valuable emotional support conducive to change. In psychotherapy, the regularity of contact should ideally allow for close monitoring of progress, treatment response, and, in the case of non-medically trained therapists, referral to a medical specialist to deal with poor medication tolerance.

Factors that may suggest the use of psychotherapeutic interventions include the presence of significant psychosocial stressors, intrapsychic conflict, interpersonal difficulties, a co-occurring personality disorder, treatment availability, and patient preference (Gautam, Jain, Gautam, Vahia, & Grover, 2017). Considerations in the choice of a specific type of psychotherapy include the goals of treatment (in addition to resolving major depressive symptoms), prior positive response to a specific type of psychotherapy, patient preference, and the availability of clinicians skilled in the specific psychotherapeutic approach (Gautam et al., 2017). As would be expected with patients who are receiving medication treatment, depressed patients receiving psychotherapy should be carefully and systematically monitored on a regular basis to assess their response to treatment and assess the patient's safety (Unutzer & Park, 2012).

Marital and family problems are common in the course of major depressive disorder, and such problems should be identified and addressed, using marital or family therapy when indicated (see Chapter 2.7). A number of common faulty cognitions, associated with depression, increase the likelihood of the person experiencing sadness, and also of continuing behaviour that reinforces this sadness. For example, a patient may avoid interaction with others because of the perception that he or she is hopeless and worthless, and is ashamed that others will see him or her in this way. The therapist can work on the faulty cognitions and encourage the patient to participate in social interaction to disprove his or her hypothesis that he or she is hopeless and worthless.

RECOMMENDED PSYCHOSOCIAL TREATMENTS

First-line treatment for patients with mild-moderate non-melancholic depression should be one of the evidence-based psychotherapies. Indeed, psychotherapy has been recommended as a first-line treatment for young people in general (Davey & McGorry, 2019), but melancholic features, substance use and medical issues need to be considered. For patients with moderate-severe depression or chronic depressive disorders, combined pharmacotherapy and psychotherapy is offered as first-line treatment. For severe melancholic and/or psychotic depression, the patient may need to improve symptomatically before they can avail themselves of psychotherapy, but behavioural activation is still useful. A fuller description of psychotherapies is provided later in this chapter and CBT and IPT are explored in greater depth (see Chapter 2.6).

Psychosocial therapies may be complementary with pharmacological treatments. A patient who might be reluctant to comply with medication might find psychoeducation of assistance in making an informed choice regarding a best treatment strategy and can be helpful in instances when pharmacological treatment alone has not yielded expected outcomes (see Section 2.6.9).

The RANZCP Clinical Practice Guidelines (CPGs) for Mood Disorders (Malhi et al., 2015) provide an overview of medication for depression and bipolar disorder, with a more detailed overview of medication for depression (Malhi et al., 2015, tables 13–15) and bipolar disorders (Malhi et al., 2015, tables 19–20); recommendations for ECT and rTMS are listed in Malhi et al., 2015, p. 44, box 4.)

The RANZCP recommendations for psychological therapy for MDD state:

- Psychological interventions should only be delivered by clinicians trained in the relevant evidence-based approach.
- Treatment should be guided by a published manual, tailored to the individual, and should pay particular attention to establishing and maintaining the therapeutic alliance.
- Patients with mild-moderate depression should be offered one of the evidence-based psychotherapies as first-line treatment.
- Patients with moderate-severe depression should be offered combined pharmacotherapy and psychotherapy as first-line treatment. (If there is a melancholic and/or psychotic depression, then psychotherapy is limited until there has been some symptomatic improvement.)

- Patients with chronic depressive disorders should be offered combined psychotherapy and pharmacotherapy as first-line treatment (Malhi et al., 2015).

Table 4.15 gives a summary of psychotherapies recommended as treatments for depression based on the NHMRC guidelines, using information from RANZCP Clinical Practice Guidelines and the Australian Psychological Society (Australian Psychological Society, 2018) review of evidence-based psychological interventions as useful for depression, while Table 4.16 provides a summary of other therapies lacking Level 1 evidence base, but is still useful in some circumstances.

Table 4.15 Brief description of therapies identified as useful for treating depression

Therapesytic intervention	Description, with level of evidence using NHMRC and criteria
Cognitive behavioural therapy (CBT)	CBT aims to modify dysfunctional cognitions and related behaviours presumed to maintain depression. There is Level I evidence for CBT, online CBT (clinician-guided and unguided), mindfulness-based cognitive therapy for acute and maintenance phases. It is useful for patients motivated enough to deal with homework and structured guidance. It also requires the ability to be able to question the underlying thought processes that have led to symptomatology. Individuals are helped to understand their disorder to enhance their therapy.
Interpersonal therapy (IPT)	IPT is a brief structured approach that addresses interpersonal issues and role transitions. It is also useful for working with grief and for people with physical illness, who are coping with challenging situations. It has Level 1 evidence in treatment and acute depression and maintenance.
Supportive psychotherapy (SPT)	SPT provides counselling that is not aimed at changing the underlying structure of the patient's thought processes, but at supporting the patient's current (positive) coping styles. The goals (Yager, 2018) include: discouraging the patient from instituting major life changes while depressed; bolstering their morale by strengthening expectations of help and hope for the future; enlisting support of others in the patient's social network while offering additional help if necessary; setting realistic and achievable goals; encouraging the patient to seek new success experiences. SPT provides opportunity for psychoeducation, monitoring suicide risk and promoting recovery (Akiskal, 1985), with Level 1 evidence for its role in the acute phase of depression.
Behavioural activation (BA)	BA (National Institute for Health Research, 2019) encourages patients to define goals and 'activity schedules' for activities they have been avoiding. It is similar to CBT but focuses on encouraging increased activity rather than analysing thought patterns. Currently, NICE guidelines recommend BA for mild-moderate depression, although the evidence base is less strong than for CBT. However, BA is useful in severe depression as an adjunct to medication, when patients are too unwell to be able to use more cognitively based therapies.
Short-term psychodynamic psychotherapy (STPP)	STPP is a brief, focal, transference-based therapy aiming to help the patient explore and work through specific intrapsychic and interpersonal conflicts (as opposed to long-term PP (see below). With Level 1 evidence for role in acute phase of non-melancholic depression.
Mindfulness-based CBT (MCBT)	Here a mindfulness component is added to CBT. This has not been evaluated as much as CBT but seems promising, particularly for those who are prone to worry. There is Level 1 evidence for preventing depression relapse (Fjorback, Arendt, Ornbol, Fink, & Walach, 2011). Source: Adapted from Malhi et al., 2015; Australian Psychological Society, 2018

Source: Adapted from Malhi et al., 2015; Australian Psychological Society, 2018

BIPOLAR DISORDER

Pharmacotherapy is the first-line treatment for bipolar disorder, both during the acute phase and for the prevention of future episodes. However, there is broad agreement that optimal treatment for bipolar disorder involves a combination of pharmacotherapy and adjunctive psychological therapy. The RANZCP Guidelines state: 'Compared with major depressive disorder, bipolar disorder is more complex and difficult to treat and polypharmacy is more common. There is no evidence for psychological monotherapy and adjunctive psychological therapies are primarily used during the maintenance phase of treatment' (Malhi et al., 2015, p. 66).

For treatment of bipolar disorder in adults:

- Level I evidence for CBT (as an adjunct to medication).
- Level II evidence supports use of family interventions, MBCT (based on one RCT and for comorbid anxiety symptoms only), and psychoeducation.
- Level IV evidence for interpersonal and social rhythm therapy (based on three studies with small sample sizes).

The APS review (Australian Psychological Society, 2018), showed that there was insufficient evidence to indicate that any of the remaining interventions were effective. These conclusions were largely in line with the most recent National Institute for Clinical Excellence guidelines (National Institute for Health and Care Excellence, 2014) for bipolar disorder which recommend high intensity psychological interventions (i.e., CBT, IPT, or behavioural couple therapy).

PSYCHOTHERAPY FOR BIPOLAR DISORDER

Psychosocial interventions are recommended (Malhi et al., 2015, p. 100) for adults with bipolar disorder who should be offered adjunctive psychosocial intervention to ameliorate residual symptoms, reduce risk of relapse and improve quality of life (Scott, Colom, & Vieta, 2007) and this should be delivered by an appropriately trained professional with experience in managing bipolar disorder, and should be guided by one of the evidence-based treatment manuals (Malhi et al., 2015). Scott's review (Scott et al., 2007) noted that interventions aimed at relapse prevention were most useful when the patient was euthymic. There is a critique of psychological treatments for bipolar disorder: with a summary of the common feature of evidence-based treatments in Table 4.16, which also illustrates important principles in management.

Table 4.16 Shared content elements of evidence-based psychological interventions

Improve ability to recognise changes in mood and signs of prodromal periods, and to respond quickly and effectively (via pre-planning to these prodromal symptoms)	Re-engage with social, familial and occupational roles
Increase knowledge about and acceptance of BD, including acceptance of, and adherence to medication regimens	Improve stress response and emotion regulation skills, especially around goals and reward activation
Encourage daily monitoring of mood and sleep	Proactively stabilise sleep/wake and other social rhythms
Improve interpersonal communication, particularly in the family	Identify and critique maladaptive thoughts and beliefs, particularly in relation to the self and the disorder
Improve significant others' understanding of BD including ability to identify and productively respond to prodromal symptoms	Reduce drug or alcohol misuse

Some specific psychological therapies used for bipolar disorder are shown in Table 4.17. There are four specific psychological interventions that can be considered as evidence-based (at least one positive RCT), with associated published manuals.

Of note, a recent meta-analysis reported that the most beneficial effects for psychotherapy came from working with the families of those with bipolar disorder (Chatterton, Berk, Barendregt, & Carter, 2017). Their results concluded that 'intensive psychosocial treatment enhances relationship functioning and life satisfaction among patients with bipolar disorder. Alternate interventions focused on the specific cognitive deficits of individuals with bipolar disorder may be necessary to enhance vocational functioning after a depressive episode.' Both FFT and IPSRT (a form of IPT for people with bipolar disorder/mood dysregulation) have an interpersonal focus and CBT and psychoeducation can incorporate families. A family-based approach has also been used successfully in adolescents (Miklowitz et al., 2014).

Table 4.17 Specific psychological interventions for bipolar disorder

Psychological intervention	Description
Cognitive behavioural therapy (CBT; Lam et al., 2010)	Focuses on the reciprocal relationships between thinking, behaviour and emotions to decrease symptoms and relapse risk.
Psychoeducation (Colom and Vieta, 2006)	Aims to assist people to become experts on managing their bipolar disorder, emphasising adherence to medication and stabilising moods. Psychoeducation is a descriptive term referring to providing information about the condition, but has been developed into manualised high intensity treatments by two groups of researchers (Bauer et al., 1998; Colom et al., 2003) and these formal interventions are the focus of the majority of the evidence base.
Family-focused therapy (FFT; Miklowitz, 2008)	Based on evidence that family stress and interactions moderate relapse, FFT aims to improve communication and problem-solving skills in the family. Although only one family member may have diagnosis of bipolar disorder, the entire family is considered 'the client'.
Interpersonal and social rhythm therapy (IPSRT; Frank, 2005)	An amalgamation of interpersonal therapy addressing losses, role conflicts and other interpersonal problems with behaviours aimed at stabilising circadian rhythms via stabilising circadian rhythms (e.g., fixing wake time across 7 days of the week).

Meta-analyses of studies looking into psychotherapy in bipolar disorder have shown that, regardless of whether the therapy is delivered in an individual or group basis, patients who receive therapy tend to fare better than patients who do not in terms of symptom relief, functioning, sense of wellbeing and quality of life (Chatterton et al., 2017). Psychotherapy appears to accelerate the recovery from depressive episodes and prevents new mood episodes (Chatterton et al., 2017). On balance, the cost-benefit analysis of carrying out psychotherapy in bipolar disorder shows that psychosocial treatments should be considered an important component of illness management in this population.

Table 4.18 Brief description of therapies that may be useful for treating mood disorders

Therapeutic intervention	Description
Psychoeducation	Involves the provision and explanation of information to people about what is widely known about characteristics of their diagnosis. Individuals are helped to understand their disorder to enhance their therapy.
Self-help: Pure self-help and self-help with minimal therapist contact	Self-help (or bibliotherapy) is used as an adjunct to traditional therapy or a stand-alone treatment. Some programs include brief contact with a clinician (guided self-help), whereas others do not (pure self-help). Individuals read books or use computer programs. CBT lends itself to this approach.

Therapeutic intervention	Description
Problem-solving therapy (PST)	PST (Pierce, 2012) involves learning or reactivating problem-solving skills. It is suitable in general practice for patients experiencing common mental health conditions. It suits those who need assistance with introducing rational and logical thinking in situations where they have tended to focus on their emotion.
Solution-focused brief therapy	Brief resource-oriented and goal-focused therapeutic approach that helps individuals change by constructing solutions. It aims to increase optimism along with experience of positive emotions to improve outcomes.
Acceptance and commitment therapy (ACT)	Individuals increase their acceptance of the full range of subjective experiences (i.e., distressing thoughts). Focuses on the context and function of psychological experiences as the target of intervention rather than on the actual form or frequency of particular symptoms. Level II evidence for face-to-face and online ACT.
Cognitive analytic therapy (CAT)	CAT aims to work with the patient to identify procedural sequences; chains of events, thoughts, emotions and motivations that explain how a target problem is established, maintained and can be changed. A second distinguishing feature of CAT is the use of reciprocal roles (RRs) to identify problems as occurring between people and not within the patient.
Family interventions—includes marital therapy (MT) and family therapy (FT)	Interventions to improve functioning of the family unit, its subsystems and/or individual members can be useful in depression and bipolar disorder. Marital and family difficulties are very common during and as a result of mood disorders and may significantly retard recovery. MT focuses on the relationship dyad as a vehicle for changes in communication. An important element is understanding the nature of the family of origin of both parties (what they have learned from their families about relationships is what they bring to their partnership). FT enables an individual's problems to be understood in a family context: it enables sharing the problem, minimising blame and seeking family-based solutions.
Narrative therapy	Based on understanding the stories that people use to describe their lives. The clinician listens to how people describe their problems as stories and helps them consider how the stories may restrict them from overcoming their present difficulties. A valuable mode to use with Aboriginal and Torres Strait Islander people.
Emotion-focused therapy	Combines a person-centred therapeutic approach with process-directive, marker guided interventions derived from experiential and Gestalt therapies. A major intervention is the empty chair technique, used to facilitate creating new meaning from bodily-felt sense to let go of anger, for instance.
Schema focused therapy	Emphasis on identifying and changing maladaptive schemas (psychological constructs that include beliefs that people have about themselves) and the associated ineffective coping strategies. It looks at the way that childhood needs were dealt with and includes experiential work with visual imagery.
Dialectical behaviour therapy (DBT)	DBT (Linehan, 1993) was developed for chronically suicidal patients who have borderline personality disorder (Level 11 evidence) but can be used more broadly in the treatment of depression. DBT focuses on dealing with emotions by concentrating on acceptance and working towards change. Emotion regulation and distress tolerance are cornerstones of this approach.
Long-term psychodynamic psychotherapy	Long-term: open ended and intensive, clarification and interpretation based and characterised by a framework in which the central elements are exploration of unconscious conflicts, developmental deficits and distortion of intrapsychic structures.

Choice of therapy

Psychotherapy can be traced back, at the very least, to ancient Greece where there was early recognition that consoling words had treatment value. English psychiatrist Walter Cooper Dendy introduced the term 'psycho-therapeia' in 1853, but the use of talking as a form of therapy was only popularised three decades later by Sigmund Freud (Haggerty, 2018).

The full benefits of psychotherapy may only be attained once the patient has improved sufficiently with psychopharmacological interventions. When acutely unwell, the failure of the patient's memory, concentration, and ability to process information limits the potential benefits of psychotherapy. The decision regarding which therapy to use depends upon patient *and* clinician preferences, and clinical need. There is little information about the side effects of psychological treatments, which can include not understanding whether the treatment is appropriate, what the goals are, and at times, whether it is being properly administered. For some, the treatment may awaken previous trauma or secrets.

The choice of therapy is often dependent upon its availability and the experience of the therapist. It is also dependent upon the depression type, and stage in which treatment is being undertaken.

DBT and IPT may not be freely available, especially in the primary care arena. However, there is an interpersonal counselling form of IPT, intended for use by primary care clinicians (see illustrative case below) and problem-solving strategies are useful per se or as preparation for CBT and DBT.

Factors that may suggest the use of psychotherapeutic interventions include the presence of significant psychosocial stressors, intrapsychic conflict, interpersonal difficulties, a co-occurring personality disorder, treatment availability, and patient preference (Gautam et al., 2017).

Considerations relevant to the choice of a specific type of psychotherapy include the goals of treatment (in addition to resolving major depressive symptoms), prior positive response to a specific type of psychotherapy, patient preference, and the availability of clinicians skilled in the specific psychotherapeutic approach (Gautam et al., 2017). As would be expected with patients who are receiving medication treatment, depressed patients receiving psychotherapy should be carefully and systematically monitored on a regular basis to assess their response to treatment and assess the patient's safety (Unutzer & Park, 2012). CBT and IPT will now be considered in more depth.

WHAT IS CBT?

In the 1960s the psychiatrist Aaron Beck identified that his depressed patients had negative ideas about themselves, the world and/or the future and developed a treatment approach aimed at changing these ideas. He called this approach 'cognitive therapy' and later 'cognitive behaviour therapy' (CBT; Benjamin et al., 2011).

CBT is a focused approach based on the premise that cognitions influence feelings and behaviours, and that subsequent behaviours and emotions can influence cognitions. The clinician works with individuals to identify unhelpful thoughts, emotions, and behaviours (see Chapter 2.6).

CBT has two aspects: behaviour therapy and cognitive therapy. Behaviour therapy is based on the theory that behaviour is learned and therefore can be changed. Examples of behavioural techniques include exposure, problem solving and goal setting, activity scheduling, a range of relaxation techniques, assertiveness training, and behaviour modification. Cognitive therapy is based on the theory that distressing emotions and maladaptive behaviours are the result of faulty patterns of thinking. Therefore, therapeutic interventions such as cognitive restructuring and self-instructional training are aimed at replacing dysfunctional thoughts with more helpful cognitions, which lead to an alleviation of problem thoughts, emotions, and behaviour. Skills training (e.g. stress management, social skills training, parent training, and anger management) is another important component of CBT.

Phases of CBT treatment intervention

Phase 1 focuses on symptom reduction, using (i) cognitive strategies to identify and challenge negative or dysfunctional cognitions; (ii) behavioural strategies to make positive changes (as noted above), and (iii) may include mindfulness training.

Phase 2 focuses on relapse prevention, with booster sessions and, where warranted, an in-depth exploration and challenging of a person's, often long held, core beliefs and schemas.

CBT is proactive, in that it endeavours to anticipate problems that may arise, and seeks to provide clients with skills to cope with them. As such, the therapist must develop hypotheses about what reinforces and maintains dysfunctional thinking and behaviour. These core beliefs cause anxiety, anger, or avoidance. Therapy is a process of guided discovery by the patient that is based on collaboration, rather than on direct confrontation by the therapist (Beck, Emery, Greenberg, & Therapy, 1985; Dobson, 1989).

More recently there have been attempts at making CBT more effective, such as by increasing the frequency of therapeutic sessions over a short amount of time, an approach known as 'massed therapy' (Bohni, Spindler, Arendt, Hougaard, & Rosenberg, 2009). Process based therapy aims to create a more individualised treatment focused on psychological processes for multiple problems which moves away from packaged treatment approaches aimed at a single issue (Frank & Davidson, 2017).

TRIALS OF CBT AND INTERPERSONAL THERAPY

Interpersonal therapy (IPT) was originally designed as an alternative time-limited psychotherapy for a trial comparing CBT to antidepressant (ADM) amitriptyline and 'treatment as usual' (TAU; Weissman, Klerman, Paykel, Prusoff, & Hanson, 1974). Two of the main investigators, Myrna Weissman (a social worker) and Gerald Klerman (a psychiatrist) proposed four interpersonal domains (grief, interpersonal sensitivity, disputes and role transition) that precipitated and maintained depressive episodes. Here IPT plus ADM was more effective than ADM alone or TAU, but IPT plus ADM had the greatest impact on acute symptom improvement and in delaying any further episodes. Their textbook on IPT is now in its second edition. IPT and CBT were then used in a multicentre trial to test the efficacy of an ADM (imipramine) with/without psychotherapy as maintenance treatment of depression. Patients in the IPT and CBT arms showed similar rates of improvement, manifest in different ways (the CBT group showed improvement in dealing with depressogenic cognitions and the IPT group, in interpersonal function). Interest in IPT was informed by a growing interest in attachment behaviour (one of the important theories underpinning IPT). Another important pair of investigators in the multicentre trial were Ellen Frank (a clinical psychologist) and David Kupfer (a psychiatrist). Thus, from the outset, IPT involved active collaboration between psychiatrists and other mental health clinicians. Thus, IPT has always been envisaged as a treatment on its own or in combination with ADM.

What is IPT?

IPT assumes that depression has an interpersonal context and that relationship problems (such as disrupted relationships or expectations of those relationships) are important in precipitating/maintaining depressive episodes. Thus IPT's goals are to (i) relieve symptoms, (ii) educate about link between symptoms and events in relationships, and (iii) improve skills in interpersonal areas that may contribute to or exacerbate the depression.

The components of IPT include:

- Induction, orientation to therapy: History taking and interpersonal formulation, discussion of depression and medical model/meaning of sick role, interpersonal inventory, identification of interpersonal domains and plan for treatment.
- Treatment in the designated domains: Patient and therapist work in treatment in domains selected, with attention to patient's affective state and interpersonal relationships.
- Termination of therapy: winding up, with acknowledgement of termination as a transition, consideration of relapse prevention and maintenance.
- Where required, a maintenance phase is added. Here, there is attention to recalling agreed goals and new roles, maintaining social network and relationships with health providers. Cognitive

approaches can be useful to identify relapse signs and 'top up' sessions are used, if required.

- Interpersonal deficits (loneliness, isolation, interpersonal sensitivity)
  - Vulnerable styles include: anxious worrying, anxious irritability, shy, perfectionistic, high personal standards; interpersonally sensitive to rejection.
  - Having longstanding difficulties making friends; standing up for self, being taken seriously.
  - Being retrenched, leaving home; developing a chronic or life-threatening illness; recovering after a long illness.
  - Material is based on domains developed for IPT (Klerman & Weissman, 1994).

Table 4.19 Identifying the four domains for IPT

Domain	Description	Example
Grief reaction	Prolonged or unresolved response to a loss	Difficulty with grief after a death due to unresolved issues surrounding the loss
	Interpersonal dispute	This may require: (1) renegotiation or (2) acceptance of an impasse or (3) recognition that the relationship has broken down
	Longstanding bitterness due to unresolved problems	Both parties 'stuck', not able to talk about problems
	Role transitions	Difficult role transitions are either unexpected, unwelcome, untimely or involve need for upheaval and change

A recent systematic review of eight RCTs involving IPT, CBT and ADM compared IPT with other standardised forms of treatment for adult outpatients with a diagnosis of major depressive disorder (van Hees, Rotter, Ellermann, & Evers, 2013). The findings mirrored the original trial results (similar efficacy for IPT and CBT, but (not surprisingly), CBT had more impact on cognitions and IPT, on social function. The inclusion of ADM made a difference in some studies but not others and varied by ADM type (i.e., venlafaxine, imipramine and nortriptyline had more effect than SSRIs), suggesting treatment choice should relate to depression type as well as personal preference.

IPT is now well accepted as an empirically validated, manualised treatment for a variety of affective disorders, anxiety disorder and eating disorders, with other uses in other psychiatric disorders still being explored (Frank, Ritchey, & Levenson, 2014). It is also available in group format (World Health Organization, 2019c). For depression, IPT's evidence base is second only to CBT and its use has continued to expand internationally with bodies such as the Interpersonal Psychotherapy Institute providing ongoing training and accreditation.

While CBT is the most commonly used psychotherapy for depression, not everyone relates to the highly structured approach and it is not always applicable. It is well suited to specific populations going through role transitions, such as entering retirement or being diagnosed with terminal illness or engaged in interpersonal difficulties (either as disputes or attachment issues) where an IPT approach lends itself more intuitively to the therapeutic process and sometimes a CBT approach may be useful for some specific issues before/after IPT. The use of an interpersonal inventory and identifying the domains of interpersonal problems provides clinicians with a framework for understanding problems and identifying patients most likely to benefit from an interpersonal approach to psychotherapy.

Interpersonal Counselling (IPC) can be used in general practice and primary care settings (Wilhelm & May, 2017). Unlike CBT, the IPC process is comfortable with prescription of ADMs, medical interventions and lifestyle modifications alongside the therapy. IPC is designed to be conducted with minimal training (by using a series of structured questions) and is suitable for use by GPs or practice nurses

WHAT IS INTERPERSONAL COUNSELLING?

Interpersonal Counselling (IPC) is a simplified and manualised form of IPT (Weissman et al., 2014) developed for use in primary care and aimed at health professionals whose backgrounds were outside of mental health. It is highly structured and provides scripts to guide clinicians through the various stages over three to six sessions, again focusing on four domains. It can be implemented with relative ease after training and aid of supportive resources. It has been used by GPs in some settings and is a good way of learning about IPT.

FURTHER APPLICATIONS OF IPT

The original model for depression has been extended to include (i) specific categories and contexts for depression (peripartum and postpartum depression, dysthymia, recurrent depression, depression in adolescence (Mychailyszyn & Elson, 2018), depression in old age with mild cognitive impairment, depression in rural African settings, depression in patients with HIV and breast cancer, depression in patients with low level criminality) and (ii) other disorders e.g., bipolar disorder (IPSRT: Interpersonal and Social Rhythm Therapy), anxiety disorders, post-traumatic stress disorder, substance use and disordered eating (anorexia, bulimia, prevention of obesity in adolescents) and these models are still being explored and evaluated (Frank et al., 2014).

Mood disorders among minority groups

People who are part of minority groups are more likely to experience depressive disorders than those in the general population. Besides the issues related to mood disorders outlined above, this increased rate occurs as a result of experiences of discrimination, prejudice, abuse and exclusion. (For a fuller discussion of these factors, see Chapters 1.2, 1.3.) In addition, the Beyondblue website has some useful handouts about minorities and disadvantaged peoples (Beyond Blue, 2019a; Beyond Blue, 2019c; Beyond Blue, 2019d). The College Clinical Practice Guidelines provide recommendations for treating mood disorders in the context of borderline personality features (pp. 114–117), anxiety disorders (pp. 111–112) substance use (pp. 113–114), pregnancy (pp. 121–127) and for children and teenagers (p. 127), Māori people (pp. 134–136) and Aboriginal and Torres Strait Islander people (pp. 138–9; RANZCP, 2020a).

GOOD PRACTICE EXAMPLES

The principles are outlined in Tables 4.17 to 4.18 and build on the information presented above.

The following case study involves a multidisciplinary group of clinicians working with a man experiencing both mental and medical health conditions and lifestyle issues, likely to lead to a metabolic syndrome. The principal clinician could be a GP working alone or in a shared care arrangement or a member of a mental health team. There is intentional mention of a number of techniques to illustrate what could be considered, although it is not assumed they would all necessarily be used! Interpersonal Counselling (IPC) is suggested as there is a framework available for use by primary or secondary care clinicians without training (unlike IPT).

PRACTICE ILLUSTRATION: COMPLICATED DEPRESSION IN MULTIDISCIPLINARY FRAMEWORK

Hugo is a 54-year-old factory manager, who is a married man with a 10-year history of type 2 diabetes (DM). He has two children (Alex 19, Sara 15), and a wife (Maria); he is working long hours and one of his close friends has recently moved interstate. Maria is also caring for her elderly mother, recently placed in a nursing home. Hugo has had a difficult relationship with his mother-in-law over the years. He acknowledges he is 'too heavy', drinks 'too much soft drink', engages in 'comfort eating', smokes 15–20 cigarettes/day and 'should do more exercise'. He has had intermittent episodes of depression and occasional panic attacks in the past.

He is seeing you because he is tired, has poor glycaemic control and has 'lost his purpose in life'.

His primary clinician makes the following plan in consultation with Hugo:

1 Review whether Hugo has a clinical depression; discuss 'sick role', including impact of depression on his daily function and DM (National Diabetes Services Scheme, 2016); undertake risk assessment. Check for medical causes of depression (see Table 4.7), including sleep apnoea, sedative medications, effects of diabetes and its complications. Also check for suicidal ideation (Kroenke & Spitzer, 2002).
2 Provide an understanding of how all the factors fit together. this can be an ongoing project and a simple outline is available (Black Dog Institute, 2019).
3 Consider whether ADM prescription useful. (He was commenced sertraline 25 mg at his second session, with a review at the third session for side effects, dosage.)
4 Introduce daily chart (Black Dog Institute, 2019a) to track mood, sleep, exercise, DM-related issues, ADM use.
5 Talk to him about current roles and identify people in his interpersonal network.
6 Discuss with diabetes service about managing DM (request assistance from dietitian for diet and weight) and access to exercise facilities.
7 Use motivational interviewing, problem-solving technique in relation to changes needed.
8 Discuss use of IPC (Judd, Weissman, Hodgins, Piterman, & Davis, 2004; Wilhelm & May, 2017) and the various domains and negotiate a domain (using role transition as focus for change from role of 'chronic, difficult patient' with little control of life and diabetes to role of 'competent self-manager').
9 An initial session on identifying the domain and sessions considering the pros and cons of staying as he is and making changes (what these changes would look like, what life would look like without any changes; who would be involved in helping him with the changes).
10 Three further sessions discussing his new roles and also how he related to his family and friends. This included Hugo deciding to involve two friends in an exercise program, discussing dietary changes with family and reviewing his relationship with his mother-in-law.
11 Continue to liaise with diabetes service.
12 Consider family/marriage functioning, and whether any further intervention required.
13 A wrap-up IPC session to review the changes and suggest that each three months, GP and Hugo will review his progress and prevent relapse.

TREATMENT CHALLENGES FOR MENTAL HEALTH WORKERS

Systemic issues

In acute situations, high turnover and pressure on getting people out of hospital and/or off the acute board can lead to a tendency to concentrate on acute situations and risk issues, without the opportunity to take or gain access to a comprehensive, inclusive history. This history should involve looking at developmental and family issues, impact of medical and mental conditions, social context and the meaning of the condition/illness to the individual (see Chapter 2.3). Achieving this takes time and resources plus acknowledgement of its importance by clinical and administrative leaders.

The other important issue here is the effect of splitting within a clinical team which refers to a process of black-and-white thinking, where the person views others as all good or all bad. This can lead to a lack of team cohesion when members or services feel pitted against each other. Splitting may be precipitated by patients, team members or even administrators. This is less likely if members have opportunities for peer review and supervision and time to reflect.

Another challenge is increased input from peer workers and community services, which may have differing languages, treatment models and expectations from clinical teams and patients and their families. It is important to have a shared appreciation and understanding of differing viewpoints and awareness that good information is available (from clinical, professional and community organisations) to improve health literacy where required.

Diagnostic issues

The concept of melancholia has been around for thousands of years and is a deeply distressing condition with high morbidity and mortality. The significance of melancholic depression has been lost as the construct of depression has broadened and overlaps with normal experience. Some mental health workers have little experience of melancholic depression and can see the problems as behavioural, leading to undertreatment and frustration for patient, family and team alike.

This has also coincided with the introduction of antidepressant medications (ADMs; see Chapter 2.5) but has also led to a dilution of their effect, in much the same way that it is hard to evaluate the efficacy of antibiotics if used for a variety of conditions for which they are not indicated (like allergies or viral conditions) and/or those that will spontaneously improve. However, ADMs are important in treating severe and/or melancholic depressions, including those with psychotic features. People in this group are generally too impaired to benefit from psychotherapy approaches, although behavioural activation is still important.

TREATMENT CHALLENGES FOR CONSUMERS

Understandability

Not surprisingly, the whole issue of mood disorders, especially depression, can be baffling for consumers. There is a literature on mental health literacy and certainly more information available in Australia, where Beyondblue and Black Dog Institute have been actively promoting education of a very high quality. There is a Men's Helpline, Lifeline and information websites for young people. There are also online treatment programs which improve access but in the case of people with long and/or complex histories, who are suicidal or have trauma histories or have severe and/or melancholic depression or bipolar disorder, this will not replace a face-to-face clinical assessment. (For a comprehensive account of Australia's mental health system and services, see Chapters 1.5, 1.6, 1.7.)

Access

General practitioners are able to access a Medicare item number for a comprehensive psychiatric assessment which is intended to provide a holistic, comprehensive plan. They can also prescribe a Mental Health Plan and may have knowledge of low-cost referral routes. (For a fuller discussion of the role of GPs, see Chapter 2.1.5.)

4.3.6 COMMENTARY AND REFLECTION

MARLIES ALVARENGA & KAY WILHELM

The optimal treatment of depression involves the management of biological, psychological, and social factors, all equally important and not treated as competing but rather different levels of inquiry. However, the weighting of these may differ according to the type and severity of the depression presentation.

Nevertheless, there are still questions about the nature of depression. Shadrina and colleagues (2018) summarise the current knowledge of depression disorders (DDs) thus: 'Despite the great medical and social significance of DDs, there is no clear conceptualisation to explain the causes and mechanisms of DD development. Several theories have been suggested to explain the onset of depression and have been confirmed by biochemical, immunological, and physiological studies'. Parallel to well-known 'monoamine, cytokine', and 'stress-induced' (hypothalamus-pituitary-adrenal (HPA) axis and stress theories) depression models, the phenomena of altered brain neural plasticity and neurogenesis and circadian rhythm desynchronosis (the chronobiological model) have been proposed to explain the onset of depression. This is a work in progress, which will be aided by critical thought about depression types and recognition that there is no one-size-fits-all approach, with the potential for exciting advances in the areas noted above.

People with some personality styles are very vulnerable to episodes of non-melancholic depression and their temperament, life experience, and personality style affects onset and course of their mood disorder. People with premorbid anxiety disorders and negative cognitive schemas are particularly vulnerable and addressing these issues in young people can help preventing onset of episodes, along with attention to lifestyle issues.

Whatever the type of mood disorder, it is best not to make definitive pronouncements about personality style while the person is in an episode, as they may be completely different or the issues are no longer so evident on recovery. However, there may be enduring traits which may need to be addressed to diminish vulnerability to further episodes. Also, some issues may come to light during the process of the episode (e.g., a family history of mood disorder or family secrets, unproclaimed trauma, substance use, eating or anxiety disorder).

This re-evaluation will identify the issues requiring psychotherapy and lifestyle approaches and the need (or not) for longer-term medication.

Treatment resistant or difficult to treat depression?

There has also been questioning of how to define what is 'enough' treatment for chronic and treatment resistant depressions (TRDs). Local guidelines, like those of the Royal Australian and New Zealand College of Psychiatrists (Malhi et al., 2015), can point out what is considered best available treatment, but it is up to experienced clinicians to decide what is enough (Wilhelm, 2019). The term 'difficult to treat' (DTT) has been proposed (Rush, Aaronson, & Demyttenaere, 2019) instead of 'treatment resistant' and Rush's paper gives a useful and comprehensive approach to DTT.

Critique of the concept

People often ask whether rates of depression are increasing. To some extent, the answer depends on how and what depression is measured. Bipolar disorder is a clearer construct and rates are more stable over time, and with no gender differences (Jongsma, Turner, Kirkbride, & Jones, 2019) but increasing the bipolar types (to include bipolar 2 and further) does blur the boundaries and lead to a greater likelihood of overlap with people with volatile personality types. Similarly, melancholic and psychotic depressions are clearer constructs and more stable over time, while the rates of the various other types of non-melancholic depression will vary with the definitions.

There is an increasing interest in the impact of some of the negative aspects of modern life on mood disorders and it does seem likely that the impact of more sedentary lifestyle, diet, substance use and more people living with complex medical conditions that in earlier times would have been fatal, will add to the rates of depression. Some of this is potentially reversible: a study of 300 000 adults in Boston, US (Choi et al., 2019) found people with higher levels of physical activity had lower odds of major depressive disorder. They reported evidence that higher levels of physical activity may causally reduce risk for depression and that replacing sedentary behaviour with 15 minutes of vigorous activity each day can reduce depression risk by roughly 25%.

Brain imaging has also led to greater understanding of the impact on the brain of both trauma and depression but also, encouragingly, highlighted brain plasticity and the impact that antidepressants and various types of psychotherapy can have.

BRIEF ORIENTATION TO DIRECTIONS OF CHANGE IN THINKING OR PRACTICE

The chapter started with how historical concepts have led to the different ways that depression has been conceptualised. This is important in terms of discussion about how depression should be treated. The evolving knowledge in areas of genetics, epigenetics, neurophysiology and neuroimaging is still being evaluated and leads to more questions about the nature of depression.

An hypothesis has been proposed that it is a nonspecific inflammatory response to stress (Berk et al., 2013; Konsman, 2019) which may be temporary or become more hardwired, leading to structural change in the context of ongoing stress and repeated episodes. We do know that depression is associated with increased cardiac excitability, reduced immunity and wound healing and that chronic depression is associated with osteoporosis, subclinical hypothyroidism, to name a few systemic effects that illustrate this point.

Mood disorders have also been described as changes in body rhythms (involving sleep, movement and hormonal cycles; Robillard et al., 2018). In all these examples, the mood states are part of the way we respond and are related to the process taking place. The statement 'there is no health without mental health' is particularly important in relation to mood disorders and points to the need for a holistic approach both at an individual and systemic level. However, this must include the notion that depression is not a homogeneous entity, any more than pain is, and that any approach needs to consider the various types of mood disorder, especially in relation to depression.

4.4

ANXIETY, FEAR, OBSESSIVE-COMPULSIVE, STRESS-RELATED AND DISSOCIATIVE DISORDERS

DANIEL FASSNACHT, ERIN PARKER, MIKE BARRY, MICHELLE BANFIELD, DARREN JIGGINS, DAVID CLARKE & MICHAEL KYRIOS

4.4.1 INTRODUCTION

DANIEL FASSNACHT, ERIN PARKER, MICHELLE BANFIELD & MICHAEL KYRIOS

At times, all of us have felt anxious or worried about something. But for some of us, this experience can become very intense.

MICHELLE'S EXPERIENCE

Living with generalised anxiety means living with a constant feeling that something is wrong. Sometimes this is a vague sense of trouble, sometimes it's a feeling of being uncomfortable in my own skin, and sometimes it escalates to uncontrollable mental practise of scenarios worrying me and active avoidance of situations that stress me. The more anxious I get, the crankier I am too. You don't want to cross me if I'm totally strung out by anxiety!

For me, it's linked to a need for control: the less control, the more anxious I feel. In one of those vicious circles, I also feel like I need to control my anxiety, leading to feelings of failure and shame when I can't.

A few times in my life, my anxiety has escalated to panic attacks. Although I've always known what they are when they hit—when my heart is pounding out of my chest, I'm having hot and cold flushes, it's difficult to breathe and I feel like I need to escape both where I am and my own body—it's hard to remember this is 'just a panic attack'. In the worst ones, I sometimes have the sense of detaching from myself and becoming an observer of my own struggle.

Since my anxiety is hitching a ride with a lot of other health problems, including bipolar disorder, it is rarely a specific focus of treatment. I have had some experience with benzodiazepines, but quickly understood why they are so addictive but ultimately not actually helpful. Instead, I have concentrated on seeking out psychological management, particularly self-management. Recognising when it is anxiety talking, using techniques like mindfulness to shortcut obsessive thoughts or grounding myself during a panic attack, and practising focused relaxation all help me to live with this unwanted hitchhiker in life.

OVERVIEW OF DISORDERS AND THEIR PRESENTATION IN THIS CHAPTER

All disorders covered in this chapter have anxiety and/or fear as a key component. In previous diagnostic classifications, obsessive-compulsive disorder and post-traumatic stress disorder were classified under the heading of 'anxiety disorders'. However, in the most recent classification systems (ICD-11 and DSM-5) disorders associated with anxiety and/or fear are grouped into three separate categories; and will be discussed as following in this chapter:

Anxiety or fear-related disorders include:

- generalised anxiety disorder
- social anxiety disorder
- panic disorder
- agoraphobia
- specific phobia, obsessive-compulsive or related disorders
- obsessive-compulsive disorder
- body dysmorphic disorder
- hypochondriasis
- hoarding disorder.

Disorders specifically associated with stress include:

- post-traumatic stress disorder
- complex post-traumatic stress disorder
- prolonged grief disorder
- adjustment disorder.

Dissociative disorders have traditionally been classified separately from anxiety disorders. This make sense in terms of the consumer's presentation—most are not seeking help for anxiety or stress and most do not initially see a connection between their dissociative experiences and stress. Nonetheless, we understand the primary cause of these dissociative experiences as being overwhelming stress. The dissociative disorders discussed in this chapter are:

- depersonalisation-derealisation disorder
- psychogenic amnesia
- dissociative neurological symptom disorder
- dissociative identity disorder.

The chapter focuses on disorders typically presenting in adulthood. Childhood anxiety-related disorders (e.g., selective mutism, separation anxiety disorder) are covered in the chapter on childhood disorders (see Chapter 3.1). The disorders in this chapter are described based on ICD-11 criteria, with any differences from DSM-5 noted where relevant.

In the next three sections, we cover phenomenology and formal diagnosis of the anxiety, obsessive-compulsive and stress disorder groups in turn. Following that, we combine these groups to present what is known about the disorders, their assessment, and the main treatments and services. Then, dissociative disorders are discussed together.

4.4.2 PHENOMENOLOGY AND DIAGNOSIS OF ANXIETY OR FEAR-RELATED DISORDERS

ERIN PARKER & MICHELLE BANFIELD

PHENOMENOLOGY

Anxiety and fear are closely related concepts; anxiety is a future-oriented state involving the anticipation of threat, while fear is the emotional/physiological response to current threat perceived or actual (American Psychiatric Association, 2013). Both anxiety and fear are normal human responses that serve an adaptive function. For instance, the physical symptoms of anxiety and fear—

often referred to as the fight-or-flight response–prepare our body to flee danger or defend ourselves in the face of danger. From an evolutionary perspective, anxiety may be considered advantageous–those who learn to anticipate danger can therefore avoid that danger and mitigate threats to survival. Even in the context of threats that are unrelated to survival, anxiety may benefit us by prompting us to perform at our best. For example, feeling anxious about an upcoming test may prompt you to study, and therefore perform better in the exam. However, when anxiety levels become too high, performance is impacted, and the opposite can occur.

The Yerkes-Dodson Law (originally described in 1908; Yerkes & Dodson, 1908) can be used to understand this relationship. It posits that there is an inverse-U-shaped association between arousal (anxiety) and performance: arousal levels at extremes of high or low result in poor performance, and optimal performance occurs at moderate levels of arousal (see Figure 4.2). In this way, anxiety and fear-related disorders can be thought of as the extreme end of a continuum of experience, rather than being categorically different from a 'normal' human response. Anxiety crosses the threshold on this continuum to become clinically significant when it is prolonged, excessive, and results in substantial impairment in functioning for the person.

Persons meeting criteria for anxiety and fear-related disorders tend to consistently overestimate the level of threat posed by anxiety-provoking situations/objects, and underestimate their ability to cope with that threat (Wells, 2013). These disorders are also characterised by symptoms in the following domains:

- mood–e.g., excessive fear/anxiety, nervousness, irritability
- thinking–e.g., difficulty concentrating, worry, catastrophising, obsessive thinking, biases toward threatening information
- behaviour–e.g., avoidance of situations, seeking excessive reassurance, lashing out at others, redundant or excessive attempts to control the environment
- physical symptoms–e.g., headaches, muscle tension, restlessness, gastrointestinal issues, increased heart and breathing rate.

Avoidance is considered the core feature of all anxiety and fear-related disorders (Rapee, 2012); in the short-term it reduces anxiety, but in the long-term avoidance leads to increased anxiety as it prevents opportunities to learn tolerance (or that feared stimuli are not dangerous) and undermines confidence (see Figure 4.3). Avoidance may take many forms, including overt avoidance of certain situations or objects, engagement in safety behaviours (such as only entering the situation with anxiolytic [anxiety-reducing] medication handy), or more covert avoidance through cognitive processes like worry.

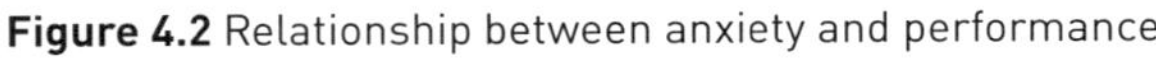
Figure 4.2 Relationship between anxiety and performance

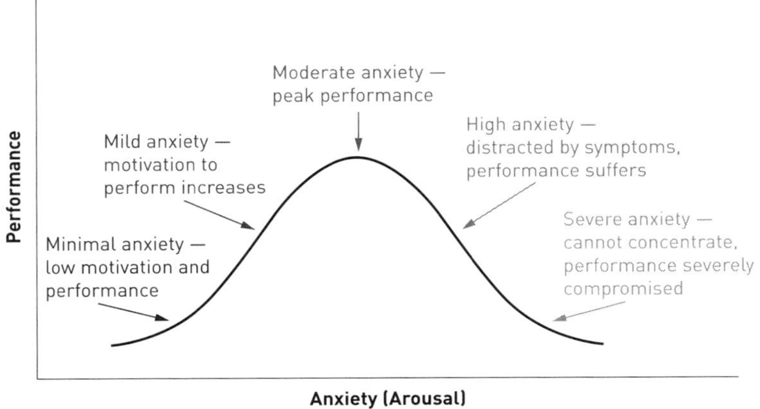

Source: Adapted from Yerkes & Dodson, 1908

Figure 4.3 Vicious cycle of anxiety

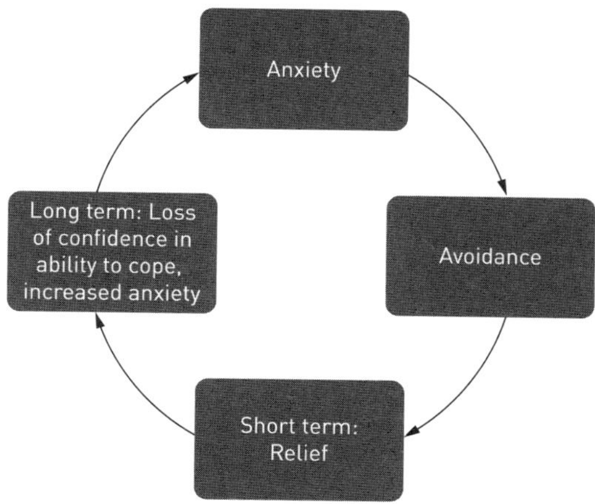

Anxiety and fear-related disorders have a high prevalence in Australia and are one of the most common presenting problems in general practice (Britt et al., 2016). They also frequently co-occur with one another as well as other disorders such as depression (Bandelow & Michaelis, 2015).

FORMAL DIAGNOSIS

Generalised anxiety disorder (6B00)

The core feature of generalised anxiety disorder (GAD) is persistent, excessive anxiety and worry about a variety of everyday events such as finances, work or school, relationships, and health. These typically take the form of 'what if' questions about the future. The worry and anxiety are associated with several physiological symptoms, such as muscle tension, restlessness, difficulties concentrating, irritability, and sleep disturbance. These features constitute the main ICD-11 criteria for GAD. However, gastrointestinal complaints (e.g., irritable bowel syndrome), headaches, and other somatic symptoms are also common (Stein & Sareen, 2015).

DSM-5 criteria require that three of six specified physiological symptoms must be present in addition to persistent worry and anxiety to diagnose GAD; ICD-11 does not specify the number of symptoms needed for diagnosis. DSM-5 criteria also include an additional symptom, 'the individual finds it difficult to control the worry', which captures a 'worry about worry' that persons with GAD tend to experience. This type of worry is referred to as Type II worry or meta-worry, and is related to beliefs that excessive everyday worries (Type I worries) are uncontrollable, dangerous, and an indicator that there is something 'wrong' (Wells, 2005).

Despite these negative beliefs, persons with GAD typically view worrying about everyday events as an effective means of problem solving about the future to avoid negative outcomes. Much like behavioural avoidance strategies, in the short-term, worrying can decrease anxiety about potential negative outcomes (Borkovec, 1994). For example, constantly worrying about being fired from your job may be considered a way of preparing yourself should this happen, which helps some individuals to feel less anxious. To some extent, this may be helpful and adaptive, but at excessive levels can leave a person unable to focus due to constant worrying. In the long-term, worrying undermines an individual's belief in their ability to cope with uncertainty, trapping them in the vicious cycle of anxiety (Borkovec, Alcaine, & Behar, 2004).

Detection of GAD can be difficult, as people often present for assistance with their somatic symptoms rather than worry (Stein et al., 2005). It is under-recognised, particularly in primary care settings (Wittchen et al., 2002). Furthermore, GAD co-occurs at high rates with depression (American Psychiatric Association, 2013), which may be identified as the cause of the person's distress without detecting the presence of an underlying anxiety disorder (National Institute for Health and Care Excellence (NICE), 2014).

Panic disorder (6B01)

Panic disorder is characterised by recurrent, unexpected panic attacks, fear and anxiety about future attacks, and behaviours intended to avoid experiencing panic symptoms. A panic attack is defined as an acute period of intense fear or discomfort in which physiological and cognitive symptoms occur (e.g., increased heart rate, chest pain, sweating, shortness of breath, fear of dying), usually reaching a peak within minutes.

Panic attacks may be present in any number of disorders, as well as in people who do not meet criteria for a specific disorder. However, in panic disorder, the attacks are uncued, meaning they are not restricted to a specific stimulus or situation (e.g., a fear of dogs in specific phobia). Panic disorder is also associated with catastrophic interpretations of panic symptoms, such as a belief that they will cause direct physical harm (e.g., a heart attack). Indeed, many of the symptoms of a panic attack may mimic that of more serious physical conditions such as a heart attack, and it is therefore common for persons with panic disorder to present to emergency departments (Deacon, Lickel, & Abramowitz, 2008). The misappraisal that panic symptoms pose a physical threat leads to fear and anxiety about the recurrence of panic attacks—sometimes referred to as a 'fear of fear'—and avoidance of situations or activities that may trigger symptoms (e.g., exercise).

Persons with panic disorder tend to be hypervigilant to internal cues that may signal a panic attack (e.g., changes in heart rate) and often monitor these closely. Paradoxically, excessive monitoring increases the likelihood of future attacks as the person views benign changes in physiology as signs of danger, which elicit a fight-or-flight response (Bouton, Mineka, & Barlow, 2001). This response is not dependent on conscious awareness of the physiological changes, which can be thought of as conditioned stimuli that elicit anxiety due to a learned associated with panic (Bouton et al., 2001).

There are small differences between DSM-5 criteria and ICD-11 criteria for panic disorder. Firstly, DSM-5 specifies a minimum number of symptoms required for a panic attack; four or more symptoms are considered a full-symptom attack, while attacks with less than four symptoms are considered limited-symptom attacks (American Psychiatric Association, 2013). The DSM-5 criteria for panic disorder then require that a person experience more than one full-symptom attack. ICD-11 does specify several symptoms and therefore does not distinguish between full- and limited-symptom panic attacks. These differences mean that a person diagnosed with panic disorder using ICD-11 criteria may not meet criteria for the disorder using DSM-5.

Agoraphobia (6B02)

The characteristic feature of agoraphobia is intense fear or anxiety in response to real or anticipated exposure to multiple situations, such as public transport, being in crowds, or being in open spaces. The fear and anxiety are related to beliefs that escape might be difficult, or help may not be available should specific negative outcomes occur (e.g., panic attacks, being embarrassed/incapacitated by other physical symptoms).

The person may avoid feared situations entirely, and in severe cases, this can result in significant functional impairment such as becoming restricted to the home (Bonham & Uhlenhuth, 2014). In other instances, the person may continue to enter into feared situations, but only through the use of safety behaviours designed to help the person manage the situation while avoiding a perceived danger (e.g., only going shopping when with a friend, only using public transport if able to sit close to an exit), or else endure them with intense fear and anxiety.

The above described symptoms constitute the main ICD-11 criteria for agoraphobia. Criteria in DSM-5 specify that anxiety and fear must be present in response to two of five specified situations to diagnose agoraphobia: 1) using public transportation, 2) being in open spaces, 3) being in enclosed places, 4) standing in line or being in a crowd, and 5) being outside of the home alone. ICD-11 is less specific, and just notes several example situations.

Agoraphobia is now recognised as a separate condition to panic disorder in both DSM-5 and ICD-11, and can, therefore, be diagnosed independently. However, agoraphobia and panic disorder commonly occur together, and both diagnoses should be assigned if appropriate (see Differential Diagnosis information later in this section).

Specific Phobia (6B03)

Specific phobias involve marked excessive fear or anxiety in response to a specific object or situation, and associated avoidance of the feared stimulus. Typically, a strong physiological response occurs in anticipation of or exposure to the feared stimulus, though the nature of this varies. For instance, it is common for those with a blood-injection-injury specific phobia to experience a vasovagal fainting response, whereas other types of phobias are associated with more panic-like symptoms (American Psychiatric Association, 2013). The majority of people who meet criteria for specific phobia fear multiple objects or situations on average (Stinson et al., 2007).

Unlike the other anxiety and fear-related disorders discussed in this chapter, specific phobias typically develop in childhood (Bandelow & Michaelis, 2015). Specific phobias may be precipitated by negative encounters with the feared stimulus (e.g., being attacked by a dog, or witnessing another being attacked), but this is not always the case. Research has demonstrated that maternal modelling of anxious responses to a stimulus can lead to toddlers acquiring a fear of that stimulus, without the child experiencing any direct negative interaction with the stimulus itself (Gerull & Rapee, 2002).

Criteria for specific phobia are very similar across DSM-5 and ICD-11, though DSM-5 has an additional criterion, 'the phobic object or situation almost always provokes immediate fear or anxiety'. DSM-5 also lists five diagnostic specifiers: animal, natural environment, blood-injection-injury, situational, and other. ICD-11 does not list specifiers but notes simple phobia, acrophobia, and claustrophobia as inclusions for this diagnosis.

Social Anxiety Disorder (6B04)

Social anxiety disorder is characterised by excessive fear or anxiety in social situations, due to concerns about being negatively evaluated by others. People meeting criteria for social anxiety disorder are typically concerned they will act in a way (e.g., saying the wrong thing), or show anxiety symptoms (e.g., being red in the face, sweating), that will elicit judgement from others. Social situations that may subject the person to scrutiny from others are therefore consistently avoided.

The focus of the anxiety may be performance-based (e.g., giving a speech), related to direct social interactions with others such as talking with peers, or being observed in public (e.g., eating or drinking, or queuing in line). The above described features constitute ICD-11 criteria for social anxiety disorder. DSM-5 diagnostic criteria are very similar, though include 'performance only' as a specifier.

Traditionally, social anxiety disorder has been thought of as a fear of negative evaluation by others, but more recent research shows that it may be associated with a fear of *any* evaluation (Heimberg & Magee, 2014). Social anxiety disorder also has many features in common with avoidant personality disorder (a DSM-5 diagnosis without an ICD-11 equivalent). The two frequently co-occur, and some models consider that people meeting criteria for both disorders may be those with severe and longstanding social anxiety disorder (Heimberg & Magee, 2014).

Differential diagnosis

In differentiating between the anxiety disorders (and other disorders where anxiety may be a feature), it is important to identify the specific focus of the anxiety or avoidance as many disorders may present similarly. Information about differential diagnoses for each anxiety disorder is listed below, and this is also discussed in Section 4.4.6.

Generalised anxiety disorder

- *Social anxiety disorder*: Social worries are frequent in GAD, though tend to focus more on ongoing interpersonal relationships (e.g., 'what if my partner leaves me?') rather than negative evaluation from others
- *Depressive disorders*: Rumination in depression can present similarly to worry in GAD. However, depressive rumination is typically past-oriented while GAD is future-oriented.

Agoraphobia

- *Specific phobia*: Situational specific phobia can have a similar presentation to agoraphobia (e.g., fear of flying). Agoraphobia is diagnosed if multiple agoraphobic situation categories are feared (e.g., public transportation and being in a crowd).
- *Social anxiety disorder*: If situations are avoided due to fear of negative evaluation from others, a diagnosis of social anxiety disorder is more appropriate.
- *Panic disorder:* When the criteria for panic disorder are met, agoraphobia should not be diagnosed unless the panic-related avoidance behaviour is present in multiple agoraphobic situations.

Panic disorder

- *Panic attack:* Panic attacks may be present in many conditions. Panic *disorder* is only diagnosed when panic attacks are uncued, and the anxiety is related to the panic attacks themselves (e.g., a fear of panic symptoms, rather than a fear of dogs which causes a panic attack)

- *Medical conditions:* It is important to rule out medical causes of panic attacks (e.g., hyperthyroidism, seizure disorders, cardiopulmonary conditions), and substance or medication-induced panic attacks (e.g., withdrawal from alcohol, intoxication with amphetamines)

Anxiety is also a feature of many other disorders such as obsessive-compulsive or related disorders (including hypochondriasis) and disorders specifically associated with stress -discussed below—as well as eating disorders (see Chapter 4.5), dissociative disorders (see Section 4.4.9) and schizophrenia spectrum and other psychotic disorders (see Chapter 4.2).

PRACTICE ILLUSTRATION: PRESENTATION AND DIAGNOSIS

Ann is a 25-year-old university student, who was referred to a psychologist from her GP because she is uncertain about many aspects of her life and is not able to stop worrying. She lives with her cat in a small apartment close to the university. Ann reports constantly thinking about 'what if' something negative would happen in the future and finds it difficult to control her thoughts. Over the past year she has been experiencing distressing intrusive thoughts in relation to harming her beloved cat; for example, she recounts recurring thoughts about suffocating her cat. She regularly engages in rituals (e.g., straightening pillows) or 'safety' behaviours (e.g., putting away her sleeping pillows) to ensure that her cat is safe. Ann also constantly worries that she will not pass her exams if she doesn't study the entire day and that her friends will judge her for 'not being good enough at university'. More recently, she has started worrying that she has not chosen the right degree and will not find a job after graduating. These thoughts result in her often feeling restless and having trouble concentrating and sleeping. Ann has stopped attending university classes and avoids meeting her friends. She considers that her worry is helpful as it prepares her for the future; however, at the same time, she acknowledges the significant impact the worry has on her life. Over the past few months Ann has spent most of her days at home worrying about her life and her future. The psychologist diagnoses GAD with comorbid obsessive-compulsive disorder.

4.4.3 PHENOMENOLOGY AND DIAGNOSIS OF OBSESSIVE-COMPULSIVE OR RELATED DISORDERS

DARREN JIGGINS & MICHAEL KYRIOS

DARREN'S LIVED EXPERIENCE

DARREN JIGGINS

Imagine you are seven years old and the fear of appearing 'bad' leads you to find comfort in completing thousands of counting rituals per day. Lily Bailey's book, *Because We Are Bad*, gives a great insight into how intensely distressing and arduous the lived experience of obsessive-compulsive disorder (OCD) can be, as it is for me.

Up until the age of 23 years, I had never heard of OCD. So, I thought that I was the strangest person in the world. This led to deep depression, yet I had the ability to hide my OCD and the depression very effectively. The unintended consequence was a 10-year spiralling depression and escalation in suicidal ideas, plans, and finally attempts.

Only after my last suicide attempt did anyone find out that I was unwell at all. I ended up in the hospital, and I was outed! Then for eight weeks, people tried to cure me to no avail. Yet every clinician would tell me that OCD was curable '...if you try hard'.

What clinicians did not know, as I found out having heard the same tale from hundreds of people with OCD, is that we are often pressured into a position where we lie about the success of the horrid treatments we have to endure in search of the elusive 'cure'. To free ourselves from the trauma of treatment, many people in the end tell their clinician 'Yes doctor, I'm fine now and I can go home' when nothing has changed.

I can say this because I listened to these tales in person in an OCD self-help group that I attended every week for 10 years. In this loving group, I learned to accept and deal with the terrible fear and anxieties of my mental illness. Acceptance and understanding empowered me to find more useful ways to manage my thoughts, especially through the help of people in my group, OCD experts and online treatments. They inspired me to adopt acceptance as a liberation from the eternal search for a cure. I now choose to 'like myself'.

PHENOMENOLOGY

Early historical records describe obsessive-compulsive symptoms as 'scrupulosity' in a religious, moral context; obsessive concerns are related to one's own sins and compulsive rituals to one's performance of religious devotion. At the beginning of the twentieth century, obsessive-compulsive phenomena were recognised as medical (psychological) conditions (e.g., termed 'obsessional neurosis'; Freud, 2008) and included a broader spectrum of obsessions and compulsions.

To date, the diagnostic conditions included in obsessive-compulsive and related disorders are heterogeneous in the presentation of their symptoms, but all are characterised by repetitive thoughts and behaviours which according to the ICD-11 (World Health Organization (WHO), 2018f) share 'key diagnostic validators'. Central to OCD are unwanted, intrusive, and uncontrollable thoughts, images, or urges (i.e., obsessions). Intrusions are observed in the general population, too, and they do not usually differ either in occurrence or content from those of people with OCD; however, those with OCD differ in the appraisal of the unwanted thoughts. Assigning personal and negative meaning or importance to the thought naturally results in anxiety. The aim to alleviate feelings of marked anxiety and distress could then lead to repetitive avoidance or checking behaviours (i.e., compulsions).

Another subset of disorders in this diagnostic category are body-focused conditions, for example, characterised by persistent preoccupations with perceived body flaws (e.g., BDD) or repetitive, habitual behaviours directed at specific body parts (e.g., hair-pulling, skin-picking, lip biting). People with body dysmorphic disorder (BDD) are preoccupied with perceived defects or flaws in their appearance which others do not or hardly notice (the flaws are often associated with facial features such as the nose, hair, eyes, chin or lips) resulting in repetitive and excessive checking (e.g., mirror checking) or avoidance behaviours (e.g., avoiding mirrors, wearing a hat). Similar to OCD, it is not the frequency of mirror checking that distinguishes a person with BDD from a person with no symptoms, but rather the cognitive bias towards the reflection; a person with BDD anticipates to see the perceived flaw, then focuses on the perceived flaw that is eventually confirmed in their mind to be defective.

In ICD-11 (World Health Organization, 2018) hypochondriasis has been moved from the somatoform disorders into the obsessive-compulsive and related disorders grouping. The psychological processes associated with health-related anxieties are considered to have similarities with those in OCD. Hoarding disorder, which was once considered a subtype of OCD, has now been recognised as a distinct clinical syndrome (World Health Organization, 2018). HD is characterised by a compulsive accumulation of possessions and difficulty and distress related to discarding them. The accumulation of possessions results in clutter usually taking over the living spaces and often compromising the safety of the home environment (Halldorsson & Salkovskis, 2017).

FORMAL DIAGNOSIS

Obsessive-compulsive disorder

The central feature of OCD is the presence of obsessions and/or compulsions. Obsessions can be defined as thoughts, images or impulses that are intrusive and unwanted and occur repetitively. In OCD, obsessions are ego-dystonic, that is individuals with OCD recognise that the content of their obsessions is incongruent with their self-view or ideas about the world. Thus, obsessions are anxiety-provoking and individuals go to great length to ignore, suppress or neutralise them by performing compulsions.

Compulsions are either overt repetitive behaviours (e.g., rituals, or avoidance strategies) or covert mental acts intended to 'neutralise' the intrusive thought or 'prevent' a dreaded, harmful event from happening. Although performing compulsions alleviates feelings of anxiety at the time, paradoxically they increase the frequency of intrusions as they strengthen the belief that the person is solely responsible for removing the threat. This repetitive cycle of intrusions leading to performing compulsions resulting in more intrusions is time consuming (the diagnostic threshold is more than an hour per day).

OCD is a clinically heterogeneous condition, with several well-established symptom dimensions, including: (i) contamination concerns with hand washing, cleaning, checking compulsions, avoidance behaviour, etc.; (ii) safety concerns, doubts and symmetry obsessions with checking compulsions and associated phenomena (e.g., avoidance, rigid rules, needing to achieve a sense of 'completeness', etc.; iii) obsessions related to morality (e.g., aggressive, sexual, religious, blasphemous or other 'forbidden' thoughts, images or urges) with checking, doubting and related neutralising (Bloch, Landeros-Weisenberger, Rosario, Pittenger, & Leckman, 2008; Nedeljkovic et al., 2009). The need to mitigate perceived personal responsibility for potential harm to self or others is a central motivation that drives and maintains OCD (Salkovskis, 1985). Whereas hoarding was commonly considered a subtype of OCD, it is now recognised as a separate disorder (see below). Comorbidity in OCD is common, not only with anxiety and mood disorders but also with impulse control disorders or disorders due to substance use (e.g., Ruscio, Stein, Chiu, & Kessler, 2008).

Body dysmorphic disorder

Most people are not happy with some aspects of their appearance. However, for some people preoccupations with an imaginary defect becomes extreme. Symptoms of body dysmorphic disorder (BDD) include persistent, excessive and disproportionate preoccupations with aspects of one's own physical appearance.

Commonly, people with BDD are preoccupied with facial features (e.g., skin, hair, nose, etc.), but any body area can be the focus of concern. Usually the perceived 'physical flaws' are minor, and despite reassurance that they are minimal or not noticeable, people with BDD are convinced that others are taking notice, judging them, or talking about the perceived defect. Often, if untreated, people with BDD have poor insight, and are more likely to consult a plastic surgeon than a mental health professional. Driven by the excessive concerns about their bodily deficit, people with BDD perform repetitive and excessive behaviours to hide (e.g., camouflaging with body position, make-up, clothes) or improve the flaw (e.g., excessive grooming, cosmetic surgery). Both excessive checking of appearance or avoidance of mirrors, reflecting surfaces or social situations due to potential stress or the shame of embarrassment are common. An ICD-11 diagnosis of BDD includes persistent preoccupations with one or more perceived defects as well as repetitive and excessive behaviours in response to these preoccupations resulting in significant distress or impairment. The ICD-11 specifically includes excessive self-consciousness, often with ideas of reference (i.e., the conviction that people are taking notice, judging, or talking about the perceived defect or flaw); but in contrast to the DSM-5 no specifier of 'muscle dysmorphia', common in males, is mentioned.

Hypochondriasis

Hypochondriasis is characterised by a persistent preoccupation with or fear about the possibility of having serious, progressive or life-threatening diseases. In the absence of a known organic pathology and despite appropriate medical evaluation and reassurance that the concerns are unwarranted, people with hypochondriasis cannot stop fearing that they are ill. They misjudge normal or commonplace bodily sensations as symptoms of a serious illness which leads them to excessive and repetitive safety behaviours such as constant self-monitoring for signs of the illness (i.e., repeatedly checking blood pressure). When preoccupations and excessive health-related or avoidance behaviours result in significant distress or impairment in personal, family, social, educational, occupational or other important areas of functioning an ICD-11 diagnosis of hypochondriasis is warranted.

The criteria for hypochondriasis (ICD-11) and illness anxiety (DSM-5) differ mildly: the preoccupations and catastrophic misinterpretation of bodily symptoms and the repetitive and excessive health-related behaviours which are included for hypochondriasis are absent in illness anxiety, however in DSM-5 a diagnosis of illness anxiety requires the presence of the symptoms for a minimum of six months.

The concept of hypochondriasis is still discussed with controversy, and confusingly differing terms are used (e.g., health anxiety or illness phobia). Although sometimes used interchangeably, hypochondriasis and health anxiety are not the same: both conditions share the fear of having a potential illness, however, hypochondriasis refers to the extreme end of health anxiety and (usually) includes the conviction that one has a serious life-threatening illness. A diagnosis of hypochondriasis can only be made in the absence of the physical illness, whereas health anxiety is often seen in conjunction with a (more or less) physical disorder. People with hypochondriasis often attend primary care due to their 'physical symptoms' where the core of the problem (i.e., the fear and rumination about the meaning, significance, or cause of the 'physical disease') is often not recognised or understood.

A recent recognised form of health anxiety is the excessive or repeated searching for health-related information using the internet, termed 'cyberchondria'. It is not a distinct type of hypochondriasis or health anxiety but can exacerbate these conditions (Starcevic & Berle, 2015).

Hoarding disorder

Hoarding disorder (HD) was introduced as a new separate diagnosis in the ICD-11. It is characterised by a strong urge to save items and/or difficulties and distress associated with discarding them, regardless of the actual value of the possessions. Among the most commonly saved items are newspapers, old clothing and bags, books, receipts and bills, greeting cards and letters, and personal and sentimental objects (Mogan, Kyrios, Schweitzer, Yap, & Moulding, 2012). As a result—and without intervention—the accumulation of possessions clutters living spaces such that their intended use and the person's safety is significantly compromised.

Difficulties in discarding items are commonly attributed to the potential usefulness, the aesthetic value, the wish to avoid creating waste, or the personal importance of the item. People with HD frequently express strong sentimental attachment towards their possessions and describe that discarding them is like 'losing a good old friend'. In severe cases the hoarding behaviour seriously poses a risk to the health of the individual and those around them including lack of sanitation, risk of fire and blocked emergency exits, as well as falling over or being trapped under clutter (Frost, Steketee, & Williams, 2000). The quality of life of people with HD is substantially affected, as are their interpersonal relationships

An ICD-11 diagnosis of HD is warranted if the excessive acquisition or the difficulty in discarding possessions (regardless of their actual value) result in accumulation of possessions and cluttering of living spaces to the point that their use or safety is compromised. Note that the diagnostic criterion of 'repetitive urges or behaviours related to amassing or buying items' is not included in the DSM-5 but instead a specifier 'with excessive acquisition' is used.

Technically, animal hoarding can be considered a form of HD; however, it is not included as a diagnostic subtype due to the limited available evidence. It is characterised by 'the accumulation of a large number of animals and a failure to provide minimal standards of nutrition, sanitation, and veterinary care and to act on the deteriorating condition of the animals (e.g., disease, starvation, death) and the environment (e.g., severe overcrowding, extremely unsanitary conditions)' (American Psychiatric Association, 2013).

Differential diagnosis

Obsessive-compulsive disorder

- Anxiety disorders: Recurrent thoughts can be also seen in anxiety disorders (e.g., specific and social phobias or GAD), but they are usually about real-life objects, situations or concerns; in OCD the content of the intrusions is often more irrational, odd and bizarre.
- Eating disorders: In anorexia nervosa concerns around food can be irrational; however, they are exclusively focused on food.
- Obsessive-compulsive personality disorder (OCPD): The pervasive and enduring behaviour is usually not driven by compulsion but by extreme perfectionism and rigid control.

Body dysmorphic disorder

BDD needs to be differentiated from social anxiety disorder, and panic disorder with agoraphobia as well as eating disorders; in BDD, people are concerned about a prominent appearance-related defect, and not about social situations (e.g., social anxiety), or body weight and shape (e.g., anorexia nervosa).

Hypochondriasis

Panic disorders also include the catastrophic misinterpretation of bodily symptoms, but the fear is immediate and instant, and not future-oriented.

Hoarding disorder

Other medical (e.g., brain injury) and mental conditions (e.g., neurocognitive disorders, schizophrenia, and depression) which can result in clutter need to be eliminated. Non-discarding that results from fears of contaminating others is considered OCD and not HD.

4.4.4 PHENOMENOLOGY AND DIAGNOSIS OF DISORDERS SPECIFICALLY ASSOCIATED WITH STRESS

MIKE BARRY

PHENOMENOLOGY

Unlike other mental health conditions, disorders specifically associated with stress are directly related to exposure to a stressful or traumatic event, or a series of such events or adverse experiences. This means that for each of the disorders in this grouping, an identifiable stressor is a necessary, though not sufficient, causal factor.

Stressful events for some disorders are within the normal range of life experiences, for example, divorce, socioeconomic problems and bereavement. Other disorders, however, require the experience of a stressor of an extremely threatening or horrific nature, that is, a potentially traumatic event. Thus, it is the nature, pattern, and duration of the symptoms that arise in response to the stressful events—together with associated functional impairment—that distinguishes the disorders.

Post-traumatic stress disorder (PTSD) is a syndrome that develops following exposure to an extremely threatening or horrific event or series of events when a person does not return to normal functioning. Throughout history, descriptions of the range of symptoms that typify post-traumatic psychopathology have often been closely linked to loss of identity, damage to a person's sense of self, or character, or a lack of courage. During World War I, 80 000 British soldiers presented with symptoms resembling PTSD (Beveridge, 1997) and this war saw the start of the formal psychological study of the human response to trauma in military and civilian populations. During World War II, PTSD-like symptoms were variously labelled 'battle fatigue', 'combat exhaustion' and 'operational fatigue' (Campise, Geller, & Campise, 2006), with terms like 'fatigue' and 'exhaustion' perhaps reflecting the overwhelming nature of the symptoms.

It was not until the Vietnam War however, that the terms post-traumatic stress syndrome and PTSD were introduced (Campise et al., 2006) and finally accepted as a formal psychiatric disorder (American Psychiatric Association, 1980). By the fourth edition of the DSM, the main criterion had expanded from actual or threatened death or serious injury, to include awareness of events that threatened others, eliciting a response that involves intense fear, helplessness, or horror (DSM-IV; APA, 2000). It has been suggested that a new diagnosis, complex PTSD, is needed to describe the symptoms of chronic trauma (Herman, 2015). The evolution of disorders in this category has not been without controversy and debate continues about several issues concerning the diagnosis of PTSD and complex PTSD.

While traumatic stress disorders relate to a person's reaction to events involving actual or threatened death or serious injury, two other disorders in this section relate to a person's response to stressful events which are within the normal range of life experiences. While it is normal to grieve following the loss of a loved one, prolonged grief disorder occurs when, after the death of a partner, parent, child, or other person close to the bereaved, there is a pervasive grief response persisting for a longer than typical period following the loss. Also, while many people experience some difficulties adapting to or coping with change, adjustment disorder is an abnormal and excessive reaction to an identifiable life stressor (within three months of the onset of the stressor lasting no longer than six months after the stressor). The reaction is more severe than would normally be expected and can result in significant impairment in social, occupational, or academic functioning.

LIVED EXPERIENCE: AUSTRALIAN PEACEKEEPER, MID-1990S

In the mid-1990s, I served as part of a multinational United Nations military force helping to re-establish peace in an African nation following a brutal civil war. As part of my role, I visited and spent time at many of the internal displaced persons camps, including one in which several thousand displaced men, women and children were killed by government troops who were trying to close the camp by force.

I visited the camp again in the aftermath of the massacre where I talked with United Nations soldiers working there, and witnessed bodies buried among the rubbish left behind by over 100 000 people who had fled following the killings, while the remaining survivors were crammed into a tiny compound, too frightened to leave. I still get upset at the memory of watching a woman washing her child with water from a puddle on the ground, surrounded by rubbish and human waste, and seeing people eating scraps of food they had picked up out of the rubbish.

For months after the event, I couldn't eat certain foods, I was triggered by smells, which took me back to the camp, and I felt disillusioned about the role of peacekeeping in a world run by political agendas. I avoided talking about my experiences to my family when I returned home, was withdrawn and distant, became rigid and 'rule-based', and was often impatient and short-tempered, especially with family and others who would be concerned about what I considered 'trivial' things. For a long time, it was hard to put my experiences into perspective, and rationalise what I had witnessed, with day-to-day life in suburban Australia.

While I was never diagnosed with PTSD, with the benefit of hindsight I recognise that many of the symptoms that I experienced met this diagnosis, and I learned how common they are in veterans, and especially former peacekeepers. In the years since those events occurred, the memories have softened, and I can talk about what I experienced more easily. Even to this day however, I avoid watching media coverage, TV series and movies depicting the events that occurred, for fear of 'poking the bear'. Part of me would like to, to get closure, but I figure, why take the chance?

I now work with veterans, many with PTSD, and find that not only do my own experiences help me to connect with them, but in connecting with them, I have found it easier to process and manage my own experiences and memories.

FORMAL DIAGNOSIS

Post-traumatic stress disorder

While it is normal to experience some change in functioning for a while following exposure to traumatic events, most people return to normal functioning within a few days or weeks. To meet criteria for a diagnosis of PTSD, a person must have witnessed, experienced or been confronted with an event or events involving actual or threatened death, or serious injury to themselves or others; and their response to the trauma must have involved intense fear, helplessness or horror. These events can include, but are not limited to, serious road accidents, violent or sexual assaults, being involved in an armed hold-up, a traumatic birth, witnessing violent deaths, involvement in military combat, being held hostage or being exposed to a terrorist attack, natural disasters or the diagnosis of a life-threatening condition. PTSD is not usually related to situations that are simply upsetting, such as divorce, job loss or failing exams.

While DSM-5 and ICD-11 differ in terms of how they group specific criteria, with the DSM dividing criteria into four symptoms clusters, while the ICD identifies three, in general terms, symptoms fall into several broad clusters:

- Re-experiencing symptoms (memories of trauma), which are distressing and intrusive; because they are unwanted, the individual cannot control when they occur and because they invoke strong negative emotions associated with the initial trauma (Resick & Calhoun, 2001).
- Avoidant symptoms, which represent the behavioural, cognitive or emotional strategies used to gain psychological and emotional distance from the trauma (Briere & Scott, 2006).
- Changes in the person's view of themselves or the world, and changes in their ability to regulate their emotions. They often feel detached from family and friends and may experience persistent and negative beliefs about blame and trust.
- Increased arousal and reactivity symptoms, which place the person in a constant state of alertness similar to the body's reaction to the actual traumatic event. In this state of alert, the individual perceives an ongoing sense of threat and is constantly prepared to react to new threats of danger, even in relatively 'safe' situations.

Complex PTSD

Complex post-traumatic stress disorder (complex PTSD) is a disorder that may develop following exposure to an event or series of events of an extremely threatening or horrific nature. These are most commonly prolonged or repetitive events from which escape is difficult or impossible for example: torture, slavery, genocide campaigns, prostitution, prolonged domestic violence, or repeated childhood sexual or physical abuse.

According to the National Centre for PTSD, US Department of Veterans Affairs, in addition to the standard PTSD symptoms, a person who has experienced a prolonged period (i.e., months to years) of chronic victimisation and control by another may also experience difficulties in the following areas:

- Emotional regulation—including persistent sadness, suicidal thoughts, explosive anger, or inhibited anger.
- Consciousness—such as forgetting traumatic events, reliving traumatic events, or having

episodes in which one feels detached from one's mental processes or body (i.e., dissociation).

- Self-perception—including helplessness, shame, guilt, stigma, and a sense of being completely different from other human beings.
- Distorted perceptions of the perpetrator—for example attributing total power to the perpetrator, becoming preoccupied with the relationship to the perpetrator, or preoccupied with revenge.
- Relations with others—including isolation, distrust, or a repeated search for a rescuer.
- One's system of meanings—including a loss of sustaining faith or a sense of hopelessness and despair.

To satisfy a diagnosis of complex PTSD, usually all of the diagnostic requirements for PTSD need to be met at some point during the course of the disorder plus changes in belief structures which impact on a person's ability to engage in relationships and regulate their mood. The DSM-5 does not include a diagnosis for complex PTSD because it was argued that the current definition of PTSD was satisfactory, whereas ICD-11 recognises this as a distinct condition.

Prolonged grief disorder

While it is normal to grieve following the loss of a loved one, prolonged grief disorder occurs when, after the death of a person close to the bereaved, there is a persistent and pervasive grief response characterised by longing for the deceased or a persistent preoccupation with the deceased, accompanied by intense emotional pain, denial, blame, difficulty accepting the death, feeling one has lost a part of one's self, an inability to experience positive mood, emotional numbness, and difficulty in engaging with social or other activities.

To satisfy criteria, the grief response needs to have persisted for a longer than typical period following the loss (more than 6 months at a minimum) and have clearly exceeded expected social, cultural or religious norms for the individual's context. Grief reactions that have persisted for longer periods but are within a normative period of grieving given the person's cultural and religious context are viewed as normal bereavement responses and are not assigned a diagnosis.

Adjustment disorder (6B43)

Adjustment disorder is a maladaptive reaction to an identifiable psychosocial stressor or multiple stressors that usually emerges within a month of the stressor. It is characterised by a preoccupation with the stressor or its consequences, as well as by failure to adapt to the stressor causing significant impairment in personal, family, social, educational, occupational or other important areas of functioning. Adjustment disorders are associated with an increased risk of suicide and suicidal behaviour, substance abuse, and the prolongation of other medical disorders or interference with their treatment. Adjustment disorder that persists may progress to become a more severe mental disorder, such as major depressive disorder.

Differential diagnosis

Post-traumatic stress disorder

Because people who experience chronic trauma often have additional symptoms not included in the PTSD diagnosis, they may be often diagnosed with another condition such as borderline personality disorder (BPD). People with complex PTSD are shown to have consistently negative self-conceptions however, while people with BPD have demonstrated self-conceptions that are unstable and changing (Cloitre, Garvert, Weiss, Carlson, & Bryant, 2014).

Adjustment disorder

In adjustment disorder, symptoms must not be of sufficient specificity or severity to justify the diagnosis of depression or GAD, and typically resolve within six months, unless the stressor persists for a longer duration.

Prolonged grief

In prolonged grief that does not have a cultural or religious context, depression could be considered as a differential diagnosis.

4.4.5 WHAT DO WE KNOW ABOUT ANXIETY, OBSESSIVE-COMPULSIVE AND STRESS-RELATED DISORDERS?

DANIEL FASSNACHT, ERIN PARKER, MIKE BARRY, MICHELLE BANFIELD & MICHAEL KYRIOS

PREVALENCE, COURSE AND IMPACT

Anxiety or fear-related disorders

At present, there are no recent large-scale studies of the Australian prevalence of these disorders. The most recent estimates based on diagnostic interview (rather than self-report) come from the last National Survey of Mental Health and Wellbeing (Australian Bureau of Statistics, 2007) conducted in 2007. As noted above, DSM-5 and ICD-11 disorders are grouped differently from in previous versions of these manuals, so disorders that were coded as anxiety disorders (i.e., OCD and PTSD) at the time this survey was conducted no longer fall in the category, and criteria for individual disorders have changed. The current Australian prevalence of anxiety and fear-related disorders is, therefore, difficult to ascertain.

The DSM-5 estimates the prevalence of anxiety and fear-related disorders to be 7% in the United States (American Psychiatric Association, 2013). Similarly, a large systematic review estimated that for European/Anglo-Saxon countries (Western Europe, North America, and Australasia) prevalence is approximately 6.4% (Baxter, Scott, Vos, & Whiteford, 2013). Prevalence rates for individual disorders in Australia are presented in Table 4.20 and have been estimated from various sources. Where more recent prevalence data could not be found, the 2007 NSMHWB rates are reported. Generally speaking, anxiety and fear-related disorders occur about twice as frequently in women as men (Bandelow & Michaelis, 2015), except panic disorder and blood-injury-injection phobias where rates are similar across genders (LeBeau et al., 2010).

Anxiety and fear-related disorders typically develop by early adulthood with GAD having the latest age of onset (de Lijster et al., 2017). Anxiety disorders are associated with long delays in help-seeking from symptom onset, particularly in the case of social anxiety disorder, GAD, and specific phobia 9.3, 10.8, and 12.5 years (Thompson, Issakidis, & Hunt, 2008). Many anxiety disorders go unrecognised in health care settings, and only a minority of people receive treatment (National Institute for Health and Care Excellence (NICE), 2014). The untreated course of these disorders tends to be chronic, reaching a peak in middle age, but then decreasing in older age (Bandelow & Michaelis, 2015). The economic and social cost is high; anxiety disorders account for a large percentage of the non-fatal disease burden in Australia (Australian Institute of Health and Welfare [AIHW], 2016a).

Obsessive-compulsive or related disorders

OCD comes in many different forms and obsessive-compulsive symptoms are heterogeneous. Although there is some variation in symptom dimensions across different cultures (e.g., there is a preponderance of washing rituals in Middle Eastern cultures; Nedeljkovic, Moulding, Foroughi, Kyrios, & Doron, 2011), lifetime prevalence rates are consistently estimated around 1%–3% across different countries (Kessler et al., 2005; Kyrios, Sanavio, Bhar, & Liguori, 2001; Wittchen & Jacobi, 2005). In Australia, the NSMHWB suggested a lifetime prevalence of 2.8% for adults, with more females being affected. Interestingly, during childhood males are disproportionately impacted by OCD, however, these differences disappear in adults. OCD is associated with substantial comorbidities with more than three quarters of people with OCD having a lifetime history of another anxiety disorder and more than 40% of depression (Ruscio, Stein, Chiu, & Kessler, 2010).

The average age of onset of OCD is in early adulthood (around 17.5–19.5 years; Brakoulias et al., 2017). Typically, the onset is gradual and, if untreated, the course is often chronic with alternating periods of aggravated and mild symptoms. Although evidence-based treatments for OCD leads to an average symptom reduction between 50% and 70% (Öst, Havnen, Hansen, & Kvale, 2015), long delays in treatment-seeking are very common (3–17 years). OCD symptoms have a devastating impact on a person's life, and lead to substantial impairments both in interpersonal and occupational domains (Huppert, Simpson, Nissenson, Liebowitz, & Foa, 2009). There is a strong link between OCD and suicidal ideation and/or attempts: a large study reports a lifetime history of suicide attempt of 9% in OCD patients (Brakoulias et al., 2017).

For the other OCD-spectrum disorders the evidence base is less robust. BDD is closely linked to OCD, with the other diagnostics categories being different conditions in their own right. Currently there is limited research on BDD. Point prevalence estimates from Australia suggest 1.7–2.3% in adolescents and young adults, while a recent systematic review reports a weighted prevalence of 1.9% of adults in the community (Veale, Gledhill, Christodoulou, & Hodsoll, 2016). However, in specific populations such as people who are undergoing cosmetic surgery the numbers are escalating up to 20% (e.g., in rhinoplasty surgery candidates). In the community, BDD is slightly more common in females, whereas in psychiatric settings the differences disappear (Veale et al., 2016). Similarly as in OCD, comorbidities with other mental disorders is very common: 75% of people with BDD report a lifetime diagnosis of major depressive disorder, 40% of social anxiety, and one-third of OCD or eating disorders (Phillips, Menard, Fay, & Weisberg, 2005). Generally there are more similarities than differences between men and women with BDD; however, in clinical settings women report more concerns with their skin, breast and legs, whereas males are more concerned with their height and excessive facial or body hair (Perugi et al., 1997; Phillips, Menard, & Fay, 2006). People with BDD fear that others judge them due to their perceived defects resulting in impaired social relationships, suicide attempts (Phillips, 2007) and an overall poorer quality of life. Typically the onset of BDD symptoms is in late adolescence with two-thirds of patients reporting an onset before the age of 18 years (Bjornsson et al., 2013). Frequently, people with BDD look for non-mental health interventions such as cosmetic or dermatological surgery or rhinoplasty for their defects in physical appearance. This leads to delayed help-seeking of mental health treatment (often more than 10 years; Phillips, Didie, et al., 2006).

For hypochondriasis, reliable prevalence data is currently lacking. A study using NSMHWB data suggests a lifetime prevalence of 5.7% of health anxiety in the adult Australian population (Sunderland, Newby, & Andrews, 2013). While these rates are consistent with other population-based studies examining health anxiety (e.g., Bleichhardt & Hiller, 2007), it might be an overestimation of the prevalence of hypochondriasis as a broader definition of health anxiety was used in these surveys. Females tend to report more health anxiety than males, although the difference is rather small. People with hypochondriasis or health anxiety have more disability days, use medical services more often and an overall lower quality of life (Ladwig, Marten-Mittag, Erazo, & Gündel, 2001). Comorbidity with other metal disorders is high (e.g., 70% diagnosis of GAD, over 40% of depression; Creed & Barsky, 2004). Typically hypochondriasis has a chronic course if left untreated (Olde Hartman et al., 2009). People with hypochondriasis are often seen and treated in primary care due to the perception of a severe physical illness. Referral to mental health professionals can be challenging as many people with hypochondriasis refuse mental health treatment.

Epidemiological evidence for Hoarding Disorder is scarce. Community surveys suggest a point prevalence between 2% and 6% (Pertusa et al., 2010); however, only one large study from the United Kingdom used strict diagnostic criteria and psychiatric interviews (Nordsletten et al., 2018). This study estimated a lower prevalence of 1.5% for both males and females. People with HD tend to be older, living on their own, and have more often a physical health condition compared to the general public. Among people with HD the most common comorbidities are GAD, depression, and OCD. Retrospective case reports suggest that typically problems with hoarding start in childhood and become more serious in the mid-20s where symptoms start to interfere with the person's daily life (Grisham, Frost, Steketee, Kim, & Hood, 2006). The most common treatment barriers in HD are the lack of recognising that there is a problem, and stigma and shame. Further, until the recent inclusion of HD in psychiatric taxonomies, affected individuals have generally been excluded from accessing mental health services for their hoarding problems. The economic and social burden of hoarding is enormous both for the individual, their direct family as well as for the communities. Excessive clutter can cause a serious health and safety risk for the individual and direct neighbours; for example, a study in the Metropolitan District of Melbourne found hoarding and/or squalor related to 54 fires between April 2013 and April 2014 (Morse, Scott, Lackie, & Homchenko, 2014).

Disorders specifically associated with stress

Recent epidemiological studies from around the world have found that while trauma exposure tends to be higher in lower-income countries compared with high-income countries, PTSD prevalence rates are largely similar across countries, with higher rates occurring in post-conflict environments. Lifetime prevalence of PTSD varies across countries with consistent rates across South Africa (2.3%), Spain (2.2%), and Italy (2.4%) compared to Japan (1.3%) and Northern Ireland (which reported the highest lifetime PTSD prevalence of 8.8%; Atwoli, Stein, Koenen, & McLaughlin, 2015). Other studies have found the lifetime prevalence ranges from 6.1–9.2% in national samples of the general adult population in the United States and Canada (Koenen et al., 2017) and between 5–10% in Australia (Phoenix Australia, 2013).

A meta-analysis of 77 studies about risk factors for PTSD found that peri- and post-trauma factors (e.g., individual factors, trauma severity, lack of social support) had a stronger influence than pre-trauma factors (Brewin, Andrews, & Valentine, 2000). Intentional and interpersonal trauma have a greater association with PTSD than traumatic events that were unintentional/non-assaultive (Kessler et al., 2014). Women are four times more likely to develop PTSD than men, after adjusting for actual exposure rates, particularly in the case of interpersonal and sexual trauma. In many cases, people do not seek treatment immediately following a traumatic event, and even after symptoms emerge, many people are reluctant to seek treatment due to fear of being stigmatised and implications for their careers, particularly in the military and emergency service personnel (Mittal et al., 2013).

Living with a person with PTSD can be difficult. People with PTSD frequently experience recurring nightmares, and can often thrash out, or call out in their sleep, they are easily startled, hypervigilant and overly security and safety conscious, and avoid social situations. They often have difficulty expressing or responding to emotions, feel more detached from others, which can impact on forming attachment bonds with children and loved ones, and often experience lower satisfaction in parenting.

Table 4.20 Prevalence rates of anxiety, fear, obsessive-compulsive, stress-related and dissociative disorders

	Lifetime prevalence	12-month prevalence	Point prevalence
GAD	5.9 [b]	2.7 [a]	
Panic Disorder	5.2 [b]	2.6 [a]	
Panic disorders/ panic attacks		2.5 [†]	
Agoraphobia	6.0 [b]	2.8 [a]	
Specific Phobia	3.5 [d] (Females)		

SAD	8.4[p]	4.2[p]	
Phobic anxiety disorders		1.3[†]	
OCD	2.8[b]	1.9[a] 1.0[c]	
BDD			1.7[f] (Adolescents) 2.3[e] (University students) 2.4[g] (Adults)
Hypochondriasis/ Health anxiety	5.7[n]		3.4[n]
HD			2.8[h] (Adult twins) 1.5[i] (Adults) 5.8[j] (Adults)
PTSD	12.2[b] 1.5[m]	6.4[a] 1.0[c]	
Complex PTSD	0.5[m]		
Adjustment disorder		0.9[o]	
Dissociative amnesia		1.8[k] 7.3[l] (Females)	
DID		1.5[k] 1.1[l] (Females)	
Depersonalisation-derealisation disorder		0.8[k]	
Depersonalisation disorder		1.4[l] (Females)	
Derealisation without depersonalisation		1.1[l] (Females)	

Lifetime prevalence = proportion of sample that at some point in their life has experienced the condition; 12 month prevalence = proportion of sample that has experienced condition in the last 12 months; point prevalence = proportion of sample that has the condition (usually) at the time of assessment

[a]National Survey of Mental Health and Wellbeing, 2007 (Slade, Johnston, Oakley Browne, Andrews, & Whiteford, 2009)
[b]National Survey of Mental Health and Wellbeing, 2007
[c]National Health Survey, 2014–15
[d]Age-stratified representative sample of Australian women (Williams et al., 2010)
[e]Australian university students (Bartsch, 2007)
[f]Australian adolescents (Schneider, Baillie, Mond, Turner, & Hudson, 2018)
[g]Adults in the United States (Koran, Abujaoude, Large, & Serpe, 2008)
[h]Australian adult twins (López-Solà et al., 2014)
[i]Adults in the United Kingdom (Nordsletten et al., 2018)
[j]Adults in Germany (Timpano et al., 2011)
[k]Adults in the United States (Johnson, Cohen, Kasen, & Brook, 2006)
[l]Female adults in Turkey (Şar, Akyüz, & Doğan, 2007)
[m]Adult sample in Germany (Maercker, Hecker, Augsburger, & Kliem, 2018)
[n]Adult sample based on NSMHW 2007 (Sunderland et al., 2013)
[o]Adult sample in Germany (Maercker et al., 2012)
[p]Adult sample in Australia (Crome et al., 2015)

Note for a, b, c: Data for 2014–15 are not comparable to earlier years due to a change in collection methodology. In 2014–15, information on mental health conditions was obtained through a new Mental, Behavioural and Cognitive Conditions module, while in previous years it was collected as part of the Long-Term Conditions module.

HOW CAN WE UNDERSTAND THE ORIGINS?

As with most mental illnesses, the development of disorders discussed in this chapter is best understood through the use of a biopsychosocial model.

Aetiological models for anxiety and fear-related disorders

The triple vulnerability theory (Barlow, 1988, 2000, 2002) is a useful way of understanding the development of anxiety and fear-related disorders in general, though specific models exist for specific disorders.

It is believed that factors such as a heritable tendency to experience negative affect and an inhibited temperament in childhood (characterised by being slow to warm up to peers, seeking proximity to caregivers, and unwillingness to explore new situations) are related to a biological vulnerability to anxiety disorders (Barlow & Craske, 2014; Fox & Pine, 2012; Rapee, 2012; Rosenbaum et al., 1993).

This biological vulnerability then interacts with social/environmental factors to produce psychological vulnerabilities. For example, children with behaviourally inhibited temperaments tend to elicit an overprotective response from their caregivers, which leads to a diminished sense of control and reduced opportunity for the child to learn anxiety can be tolerated (Barlow & Craske, 2014). In general, parenting factors and family environment are believed to play a large role in the development of anxiety disorders for those with an existing biological vulnerability (Rapee, 2012). Insecure child-caregiver attachment style has also been repeatedly linked to the development of anxiety disorders, with some studies demonstrating that this predicts later anxiety to a greater degree than temperament (Warren, Huston, Egeland, & Sroufe, 1997). Overall, it is believed that such factors create a generalised psychological vulnerability to anxiety and fear-related disorders.

Specific early learning experiences may then focus anxiety on a particular area of concern, creating a specific psychological vulnerability to a particular disorder (Barlow & Craske, 2014). Learning can occur through multiple pathways—direct experiences with a threat, straightforward information transmission about a potential threat, and vicarious (observational) learning have all been demonstrated to impact the development of anxiety (Antony & Stein, 2008). For example, development of social anxiety disorder is associated with the direct experience of being bullied in childhood (Heimberg & Magee, 2014), as well as modelling of social anxiety and direct information transmission from caregivers about the potential dangers of being socially evaluated (Barlow, 2002).

Aetiological models for obsessive and compulsive-related disorders

Biological models

There is evidence that OCD has a biological base. Twin and family studies suggest that the risk for OCD increases proportionally to the degree of genetic relatedness (Mataix-Cols et al., 2013). In BDD, twin studies suggest a moderate heritability (Monzani, Rijsdijk, Harris, & Mataix-Cols, 2014). Heritability rates for hoarding range from 38–50% (Iervolino et al., 2009); a study using the Australian Twin Registry suggests a stronger genetic influence on hoarding symptoms in females compared to males (López-Solà et al., 2014).

Neurocognitive functioning

Evidence from neuropsychological studies in OCD support specific deficits relative to clinical and healthy controls, particularly in impaired planning and strategy, non-verbal memory, slowed response speed (Purcell, Maruff, Kyrios, & Pantelis, 1998), and inhibition control (Yücel et al., 2007). Interestingly, studies found changes in neuropsychological deficits following cognitive behavioural treatment (Nedeljkovic, Kyrios, Moulding, & Doron, 2011), potentially neutralising support for a trait model of neurocognitive deficits in OCD.

While preliminary evidence suggests that people with BDD have poorer executive functioning (Dunai, Labuschagne, Castle, Kyrios, & Rossell, 2010), and emotional processing deficits (Buhlmann, Etcoff, & Wilhelm, 2006), results need to be replicated (Feusner, Neziroglu, Wilhelm, Mancusi, & Bohon, 2010). Similarly in HD, neurocognitive processes, such as deficits in problem solving, visuospatial ability, attention, and organisation may contribute to the overvaluing of objects and the associated difficulties in discarding (Woody, Kellman-McFarlane, & Welsted, 2014).

PSYCHOLOGICAL MODELS

Salkovskis's cognitive behavioural approach (Salkovskis, 1985) and revised models based on his framework (e.g. Freeston, Rheaume, & Ladouceur, 1996; Frost & Steketee, 2002) argue that obsessions and compulsions arise from a dysfunctional belief system—especially the dysfunctional appraisal of intrusions (e.g., 'sticking thoughts' such as 'Did I check my apartment?'). Only when intrusive thoughts are seen as a threat for which the person is personally responsible, will the intrusion develop into a clinical obsession (e.g., 'When I don't check my front door, my apartment is not a secure and safe place'). There is evidence supporting that intrusions are no different in occurrence and content in the general population compared to individuals with OCD, although clinical obsessions might be experienced in greater frequencies, more spontaneous, and are often more violent/aggressive or bizarre (Berry & Laskey, 2012). But why are some people misinterpreting intrusions as significant, meaningful and important? Rachman (1998) argues that 'obsessions are caused by catastrophic misinterpretations of the significance of one's thoughts (images, impulses)' (p. 793). The Obsessive-Compulsive Cognitions Working Group (OCCWG; Frost & Steketee, 2002) identified six types of dysfunctional beliefs associated with onset and maintenance of OCD: inflated responsibility, overimportance of thoughts (i.e., thought-action fusion), need to control thoughts (it is both essential and possible to have total control over one's own thoughts), overestimation of threat, perfectionism, and intolerance for uncertainty. Others have additionally argued that such cognitions emerge from compromised early attachment patterns and are associated with compromised self-construals (Bhar & Kyrios, 2007; Doron, Moulding, Kyrios, Nedeljkovic, & Mikulincer, 2009; Guidano & Liotti, 1986; Kyrios et al., 2016).

In BDD, a cognitive behavioural model has been proposed (Veale, 2004) that highlights a dysfunctional belief system, too. People with BDD see themselves as an 'aesthetic object' and their core belief is that their body parts are 'flawed'. This distorted mental image of themselves develops through selective attention to aspects of one's appearance wherein individuals are looking for confirmation of perceived flaws. Then negative appraisal of 'flaws' led to avoidance including attempts to hide or camouflage them. A behavioural model of BDD which highlights the importance of early experiences that positively reinforce an individual for appearance has been proposed (Neziroglu, Roberts, & Yaryura-Tobias, 2004). More recently, BDD has also been associated with self-ambivalence (Labuschagne, Castle, Dunai, Kyrios, & Rossell, 2010).

The cognitive behavioural model of hoarding by Frost and Hartl (1996) postulates both information processing deficits and erroneous beliefs about the nature of possessions are aetiological and maintenance factors in HD (Kyrios, Mogan, et al., 2018). Problems in forming emotional attachments are also thought to result in compensatory attachments to objects leading to difficulties in discarding objects. Finally, as seen in other anxiety disorders, behavioural avoidance is a key factor in HD: saving an item allows the person with HD to avoid a decision about the possession. This indecisiveness is strongly related to the concern of making mistakes (e.g., by discarding the item and realising later that it is still needed).

Theoretical models of PTSD

Early theoretical efforts to understand the nature of PTSD included models which were based on conditioning processes, and on information processing during and after the traumatic experience, while more recently, diathesis-stress models focused on psychological, social and biological vulnerabilities.

Basic conditioning theory suggests that a traumatic event acts as an unconditioned stimulus leading to an unconditioned response, fear (Mowrer, 1960), while the unconditioned stimulus may also be linked to contextual cues that can become conditioned stimuli to fear, and that act as learned alarms (Orr et al., 2000).

Information processing approaches

There are conflicting views on how the processing of trauma-related information influences post-trauma reactions. One common view is that information fails to be processed when it conflicts with the dominant view of the self, and thus cannot be readily incorporated within the autobiographical knowledge base (Brewin & Holmes, 2003) An opposing view however, suggests that the traumatic memory stays highly accessible, and acts as a reference point for the organisation of autobiographical knowledge, because of its distinctive nature and high emotional impact (Berntsen & Rubin, 2007). According to the latter view, it is the *enhanced* integration of trauma memories into one's identity that appears to be a key factor in predicting PTSD symptomatology, rather than poor integration. This would suggest that it is assimilated to create or reinforce negative self-schemas (Dalgleish, 1999; Foa & Rothbaum, 1998), negative beliefs (Ehlers & Clark, 2000) or negative identities (Brewin, 2003).

Vulnerability approaches

Diathesis-stress models focus on vulnerability factors and propose that there are predisposing variables, or diatheses, creating vulnerability for any given psychological disorder. Ingram and Price (2001) suggest that three themes emerge when examining vulnerability: vulnerability as a trait; the endogenous and latent nature of vulnerability; and the role of stress. Trait-like factors exist even in the absence of a disorder, creating a diathesis or premorbid risk factor on which daily stresses act. Each individual's 'breaking-point' varies, depending on the interaction between these risk factors and the degree of stress being experienced (Monroe & Simons, 1991).

4.4.6 ASSESSMENT OF ANXIETY, OBSESSIVE-COMPULSIVE AND STRESS-RELATED DISORDERS

DANIEL FASSNACHT, ERIN PARKER, MIKE BARRY, MICHELLE BANFIELD & MICHAEL KYRIOS

GOOD PRACTICE IN DISORDER-SPECIFIC ASSESSMENT AND HELPFUL ASSESSMENT INSTRUMENTS AND GUIDES

Anxiety or fear-related disorders

As noted above, avoidance is the key maintaining factor in anxiety and fear-related disorders and therefore a primary target of treatment, irrespective of the treatment approach used. A thorough assessment of avoidance behaviours is therefore crucial to the successful treatment, including assessment of safety behaviours (e.g., using public transport but always sitting close to the door, keeping a benzodiazepine in your pocket 'just in case').

Assessment of maladaptive anxiety and fear-related cognitions (including worries in GAD) is also vital, as these cognitions perpetuate anxiety by fuelling avoidance behaviours and increasing emotional and physiological anxiety symptoms (Wells, 2013).

Finally, several physical illnesses produce symptoms of anxiety (e.g., hypoglycaemia, thyroid or cardiac conditions) so excluding an underlying medical cause is important (Kyrios, Mouding, & Nedeljkovic, 2011). However, anxiety disorders have high rates of co-occurrence with physical illnesses (Roy-Byrne et al., 2008), so identification of a related medical condition does not rule out the presence of an anxiety disorder.

The Depression Anxiety Stress Scale-21 (DASS-21; Lovibond & Lovibond, 1995) may be useful as an initial screening tool to identify whether anxiety is a primary concern, as it produces separate subscale scores for depression, anxiety, and stress. However, it assesses physiological and emotional anxiety symptoms rather than cognitive symptoms (i.e., worry). For this reason, if GAD is suspected, it may be useful to use a disorder-specific instrument such as the GAD-7 (Spitzer, Kroenke, Williams, & Löwe, 2006), which was developed for use in primary care settings. A list of other disorder-specific measures that are freely available can be found in Appendix I of the Australian Clinical Practice Guidelines (Andrews, Bell, et al., 2018).

In addition to psychometric measures, the flow chart in Figure 4.4 has been adapted from Kyrios and colleagues (2011) as a tool to assist in the differential diagnosis of anxiety disorders.

Obsessive-compulsive or related disorders

For treatment planning it is important to assess the obsessional thoughts, ideas, impulses, and the stimuli or situations that trigger these obsessions, as well as the rituals and avoidance behaviour which is performed to alleviate anxiety associated with the obsessions. Another important area of assessment is the link between obsessions and compulsions (i.e., what are the anticipated harmful consequences of confronting feared situations without performing rituals?). The Yale-Brown Obsessive-compulsive Scale (YBOCS), can be both used as a semi-structured, clinician-administered interview or a self-report instrument (Goodman, Price, Rasmussen, Mazure, Delgado, et al., 1989; Goodman, Price, Rasmussen, Mazure, Fleischmann, et al., 1989). It includes a symptom checklist to identify the patient's obsessions and compulsions and a 10-item scale which assess the severity of these obsessions and compulsions. There are several self-report measures available to assess OCD symptoms; for example, the Dimensional Obsessive-Compulsive Scale (DOCS), a 20-item instrument developed to measure the severity of the four most common dimensions of OCD symptoms (contamination, responsibility for harm and mistakes, symmetry/ordering, and unacceptable thoughts; Abramowitz et al., 2010).

The use of a screening measure can facilitate the diagnosis of BDD, as patients usually do not reveal their appearance concerns immediately. The brief, 4-item self-report Body Dysmorphic Disorder Questionnaire has excellent sensitivity to correctly identify BDD symptoms (Phillips, 2009). The Yale-Brown Obsessive-Compulsive Scale Modified for Body Dysmorphic Disorder (BDD-YBOCS) is a 12-item, clinician rated instrument that assesses BDD severity during the past week (Phillips et al., 1997). It measures both the obsessional preoccupations about the perceived appearance flaw, and the repetitive behaviours related to these preoccupations such as excessive grooming or mirror checking.

Assessment of patients presenting with possible hypochondriasis initially includes a medical history. Self-report instruments like the 7-item Whiteley Index can be used to assess excessive thoughts, worrying, or behaviours related to the health concerns (Fink et al., 1999). Both the 14- and 18-item versions of the Short Health Anxiety Inventory (Alberts, Hadjistavropoulos, Jones, & Sharpe, 2013; Salkovskis, Rimes, Warwick, & Clark, 2002) can be used to assess symptoms of hypochondriasis or health anxiety.

The Savings Inventory-Revised (SI-R; Frost, Steketee, & Grisham, 2004), the current gold standard measure for hoarding symptoms in treatment trials, is a 23- item self- report scale that measures the severity of each of three major features in the definition of HD. The Hoarding Rating Scale, available in an interview and self-report version, is a 5-item instrument assessing key features of compulsive hoarding: clutter, difficulty discarding, acquisition, distress, and impairment. It can reliably identify hoarders (Tolin, Frost, & Steketee, 2010).

Disorders specifically associated with stress

When assessing PTSD, it is important to understand the difference between a PTSD measure and a trauma exposure measure. A PTSD measure assesses PTSD symptoms related to one or more traumatic events, while a trauma exposure measure identifies what traumatic events an individual has experienced.

Figure 4.4 Anxiety disorder differential diagnosis flowchart

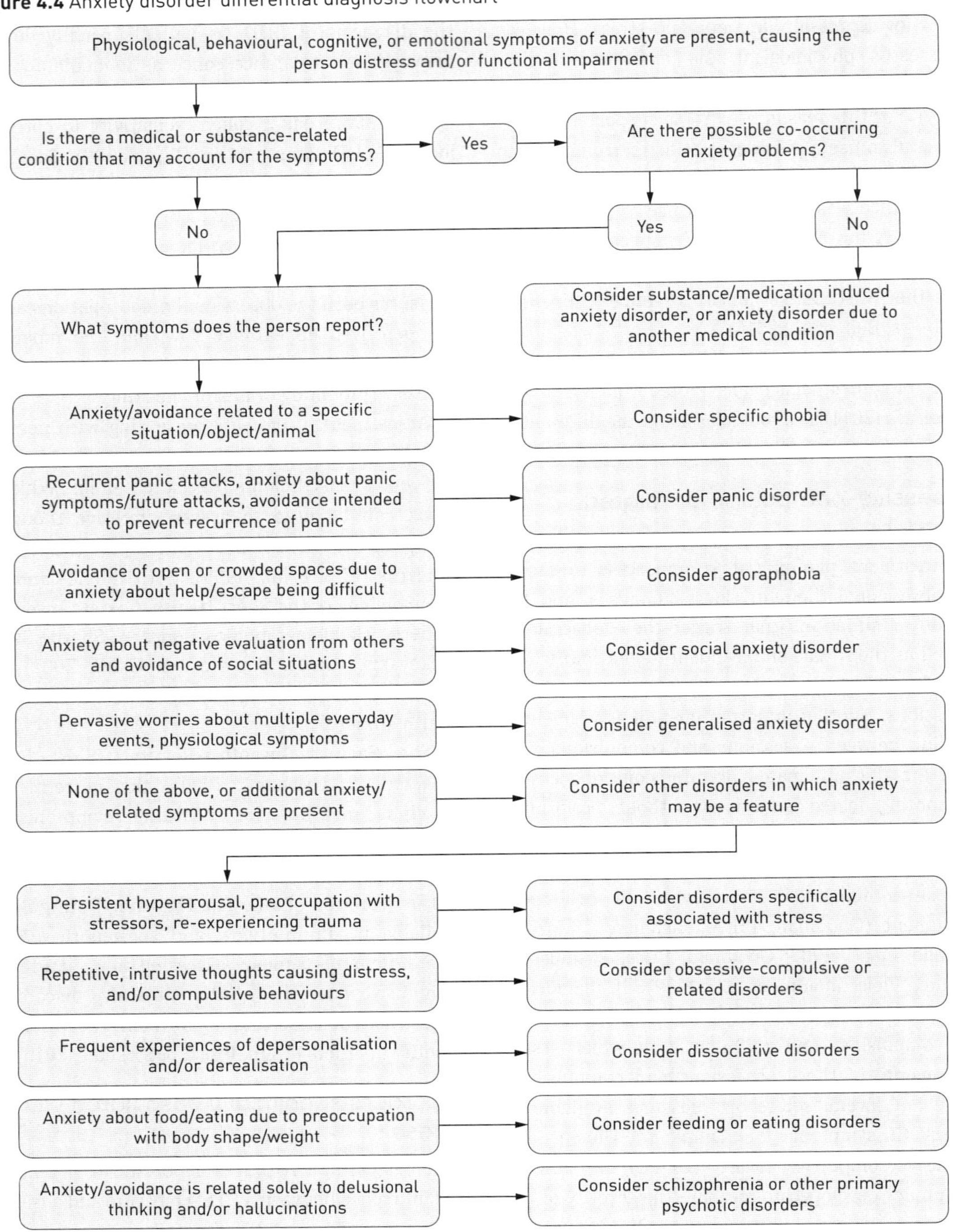

Source: Adapted from Kyrios et al., 2011

PRACTICE ILLUSTRATION: INITIAL TREATMENT

After discussing the treatment options with Ann, the psychologist suggests working on Ann's worries first by using a cognitive-behavioural approach. The first sessions focus on explaining how excessive anxiety and worries are developed and maintained, introducing self-monitoring strategies (e.g., a worrying outcome journal), progressive muscle relaxation techniques to help her manage her anxiety and controlled worry strategies. Ann is then progressively exposed to anxiety-provoking stimuli with the support of the psychologist preventing her from typical avoidance or safety behaviours. After a few sessions, Ann has started managing her worries and, using a similar exposure-based and cognitive therapy approach, she is now ready to address the intrusive thoughts about her cat and management of her rituals.

- *Clinician-Administered PTSD Scale for DSM-5 (CAPS-5).* The gold standard assessment instrument for assessing PTSD is the Clinician-Administered PTSD Scale for DSM-5 (CAPS-5). This 30-item structured interview can be used to make a current diagnosis, determine lifetime diagnosis, or assess PTSD symptoms over the previous week (Weathers et al., 2013).
- *PTSD Checklist for DSM-5 (PCL-5).* While the gold standard for diagnosing PTSD is a structured clinical interview such as the CAPS-5, the PCL-5 is of more practical use in a clinical setting and is a 20-item self-report measure that assesses DSM-5 symptoms (Weathers et al., (2013b).) The PCL-5 takes approximately five minutes to complete and can be used make a provisional diagnosis for PTSD. A total symptom severity score (range—0-80) can be obtained and a score of 33 is recommended as a cut-off for indicating PTSD.
- *Life Events Checklist for DSM-5 (LEC-5).* The Life Events Checklist for DSM-5 (LEC-5) is a self-report measure designed to screen for potentially traumatic events in a respondent's lifetime (Weathers, 2013). The LEC-5 assesses exposure to 16 events known to potentially result in PTSD or distress and includes one additional item assessing any other extraordinarily stressful event.

COMMON ISSUES AND DILEMMAS IN ASSESSMENT

In Australia, assessment of anxiety disorders commonly occurs in general practice (Australian Bureau of Statistics, 2007), where general medical practitioners (GPs) face barriers to accurate diagnosis. Within short consultation times GPs need to differentiate anxiety disorders from medical causes and other mental health conditions and identify possible co-occurring problems. Furthermore, persons with an anxiety disorder will often present to general practice seeking help for the physical symptoms of their anxiety rather than anxiety itself (Stein et al., 2005).

Some people with OCD lack insight while, in HD, poor insight is very common. People do not see themselves as having a problem or they fail to acknowledge the severity of the hoarding problem and associated consequences, making assessment and help-seeking challenging.

As expected, assessing for traumatic exposure can be distressing for the individual being assessed. Because discussing the trauma itself is often distressing, clients can be reluctant to talk about their memories and experiences for fear of being retraumatised. In addition, their memories may be fragmented, so they may feel unable to provide an accurate account of their experience, and they are likely to have spent months or even years actively trying to avoid recalling their experience. It is important for the clinician to establish trust with the client so that they feel safe enough to expose themselves to their memories. If they are still in an environment in which they do not feel safe, for example they are living in an abusive relationship, then it can be difficult to assess for past trauma, as they are potentially still being exposed to new trauma. Sometimes it is necessary to provide the client with grounding and arousal management strategies, prior to doing an assessment, so that they feel confident that they can manage any increased arousal or distress that they may have.

4.4.7 EVIDENCE-BASED AND OTHER TREATMENTS FOR ANXIETY, OBSESSIVE-COMPULSIVE AND STRESS-RELATED DISORDERS

DANIEL FASSNACHT, ERIN PARKER, MIKE BARRY, MICHELLE BANFIELD & MICHAEL KYRIOS

MAIN TREATMENTS AND STRENGTH OF EVIDENCE

Updated Australian Clinical Practice Guidelines for the treatment of social anxiety disorder, panic disorder, and GAD were published in 2018 (Andrews, Bell, et al., 2018). These guidelines state that anxiety disorders should be treated using a stepped care model including psychological interventions (online and face-to-face), pharmacological interventions, and their combination. An overview of the recommendations for the management of anxiety disorders, taken from the Australian practice guidelines can be seen in Figure 4.5. It should be noted that despite recommendations for the combination of psychological and pharmacological interventions in severe cases, the evidence for this is limited (Andrews, Bell, et al., 2018).

Psychological treatments

Anxiety and fear-related disorders

Psychological therapy, and cognitive behavioural therapy (CBT; see Section 2.6.11) in particular, is effective for anxiety disorders and is considered a first-line treatment (Andrews, Bell, et al., 2018; National Institute for Health and Care Excellence (NICE), 2005b). Mindfulness and acceptance-based therapies (see Section 2.6.12) such as acceptance and commitment therapy are also increasingly used in the treatment of anxiety disorders and are supported by an emerging body of evidence (e.g., Forman, Herbert, Moitra, Yeomans, & Geller, 2007; Hofmann, Sawyer, Witt, & Oh, 2010), though are less well-researched than traditional CBT.

The specific CBT techniques used to treat anxiety vary for each disorder, and a wide variety of strategies may be used within disorders. However, a key component of treatment across the board is the inclusion of exposure techniques. Exposure therapy involves graduated exposure to feared stimuli to both decrease levels of, and build tolerance to, anxiety. Other components that should form part of any CBT-based anxiety treatment regimen are listed below (Andrews, Bell, et al., 2018):

- psychoeducation about the nature of anxiety, including the fight-or-flight response (particularly in panic disorder) and the maintenance role of avoidance
- arousal reduction strategies (e.g., deep breathing, mindfulness, relaxation techniques)
- cognitive strategies (e.g., challenging catastrophic beliefs, structured problem solving)
- behavioural strategies (predominantly exposure techniques, usually graded exposure).

Treatment of GAD differs slightly from other anxiety disorders, as it is less behavioural in nature (although, engagement in worry can be viewed as a behaviour) and anxiety triggers are more diffuse (i.e., about a wide variety of everyday events). That being said, reducing behavioural avoidance remains a goal of treatment. Behavioural strategies may involve graded exposure to internal experiences of anxiety themselves (i.e., worries, emotions, and physiological symptoms; (Roemer & Orsillo, 2014), as well as engaging in unplanned activities without over-preparing (Andrews, Bell, et al., 2018)). Furthermore, problem-solving skills are often also taught as part of treatment for GAD, with a focus on helping the person identify the difference between effective problem solving and the ineffective use of worry as a problem-solving technique.

CBT can be self-guided (such as through self-help books), delivered online (e.g., smartphone app, computer), or in a traditional face-to-face setting (either individually or in a group). Individually delivered, face-to-face CBT is the most widely studied method, though there is also good evidence for online CBT-based programs in the treatment of anxiety disorders (e.g., Andrews, Basu, et al., 2018; Olthuis, Watt, Bailey, Hayden, & Stewart, 2016). (Information about disorder-specific online treatment programs in Australia can be found at www.headtohealth.gov.au.)

OBSESSIVE-COMPULSIVE OR RELATED DISORDERS

CBT is recommended for OCD and BDD at all levels of symptom severity (National Institute for Health and Care Excellence, 2005). The evidence for treatment guidelines for hoarding (Tolin, Frost, Steketee, & Muroff, 2015) and hypochondriasis/health anxiety (Olatunji et al., 2014) is emerging but still less clear.

Salkovskis' cognitive behavioural model of OCD (Salkovskis, 1985) leads to specific treatment targets: for example maladaptive beliefs (e.g., that 'something bad' will happen) and the appraisal of inflated responsibility (e.g., if 'something bad' happens I'm personally responsible) are challenged. Further, avoidance and safety-seeking behaviours (e.g., performing rituals to avoid 'something bad' happening) that prevent the self-correction of maladaptive beliefs are targeted.

Psychoeducation and cognitive strategies to change dysfunctional core beliefs (e.g., 'I'm worthless') are used in CBT for both OCD and BDD. However, the essential component is exposure and response prevention (Kyrios, Moulding, & Bhar, 2014). During exposure the therapist guides the patient through repeated and prolonged situations that usually provoke obsessional fears (i.e., exposure) without allowing any compulsive or avoidance behaviours (i.e., response prevention). This helps the person to learn that the obsessional situation is not realistically dangerous, and that the anxiety naturally diminishes. Behavioural experiments can be used throughout the exposure sessions to 'test' the obsessional fear: for example, a person with contamination fear can test whether they get 'seriously sick' when they eat a cookie after they have touched a 'dirty' money note. CBT for OCD can be disseminated effectively in face-to-face individual and group settings, as well as online or digital modalities (Kyrios, Ahern, et al., 2018).

Similar strategies are used in CBT for BDD (Wilhelm, Phillips, & Steketee, 2012): patients practice exposure to the social situations that they would usually avoid due to their perceived appearance defect without performing the usual rituals (e.g., repetitive mirror checking) or avoidance behaviours (e.g., actively avoiding seeing their own reflection in mirror).

Psychoeducation is also an essential part of CBT for hypochondriasis or health anxiety (e.g., explaining that some somatic sensations that worry the person are normal aspects of bodily functions). The behavioural exposure-based component of CBT targets maladaptive behaviours (i.e., excessively checking oneself for signs of illness or seeking reassurance from doctors) whereas cognitive strategies address dysfunctional beliefs about health and selective attention to information.

Ideally treating HD involves a multimodal, psychosocial intervention team including mental health professional trained in CBT for hoarding as well as community service workers (e.g., council or housing board) who can help to maintain the health and safety of the person. The cognitive behavioural based treatment consists of the following components:

- motivational interviewing to address ambivalence about therapy
- psychoeducation
- skills training in organising, decision making, and problem solving
- strategies to stop excessive acquisition (e.g., go to flea market without buying anything)
- exposure to not acquiring, sorting and discarding possessions
- cognitive strategies to challenge erroneous thinking (e.g., How many items do you really need of this?)

Cognitive remediation techniques can be used to improve neuropsychological functioning and

Figure 4.5 Overview of the management of anxiety disorders

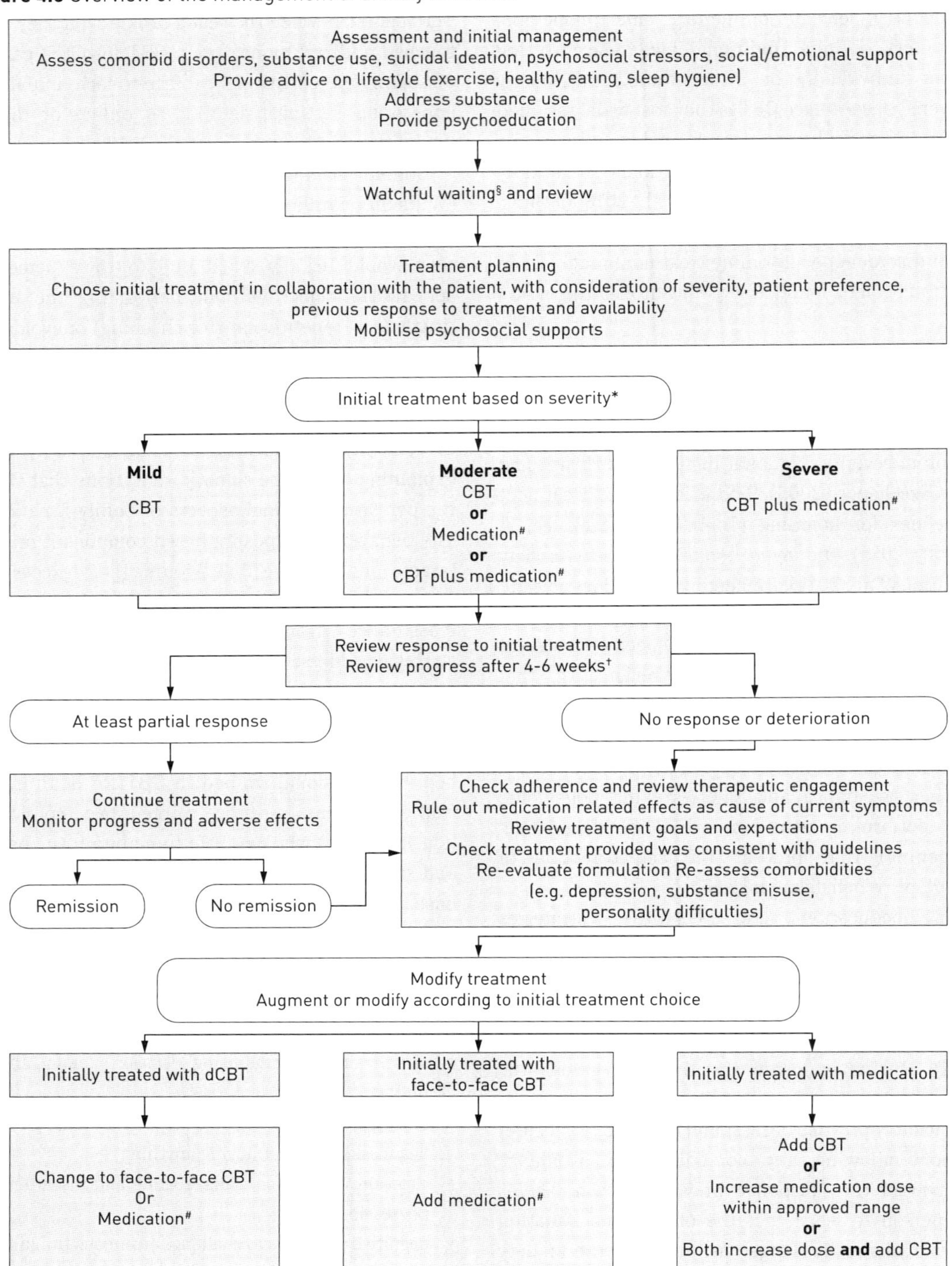

Source: Adapted from Andrews, Bell, et al., 2018

information processing deficits in people with hoarding difficulties through repeated task practice for example in attention, categorisation, or memory. There is some limited evidence that mutual support counselling groups such as the 'Buried in Treasures Workshop' which is a peer-led group treatment consisting of 15 sessions spread over 20 weeks facilitated by a nonprofessional (who may have, or have had HD) leads to symptom reductions in people with hoarding difficulties (Frost, Ruby, & Shuer, 2012).

DISORDERS SPECIFICALLY ASSOCIATED WITH STRESS

In the early aftermath of a traumatic event, routine psychological debriefing is not recommended. The best approach to helping people following a potentially traumatic experience is to offer practical and emotional support and encourage the use of helpful coping strategies and social supports. The goal here is to enhance the person's natural resilience and coping ability in the face of trauma.

Not everyone who experiences a traumatic event will develop a diagnosable disorder. Many people will experience only subthreshold symptoms and others will not experience significant symptomatology at all. A stepped care service model may be helpful to ensure that people receive care according to their need. The approach involves ongoing monitoring of people who are more distressed and/or at heightened risk of poor psychological adjustment, with increasingly intensive interventions delivered as indicated.

According to the Australian Guidelines for the Treatment of PTSD and ASD (Phoenix Australia, 2013), adults with PTSD should be offered trauma-focused psychological interventions, trauma-focused cognitive behavioural therapy (TF-CBT) or eye movement desensitisation and reprocessing (EMDR).

TF-CBT is a short-term, structured psychological intervention that aims to address the emotional, cognitive and behavioural sequelae of exposure to traumatic events (Phoenix Australia, 2013). Although it often includes additional interventions such as psychoeducation and symptom management strategies (notably arousal reduction), the two core interventions are:

- Exposure therapy–which involves confronting the memory of traumatic experiences in a controlled and safe environment (imaginal exposure), as well as confronting trauma-related avoided situations and activities through *in vivo* exposure
- Cognitive therapy–which helps the individual to identify, challenge and modify any biased or distorted thoughts and memories of their traumatic experience, as well as any subsequent maladaptive or unhelpful beliefs about themselves and the world that they may have developed.

Cognitive processing therapy (CPT) is a form of cognitive therapy developed specifically for the treatment of PTSD (Resick, Monson, & Chard, 2017). It helps the person to identify unhelpful thoughts and beliefs ('stuck points'), challenge them, and replace them with rational alternatives in an adaptation of standard cognitive therapy approaches. It has a smaller exposure component than traditional exposure therapy (restricted to writing an account of the experience) and is therefore potentially more acceptable to patients or practitioners seeking alternatives to purely exposure-focused treatments.

Eye Movement Desensitisation and Reprocessing (EMDR) therapy was initially developed in 1987 for the treatment of PTSD and is guided by the Adaptive Information Processing model (Shapiro, 2007). EMDR is based on the assumption that, during a traumatic event, overwhelming emotions or dissociative processes may interfere with information processing. This leads to the experience being stored in an 'unprocessed' way, disconnected from existing memory networks. In EMDR the person is asked to focus on trauma-related imagery, negative thoughts, emotions, and body sensations while simultaneously moving their eyes back and forth following the movement of the therapist's fingers across their field of vision for 20–30 seconds or more. This process may be repeated many times. Over time, EMDR has increasingly included more treatment components that are comparable with cognitive behavioural therapy (CBT) interventions including cognitive interweaving (analogous to cognitive therapy), imaginal templating (rehearsal of mastery or coping responses to anticipated stressors), and standard in vivo exposure.

In complex PTSD, more integrated approaches are needed to include emotion regulation and interpersonal functioning strategies, as well as treatment for traumatic memories (Ingenhoven, 2015). Due to the added impact on identity, treatment for complex trauma tends to focus more on adjusting underlying belief mechanisms and developing new coping responses. Especially when childhood sexual or physical abuse involved attachment figures, and when emotional support was lacking, the impact on personality development is such that other treatment efforts are necessary to establish a trustful therapeutic relation prior to starting active therapy. Dialectical Behaviour Therapy (DBT; Heard & Linehan, 1994) and Schema Focused Therapy (SFT; Young, Klosko, & Weishaar, 2003) are widely used in treating people with complex PTSD.

In DBT, as soon as the patient is stabilised, cognitive behavioural approaches such as imaginal exposure will be introduced. In the mid-phase of treatment, the theme of abuse will be activated. Identification with both victim and perpetrator is elaborated, and sexual and aggressive impulses should be disentangled, with the purpose of resolving inner conflicts, fostering identity integration, and enhancing adaptive functioning. Similarly, in SFT, the first phase of treatment involves identifying maladaptive schemas and building up adaptive capacities. SFT uses specific strategies drawn from Gestalt Therapy for treating traumatic experiences, such as chair work to challenge and modify internalised negative voices; and imagery-based rescripting in which the person recounts the traumatic memory, and then confronts the perpetrator of the abuse within the memory, gains control over the traumatic situation, and comforts and provides support to their younger self.

PHARMACOLOGICAL TREATMENTS

Anxiety and fear-related disorders

Pharmacological treatments for anxiety disorders have advantages in terms of cost and ease of access, as these can be prescribed by a general practitioner. However, pharmacotherapy should always be accompanied by psychoeducation about anxiety and instructions for graded exposure (Andrews, Bell, et al., 2018).

Antidepressants

Antidepressants are effective for anxiety disorders, in particular, selective serotonin reuptake inhibitors (SSRIs) or serotonin and noradrenaline reuptake inhibitors (SNRIs), which are the recommended first-line medications (Andrews, Bell, et al., 2018). Tricyclic antidepressants (TCAs) and monoamine oxidase inhibitors (MAOIs) can be useful where first-line treatments have not been successful, though these medications are not recommended in the first instance due to adverse effects and danger in overdose (Ravindran & Stein, 2010). Adjunctive therapy with anticonvulsants or atypical antipsychotics may also be considered for those who have not responded to first-line treatment (Ravindran & Stein, 2010).

Benzodiazepines

Benzodiazepines are no longer recommended as a first-line treatment for anxiety disorders due to the risks associated with long-term use, particularly dependence (Andrews, Bell, et al., 2018; National Institute for Health and Care Excellence (NICE), 2014). Furthermore, in clinical settings, it is well recognised that benzodiazepines can perpetuate anxiety disorders through their use as a safety behaviour. They can interfere with recovery by undermining the person's ability to cope and learn that anxiety can be tolerated (e.g., 'I was only able to get on the bus because I knew I had diazepam in my pocket'), and may impair fear extinction (Hart, Panayi, Harris, & Westbrook, 2014; Westra, Stewart, & Conrad, 2002). This may be particularly true for panic disorder, where physiological anxiety sensations themselves are the feared stimuli–the exposure to which is avoided through the use of benzodiazepines. These medications should therefore only be used on a short-term basis (2-4 weeks) for acute anxiety, as an adjunct to first-line treatments such as in the initiation phase of an SSRI or SNRI (Ravindran & Stein, 2010).

OBSESSIVE-COMPULSIVE OR RELATED DISORDERS

Not many studies have directly compared psychotherapy vs. pharmacotherapy for OCD; one RCT suggests that 12-week exposure and response prevention was superior compared to a tricyclic antidepressant (i.e., 200 to 250 mg/day of clomipramine) for non-comorbid OCD (Foa et al., 2005). For BDD, hypochondriasis or HD, no RCTs have directly compared CBT to pharmacotherapy. Thus, the presented evidence for pharmacological treatments should be considered as an augmentation strategy for psychotherapies such as CBT, or as a monotherapy if this is the patient's explicit preference or access to evidence-based psychotherapies is not available. For all obsessive-compulsive or related conditions discussed here selective serotonin reuptake inhibitor (SSRI) antidepressants have the strongest evidence in alleviating symptoms.

For OCD, meta-analyses of SSRIs (e.g., fluoxetine) and tricyclic antidepressant (e.g., clomipramine) compared to placebo suggests that they are efficacious (Ackerman & Greenland, 2002; Soomro, Altman, Rajagopal, & Oakley Browne, 2008); however, no individual medication was found to be more efficacious. Serotonin-norepinephrine reuptake inhibitors (SNRIs) have a similar mechanism of action as SSRIs, but research on their use for OCD is limited. Generally, the use of these medications as stand-alone intervention led to 20–40% reduction in OCD symptoms (e.g., Pigott & Seay, 1999), thus offering amelioration rather than full elimination of symptoms.

For BDD the first-line treatment is CBT, and for severe and treatment resistant cases, this is often augmented with medication. A recent systematic review reports that both SSRIs and SNRIS (i.e., fluoxetine, desipramine) as well as clomipramine were effective in reducing BDD symptoms compared to a placebo (Phillipou, Rossell, Wilding, & Castle, 2016). Similarly, in hypochondriasis, where the recommended first-line treatment is CBT, antidepressant medication can be used for augmentation or if other interventions are not available. For HD, only uncontrolled studies of pharmacotherapy have been conducted: a recent meta-analysis reports preliminary evidence for the efficacy of SSRIs (e.g., venlafaxine) in reducing hoarding symptoms (Brakoulias, Eslick, & Starcevic, 2015).

DISORDERS SPECIFICALLY ASSOCIATED WITH STRESS

Medication should not be used as a routine first-line treatment in preference to trauma-focused psychological therapy. Where medication is considered for the treatment of PTSD in adults, selective serotonin reuptake inhibitor (SSRI) antidepressants should be considered the first choice for practitioners (Phoenix Australia, 2013).

TREATMENT CHALLENGES FOR MENTAL HEALTH WORKERS

Facing your fears can be very challenging and unpleasant; thus, it is not surprising that people seeking help are often reluctant to engage in exposure therapy and might drop out from treatment—especially in online settings. As it is imperative that consumers engage effectively with the rationale of the exposure-based approach, any ambivalence experienced by the consumer needs to be understood, normalised and accepted.

One of the major treatment challenges for mental health professionals using PTSD is the reluctance of the person to access the traumatic memory for fear of reliving the event and being retraumatised. It is essential that time is taken to develop and establish trust, before working on the trauma, and that the person be provided with arousal management and coping strategies to assist them to cope with the increased distress caused by accessing the memories in the short-term.

In addition, it is important for the person to feel safe, and stable before engaging in active trauma-based intervention. If a person remains in a threatening environment, for example, in the case of domestic violence, then it will be difficult for them to feel safe enough to focus on their traumatic memories.

TREATMENT CHALLENGES FOR CONSUMERS

Navigating the mental health care system can be challenging. Mental health professionals are often not available for people seeking help for their anxiety or obsessive-compulsive symptoms. Living in remote rural areas or not having the financial means to pay for private treatment sessions can be serious obstacles to successful treatment. Even in larger cities it can be difficult to find appropriate treatment for conditions like BDD, hoarding or complex PTSD, as trained experts are often not available or have long waiting lists. Stigma is also a serious barrier to help-seeking and often continues during treatment. Exposure to anxiety-provoking stimuli or situations can be daunting; disclosure of trauma very difficult, especially if the health service is not trauma-informed.

GOOD PRACTICE EXAMPLES

Exposure therapy

Adequate preparation for exposure is an essential component of good practice (see, Kyrios, 2003). Preparation helps establish a safe environment where exposure therapy can be conducted systematically and with a sense of security and trust. Prior to undertaking exposure work, clients should be provided with appropriate arousal reduction and grounding strategies to enable them to regulate their arousal between sessions, as well as appropriate education about the process of treatment. Appropriate time should be spent developing a hierarchy of fears collaboratively, involving a thorough exploration of feared stimuli to ensure each step on the hierarchy is meaningful to the client. It is important to remain flexible, as the hierarchy may need to be adjusted following initial exposure tasks.

Mental health professionals should help clients identify subtle forms of avoidance that may undermine the effectiveness of therapy, such as rushing through exposure tasks or using distraction to avoid feelings of anxiety during a task. Mindfulness techniques (e.g., 'Can you describe how you feel at the moment?'; 'What is that anxiety like in your body?') can be employed to help the person engage fully with feared stimuli. However, overly focusing on feared stimuli should be done with caution as it may excessively increase distress.

Allowing adequate time to debrief at the conclusion of sessions that involve exposure tasks is crucial. This allows the person to reflect on their coping skills and strengths, and for the therapist to shape attributions of progress (i.e., helping the client attribute successful exposure to themselves rather than medication or the therapist, problem solve barriers to make the next attempt more successful). If possible, within the constraints of the service, it is desirable to plan longer sessions (1.5 hours) for exposure.

Working with trauma

As with other disorders, treatment choice when treating PTSD is influenced by the nature of the trauma being treated, for example: single event versus multiple events; interpersonal trauma versus more general trauma; the client's personality and preference; and, clinician expertise.

It is important to provide the client with appropriate psychological education about the treatment options, so that they can make informed decisions about which approach best suits their goals. Exposure therapy for PTSD aims to reduce the emotional impact of the traumatic memory, while also often providing more clarity and 'filling in' some of the gaps in the memory through the accessing of new or blocked information. EMDR by comparison, changes how the brain processes, the memory, and may cause aspects of the memory to be lost or changed. Some clients may wish to be able to recall the incident with more clarity but less distress; while others may wish to change their recollection of the memory.

For exposure therapy, when conducting treatment sessions focusing on accessing the traumatic memory itself, as opposed to providing education or arousal reduction strategies, it is usual to schedule longer sessions. This is especially important when working with trauma as it provides enough time for grounding, debriefing and processing after the active memory work.

KEY RISKS OF HARM IN TREATMENT ATTEMPTS

Over the last decades the empirical evidence has shown that psychological interventions have beneficial effects and should be included in health care systems; however, psychotherapy can be associated with inadequate responses and can also have harmful effects. Unfortunately, the study of adverse or side effects of psychotherapy is still limited, as these effects are hard to recognise and difficult to study (Barlow, 2010). In comparison to side effects of psychopharmacological medication, adverse outcomes in psychotherapy are often iatrogenic as they are directly related to the therapist's actions (e.g., inappropriate treatment planning and preparation, inadvertent reinforcement of maladaptive habits).

In other instances, it can be difficult to distinguish a harmful effect caused by the psychological treatment or the interaction with the therapist from an unavoidable deterioration (e.g., caused through a negative life event). Studying negative outcomes of psychotherapy seems crucial in order to further improve psychological treatments; focusing on individual clients' experiences rather than on the aggregated average improvement in randomised controlled trials is needed.

The side effects of psychopharmacological medications are generally well-described. For example common side effects of SSRIs include sexual dysfunction, drowsiness, weight gain, insomnia, anxiety, dizziness, headache, and dry mouth (Schatzberg & Nemeroff, 2017). As noted in the section on pharmacological treatments above, benzodiazepines carry risks of both physiological and psychological dependence and may in fact prolong anxiety disorders if used alone.

PRACTICE ILLUSTRATION: OUTCOME AND TREATMENT OVER TIME

After terminating the treatment, Ann was able to incorporate many of the techniques she had learnt during therapy (e.g., how to relax when she feels anxious and distressed, how to focus on small goals and to celebrate the little successes, how to use self-monitoring of intrusions and worries, how to use cognitive reappraisals to manage her fears). She graduated from university and started working in a small company. Ann continues to experience anxiety, particularly if she is in unfamiliar situations, but she feels more able to manage the worries. Recently, she started going to a support group for people with anxiety to share her own experience and help others on their way to recovery.

4.4.8 WHERE AND HOW DO PEOPLE GET HELP FOR ANXIETY, OBSESSIVE-COMPULSIVE AND STRESS-RELATED DISORDERS?

DANIEL FASSNACHT, ERIN PARKER, MIKE BARRY, MICHELLE BANFIELD & MICHAEL KYRIOS

Anxiety-related disorders, like other mental illnesses, are managed predominantly within primary care (Burgess et al., 2009). General practitioners (GPs) are often the first professional a consumer may see about their mental health (Australian Bureau of Statistics, 2007; Australian Institute of Health and Welfare, 2017). GPs can serve as the primary treating professional or provide referrals to mental health professionals in secondary care services (e.g., private psychologists, public mental health services). There are federal and state-based mental health organisations which provide educational material about, and contact details of health professionals with the conditions discussed in this chapter; some of these also offer mutual or peer-to-peer support. Below is a non-exhaustive list:

- WayAhead (WayAhead, 2016) is funded by the Mental Health Commission of NSW and offers support groups mainly in the metropolitan area of Sydney.

- Anxiety Disorders Association of Victoria (ADAVIC, 2014) is a not-for-profit, self-funded organisation holding support group meetings in Melbourne.
- Anxiety Recovery Centre (ARCVIC, 2020) is a state-wide, specialist mental health organisation offering support groups for anxiety disorders and OCD, hoarding, etc.
- Phoenix Australia (Phoenix Australia, 2019) at the University of Melbourne is the Australian Centre of Excellence for Research and Treatment of Posttraumatic Mental Health.
- The Traumatic Stress Clinic (Traumatic Stress Clinic, 2020) in Sydney provides evidence-based treatments and undertakes research for PTSD and prolonged grief.
- Open Arms Veterans and Veterans Families Counselling (Open Arms, 2020) provides support for current and ex-serving Australian Defence Force personnel and their families.
- 1800Respect—National sexual assault, domestic family violence counselling service (1800Respect, 2020) provides support to people impacted by sexual assault, domestic or family violence and abuse.

There are evidence-based online programs available for the treatment of GAD, SAD, panic, OCD and PTSD:

- Mental Health Online provides free of charge 12-weeks online treatment for GAD, SAD, panic disorder, OCD and PTSD (Mental Health Online, 2020). It is an initiative of Swinburne University's National eTherapy Centre (NeTC) funded by the Federal Department of Health.
- The eCentre Clinic is a not-for-profit initiative of Macquarie University and offers free online courses for OCD and PTSD (eCentre Clinic, 2019). Their courses can also be accessed via (MindSpot, 2020).
- The online self-help program moodgym, which was developed at the Australian National University, helps to manage symptoms of depression and anxiety (moodgym, 2020).

4.4.9 DISSOCIATIVE DISORDERS

DAVID CLARKE

WHAT IS THIS GROUP OF MENTAL HEALTH EXPERIENCES LIKE?

The language of dissociative disorders is unusual in psychiatric nosology because it is both descriptive of the observed mental phenomena *and* of the presumed mechanism. Diagnostic nomenclature in psychiatry is mostly the former. So for instance, dissociative amnesia is immediately distinguished from an amnestic syndrome caused by organic brain disease.

Dissociative disorders involve the splitting off from consciousness of some mental or neurological function, which therefore leads to a loss of integration of these elements—in a sense, a breaking up of the integrity of the person or of the experience of being a person.

To understand this, we may consider what it means to be conscious and human; how do we know who we are, where we are, and what we are doing? How do we know what we value and what we believe? How do we plan for the future? First, we need to be awake, or conscious; second we need to be receiving stimuli from the environment and from our body (perception); third we need to be integrating and interpreting all of this information, 'making sense' of it; and fourth, we need to be able to remember it all. Our sense of who we are is not just about present experience but importantly about the continuity of experiences over time. All of this we put together into a coherent story, and on the basis of our integration of all these elements we have a sense of who we are in the world—we make decisions, imagine and plan a future, and have a sense of agency. From this we develop our sense of identity and self-esteem, as shown in Figure 4.6.

Each of these four components of mental function can be disturbed by psychiatric illness; for instance, a psychotic illness like schizophrenia causes hallucinations or thought disorder, an organic

Figure 4.6 Developing a sense of self

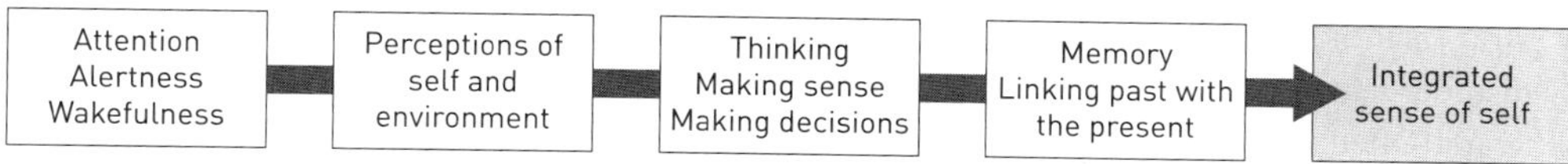

brain disease such as Alzheimer's disease causes loss of memory, or of time or spatial awareness. And of course drugs can cause impairment in any of these areas. Dissociative disorders describe a loss of these functions in the absence of any of these 'biogenic' explanations, and are understood to be 'psychogenic'—that is, directly a result of stress or psychological insult.

Dissociation is of course an everyday experience, as when we 'daydream', or we unthinkingly drive the car a familiar route rather than the correct route. It is not possible to be aware of everything that is happening all the time, or to remember everything; we are distracted, and often work on 'automatic pilot'. Dissociation is more common when we are stressed or our mind is overloaded. Dissociative symptoms also occur commonly with other psychiatric disorders, such as post-traumatic stress disorder, anxiety disorders and some personality disorders. Normal everyday dissociation is transient and can be interrupted; dissociative disorders are strong and persistent, and usually distressing.

Historical development of the concept

The concept of dissociation (the splitting off of mental functions) was developed late in the nineteenth century when a group of French neurologists began studying the phenomena of 'hysteria' (Meares, Hampshire, Gordon, & Kraiuhin, 1985). Paul Briquet studied and described several hundred patients with multiple chronic somatic symptoms. Jean-Martin Charcot, another prominent physician, experimented with hypnosis as a cure for hysteria. Both Sigmund Freud and Pierre Janet studied with Charcot and went on to make significant contributions in this area. When Freud returned from Paris to Vienna he worked with the physician Joseph Breuer to write what became a classic account of hysteria (Breuer & Freud, 1893-1895/1955). They described a patient known as Anna O, who had an illness involving multiple somatic symptoms as well as dissociation. She had weakness and gait disturbance, visual disturbance, sensory disturbance, mood shifts and alterations of consciousness. It was as if she had 'two entirely distinct states of consciousness' they said (Breuer & Freud, 1893-1895/1955, p. 24). This publication contained the first use of the concept of conversion 'to signify the transformation of psychical (mental) excitation into chronic somatic symptoms'; and it was also the first report of the 'talking cure'; (Breuer & Freud, 1893-1895/1955, p. 86).

This period of history is important because it was when the main theories of trauma and dissociation developed. Janet studied patients with multiple unexplained physical symptoms and came to see them as being representations of past trauma (Janet, 1889), an idea that continues to have validity in the current day—'the body keeps the score' (vanderKolk et al., 1996). Freud, similarly, came to the conclusion that hysteria was caused by negative early life sexual experiences, where memory of the events had been repressed (dissociated or cut off from consciousness), such that cure would come by transforming these unconscious memories into conscious ones (Freud, 1896/1962). However, Freud fairly quickly withdrew from this idea, instead proposing that symptoms of hysteria were caused by the repression of unacceptable sexual fantasies from childhood, rather than of actual sexual abuse. This switch laid the groundwork for the 'memory wars' (Crews, 1997) that have persisted since in regard to recovered memories, in which there has been vigorous debate about whether the recollection of previously unremembered traumatic events by patients in therapy should be accepted as necessarily fact.

Phenomenology

People experiencing these dissociative conditions may present directly seeking treatment, although frequently they do not. Commonly, dissociative symptoms present in the course of other considerations: dissociative neurological symptoms often after investigations by a neurologist have proven negative; depersonalisation-derealisation phenomena may be part of another anxiety disorder; dissociative identity disorder may reveal itself during a course of psychotherapy. Often they are slow to be recognised for what they are, by both the one experiencing them and clinicians. For instance, what does a therapist make of the patient who pulls her legs up and sits quietly in the chair in a foetal position. Is she being thoughtful, a little bit anxious and fearful, wanting comfort; or could she be dissociating. Dissociative phenomena generally, that is altered conscious states, gaps in memory etc, can of course be caused also by alcohol or other drugs and by organic brain disease.

As described above, dissociative disorders involve the splitting off from consciousness of some important mental or neurological function. Hence, the core phenomena for each disorder are specific to that component of mental function.

Table 4.21 Functions split off from consciousness for each dissociative disorder

Depersonalisation-derealisation disorder	Impaired consciousness or awareness affecting the perception of self (being strange or unreal) and/or the environment (being strange or unreal).
Psychogenic amnesia	Loss of memory. Not just patchy memory, but usually whole blocks of events.
Dissociative neurological symptom disorder	Loss of sensory (numbness of skin to touch, prick or pain; blindness) or motor function.
Dissociative Identity disorder	A global dissociation leading to a sense of being a different person, perhaps in a different place or a different time.

Depersonalisation-derealisation disorder (6B66)

The core feature of depersonalisation is the altered perception of the self–as being different to usual, strange or unreal. Patients describe it sometimes as being not fully alert or engaged; more like being an outsider watching what is going on but not being involved.

The core feature of derealisation is an altered perception of the environment–as being strange or unreal, different from usual. Patients will describe the environment as if the life and colour has gone out of it, moving slowly, lifeless.

The two aspects of depersonalisation and derealisation often, but not always, go together, and the descriptions patients give are often not detailed–in fact, the detail of the environment is often lost. It is more often a general sense that things are different.

ICD-11 criteria for depersonalisation-derealisation disorder (6B66)

Characterised by:

- Persistent or recurrent experiences of depersonalisation, derealisation, or both.

Depersonalisation is characterised by:

- Experiencing the self as strange or unreal, or feeling detached from, or as though one were an outside observer of one's thoughts, feelings, sensations, body, or actions

Derealisation is characterised by:

- Experiencing other persons, objects, or the world as strange or unreal (e.g., dreamlike, distant, foggy, lifeless, colourless, or visually distorted) or feeling detached from one's surroundings.

During experiences of depersonalisation or derealisation, reality testing remains intact.

Experiences of depersonalisation or derealisation do not occur exclusively during another dissociative disorder and are not better explained by another mental, behavioural or neurodevelopmental disorder.

Experiences of depersonalisation or derealisation are not due to the direct effects of a substance or medication on the central nervous system, including withdrawal effects, and are not due to a disease of the nervous system or to head trauma.

Symptoms result in significant distress or impairment in personal, family, social, educational, occupational or other important areas of functioning.

Dissociative amnesia (6B61)

The core feature of dissociative amnesia is the loss of memory of events. This is not just a patchy loss of memory but a loss of a whole block of memory of a specific event (autobiographical or episodic or declarative memory). Loss of blocks of memory can also be caused by acute drug or alcohol intoxication—as when someone has a 'blackout' of events of the night before when they were intoxicated. Amnesia can also be consciously feigned for secondary gain purposes.

ICD-11 criteria for dissociative amnesia (6B61)

Characterised by:

- Inability to recall important autobiographical memories, typically of recent traumatic or stressful events that is inconsistent with ordinary forgetting.
- Amnesia does not occur exclusively during another dissociative disorder and is not better explained by another mental, behavioural or neurodevelopmental disorder.
- Amnesia is not due to the direct effects of a substance or medication on the central nervous system, including withdrawal effects, and is not due to a disease of the nervous system or to head trauma.
- Amnesia results in significant impairment in personal, family, social, educational, occupational or other important areas of functioning.

Dissociative neurological symptom disorder (6B60)

Dissociative neurological symptom disorder describes what has previously been called conversion disorder. It presents as an apparent impairment of neurological functioning (e.g. with paralysis or sensory deficit) but where no objective neurological deficit can be found. Examples include blindness, paralysis of a limb, inability to speak, difficulty swallowing ('globus hystericus'), unusual chorieform motor movements, facial spasms, and non-epileptic seizures.

Usually these cases are sent to mental health professionals only after a long history of medical investigation and intervention and despite having had normal test results. Unfortunately, the often obsessional string of investigations serves only to confirm for the patient that there is a physical cause to their malady—'why else would the doctors have done all the tests?' Strong illness anxiety, belief and conviction often accompany dissociative neurological disorders.

Dissociative neurological disorders are considered to be acute events. Sometimes of course they persist, and then they become part of a chronic form of somatisation. Dissociative neurological symptom disorders are therefore closely related to somatoform disorders (Nijenhuis, 2001).

ICD-11 Criteria for Dissociative Neurological Symptom Disorder (6B60)

Characterised by:

- Presentation of motor, sensory or cognitive symptoms that imply an involuntary discontinuity in the normal integration of motor, sensory or cognitive functions and are not consistent with a recognised disease of the nervous system, other mental or behavioural disorder, or other health condition.
- Symptoms do not occur exclusively during another dissociative disorder and are not due to the effects of a substance or medication on the central nervous system, including withdrawal effects, or a sleep-wake disorder.
- Symptoms result in significant impairment in personal, family, social, educational, occupational or other important areas of functioning.

Dissociative identity disorder (6B64)

Dissociative identity disorder is a severe form of dissociation in which the person appears to have more than one distinct personality. The person may switch between identities, and within each identity not be aware of the other identity. Sometimes the level of differentiation is not as clearcut as this and the person is aware of the different dissociative states.

Persons with dissociative identity disorder also experience the other elements of dissociation. However, instead of splitting off a part of previous memory, or somatic experience, or consciousness, they are splitting off the whole experience—their memory, their emotions, their sensations and their behaviours of a previous time. It is as if they are someone else, or perhaps themselves at a previous time.

ICD-11 Criteria for Dissociative Identity Disorder (6B64)

Characterised by:

- Disruption of identity in which there are two or more distinct personality states (dissociative identities) associated with marked discontinuities in the sense of self and agency.
- Each personality state includes its own pattern of experiencing, perceiving, conceiving, and relating to self, the body, and the environment.
- At least two distinct personality states recurrently take executive control of the individual's consciousness and functioning in interacting with others or with the environment, such as in the performance of specific aspects of daily life such as parenting, or work, or in response to specific situations (e.g., those that are perceived as threatening).
- Changes in personality state are accompanied by related alterations in sensation, perception, affect, cognition, memory, motor control, and behaviour.
- Typically episodes of amnesia, which may be severe.
- Symptoms are not better explained by another mental, behavioural or neurodevelopmental disorder and are not due to the direct effects of a substance or medication on the central nervous system, including withdrawal effects, and are not due to a disease of the nervous system or a sleep-wake disorder.
- Symptoms result in significant impairment in personal, family, social, educational, occupational or other important areas of functioning.

WHAT DO WE KNOW ABOUT THESE DISORDERS?

Prevalence

Discrete dissociative disorders are not commonly identified in clinical practice, and they have not been included in any of the major psychiatric epidemiological studies, so the exact prevalence is not known. Dissociative phenomena, however, are not uncommon. They occur in everyday life; they can be part of the clinical picture with other anxiety disorders and post-traumatic stress disorders; and they can present in people with borderline personality disorder or appear during the therapy of people with past trauma.

Brief experiences of depersonalisation are said to occur in between 25% and 75% of the population (Hunter, Sierra, & David, 2004). The lifetime prevalence of depersonalisation-derealisation, on the other hand, is of the order of 1-2% of the population (Johnson et al., 2006).

The prevalence in the community of dissociative amnesia is also small—around 1-2% (Johnson et al., 2006). However in war veterans and people with histories of child abuse amnesia has been noted in up to about 30% (Sargant & Slater, 1941; Gleaves, Smith, Butler, & Spiegel, 2004).

The prevalence of conversion disorder (the previous descriptor for dissociative neurological symptom disorder) is probably small in the community, but unknown. In general medical settings the prevalence of unexplained medical symptoms is high, around 25% (Kroenke et al., 1994). The specific diagnosis of conversion disorder in neurological clinics is estimated to be about 5% (Feinstein, 2011).

The prevalence of dissociative identity disorder is difficult to quantify because it is a relatively new diagnosis. The book, *The Three Faces of Eve*, was published in 1957, supposedly representing the first reported case (Thigpen & Cleckley, 1957). In 1980, it was estimated that there were approximately 200 cases reported in the literature. In 2011, a study in Turkey found rates of between 0.4% and 3.1% (Şar, 2011). There has been debate in the literature about whether dissociative identity disorder is being over diagnosed or underdiagnosed and this debate will continue for a while.

How can we understand the origins (aetiology)?

The prevailing theory of the aetiology of dissociative disorders is that they are stress-related, and the more severe ones clearly posttraumatic in nature. Cognitive behavioural models provide a framework for how increasing anxiety and dissociation occur (Hunter, Phillips, Chalder, Sierra, & David, 2003). Biological understandings also explain how the stress system affects brain structures leading to impairment of declarative memory and the spatiotemporal context of emotional events.

The most common immediate precipitants of depersonalisation and derealisation are extreme stress, depression, anxiety and substance abuse (Hunter et al., 2003).

Recent literature has focused on the role of the hippocampus in the laying down of memories. Severe stress is thought to be associated with a shutdown of the hippocampus, and high cortisol levels are also observed to be detrimental to the hippocampus (Kim, Pellman, & Kim, 2015). This would explain why the specific declarative memory of a traumatic event may be lost, while the emotional and sensory aspects (non-declarative memory mediated in the amygdala) are preserved.

Dissociative identity disorder seems to be overwhelmingly associated with severe trauma occurring in childhood, with some studies reporting rates of 98% (Gleaves, 1996). Trauma is probably necessary, but not sufficient. Other factors may also contribute. Kluft (1994) identifies a number of other possible contributors to the development of dissociative identity disorder: for instance, whether the person has a biological predisposition to dissociate (similar to hypnotisability); a lack of soothing experiences in childhood that have left the child to develop their own coping mechanisms. In addition, the nature of the alternate identity may be influenced by a variety of personal, social and cultural factors.

Dissociative identity disorder has been a controversial area, and there have been what we might call 'non-trauma' theories of its development (Simone Reinders, Willemsen, Vos, den Boer, & Nijenhuis, 2012). These theories include iatrogenesis—i.e. that dissociative identity disorder is a product of therapy (Merskey, 1992)—and the Fantasy Model, that says people with Dissociative Identity Disorder are highly fantasy-prone (Giesbrecht, Lynn, Lilienfeld, & Merckelbach, 2008) Although there is not substantial evidence for these non-trauma theories, not fully reviewed here, they do highlight some potential difficulties in working therapeutically in this space.

ASSESSMENT

The recognition of dissociation can initially be difficult as patients are not always forthcoming in their descriptions of them. The differential diagnosis of dissociative disorders included PTSD, generalised anxiety disorder, psychosis and borderline personality disorder. The latter group are prone to dissociate under stress because of their lack of integration of mental functions, and their fragile sense of self and self-esteem.

Organic disease must be excluded, and the possibilities of a drug-effect and feigned illness need also to be considered.

Memory disturbance can be hard to assess, unless there is a verifying source, and denial of events or mimicking amnesia are always a possibility.

EVIDENCE-BASED AND OTHER TREATMENTS AND SERVICES

There is very little evidence base for treatments of dissociative disorders, although there is some research and rationale to guide treatment.

In depersonalisation-derealisation disorder a number of medications have been trialled, including: fluoxetine, an SSRI (Simeon, 2004); naltrexone, an opioid antagonist (Simeon & Knutelska, 2005); and lamotrigine, an anti-epileptic drug (Aliyev & Aliyev, 2011). At present the evidence is weak and no medication is recommended as treatment of choice. CBT, on the other hand, has been shown to be as effective as in other anxiety disorders (Hunter, Baker, Phillips, Sierra, & David, 2005).

In dissociative amnesia, where there is complete amnesia, there may be no imperative to treat, although hypnotic or drug-assisted interviews have been used occasionally to uncover repressed memories. When amnesia is partial, usually associated with PTSD, then imaginal exposure to the traumatic event will help to uncover the memory as well as adjust to it emotionally (Barlow & Durand, 2012).

Dissociative neurological symptom disorder is generally understood as an acute disorder precipitated by a stressor. An exploratory interview, or a number of interviews, may start to uncover what is going on that might be related to the symptom formation. From this, an hypothesis or formulation can be developed. This formulation, together with information and education, may be enough to shift the symptoms. Physical therapy (physio-, occupational or speech), relaxation and stress reduction will also assist recovery. Some neurological symptoms persist, reinforced by a strong somatic conviction. The principles of treatment for these are as for other chronic somatising conditions (see Section 4.6.3).

The treatment of Dissociative Identity Disorder is psychotherapy. The first challenge is establishing a safe therapeutic engagement in which the patient can cope with distressing feelings. Following this, traumatic memories will be worked through in a similar way as is used with PTSD—with an important difference being that with Dissociative Identity Disorder the additional emphasis will be on integrating the memories and experiences into the one personality. Treatment guidelines for this have been published (International Society for the Study of Trauma Dissociation, 2011).

4.4.10 THE IMPLICATIONS OF THE DIVERSITY OF AUSTRALIA

DANIEL FASSNACHT, ERIN PARKER, MIKE BARRY, MICHELLE BANFIELD & MICHAEL KYRIOS

Australia's cultural and linguistic diversity including Aboriginal and Torres Strait Islanders and the one in four people who were born overseas (Australian Bureau of Statistics, 2016) requires mental health professionals to be culturally competent: acknowledging that people with a culturally diverse background differ in the way they experience mental health symptoms or look for professional help, is crucial to establishing good rapport and a valuable therapeutic relationship (Gopalkrishnan, 2018). Furthermore, the availability of mental health services varies in different parts of the country and to different populations. For example, rural living is associated with long delays in seeking treatment for anxiety disorders, particularly for those with SAD (28 years on average; Green, Hunt, & Stain, 2012).

There is also a lack of culturally appropriate mental health services for Aboriginal and Torres Strait Islander peoples. Mental health needs in Indigenous communities are significantly higher (Australian Bureau of Statistics, 2014b) with suicide rates twice as high than those of other Australians (Australian Bureau of Statistics, 2016a). Health professionals who work with First Australians need to be conscious of the intergenerational trauma and how this affects their mental health. Other groups who experience significantly poorer mental health are the LGBTIQ communities. LGBTIQ people report that accessing mental health services is challenging (Rosenstreich, 2013) as they are often not inclusive or do not address LGBTIQ specific issues (e.g., the process of coming out). (See Parts 1 and 2 for further background and practice principles for working with diverse populations.)

4.4.11 COMMENTARY AND REFLECTION

DANIEL FASSNACHT, ERIN PARKER, MIKE BARRY, MICHELLE BANFIELD & MICHAEL KYRIOS

Developing and updating the Australian guidelines and resources for practice for the conditions discussed in this chapter is needed. While the Clinical Practice Guidelines for the treatment of anxiety disorders (i.e., panic disorder, SAD and GAD) have been recently updated (Andrews, Bell, et al., 2018), for other conditions they are outdated (i.e., PTSD) or non-existent (i.e., OCD).

More generally, a debate about the usefulness of our current diagnostic systems is needed. While diagnostic frameworks such as the ICD-11 or DSM-5 might be helpful tools to categorise and study mental health conditions, they have major limitations and have been strongly criticised for their lack of validity and the processes of medicalisation (Pickersgill, 2014). However, these systems represent the most utilised information currently available. It has been argued that it is time to be moving from an exclusively categorical taxonomy (i.e., listing a series of criteria for a diagnosis) to a dimensional diagnostic system (i.e., rating symptoms on a quantitative dimension; e.g., severity).

4.5

FEEDING OR EATING DISORDERS

PHILLIPA HAY, STEPHEN TOUY, JUNE ALEXANDER & SALLY MORRIS

4.5.1 WHAT IS THIS GROUP OF MENTAL HEALTH EXPERIENCES LIKE?

LIVED EXPERIENCES

JUNE ALEXANDER

At 11, I became intensely anxious and developed restricting type anorexia nervosa [AN]. Eighteen months later I transitioned to a binge-purge-restrict pattern, gained weight and was considered 'normal'. Traumatic factors adding complexity to my ED included birth trauma, childhood sexual abuse, emotional abuse and road trauma physical injuries at age 20.

At 16, 'I'm depressed' appeared in my diary. Calorie counting was my gear-stick for daily life. I married at 20. I looked okay, was expected to be okay but was moody, self-harming, unable to settle. At 28, fearing madness, I disclosed suicidal thoughts with a GP for the first time.

Misdiagnosis and incorrect treatment ensued. At 32, a psychiatrist diagnosed AN, chronic anxiety and depression. He established trust and provided hope. This psychiatrist saved my life, partly by calming my brain with prescription drugs, allowing time to work through layers of issues, and learn new thinking processes and coping skills. At 47 I learnt the critical concept of identifying and separating illness thoughts from healthy-self thoughts. Until then thoughts confirmed daily I was weak.

The slow and gruelling healing process incurred the loss of both my marriage and family of origin. I believe if PTSD and dissociative symptoms had been noted sooner my health challenges might have been treated more quickly and effectively. No specialist early on inquired about childhood sexual abuse or other traumatic events, which contributed greatly to my anxiety and ED. In my experience, the therapeutic alliance, i.e., the trust between therapist and patient is as important as the treatment itself. Diary-writing has helped to maximise benefits of this trust. Writing about the traumas and discussing this with my treatment team has allowed painful experiences to be revealed, processed and revised to promote self-growth. At 55, my mind and body became reintegrated as one self-loving, loving-life entity.

HISTORICAL DEVELOPMENT OF THE CONCEPT

PHILLIPA HAY

Anorexia nervosa has a long history, with forms being recognised perhaps as early as the seventeenth century. It was in the nineteenth century that Gull (1816–1890) and Lasègue (1816–1883) provided the first convincing accounts of what is known today as 'anorexia nervosa' (Gull, 1874; Lasègue, 1873). Gull proposed the term 'anorexia nervosa' and described it as a syndrome of relentless self-starvation, not due to an organic lesion but rather a 'morbid mental state'. Binge eating on large amounts of foods was also sometimes reported in these early cases. For a period in the first half of the twentieth century, anorexia nervosa was considered to be a form of 'functional hypopitutarism' but a careful review by Sheehan and Summers (1949) showed that the clinical features of anorexia nervosa and hypopitutarism were in fact distinct. This preceded the revival of interest in anorexia nervosa as a psychiatric disorder, and the major contribution of Hilda Bruch. She synthesised analytic and descriptive approaches, and distinguished the disorder from anorexic syndromes secondary to other disorders (Bruch, 1962; Bruch, 1974). Diagnostic criteria used in this period were, however, loosely defined, and the term anorexia nervosa tended to be used to embrace all forms of weight loss not attributable to an organic aetiology until the landmark criteria proposed by Gerald Russell in 1970 that influenced subsequently both DSM and ICD diagnostic schemes (Russell, 1970).

'Bulimia' is derived from two Greek words, *'bous'* ('an ox') and *'limos'* ('hunger'). In the nineteenth century, clinical descriptions of *'boulimie'* or 'bulimia' appeared where food was a major preoccupation, and enormous quantities were consumed (Habermas, 1989) and at the end of the nineteenth century references to bulimia appeared in textbooks. Bulimia nervosa, however, is a twentieth-century disorder with the first case report of a syndrome of uncontrolled overeating associated with vomiting and laxative misuse, namely Binswanger's account of 'The Case of Ellen West' in 1944 (Binswanger, 1958). This was followed with accounts of binge eating followed by vomiting in college women termed 'bulimarexia' (Boskind-Lodahl, 1976). Then in 1979 Russell published a further landmark paper titled *'Bulimia nervosa: An ominous variant of anorexia nervosa'*, and this also influenced the criteria adopted for bulimia nervosa in the 1987 revision of the DSM and the 10th revision of the International Classification of Disease (ICD) scheme (Russell, 1979).

Binge eating was first described in the context of a failure of satiety associated with weight disorders and 'night-eating' by Stunkard and colleagues in the early 1950s. Patients described an overwhelming difficulty in stopping eating, but not hunger and would not necessarily search out food if it was not available. Stunkard (1959) termed the uncontrolled overeating of large amounts of food 'binge eating' based on its similarity to alcoholic binges. The introduction and definition of the term binge eating contributed to the development of diagnostic criteria for the broadly defined bulimia in the 1980 DSM-III and were later incorporated in the proposed binge eating disorder in the 1994 DSM-IV. It was not until 2013 that binge eating disorder (BED) reached full status in the DSM-5 scheme (American Psychiatric Association, 2013) and 2019 in the ICD-11 revisions (World Health Organization, 2019d) scheme.

Feeding disorders were first included with eating disorders in the DSM-5 (American Psychiatric Association, 2013). These included Avoidant/Restrictive Food Intake Disorder (ARFID) and disorders of childhood feeding such as pica (see Section 1.2.4). ARFID had been recognised in the earlier WHO ICD-10 scheme as a nonspecific category of 'feeding disorder of infancy or early childhood'. However, the DSM-5 and ICD-11 ARFID diagnosis significantly expanded the defining features to include cases across the lifespan where the food restriction or avoidance is not motivated by disturbance in body image or significant concerns with weight and shape as in anorexia nervosa or bulimia nervosa.

PHENOMENOLOGY

Anorexia nervosa in essence is a disorder of self-maintained starvation and severe weight loss associated with body image concerns, and extreme fear of weight gain leading to behaviours such as compulsive exercise or vomiting after meals. The fear of weight gain may be overt or covert, that is, is elicited only when re-feeding is commenced. In addition many, but not all, with anorexia nervosa, have body image distortion: an insistence that they are normal or overweight in spite of evidence to the contrary. Although the name 'anorexia' implies loss of appetite, this is not actually the case, and people may use strategies such as excessive water drinking to help suppress hunger.

Bulimia nervosa is characterised by recurrent episodes of binge eating (uncontrolled eating of excessive or unusually large quantities of food), extreme weight and shape concerns and compensatory behaviours, such as self-induced vomiting or laxative misuse (purging form), or fasting or excessive exercise (non-purging form). Patients with bulimia nervosa are of normal or above normal weight by definition. If underweight, the diagnosis is of anorexia nervosa binge eating or purging subtype. As for anorexia nervosa, people have an over-evaluation of weight and/or shape to their self-view.

BED is also characterised by recurrent binge eating in the absence of regular extreme weight control behaviours. People often have high body weight, but equally can be of normal weight. Binge eating diagnoses have quality specifiers such as marked distress and a range of emotions including guilt and disgust that are often experienced following binge eating.

The fourth main disorder is ARFID which is characterised by food restriction and/or avoidance which has notable physical or mental health consequence(s) and is not driven by body image concern or weight/shape over-evaluation. The remainder of eating disorders comprises people whose (a) symptom severity excludes them from a diagnosis of bulimia nervosa, anorexia nervosa or BED; for example, they fail to meet the frequency requirement for binge eating episodes; or (b) a range of disorders characterised by extreme weight control methods (World Health Organization, 2019d).

FORMAL DIAGNOSIS

Box 4.3: ICD-11 descriptors

Anorexia nervosa 6B80

Anorexia nervosa is characterised by significantly low body weight for the individual's height, age and developmental stage (body mass index [BMI] less than 18.5 kg/m2 in adults and BMI-for-age under fifth percentile in children and adolescents) that is not due to another health condition or to the unavailability of food. Low body weight is accompanied by a persistent pattern of behaviours to prevent restoration of normal weight, which may include behaviours aimed at reducing energy intake (restricted eating), purging behaviours (e.g., self-induced vomiting, misuse of laxatives), and behaviours aimed at increasing energy expenditure (e.g., excessive exercise), typically associated with a fear of weight gain. Low body weight or shape is central to the person's self-evaluation or is inaccurately perceived to be normal or even excessive.

Bulimia nervosa 6B81

Bulimia nervosa is characterised by frequent, recurrent episodes of binge eating (e.g., once a week or more over a period of at least one month). A binge eating episode is a distinct period of time during which the individual experiences a subjective loss of control over eating, eating notably more or differently fro, usual, and feels unable to stop eating or limit the type or amount of food eaten. Binge eating is accompanied by repeated inappropriate compensatory behaviours aimed at preventing weight gain (e.g., self-induced vomiting, misuse of laxatives or enemas, strenuous exercise). The individual is preoccupied with body shape or weight, which strongly influences self-evaluation. The individual is not significantly underweight and therefore does not meet the diagnostic requirements of anorexia nervosa.

Binge eating disorder (BED) 6B82

Binge eating disorder is characterised by frequent, recurrent episodes of binge eating (e.g., once a week or more over a period of several months). A binge eating episode is a distinct period of time during which the individual experiences a subjective loss of control over eating, eating notably more or differently from usual, and feels unable to stop eating or limit the type or amount of food eaten. Binge eating is experienced as very distressing, and is often accompanied by negative emotions such as guilt or disgust. However, unlike in bulimia nervosa, binge eating episodes are not regularly followed by inappropriate compensatory behaviours aimed at preventing weight gain (e.g., self-induced vomiting, misuse of laxatives or enemas, strenuous exercise).

Avoidant/restrictive food intake disorder (ARFID) 6B83

Avoidant-restrictive food intake disorder (ARFID) is characterised by abnormal eating or feeding behaviours that result in the intake of an insufficient quantity or variety of food to meet adequate energy or nutritional requirements. The pattern of restricted eating has caused significant weight loss, failure to gain weight as expected in childhood or pregnancy, clinically significant nutritional deficiencies, dependence on oral nutritional supplements or tube feeding, or has otherwise negatively affected the health of the individual or resulted in significant functional impairment. The pattern of eating behaviour does not reflect concerns about body weight or shape. Restricted food intake and its effects on weight, other aspects of health, or functioning is not better accounted for by lack of food availability, the effects of a medication or substance, or another health condition.

Source: Adapted from http://id.who.int/icd/entity/263852475

Feeding and eating disorders criteria are specified in Chapter 6, 'Mental, behavioural or neurodevelopmental disorders', of ICD-11 (World Health Organization, 2019d). They are described as disorders that 'involve abnormal eating or feeding behaviours that are not explained by another health condition and are not developmentally appropriate or culturally sanctioned. Feeding disorders involve behavioural disturbances that are not related to body weight and shape concerns, such as eating of non-edible substances or voluntary regurgitation of foods. Eating disorders include abnormal eating behaviour and preoccupation with food as well as prominent body weight and shape concerns' (World Health Organization, 2019). (Pica and rumination/regurgitation disorder are also included within this ICD chapter and are further addressed in Chapter 3.1.)

ICD-11 also contains codes for 6B8Y, other specified feeding or eating disorders (OSFED; 6B8Y) and 6B8Z, feeding or eating disorders, unspecified (FEDU; 6B8Z). In the DSM-5 scheme, the OSFED category contains atypical anorexia nervosa (people who are not underweight), subthreshold (low frequency and/or duration) bulimia nervosa and BED, purging disorder (purging without recurrent binge eating) and night-eating syndrome (binge eating at night in clear consciousness). UFED comprises any other subthreshold feeding or eating disorders with no specific criteria.

ICD-11 differs from the DSM-5 in its definition of binge eating. In the ICD scheme a binge is a subjective experience of overeating with loss of control, although it may not be a large amount of food that is consumed. This is broader than the DSM-5 definition, which requires the eating episodes also to be an objectively large amount of food. In other respects ICD-11 criteria resemble those of the DSM-5 with the caveat that ICD-11 is more flexible and allows a greater degree of clinical judgement.

ASSESSMENT TIPS

The underweight patient: People who are underweight present in a variety of ways and settings, and up to 50% may never present at all (Keski-Rahkonen et al., 2007), or present with poor motivation and at a precontemplative stage of change (Casasnovas et al., 2007). Primary and secondary health care professionals thus need to be alert to the underweight patient, presenting with other problems, for example unexplained hypogonadism and infertility, osteopenia and stress fractures or dental caries (from vomiting). Younger patients are most usually brought to attention by concerned parents and/or school counsellors. Similarly, athletes may present with physical debility or collapse while training. Sometimes the eating disorder follows another health problem with inadvertent weight loss, and the latter's positive effects on self-view fuelled by societal praise.

All patients, whether or not they ascribe to fear of fatness or weight gain, will be in the grip of a relentless and self-imposed state of starvation. This in turn has notable psychological consequences of depression and mood lability, irritability and compulsive behaviours, including non-eating related, such as excessive cleaning. There can also be hoarding of food and eating rituals, and binge eating followed by compensatory behaviours like vomiting. Patients became isolative and withdrawn, with food and eating replacing all other interests and activities (Keys, 1950). In addition, brain volume reduces, cognitive style becomes inflexible and executive function is impaired (Hay & Sachdev, 2011). This, as well as commonly an alexythymic personality, may make it hard to engage the underweight patient in psychological therapies, and thus the focus early in treatment is often on nutrition and supportive approaches (Treasure & Russell, 2011).

The normal weight patient: People who are not underweight usually present at an older age than underweight patients, being in their young adulthood or mid-life years (Hudson, Hiripi, Pope, & Kessler, 2007). They are most likely to suffer from bulimia nervosa, BED or OSFED of a bulimic type with, for example, extreme weight and shape concern and behaviour to prevent weight gain or compensate for perceived binge eating, whether or not the bingeing is on large quantities. Despite not being underweight they often have large shifts in weight. Although motivation to change may be stronger than in those with anorexia nervosa, disgust with the eating disorder behaviours is associated with reluctance to seek help, and delays of a decade or more in presenting for help are common. Psychiatric comorbidity is very common, including depression, other impulse control, substance use and/or personality disorder of Cluster B type.

In general practice, around one in 20 women and one in 100 men attendees will have an eating disorder of bulimia nervosa or similar OS/UFED type (Hay, Loukas, & Philpott, 2005). They most often, however, are not seeking help for their eating problems, but rather seeking help for either an unrelated problem, or if they do seek help around eating and weight issues, it is for help in weight control (whether or not they are normal or overweight) or another mental health problem, such as depression. Like people with anorexia nervosa, they may also present with physical problems, such as infertility, oligomenorrhoea, dental caries and nonspecific gastrointestinal symptoms.

The patient with a high BMI: There is a noted overlap between weight disorders and eating disorders. Around one-third of people with a BMI over 30 have BED or a similar eating disorder, and up to one-half or more of those with BED or bulimia nervosa will have BMI>27. As noted above, most often people will be seeking help for the weight disorder rather than the eating disorder. It is still far too common for people to undergo many years of treatment for weight disorder, including bariatric surgery, without problems of binge eating and extreme weight and/or shape concerns being identified. This is a problem, as although weight management programs may be helpful in stabilising disordered eating, their longer-term efficacy in improving psychological features of the eating disorder is less clear.

4.5.2 WHAT DO WE KNOW ABOUT THESE DISORDERS?

PHILLIPA HAY & STEPHEN TOUYZ

PREVALENCE

Eating disorders are common and eating disorder symptoms are increasing in Australia (da Luz et al., 2017; Hay et al., 2005). The Australian adult general population point prevalence of anorexia nervosa is unknown, sub-syndrome anorexia nervosa and ARFID are about .5% each, bulimia nervosa about 1%, BED about 1.5% and OSFED around 3% (Hay et al., 2017). A nationally representative study of all eating disorders was undertaken in the United States in 2001–03 (Hudson et al., 2007). Lifetime prevalence of (a) anorexia nervosa was 0.9% in women and 0.3% in men; (b) bulimia nervosa was 1.5% in women, 0.5% in men; and (c) BED was 3.5% in women and 2.0% in men.

The prevalence of eating disorders is higher in women and adolescents/young adults compared to men and older people (Micali et al., 2017; Allen, Byrne, Oddy, & Crosby, 2013). However they occur throughout all age, gender and socioeconomic groups in the community (Mulders-Jones, Mitchison, Girosi, & Hay, 2017). The peak age of onset of anorexia nervosa is in early to mid- adolescence, but it can start in childhood, where the gender balance is more even (Madden, Morris, Zurynski, Kohn, & Elliot, 2009). The reasons for the greater number of boys presenting in childhood years are unclear. In bulimia nervosa and BED, onset is in later adolescence and young adulthood (Stice, Killen, Hayward, & Taylor, 1998). In addition, eating disorders often go undiagnosed and untreated. Thus it is common for adults to present for treatment many years after onset, even into late middle age.

HOW CAN WE UNDERSTAND THE ORIGINS?

Social determinants

The strongest risk factor for having an eating disorder continues to be being of female gender and being from the developed world, where the 'thin ideal' predominates. Migrants from the developing world seem to be at particular risk. Also at risk are those living in urban areas and undertaking life pursuits, such as classical ballet dancing and elite sports, where body image concerns predominate.

Genetics and other biological factors

In all eating disorders there is an increased heritability (genetic risk) and increased frequency of a family history or both eating, mood and anxiety disorders. A family history of leanness is associated with anorexia nervosa, and a personal or family history of obesity with bulimic-type eating disorders. Early menarche (controlling for body weight) also increases risk. Heritability estimates have a wide range for anorexia nervosa and even wider range (5–60%) for other eating disorders (Mitchison & Hay, 2014).

Psychological determinants—stress and trauma.

Psychological determinants of eating disorders are important, as they are most amenable to targeted and indicative prevention strategies. They include a milieu of weight concern in formative developmental years, often where there is familial weight disorder and overt repeated critical appraisal of the child's weight. Specific personality traits are also relevant, mostly notably low self-esteem for all, high levels of clinical perfectionism for those with anorexia nervosa and impulsivity for bulimic disorders. Adverse experiences, including emotive and sexual child abuse, increase personal vulnerability, most likely through impeding a robust sense of self-worth and adaptive coping.

In addition, family issues about control and approval can be played out in dieting behaviour, which provides a sense of self-control for the individual and attains peer approval. In anorexia nervosa, delayed pubertal development and amenorrhoea may help contain and hold the person emotionally in adolescence (see Stice, 2002, for a comprehensive review).

The pathway into an eating disorder is usually a complex of personal and familial vulnerabilities together with environmental exposure to the admiration of thinness and adversities in formative years. These most often precede triggering events such as public weighing and weight criticism.

Factors influencing prognosis

An earlier age of onset and presentation, less severe weight loss and faster weight regain during treatment, good parent-child relationships and having children (in women) are associated with better outcomes for people with anorexia nervosa. Poorer outcomes are found in people with more severe body image disturbance at presentation, those who use purgative methods of weight control, who have childhood developmental problems including disordered eating, who have psychiatric comorbidity and/or obsessive-compulsive personality trait/disorder (Hay & Claudino, 2010; Vall & Wade, 2015).

Having a history of anorexia nervosa, child or adult high BMI, substance-use disorder, mood intolerance and failing to attain binge eating abstinence in therapy may predict a poorer outcome for people with bulimia nervosa and similar eating disorders such as BED although less is known about the latter (Vall & Wade, 2015). The long delays from illness onset to presentation likely also contribute to poorer outcomes. There are many personal and external barriers to treatment including stigma, poor access to care and also the fear of negative experiences in treatment particularly for gay and gender diverse peoples (Duffy, Henkel, & Earnshaw, 2016).

COURSE AND IMPACT

A systematic review of 119 studies of 5590 people with anorexia nervosa between one and 29 years reported that, although around half of people recover (range 0–92%) and a further third improve (range 0–75%), a small number will die (5%) and one-fifth develop a chronic eating disorder (range 0–79% ; Steinhausen, 2002). In contrast, the majority of people with bulimia nervosa, BED or similar eating disorders make a good outcome in long-term follow-up studies, with up to 50% or more patients free of symptoms at five years or more (Fairburn, Cooper, Doll, Norman, & O'Connor, 2000; Steinhausen & Weber, 2009).

All eating disorders are associated with poor health-related quality of life and impairments in home, work, personal and social life (Hay et al., 2017). Eating disorders also frequently co-occur with other mental health disorders, particularly anxiety disorders and depression (Hudson et al., 2007). There is a notable burden on families and carers as well as broader societal costs. The cost of informal care for people in Australia with eating disorders in 2012 was estimated to be $8.5 million and the 'burden of disease' estimated to be $52.6 billion in Australia (Paxton et al., 2012). Families and carers report high levels of personal stress and poorer health.

Health literacy with regard to identification of eating disorders is mixed, with generally a better community understanding of anorexia nervosa and bulimia nervosa compared to BED and available evidence-based treatments for the latter (Reas, 2017). Poor health literacy and favourable regard for weight loss in the community may well contribute to the treatment gap for people with normal or above normal weight eating disorders (Ali et al., 2017).

PRACTICE ILLUSTRATION: ENTERING TREATMENT

Julie, an 18-year-old adolescent, attended her local GP complaining of general lethargy and leg pain. The GP noted that she was very thin. On examination, she showed some signs of starvation and her BMI was 17. She seemed reluctant to answer questions, and just wanted the doctor to give her some medication to help her feel better.

The GP explained that it was important to undertake a range of tests to ensure that there were no physical problems, and asked Julie to return in a few days for a longer appointment. Julie attended the second appointment. While the tests indicated no immediate health worries, the GP asked Julie if she would complete the SCOFF Questionnaire. Her score of three on the questionnaire indicated that she may have an eating disorder, and provided an opportunity to discuss with Julie her food intake and her use of laxatives and induced vomiting. The GP offered a referral to a psychiatrist or a psychologist, but Julie refused. She did however agree to see a dietician and meet with the GP on a regular basis.

In this situation the GP did not immediately push for specialist referral as Julie was not ready to agree with this and there were no urgent health concerns. The GP elected instead to keep Julie engaged in treatment with a view to helping her become more motivated to accept more active care.

4.5.3 ASSESSMENT

PHILLIPA HAY & STEPHEN TOUYZ

GOOD PRACTICE IN DISORDER-SPECIFIC ASSESSMENT

In assessment it is essential to explore core beliefs about eating, food, weight and shape and to document current eating patterns and diet, including episodes of binge eating, compensatory (purging) behaviours and presence of driven or compulsive exercise. In addition to a comprehensive psychological appraisal, it is imperative that a full medical history be taken and a physical examination done.

The physician should assess objective height and weight, calculate body mass index (kg/m^2; BMI) and check for signs of dehydration and cardiovascular instability, most often bradycardia, increased variability of heart rate, postural hypotension and other indicators of purging; for example, dorsal hand calluses. In underweight patients, signs of starvation (for example, lanugo hair, hypothermia, muscle wasting and delayed pubertal development) will be present. Other physical problems include mitral valve prolapse (usually a benign condition whose association with starvation is poorly understood); oedema (may be a result of starvation itself, re-feeding, low protein and/or cardiac failure); stress fractures; thyroid hypofunction; and an irregular heart rate.

Table 4.22 Core medical investigations

All patients	The underweight patient
Full blood screen Urea and creatinine Serum electrolytes: • sodium • potassium • magnesium • phosphate Liver function	Fasting glucose, B_{12}, folate Iron studies Thyroid function Electrocardiogram Bone densitometry*

*If amenorrhoeic greater than six months or other evidence of hypogonadism

Recommended core investigations are listed in Table 4.22. An electrocardiogram is indicated, particularly as if a prolonged QT interval is present, it may presage an arrhythmia. A comprehensive assessment of endocrine status is not mandatory. Although there is a well-known association between starvation and anovulation, thyroid hypofunction and raised plasma cortisol and growth hormone, this requires no specific intervention apart from re-feeding. However, specific treatment for osteopenia with supplementary calcium and vitamin D, and even bisphosphonates, may be indicated.

COMMON ISSUES AND DILEMMAS IN ASSESSMENT

Practitioners need to have a heightened level of suspicion of an eating disorder in young people presenting for help with perceived or actual weight disorder and/or psychological distress. The initial assessment is then an important opportunity to engage ambivalent patients, the majority, in treatment. Although it is essential to discuss medical and psychological consequences of the eating disorder, the clinician should not anticipate a full appreciation of the need for change and (in the underweight) weight regain. In patients with more longstanding illness this can take several months, if not longer, and for some several years.

Normal or overweight patients should be reassured that with psychological therapy their weight will stabilise and not usually change with regularised eating patterns. They can be advised that resuming normal eating will decrease food preoccupation, reduce urges to binge, attenuate tiredness and depression and facilitate improved family and peer relationships.

HELPFUL ASSESSMENT INSTRUMENTS AND GUIDES

The SCOFF Questionnaire (see Table 4.23; Luck et al., 2002) has been developed as a useful and validated tool in screening for eating disorders, particularly anorexia nervosa and bulimia nervosa in primary care settings. A useful self-report measure for assessment and/or rating outcomes is the Eating Disorder Examination-Questionnaire (Fairburn, 2010, pp. 309-13).

Table 4.23 The SCOFF Questionnaire

Do you ever make yourself Sick because you feel uncomfortably full?
Do you worry you have lost Control over how much you eat?
Have you recently lost more than One stone in a three-month period?
Do you believe yourself to be Fat when others say you are too thin?
Would you say that Food dominates your life?

*One point is given for every 'yes' answer. A score of two or more indicates a possible eating disorder.

Note: 1 stone is approximately 6.35 kg.

Source: Luck et al., 2002

4.5.4 EVIDENCE-BASED AND OTHER TREATMENTS AND SERVICES

PHILLIPA HAYS & STEPHEN TOUYZ

MAIN TREATMENTS AND STRENGTH OF EVIDENCE

Nutritional management

In all patients, but especially those who are underweight, eating must be addressed, and the collaboration of a dietitian is valuable. Records of food consumed, and whether the diet includes essential nutrients, are made. Psychoeducation about normal eating and dietary guidelines is very important, and reference can be made to Australian guidelines (National Health and Medical Research Council, 2003).

Box 4.4: The re-feeding syndrome

The re-feeding syndrome is a potentially fatal medical emergency. It is precipitated by the sudden introduction of larger amounts of food in the starved patient. This leads to a demand for intracellular metabolic electrolytes (potassium, phosphate, magnesium), which is met by drastically reducing plasma levels.

People at increased risk include those with recent, rapid weight loss, minimal energy intake, low glucose and high serum urea. It is essential to monitor and replace as indicated phosphate, magnesium and/or potassium.

Clinical features comprise cardiac failure or arrhythmia, oedema, seizures, paraesthesia, delirium and coma.

Patients who are underweight are in a negative energy balance, and thus they need to eat more than normal to regain healthy nutritional status. Outpatient sessions need to be regular, and most often weekly, until substantial improvement occurs. Weight is recorded on each occasion. The first step is to stop losing weight, and then aim for increase at about half a kilogram per week as an outpatient, or up to one kilogram per week for inpatients. Physical exercise, although usually done to lose weight, can be a good thing if moderated; for example, yoga is preferable to running. Moderate exercise may help preserve lean body mass (muscle) and prevent osteoporosis (strengthen the bones), and improve mood. Vitamin supplements are advised, especially in hospital, where phosphate and B group multivitamins, including thiamine, should be prescribed to avoid re-feeding syndrome (see Box 4.3). They are generally less essential as an outpatient unless the patient is a very strict vegetarian and/or otherwise deficient.

Psychotherapy

This is the core of treatment RANZCP Guidelines (Hay et al., 2014). The therapies with best evidence for effectiveness are cognitive behaviour therapy in adults with bulimia nervosa, and family-based therapy in children and adolescents with anorexia nervosa (see Part 2; see also Chapter 4.3). In children and adolescents with anorexia nervosa, the approach is to empower the family to assist in the re-feeding and supervision of meals. Psychological therapy is provided to the family as a whole, although additional individual sessions may be useful. If the patient has left school and is living apart from the family, then individual therapy is probably more appropriate, although some contact with the family may be helpful (as is some contact with spouse or partner for adults having individual therapy).

Maudsley family-based therapy

The manualised Maudsley family-based therapy for children and adolescents with anorexia nervosa (Lock, Grange, Agras, & Dare, 2001) has become the recommended approach in Australia. It is conducted over three phases, following an important first session. In this first meeting the clinician evaluates the family's strengths and weaknesses, and ensures that a positive comment is conveyed to each member as the session closes. If there are emergent major problems, such as physical or sexual abuse, substance abuse or difficulties with another child (for example, substance abuse or disturbed behaviour), the family should be referred to a specialist family therapist. Most families, or at least the parents, are then offered regular sessions, with the aim being to elicit the family's assistance in helping the member with anorexia nervosa.

The three treatment phases of the Maudsley approach comprise: *parental empowerment* to facilitate re-feeding the patient (including having a family meal); negotiations for a *new pattern of relationships*; and the establishment of a *healthy adolescent or young adult relationship* with the parents, in which the disordered eating does not constitute the basis of interaction, and there is increased personal autonomy for the adolescent. It is important to note that family-based therapy challenges the practical factors maintaining the illness, such as allowing the ill adolescent to make his or her own food choices, and makes no assumptions about the cause of anorexia nervosa. It thus does not presuppose a familial pathology, but rather aims to reduce parental and patient self-blame.

Treating adults with anorexia nervosa

For adults with anorexia nervosa there is no best evidence therapy; however, specialist care has better outcomes than non-specialist care (Lock & Fitzpatrick, 2009). Psychotherapy is medium to long-term, but 20 sessions is minimal and up to 40 usual. All approaches benefit from application of motivational enhancement strategies, such as decisional analysis (debating the pros and cons of having anorexia nervosa), and are integrated with nutritional counselling and monitoring of physical state within a team model. Forms of cognitive behaviour therapy (CBT) have become first-line in Australia, and include the transdiagnostic CBT-Enhanced (CBT-E; see Chapter 4.3) and CBT-AN.

Cognitive behaviour therapy specific for anorexia nervosa (CBT–AN)

Pike and colleagues have produced a manualised cognitive behaviour therapy specific for anorexia nervosa (CBT-AN). It has been found effective in improving symptoms (Hay et al., 2018) and in reducing relapse in one randomised trial (Pike, Walsh, Vitousek, Wilson, & Bauer, 2003) and one non-randomised trial (Carter et al., 2009). The main aim of CBT-AN is normalisation of eating behaviour, ensuring steady weight gain and medical stability. This is to achieve a healthy weight while addressing the interaction between the thoughts, emotions and behaviours that are the driving force of anorexia nervosa. It is built on the seminal work of Garner and colleagues (Garner, Vitousek, & Garfinkel, 1997) who postulated the following principles of CBT in anorexia nervosa:

> (i) the acceptance of conscious experience rather than unconscious phenomena; (ii) focus upon belief, assumptions, schematic processing and meaning systems as mediating variables for maladaptive behaviours and emotions; (iii) the employment of questioning as a prominent therapeutic strategy; (iv) active participation by the therapist in treatment; and (v) the essential contribution of homework sessions including self-monitoring.

The manualised CBT-AN of Pike and colleagues (Pike et al., 2003) follows three clearly defined phases of treatment. The first phase aims to achieve trust and a positive alliance, and to set treatment parameters. The key features of the eating disorder are explored, there is education about starvation symptoms and other related topics (as above), a rationale and advice for restoring normal nutrition and body weight is provided, and regular eating patterns prescribed with a gradual increase in portion sizes. This phase incorporates motivational enhancement therapeutic strategies. Behavioural experiments are introduced to increase the range and quantity of foods and reduce behaviours such as driven exercise. The second phase centres around changing beliefs related to food and weight (examples are found in Table 4.24), and then broadening the scope of therapy. There is continued emphasis on weight gain and normalising eating, and how to bring these about by reframing relapse, identifying dysfunctional thoughts, exploring negative schema and thinking patterns, developing cognitive restructuring skills, modifying self-concept and developing an interpersonal focus in therapy. The final phase involves relapse prevention and termination. Here the therapist revisits the changes the patient has made, and prepares the patient for residual problems that may be found once therapy has concluded.

Table 4.24 Common beliefs and misconceptions in people with eating disorders

Undue influence of shape and/or weight on self-view or self-worth: *key diagnostic feature*
Extreme fear of weight gain or fatness: *diagnostic in anorexia nervosa*
Believing one has binged on small or normal amounts of food; subjective binges: *seen often in anorexia nervosa*
All-or-nothing or black-or-white reasoning; for example, it is a 'fast' or a 'binge' day; foods are either 'good' or 'bad'
Magical thinking around certain weights in anorexia nervosa: 'I can only be happy with a weight under 45 kg'
Having to be perfect at everything; for example, 'An A– grade is not good enough; it has to be an A'
Belief that taking laxatives and diuretics removes fats and not just fibre and water
Believing that muscle that is not exercised will turn into fat

Third-wave and other new therapies

Researchers in the field have also turned their attention to the newer 'third-wave' therapies, such as acceptance and commitment therapy (ACT). This is a recent mindfulness-based behaviour therapy (see Part 2; see also Chapter 4.3) which has been shown to be effective with a diverse range of clinical conditions. However, the effectiveness of this therapy in the treatment of anorexia nervosa is unknown.

Cognitive remediation therapy has been widely researched at Kings College London and now forms part of their novel Maudsley Anorexia Nervosa

Treatment for Adults (MANTRA) treatment program. This is an alternate to CBT and has been found effective in controlled trials.

Cognitive behaviour therapy for bulimia nervosa and enhanced (CBT-BN and CBT-E)

In normal and overweight patients with bulimia nervosa, BED or other eating disorders, the recommended approach is CBT for bulimia nervosa (CBT-BN), as developed by Fairburn (2010). However, other focused psychotherapies, such as interpersonal psychotherapy or dialectical behaviour therapy, have shown some success in trials. CBT-BN has since been enhanced (CBT-E) to a transdiagnostic therapy incorporating modules utilising such other techniques and addressing specifically maintaining factors of mood intolerance, low self-esteem, clinical perfectionism and interpersonal deficits (Fairburn, 2010). Core CBT-BN is conducted over a series of 20 sessions. It is recommended that they begin twice weekly, decreasing to weekly and then having one or two follow-up sessions over a period of around four months. There are four stages, the first psychoeducation, the second monitoring of eating behaviours, the third introducing behavioural experiments to prevent eating disorder behaviours and promote self-control, and the fourth comprising cognitive challenging of body image, weight–shape concerns and other attitudes and beliefs common in people with eating disorders.

In the first phase, in addition to information about eating disorders, a personalised CBT formulation is drawn out, with the diet–binge–purge cycle at its core. Examples of such formulations can be found at <www.psych.ox.ac.uk/research/researchunits/credo>. Specific discussion addresses the role that extreme dietary restriction plays in promoting binge eating, which often includes results of research studies of starvation. Patients are usually very positive and relieved when given such an understanding of the antecedents to binge eating, together with insights into the way early life experiences or their social and interpersonal context have contributed to the development of their eating disorder.

The second phase of therapy introduces behavioural monitoring and recording of eating and weight control behaviours. Patients often find keeping this aversive, and its core role needs to be emphasised. Forms are standardised, but can be adapted into journal format and can be downloaded from the website. Records are reviewed at each session. The next step is instituting a meal plan of regular eating; for example, three meals and two snacks per day combined with dietary education. It is essential to avoid long periods without eating, as this exacerbates the diet–binge cycle. The third phase of therapy focuses on cognitive strategies, such as Socratic questioning and challenging of beliefs and attitudes that reinforce eating disorder behaviours (see Table 4.24). Problem solving is also usually incorporated here, comprising the five steps: defining the problem; generating a solution; listing advantages and disadvantages of each; choosing a solution; and trying it out and reviewing it and, if unsuccessful, revisiting other solutions. A useful supplementary book for patients at this stage is the CBT self-help manual by Waller et al. (2007) which also is a useful guide through therapy for carers.

The final phase of CBT-BN involves relapse prevention and review of 'lapses'. Here it is important to stress that lapses will always occur, but the patient will not revert to baseline levels of binge eating and purging. Patients may compile a record of strategies that have successfully helped them, such as monitoring and distractions at times of vulnerability to binge eating. The use of relaxation, slow breathing and other anxiety management and coping strategies can also be usefully introduced during these later points in therapy.

Patients with problems related to a high BMI

Patients who are overweight or obese and have an eating disorder, such as BN or BED, will also benefit from CBT-BN as described above. They may also need a supported weight loss program particularly if they have weight-related metabolic, cardiovascular or musculoskeletal/mobility problems, such as diabetes or high blood pressure. In many cases, even a small weight loss, such as 5–10% body weight, can reduce the risk of developing diabetes or other cardiac problems (National Health and Medical Research Council, 2003; Vidal, 2002). Patients should be encouraged to set modest weight loss goals, mindful of studies investigating weight regain following obesity treatment. This research has found that those people who regain weight were the ones who set unrealistic weight goals and did not reach these goals (Byrne, Cooper, & Fairburn, 2003).

The following strategies may assist people achieve modest weight loss: increasing physical activity that is not compulsive but enjoyable and preferably sociable (for example, tennis versus solitary gym exercise); modifications of meal and snacks choices to ensure meal patterns and portion sizes accord with dietary guidelines; education on how to read nutrition information panels on supermarket foods to enable informed decisions when choosing between products; and strategies to modify unhealthy dietary patterns, such as eating when stressed, or habitually overeating when not hungry. A helpful book incorporating these and other strategies, such as mindful eating, is Kausman's book, *If Not Dieting, Then What?* (2004) Core to this is promoting the position that physical health and a healthy diet are not attained by any absolute weight but may be found within a wide range of BMI.

Pharmacological therapies

Although psychotherapy is generally the main approach, medications can be helpful as adjunctive or additional therapy, or where access to psychotherapy is delayed or otherwise problematic. Antidepressants (see Chapters 2.5 and 4.3) are indicated for eating disorders where there is comorbid major depression or where binge eating is severe. In particular, high-dose fluoxetine (60 mg/day) has been found more efficacious than low dose (20 mg/day) in reducing binge eating in bulimia nervosa (Hay & Claudino, 2010). Other agents that reduce binge eating in the short term are the anticonvulsant topiramate and the stimulant lesdexamfetamine. The long-term effects are unclear.

In anorexia nervosa, tricyclic antidepressants are to be avoided, because they may affect cardiac conduction, particularly in overdose. Cisapride (given formerly to improve gastric motility) is not used for the same reason. A benzodiazepine or small dose of an atypical antipsychotic (such as olanzapine 2.5–5 mg) may also be helpful in assisting people with acute anorexia nervosa with emotive arousal and ruminations. This is most relevant to the early re-feeding phase of care.

Self-help approaches

Self-help in eating disorders has become increasingly popular as a way of improving access to care and as a first step while waiting for treatment. There are a number of self-help books about weight and eating problems, but few provide a treatment approach or program that the person is able to apply for themselves. Particularly helpful are those for bulimic disorders that have translated CBT-BN or similar manualised therapy into a self-help form. On the whole, pure self-help approaches have been found to be less efficacious than guided self-help or full therapy with a trained therapist (Perkins, Murphy, Schmidt, & Williams, 2006; Stefano, Bacaltchuk, Blay, & Hay, 2006). It seems that most patients prefer to have a therapist, even if that therapist may be at the end of a telephone or videoconference link.

In addition to self-help books, there are also many websites related to eating disorders and including, unfortunately, a myriad pro-anorexia nervosa and pro-eating disorder websites. Around Australia there are a number of reputable websites, well supported by expert advice and opinion, and these include:

- Butterfly Foundation: www.thebutterflyfoundation.org.au
- Eating Disorders Association of Queensland: www.uq.net.au/eda
- Victorian Centre of Excellence in Eating Disorders: www.rch.org.au/ceed
- InsideOut Institute: insideoutinstitute.org.au.

TREATMENT CHALLENGES FOR MENTAL HEALTH WORKERS

Therapists can be challenged by the egosyntonicity and intractability of anorexia nervosa, and often very slow rate of progress. When and how to use the Mental Health Act for medical and psychiatric safety is challenging, and supervision and/or a team approach is invariably helpful. Therapists should be mindful that a cognitive shift to accepting the need for change can occur unpredictably, and is often a 'road to Damascus' type experience, such as typified by Clare Park, a talented photographer. She described the exact moment when she was released from a view of herself whereby 'the outward visual appearance is of utmost importance. And these pictures [of herself] are all about how you feel ugly inside... It was almost an out of body experience ... I saw myself for a split second in a mirror. And I actually stopped for one second, thinking I was too fat, I saw what I had become–like something out of Belsen (Park, 1991).

PRACTICE ILLUSTRATION: TREATMENT CHALLENGES

Over the next three months Julie continued to visit the GP on a fortnightly basis. She had had three visits to the dietician and had found them useful. She had also brought her parents along to two meetings with the GP, and they expressed their concerns about Julie and her impact on the family. She had gained a small amount of weight and generally was feeling better.

However, three months into her treatment, she became depressed after a conflict with one of her friends, increased her purging and lost 5 kg within a very short period. Her GP became concerned, and again raised the issue of a referral to a specialist eating disorder service. With some encouragement from her family, Julie agreed to accept the referral.

Sadly, up to one-fifth of patients may develop a longstanding illness with a history of negative treatment experiences and repeated treatment failures. In this situation, the patient and their therapist experience a sense of hopelessness. Strober (2010) has argued the need to move beyond targeting core eating disorder pathology (primarily weight restoration) in these patients. He advises a supportive approach that aims to minimise harm and reduce the personal and social costs of chronic illness, such as medical morbidity, the burden on health services, poor quality of life, frequent depression and profound social isolation. Less intensive psychotherapies, such as *specialist supportive clinical management* (SSCM; McIntosh et al., 2005; Touyz et al., 2013), may be helpful in these patients with severe and enduring illness.

TREATMENT CHALLENGES FOR CONSUMERS

While the recognition of mainstream eating disorders such as anorexia nervosa and bulimia nervosa is good, BED and ARFID are less well known. Further, understanding of the effectiveness of psychological treatments is not as good and access in Australia is often difficult. Publicly funded centres offering treatment are increasing but are by no means universal and access to privately funded psychological therapy is expensive.

PRACTICE ILLUSTRATION: TREATMENT OUTCOMES

Eighteen months later, Julie successfully completed her first year of university. While initially reluctant, she had found the psychotherapy sessions provided by her clinical psychologist very helpful. A psychiatrist had diagnosed her with depression, and her GP had agreed to monitor her antidepressant treatment on the proviso that she attended regular sessions with the psychologist. She had ceased purging, and managed to improve her weight to a BMI of 20 but continued to be restrictive in her eating with fears of binge eating. The psychologist also provided support for her parents, assisting them to respond to her eating issues in different ways and encourage her independence.

Over the next 12 months Julie continued in therapy and her fears of loss of control over eating and weight had receded. She was very happy in a new relationship and for the first time in years she said her life was 'no longer dominated by thoughts of food, weight and eating'.

GOOD PRACTICE EXAMPLES

The case described in the Practice illustration of Julie's situation exemplify the need for a multidisciplinary approach. This is usually coordinated by the family doctor and incorporates medical, nutritional and psychological therapy. It shows the need to be patient especially but not only in the care of people with anorexia nervosa.

KEY RISKS OF HARM IN TREATMENT ATTEMPTS

The main risks of harm in the care of people with an eating disorder is not recognising and undertreating the physical effects of starvation and/or purging. Identifying suicidal and self-harm ideation is equally an imperative. Balancing the need to ensure safety as well as respecting autonomy and providing care in the least restrictive setting is often not easy. Sometimes a community treatment order may be used for people with intractable illness as an alternative to repeated hospital admissions but the goals of such orders are necessarily limited.

4.5.5 WHERE AND HOW DO PEOPLE GET HELP?

The majority of people with an eating disorder are treated in the community by a clinician trained in specialist psychological therapy with care-coordinated by a family doctor. The doctor's role is to also arrange dietetic and more intensive specialist psychiatric and medical care, and day or inpatient care as appropriate. The RANZCP Guidelines recommend a recovery orientated stance with care in the least restrictive setting. There is increasing evidence for the role of peer mentoring from people who have recovered and support led by people with the lived experience can be invaluable for the patient and those who care for them.

4.5.6 THE IMPLICATIONS OF THE DIVERSITY OF AUSTRALIA

SALLY MORRIS, PHILLIPA HAY & STEPHEN TOUYZ

Access to care for an eating disorder in Australia is poor outside major metropolitan centres. Migrants and Aboriginal and Torres Strait Islander peoples experience eating disorders to the same or greater degree than other Australians. Eating disorders are also under-recognised and treated in people with socioeconomic disadvantage. There are major gaps in the development of gender (Thapliyal, Hay, & Conti, 2018) and culturally informed treatment services.

Research into LGBTIQ people's experiences of eating disorders is still in its infancy. Limited research to date shows that different gender and sexuality subgroups that make up the 'LGBTIQ' acronym have different contributing factors and experience eating disorder in specific and particular ways (McClain & Peebles, 2016; Feldman & Meyer, 2007).

In particular, gay and bisexual men have greater body dissatisfaction, and more frequently report engaging in unhealthy weight control practices and disordered eating behaviours (McClain & Peebles, 2016; Feldman & Meyer, 2007).Conversely, lesbian and bisexual women are not more likely to have an eating disorder than their heterosexual counterparts, however are more likely to be obese (McClain & Peebles, 2016).

Transgender and gender diverse people particularly have a higher rate of eating disorders, with a study of 452 transgender people showing that 7.4% self-reported having an eating disorder (Diemer et al., 2018). A review of literature highlighted that body dissatisfaction of their gender identity not aligning with their bodily appearance is core to the distress of transgender people, which may put some people at risk for disordered eating (Jones, Haycraft, Murjan, & Arcelus, 2016). Just as there was variation across the LGBTIQ population (Diemer et al., 2018) demonstrated that eating disorder diagnoses are unevenly distributed across transgender men, transgender women, and gender non-conforming sub-groupings (Diemer et al., 2018). People with a nonbinary gender were significantly more likely than participants with a binary gender identity to report an eating disorder diagnosis.

While insufficient research has been conducted on the eating disorders within an intersex population, there is a culture of stigma that surrounds intersex bodily variations that impacts how intersex people feel about their bodies. Engaging with other people with intersex variations helped improve body image and self-esteem (Jones, Hart, & Carpenter, 2016).

LGBTIQ young people are particularly vulnerable to eating disorders, as adolescence is a crucial period for emerging sexual orientation and gender, the time when eating disorders are also most likely to develop (McClain & Peebles, 2016). A survey of 1034 LGBTIQ young people aged 13–24 revealed that a significant 54% had been diagnosed with an eating disorder. Of those who had not being diagnosed with an eating disorder, half of these suspected that they had an undiagnosed eating disorder (The Trevor Project, 2018).

The experiences of eating disorders among LGBTIQ populations demonstrates that the diagnosing and treatment of eating disorders within a traditional gender binary male/female approach is not useful (Diemer et al., 2018). Clinicians lack of knowledge of gender diversity and competence in supporting transgender people may result in the treatment being ineffective, and potentially harmful (Duffy et al., 2016). Successful treatment of eating disorders with LGBTIQ people are required to be tailored, and should take into account the unique stressors that LGBTIQ people encounter, along with the resilience within LGBTIQ populations (Goldhammer, Maston, & Keuroghlian, 2019).

4.5.7 COMMENTARY AND REFLECTION

PHILLIPA HAY & STEPHEN TOUYZ

Eating disorders are common disorders that are generally responsive to psychological treatments. Despite arguments to the contrary, eating disordered patients, although often challenging, can be very rewarding to treat. Many do go on to make a full recovery, in every sense of the word, despite the turbulent journey that many undertake often lasting several years. When treating such patients it is very important never to lose hope. One can never be quite sure when the person may decide to embrace treatment with the benefits that may arise from this. However, what we do now know, especially with respect to anorexia nervosa, is that early identification and diagnosis are critical, as there is much greater likelihood of complete recovery if treatment is initiated within three years of onset.

As the window into the mind, through neuroimaging and neuropsychological studies, gains momentum, so will diagnostic understanding evolve and be informed by neuroscientific investigation. It is possible the current 'splitting' of diagnoses could be replaced by fewer categories delineated by genetic and cognitive correlates as much as by presenting symptoms. For example, eating disorders characterised by a genetic predisposition to leanness, weak central coherence and clinical perfectionism may replace current conceptualisations of anorexia nervosa and include people who are not underweight (Treasure & Schmidt, 2013).

4.6

DISORDERS OF BODILY DISTRESS OR BODILY EXPERIENCE, FACTITIOUS DISORDERS, AND PSYCHOLOGICAL OR BEHAVIOURAL FACTORS AFFECTING DISORDERS OR DISEASES

AKSHAY ILANGO, DAVID CLARKE & GRAHAM MEADOWS WITH GRAEME SMITH

4.6.1 INTRODUCTION

People put a lot less effort into picking apart evidence that confirms what they already believe.

Peter Watts, Echopraxia

People are always clinging to what they want to hear, discarding the evidence that doesn't fit with their beliefs, giving greater weight to evidence that does.

Paula Stokes, On Confirmation Bias

Bodily symptoms, particularly if mild or transient, may not lead to presentation to health care. Reported symptoms may be seen as being directly related to a physical illness in a way that is clinically typical and understandable. However, there are times when symptoms do not fit neatly into any one diagnostic category, with potential for overlap (and blurred diagnostic boundaries) between medical disciplines and psychiatry. Diagnoses grouped by organ system are to be found in the various major sections of ICD-11 outside ICD's Chapter 6, where mental, behavioural or neurodevelopmental disorders are described.

Bodily symptoms represent expression of psychological and social factors through a process of somatisation. Somatisation can involve various mechanisms which are important to understand and will be described in some detail.

- Bodily symptoms may present as a disorder of bodily distress or bodily experience. Disorders of bodily distress represent a broad category of disorders and subsume two diagnostic groups. Namely, bodily distress disorder (BDD) and body integrity dysphoria (BID). ICD-11 BDD (see Section 4.6.3), replaces ICD-10 Somatoform Disorders and Neurasthenia and is seen as being equivalent to somatic symptom and related disorders (DSM-5). BDD is a relatively new diagnostic label and therefore literature from somatoforms disorders has been drawn upon. The body may rarely be a focus in presentation where someone has an intense and persistent desire to become physically disabled, a condition described as body integrity dysphoria (covered in Section 4.6.4).
- A common set of challenges for mental health care arise where there is a recognisable underlying pathophysiological or physical disease process, and there are significant behavioural and psychological factors contributing or exacerbating the underlying medical condition. (The process of understanding these challenges is described in Section 4.6.6.)

Bodily symptoms, among others, may occasionally be induced, aggravated or falsified in the person or another in what is described as 'factitious disorder'. (See Section 4.6.7. This is the next focus area for this chapter, along with brief coverage of the issue of malingering covered in Section 4.6.8.)

Bodily symptoms may represent other psychiatric disorders, outside the BDD group:

- Mental disorders including anxiety and mood disorders may have prominent features related to physical symptoms. These may sometimes be salient aspects of the clinical presentation, the physical features may be recognisable and explicable as part of a diagnosis, in this case a psychiatric one. Diagnostic considerations are addressed in ICD-11's Chapter 6 and in Chapters 4.3 and 4.4.
- Hypochondriasis, with its strong implication of preoccupation, fear and distress regarding physical illness, in ICD-11 is located in the obsessive-compulsive and related disorders category and is described in Chapter 4.4. Also grouped in obsessive-compulsive or related disorders is body dysmorphic disorder, characterised by persistent preoccupation with flaws in appearance. Body dysmorphic disorder shares an acronym with Bodily distress disorder (BDD) but in this chapter the second usage is intended. In the Anxiety disorders section of ICD-11 are a group of conditions where neurological symptoms are presenting features but in ways not consistent with currently recognised neurological condition; these are referred to as dissociative disorders (see also Chapter 4.4). In ICD-10 and DSM-5 the term 'conversion disorder' also was used for these conditions and may often still be encountered.
- In a watershed area between physical and mental disorders lie the functional somatic syndromes (FSS). FSS may present with a single symptom or a cluster of symptoms. These syndromes are identified either through the system involved, for instance, Irritable Bowel Syndrome (IBS) is diagnosed when the presenting system relates to the gastrointestinal system. Alternatively, syndromes may be identified based on the nature of the presenting symptom, for instance, severe fatigue and widespread pain are the presenting symptoms of chronic fatigue and fibromyalgia respectively. This group of diagnoses resurrect the age-old debate: are these presentations organic or psychogenic? At one end of the spectrum is the view that these are as yet to be fully understood and that biological evidence will accumulate over time. On the other end of the spectrum is the notion that these disorders are quasi-diagnoses and they arise from complex psychological and social struggles. It is important to avoid finding oneself at polar ends of the organic versus psychogenic debate. In this context, a pragmatic

way forward is to maintain a holistic perspective on aetiology, with attention to biological, psychosocial and cultural factors. The concept of central sensitisation has been particularly researched in pain syndromes and the concept is truly biopsychosocial in that it acknowledges the impact of various biopsychosocial factors on the central nervous system. Peripheral sensory inputs through central sensitisation interact with brain networks (including those involved in thinking and feeling), within a psychosocial context. This concept has also been applied to IBS and fibromyalgia (Guo, Kleinstauber, Johnson, & Sundram, 2019). While the extent of organic versus psychogenic underpinnings may be a matter of investigation and debate, psychological stress is seen as making a contribution to their occurrence and exacerbation. Importantly, the diagnosis of chronic fatigue does not preclude a comorbid diagnosis of BDD. Comorbidity with other psychiatric disorders, such as anxiety disorder or mood disorder is also common, further complicating diagnostic considerations and management. The major specialist textbooks on this topic are by Crone, Lackamp and Alkis (2018) and Sharpe and O'Malley (2018). For a detailed description of the above-named syndromes and management of functional somatic syndromes, see Henningsen, Zipfel and Herzog (2007, p. 55). Interpersonal psychotherapy has been shown to reduce both physical and mental symptoms in chronic fatigue syndrome and irritable bowel syndrome (Guthrie, Creed, Dawson, & Tomenson, 1991; Sharpe et al., 1996). Henningsen and colleagues have provided a detailed review of the literature on the treatment of functional somatic syndromes, and it is important to note that the psychological therapies such as CBT, hypnotherapy and Mindfulness-Based Therapy have low to moderate efficacy in IBS (Henningsen, Zipfel, Sattel, & Creed, 2018). Notwithstanding the above, there appears to be a clear signal that psychotherapy has a role in these patients presenting with persistent physical symptoms, hence offering hope.

4.6.2 BODILY SYMPTOMS, MENTAL PROCESSES AND DISORDERS

INTRODUCTION

The term 'somatisation' has roots grounded in psychoanalytical and psychodynamic theory and the historical definition of somatisation relied upon a prerequisite absence of medical condition and involved processes such as denial of conflict, repression of impulses and somatisation (an embodying) of the underlying emotional conflicts. This chapter will not cover the details of the psychodynamic tradition. DSM-5 and ICD-11 have reformulated disorders of somatisation.

Somatisation (see Figure 4.8) is a process by which normal physiological, psychological and social factors become converted into, and are expressed as physical symptoms. This is a process, not a diagnosis and it is unconscious (out of personal awareness). Somatisation occurs in a biopsychosocial context and includes a number of different elements: the *perception of physical symptoms*; the *attribution* of these symptoms to a physical disease or cause; *illness concern*, that is, concern or worry about having an illness; and *illness behaviour* which is the seeking of remedial help. The severity of somatisation presentation varies remarkably, ranging from mild symptoms (without impairment) through to severe impairment and disability. Presentations encountered in practice may be complex—a common finding for instance is the co-occurrence of known medical condition with a superimposed psychological component, for example, a person may present with acute or chronic abdominal pain on a background of alcohol-related chronic pancreatitis in the context of a breakdown of a marital relationship and comorbid depression. Firstly in the examination of somatisation we will set out a pragmatic approach to how somatisation can be understood, then we will explore the evidence and relevant understandings around the mechanisms operating in this context, beginning here to consider how these understandings may be applied in mental health care for people with such problems.

PHYSICAL SYMPTOMS: PERCEPTION AND RESPONSE

Context and attention

The experience of any symptoms is mediated through an interplay between biology, psychology and sociocultural context. The flourishing biological literature on perception of symptoms, pain in particular, has shed light on the complex interplay between the body and the mind. Detailing the biological research is beyond the scope of this chapter, however, the psychological and sociocultural factors will be explicated. A serious injury gained during the rush of a sporting match may not be felt until much later and yet an apparently trivial injury at work may result in persisting symptoms and severe disability. The experience of a bodily symptom is determined, in part, by the level of consciousness and attention given to it, as well as to the 'attribution' of symptoms.

Attribution

Here the individual seeks to answer questions such as: What has caused my symptoms? Is it a result of some stress in my life? Or is it caused by a serious physical disease?

Attribution occurs at a conscious level, but is influenced by a range of social, cultural and personal values. Some of these will be consciously held, but many will be held outside conscious awareness. In 'somatisation' there is a premature and persistent judgement made of a physical attribution of cause. Studies indicate that patients with a physical/somatic attributional style report fewer emotional problems to the doctor and reporting more obscure somatic complaints (Kirmayer & Robbins, 1996). In turn, doctors are more likely to diagnose a psychological problem when patients attribute their symptoms to a psychological cause (Greer, Halgin, & Harvey, 2004), and as a corollary, search for a physical cause when the patient presents a physical attribution. In other words, patient attribution style is very important in determining the trajectory of medical care. Similarly, clinicians are at risk of falling victim to confirmation bias, seeking only information that confirms their hypothesis.

Illness concern

Attribution determines the level of concern and how much the person will worry. It involves an affective component (anxiety) as well as cognitions (thoughts and worry). The combination of worry about getting or having an illness, a preoccupying concern about bodily symptoms, and a somatic attributional style underpin somatisation.

Illness behaviour

Finally, the illness concern determines what the person will do about the symptoms (behavioural component). Do they take on the 'sick role', go to bed, take time off work or visit the doctor? Do they ignore the symptom stoically and continue to work despite the pain? The concept of the sick role and illness behaviour (see Table 4.25) come from the sociological literature.

> I told you I was ill.
>
> *Spike Milligan, as inscribed on his tombstone*

Figure 4.7 The process of somatisation

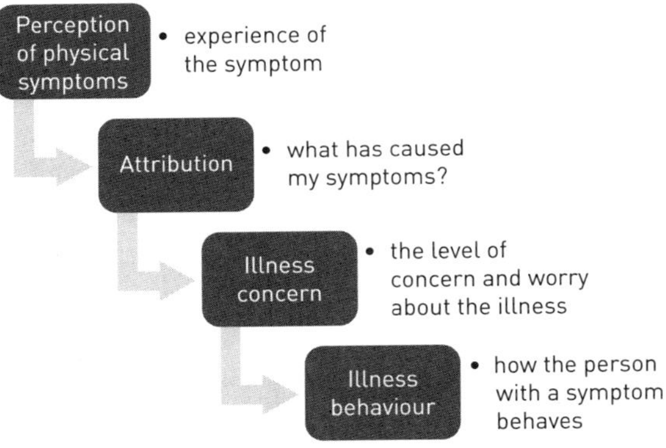

In the process of somatisation, there may be amplification in one or more of the steps and this may in turn lead to behaviours that are viewed as normative

Table 4.25 Definitions of concepts

Somatisation A process by which emotional distress (psychological and social factors) becomes converted into, and expressed as, physical symptoms. Somatisation is a process of which the individual has no conscious knowledge. It is not a syndrome nor a diagnosis. It may be a trait phenomenon—a natural disposition of somatic concern—or a state phenomenon, as is often found in the acutely depressed person.
Sick role When disease occurs in a previously well individual, that person is granted certain privileges (exemption from work and other responsibilities, is offered care) but also has obligations (to seek and accept appropriate treatment and to get better). This is a sociological concept, and the specifics of the sick role will be determined by the sociocultural context.
Illness behaviour In the sociological literature, 'illness behaviour' is used to describe the whole process, being defined as 'the ways in which individuals experience, perceive, evaluate and respond to their own health status' (Mechanic, 1968). Put simply, it describes the behaviour of the sick person, the one in the sick role. Some people will be stoical, others dramatic. Some may seem to minimise symptoms, others exaggerate them.
Abnormal illness behaviour The concept of *abnormal illness behaviour* is very useful in considering somatisation (Kirmayer & Robbins, 1996). This is defined as 'an inappropriate or maladaptive mode of experiencing, evaluating or acting in relation to one's own state of health' (Pilowsky, 1997). 'Inappropriate' and 'maladaptive' is always a matter of judgement and dependent on the context. Often there is a discrepancy between what the patient thinks is wrong with them and what the clinician's appraisal is of the problem; this discrepancy is exemplified in the somatoform disorders. An example is someone who accepts the benefits of the sick role without meeting the other obligations of being a patient.
Alexithymia People who are unable to put words to their feelings (and distress) and so the distress is expressed in somatic terms. They focus on the details of external events while having great difficulty describing the internal emotional experience.

at one end of the spectrum to maladaptive at the other. Note also, what is adaptive in one context may be inappropriate in another. For example, a 9-year-old may complain of tummy pains and ask for a day off school because the school bully is back on the prowl, so will not meet the diagnostic threshold for disorder. A middle-aged man wakes up in the morning with severe chest pain. The first thing that comes to mind is that it is probably a heart attack. His father died of a heart attack and he is the right age for it and, yes, he has been under stress at work. He is, reasonably, concerned, shares that concern with his wife and they decide to call an ambulance. Here somatisation is not so much 'abnormal' but rather involves a distortion or exaggeration in elements of the process.

This is a good time to remind ourselves of the words of Engel: 'the inclusion of somatic and psychosocial factors is indispensable (in health care) and central to our understanding of human experience of health and illness' (Engel, 1977). Social status, social supports, education, socioeconomic status and issues of access to health care need to be borne in mind at all times. Cultural factors have been implicated in the experience of symptoms such as pain and menopause, delay in health care seeking and the doctor-patient relationship being influenced by gender. The interested reader is directed to the work of Uskul (2010), who articulated in detail the role of sociocultural aspects of health and illness.

4.6.3 BODILY DISTRESS DISORDER

FORMAL DIAGNOSIS

Bodily distress disorder (BDD) involves bodily symptoms that are distressing–sometimes single symptoms but often multiple symptoms–varying over time but present most days for some months. Excessive attention is drawn to these symptoms, often with repeated contact with health care providers, with secondary impairment, anywhere from mild to severe. Whether or not these are related to an identified health condition, the attention to them is excessive. A person may experience symptoms and significant emotional distress and/or result in significant disability when an underlying pathology is either absent or elusive. Further, even where pathology is present, the symptoms may not fully be explained, or symptoms may persist despite treatment of the underlying condition. In summary, the key features include excessive worry and associated behaviours and the presence or absence of organic pathology is less relevant and not necessary to make a positive diagnosis. There is an equivalent diagnosis, Bodily Stress Syndrome (BSS) intended for use in primary care (ICD-11 PHC) to allow for patients who may only have one or two symptoms and a more conservative concept than BDD (Ivbijaro et al., 2019).

WHAT DO WE KNOW ABOUT BDD?

Prevalence, including comorbidity and public health impact

Prevalence data on the bodily distress disorder category is emerging at present but as stated previously, the ICD-11 diagnosis of bodily distress disorder encompasses most of the diagnoses subsumed under the umbrella term of somatoform disorders (with the exception of hypochondriasis and conversion disorder; see Chapter 4.4) and, therefore, it is likely that the prevalence rates will be in the order of that described for the somatoform disorders. In a review of prevalence rates of somatoform disorders in a primary care setting across 24 countries (Haller, Cramer, Lauche, & Dobos, 2015), about 40-49% had at least one medically unexplained symptom, 26-35% met the criteria for at least one somatoform disorder and 0.8-5.9% had the strictly defined severe and chronic form of somatisation disorder, the most severe form of the disorder (Haller et al., 2015). In a study of general medical ward admissions, one in five patients met the diagnostic criteria for somatoform disorder (ICD-10 or DSM-IV), and comorbidity with another psychiatric disorder was common (Fink, Hansen, & Oxhoj, 2004).

A recent Danish cross-sectional study found 16% of the general population had a bodily distress syndrome and 16% had at least one functional somatic syndrome (Petersen et al., 2019). BDD is associated with higher health care costs and longer-term disability and this is particularly so for those with multiple symptoms (Rask, Ornbol, Rosendal, & Fink, 2017; Creed et al., 2013).

Anxiety and depressive disorders are three times more likely and a quarter of somatoform disorder patients also have an anxiety or depressive disorder. Interestingly more than 50% of individuals with a primary anxiety or depressive disorder also met the criteria for a somatoform disorder (de Waal, Arnold, Eekhof, & van Hemert, 2004). Personality disorders, especially the paranoid, obsessive-compulsive and histrionic subtypes, were also found to be frequently comorbid (Garcia-Campayo, Alda, Sobradiel, Olivan, & Pascual, 2007). One in three persons with a borderline personality disorder (BPD) were found to also have a somatoform disorder and one in six persons with a somatoform disorder were found to also have a BPD (Schmaling & Fales, 2018). In summary, comorbidity is common and there is substantial overlap with other psychiatric disorders.

PRACTICE ILLUSTRATION: ENGAGEMENT AND ASSESSMENT

Maria, a 59-year-old woman, attends the emergency department complaining of pain in her legs. She has presented three times in the past two months with the same symptoms. Each time she has seen a different doctor, and a variety of investigations have been conducted with no clear cause of her symptoms identified. Maria does have a history of diabetes and ischaemic heart disease. She has no history of mental disorders. On this visit to the emergency department, she is accompanied by her husband and daughter. While Maria has fair English, when she is stressed her comprehension seems to diminish and she misunderstands what is said to her. The physical examination, on this occasion as before, is normal, and her diabetes and heart disease appear well controlled. The doctor speaks to the mental health worker in the emergency department, who agrees to speak with Maria. The mental health worker interviews Maria in the emergency department and obtains the following story. Maria migrated to Australia from Italy when she was 22 years old. She met her husband, who had been born in Australia to Italian parents, shortly after she arrived, and they married 12 months later. They have four children, all of whom have left home, although only her eldest daughter is married. There are no grandchildren. She describes her husband as a 'good provider' and says that their marriage is happy. She frequently comments on the marital status of her children and the lack of grandchildren, and wonders if she has been a bad mother. Her husband has recently retired, and she finds it stressful to have him around the house all the time. She has a small number of close friends but has been finding it difficult to leave the house and visit them, feeling a responsibility for looking after her husband while he is at home. Maria is very worried about the pain in her legs and feels that the doctors have not been listening to her. She does not have a regular GP and attends a large general practice clinic for the monitoring of her diabetes and heart disease, where she sees a different doctor each time she attends.

HOW CAN WE UNDERSTAND THE ORIGINS?

Biological findings

Approximately 30% of the genetic variance in somatic distress has been found to be secondary to genes unrelated to those linked with depression and anxiety (Gillespie, Zhu, Heath, Hickie, & Martin, 2000). A family history of functional syndromes and bodily distress is commonly encountered in practice, likely a combination of genetics and modelling influences (Osborne & Hatcher, 1989; Levy et al., 2004). MRI findings of somatoform disorder patients suggest selective impairments in specific cortico-limbic regions associated with the neuromatrix of pain and the emotion regulation system (Delvecchio et al., 2019). Research also suggests other neurobiological mechanisms including: failure of habituation (habituation being the diminution of response of neurones following repeated stimuli; Horvath, Friedman, & Meares, 1980), or somatosensory amplification (experiencing everyday sensations as intense and noxious; Barsky, Goodson, Lane, & Cleary, 1988).

Individual psychological factors

A family history of medical illness may serve as a model for the specific illness expression. Considering the developmental and family context, typically, there may be a history of emotional deprivation, in which authentic emotional expression was discouraged but physical illness was attended to. The child learns not to report emotional matters, instead reporting symptoms to secure a caring response. Carrying forward this relational style into adulthood, what can emerge is a pattern of emotional expression and ways of relating to others through expression of illness. There may be a history of childhood chronic medical conditions and frequent hospitalisations. Hospitalisation is a very emotional event involving separation from parents (with resulting feelings of abandonment and loss of attachment). On the other hand, the child may receive special care from health care staff and concerned parents while in hospital. Childhood sexual abuse, which often induces feelings of guilt and low self-esteem, is associated with somatisation (Morrison, 1989), especially in functional neurological disorders (Karatzias et al., 2017). As stated previously, personality disorder may also predispose to BDD and related problems; paranoid, obsessive-compulsive and histrionic personality disorder have been found frequently to co-occur with somatisation (Garcia-Campayo et al., 2007)

Immediate family factors

Around the time of onset of the medically unexplained symptoms there is often a significant change in the nature and quality of relationships within the family. The precipitating event may be the loss or the threat of loss of a relationship or a response to a family crisis. Abandonment or estrangement are common precipitants. And so, the symptoms may represent the person's (unconscious) attempt to either solve or avoid a significant family crisis or conflict. At the very least, the symptoms 'halt the progression of time' so as to allow the person time to work through the family crisis. Enquiring about this person's place in the family may be central to understanding the meaning and function of the symptom. For instance, the young person with chronic abdominal pain may be able to keep her parents' fragile marriage intact and giving up the symptom may mean risking the integrity of the family unit. Conversely, the parents may focus on the pain as a distraction from a loveless marriage. Notwithstanding the potential aetiological role of family, they are also the vehicle for change. Addressing family dynamics can therefore be crucial for recovery.

Sociocultural factors

The value a person attaches to an illness will depend on the traditions and values of the society. Physical illnesses legitimise the sick role (to be cared for and to be absolved of societal expectations to study, to form relationships or to earn a living). Often conflict in the workplace sets the stage for an illness which offers the opportunity for a quick exit from the situation. Over time, the illness allows the person a face-saving strategy to avoid returning to their workplace where they were perhaps bullied.

IATROGENIC FACTORS

The health sector can also perpetuate such conditions. Implicit in the doctor-patient relationship is the notion that the relationship will continue so long as there is suffering (the symptom) and when the symptom is alleviated this relationship will end. Giving up the symptom also means giving up this sometimes crucial relationship. Additionally, the more a person feels invalidated or stigmatised by clinicians the more likely they will somatise. It is not uncommon for people to feel unheard in the medical context and it is vital to remain empathic and professional at all times. The person may be driven to prove the existence of physical illness and feel the need to dismiss any associated psychosocial factors. If the person is absolved of legal sanction or likely to gain financially they may have a protracted course. For instance, if the person has income protection that is contingent on a certain level of disability it is easy to imagine the pressure this person may be under. Recovery may come at a substantial cost, and risks putting the individual in very same context in which the symptoms initially emerged. In terms of financial losses, BDD and related problems can be difficult to differentiate from factitious disorders and the rare event of malingering.

PRACTICE ILLUSTRATION: TREATMENT

After discussing Maria's symptoms with the medical registrar, the mental health worker comes to the conclusion that they are likely to be stress-related. The symptoms have both a symbolic and real effect of getting her out of the house and receiving care. Little is known about Maria's family of origin at this stage, and a reminder note is made to inquire about this, as this may help to understand the fears and disappointments that Maria is experiencing associated with her children leaving home and her husband retiring. In addition, her early illness experiences (her own or her family's) may provide a model for her present condition and explain the meaning of illness for her.

The mental health worker discusses with Maria the impact of stress on her physical health and arranges for Maria to attend the local community health centre, which has a general practitioner who speaks Italian. In addition, Maria is able to speak with a counsellor about her worries and is encouraged to talk with her husband about her feelings. Maria's husband also attends some sessions with the counsellor and identifies his fear that he no longer has a useful role now that he is retired. The counsellor arranges for him to become a volunteer at a local aged care facility, where he is able to assist with minor repairs to the buildings.

SOME POINTS OF SYNTHESIS

Some key points then are offered arising from this review regarding causality and implications for approach to care for people with BDD and related problems.

Aetiology and clinical presentation can be heterogeneous and identification of comorbidities, such as depression, drug abuse and relationship difficulties is vital. It is important to understand predisposing and precipitating factors, noting that these factors, if unaddressed, quickly become perpetuating factors. Perpetuating factors perhaps require the most attention because they may offer a roadmap to remediation, recovery and prevention.

A somatic focus is supported by cognitions, illness worry, learnt behaviours and eventually the wider system of family, health care practitioners and systems of compensation. In some circumstances, legal and compensation issues become superimposed, which further maintain the illness behaviour. While in some ways the person pays a heavy price for the symptoms/illness through impairment and disability, the hope of recovery may also come with fear—it invariably involves yet another change to the status quo and may mean giving up some gains as well resulting from the somatisation process.

ASSESSMENT

Broadly understanding the BDD presentation

An important consideration in any disease presentation is the extent to which psychological factors play a role. Identifying an illness as either psychogenic or biogenic can be overly simplistic in ignoring interactions between multiple biopsychosocial factors. Aetiology is complex and multifactorial, and can be considered from a number of points of view.

Clinician practice in assessment of possible BDD

Practice challenges in recognition

While this is a common medical problem, clinicians need to be aware of the barriers in making a positive diagnosis in primary care, as shown in Table 4.26.

Full and proper evaluation of the physical problem

Taking a detailed medical history with a biopsychosocial approach is vital as is a thorough physical examination. In addition, patients need to know that reasonable care has been taken to exclude physical disease. Knowing how far to go with investigations, and when to stop, is part of the 'art' of management. Suggest necessary tests and discuss the results in a reassuring manner being mindful to not come across as trivialising. This approach engenders confidence in the patient (and the clinician) that the right diagnosis will be made and it then gives the clinician credibility when a mental health diagnosis is ultimately made.

Understanding the factors beyond the symptom

Alongside the evaluation of the physical symptom and the patient narrative, the clinician should ask the question, 'What else is going on here?' Michael Balint, a great student of general practice and a psychoanalyst,

Table 4.26 Barriers to making a diagnosis

Factor	Example(s)
Patient related	The history is presented in a manner that overwhelms the doctor or cannot be integrated, the patient holds a biomedical view or feels that it would be inappropriate to bring up psychological factors during the consultation
Primary Care Physician	Entrenched dualistic thinking (either mental or physical) rather than mind and body (Henningsen et al., 2018) Inability to fully explore the psychosocial context. Internal attitudes towards patients who somatise and lack of confidence Interestingly, confirmation bias may lead the clinician to make a premature diagnosis or a delayed diagnosis
Doctor-Patient Interactional	Something happens in the interaction that may lead to over-investigation and a premature diagnosis of a medical disorder and avoidance of exploring the context of the symptom. Difficulty in finding common ground when there is a fundamental disagreement on the causation of the symptom
Situational	Brief appointment times, nonspecific symptoms, complexity, problem of comorbidity (with physical illness and other psychiatric disorders)
Conceptual and Operational	Physical illness is seen as more acceptable as psychosocial suffering, mind-body dualism, and blurred diagnostic boundaries

Source: Adapted from Murray, Toussaint, Althaus, & Löwe, 2016

has made the point that every illness is also the 'vehicle' for attention and care; that is, the presenting symptom is not necessarily the real problem—there may be a broader issue. The physical symptom is just the ticket for entry and the physical illness is simply the form of communication (Marinker, 1970, p. 80).

It is important to aim to answer the question, 'Why is this person presenting in this way at this time?' that is, create a biopsychosocial formulation. The formulation will be discussed between doctor and patient as part of 'finding the common ground', discussed below. It will also direct the doctor in management and facilitate the process of reducing the somatic focus and developing a broader perspective on the problem. Helpful for this may be consideration of Table 4.27, which highlights key risk factors that make a person vulnerable to experiencing bodily symptoms and somatoform disorders. Often there is a triggering event such as a loss or threat. The 'event' occurs in a social milieu which also needs to be considered. Symptoms may become chronic if the context in which the symptoms arose is not understood and appropriately managed.

PRACTICE ILLUSTRATION: OUTCOME

Six months later, Maria is feeling much better. The bodily symptom occurs only occasionally. The GP is monitoring her diabetes and heart disease, and she has not felt the need to attend the emergency department. She is more satisfied now she is seeing the same doctor regularly. Maria also finds it useful that the GP is able to speak Italian, so that she is able to express her problems more clearly. She is no longer seeing the counsellor, but often drops in to say hello when she is visiting the community health centre. Maria is very happy that her husband is now volunteering at an aged care facility; she feels he is more independent and that she can return to her usual activities. She continues to lament the absence of grandchildren but is hopeful that her daughter will become pregnant soon.

Table 4.27 Framework for understanding the presentation

	Biological	Individual	Social
Predisposing factors	Factors that make a person vulnerable. These are remote or historical factors		
	Female adolescent Genetics Underlying medical condition Failure of habituation Somatosensory amplification Dysregulation of neuromatrix of pain and emotional regulation	Early modelling Abuse/neglect Anxiety and tendency to worry Personality and personality disorder	Low education Societal view of mental illness, and the legitimacy of physical illness Modelled behaviour of medical condition
Precipitating factors	Factors that temporally correlate with the onset of the symptom. Ask the question 'What was happening in your life when you first started to feel ill?'		
	Infective (viral or bacterial) illness can precipitate IBS or CFS suggestive of an inflammatory process Progression of underlying medical condition Physical injury	A life event that has meaning for the person or a change in the nature and quality of a key relationship The event may evoke feelings of threat and loss Anger, shame, guilt may emerge and these feelings need to be managed; the symptom may provide a solution to the problem	The illness achieves some form of homeostasis in relationships at a time of dysfunction The illness removes person from a dreaded situation e.g. work stress Or manages a family problem or diverts family attention Creates a dependent relationship Financial compensation or freedom from legal sanction
Perpetuating factors	Factors that lead to ongoing distress and impairment or chronicity. Over time, a kind of homeostasis is achieved which maintains the status quo		
	Ongoing medical illness Comorbid depression or anxiety	Ongoing chronic stressors High health anxiety, catastrophic thinking, body checking, illness conviction and avoidance or reassurance seeking behaviours Experience of shame and loss and the illness helps avoid shame Anxiety, depression and demoralisation	Reinforcing effects of family behaviour towards their illness, financial compensation, the health care system which may perpetuate the condition Poor access and inequity in service distribution
Protective factors	These are mitigating factors		
	Few symptoms Short duration	Psychological mindedness Coping strategies and problem-solving skills Motivation to improve their situation	Supportive family system

From a cognitive behavioural perspective, the person may exhibit substantial health anxiety and worry. They may be distressed by catastrophic thinking and feel the pressure to repeatedly scan their bodies and check for evidence of disease or avoid doing what they perceive to be exacerbating factors. They may seek reassurance by seeking frequent medical reviews or request investigations. These behaviours perpetuate their distress and impairment. While it may be that the person is deeply distressed by the symptom which is attributed purely to a physical condition and psychological factors are minimised or denied, it may also be that the bodily symptom is overshadowed by the degree of emotional distress and concern—or the person may appear relatively unconcerned by symptoms causing (described psychodynamically as *'la belle indifference'*). Searching for a temporal correlation between the onset of the symptom and a life event and identifying a significant change in key relationship may help the clinician understand the person's experience and also the underlying feelings of threat or loss (real or perceived), for example, domestic violence may present bodily symptoms. Not uncommonly, there are deeper feelings of dependency, anger, shame and guilt but these are kept at bay, and embodied in the physical symptom. Somatisation may serve a homeostatic self-regulatory function (to maintain psychological integrity) or reflect an attempt to manage the dynamic with another. The symptom may serve a function to control or punish another, or fulfil a need to punish oneself (in response to feelings of guilt or shame). During the assessment, it would be useful to enquire about the thoughts and feelings about the symptom and observe their behaviours in relation to the symptom, also asking oneself, 'How does the symptom change the way the person sees themselves and the impact on the relationship?'

EVIDENCE-BASED AND OTHER TREATMENTS

The key management issues are to:

- engage the person and focus on the therapeutic relationship
- formulate the presentation (perpetuating factors in particular)
- adopt a stepped care approach based on severity
- encourage a rehabilitative approach rather than focus on a symptom cure and
- avoid a range of forms of iatrogenic harm (see also Chapter 1.5).

Reattribution and reassurance

The therapeutic technique of making a link between the physical symptom and the context is called 'reattribution', the main steps of which are listed in Table 4.28. The aim of reattribution is to reduce the somatic preoccupation, encourage the patient to think about psychological issues, and link the physical symptoms with emotions and life events. This gives an explanation of the physical symptoms to the patient, and also serves to educate him or her about their body and bodily symptoms.

Table 4.28 Steps in reattribution

Step 1: Making the patient feel understood This is done by taking a careful history, evaluating the physical symptoms thoroughly, and exploring the psychosocial context to formulate the problem.
Step 2: Broadening the agenda In the patient with physical symptoms broaden the agenda by sharing the formulation with the person and asking them to wonder whether their physical symptoms could be due to their stress, depression or anxiety. If they are willing to consider this, one then goes on to indicate the evidence for that proposition. 'What was happening in your life when you first started to feel ill?'
Step 3: Making the link Give a simple explanation of how these different aspects are related.

Source: Adapted from Gask, 1995

After reattribution the person needs more reassurance and further explanation, and reinforcement of the changed attribution will need to be given. Addressing the key precipitating and perpetuating biopsychosocial factors is central to recovery.

Building an alliance: finding common ground

Underpinning the problem with communication is an even more basic problem: a disagreement about what the problem is. The patient may be convinced that he or she has a primarily physical disease. The doctor and other health practitioners may think that it is primarily psychological. Indeed, health practitioners may not agree. The correct answer is most probably somewhere in the middle; that is, there are both physical and psychosocial contributions. For a doctor and patient to work together, there has to be some agreement. This is called 'finding common ground', and is part of developing a treatment alliance. Time needs to be spent discussing with the patient what each thinks is the nature of the problem, finding the common ground and making an alliance in the pursuit of moving forwards. Often, whether the problem is primarily physical or psychological cannot be agreed upon, and it is unwise to focus on this disagreement. What can be agreed is that the pain or other symptom is disabling. Doctor and patient can then work towards developing realistic goals of ameliorating symptoms and maximising the level of functioning.

Remaining therapeutic

Good routine medical care can prevent acute bodily symptoms from becoming chronic (Mayou, 2014). A breakdown of the therapeutic relationship can be traumatic for the person and often this means that the person has to consult yet another unfamiliar clinician. Reminding oneself that the patient is not feigning the symptoms, and remembering that stress can lead to physical symptoms will influence how we approach the symptom and the person's experience of the consultation. Much like the person who goes through a roller coaster of emotions in this complex journey, so does the clinician. Fear of missing a diagnosis (which fosters litigation concerns), self-doubt, anger and therapeutic nihilism may impact on the clinician's ability to remain therapeutic. Conflict with other health professionals needs to be avoided. Support the persons request for complementary therapies but also encourage self-management.

Case management: communication and coordination

Some patients, of course, do not respond to reattribution or reassurance; symptoms persist, and somatisation becomes chronic. The general practitioner plays a pivotal role as mediator, coordinator and communicator. Case management and good communication between health practitioners, family and welfare agencies become the most important aspects of successful management. The language used needs to be geared towards a mind-body interaction rather than suggest dualistic mindset. Suggest that psychosocial contextual factors amplify rather than cause the symptom. Schedule regular appointments for review to avoid a situation where the patient needs to have a symptom in order to have an appointment with their doctor (Kurlansik & Maffei, 2016).

Goal setting

It is important to set realistic and achievable goals, particularly goals the patient values coupled with a comfort rather than cure stance. Avoid myopic goals that are contingent upon symptom resolution or ones that suggest an overinvestment in medications. Instead encourage and maintain a broader biopsychosocial lens. Suggest relaxation, exercise, good diet and graded exercise.

General counselling

Reattribution and general psychological intervention is a very important aspect of the medical management. Attention and empathy can themselves be therapeutic and satisfying their need for care and convey realistic hope. Negative or pessimistic thoughts can also be identified and corrected using methods of cognitive therapy. Helping the patient see any links between events, emotional state and level of physical symptoms can be enlightening, enabling an understanding of how the physical symptoms are related to emotions.

Role of family

The family are a source of collateral information that will inform the formulation and, therefore, management. An explanation given to the family about the nature of the problem will help allay fears and recruit support. As conditions become chronic, family members frequently become fatigued and uninterested in the patient's state, and reduce their interest and support.

Psychotherapy

Treatment as usual involves building an alliance, remaining therapeutic, goal setting, general counselling, care coordination as described above. A key question is whether the patient requires formal psychotherapy or is 'treatment as usual' (TAU) good enough? The answer isn't straightforward: for some people, TAU may be good enough; for others, formal psychotherapy may yield better outcomes.

In a meta-analysis, Koelen et al. (2014) demonstrate significant reduction in physical symptoms and functional impairment in patients treated with psychotherapy in comparison to treatment as usual (TAU), for severe disorders in secondary and tertiary care. Also, there were clinically meaningful, but not statistically significant, improvements in psychological symptoms in both groups. A recent meta-analysis, concluded that cognitive behaviour therapy (CBT) was a more effective treatment than treatment as usual for somatoform disorders and medically unexplained physical symptoms (Liu, Gill, Teodorczuk, Li, & Sun, 2019) in reducing severity of symptoms of anxiety and depression but the improvement in physical functioning was less robust and the study was unable to demonstrate a change in social functioning or a change in the number of doctor visits (Liu et al., 2019). Mindfulness-based therapy (Lakhan & Schofield, 2013) and psychodynamic psychotherapy (Koelen et al., 2014) were all effective.

In the context of being uncertain on which treatment modality to apply, the clinician must turn to medical ethics as a guide. Principles of beneficence and respect for autonomy must guide our choice, and as such the patient should make an informed choice on the treatment modality that best suits their needs. Pragmatically speaking, a stepped care approach is suggested with TAU as first-line for the milder forms and formal psychotherapy (of any modality) as first-line for the more severe forms or in cases with a comorbid anxiety or depressive disorder.

Medication

Analgesics and hypnotics are prone to overuse leading to tolerance and dependence while narcotic analgesics should not be used for chronic pain of unknown aetiology. Antidepressants have been found to have some useful effects in medically unexplained symptoms (O'Malley et al., 1999). Tricyclics (of which amitriptyline was the most researched) were more effective than selective serotonin reuptake inhibitors (fluoxetine was most efficacious of these) in pain and in improving functional status. There is modest evidence for the usefulness of antidepressant medication in the severe and chronic somatisation disorder (Kroenke, 2007) which would now be classed within BDD in ICD-11. Antidepressants can augment analgesics especially in those with comorbid depression in combination with psychotherapy.

Physical and behavioural therapies

Physical therapies (such as physiotherapy, exercise and massage) aimed at improving physical functioning and healing soft-tissue injuries are obviously important in the treatment of pain syndromes. Because there is no cure, consider only simple, non-invasive interventions. Invasive investigations reaffirm the sick role and set unreasonable expectations that only lead to disappointment. Treatments that focus on improving functioning, such as physiotherapy combined with gentle, patient-initiated exercise such as swimming, are particularly important.

Chronic disorders require physical therapy (such as physiotherapy and hydrotherapy) combined with behavioural interventions. Formally structured rehabilitation programs are useful for people with chronic illness and disability, and this is just as true when the diagnosis is a somatoform as it is for rheumatoid arthritis. Behavioural interventions usually consist of a program with graded targets of improved functioning: there is a reduced focus on symptoms (such as pain) and more on functioning. A diary will help identify the pattern of discomfort or disability as well as the level of analgesic use. The current level of functioning should be ascertained, and goals set for increasing the level of functioning; for instance, distance walked, distance swum and time spent out of bed. Sleep may be a problem, and again a diary may assist to clarify the issues here. Attention to sleep hygiene (such as through improved diet and exercise, and reduced coffee and stimulation) might be relevant. Because much of the time patients are preoccupied with the physical symptoms and disability, exploring with them opportunities for enjoyable activities might be a beneficial strategy. This will help patients rediscover important things in life apart from their illness.

Dealing with treatment resistance and chronicity

Acute somatisation, such as the functional neurological disorder, often gets better with usual medical attention and care. The common somatisation presenting to general practitioners can often be dealt with easily by reattribution, and attention to the depression or other emotional issues in the manner described. Chronic somatisation is, on the other hand, by definition, chronic and difficult to treat. Such cases are very difficult for doctors, who can feel the same impotence, shame and failure that the patient may feel. They may resent the demands of the patients, or be inclined to seek relief by referral to yet another clinician. All these emotions must be contained. For this reason, it is important to have good support and good communication between the different health carers. When things seem difficult, it is time to have a case conference or at least a telephone conversation. Remember that the way the health professional feels is only a small reflection of what the patient and family are feeling. Managing chronic BDD patients is similar to managing patients with other chronic conditions, such as rheumatoid arthritis and asthma, except that expectations are frequently different. (Once a symptom is determined to be psychogenic, patients are often given the expectation that their distress is exaggerated or invalid and they should get better.) Symptoms will wax and wane. They will not respond fully to treatment, and doctors, carers and patients must be prepared for this.

4.6.4 BODY INTEGRITY DYSPHORIA

In ICD-11, body integrity dysphoria (BID) is characterised by an intense and persistent desire to become physically disabled in a significant way (e.g., a wish to become a major limb amputee, paraplegic, paralysed, blind), with onset by early adolescence accompanied by persistent discomfort, or intense feelings of inappropriateness concerning current non-disabled body configuration. The person acknowledges the presence of the body part as being present on their person; however, the body part is seen as 'separate' or is disowned. The desire to become physically disabled results in harmful consequences, as manifested by a substantial period of time being spent as a disabled person e.g. by bandaging up the limb rendering it unusable and/or a preoccupation with the desire for amputation.

Little is known about the specific aetiology of this complex condition including why a person would choose one symptom over another or why a person would be driven to become disabled. For the purpose of this chapter the focus here is on the person requesting an amputation. Money and colleagues argued that BID is a condition wherein the stump, crutches or the wheelchair is eroticised and that amputation leads to sexual gratification (Money, Jobaris, & Furth, 1977). However, the sexual gratification theory is insufficient on its own to explain the disorder. Braam and colleagues hypothesise that this disorder is an amalgamation of obsessive-compulsive disorder (OCD), a body dysmorphic disorder and an identity disorder (Braam, Visser, Cath, & Hoogendijk, 2006). The key differences between body dysmorphic disorder and BID lie in the focus of the preoccupation. In BID, the focus is on the 'non-belonging' of the limb (e.g. the arm does not belong) and not a part of the self and hence driven to have it removed (amputated) from the body. In body dysmorphic disorder, the focus is on a perceived defect in appearance (e.g. the arm is seen as part of the self but is seen as being ugly) and hence undergo corrective cosmetic surgery. First (2005) argued that BID is more of a disorder of identity because many of the patients seeking amputation were in fact seeking their 'true identity' and their internal sense of who they were (sense of self) was at odds with their anatomy. Bruno (1997) has suggested that BID may a variant of factitious disorders given that some patients are driven to a state of disability or simulate disability in order to be cared for.

In addition to the above psychological theories there are some neurobiological ones as well. These theories have emerged from the phantom limb literature, suggestive of similar biological underpinnings. Body image is a consciously accessible representation of one's body (with continual inputs from visual, tactile, vestibular, motor and proprioceptive impulses). Body image combined with a perception of being in control of the body (sense of agency) which in turn form the basis of one's belief about body ownership (embodiment) and oneself (body identity; Bayne & Levy, 2005; Giummarra, Bradshaw, Nicholls, Hilti, & Brugger, 2011). A failure to represent a body part or a misrepresentation of the body part and/or the failure of multisensory integration can potentially lead to a mismatch between the afferent and efferent information systems and hence BID. There are post-war case reports after a peripheral injury to the limb, suggesting that the injury can lead to alienation and BID. Right parietal lobe lesions are also associated with similar alienation syndromes (with a desire for amputation on the left). Such lesions are hypothesised to 'decouple' the body map in the brain and the body itself as are lesions of the corpus callosum or medial frontal cortex (from tumour or stroke; Müller, 2009). The observation of childhood onset has led some researches to hypothesise that there may be neurodevelopmental antecedents (from a blood vessel anomaly or birth trauma).

There is no single aetiology and no known effective treatment. Traditional psychotherapies and antidepressants have not been found to be helpful. There are case reports of amputation of the desired limb leading to a remission of symptoms and an improvement in quality of life (Blom, Hennekam, & Denys, 2012) but not in others. Bayne and Levy (2005) argue that elective amputation can be ethically justified, however, the contrary position has also been argued.

4.6.5 LIVED EXPERIENCE

ANONYMOUS

I am a 38-year-old lady who currently lives independently. I am a qualified Chartered Accountant and have three Commerce degrees, including a Master's degree in International Accounting. I immigrated to Australia for a job opportunity in 2008, from South Africa where I grew up. My dream was to live in Australia after spending 12 months in Australia as a Rotary Exchange Student. In my early years, I lived with my parents, older sister and two dogs. I started competing as an elite swimmer at the age of 10 years and competed at the national level when I was 15 years old. I was required to train 3-5 hours per day throughout my schooling. I loved sport and played state cricket, club tennis, school volleyball, hockey and water polo. Due to the elite level of swimming I competed in, I was expected to be very disciplined with my time, diet and schoolwork. I was rarely allowed to go out and socialise with my friends due to training and competing. I was sexually assaulted by a family relative when I was 5 years old. I didn't know how to deal with this at the time so I immersed myself in sport and school work to try push any feelings away. I spent my entire childhood running from the trauma. Sport became my coping mechanism.

After moving to Australia, prior to my spinal injury, I lived a very full and active lifestyle. I worked very long hours for large financial companies and the Australian Government, as well as trained most days as a competitive rower, attended church and volunteered for several charitable organisations. I was strong, fit and healthy, and ignorantly thought I was untouchable. I used to push myself to be successful in all areas of my life. I didn't realise prior to my spinal injury I was filling my days with busyness to keep me from focusing on the trauma and pain of my childhood. Reflecting back on it I think I used sport to help me survive.

In 2012, I sustained a cervical spinal injury while racing in a rowing competition. I required spinal surgery, which didn't go according to plan. I was left with acute complications, which impacted my rehabilitation post operatively. Due to poor management of my spinal injury and rehabilitation I developed Complex Regional Pain Syndrome (CRPS) down my right side, lost function and I became totally immobilised. My bladder and gastrointestinal tract were compromised resulting in me being catheterised and wearing nappies. While in this state, I was sexually assaulted several times by a male nurse in the hospital. Consequently, I now struggle with poor sleep, anxiety and lose consciousness unpredictably. My physical condition as well as the trauma significantly impacted my ability to cope with the distress from such sudden life changing events. I spent four years in hospital in rehabilitation, medical and mental health wards. During this I became very frightened, was experiencing flashbacks and was sensitive to noise and light. My inability to cope caused me to attempt to commit suicide several times while in hospital. I was fragile, broken, on edge, sleep deprived, felt unclean and didn't want to carry on with life.

Although I have experienced several traumatic events in my life, I've learned that you can't let bad things define you. I'm not saying it is easy to just overcome traumatic events. It is a matter of putting things in place that are of importance to you to help you survive and heal. I chose to get up every day and do everything I possibly can to improve my physical and mental health and experience the best quality life. I am now able to walk unaided after being told in 2014 that I wouldn't walk again. Doing things I enjoy prevents me from getting disappointed and disheartened by the things I cannot yet do. Things I enjoy doing that help give me a sense of purpose and help manage my anxiety include hydrotherapy, physiotherapy, psychology sessions, art therapy, practising mindfulness, looking after my puppy whom I'm training to become an assistance dog, catching up with friends for a coffee, going for a walk at the beach, attending church, volunteering my time for causes that are important to me and studying Anatomy and Physiology so I can complete a Master's degree in occupational therapy. Although I'm not yet able to return to work or full-time study, I've learned to find pleasure in the small things such as sitting in the sun, listening to the birds, gardening, playing my harp and walking my puppy. I remind myself every day that no matter how bad life is there is always something to be grateful for.

4.6.6 PSYCHOLOGICAL OR BEHAVIOURAL FACTORS AFFECTING DISORDERS OR DISEASES

Psychological and behavioural factors may adversely affect the manifestation, treatment, or course of the disorder or disease by: interfering with the treatment of the disorder or disease by affecting treatment adherence or care seeking; constituting an additional health risk; or influencing the underlying pathophysiology to precipitate or exacerbate symptoms or otherwise necessitate medical attention. Such psychological factors may be thought to predispose, precipitate or exacerbate the condition in some significant way, interfere with the successful treatment or lead to exaggerated illness behaviour. Examples of psychological factors are stressful life events or an episode of depression. Behavioural factors that affect the disease process, such as drug abuse and noncompliance, are also examples of factors that could be considered under this term. This additional diagnosis should be assigned only when the factors increase the risk of suffering, disability, or death *and* represent a focus of clinical attention, and should be assigned together with the diagnosis for the relevant other condition.

This is a particularly cumbersome term, but one that has validity. It is derived from the concepts of psychosomatics, where there were certain disorders considered to be psychosomatic or psychophysiological. These included atopic dermatitis, hypertension, thyrotoxicosis, ulcerative colitis, peptic ulcer, rheumatoid arthritis and asthma. The concept that some diseases are psychosomatic and others not is outdated. Although there may be psychosocial factors involved in the genesis of these conditions, we also know a lot more about other biological and genetic risk factors. Similarly, we also now appreciate that psychosocial factors can contribute to the onset or progression of any disease.

While each case must be treated individually, there is a substantial literature now describing the psychological contributions commonly encountered in respect of particular medical disorders (Clarke & Currie, 2009). We should also note that depression and anxiety are very common in people with physical illness. It can be difficult to tease out the direction of causality in this situation, although there is evidence that causality works in both directions. Certainly, having a physical illness is a strong risk factor for depression. Causality is worked out in the individual case by listening to the patient narrative, understanding the sequence of events, and listening to what sense the patient makes of these.

While a comprehensive review of the literature is beyond the scope of this chapter, the following diseases illustrate the complex relationship between physical and mental disorders. The co-occurrence of a psychiatric disorder and a medical condition warrant assertive treatment of both conditions concurrently.

ISCHAEMIC HEART DISEASE

The heart has for a long time been closely identified with emotions, and it is therefore not surprising that it has attracted psychosomatic interest. The focus of attention has been on the effects of stress (acute and chronic) and depression. Chronic stress is an independent risk factor for coronary heart disease (and poor cardiovascular prognosis) and acute stress has been known to precipitate acute coronary events. Stresses (acute and chronic) lead to an upregulation of the sympathetic nervous system (increasing catecholamines) and upregulation of the hypothalamic pituitary adrenal axis (increasing cortisol and reducing glucocorticoid sensitivity). The downstream effects include an acute immune response and inflammation of the (coronary) blood vessels (Wirtz & von Kanel, 2017). More recently, attention has turned to clinical depression, which has also been shown to be a risk factor for coronary artery disease. Depression is also common after myocardial infarction, occurring in around 20% of patients, and confers an increased mortality of between two and four times in the year following infarction, the risk being proportional to the severity of depression (Wulsin, 2004). The physiological mechanisms linking stress, depression and cardiac death appear to be related to changes in autonomic activity (measured by heart rate variability), inflammation and platelet reactivity (Stapelberg, Neumann, Shum, McConnell, & Hamilton-Craig, 2011).

STROKE

Depression is a potent and possibly independent risk factor for stroke. Diabetes, small vessel disease and hypertension are perhaps confer cumulative risk (Dong, Zhang, Tong, & Qin, 2012). Furthermore, for patients with stroke, the presence of depression confers an increased risk of death and poorer rehabilitation.

DIABETES MELLITUS

There is a bidirectional association between depression and diabetes complications. People with depression are more likely to develop diabetes through various biological and lifestyle mechanisms and people with diabetes are more likely to develop depression, although this association is weaker than the former. When depression is comorbid with diabetes, vascular complications of diabetes and non-adherence are more likely (Nouwen et al., 2019).

CANCER

Historically there was some interest in linking personality style, adverse life events and depression as risk factors for developing cancer. This is yet to be proven (McKenna, Zevon, Corn, & Rounds, 1999). The literature, however, provides stronger support for the role of psychosocial factors in cancer progression (as opposed to onset). Researchers have shown that patients exhibiting a 'fighting spirit', as opposed to hopelessness and helplessness, survive longer (Watson, Haviland, Greer, Davidson, & Bliss, 1999), and that depression is associated with noncompliance with cancer treatment and poorer outcomes (DiMatteo, Lepper, & Croghan, 2000).

4.6.7 FACTITIOUS DISORDER

While most people who present for health care accurately report their experience of symptoms, some patients deny or exaggerate symptoms and an even smaller number simulate or feign them. Factitious disorders, in ICD-11, are characterised by intentionally feigning, falsifying, inducing, or aggravating medical, psychological, or behavioural signs and symptoms or injury (see Table 4.29). This can be observed in the person presenting or someone else who is presented as the person who is unwell, most commonly a child dependent. Where a pre-existing disorder or disease is present, the person intentionally aggravates existing symptoms or falsifies or induces additional symptoms. For people with factitious disorders, the goal is to receive care and to be cared for through adopting the role of the patient. There is no other obvious external gain. While the person may be fully aware of their illness behaviours, they may not be entirely aware or are unaware of their motivations for such behaviours, that is, to be cared for (the sick role). Most the available literature understandably focuses on those presenting with physical symptoms. Patients with factitious psychiatric or psychological symptoms are particularly difficult to diagnose. McCullumsmith and Ford (2011) identified three subsets of factitious disorders. First, the common factitious disorder (which is discussed here). The second, Munchausen syndrome subset, refers to patients who simulate their symptoms, who report a complex medical history with grand tales of travel and achievements (pseudologia fantastica) despite the illness and a history of care in multiple hospitals often in many states. Lastly, there is the Munchausen by proxy subset, which is typically a mother who presents her dependent child as the person who is sick.

Table 4.29 Differentiation of bodily distress and factitious disorders and malingering

	Illness behaviour	Motivation	Management
Bodily distress disorder	The person is unaware of the cause of symptom	The person is unaware of their need for care	See Section 4.6.3
Factitious disorders	Simulated illness and the patient is aware of their role in the illness	The person is aware of some gains arising from the illness but are unaware of their need for care	See Section 4.6.7
Malingering	Simulated illness	There are clear external gains for the person	See Section 4.6.8 for a consideration of the ABCs

True prevalence rates of factitious disorder in primary care are difficult to ascertain partly because people with factitious disorder are driven to be seen as unwell or ill and are referred to specialist clinics for diagnostic clarification. Hence, under-diagnosis in primary care is likely to be a problem and prevalence rates are likely to be higher in specialist clinics. A survey of a 100 physicians and surgeons in private practice and hospital settings estimated 1-year prevalence of factitious disorder of about 1.3% (Fliege et al., 2007; Gieler & Eckhardt-Henn, 2004).

Females in their mid-30s are predisposed and 22% have worked in health care/laboratory profession, often nurses. Comorbidity with depression and borderline personality disorder were common, almost 40% and suicidal behaviours are observed in 14%. It is important to note that most patients elected to self-induce injury or illness and are at high medical risk. Only 20% simulate and 20% falsely report their symptoms (Yates & Feldman, 2016; Caselli et al., 2018).

For the assessment of people with factitious disorders, it will be helpful to take a biopsychosocial approach to understand 'why this patient is presenting in this way at this time'. Table 4.30 provides a guide to information and observations which can inform diagnosis.

Table 4.30 Factors leading to a diagnosis of factitious disorder

First, exclude medical and psychiatric causes for the presentation before making FD diagnosis	
Past health care service use	Multiple hospitals, multiple investigations, often from an early age
Information provided by the patient	The account is inconsistent, contradictory, fragmented, attempts to collate the information may be resisted (refusal to consent to the sharing of information and opt out of health information linkage initiatives)
Atypical presentation	Symptoms may occur when being observed and abate when being viewed unobtrusively. The illness does not follow known natural trajectory and the patient presents as a diagnostic dilemma; the multiple investigations are inconsistent or contradictory in their findings
Investigations	Unremarkable, inconsistent or contradictory. Investigations may reveal fabrication
Evidence of fabrication	Revealed through search or directly witnessed
Patient behaviour	Use of medical jargon, seeking investigations and referrals, non-adherence to proposed treatments, refuse having definitive diagnostic tests, deterioration of condition prior to discharge/transfer, decline referral to psychiatry
Therapeutic relationship	The ambivalent relationship ranges from one of collaboration (while investigations and further referrals are being pursued) to a breakdown in the relationship
Treatment failure	Failure of known treatments, emergence of new symptoms after apparent resolution of symptoms, unexpected worsening

Source: Adapted from Yates & Feldman, 2016; Bass & Halligan, 2014

Making an accurate cross-sectional diagnosis can be difficult and having access to detailed past medical records that highlight the inconsistencies is crucial. Record linkage including through the MyHealth platform might make this easier; however, patients with these conditions may opt out. Conclusive evidence, for example, the finding of an undisclosed vial of insulin may help the assessment of recurrent hypoglycemia which would help make a definitive diagnosis. Such evidence is discovered in only one in three suspected cases (Caselli et al., 2018). Therefore, speaking to previous clinicians who may have suspected the disorder and family will help put the pieces of the puzzle together.

It is hypothesised that vulnerable individuals, at times of stress, adopt unhelpful behaviours (as alluded to above) in order to cope with their situation. The first step involves excluding comorbid medical and psychiatric diagnoses that may better explain the presentation. Next, gathering definitive information about the nature of the problem and collection of clear evidence of fabrication before making a positive diagnosis. There is no definitive treatment modality for this disorder. However, there are some general management principles suggested by McCullumsmith and Ford (2011). The first phase of management includes the management of the acute presentation in the emergency or clinic, followed by the second phase of engaging the patient in longer-term therapeutic treatment. In both phases the focus remains on arriving at a shared understanding of the diagnosis and engaging the patient in a therapeutic treatment plan. Providing feedback to the patient can be challenging for the clinician and planning the consultation is important. There is a risk that clinicians may feel misled and therefore angry. Arranging a care team meeting, consultation with the primary care physician (and a psychiatrist, if available) may help in developing an approach to the feedback session. Maintaining a focus on the psychosocial factors driving the presentation offers the patient a 'face-saving exit' from the sick role. Direct confrontation carries the risk of the patient rejecting the diagnosis, signing themselves out against medical advice, deterioration in their mental health or even litigation. McCullumsmith and Ford (2011) suggest a framework for providing feedback to the patient, as shown in Table 4.31.

Table 4.31 Framework for providing feedback to the person with FD

Step 1	Provide the inexact interpretation	Stressors are identified and simply mentioned as being temporally correlated with the onset of symptoms. No attempt is made to make a definitive causative link between the stressors and the simulation of symptoms.	'It sounds like your loss of job and housing is putting you under a tremendous amount of stress.'
Step 2	Therapeutic use of the double-bind	It is important to mention that the team are considering FD as one of many diagnoses being considered.	'We are considering a number of interpretations of your diagnoses. While one possibility is that you have an unusual cause for your hypoglycemia that we cannot identify, another possibility is that your anxiety and need for help have led you to create these symptoms.'
Step 3	Offer a 'face-saving' exit	Suggest strategies that allow the patient to lose the factitious symptom without losing face, like hypnosis.	'Sometimes we find that problems like the ones you are having can be helped by a short course of therapy.'

Source: Adapted from McCullumsmith & Ford, 2011

The 'constructive confrontation' involves at least two staff members who focus on what can be done to help the patient, taking a 'non-judgemental and non-punitive approach rather than 'confronting' the person about their role in causing the illness (Bass & Halligan, 2014; Eisendrath & Feldman, 1996). Accurate documentation of the meeting and then communicating with the broader health care team (including the primary care physician) is vital. Keeping in mind recovery-oriented practice, clinicians need to be mindful of the language used to communicate with the person about their condition and how clinicians communicate with each other. Language sets the scene for hope. Finally, clinicians will need to consider medicolegal and ethical factors.

4.6.8 MALINGERING

Malingering is a differential diagnosis to factitious disorder. The signs and symptoms are consciously simulated and their illness behaviour is motivated by external incentives or rewards. Examples are: gaining financial benefit; getting medications or drugs; release from incarceration, the avoidance of punishment, work or school, or some type of service such as the military or jury duty. Malingered neurological symptoms and some endocrine symptoms can be objectively determined but clinicians have no objective measures to rely upon when differentiating FD and malingering when the symptoms involved are of a psychological nature. Clinically, it can be challenging to assess the extent to which the patient is aware of their contribution in the creation of these symptoms (intentionality) and their motivation/intent for doing so.

A referral to a clinical psychologist or neuropsychologist may assist with diagnostic clarification through the use of objective testing. Exaggerated or inconsistent reporting can be revealed through both specific tests such as the Minnesota Multiphasic Personality Inventory (MMPI) and the pattern of responding within and across tests. The reader is referred to McCullumsmith and Ford (2011) for a detailed description of factitious disorder, Munchausen syndrome by proxy and malingering. For the management of malingering, LeBourgeois (2007) suggests using the 'ABCs' approach, where the 'A' is 'Avoid accusations of lying', the 'B' is 'Beware of your own attitudes and feelings towards the person', the 'C' is 'seek Clarification' and the 'S' is 'Security measures for staff'.

4.6.9 WHERE AND HOW DO PEOPLE GET HELP?

These disorders are incredibly heterogeneous in their presentation and range in severity. At the mildest end of the spectrum, the person may not present to health care, suffering mild symptoms without observable disability or loss of function. Such patients may present to primary care and will inevitably be worked up to exclude underlying organic causes. If an underlying organic cause is found, any associated distress is likely to be attributed to the underlying condition and viewed as being a normal adjustment to the underlying condition. If an underlying organic cause if not found or is elusive, the clinician is more likely to consider an appropriate psychiatric diagnosis, reflective of a dualistic decision making tree. In reality, a person may be diagnosed with BDD whether or not there is an underlying organic cause. The likelihood of making a diagnosis of BDD is contingent upon on the degree of emotional distress communicated to the clinician. Primary care physicians may be able to sit with a level of distress and assist the patient. However, there is a threshold, and it differs from one clinician to another, beyond which the clinician may make an onward referral to a psychologist or psychiatrist for diagnostic clarification and/or management.

At the more severe end of the spectrum, the patient may have multiple symptoms across multiple systems and suffer extreme distress and be significantly impaired. These severely impacted patients are typically found in specialist clinics and tertiary care. The level of distress experienced by the patient may be mirrored by the experience of the clinicians. The prognosis for the more severe and persistent symptoms is not as good as it is for those who have milder or fewer symptoms. A key related issue is that of access and social determinants of health (see Chapter 1.2). People in poorer areas are much less likely to be able to access mental health services despite higher levels of distress (see Chapter 1.5). In contrast, in well off areas, the rates of distress (and anxiety and depressive disorders) is lower but the rate of access to mental health services is relatively higher. Along a similar vein, access to mental health services is highest in major urban areas in comparison to regional and remote areas despite high levels of distress. This has direct implications for the location of the patient and the clinician. In a regional or remote area, where specialist clinics or specialist mental health services may be sparse/absent, it is more likely that the primary care physician may be the only clinician involved in the patients' recovery journey, irrespective of the severity of their condition.

4.6.10 CONSIDERATION OF THE DIVERSITY OF AUSTRALIA

In the Australian context, it is also important to bear in mind in Australia's First Peoples. (Chapter 1.3.2 provides a detailed perspective on the conceptualisation of health and wellbeing.) When meeting a patient with physical symptoms, it is important to understand that Western notions of health and illness must take into account the deeper and broader perspective held by our Aboriginal and Torres Strait Islander peoples. The National Strategic Framework for Aboriginal and Torres Strait Islander Peoples' Mental Health and Wellbeing 2017–2023 (National Indigenous Australians Agency (NIAA), 2017) articulates the key principles that are borne in mind when assisting the patient. Clinicians have a responsibility to be culturally responsive, we need to invest time and energy in our training, and in the absence of such training, we are guided by key ethical principles articulated (see Chapter 1.5). Dispossession and intergenerational trauma need to factor into our thinking. Drawing upon the strengths and resources of the person and involving community Elders and linking people in with Indigenous Services are central to a successful outcome. Finally, and perhaps most importantly, we need to examine our own attitudes and adopt a reflective stance.

As we think about our internal attitudes and biases, the care of the LGBTIQ community also needs to be reflected upon because the assessment and management of the disorders listed in this chapter depend as much on the quality of the therapeutic relationship as they do on sound clinical judgement. Chapter 1.3 highlights the increased rates of mental health conditions and poorer outcomes in this community, which has faced discrimination, deprivation and abuse. As health care providers, we need to acknowledge that this is a vulnerable community, maintaining application of sound clinical algorithms. Given sometimes blurred diagnostic boundaries in the realm of somatoform disorders, risks of confirmation biases (see Chapter 2.3), if we also are influenced by internal stigmatising attitudes, we may be doomed to fail in our task.

4.6.11 COMMENTARY AND REFLECTION

This chapter aims to bring together various threads that make working in this area of medicine both challenging and potentially rewarding.

Firstly, historically the area of somatoform disorders has been plagued with primitive debates of organic versus psychogenic. ICD-11 has seemingly somewhat addressed this by de-emphasising the need to exclude organic causes in making a positive diagnosis of BDD. This is an extremely heterogeneous disorder, varying in presentation, severity and complexity. At the milder end, primary care physicians are the first port of call, and indeed, ideally placed to help these patients. At the more severe end of the spectrum, there is greater distress and psychiatric comorbidity needs management. Access to mental health services is inequitable in Australia, with primary care and mental health services concentrated in urban areas. Inequity of services brings into focus other inequities and injustices, such as the marginalisation of LGBTIQ communities and inequities for our First Australians. The former group are beginning to get the much needed attention, in contrast to the latter group who have a host of services but remain disadvantaged in multiple domains in health care.

Secondly, the traditional medical model is incompatible with these disorders. The disorders discussed in this chapter require the clinician to maintain a broad biopsychosocial and cultural perspective. Often the perpetuating psychosocial factors need to be identified and remediated to reduce suffering and disability. Iatrogenic harm is a risk to manage in this population. Fortunately, there are treatments available and with the right systems of care in place positive outcome are observed.

BDD is a relatively new diagnosis and not much is known about the aetiology and treatment. On the other hand, factitious disorder and malingering are well known differential diagnoses for those presenting with functional somatic symptoms. Therefore, there is a real risk of misdiagnosis. Clinicians also need to monitor their own internal emotional state and feelings towards the patient and recognise moments when the therapeutic relationship is breaking down or when therapeutic nihilism is beginning to set in. If this is not recognised, the clinician may be drawn to making diagnoses of factitious disorder or malingering. Finally, confirmation bias and our internal attitudes have a substantial bearing on how we understand the patients presenting problems. A strong focus on therapeutic relationship and ethical practice will ground the clinician at times when they feel lost.

4.7

SUBSTANCE USE DISORDERS

MAREE TEESSON, LOUISE MEWTON & ANDREW BAILLIE

4.7.1 LIVED EXPERIENCE

JACK NAGEL

When I first tried ice at 18, I was in a stereotypical stage of my life, I guess, where I was going through finding my identity, rebelling against my parents a little bit and, I guess, conventional thinking and questioning various different things. And I remember quite clearly, ice had just started to come out in a bit more prevalence, at that time.

It sounds strange to some people but anytime I've ever done something that I've liked, I've wanted to do it to the best and almost had this competitive attitude with other people. And that's what started to happen with me and my friends and drug use, we started to push the limits, and it almost became a bit of a competition about who could use more and different types of drugs, and all that kind of stuff. So that definitely played a big part into it turning into a more frequent thing and turning out of control.

Because it was so powerful and my dependence became so strong to it, it really brought me to my demise really quickly which was, actually, a good thing because I didn't go through years and years of suffering. But it was obviously a bad thing because I started to experience really negative consequences, really quickly. So not having any money and, I guess, I became increasingly desperate to get drugs and to get ice. And I started to push my moral boundaries, my day-to-day life started to fall apart, and I wasn't able to manage simple tasks like going to work. And all the different things that you just do in an average day I couldn't do anymore, because my life started to become solely about the getting and using of ice.

It took me a while, and a major function of my problem was this extreme denial that I had about my situation. And I think that's the really scary thing that happens with addiction, but for me with my ice use was that abnormal and crazy situations in life became normal. I actually had a suicide attempt one night where I was hanging around people that had, basically, just come out of prison and the house was like a chemist. And I took a bunch of different drugs and actually, yeah, died in their house.

And then they left me in an alleyway just to die because they were scared of the consequences. I was very lucky, I got taken to hospital, and revived, and I was in hospital for three days. But then what happened was when I woke up and sort of came to, despite what had happened with those people leaving me in the alley and all that kind of stuff, I knew that they had drugs, and I went straight back to them to score.

And then once I use the drugs have walked away, that was one of the first times when I when, 'Hold on, this is a real problem. You just had this experience where these people essentially left you the die and don't actually care about you. And because your need for drugs is so high, you're going back to those compromising positions and using with those same people three days later, that's crazy.' And that was ... Yeah, it took situations like that for me to really realise how bad my problem was and that I needed help.

I was really lucky to have my family behind me who had done some research into rehab centres and things like that. And I'd spoken to different professionals before, but this time was really profound and unique for me because the person that I met, this time, had actually been treated for addiction, themselves, and had come out the other side. And it wasn't so much hearing their story that really gave me the hope, it was because that person was able to, intimately, describe to me how I was thinking and feeling. And it completely blew my mind, because I'd never heard anyone talk like that before, and I thought I was the only one on the whole planet that thought the way and felt the way that I did.

And I guess, in that moment of hearing that and talking to that person, who was a professional as well as having that lived experience, really gave me this massive sense of hope that maybe it was possible in my life, to really change things up as well. In that program it was pretty much all day therapy, if you like, and educational workshops and presentations, and was medically assisted.

And so we would do individual counselling, group therapy, psychotherapy; lots of therapy which was incredibly challenging for me. Because as I said, that was all the stuff that I was running from, it actually had turned into this vicious cycle. So I would use drugs, do different things that I would regret, have lots of different mental health stuff happen, and all that stuff would build up as underlying problems for me.

So anytime I tried to stop using drugs, all that emotional baggage would come simmering to the surface. And I wasn't conscious of this at the time, but then my solution to make all that go away was using drugs. The recovery process for me, actually, was focusing on processing and dealing with all those underlying issues. And then from there, I went and stayed at a rehabilitation program/supported accommodation. And I actually stayed there for 18 months, so all up, the process was nearly two years of me being in services and supportive environments.

I am extremely hopeful for the future, and I think it's something that we have to talk about more in the general conversation when we talk about these issues with addiction and other social problems in society. We tend to focus on the negative stuff a lot, and the really bad stuff that can happen, and we really forget about all the amazing things that can happen and can change as a result of getting some help and getting some support; because it actually does happen to a lot of people.

That's the biggest problem that I see with change in Australia and in the addiction treatment space is not actually the services that are available, not actually people's attitudes, but definitely, I guess, the political conversation around it. And also, I think one of the key areas that really has to change and be addressed is the way that drugs and alcohol are reported on in the media. And the way that drug and alcohol problems and social issues are portrayed to people. I think, if that can be an area that is focused on the most, I think it's going to dramatically change the conversation in society around drugs and alcohol and treatment and have positive impacts on everyone.

Source: www.mydr.com.au/addictions/video-ice-addiction-jacks-story

4.7.2 SUBSTANCE USE DISORDERS

MAREE TEESSON, LOUISE MEWTON & ANDREW BAILLIE

DRUG AND ALCOHOL USE IN AUSTRALIA

According to the 2016 Australian National Drug Strategy Household Survey (NDSHS), 77% of Australians over the age of 14 years drink alcohol (Australian Institute of Health and Welfare, 2018f; see also Table 4.32) and a significant number (15.4%) had consumed 11 or more standard drinks on a drinking occasion in the past 12 months. Tobacco use is also common in Australia, with 12.2% of the population being current daily smokers in 2016. A significant proportion of Australians (15.6%) over the age of 14 reported having used an illicit drug in the past 12 months. Cannabis was the most frequently used, with just over one in 10 Australians over the age of 14 reporting cannabis use in the past 12 months.

Table 4.32 Percentage of Australian population reporting drug use in past 12 months (2016)

Substance	Reporting use (%)
Alcohol	77.5
Tobacco	12.2
Cannabis	10.4
Ecstasy	2.2
Methamphetamines	1.4
Cocaine	2.5
Heroin	0.2
Hallucinogens	1.0
Inhalants	1.0
Nonmedical use of pharmaceuticals	4.8

Data are percentages of people in Australia aged 14 years and over. Nonmedical use of pharmaceuticals refers to the use of pain medicines (3.3%), tranquilisers (1.6%), steroids (0.1%), methadone/buprenorphine (0.2%) and other opiates/opioids (0.4%) for a nonmedical, non-prescribed use. It excludes paracetamol, aspirin and other non-opioid over-the-counter pain-killers/analgesics.

Source: Australian Institute of Health and Welfare, 2018b

SUBSTANCE USE DISORDERS

Substance-use disorders are characterised by:

- a desire to take alcohol and/or other drugs
- difficulty in controlling use
- associated problems that are the result of alcohol and/or other drug use.

The key feature of substance-use disorders is a desire to take psychoactive drugs, alcohol or tobacco. The desire is often strong, and sometimes overpowering. The psychoactive drugs may or may not have been medically prescribed. There may also be evidence that individuals who return to substance use after a period of abstinence experience a rapid return to dependence compared to individuals who were not dependent.

Individuals who are experiencing substance-use disorders may present with physical complaints (for example, liver damage) or psychological complaints (depression), but may not attribute these problems to their substance use. Substance use is a risk factor for many physical and psychological complaints, and a full alcohol and drug assessment is necessary to ascertain its role in the presenting problems.

Individuals do not need to be drug-free before treatment for mental disorders is commenced.

DEPENDENCE

According to ICD-11, dependence is a disorder of regulation of drug use arising from repeated or continuous use. The diagnosis of dependence should usually be made only if there is a strong internal drive to use alcohol or drugs, which is manifested by impaired ability to control use, increasing priority given to use over other activities and persistence of use despite harm or negative consequences. These experiences are often accompanied by an urge or craving to use substances. Physiological features of dependence may also be present, including:

- tolerance to the effects of alcohol
- withdrawal symptoms following cessation or reduction in use of substances or
- repeated use of substances to prevent or alleviate withdrawal symptoms.

The features of dependence are usually evident over a period of at least 12 months but the diagnosis may be made if alcohol use is continuous (daily or almost daily) for at least one month.

HARMFUL USE

The diagnosis of harmful use should usually be made when an individual experiences a pattern of substance use that has caused damage to a person's physical or mental health or has resulted in behaviour leading to harm to the health of others. The pattern of substance use is evident over a period of at least 12 months if substance use is episodic or at least one month if use is continuous. Harm to health of the individual occurs due to one or more of the following: (1) behaviour related to intoxication; (2) direct or secondary toxic effects on body organs and systems; or (3) a harmful route of administration. Harm to health of others includes any form of physical harm, including trauma, or mental disorder that is directly attributable to behaviour related to alcohol intoxication on the part of the person to whom the diagnosis of harmful pattern of use of alcohol applies.

The experience of dependence and harmful use of a drug can be very different for different individuals, and across different drug classes. Drug use can be sporadic or more chronic and long-term.

There are some important differences between ICD and DSM conceptualisations of substance use disorders. The DSM-IV included two broad categories: substance abuse and substance dependence. However, problems with these two categories, including low reliability and results of studies suggesting that the criteria fit better in one category rather than in two, led to revisions in DSM-5. The DSM-5 has just one category: substance use disorder. Severity is indicated through the number of symptoms met, with individuals meeting six or more of the diagnostic criteria being considered to have a severe substance use disorder. Also new to DSM-5 is the inclusion of gambling disorder (see Chapter 4.8).

The 2009 National Health and Medical Research Council (NHMRC) guidelines for reducing health risks associated with the consumption of alcohol state that, for healthy men and women, 'drinking no more than two standard drinks on any day reduces the lifetime risk of harm from alcohol-related disease or injury'.

The 2009 NHMRC guidelines also advise that on a single occasion of drinking, the risk of alcohol-related injury increases with the amount consumed. For healthy men and women, 'drinking no more than four standard drinks on a single occasion reduces the risk of alcohol-related injury arising from that occasion'.

4.7.3 WHAT DO WE KNOW ABOUT THESE DISORDERS?

LOUISE MEWTON, MAREE TEESSON & ANDREW BAILLIE

PREVALENCE

The most recent statistics on the prevalence of substance use disorders in the Australian population come from the 2007 Australian National Survey of

Mental Health and Wellbeing (NSMHWB; Slade, Johnston, Oakley Browne, Andrews, & Whiteford, 2009). The survey interviewed a representative sample of 8841 Australian adults (aged 16 years or older), and assessed lifetime and 12-month symptoms of the affective, anxiety and substance-use disorders. Disorders were defined in terms of ICD-10 and DSM-IV diagnostic criteria. Substance-use disorders included harmful use and dependence on alcohol, and harmful use and dependence on four classes of drug: cannabis, stimulants, sedatives and opioids.

The survey found that 24.7% of Australians aged 16 years and over had a lifetime ICD-10 substance-use disorder. In the past 12 months, 4.3% of Australians had an ICD-10 alcohol use disorder, and 1.5% had another drug-use disorder. More males than females had an alcohol and other drug use disorder: 6% of males and 2.8% of females met criteria for an alcohol use disorder, and 2.2% of males and 0.9% of females met criteria for other drug-use disorder within the past 12 months. Although it appears that the prevalence of substance-use disorders is much higher in the NSMHWB when compared to other international surveys, it should be noted that the international surveys did not assess dependence in the absence of symptoms of abuse. Per capita alcohol consumption places Australia 17th in OECD rankings, higher than the United Kingdom, New Zealand and the United States (OECD, 2019).

According to the 2007 survey, alcohol use disorders are especially frequent among young adults in Australia. Over one in ten young adults (aged 16–24 years) met criteria for an alcohol use disorder in the previous 12 months (Mewton, Teesson, Slade, & Grove, 2011). According to the 2016 NDSHS, young adults are also more likely to drink at levels that put them at risk of injury on a single occasion of drinking (four or more drinks on a single occasion) when compared with their older counterparts (Australian Institute of Health and Welfare, 2018f). Young adults are also more likely to consume 11 or more standard drinks on a single occasion. However, recent decades have seen some improvements in alcohol consumption among young people. Abstaining has increased in adolescents (aged 12–17 years) from 54.3% in 2004 to 81.5% in 2016. Single occasion risky drinking (5+ drinks/occasion) has decreased significantly for young adults (aged 18–30 years) over that same period. Meanwhile, the average age of alcohol initiation has increased significantly, from 14.7 years in 2004 to 16.2 years in 2016. According to the 2016 NDSHS, males in their 40s and females in their 50s are more likely to drink at levels that put them at risk of alcohol-related harm over their lifetime, defined as consuming more than two standard drinks per day on average, when compared with all other age groups.

In general, more men than women have problems with alcohol, though this varies by age. International evidence also indicates that the gap between men and women is closing in terms of alcohol use and related harms. In a review of 68 studies around the globe, it was found that in the early 1900s men were twice as likely as women to consume alcohol and three times as likely to experience alcohol-related problems (Slade et al., 2016). However, in more recent cohorts the rates of consumption and alcohol-related problems were nearly equalised among men and women. These findings suggest that young women in particular should be the targets of early intervention efforts. To date these have traditionally focused on males.

The prevalence of alcohol use disorders differs by ethnicity and country of birth. Those born in Australia and other English-speaking countries are over three times as likely to meet criteria for an alcohol use disorder (Teesson et al., 2010) when compared to people born in a non-English-speaking country. Indigenous Australians are more likely than their non-Indigenous counterparts to abstain from alcohol (Australian Institute of Health and Welfare, 2018b). However, those who do consume alcohol are often more likely to drink at levels that put them at risk for short-term injury and long-term harm.

Alcohol-use disorders are highly comorbid with mental and other substance use disorders. According to the 2007 NSMHWB, one in five people with an alcohol use disorder also met criteria for another disorder, compared with 8% of the rest of the sample (Teesson et al., 2010). When compared with the rest of the population, those with an alcohol use disorder were nearly 20 times as likely to meet criteria for a comorbid substance use disorder and over two and a half times more likely to meet criteria for a comorbid anxiety disorder. The rates of affective disorders are similar among those who had met criteria for an alcohol use disorder and those who had not.

The rates of daily smoking among Australians aged 14 years or older have decreased significantly in recent decades, reducing from 20.9% in 2001 to 12.2% in 2016 (Australian Institute of Health and Welfare, 2018b). Nevertheless, tobacco use remains the leading risk factor contributing to burden of disease in the Australian population (Australian Institute of Health and Welfare, 2016b). E-cigarette use has grown rapidly in parts of the world, particularly in the United Kingdom and United States. However, the prevalence of e-cigarette use in Australia is not well documented. According to the 2016 NDSHS, 1.2% of people aged over 14 years currently use e-cigarettes, while almost a third (31%) of smokers aged 14 years or older reported that they had used an e-cigarette in their lifetime. Younger smokers are more likely to have used an e-cigarette than older smokers (Australian Institute of Health and Welfare, 2018f).

Drug use disorder prevalence in Australia is highly related to the drugs used (see Table 4.33). As noted, cannabis is the most frequently used illicit drug. In 2016 6.6 million people (or 35%) of people aged 14 or older reported using cannabis in their lifetime, and about 1.9 million (or 10.4%) had used cannabis in the previous 12 months (Australian Institute of Health and Welfare, 2018b). According to the 2007 NSMHWB, the prevalence of cannabis use disorder in the previous 12 months is just over 2% (Slade et al., 2009). The 2007 NSMHWB estimated that the 12-month prevalence of opioid dependence in the Australian population was 0.1% (Slade et al., 2009). In Australia, 1.3 million people (7.0%) aged 14 years and over had used amphetamines in their life, and 2.1% had used them in the previous 12 months (Australian Institute of Health and Welfare, 2018b). Of those who had used amphetamines, 50.4% report crystal methamphetamine as the main form of the drug used. After cannabis, ecstasy is the most commonly used illicit drug (10.9% of Australians over the age of 14 years; Australian Institute of Health and Welfare, 2018b). In 2016, 2.2% of Australian aged over 14 years reported using ecstasy in the previous 12 months.

According to the 2007 NSMHWB, relatively few people with a substance-use disorder had sought assistance with their substance-use problem from a mental health professional. Among those with a substance-use disorder, 24% had used services for mental health problems in the previous 12 months. Higher levels of service use were observed among those with dependence disorders compared to those with harmful use disorders. Moreover, there was a trend for higher service use among people with drug harmful use or dependence compared to people with alcohol harmful use or dependence. One-half (52.4%) of people diagnosed with drug dependence and one in four (24.1%) with drug harmful use had used services in the 12 months prior to interview, whereas one-third (35.5%) of people with alcohol dependence and one in six (15.5%) with alcohol harmful use used services in the previous 12 months (Slade et al., 2009).

HOW CAN WE UNDERSTAND THE ORIGINS?

Many people begin with using alcohol and drugs for the positive effects (e.g. relaxation), then begin using it regularly, then use it heavily, and finally become dependent on it. Although applicable in many cases, this developmental process approach does not account for all cases of the development of substance use disorders. For example, some people have periods of heavy use of a substance—for example, alcohol—and then are able to return to moderate use. The origin of substance use disorders is complex and based in genetic, neurobiological, psychological, and sociocultural factors.

Genetic factors

Much research has addressed the possibility that there is a genetic contribution to drug and alcohol use disorders, in particular gene-environment relationships in alcohol and drug use disorders (Kendler, Myers, &

Prescott, 2007). Among adolescents, peers appear to be particularly important environmental variables. For example, a large twin study found that heritability for alcohol problems among adolescents was higher among those teens who had a large number of peers who drank compared to those who had a smaller number of peers who drank (Dick et al., 2007).

Neurobiological factors

A major focus of neurobiological research has been the dopamine system. Nearly all drugs, including alcohol, stimulate the dopamine systems in the brain particularly the mesolimbic pathway (Koob & Le Moal, 2008). It remains unresolved whether problems in the dopamine system may increase the vulnerability of some people to becoming dependent on a substance, sometimes called the 'vulnerability model', or whether problems in the dopamine system are the consequence of taking substances (the 'toxic effect model'). For many people, they continue to take drugs to avoid the negative feelings associated with withdrawal. A substantial body of research with animals supports this motivation for drug-taking behaviour (Koob & Le Moal, 2008).

Psychological factors

There are three major groupings of psychological factors associated with substance use disorders. The first is the potential tension-reducing effect. Second, expectancies about the effects of substances on behaviour. Third, personality traits that may make it more likely for some people to use alcohol or drugs.

It is generally assumed that one of the main psychological motives for using drugs is to alter mood or emotion—that is, drug use is reinforced because it enhances positive moods or diminishes negative ones. For example, most people believe that an increase in tension leads to increased alcohol consumption and it has been demonstrated that alcohol reduces self-reported and physiological indicators of anxiety (Bradford, Shapiro, & Curtin, 2013). Other research has shown that expectancies about a drug's effects predict increased drug use in general (Stacy, Newcomb, & Bentler, 1991). Similarly, 'drinking to cope' or people who believe that alcohol will make them seem more socially skilled are likely to drink more heavily than those who accurately perceive that alcohol can interfere with social interactions (Stapinski et al., 2016). Finally, personality factors appear to be important in predicting the later onset of substance use disorders. Personality traits related to anxiety and depression appear to be linked to substance use through negative reinforcement motives. In contrast, disinhibitory personality traits, such as impulsivity and sensation-seeking, appear to be linked to substance use through positive reinforcement pathways (Nair et al., 2016; Newton, Barrett, et al., 2016). In this pathway, substance use is thought to enhance positive affect. Recent research has focused on specific neurotic and disinhibitory personality dimensions that appear to be consistently linked with the initiation and maintenance of substance use; namely, hopelessness, anxiety sensitivity, impulsivity and sensation-seeking (Newton, Conrod, et al., 2016; Woicik, Stewart, Pihl, & Conrod, 2009). Recent research has shown that these personality traits were among the strongest predictors of adolescent binge drinking (Whelan et al., 2014), with an Australian trial showing that a personality targeted intervention can have long-term effects in reducing alcohol and related harms (Newton, Conrod, et al., 2016).

Sociocultural factors

Sociocultural factors play a widely varying role in substance use disorders. People's interest in and access to drugs are influenced by peers, the media, and cultural norms about acceptable behaviour. Ready availability of the substance is also a factor. Findings from the Monitoring the Future Study, an ongoing study begun in the 1960s that surveys over 50 000 high school students in the United States every year, indicate that the greater reported availability of particular drugs or alcohol corresponded to greater use of those drugs (Johnston, O'Malley, Bachman, Schulenberg, & Miech, 2014). Meanwhile, Australian research also shows that increased alcohol outlet density and extended alcohol trading hours are correlated with increased alcohol use and alcohol-related harms (Chikritzhs, Catalano, Pascal, & Henrickson, 2007). Indeed, increasing the price of alcohol and cigarettes has been robustly associated with decreases in their use internationally (Wagenaar, Salois, & Komro, 2009; Wakefield et al., 2014).

COURSE AND IMPACT

PRACTICE ILLUSTRATION: TREATMENT TRAJECTORY

Jim is a 26-year-old male, who presented to his general practitioner because he had been missing work as a result of hangovers from his alcohol use. He is married with two children. His wife encouraged him to ask his general practitioner about his drinking.

Jim had begun drinking at the age of 15, and started regular consumption at 18. By the time he was 20 years old, he was drinking four to six beers regularly through the week and on Friday and Saturday nights. In the last year, he had begun binge drinking, drinking up to 15 or more standard drinks. He was also drinking the next day in order to recover.

His recent alcohol use was two standard drinks of beer before work, eight at lunch and another five standard drinks of beer after work. His GP did a medical examination, and had some liver enzyme levels analysed. While Jim's liver was not enlarged, there were elevated levels of a number of liver enzymes, confirming Jim's heavy drinking.

While Jim is initially ambivalent about acknowledging that he has an alcohol problem, he agrees to see a clinical psychologist to discuss his drinking. Jim discovers that the regular visits to his clinical psychologist are helpful. He does not feel judged, and he has given him some useful suggestions to reduce his drinking by, for example, switching to a lower alcohol beer. Jim also finds it useful to discuss other problems in his life, including the conflict with his wife and stress at work. After visiting his clinical psychologist for three months, Jim begins to think it might be useful to reduce his drinking further. His treatment plan includes teaching Jim strategies to refuse alcohol when he is with his friends, assertiveness and communication skills. Jim's wife also agrees to attend some sessions to discuss their relationship.

Two years later, Jim has reduced his alcohol drinking, his physical health has improved and the arguments with his wife have reduced. He regularly visits his GP to monitor his physical health and talk about how he is managing. Jim worries that he may begin drinking heavily again, although he does feel prepared should this happen. His clinical psychologist has explained to him that relapse is common, and that having one night of heavy drinking would not necessarily result in a return to his previous heavy drinking patterns. The clinical psychologist has also encouraged him to return to treatment if he feels that he needs further assistance in the future.

4.7.4 ASSESSMENT

MAREE TEESSON, LOUISE MEWTON & ANDREW BAILLIE

This chapter outlines evidence for the effective clinical practice related to all substance-use disorders, whether the substance be alcohol or another drug. This comprehensive approach was taken because, in real life, it is uncommon for individuals seeking treatment to have a problem with only one substance, therefore the techniques described are applicable across all alcohol and drugs.

PRACTICE ILLUSTRATION: THE PROBLEM EMERGES

It was Tom's friends who first noticed he was drinking more and that he was often drinking a lot more than they did. In his early 20s, Tom would go out on most weekends with his friends. He would always drink when he went out. Tom didn't usually drink much during the rest of the week (2–3 drinks a day) but on nights during the weekend he was regularly drinking around 20 drinks a night (over a period of 8–10 hours). Sometimes he drank so much on the weekend that he was unable to get home and had little memory of what had happened that night. Tom's family are concerned for him. Recently, Tom was hospitalised after falling and hitting his head. He remembers starting the night at a local bar listening to his favourite band and thinking that he would only have a few drinks. At the end of the fourth drink he didn't stop drinking and by the end of the night he was shouting and threatening his girlfriend. His girlfriend had asked him to stop drinking. Security guards intervened and escorted him out of the bar as they were concerned for his girlfriend's safety. He could not manage the stairs on the way up to his house, tripped and fell. When he was assessed in the emergency department of the hospital he realised that he was drinking a lot more than he used to drink. He didn't ask for help for his drinking as he thought he should be able to reduce his drinking by himself. He didn't think he had a problem, he felt like his girlfriend was being unreasonable and that he had simply not judged the stairs and slipped. He felt he was just unlucky he had hit his head. After a few months of weekends like this he started to notice that he was getting strong urges to drink during the week and that he was now drinking five or more drinks every night. His girlfriend has stopped seeing him and he is at risk of losing his job because he has been turning up late to work. He still thinks he can stop whenever he wants.

DIAGNOSIS

The key feature of substance dependence is a desire to take psychoactive drugs, alcohol or tobacco. The desire is often strong, and sometimes overpowering. The psychoactive drugs may or may not have been medically prescribed. Individuals who are experiencing substance-use disorders may present with physical complaints (for example, related to the liver) or psychological complaints (depression), but may not attribute these problems to their substance use. Substance use is a risk factor for many physical and psychological complaints, and a full alcohol and drug assessment is necessary to ascertain its role in the presenting problems. Individuals do not need to be drug-free before treatment for mental disorders commences.

ASSESSING SEVERITY

The assessment of substance-use disorders will involve a review of the quantity of substance being consumed and the consequences of such use. An important aspect of the assessment process is to provide feedback to the individual, and develop a rapport between the assessor and the individual. Individuals with substance-use disorders are often reluctant to commence treatment.

Some individuals may be ready to accept treatment for substance dependence. However, if the individual is not committed to treatment, failure is likely. The outcome of treatment in substance dependence may depend on how ready the individual is to change his or her drinking or drug-taking behaviour, so this forms an important component of the assessment. A useful structure for assessing an individual's willingness to change his or her behaviour is that of stages of change, which sees an individual progressing through the following stages: precontemplative stage; contemplative stage; preparation stage; action stage; and maintenance stage (Prochaska & DiClemente, 1982). An individual needs to progress to the stage of contemplation in order to be ready to change according to the model.

The patterns and context of drinking of the individual should be assessed. This assessment should include the following:

- Alcohol use:
  - ask the individual how frequently he or she drinks and how much alcohol he or she drinks per week; on a typical drinking day; and on a heavy drinking day
  - ask about the sequence of events on a typical drinking day; the time when the individual starts to drink; where and with whom he or she usually drinks; the period of time spent drinking; the amount and type of alcohol consumed; and when and how they stop drinking
- Drug use:
  - for injecting drug use, it may also be useful to ask, in addition to the above questions, whether the individual typically injects.
- Some useful instruments include a day diary in which an individual records:
  - day, date and times of drinking or drug taking
  - the amount and type of drink or drugs taken; the context of drinking or drug taking (for example, where, with whom, doing what)
  - number of standard drinks or drugs taken
  - thoughts before drinking or drug taking
  - behaviours, thoughts and consequences after drinking or drug taking.

Measuring the level of dependence of an individual is also important in treatment planning. Seven factors are regarded as important in assessing dependence:

- narrowing of the drinking repertoire; salience or importance of drinking
- subjective awareness of a compulsion to drink
- increased tolerance to the effects of alcohol
- repeated withdrawal symptoms
- relief or avoidance of withdrawal symptoms by further drinking
- reinstatement of dependent drinking after abstinence.

The questionnaires in Table 4.32 were developed to assist with the assessment of substance-use disorders.

The Alcohol Use Disorders Identification Test (AUDIT; Saunders, Aasland, Babor, De la Fuente, & Grant, 1993) is a 10-item screening instrument designed to screen for a range of drinking problems and, in particular, for hazardous and harmful consumption. A score of 8–10 is associated with harmful or hazardous drinking; a score of 13 or more is likely to indicate alcohol dependence.

The Opiate Treatment Index (OTI) is an instrument that uses a structured interview covering six independent outcome areas: drug use; HIV risk-taking behaviour; social functioning; criminality; health status; and psychological adjustment (Darke, Hall, Wodaki, Heather, & Ward, 1992). It takes 20–30 minutes to administer, and is available from the website of the National Drug and Alcohol Research Centre, University of New South Wales (https://ndarc.med.unsw.edu.au).

Several scales have been developed to assess level of dependence. These scales include the Severity of Alcohol Dependence Questionnaire Form C (SADQ-C; Stockwell, Sitharthan, McGrath, & Lang, 1994), the Severity of Opiate Dependence Questionnaire (SODQ; Sutherland et al., 1986) and the Severity of Dependence Scale (Gossop et al., 1995).

ASSESSING RISK

Assessment of risk differs for those who have primarily an alcohol problem and for those individuals with drug-use disorders. Assessment of the risk of HIV infection in those who are injecting drug users is important. Individuals who inject drugs are at risk for poor nutrition, dental caries, respiratory illnesses, and hepatitis C and B.

Individuals with alcohol use disorders are at greater risk of liver dysfunction, pancreatitis, problems with the heart and blood circulation, poor nutrition and, in the case of excessive use, alcohol-related brain damage. Liver function tests can be used to measure the effects of alcohol use. Another common blood test is a measure of mean corpuscular volume (MCV); when elevated this may indicate liver disease.

Table 4.33 Alcohol Use Disorders Identification Test (AUDIT)

Please circle the answer that is correct for you:				
1 How often do you have a drink containing alcohol?				
Never	Monthly or less	2–4 times a month	2–3 times a week	4 or more times a week
2 How many standard drinks containing alcohol do you have on a typical day when you are drinking?				
1 or 2	3 or 4	5 or 6	7 to 9	10 or more
3 How often do you have six or more drinks on one occasion?				
Never	Less than monthly	Monthly	Weekly	Daily or almost daily
4 How often during the last year have you found that you were not able to stop drinking once you had started?				
Never	Less than monthly	Monthly	Weekly	Daily or almost daily
5 How often during the last year have you failed to do what was normally expected from you because of drinking?				
Never	Less than monthly	Monthly	Weekly	Daily or almost daily
6 How often during the last year have you needed a drink in the morning to get yourself going after a heavy drinking session?				
Never	Less than monthly	Monthly	Weekly	Daily or almost daily
7 How often during the last year have you had a feeling of guilt or remorse after drinking?				
Never	Less than monthly	Monthly	Weekly	Daily or almost daily
8 How often during the last year have you been unable to remember what happened the night before because you had been drinking?				
Never	Less than monthly	Monthly	Weekly	Daily or almost daily
9 Have you or someone else been injured as a result of your drinking?				
Never	Yes, but not in the last year		Yes, during the last year	
10 Has a relative or friend or a doctor or other health worker been concerned about your drinking or suggested you cut down?				
Never	Yes, but not in the last year		Yes, during the last year	

Source: Saunders et al. 1993 © Taylor & Francis. Reproduced with permission.

Alcohol withdrawal can develop in individuals who are dependent on alcohol within six to 12 hours of last drinking. There are three main sets of symptoms of withdrawal:

- autonomic nervous hyperactivity, such as restlessness and tremor
- neuronal excitation, such as seizures and delirium tremens, including loss of insight and severe disorientation
- sleep disturbance.

In most cases, withdrawal does not require medical attention, and will resolve within seven days. However, in the case of severe withdrawal, medical care should be sought.

4.7.5 EVIDENCE-BASED AND OTHER TREATMENTS AND SERVICES

MAREE TEESSON, LOUISE MEWTON & ANDREW BAILLIE

Treatment aims to assist the individual to control or manage his or her drug use, and deals with the physiological, psychological and social implications arising from an individual's drug abuse.

The aims of treatment are to:

- reduce illicit and licit drug use
- reduce the hazard, harm and disability associated with illicit and licit drug use
- decrease the public health, social burden and public safety threats associated with illicit and licit drug use.

4.7.6 PHARMACOTHERAPIES

MAREE TEESSON, LOUISE MEWTON & ANDREW BAILLIE

ALCOHOL

Until recently, the main pharmacotherapy available for alcohol use disorders was antidipsotropic drugs, such as disulfram and calcium carbamide. These drugs inhibit the enzyme that catalyses the breakdown of acetaldehyde in the blood. Injection of alcohol raises the acetaldehyde levels, which, if allowed to build up in the system, cause symptoms of nausea, vomiting and shortness of breath. These drugs have been mostly used with individuals who are dependent on alcohol. More recently, with improved understanding of brain neurobiology, pharmacological treatments have been developed. These developments have focused mainly in the area of relapse prevention.

Approximately 50% of people who are alcohol dependent relapse within three months of treatment. The efficacy of acamprosate and naltrexone in preventing relapse in people with alcohol dependence has been demonstrated in randomised controlled trials (Rösner et al., 2010). Naltrexone has been shown to reduce the rates of relapse and increase periods of abstinence in people with alcohol dependence (Haber, Lintzeris, Proude, & Lopatko, 2009). Evidence is mixed regarding whether this drug is more effective than a placebo in reducing drinking when it is the only treatment (Krystal, Cramer, Krol, Kirk, & Rosenheck, 2001). A review of data from all published double-blind, placebo-controlled clinical trials of acamprosate for people dependent on alcohol suggests that it is highly effective (Mason, 2001). A meta-analysis comparing the effectiveness of acamprosate and naltrexone found them to be equally effective (Kranzler & Van Kirk, 2001). Acamprosate and naltrexone can be administered simultaneously, with evidence suggesting that the combination may be better than acamprosate alone, but not more effective than naltrexone alone (Haber et al., 2009). A relatively new drug, topiramate, also appears to be promising in treating alcohol dependence (Johnson et al., 2008; Johnson et al., 2007).

However, one important limitation to any pharmacological treatment is patient compliance. This has long been the problem with older pharmacotherapies, such as disulfiram. A robust treatment effect size for naltrexone relative to placebo has been shown for compliant subjects, but not for subjects who are not compliant with the treatment. Studies have shown successful outcomes for a brief intervention aimed at addressing compliance with acamprosate (Reid, Teesson, Sannibale, Matsuda, & Haber, 2005; Teesson et al., 2003). Compliance therapy for alcohol dependence consists of four to six individual sessions lasting approximately 60 minutes each. In the first phase of compliance therapy (sessions 1 and 2), patients' beliefs about their alcohol dependence and the role of treatment (medication and psychological therapy) are explored. In the second phase (sessions 3 and 4), treatment experience is addressed, with a review of side effects and symptoms; ambivalence towards treatment is explored; and the benefits of treatment versus return to drinking are compared. In the third phase (sessions 5 and 6), the need for treatment maintenance and relapse prevention is addressed, and self-efficacy is enhanced. Compliance therapy significantly increased the average time on medication and number of days to relapse compared with just usual medical care as offered in a conventional outpatient setting.

OPIATES

Methadone maintenance is a well-accepted intervention for opioid dependence, and is widely used in Australia (Hall & Mattick, 2007). At present, it is the most effective intervention for individuals suffering from heroin dependence (Mattick, Breen, Kimber, & Davoli, 2009, 2014).

Buprenorphine is a partial opioid agonist increasingly used in Australia in opioid maintenance therapy and for the treatment of opioid withdrawal. Buprenorphine has less euphoric and sedating effects when compared with pure opioid agonists, such as heroin and methadone, and is longer acting and easier to withdraw from. When compared with methadone, there is also less risk of overdose from buprenorphine. Reviews of the efficacy of buprenorphine have shown that medium-to-high doses of buprenorphine improve treatment outcome and illicit opioid use when compared with placebo. However, it was found to be less effective than methadone, indicating that methadone should be the treatment of first choice in most treatment settings (Mattick et al., 2014).

Naltrexone is a long-acting (up to 72 hours, depending on dose) opioid antagonist, which is used as an abstinence-based treatment for opiate dependence. Naltrexone blocks both the analgesic and euphoric effects of opioids, it can be administered orally and it has no major side effects, making it a potentially useful maintenance drug. Naltrexone has been the subject of much research, and there are a number of controlled trials comparing naltrexone with methadone or placebo (Johansson, Berglund, & Lindgren, 2006; Lerner et al., 1992; O'Brien, Greenstein, Mintz, & Woody, 1975; Rawson & Tennant, 1984a; San, Pomarol, Peri, Olle, & Cami, 1991; Shufman et al., 1994).

The results to date are equivocal. A review of naltrexone concluded that there is insufficient quality research to assess the efficacy of naltrexone maintenance (Minozzi et al., 2011). Again, as with alcohol, one important limitation to any pharmacological treatment is patient compliance. Many of the programs using naltrexone report substantial dropout rates and poor compliance with treatment (Johansson et al., 2006; Tucker, Ritter, Maher, & Jackson, 2004). The findings are therefore often based on small numbers. Sustained-release depot injections and implants have recently been investigated as a means of improving compliance. When compared with oral naltrexone, it has been found that sustained-release naltrexone was more effective at preventing relapse to heroin use (Kunoe et al., 2009). However, longer-term outcomes are less clear. Although retention rate in naltrexone maintenance has proven difficult with illicit-drug-using individuals, other research supports the value of naltrexone maintenance for at least some patients (Johansson et al., 2006; O'Brien et al., 1975; Rawson & Tennant, 1984b). Naltrexone has a potential maintenance role, particularly with highly motivated patients. Naltrexone may also act as a method of withdrawing those patients who wish to cease all maintenance therapy.

As with pharmacotherapies for alcohol use disorder, compliance is one of the key factors in the effectiveness of medications for opiates. Both clinical effectiveness and treatment compliance can be increased by adding a contingency management component to the therapy (Carroll et al., 2001). Giving people vouchers that they can exchange for food and clothing in return for taking naltrexone and having drug-free urine samples markedly improves effectiveness. In one randomised controlled trial (Pierce et al., 2006), people receiving methadone from a clinic could draw for prizes each time they submitted a (carefully supervised and obtained) urine sample that had no trace of illegal drugs or alcohol. Prizes ranged from praise to televisions. People who were in the contingency management group were more likely to remain drug-free than those people who received only usual care from the methadone clinic. Of course, it remains to be seen whether such abstinence gains can be maintained after treatment ends and therapists are no longer providing such incentives.

NICOTINE

Reducing a smoker's craving for nicotine by providing it in a different way is the goal of nicotine replacement treatments (NRT). Attention to nicotine dependence is clearly important because the more cigarettes people smoke daily, the less successful they are at quitting. Nicotine may be supplied in gum, patches, inhalers, or e-cigarettes. The idea is to help smokers endure the nicotine withdrawal that accompanies any effort to stop smoking. Abstinence rates for NRT are about 50% at 12-month follow-ups. In addition, these types of nicotine replacement treatments may be less effective with adolescents (Curry, Mermelstein, & Sporer, 2009).

NRT enhanced with medication or psychological treatment appears to be more effective than NRT alone (Rose & Behm, 2014). For example, combining the antidepressant medication buproprion and nicotine patches yielded a 12-month abstinence rate of 35% in one study (Jorenby et al., 1999) but there were less promising results in other studies (Hughes, Stead, Hartmann-Boyce, Cahill, & Lancaster, 2014). Another drug, varenicline, may be effective in combination with behavioural treatment, and even more effective than buproprion (Cahill, Stead, & Lancaster, 2009).

There is a current debate about whether e-cigarettes are an effective form of NRT. Results from one longitudinal study found that only 10% of people using e-cigarettes had quit smoking one year later (Grana, Popova, & Ling, 2014). An internet survey of over 400 people who used e-cigarettes found that 22% of people had stopped smoking after one month and 46% had stopped at the one-year follow-up (Etter & Bullen, 2014). A randomised controlled clinical trial assigned people who wanted to quit smoking to either e-cigarettes, the nicotine patch, or placebo e-cigarettes. The numbers of people who quit smoking were very small in all three groups, so small in fact that the researchers did not have the statistical power to detect any significant differences between the groups (Bullen et al., 2013). Clearly, more research is needed, but thus far, e-cigarettes do not appear to be more effective than other forms of NRT.

4.7.7 PSYCHOTHERAPIES AND SOCIAL INTERVENTIONS

BRIEF INTERVENTIONS

Brief interventions can be delivered in five to 30 minutes, and typically involve a single-session intervention. Brief interventions are appropriate for individuals with few medical problems associated with that use. They often include a self-help manual, with brief support and guidance from the clinician. They aim to produce enough assistance to ensure the individual achieves his or her desired behaviour change.

There are two steps to brief interventions:

- screening to detect excessive alcohol or drug use
- advice to individuals to reduce consumption of alcohol and drug taking to safe and responsible levels.

DRINK–DRUG REFUSAL SKILLS

Inevitably, individuals with substance-use disorders will be confronted with a situation in which they will be asked to drink or take drugs. Drink–drug refusal skills allow the development of skills that enable the individuals to refuse the offer. Role-plays are a useful technique in teaching drink-drug refusal skills.

The basis of drink–drug refusal skills are that:

- almost everyone is placed, at some time, in a situation in which he or she will be offered drinks or drugs
- it is impossible to avoid all situations where drink or drugs may be offered
- there are strategies that make it easier to refuse alcohol or drugs. These strategies include the use of appropriate body language and tone of voice, and the use of direct statements to refuse the offer of alcohol or drugs
- a confident refusal is more likely to be accepted than a hesitant refusal. Confidence skills include speaking in a firm and unhesitating manner, making direct eye contact and standing or sitting straight (Teesson, 1998).

STRUCTURED PROBLEM SOLVING

Individuals will encounter events and life experiences that may challenge their commitment to changing their patterns of drinking and drug use. The technique of structured problem solving provides a method for the individual to deal with such events. Instead of turning to alcohol or drugs whenever problems arise, problems can be managed more effectively with the use of structured problem solving, which include the following steps:

- define the problem or problems
- encourage the individual to seek as wide a range of options as possible
- define solutions in terms of current resources
- carefully consider any practical constraints that are involved in applying a possible solution.

ASSERTIVENESS TRAINING AND COMMUNICATION SKILLS

The aim of assertiveness training is to assist individuals who have difficulty in expressing their emotions. Some individuals, instead of taking control of difficult situations by expressing their thoughts, may become angry and distressed, and this may in turn contribute to excessive drinking and drug use. Communication skills training overlaps with assertiveness training. The aim of communication skills training is to teach individuals how to discuss their thoughts constructively. Not everyone will need such types of interventions.

CHALLENGING THOUGHTS

The urge to use drugs and alcohol is one of the distinguishing features of dependence on alcohol and drugs. Cognitive restructuring involves teaching the individual to identify and challenge thoughts and feelings that may lead to drinking and drug taking (McHugh, Hearon, & Otto, 2010; Teesson, 1998).

The aim of cognitive restructuring is to help the individual to recognise when he or she is thinking in a way that could lead to drinking or drug use. The individual is taught to stop or interrupt such a train of thought and challenge the unproductive thoughts. He or she is then taught to replace them with more reasonable thoughts. A method for implementing the challenging of thoughts is outlined below (Teesson, 1998):

- identify as many negative or automatic thoughts as possible with the individual; discussing a recent drinking situation is a useful technique in eliciting negative thoughts
- the individual uses a day diary to keep a record of thoughts and identify thoughts in specific situations; the diary should be completed by the individual at a suitable time each day
- with the individual, identify negative thoughts from the diary
- train the individual to challenge the thoughts in the diary; the steps are:
    - assess the evidence for the thought
    - produce a reasonable alternative to the thought
    - ask whether the thought is helpful
    - identify the thinking error.

ENCOURAGING SELF-MANAGEMENT

Self-management can be a useful technique when the aim of the intervention is moderation, and the individual does not have any serious physical consequences from alcohol or drug use. Self-management involves:

- self-monitoring
- setting drinking limits
- controlling rates of drinking
- drink-refusal skills
- problem solving
- identifying risk situations
- learning coping skills
- self-reward.

The aim of behavioural self-management is to assist the individual to reduce drinking to levels that minimise both physical health and social problems by using specific skills.

The rationale is that eventually the individual will learn these skills to help him or her cut down and maintain his or her drinking at a harm-free level.

BEHAVIOURAL SELF-MANAGEMENT STEPS

The steps in order to achieve behavioural self-management include: daily self-monitoring; setting limits on drinking; maintaining set limits; identifying high-risk situations; and utilising skills for coping with high-risk situations (Teesson, 1998).

BUILDING ALLIANCES

Engagement in treatment is of particular concern in the treatment of the substance-use disorders, as individuals will often present for treatment ambivalent about their desire to change their drinking or drug taking. Motivational interviewing techniques (Miller & Rollnick, 2012) are particularly useful in the substance-use disorders for building strategic alliances. The aim of motivational interviewing techniques is to encourage the individual to decide that change in his or her drinking or drug-taking behaviour may be advisable. The techniques are based on the assumption that most individuals are still ambivalent about changing their drinking or drug taking when they consult for help. It is therefore possible that diagnosis of a problem or confrontation leads to defensive reactions. Motivational interviewing, by contrast, aims to assist individuals themselves to be aware of the reasons for change.

During motivational interviewing, the therapist facilitates changes in behaviour using non-confrontational approaches. Motivational interviewing can be delivered as a stand-alone treatment or as an adjunct to other psychosocial or pharmacological treatments. A recent meta-analysis indicated that among young drinkers, motivational interviewing is only minimally effective (Foxcroft, Coombes, Wood, Allen, & Almeida Santimano, 2014).

The implementation of motivational interviewing techniques is varied, and should reflect the treatment goals of the individual. There are three key strategies that can each take between five and 15 minutes and may need to be repeated. They are, in order:

- exploring good and less good aspects of drinking or drug use
- life satisfaction, or discussing the discrepancy between how things are and how they could be
- helping with decision making or assisting the individual with taking action

4.7.8 EDUCATION

Education is a crucial aspect of treatment, especially as individuals will vary in the extent of their knowledge about safe drinking levels. Education provides a knowledge base that can give the individual a sense of greater control over his or her problems. This can in turn lead to a reduction in feelings of helplessness.

Education aims to facilitate understanding about the problem and its management as relevant to each individual. The following information will be important in education sessions with individuals with substance-related disorder:

- abstinence may not be the only goal
- treatment is effective, and many treatment options are available
- the ultimate goal of treatment is to improve health and wellbeing
- the physical and psychological consequences of alcohol and drug use.

The education process should be thought of as a two-way interaction. The individual not only receives information but also educates the clinician about his or her unique experience of the problem.

4.7.9 SETTING GOALS

Planning goals is important, because it provides a link between assessment and the intervention. Negotiation with the individual should ensure that the goals are realistic, achievable, specific, broken down into small steps and owned by the individual.

There are three possible overall goals in the treatment of substance-related disorders: abstinence, moderated drinking or drug taking, and attenuated or reduced drinking or drug taking.

In moderated drinking or drug taking, the individual moderates his or her drinking to harm-free levels. In attenuated drinking or drug taking, the individual moderates his or her drinking or drug taking so as to reduce the harm to him- or herself. The latter is obviously not an ideal goal, but may be the only goal an individual is willing to work towards.

A number of factors should be considered when deciding on the most appropriate goal:

- the physical health of the individual, and the risk to him- or herself of further drinking or drug taking. Significant health problems may indicate abstinence as a goal

- the presence of brain damage, impaired cognitive functioning, or HIV may indicate an abstinence goal
- highly dependent individuals may be less able to moderate their drinking or drug taking than independent individuals (Mattick & Jarvis, 1993).

Available research suggests that, irrespective of stated treatment goals or amount of drinking skills training, the most likely positive outcome of treatment for low-dependence drinkers is controlled drinking, while for high-dependence drinkers the goal most likely to be effective is abstinence (Sobell & Sobell, 1995). There is also evidence that factors such as social support and poor vocational history may be more important in deciding treatment aims than consideration of levels of dependence (Sobell & Sobell, 1995).

Individuals with injecting drug use disorders are at risk of a number of bloodborne viruses. Goals in opioid and polydrug use are therefore particularly concerned with reducing risk of infection from the human immunodeficiency virus (HIV) and other infectious diseases such as hepatitis B, C and D. The focus is on reducing unsafe injecting practices and unsafe sexual practices (Baker, Heather, Stalwart, O'Neill, & Wodak, 1996). The following goals should be considered with injecting practices:

- cleaning and sterilising needles before use
- using only clean or new needles
- reducing unsafe sexual practices.

IMPLEMENTING THERAPIES: MANAGEMENT PLAN

The substance-related disorders have much in common across the different drug classes. In addition, people often present with problems with more than one drug. The first stage of implementing therapy is to assess the individual's motivation to change. The management plan should follow a thorough assessment of the relevant problems, target all relevant problems and be based on specific strategies. It is important that the management plan be understood by the individual, and that it is regularly evaluated for both positive and negative consequences. The following is a useful outline for putting all the aspects of intervention together:

1. Conduct a thorough assessment:
   - stages of change
   - patterns and context of drinking or drug use
   - severity of dependence
   - risk-taking behaviour
2. Engagement and building rapport:
   - motivational interviewing
   - education
3. Assist the individual to plan goals
4. Implement interventions:
   - pharmacotherapies (where appropriate)
   - brief intervention
   - drink–drug refusal skills
   - structured problem solving
   - assertiveness training and communication skills
   - challenging thoughts
   - encourage self-management
5. Maintain change in substance use and relapse prevention.

RELAPSE PREVENTION AND DEALING WITH TREATMENT FAILURES

It is highly likely that individuals will experience relapses, especially if they are attempting to change longstanding behaviours. The general aim of relapse prevention training is to provide the individual with skills to avoid lapses and prevent lapses from becoming relapses to alcohol or drug use. It also aims to teach strategies and beliefs to reduce the negative consequence of relapse (see www.verywellmind.com for a helpful diagrammatic presentation of the stages of change).

When relapses occur, individuals may find it helpful to remind themselves of positive changes they had achieved before relapse. By focusing on positive changes before relapse and strengths and coping skills used before relapse, the individual is in a better position to be motivated to continue to attempt to change.

Relapse can often be as a consequence of external factors. Therefore relapse prevention training also involves examining lifestyle factors that can either hinder or support behaviour change.

Relapse prevention training can be divided into the following areas:

- enhance commitment to change
- identify causes of relapse
- reintroduce useful strategies
- prepare for relapse
- emphasise lifestyle issues important to maintaining initial change (Jarvis, Tebbut, & Mattick, 1995).

Commitment to maintaining behavioural change is an essential component in relapse prevention training. The individual may benefit from reviewing the negative aspects of drug or alcohol use and the reasons for changing his or her use patterns.

Comorbid psychiatric conditions such as depression (see Chapter 4.3) have been found to influence treatment outcome in addiction.

The comorbid condition may play a role in maintaining the substance use disorders and therefore should be considered.

Ongoing short-term follow-up will often be helpful for encouraging and supporting adherence to treatment achievements. Follow-up sessions allow the individual to discuss problems or relapses that may have occurred and discuss strategies for coping with these. The time and length of follow-up is best determined by the individual and the clinician, and depends on the initial severity of the problem and the level of functioning achieved after treatment. However, it is important that sessions are arranged in advance and that, when individuals do not attend, they are followed up.

4.7.10 WHERE AND HOW DO PEOPLE GET HELP?

In the most recent census of help provided for alcohol and drugs in Australia, approximately one in 200 people sought treatment. This treatment was provided through over 850 alcohol and other drug treatment services and to around 115 000 people in total (Australian Institute of Health and Welfare, 2014b). Two-thirds of those seeking treatment were males, and 15% were Indigenous. The main drugs of concern were alcohol (38% of treatment episodes) and cannabis (24% of treatment episodes), followed by amphetamines (20% of treatment episodes) and heroin (6% of treatment episodes). Importantly, more than half of respondents were concerned about more than one drug. While help-seeking differs across different substances, the main treatment delivery setting is a non-residential treatment facility, followed by residential treatment facilities and outreach treatment facilities. Types of alcohol and drug treatment services provided included counselling, non-residential, residential and hospital-based withdrawal services, residential and therapeutic day rehabilitation, care and recovery coordination, as well as pharmacotherapy. There are also services available that are specific to youth and Indigenous populations. Most services in Australia adopt a harm minimisation, rather than an abstinence-based, approach to treatment. In Australia, the delay to seek treatment is considerable, especially for alcohol use disorders. Data from the 2007 NSMHWB indicate that one in five people who met criteria for an alcohol use disorder in the previous 12 months had sought treatment (Teesson et al., 2010), and this reduced to one in ten among those aged 16–24 years (Mewton et al., 2011). Among those with a lifetime alcohol use disorder, the median delay to first treatment was 18 years (Chapman, Slade, Hunt, & Teesson, 2015).

There is a high prevalence of mental disorders among individuals with substance use disorders in the Australia general population (Teesson et al., 2012). Overall, 35% of individuals with a substance use disorder (31% men and 44% of women) will also have at least one co-occurring affective or anxiety disorder (see Chapters 4.3 and 4.4). This represents nearly 300 000 Australians. The prevalence of comorbidity is even higher in those entering treatment (Slade et al., 2009). The National Guidelines on the management of co-occurring alcohol and other drug and mental health conditions in alcohol and other drug treatment settings (Marel, Mills, Deady, & Teesson, 2009) provide up-to-date evidence-based information on the management of comorbid mental health conditions. They are based on extensive literature reviews and draw upon the extensive knowledge of clinicians, researchers and those with lived experience.

4.7.11 THE IMPLICATIONS OF THE DIVERSITY OF AUSTRALIA

Overall, interventions and treatments for substance use disorders have been developed with urban city dwelling, predominantly male populations. The implication of diversity is that approaches may need to be adapted, depending on individual characteristics. Three main areas of consideration with specific implications for substance use disorders are covered including Indigenous peoples, culturally and linguistically diverse groups and gay, lesbian, bisexual, transgendered and intersex individuals.

INDIGENOUS PEOPLES

Physical and mental health among Indigenous Australians is poor in comparison with the Australian community. Indigenous Australians are more likely than their non-Indigenous counterparts to abstain from alcohol (Australian Institute of Health and Welfare, 2015c). However, those who do consume alcohol are more likely to drink at levels that put them at risk for short-term injury and long-term harm. It is possible that heavy risky drinking may be normalised within some communities and this could be a barrier to people seeking help (Conigrave et al., 2012). In regards to drugs, just under one in four Indigenous Australian adults reported 12 month use of any illicit drug (Australian Institute of Health and Welfare, 2015). The most commonly used substances among Indigenous Australians were cannabis (17%), non-prescription analgesics (5%) and amphetamines (4%). Volatile substance misuse and petrol sniffing among remote Aboriginal communities of Central Australia are significant health issues (d'Abbs & MacLean, 2008). Tobacco use is also significantly higher in Indigenous peoples with 45% reporting current smoking (Australian Institute of Health and Welfare, 2015). Indigenous Australians were 2.5 times as likely to smoke daily when compared with their non-Indigenous counterparts (32% compared with 12.4%). Unlike their non-Indigenous counterparts, the rates of daily smoking did not decline among Indigenous Australians between 2010 and 2013. (See Chapters 1.2 and 1.3.)

The destruction of social infrastructure, poverty, cultural alienation, loss of identity, negative early life events (domestic violence, physical and sexual abuse) have all been reported to be associated with early initiation of alcohol and drug use (Lee, Harrison, Mills, & Conigrave, 2014). The trauma of stolen generations has a direct impact on the mental health and substance use disorders in Indigenous peoples (Nagel, 2006; Nagel et al., 2011).

The Alcohol and Other Drugs Knowledge Centre, established by the Australian Indigenous *HealthInfoNet* (see https://healthinfonet.ecu.edu.au), has high quality, relevant and up-to-date information and is a significant national resource. The Centre builds the capacity of the Alcohol and Drugs workforce, promotes evidence-informed practice, and encourages greater integration between policy, practice and research. The Centre's mission is to contribute to improving the health of Australia's Aboriginal and Torres Strait Islander peoples and assist in closing the gap by providing the evidence base to help reduce the harmful use of alcohol and other drugs (see further https://aodknowledgecentre.ecu.edu.au).

4.7.12 CULTURAL AND LINGUISTIC DIVERSITY GROUPS

The prevalence of alcohol problems differs by ethnicity and country of birth (see Chapter 1.3). When compared to people born in a non-English-speaking country, those born in Australia and other English-speaking countries are over three times as likely to meet criteria for an alcohol use disorder (Teesson et al., 2010). Research also demonstrates the significance of ethnicity in nicotine addiction. While the rates of daily smoking reduced among those who speak English at home between 2010 and 2013, the rates increased among those people who speak a language other than English in the same time period (Australian Institute of Health and Welfare, 2014b). Rates of tobacco smoking have been identified as particularly high among men of Chinese, Arabic and Vietnamese backgrounds. Indigenous Australians are more likely to die of smoking-related illnesses. Despite the high rates of some drug use in culturally and linguistically diverse populations, ethnic groups are under-represented in treatment services. Significant barriers to treatment include shame and guilt, fear of stigmatisation, cultural differences between therapists and individual seeking help, confusion, lack of education, language difficulties (Marsh, O'Toole, Dale, Willis, & Helfgott, 2013).

It has been suggested that information about three aspects of an individual's experience is crucial to address treatment for alcohol and drug use in those who are culturally and linguistically diverse:

- context of migration including why they left their country, how they arrived in Australia, their legal status, whether they have residency, trauma experiences in the context of their country of origin.
- subgroup membership including ethnicity, gender, sexual orientation, area in which they live.
- Degree of acculturation including traditional (beliefs, values predominantly from country of origin), bicultural (mix of new and old beliefs) and acculturated (modified beliefs; Marsh et al., 2013).

There are few screening tools and interventions developed specifically for culturally and linguistically diverse individuals (Drug and Alcohol Multicultural Education Centre, 2014).

LESBIAN, GAY, BISEXUAL, TRANSGENDERED, INTERSEX AND QUEER INDIVIDUALS

There is a lack of research into substance use disorders in lesbian, gay, bisexual, transgendered, intersex, queer individuals (LGBTIQ; Ritter, 2015). Overall, there is evidence that LGBTIQ individuals experience higher rates of substance use and substance use disorders than heterosexual individuals (Ritter, 2015). Treatment and interventions for substance use disorder in LGBTIQ individuals follows the same principles as for any other client group and should focus on the individual needs. Specific individual issues which should be considered are that same-sex attracted identity usually occurs within a context of internal pressure and stigma (Lea, de Wit, & Reynolds, 2014). This can result in social isolation, guilt, loss of social support, all increasing the risk of substance use disorders. Ritter and colleagues (Ritter, 2015) have identified several key features for working with LGBTIQ individuals that are associated with more positive outcomes: welcoming non-judgemental environment, an accepting and affirming approach, use of culturally sensitive language, staff awareness of LGBTIQ support services, high regard for confidentiality and affirmation of non-traditional family networks (see Chapter 1.3).

4.7.13 COMMENTARY AND REFLECTION

Substance use disorders are determined by multiple interacting factors. It is clear that genetic and environmental factors can play significant roles in initiation and maintenance of alcohol and drug use. It is also clear that learning within a sociocultural context is important and that changing this context can be a way of treating drug and alcohol problems. There is no doubt that substance use disorders cause a considerable burden to individuals and to society. Alcohol and drugs are major contributors to the burden of disease in Australia. Motivational factors and individual preference for treatment type are important factors in determining treatment effectiveness. We need a better understanding of the impact of comorbid psychological and physical illnesses. While evidence in this area is growing, there remain significant gaps. That said, assessing and effectively treating these comorbid disorders, has led to improved outcomes in drug and alcohol treatment. In general a stepped care approach is recommended where less intensive interventions are used before more costly psychological and medical interventions.

The illegality of some drugs of addiction will continue to present both moral and logistical issues in our treatment response. In particular, the use of illicit drugs for the treatment of dependence remains a challenge in the addictions. For example, there has been considerable controversy over the use of injectable heroin for those people for whom other treatments are ineffective. However, research continues to be carried out on this treatment because of the significant need of the chronically heroin dependent people in our communities.

A growing understanding of the neurobiology of alcohol and drug addiction may lead to new and better pharmacological treatments of alcohol and other drug dependence. A combination of biological, social and psychological perspectives on drug use and disorders is required if we are reduce the burden and disability of substance use disorders.

4.7.14 FUNDAMENTAL ISSUES IN ASSESSMENT

The assessment of substance-use disorders will involve a review of the quantity of substance being consumed and the consequences of such use. An important aspect of the assessment process is to provide feedback to the individual, and develop a rapport between the assessor and the individual. Individuals with substance-use disorders are often reluctant to commence treatment.

ETIOLOGICAL FACTORS IN SUBSTANCE USE DISORDERS

A number of etiological factors have been proposed regarding substance use disorders, and some have more support than others. Several studies show how genes interact with the environment for smoking and alcohol problems. Psychological factors have also been evaluated. Expectancies about the effects of drugs, such as reducing tension, helping to cope with emotions and increasing social skills, have been shown to predict drug and alcohol use. Studies of personality factors also help us understand why some people may be more prone to abuse drugs and alcohol. Sociocultural factors play a role, including the culture, availability of a substance, family factors, social settings and networks, and advertising.

Approaches to treating substance use disorders

For heavy alcohol users, withdrawal management is often necessary. There is some evidence that cognitive behavioural based interventions, including couples therapy and motivational interviewing, are of value. Self-help programs may also be effective in the treatment of alcohol use disorders. Medications for alcohol use disorder treatment include naltrexone, acamprosate and disulfiram. There is some evidence that CBT is an effective treatment for cocaine dependence. Residential treatment homes have not been adequately evaluated for their efficacy, though they are a common form of treatment. The use of heroin substitutes, such as methadone or naltrexone, is an effective treatment for heroin use disorder.

4.8

GAMBLING AND GAMING DISORDERS

STEPHANIE MERKOURIS, DANIEL KING, CHLOE HAWKER, KATE SOMMERVILLE & NICKI DOWLING

4.8.1 WHAT IS THIS GROUP OF MENTAL HEALTH EXPERIENCES LIKE?

KATE SOMMERVILLE

LIVED EXPERIENCE

My pokie gambling was medically induced by dopamine agonists prescribed for a neurological condition. At the time, the medical profession was unaware that this medication causes compulsive behaviours by changing dopamine pathways in the brain's reward system. Pokie gambling is now a known high risk for those on this medication.

In 2001, I was exposed to pokies through my work as a social planner in local government. The machines mesmerised me from the beginning, which is their purpose. All my money went on the machines. I became confused and fearful about the changes in my thinking and behaviour. My life quietly spiralled out of control and memories of that time are still painful. Years later, I realised that I began to disassociate from my action to survive. As a professional working in the gambling policy field, my fear and shame were profound.

After 12 months, I confided in my partner, consulted with a nurse, and visited a psychiatrist. The visit to the psychiatrist was unhelpful, and I felt uncomfortable with him. He did not ask about my general health or medical conditions. I was deeply afraid. Eventually, I lost a job because my work performance worsened. I sought help from a psychologist and a spiritual advisor. The latter took me into her development group which helped. By this time, I sensed there was something wrong with the medication and stopped using it so the urge to gamble lessened.

My path to recovery began when I got a new position that I loved in disability policy and soon after discovered the role that dopamine agonists had played in my gambling. I had many lapses before stopping. This is common. My neurologist at the time told me that my brain may have changed permanently. During a class action regarding the medication, a psychiatrist diagnosed me with post-traumatic stress disorder (PTSD), but at the time I did not understand what this meant. I kept working because work provided meaning and purpose. It took me a long time to realise that what I thought were 'normal' reactions and thinking were not. I still have flashbacks and anxiety, but both have decreased.

My gambling removed everything that I valued: friends, partner, family, identity and huge amounts of money. I also lost a sense of internal order and time. Facing and accepting the consequences and sadness from these losses is an ongoing part of my recovery. As an older person, recovery was difficult because there seemed little reason to hope. In hindsight, shame and lack of trust prevented me from asking for help. The ability to concentrate took a long time to return. I doubted that I would ever recover. I couldn't sleep either. It was a tough journey.

What helped? Years later I can say that living in the present moment, working with others and gratitude for what I have all help me maintain some balance and peace. I have known six people who suicided, and I did not want to make this choice. Nor did I want to live my life as a victim. Through reflection, I've learned to retrieve memories of positive achievements and times of happiness and I now define myself through those. Reading, writing, walking, photography and music also bring pleasure and happiness.

Finding meaning in difficult experiences can enhance recovery. My professional training and experience allowed me to become a community educator and an advocate for better services for people who have a lived experience of gambling harm. I believe that compulsive gambling has societal causes and a neurological basis and that understanding both these factors facilitates recovery. They mitigate the shame. We need time to grow again, and we also need to be alert for people and opinions that confine us to lives of victimhood. Community attitudes towards prevention, healing and support still need to change. The political and mercenary nature of the gambling industry makes healthy changes harder for individuals and communities and I believe that understanding and accepting that gambling reform as a long-term challenge is also important.

HISTORICAL DEVELOPMENT OF THE CONCEPT

STEPHANIE MERKOURIS, DANIEL KING, CHLOE HAWKER, KATE SOMERVILLE & NICKI DOWLING

Phenomenology

Prior to the nomenclatural recognition of gambling and gaming disorders, researchers had recognised the general phenomenon of 'compulsive gambling' and 'problematic gaming'. Descriptions of compulsive gambling first appeared in the psychological literature in the 1950s, while the first descriptions of problematic gaming appeared in the early 1980s. These behaviours were often formulated as 'compulsive', 'dependency' or addictive phenomena that could vary in severity and course. Individuals who gambled or played video games excessively were often described as displaying similar symptoms as those with substance use disorders (Fisher, 1994).

Gambling disorder and gaming disorder have been considered behavioural addictions, characterised by impaired control rather than physiological dependence. It has been extensively argued that these disorders share features across diagnostic, clinical, physiological, and behavioural domains (Wareham & Potenza, 2013). The inclusion of behavioural addictions in diagnostic systems has stimulated research, promoted industry regulation, and enhanced diagnosis, prognosis, treatment opportunities, and prevention efforts (Kuss & Griffiths, 2012). Their inclusion has, however, been controversial due to the lack of an ingested psychoactive substance (Hodgins & Makarchuk, 2003) and concerns raised about a 'slippery slope' of viewing almost any human activity as a potential addiction (Shaffer, Hall, & Vander Bilt, 2000). These concerns reflect ongoing debate regarding the definition of addiction, whereby traditional models focusing on physical dependence, biological changes, and neuroadaptation contrast with contemporary models that emphasise impairment of control (Grant, Potenza, Weinstein, & Gorelick, 2010).

Pathological Gambling was first officially recognised as a psychiatric disorder in the ICD-9 and the DSM-III, in which it was categorised as a Disturbance of Conduct and an Impulse Control Disorder (Not Elsewhere Classified) in 1979 and 1980, respectively (American Psychiatric Association [APA], 1980; World Health Organization [WHO], 1979). The DSM-5 has renamed the diagnosis 'gambling disorder' and reclassified it as an addiction and related disorder, alongside alcohol and substance use disorders. Consistent with this change, gambling disorder is now included in the Substance Use and Related Disorders chapter of the ICD-11. While the term problem gambling is often used in psychiatric settings to describe subclinical presentations of gambling disorder, many jurisdictions, including Australia, use this term to describe any individual with difficulties in restricting money and/or time spent gambling which impacts themselves and others (Korn & Shaffer, 1999; Neal, 2005). This definition reflects a public health approach, in which gambling problems are conceptualised across a continuum of risk, ranging from no risk (gambling not associated with health or social problems) to extreme risk (gambling associated with serious problems; Korn, Gibbins, & Azmier, 2003). In contrast, gaming disorder was officially adopted at the World Health Assembly in May 2019 as a diagnosis in the ICD-11 following a provisional status for internet gaming disorder in the DSM-5.

Formal diagnosis

In the ICD-11, the diagnostic criteria for gaming disorder are comparable to those of gambling disorder. These disorders are defined as a pattern of persistent or recurrent gambling or gaming behaviour (i.e., digital gaming or video gaming) leading to significant distress or impairment in important areas of functioning (e.g., personal, social, occupational). These disorders are typically characterised by: (1) impaired control over gambling or gaming (e.g., onset, frequency, intensity, duration, termination, context; (2) increasing priority given to gambling or gaming to the extent that they take precedence over other life interests and daily activities; and (3) continuation or escalation of gambling or gaming despite negative consequences. Gambling or gaming behaviours may be continuous or episodic and recurrent. The gambling or gaming behaviour are normally evident over a period of at least 12 months, but this may be shortened if all diagnostic requirements are met and symptoms are severe. The ICD-11 applies an exclusion of hazardous gambling or betting and bipolar type I and II disorder for gambling disorder, and hazardous gaming for gaming disorder. Both gambling and gaming disorder may include online, offline, or unspecified types, although the offline variant is considered much more common for gambling disorder and the online variant is considered much more common for gaming disorder.

The diagnostic criteria for gambling and gaming disorder are similar across the ICD-11 and DSM-5, in that they both refer to persistent and recurrent patterns of behaviour leading to clinically significant impairment or distress. In the DSM-5, gambling disorder is indicated by four or more of the following nine diagnostic criteria in a 12-month period: tolerance, withdrawal, loss of control, preoccupation, escape or mood relief, chasing losses, deception, interference, and bailout; and includes an exclusion criteria of a manic episode, as well as specifiers for course (episodic, persistent), remission (early remission, sustained remission), and current severity (mild, moderate, severe). Similarly, internet gaming disorder is indicated by meeting five or more of the following criteria in a 12-month period: preoccupation, withdrawal, tolerance, loss of control, loss of non-gaming interests, gaming despite harms, deception, escape or mood relief, and interference; and only refers to persistent and recurrent use of online forms of gaming but not offline forms.

4.8.2 WHAT DO WE KNOW ABOUT THESE DISORDERS?

PREVALENCE

Epidemiological research on gambling disorder and gaming disorder has improved greatly over the last decade, with numerous high quality population cohort studies and many large-scale studies assessing these disorders. These developments have led to more precise estimates of the population level harms related to these disorders. There is, however, substantial variation in prevalence rates arising mainly due to differences in sample characteristics (e.g., age, gender), cultural and regional differences (e.g., Asian vs non-Asian countries, urban versus rural locales), choice of screening tools, and cut-off scores.

Gambling disorder

Worldwide prevalence rates for problem gambling range from 0.5% (Denmark and Netherlands) to 7.6% (Hong Kong), with a global average of 2.3% (Williams, Volberg, & Stevens, 2012). Generally, the highest prevalence rates of problem gambling are observed in Asia, with intermediate rates identified in North America and Australia, and the lowest prevalence rates occurring in Europe. In Australia, 0.4–0.6% of adults report problem gambling, with an additional 1.9–3.7% reporting moderate-risk gambling and 3.0–7.7% reporting low-risk gambling (Dowling et al., 2016; Gainsbury, Russell, Hing, Wood, & Lubman, 2014). Despite these relatively low prevalence rates, gambling is associated with a large burden of harm across the gambling risk continuum, which is of a similar magnitude to alcohol use and dependence (see Chapter 4.7) and major depressive disorders (Browne, Greer, Rawat, & Rockloff, 2017; see Chapter 4.3). Recent research has shown that approximately 85% of this burden of harm is attributable to low- and moderate-risk gamblers, due to their greater prevalence in the population (Browne et al., 2017); however, this figure has been critiqued (see Delfabbro & King, 2017).

Gaming disorder

Gaming disorder prevalence rates generally fall between 1–2%. Most of the robust prevalence studies have been conducted in Europe, such as Rehbein and colleagues' (2015) state-representative school survey of 11 003 adolescents aged 13–18 years, which reported a prevalence of 1.2% using the DSM-5 criteria for internet gaming disorder. Furthermore, Müller and colleagues (2015) examined gaming disorder in seven European countries based on a representative sample of 12 938 adolescents between 14 and 17 years, reporting that 1.6% of the sample met the criteria for internet gaming disorder, with a further 5.1% at risk for internet gaming disorder by meeting up to four criteria. Other studies have reported comparable figures, including: 0.6% of 816 Norwegian adolescents (Mentzoni et al., 2011); 1.3% in a nationally representative panel of 902 Dutch gamers (Haagsma, Pieterse & Peters, 2012); and 1.5% of Dutch adolescents (van Rooij et al., 2011). These figures appear comparable with prevalence estimates reported for similar disorders, such as gambling disorder (Calado & Griffiths, 2015). Numerous studies, however, have reported much higher gaming disorder prevalence estimates, including rates in excess of 15–20% which seem to defy logic (Sosso et al., 2020; Seok & DaCosta, 2012; Wang et al., 2014; Xin et al., 2018) and raise concerns about the validity of instrumentation and associated risks such as false positives.

HOW CAN WE UNDERSTAND THE ORIGINS?

Gambling disorder

There is growing evidence for numerous psychosocial determinants (see Chapter 1.2) of gambling disorder, including depression, male gender, substance use (alcohol, illicit, and tobacco), impulsivity, problem gambling severity, sensation-seeking, violence, under-controlled temperament, antisocial behaviours, and poor academic performance, while factors such as socioeconomic status, parent supervision and social problems serve as protective for developing gambling problems (Dowling et al., 2017a). There is also growing evidence for genetic (50%) and non-shared environmental (50%) determinants, which suggest that genetics plays a larger role for men (compared to women) and adults (compared to adolescents; Xuan et al., 2017).

While many aetiological models seek to explain the development of gambling problems, no model adequately accounts for its psychological, social, and biological determinants. Psychological formulations posit that gambling is a learned maladaptive behaviour that results from a combination of personal reinforcement history and prevailing reinforcement contingencies (behavioural theory) and that gamblers hold invalid beliefs that are based on false assumptions and are maintained by a biased interpretation of the evidence (cognitive theory). Numerous neurochemical systems, such as the dopaminergic system (i.e., reward and reinforcement) and the serotonergic system (i.e., regulation of behavioural inhibition), as well as reward-related brain regions (e.g., ventral prefrontal, ventral striatal and limbic regions) have also been associated with the development of gambling disorder (Gyollai et al., 2014; Potenza, 2013). Broader contextual factors, which influence the availability of gambling and gambling advertising, include regulatory environments and the commercial practices of the gambling industry (Deans, Thomas, Derevensky, & Daube, 2017).

Several aetiological models incorporate components of the diathesis-stress-coping model, which posits that stress leads to greater arousal and dysphoric mood in individuals with psychological/physiological vulnerabilities (e.g., impulsivity) due to inadequate coping skills and a tendency to engage in escape and avoidant behaviour (e.g., gambling). For example, Sharpe's (2002) model proposes that a genetic vulnerability to gambling disorder could be conferred through biological changes in neurotransmitters or through psychological traits such as impulsivity. This genetic vulnerability is likely to be compounded by early experiences that result in a psychological vulnerability in the form of positive gambling attitudes, impulsivity, and poor coping skills. Membership in gambling subcultures and a pattern of early wins combine to produce a perceptual filter through which wins and losses are interpreted. These factors contribute to the development of cognitive biases, and to the association between gambling and arousal. As the frequency of gambling increases, the association between gambling, cognitive biases, and arousal becomes more automatic.

Finally, the pathways model (Blaszczynski & Nower, 2002), which attempts to account for the heterogeneous nature of gambling disorder, posits that there are three different subtypes based on biological, psychological and environmental vulnerabilities. All three pathways have common processes or qualities, including increased accessibility to gambling, impact of classical and operant conditioning, and cognitive schemas. Pathway 1 (i.e., behaviourally conditioned pathway) is also characterised by a lack of premorbid psychopathology and impaired control, whereby gambling occurs due to cognitive distortions and poor decision making. Pathway 2 (i.e., emotionally vulnerable pathway) gamblers present with psychosocial and biological vulnerabilities, such as anxiety, depression, adverse life events and poor coping or problem-solving skills. Pathway 3 (i.e., antisocial impulsivist pathway) adds to these characteristics via features of antisocial personality disorder and impulsive traits. There is increasing empirical support validating aspects of this model (Ledgerwood & Petry, 2006; Turner, Jain, Spence, & Zangeneh, 2008; Vachon & Bagby, 2009).

Gaming disorder

Gaming disorder involves continued gaming despite resultant harms, often with unsuccessful attempts to reduce or stop gaming, with poor behavioural control central to gaming disorder. The Interaction of Person-Affect-Cognition-Execution model (I-PACE model; Brand et al., 2019) of behavioural addiction posits involvement of complex interactions between predisposing risk factors (e.g., genetics, personality, upbringing), maladaptive psychological responses (e.g., cognitive and attentional biases), and executive functions (e.g., poor control and decision making). Shared mechanisms underlying neuropsychological features of gaming disorders exist including decreased loss sensitivity, enhanced reactivity to activity-specific cues, greater choice impulsivity, and aberrant reward-based learning.

Excessive gaming may involve controlled, planned, and conscious psychological processes being overridden by implicit, effortless, and automatic processes that underlie habitual responses to gaming stimuli. Neurobiologically, fronto-striatal circuits involving the ventral striatum have been proposed to be involved in early stages of gaming disorder and fronto-striatal circuits involving the dorsal striatum have been proposed to contribute to habit formation in gaming disorder (Yao et al., 2017). Both functional and structural differences in these and other regions have been implicated in gaming disorder. Longitudinal research has linked fronto-striatal activations to gaming cues to transitions in gaming disorder, including recovery (Dong, Liu, Zheng, Du, & Potenza, 2019).

Psychological learning theories emphasise reinforcing stimuli of gaming activities. Individuals with gaming disorder may develop learned associations between predictable and variable in-game rewards in the form of praise, virtual items, and higher status among players, and may thus experience positive affect and/or relief of negative mood (King, Delfabbro, & Griffiths, 2011). Habitual immersion in gaming may create emotional detachment from the real world that is compounded by depressive mood states related to sedentary activity, poor diet, and sleep deprivation. Additionally, depression may precede gaming disorder given negative reinforcement motivations. Games linked to gaming disorder often involve complex design and socially driven, seemingly endless play. These games have design features that may entice players and satisfy various motivational drives. Games may escalate time and skill requirements, as well as financial commitment (e.g., 'loot boxes'), to attain desired in-game outcomes (King et al., 2019).

COURSE AND IMPACT

Gambling disorder

Gambling disorder is a major public health issue in Australia, costing between $4.7 and $8.4 billion per year (Productivity Commission, 2010). Gambling disorder has a wide impact on individuals, with evidence to suggest harms including financial harm, relationship dysfunction, emotional difficulties, health concerns, cultural harm, decreased work or academic performance, and criminality (Langham et al., 2016). The gambling problems of an individual has also been shown to impact at least six others (i.e., family members and friends), with low-risk and moderate-risk gambling affecting one and three others, respectively (Goodwin, Browne, Rockloff, & Rose, 2017). It has generally been assumed that gambling disorder is persistent and progressive. Recent longitudinal research, however, suggests that there is considerable movement between gambling risk categories and that the likelihood of improvement for people classified at the highest severities of gambling problems is high (LaPlante, Nelson, LaBrie, & Shaffer, 2008).

Gaming disorder

Gaming-related harms have received much less attention in Australia than abroad. Nevertheless, problems associated with excessive gaming are internationally recognised on public health agendas, particularly in Asia and Europe. Individuals with gaming disorder are negatively impacted by their extreme time investment in gaming (i.e., 8-12 hours per day; Baggio et al., 2016). This results in missed opportunities and the interference with, and displacement of, normal routine and functioning, including basic activities (i.e., sleep, eating, personal hygiene); real world social interaction (i.e., talking to people, meeting friends face-to-face, visiting family); and important responsibilities (i.e., school, work, child care). There are currently mixed longitudinal research findings on the stability of gaming disorder. Despite some preliminary evidence suggesting that problematic gaming may be highly stable (Gentile et al., 2011), some recent studies suggest that the condition may be much more transient despite relatively low treatment-seeking (Thege, Woodin, Hodgins, & Williams, 2015) as long-term cases of gaming disorder are quite rare (Baysak, Yertutanol, Dalgar, & Candansayar, 2018; Scharkow, Festl, & Quandt, 2014).

4.8.3 ASSESSMENT

GOOD PRACTICE IN DISORDER-SPECIFIC ASSESSMENT

Good practice in gambling disorder assessment includes measuring:

1 gambling symptom severity
2 gambling behaviour (e.g., frequency, expenditure, and time)
3 gambling harms (e.g.., psychiatric, financial, relationship, quality of life)
4 processes/mechanisms of change (Walker et al., 2006).

Good practice in gaming disorder assessment includes measuring:

1 gaming symptom severity
2 gaming behaviour (e.g., frequency, time, expenditure for games with monetisation features)
3 context of gaming and types of games and
4 gaming beliefs and motivations; and activities that support gaming.

COMMON ISSUES AND DILEMMAS IN ASSESSMENT

Many self-report measures and clinician-administered diagnostic interviews have been developed to assess gambling disorder (Stinchfield, 2014) and gaming disorder (King et al., 2020). There has also been an increase in the number of available brief screening instruments with recent systematic reviews identifying 20 brief screening instruments (1-5 items) for gambling disorder (Dowling et al., 2019a) and 32 screening tools for gaming disorder (King et al., 2020). Many of these instruments are based on items used to assess substance-based disorders. Important considerations for selecting assessment measures include:

1 classification accuracy
2 timeframes employed (current vs lifetime) and
3 the purpose for which they were originally developed (population-level vs clinical settings; Dowling et al., 2019a).

HELPFUL ASSESSMENT INSTRUMENTS AND GUIDES

Gambling disorder

Self-report measures such as the Problem Gambling Severity Index (PGSI; Ferris & Wynne, 2001), South Oaks Gambling Screen (SOGS; Lesieur & Blume, 1987), NORC DSM-IV Screen for Gambling Problems (NODS; Gerstein et al., 1999) and DSM-criteria tend to be used for assessing gambling problems and treatment outcomes. These measures typically assess past year or lifetime symptomatology. However, shortened timeframes have been developed for some of these instruments (e.g., SOGS and NODS; Wulfert et al., 2005). The Gambling Symptom Assessment Scale (G-SAS; Kim, Grant, Potenza, Blanco, & Hollander, 2009) is recommended for measuring treatment outcomes as it employs a past-week timeframe and was specifically designed to measure change during treatment. Similarly, the Pathological Gambling–Yale-Brown Obsessive-Compulsive Scale (PG-YBOCS; Hollander et al., 1998) and the Clinical Global Impression Scale (Hollander et al., 1998) are suitable for measuring treatment outcomes over a short time period. Finally, indices of gambling behaviour (frequency, expenditure, duration) are also often primary outcomes in this literature but these are usually assessed using single author-derived items.

Despite its intended use in epidemiological research, the PGSI is one of the more frequently employed measures for assessing gambling problems in treatment settings. Research, however, has shown that when employing the problem gambling cut-off of 8 or more, 92–94% of individuals seeking help for gambling meet the criteria for problem gambling (Dowling et al., 2019; Waluk, Youssef, & Dowling, 2016). Instead, a cut-off of 19 or more on the PGSI distinguishes between lower and higher problem gambling severity; this cut-off can assist gambling services with treatment planning and improved client outcomes via identification and delivery of targeted treatment options (Merkouris et al., 2020).

Other relevant constructs for treatment planning include:

1 cognitive distortions (e.g., Gambling-Related Cognitions Scale; Raylu & Oei, 2004a)

2. gambling motives (e.g., Gambling Motives Questionnaire–Financial; Dechant, 2014)
3. gambling expectancies (e.g., Gambling Expectancies Questionnaire; Gillespie, Derevensky, & Gupta, 2007)
4. gambling urges (e.g., Gambling Urge Scale; Raylu & Oei, 2004b)
5. high-risk situations (e.g., Inventory of Gambling Situations–Short Form; Smith, Stewart, O'Connor, Collins, & Katz, 2011)
6. readiness to change (e.g., Ready Willing and Able; Rodda, Lubman, Iyer, Gao, & Dowling, 2015)
7. self-efficacy (e.g., Brief Situational Confidence Questionnaire; Breslin, Sobell, Sobell, & Agrawal, 2000)
8. gambling attitudes (e.g., Attitudes Towards Gambling Scale; Canale, Vieno, Pastore, Ghisi, & Griffiths, 2016) and
9. gambling harms (e.g., Short Gambling Harms Scale; (Browne, Goodwin, & Rockloff, 2018).

GAMING DISORDER

There are numerous general-purpose internet addiction tools used to measure gaming-related problems, such as the 20-item Young Internet Addiction Test, which is the most frequently employed measure of problematic gaming. New tools for problematic gaming or gaming disorder have been published every year since 2012. Some noteworthy measures with stronger evidential support include the Internet Gaming Disorder Test-10 (IGDT-10; Kiraly et al., 2017) and the Scale for Assessment of Internet and Computer game Addiction (AICA-S) gaming module (Wolfling, Beutel, & Müller, 2012), with the latter used in many clinical trials (Wolfling et al., 2019).

Assessment of gaming disorder is a part of the therapeutic process in which the clinician helps the client with gaming disorder to begin to understand the links between gaming behaviours and resultant harms. To gather a more complete picture of the client's gaming behaviour and associated lifestyle problems, and to help the client begin to develop more awareness of their gaming problems, additional questions and exploration in the following areas may be beneficial and complement the standard clinical interview. Some specific issues to consider include:

1. Frequency of gaming behaviour. How often gaming occurs, how much time is spent gaming and how much money is spent on gaming? Some games have monetisation features (e.g., loot boxes or micro-transactions) that enable endless spending (King, Delfabbro, et al., 2019).
2. Context of gaming and types of games. How and where does gaming typically occur (e.g., at home and/or elsewhere)? This information can help to build a picture of the client's level of commitment to gaming, the extent to which the client feels unable to be without gaming opportunities, and the co-occurrence of gaming with other daily activities.
3. Client beliefs and motivations. What is the meaning and significance of gaming activities and their link to gaming-related schema (e.g., 'What makes the game special for you?' and 'What is your strongest memory from playing the game in general?').
4. Activities that support gaming. What activities and other influences (e.g., peer influences) support and maintain gaming? These activities are important to identify because they may act as triggers or maintaining factors for gaming, or create or exacerbate other problems (e.g., low mood, inactivity, or social isolation).

PRACTICE ILLUSTRATION: PROBLEM BEGINNINGS

Brendan is a 45-year-old male who lives with his partner of 18 months in a country town. Brendan's three teenage children live with their mother (his ex-wife) and visit on weekends. Brendan retired from his successful plumbing business six months ago, which he described as 'well deserved' after working his way up the business from an apprentice to the owner, with 'decent coin in the bank' for retirement.

Brendan's retirement was reportedly relaxing for the first few months, but things took a downturn two months ago when his dad was diagnosed with pancreatic cancer. Brendan described his father as a 'hard man', who never showed his emotions. Brendan found his father's diagnosis particularly distressing, as none of his family of origin were alive, with his mother dying 10 years ago and his brother dying by suicide six years ago. Following his father's diagnosis, Brendan found himself at the local pub, gambling $200–300 on greyhound races over a few hours, 3–4 times per week.

In the last month, his gambling escalated to a daily occurrence, with losses of up to $1000 per day. In the past, Brendan very occasionally dabbled on the greyhound races with his mates but reported no difficulty in limiting his gambling. Brendan had not told anyone about his current gambling, as he felt ashamed and panicked about his dwindling retirement funds and apparent inability to quit gambling despite repeated attempts. He found himself lying awake at night, with his heart and mind racing. Following another loss, Brendan presented to the emergency department with a suspected heart attack, as he reported sharp pains in his chest, shortness of breath, and 'clammy' skin. Following medical tests, Brendan was cleared of any physical health concerns and referred for a psychology assessment. During this assessment, Brendan revealed the extent of his gambling problems and scored in the problem gambling category on the Problem Gambling Severity Index, resulting in a referral to the closest gambling service.

Assessment

The closest gambling service was over an hour away from Brendan's house, which would make it hard for him to get to treatment. Regardless of the travel, Brendan was reluctant to engage in treatment, as he had been brought up with a 'stiff upper lip' attitude. Deep down, Brendan was also afraid that a psychologist would talk about his brother's suicide and his father's recent diagnosis because he experienced chest pains whenever he thought about them. Brendan was also fearful of his partner finding out about his gambling because he did not want another 'failed relationship', nor his children because he 'couldn't face their disappointment'.

Brendan showed up to the first appointment, 'rattled' by his emergency presentation and feeling hopeless about any chance of treatment success. At this intake appointment, Brendan scored in the severe gambling symptom range on the Gambling Symptom Assessment Scale. Brendan's psychologist utilised motivational interviewing techniques during the appointment, in which Brendan realised that the pros of engaging in treatment (e.g., salvaging his retirement) far outweighed the cons (e.g., inevitable impact on others). They also discussed positives of travelling to a psychologist, such as a sense of anonymity and reduced time available to gamble. Brendan agreed to a course of CBT for gambling problems comprising six weekly sessions, subsidised with a mental health care plan, before reviewing treatment progress. Brendan's psychologist also gave him the details for helplines and self-help resources for in between appointments, and offered the option of designating 'off-topics' which they would not discuss without Brendan's permission.

Treatment

Brendan found treatment hard at first, as he was not used to talking about his thoughts and feelings and he felt shame for gambling with his retirement funds. His psychologist used motivational interviewing techniques at the start and end of sessions to connect Brendan with his reasons for engaging in treatment. Brendan's psychologist also encouraged him to join an online forum, using a pseudonym, to show him that he was not alone in his troubles. Brendan found this forum validating and normalising, and he gradually gained the confidence to tell his partner about his gambling problems and to ask for her support in treatment. Brendan found behavioural techniques most helpful, as he enjoyed filling his time with activities involving his partner, mates, and children and he enjoyed the positive impact this was having on his relationships; he also found it much harder to avoid gambling when he had a lot of spare time.

Brendan consistently cut down his gambling behaviour over the course of treatment and, by his six-session review, he had made significant treatment gains. His Gambling Symptom Assessment Scale score had reduced to the mild gambling symptom category and he had not experienced a panic attack in over a month. Brendan was finding it harder to ignore his grief about his brother's death, however, particularly as his father's health was deteriorating. Brendan knew that he needed longer-term help for grief, as he feared a relapse when his father inevitably passed. Brendan's psychologist extended his appointments to occur every three weeks and they found a local grief counsellor for therapy between their sessions. As a team, Brendan, his psychologist, and grief counsellor worked together until he felt he no longer needed gambling treatment.

4.8.4 EVIDENCE-BASED AND OTHER TREATMENTS AND SERVICES

MAIN TREATMENTS AND STRENGTH OF EVIDENCE

Gambling disorder

The Australian Government's National Health and Medical Research Council (NHMRC) developed an evidence hierarchy to allocate interventions to grades of evidence of support for their use (from Grade A–D). By definition, Grade A evidence can guide practice, Grade B evidence can guide practice in most situations, Grade C evidence provides some support but caution is required, and Grade D evidence is weak and recommendation must be applied with caution (Problem Gambling Research and Treatment Centre, 2011).

NHMRC-endorsed treatment guidelines recommend psychological therapies delivered face-to-face, including cognitive behaviour therapy (CBT), motivational interviewing, motivational enhancement therapy, and practitioner-delivered interventions as first-line treatment options based on Grade B evidence (see also Chapters 1.4, 1.5; Cowlishaw et al., 2012; Problem Gambling Research and Treatment Centre, 2011; Thomas et al., 2011; Yakovenko, Quigley, Hemmelgarn, Hodgins, & Ronksley, 2015). A Cochrane review (Cowlishaw et al., 2012) revealed that relative to control groups, participants randomised to CBT demonstrated medium to very large short-term reductions in gambling behaviour and psychological functioning, but that the durability of effects from CBT gambling treatments remains unknown. In contrast, this review suggested beneficial effects from motivational interviewing that are limited to gambling behaviour and which do not extend to other symptoms of disordered gambling. In addition, there is Grade C evidence for psychological interventions delivered in a group format. Recently, there has also been growing evidence for mindfulness-based interventions (Maynard, Wilson, Labuzienski, & Whiting, 2015) and self-help interventions (e.g., Casey et al., 2017; Dowling et al., 2017) with some evidence that structured online CBT programs may be as effective as face-to-face interventions (Goslar, Leibetseder, Muench, Hofmann, & Laireiter, 2017). Self-help interventions may be a promising avenue for treatment, as only a minority of people (8–17%) access face-to-face services for gambling problems (Productivity Commission, 2010).

There is also Grade C evidence for naltrexone as a pharmacological intervention to reduce gambling severity. A recent Cochrane review of pharmacological interventions for gambling disorder (Dowling, Merkouris, et al., 2020) revealed evidence of a consistent medium beneficial effect of opioid antagonists (naltrexone, nalmefene) relative to placebo for gambling behaviours, psychopathology, and functional impairment immediately following treatment. Pharmacotherapies classified as mood stabilisers (including mood stabilisers, anticonvulsants, and atypical antipsychotics) also displayed a medium to large effect on gambling symptom severity relative to placebo conditions immediately post-treatment; but the effect of these pharmacological agents did not extend to other indices of gambling behaviour, psychological functioning, or functional impairment.

Gaming disorder

Gaming disorder is a complex disorder, frequently exhibiting multiple features requiring attention in treatment (Griffiths, Kuss, & Pontes, 2016; King et al., 2017; Zajac, Ginley, Chang, & Petry, 2017). To date, studies of psychological treatments for gaming disorder outnumber those involving pharmacological treatment by a factor of 3:1, with the majority of this psychological treatment literature exploring the efficacy of CBT. A recent meta-analysis examined 12 independent CBT studies for gaming disorder (Stevens, King, Dorstyn, & Delfabbro, 2019), with CBT demonstrating high efficacy in reducing gaming disorder symptoms and depression, and moderate efficacy in reducing anxiety, in the short-term. It was unclear, however, whether CBT reduced time spent gaming. CBT for gaming disorder may be an effective short-term intervention for reducing gaming and depressive symptoms, but more studies with follow-up are needed to assess longer-term gains.

As such, current recommended psychological treatment involves a combination of cognitive behavioural therapy (CBT) and adjunctive strategies that:

1 modify maladaptive cognitions (attitudes, beliefs, biases) that initiate and maintain excessive gaming
2 foster coping strategies to reduce withdrawal and other unpleasant mood states (depression) when not gaming and
3 develop social skills and establish new behavioural routines, including physical activities, in place of gaming activities.

TREATMENT CHALLENGES FOR MENTAL HEALTH WORKERS

Mental health workers in both the gambling and gaming fields face various treatment challenges, including high rates of drop out and relapse during treatment, low compliance with therapeutic guidelines, and a need to adapt indicated treatments for each individual given the heterogeneity of presentations (Menchon, Mestre-Bach, Steward, Fernández-Aranda, & Jiménez-Murcia, 2018). In the gaming field, mental health workers face the obvious challenge of not having a set of treatment recommendations or guidelines to follow when supporting someone with gaming disorder due to a lack of an evidence base.

TREATMENT CHALLENGES FOR CONSUMERS

Gambling treatment consumers face numerous barriers to accessing treatment, including shame, denial, stigma, a desire to deal with one's own problem, a lack of available services and trained clinicians, geographic barriers, cost, and/or the necessity of abstinence as the goal of treatment (Suurvali, Cordingley, Hodgins, & Cunningham, 2009; Suurvali, Hodgins, Toneatto, & Cunningham, 2008). Gaming treatment consumers likely face many of the same barriers, as well as a lack of recognition of gaming disorder as a mental health disorder and a lack of an evidence base for treatment (Wang, Ren, Long, Liu, & Liu, 2019). In both fields, consumers may benefit from a multi-pronged treatment approach (e.g., a combination of professional support, peer support and self-exclusion), and recovery can be a long process in which multiple treatment attempts may be needed.

KEY RISKS OF HARM IN TREATMENT ATTEMPTS

Harms associated with the psychological treatment of gambling disorder have not yet been investigated. However, there is some evidence that some minor adverse effects, such as nausea, headaches, diarrhoea, constipation, dry mouth, insomnia, dizziness, sedation, and somnolence, are associated with pharmacological interventions for gambling disorder (Bullock & Potenza, 2013). Harms associated with treatment attempts for gaming disorder are also largely unknown given the fledgling state of the literature, which indicates that treatment ought to be conducted with caution.

4.8.5 WHERE AND HOW DO PEOPLE GET HELP?

GAMBLING DISORDER

People seeking help for gambling in Australia can access free government-funded services specialising in gambling treatment, including face-to-face, telephone, and online counselling, financial counselling, peer support (e.g., online forums, blogs, and support groups), peer counselling, legal services (in selected jurisdictions), and self-help resources. Due to the low rate of treatment-seeking in this population, many jurisdictions are currently investing in the development of online and mobile self-help interventions. Most of the government-funded services also provide support for people affected by someone's gambling. Peer support through Gamblers Anonymous is also available in most Australian states and territories. Australian gambling providers also offer free self-exclusion programs, in which people can opt to exclude themselves from specific providers for an agreed period of time. Mental health care plans can also be received for subsidised appointments with a mental health professional.

GAMING DISORDER

In contrast, there are very few specialised treatment options for gaming disorder in Australia. Those seeking help for gaming disorder and problematic gaming may be referred to psychological and/or counselling services, including those which specialise in addiction. Psychiatrists may prescribe medications (typically, an antidepressant such as bupropion) to improve engagement in these therapies. For adolescents and emerging adults, it is recommended that supportive parents or other family members also attend therapy. Some treatment centres provide brief voluntary retreats, which typically involve abstinence from digital technologies, group therapy and social activities, but these options may be financially burdensome and have limited evidence for their long-term efficacy. Self-help support groups are also available online internationally.

4.8.6 THE IMPLICATIONS OF THE DIVERSITY OF AUSTRALIA

RURALITY

For people living in rural Australia, it is difficult to access evidence-based treatment for gambling or gaming problems (Oakes, Gardiner, McLaughlin, & Battersby, 2012). Often, people need to travel to urban areas for treatment, which poses time and financial barriers. Some gambling services have partnered with rural providers to upskill local staff in the treatment of gambling problems; however, most rural areas are severely underserviced (Gannon, Delfabbro, & Sutherland, 2020). To overcome geographical service barriers, helpful treatment options may include online or telephone counselling or self-directed interventions.

AREAS OF DISADVANTAGE

Helpful gambling or gaming treatment services for people from areas of disadvantage likely include free or low-cost service options, such as free online or telephone counselling or self-directed interventions. Given evidence of higher gaming machine density and expenditure per capita in areas of socioeconomic disadvantage (Barratt & Livingston, 2015), there is a clear need for gambling treatment options among these communities.

INDIGENOUS PEOPLES

Indigenous peoples are often reluctant to seek help from mainstream services for gambling or gaming due to significant barriers to accessing help. These barriers include shame, stigma, denial, confidentiality concerns, ambivalence about counselling (as it is a distinctly Western concept) and a lack of culturally appropriate interventions (Hing & Breen, 2014). Typically, Indigenous peoples attempt to deal with the problem themselves, before seeking informal support from family, friends, and community elders, and only seek professional support (ideally from Indigenous providers) once all other options are exhausted (Breen, Hing, Gordon, & Holdsworth, 2013; Hing & Breen, 2014; McMillen & Donnelly, 2008). There are a small number of professional Indigenous gambling support services offering telephone, email, and face-to-face counselling and workshops, outreach programs, health services, and health promotion resources. Professional gaming support services for Indigenous support services have yet to be developed. While Indigenous peoples can also access mainstream services, their appropriateness has been questioned (Breen et al., 2013). Cultural considerations for treatment include developing appropriate interventions within the community, rather than imposed from outside, and utilising a holistic approach to address other issues (e.g., housing, employment), spirituality, kinship, and information sharing via traditional narrative methods (McMillen & Donnelly, 2008).

CULTURAL AND LINGUISTIC DIVERSITY

While culturally and linguistically diverse (CALD) communities tend to gamble less than the overall population in Australia, they often experience more problems when they do gamble (Dickins & Thomas, 2016; Dowling, Brown, Aarsman, & Merkouris, 2020). There is also a higher prevalence of problematic video gaming in the East Asian population, as compared to Western European, North American and Australian populations (King, Delfabbro, & Griffiths, 2012). As with other minority populations, there are numerous barriers to help-seeking for gambling or gaming problems, such as shame and stigma, which often affects the entire family system, particularly among collectivist cultures, as well as cultural mores which preclude seeking professional support (Dickins & Thomas, 2016). Hence, people from CALD communities typically deal with the problem within the family, only seeking professional help if the problem exceeds their coping capacity.

Although CALD-specific services are generally unavailable for gaming disorder, there are some CALD-specific professional support services available for gambling disorder. These services offer counselling, information, support groups, and outreach clinics to individuals with gambling problems and their families in numerous different languages. There are also services for specific cultural groups. Some mainstream services also offer resources translated into various languages, as well as telephone counselling with the aid of an interpreter service. Cultural considerations for treatment involving CALD communities may be highly individual; for example, some individuals may prefer a counsellor outside of the community to avoid bringing shame on the family, while others prefer to involve family in treatment. Nevertheless, it is likely helpful for treatment to involve speaking to someone who speaks their first language and understands their background.

REFUGEES

There are few gambling or gaming support services specifically tailored to migrants and refugees, despite being identified as an at-risk group for gambling disorder (Dickins & Thomas, 2016) and gaming disorder (Griffiths, 2000; Saquib et al., 2017). There are general mental health services for migrants and refugees; however, their training in the treatment of gambling and gaming problems is unclear. Cultural considerations for treatment may overlap with those from CALD communities, plus potentially added considerations, such as the management of trauma and uncertain migrant status.

LGBTIQ COMMUNITY

There are virtually no gambling or gaming treatment services specifically developed for the LGBTIQ community, due to scant research in this area, despite emerging evidence of higher risk gambling (Hershberger & Bogaert, 2005; Richard et al., 2019; Rider, McMorris, Gower, Coleman, & Eisenberg, 2019) and gaming (Broman & Hakansson, 2018) behaviour compared to cisgender and heterosexual individuals. Mental health services for LGBTIQ people often utilise affirmative counselling and peer support frameworks, which typically provide support for issues relating to sexual and/or gender diversity. None of these services, nor mainstream gambling services, provide specialised adjunctive support for gambling problems and issues relating to sexual and gender diversity. There is evidence that LGBTIQ people, particularly young people, prefer to access support via the internet (Lucassen et al., 2018; McDermott, Hughes, & Rawlings, 2016). Hence, helpful services may include online services which claim to be inclusive. Some general treatment considerations may include providing affirmative services, understanding terminology, and avoiding a one-size-fits-all approach among this diverse community.

4.8.7 COMMENTARY AND REFLECTION

The gambling and gaming disorder fields are growing rapidly. However, there is a continued need for high quality epidemiological and longitudinal studies to establish the risk and protective factors across individual, peer, family, and community domains for each disorder. Intervention studies that move beyond the delivery of cognitive behavioural interventions and attempt to identify the mechanisms underlying the efficacy of interventions and subgroups for whom interventions are effective are required. Empirical research should include consistent measures of comorbidity (e.g., to address questions regarding the presence of other mental disorders, such as depression, anxiety, attention deficit/hyperactivity or other factors such as past trauma that may affect risk of these disorders). Similarly, future work should consider not only addictive aspects of these behaviours (King, Koster, & Billieux, 2019), but also other relevant perspectives and concepts related to understanding repetitive behaviours, notably impulsivity and compulsivity, in further developing and refining instruments and diagnostic criteria. Non-problematic gambling and gaming habits, as well as diagnostically subthreshold entities such as 'hazardous gaming' (QE22) in the ICD-11 and low- to moderate-risk gambling, deserve closer attention (Potenza, 2018). Finally, the introduction of the public health perspective, which positions gambling and gaming within a whole of population approach that can inform policy for prevention and intervention practices (Korn & Shaffer, 1999), has resulted in another wave of conceptual confusion, in which the symptomatology and characteristics of the disorder are conflated with the potential negative consequences of the behaviours (Browne et al., 2016; Productivity Commission, 2010).

4.9

PERSONALITY DISORDERS

SATHYA RAO, JAYDIP SARKAR, JILLIAN BROADBEAR, RITA BROWN, FLICK GREY & DANIELLE JAEGER WITH BRUCE FALCONER

4.9.1 LIVED EXPERIENCE

FLICK GREY

My name is Flick Grey.

My diagnosis is borderline personality disorder.

No, wait, borderline is not mine.

While it may be a fairly accurate description of my behaviour

when I am overwhelmed with shame and inarticulable distress,

(which for many years was much of the time),

it's a profoundly cruel diagnosis

and not how I would describe my suffering

if I were really listened to.

Seeking understanding, healing and a way forward,

I read what is written about us.

I read voraciously. And it is shattering.

We do not deserve ...

I have become aware

that borderline is an unexplanation.

It not only fails to offer meaningful explanation

for my distress,

it not only fails to articulate the experience,

—my experience, not the experience of those observing me—

it not only fails to open up deep healing and empathic support,

it stands in the way.

Seeking support, healing and a way forward,

I turn to the mental health system.

I reveal my private shames, disclose my intimate relationships with blades, liquor, traffic, trains.

But the signs are not 'serious' enough.

Seeking attention is inappropriate?

I don't yet have a vocabulary to articulate this experience.

I know in my body that trauma can pale next to this ...

Insignificance? Invalidation? Incongruence?

My childhood knew overt trauma

which paled next to other things:

abandonment, inconsolable anxieties,

disorganised attachment,

emotional resonances that I am still disentangling

and finding words for,

words that could do justice to the complexities,

words that could be mine.

The supports that are offered

in the cracks we don't fall through

have taught me to behave OK.

I've been taught to do OK really well.

So long as I'm not cutting

or screaming at my mother,

(sorry mum)

everyone's OK.

So long as the pain is invisible, it's not 'serious'.

Resisting the temptation to play the blame game,

(and we are usually blamed)

I wonder what has worked, for me.

Time—I could never get enough—

relationships, connection, care,

non-shaming boundaries.

and joy, creativity, belonging, love.

And finding my voice.

Sometimes it seems as simple as being really heard.

So thank you,

thank you

for trying to hear me.

4.9.2 INTRODUCTION

SATHYA RAO

PERSONALITY DISORDERS

The science of personality disorders has taken centre stage in mental health during the last two decades. Personality disorders are the most stigmatised, misunderstood and underdiagnosed conditions in psychiatry; a generation of mental health professionals has not been trained to treat and manage people with personality disorders. At present, evidence-based treatments are only available for borderline personality disorder.

Personality disorder describes pervasive and persistent patterns of thoughts, emotions and behaviour that deviate markedly from cultural expectations and cause clinically significant distress or impairment. It is vital to develop a comprehensive understanding when an individual has a disordered personality, as its consequences are distressing not only to the person but also to people around them and may lead to profound functional impairment. Personality disorders (PD) often influence the course and outcome of coexisting mental health conditions.

Personality disorders occur frequently in the community, impacting approximately 6% of the world population (Huang et al., 2009). 6.5% of Australian adults meet diagnostic criteria for at least one personality disorder (Jovev & Jackson, 2006). Unfortunately, personality disorders have received limited recognition as a public health issue to date. Consequently, people with personality disorders have limited access to care and are often discriminated against in health care settings. These individuals carry a high risk of suicide and experience high rates of comorbid mental health disorders (Grenyer, Ng, Townsend, & Rao, 2017).

Thirty-one to 45% of psychiatric patients meet criteria for at least one personality disorder (Zimmerman, Chelminski, & Young, 2008). Personality disorder accounted for just over 7% of all admissions to general adult psychiatric beds in 2001 (Dasgupta & Barber, 2004). People with disorders (such as schizoid personality disorder) are very unlikely to present for assistance, whereas people with borderline personality disorder are most likely to come to the attention of services. People who have personality disorders experience difficulties in interpersonal relationships, are often single, tend to be less educated, often unemployed and may have problems with substance use. These contribute to poorer quality of life which worsens as more personality disorder criteria are met (Cramer, Torgersen, & Kringlen, 2006). A large component of community services and resources within the psychiatric, social welfare, public health and prison services are directed towards people who have personality disorder: despite this, adequate and appropriate psychological interventions are rarely delivered (Cloninger & Svrakic, 2009).

Clients and medical professionals often perceive a diagnosis of personality disorder as a pejorative label, one that carries negative, blaming, attacking and disrespectful connotations (Henry & Cohen, 1983). For professionals, diagnostic difficulties arise due to issues of classification and the lack of clarity in relation to diagnosis. The paucity of evidence-based research and treatment approaches for most personality disorders limits guidance for assessment and therapy. These difficulties and attendant controversy raise many issues, not the least of which is defining what constitutes a 'normal' personality and the point at which it becomes a disordered personality. The challenge for clinicians is to develop an understanding of the person within his or her context, taking into account the unique factors that define the person and the nature of their difficulties and distress. The contributions to this chapter from Flick Grey, Danielle Jaeger and Rita Brown clearly illustrate how misunderstanding, stigma and discrimination magnify the difficulties facing people who have personality disorders, particularly borderline personality disorder, and that being listened to and taken seriously is central to being able to utilise help.

LIVED EXPERIENCE: A CARER

RITA BROWN

The mental health system calls me a 'carer'. The term carer is not a term I particularly like—yet I am unaware of another word that is inclusive of all the various care/support relationships that exist. To me, the term 'carer' gives the perspective of 'doing for' rather than 'supporting'. It is important for us to understand that as family members and friends, our primary role is to support and empower the person with BPD in their recovery journey although there will be times when, due to acute unwellness, we will need to do things for them. We need to stay mindful that it is important to give back these responsibilities as soon as possible so that they can maintain ownership of their recovery. In addition, to me my relationship with the person is of prime importance and I would rather be regarded as a mum or sister or partner whatever happens. Sometimes, unfortunately, to access the supports I/we need, I need to identify as my daughter's carer.

My daughter took her first overdose at the age of 15. Later she told me that she started self-harming about the age of 10. I knew she was struggling... something wasn't right... and she and I were totally alienated. I was also struggling. As a loving mum, I felt it was my responsibility to protect her, to ease her pain and keep her safe. I felt totally helpless not knowing how to help her. Whatever I tried seemed to be wrong, It seemed no matter how much I tried to be there for her, to support and to love, it wasn't enough. I felt totally powerless and questioned my parenting... what have I done/what have I missed? By friends and even a school counsellor I was told, 'Oh don't worry about her...she's fine.... she'll grow out of it'. How negating this was of how she was feeling and of my concerns.

Fortunately, a family friend made me aware of this diagnosis called BPD and it seemed to offer an explanation. It took many more years of pain and incorrect diagnoses (and treatment) before her main therapists agreed on the diagnosis of BPD and she was able to access appropriate services.

To me, accessing my own professional support and finding a support group were essential for my own wellbeing and helped me to get through each day. I felt less alone knowing someone understood my pain and distress.

I learnt to accept that while my daughter had BPD it did not define who she was. I realised that she was doing the best she could at any particular moment and to hold some hope for her (and us) for a better future.

4.9.3 CLASSIFICATION AND DIAGNOSIS OF PERSONALITY DISORDERS

JAYDIP SARKAR

INTRODUCTION

Clinicians have two systems of classifications at their disposal: the Diagnostic & Statistical Manual (DSM), which was developed for research and clinical practice in North America, and the International Classification of Diseases (ICD), which is promulgated by the World Health Organization and used worldwide. The ICD-10 and DSM-IV revealed several inherent problems in the validity and reliability of personality disorder diagnosis since both rely upon a categorical approach, i.e. that a person either had or did not have a personality disorder (Livesley, 2007; Tyrer et al., 2007). Neither system envisioned personality disorder as representing the extreme position on a continuum, with the other pole representing normal personality, nor the notion that normal merges imperceptibly into the disordered state; the dimensional position. These differences are due to philosophical and theoretical approaches that distinguish the biological and the social sciences: medical systems belong to the categorical school and psychology to the dimensional one (Sarkar & Duggan, 2010).

DEFICITS OF CATEGORICAL SYSTEM

Some deficits of the categorical approach taken by ICD-10 (World Health Organization, 1992) and DSM-5 (APA, 2013) to diagnosing personality disorders include:

- **a** no evidence of there being 10 discrete personality disorder diagnoses
- **b** problems of overlap or diagnostic heterogeneity (individuals may fulfil several personality disorder diagnoses)
- **c** inadequate capture of important clinical aspects of personality pathology (e.g. sadistic and passive-aggressive traits; Westen & Shedler, 2000)
- **d** insufficient discrimination of categories or within-disorder heterogeneity, when traits of multiple disorders found in one person led to diagnosis of 'personality disorder not otherwise specified' or PD-NOS (Verheul & Widiger, 2004)
- **e** classificatory schemes being unhelpful in treatment selection (Livesley, 2007; Sanderson, Swenson, & Bohus, 2002).

DIMENSIONAL SYSTEMS

Subsequently, both the DSM-5 and ICD-11 (WHO, 2019e) have offered a dimensional option. While the ICD-11 is entirely dimensional in its approach, the DSM-5 has retained the categorical approach in its main body along with an Alternative Model of Personality Disorders (AMPD), which is dimensional in nature. Both versions comprise two dimensions. The ICD-11 has a) a *severity* dimension which reflects a psychodynamic understanding of personality dysfunction, and b) a *five-trait domain model* which corresponds to the pathological 'poles' of the well-known and widely validated five-factor model of personality (Rothmann & Coetzer, 2003). Trait domain qualifiers describe the characteristics of a personality that are most prominent and that contribute to personality disturbance. These are not diagnostic categories but are continuous with normal personality characteristics, representing a set of dimensions that correspond to the underlying structure of personality. Individuals with more severe personality disturbance tend to have a greater number of prominent trait domains.

There are five-trait domains (negative affectivity, detachment, dissociality, disinhibition and anakastia) and a single pattern (the borderline pattern). Their core features are as follows:

- *Negative affectivity*: tendency to experience a broad range of negative emotions with a frequency and intensity out of proportion to the situation; emotional lability and poor emotion regulation; negativistic attitudes; low self-esteem and self-confidence; and mistrustfulness. This trait corresponds with borderline personality of the categorical approach.
- *Detachment*: tendency to maintain interpersonal distance (social detachment) and emotional distance (emotional detachment) manifested as lack of friendships, avoidance of intimacy, reserve, aloofness, and limited emotional expression and experience. This domain corresponds to schizoid personality of the categorical approach.
- *Dissociality*: involves the disregard for the rights and feelings of others, self-centredness and lack of empathy, a sense of entitlement, expectation of others' admiration, positive or negative attention-seeking behaviours, indifference to causing hurt to others by being deceptive, manipulative, and exploitative, being mean-spirited and physically aggressive, callousness in response to others' suffering, and ruthlessness in obtaining one's goals. This domain corresponds to a combination of antisocial personality (psychopathy in its more extreme form) and narcissistic personality of the categorical approach.
- *Disinhibition*: the tendency to act rashly based on immediate external or internal stimuli (i.e., sensations, emotions, thoughts), without consideration of potential negative consequences, commonly manifested by impulsivity; distractibility; irresponsibility; recklessness; and lack of planning. This domain is a combination of borderline, antisocial and histrionic personalities of the categorical approach.
- *Anakastia*: is a narrow focus on rigid standards of perfection, of right and wrong, and on obsessive insistence of adherence of one's own and others' behaviour to these standards. Common manifestations include: a desire for perfectionism with social rules, obligations, norms of right and wrong, attention to detail, rigid, systematic, day-to-day routines, hyper-scheduling as well as rigid control over emotional expression, stubbornness and inflexibility, risk-avoidance, perseveration, and deliberativeness. This domain corresponds to obsessive-compulsive personality from the categorical approach.
- *Borderline pattern*: characterised by a pervasive pattern of instability of interpersonal relationships, self-image, and affect, with marked impulsivity. The descriptive features of this pattern are similar to previous borderline personality criteria, although its inclusion is not intended to imply a unique ontological status. Since borderline personality disorder (BPD) is the most frequently diagnosed PD in ICD-10, its inclusion is specifically intended to facilitate the transition from a categorical to a dimensional PD model by providing clinicians with tools for documenting the variability in presentation of people previously considered to have BPD (Clark, Cuthbert, Lewis-Fernández, Narrow, & Reed, 2017).

The Alternative DSM-5 Model for Personality Disorders (AMPD) is conceptually similar to the ICD-11 (they are compared in Table 4.34). Given their similarities, a legitimate question might be 'Which system to use?' While the AMPD personality disorder traits can be used for describing ICD-11 personality disorder domains, the ICD-11 is parsimonious, 'simple' and feasible for 'busy' practitioners while aligning with the domains of the more comprehensive AMDP. For services with specialist interest and expertise, the AMDP is more comprehensive, more aligned to research evidence and likely to be useful in allocation of clinical resources, as well as in legal and research settings.

The definitions and diagnostic criteria for the ICD and DSM systems are summarised in Table 4.34.

Table 4.34 Evolution and comparison of the ICD and DSM systems

Revisions	ICD-10 (categorical)	ICD-11 (dimensional)	DSM-5 (categorical)	Alternative model (AMPD; dimensional)
Definition of personality disorder	Conditions not directly attributable to gross brain damage or disease, or to another psychiatric disorder; abnormal pattern is enduring and not limited to episodes of mental illness Disturbance in several areas of functioning, e.g. affect, arousal, impulse control, ways of perceiving or thinking, and interpersonal conduct Behaviours maladaptive to a broad range of personal and social situations Developmental onset and continue into adulthood with considerable personal distress Different sets of criteria needed for different cultures with regard to social norms, rules and obligations Usually but not invariably, associated with significant problems in occupational and social performance	Characterised by problems in identity, interpersonal dysfunction, disturbance in cognition, emotional experience and expression Maladaptive behaviours across a range of social and personal situations Cannot be explained by cultural or social factors; not developmentally appropriate Disturbance associated with significant impairment in personal, family, social, educational, occupational or other important areas of functioning	Deviation is not explained by other mental disorders or organic brain disease or drug abuse Characteristic and enduring patterns of inner experience and behaviour that deviates markedly from the cultural norm in terms of cognition, affect, impulse control and need gratification, and interpersonal relationships Behaviour is inflexible, maladaptive or otherwise dysfunctional across a range of personal and social situations Abnormal pattern is stable, having onset in late childhood or adolescence Behaviour that deviates markedly from the cultural norm There is personal distress and/or adverse impact on social environment	Condition not better explained by another mental disorder nor solely attributable to physiological effects of a substance or another medical condition (e.g. head trauma) Moderate or greater impairment in personality. [self (identity and self-direction) and interpersonal (empathy and intimacy)] Impairments in personality functioning and trait expression are relatively inflexible and pervasive across a broad range of personal and social situations Relatively stable and can be traced back to adolescence or early childhood Not understood as normal for an individual's developmental state or sociocultural environment
Description of the system	**Categories** Paranoid, schizoid, dissocial, emotionally unstable (impulsive & borderline type), histrionic, anankastic, anxious-avoidant, dependent, other specific, unspecified	**Severity dimension** Difficulty, mild, moderate, severe **Prominent traits or patterns** *Traits (5 domains):* negative affectivity, detachment, dissociality, disinhibition, anakastia **Pattern:** borderline pattern	**Categories** Cluster A: paranoid, schizoid, schizotypal Cluster B: antisocial, borderline, histrionic, narcissistic Cluster C: avoidant, dependent, obsessive-compulsive	**Pathological personality traits** (5 domains with 25 trait facets) negative affectivity, detachment, antagonism, disinhibition and psychoticism **Specific personality disorders** antisocial, avoidant, borderline, narcissistic, obsessive-compulsive, schizotypal and trait specified

BENEFITS OF A DIMENSIONAL APPROACH

Defining personality disorder in terms of personality functioning and traits provides an efficient stepwise approach to personality disorder assessment. The AMPD system enables the diagnosis of five specific personality disorder categories or 'personality disorder-trait specified' for all other presentations. The ICD-11 system enables the determination of a severity level such that a person can have different severities at different points in life or during different stressful periods and acknowledges that personality can manifest different domains and a borderline pattern.

DEFICITS OF THE DIMENSIONAL MODEL

The main criticism of the AMPD is that it is too complicated for general clinical use, although the evidence is contrary to this perception. The reliability of BPD diagnosis was comparable to bipolar I disorder and exceeded schizophrenia and major depressive disorder (Clark et al., 2017).

The critique of the ICD-11 refers to the imprecise definition of degrees of impairment and use of personality domains without facet specification. This could lead clinicians to equate domains in ICD-11 with disorder in ICD-10, e.g. equate 'negative affectivity' with 'what we used to call BPD'. Moreover, high-order, highly stable personality dimensions are of limited clinical utility for treatment selection and prediction of response; guidelines regarding how such broad domains can be utilised in meaningful ways are not available.

CONCLUSION

The newer versions of the ICD and DSM classificatory systems provide a more empirically based, clinically useful system that is likely to enable more appropriate choice of treatment options. The dimensional systems are not free from deficits either and only time will show the extent to which these criteria are adopted by clinicians.

4.9.4 ETIOLOGY AND COMORBID FEATURES OF PERSONALITY DISORDER

SATHYA RAO

ETIOLOGY

While it is self-evident that personality develops from birth to adulthood, less obvious is that experiences throughout life engender continuous change and development of personality in both the healthy and pathological ranges, through the interaction of inherited characteristics with environmental factors (Newton-Howes, Clark, & Chanen, 2015).

Research into the genetic heritability of personality disorders has attracted a lot of attention during the past two decades, concluding that about half of the variability seen in personality function is directly attributable to genetic differences among individuals. While it is unlikely that specific genes associated with personality pathology or personality disorders will be identified, multivariate genetic analyses may clarify the nosology of personality disorders (Livesley & Larstone, 2018).

A significant number of people (up to 85%) diagnosed with BPD report history of trauma (physical, emotional or sexual) during childhood. About five million Australian adults report childhood trauma including abuse affects (Kezelman, Hossack, Stavropoulos, & Burley, 2015). However, community studies have demonstrated that childhood trauma doesn't result in personality disorders or other mental illnesses in most people (Browne & Finkelhor, 1986; Rind & Tromovitch, 1997). It was previously believed that adverse childhood experiences played a causative role in the formation of personality pathology. The current understanding is that childhood trauma is not essential for formation of borderline personality pathology, but it is a significant risk factor (Paris, 2008). Perhaps a complex set of interactions between genetic vulnerability, attachment issues and life experiences play a role in the aetiology of personality disorders.

COMORBIDITY

There is widespread comorbidity between major psychiatric diagnoses and personality disorders, with up to half of psychiatric patients seeming to have personality disorder (Tyrer, Gunderson, Lyons, & Tohen, 1997). The considerable overlap with affective disorders, particularly major depression, means that very few people receive a single personality disorder diagnosis (Zimmerman, Pfohl, Coryell, Corenthal, & Stangl, 1991). Personality disorder diagnosis is often missed or mistaken for other mental illnesses; for example, treatment resistant major depression is diagnosed instead of borderline personality disorder (Fava, 2003).

There is considerable overlap of personality disorders with depression, anxiety, drug and alcohol problems, post-traumatic stress disorders (PTSD) and eating disorders. Complicating this, a majority of people who meet criteria for a particular personality disorder also meet criteria for another personality disorder (Barbato & Hafner, 1998; Lenzenweger, Lane, Loranger, & Kessler, 2007).

4.9.5 OUTCOME AND TREATMENT

BRUCE FALCONER & SATHYA RAO

OUTCOME STUDIES

> Personality disorders are amalgams of traits and symptoms, and even when symptoms remit, problematic traits can produce difficulty. That is probably why remission is more common than full recovery.
>
> *Joel Paris*

Personality disorders have traditionally been seen as difficult to treat. Clinical wisdom and longitudinal studies indicate that in general, personality disorders tend to improve over time or at least the symptoms become less severe as the individual ages (reviewed in Beatson et al., 2016). However, there is a paucity of long-term studies that have adequately investigated the course and outcome of personality disorders, with the single exception of borderline personality disorder (Temes & Zanarini, 2018).

TREATMENT

In the past, personality disorders were considered unresponsive to treatment, with the appropriateness of providing any treatment being questioned. This view arose in part from the belief that the personality is predetermined and immutable. Clinical research has subsequently validated various treatment modes that focus on identifying and targeting symptom reduction. The application of these treatments can be complex and depends on the skills and experience of the clinician, the clinician's aetiological view of the disorder, the motivation of the patient to engage and be responsive to psychological therapy, and the presence of comorbid symptomatology.

Dixon-Gordon and colleagues (2011) identified 33 randomised controlled trials evaluating the efficacy of psychosocial treatments of personality disorders (reported using DSM-IV diagnoses), 19 of which focused on borderline personality disorder and five on Cluster C personality disorders; none focused on Cluster A personality disorders. Although the outlook for effective treatments for personality disorders is hopeful, there is insufficient research to validate specific treatments for personality disorders other than borderline (Dixon-Gordon, Turner, & Chapman, 2011; Levy & Johnson, 2016). Nonetheless, successful clinical management of personality disorders generally entails adherence to the treatment principles outlined in Table 4.35.

Table 4.35 General principles of management of personality disorders

- Well-structured treatment approach
- Clear focus
- Coherent theoretical basis
- Long-term focus
- Well integrated and coordinated, with other services available to clients
- Clear therapeutic alliance
- Treatment undertaken by trained staff who are well supervised

Source: Adapted from Bateman and Tyrer 2002

4.9.6 ASSESSMENT AND TREATMENT OF COMMONLY PRESENTING PERSONALITY DISORDERS

A range of validated instruments assist with screening and diagnosis of personality disorder, though at time of writing these have not been validated for ICD-11. Two well-known structured clinical interviews that incorporate all currently recognised personality disorders are (i) the International Personality Disorder Examination (IPDE), which reflects the diagnostic criteria outlined in the ICD-10 and (ii) the Structured Clinical Interview for DSM-IV Axis II Disorders (SCID-II). With respect to screening for BPD, the self-report McLean BPD Questionnaire and clinician-scored ZAN-BPD are useful instruments when BPD is suspected. For diagnosing BPD, a commonly used assessment instrument is the Borderline Personality Questionnaire (BPQ) which is based on the DSM-IV description. For longitudinal assessment of BPD symptom severity and clinical change, the self-report Borderline Evaluation of Severity over Time (BEST) is a useful tool.

GOOD PRACTICE IN PERSONALITY DISORDER CLINICAL ASSESSMENT

- All psychiatrically unwell patients should be assessed for clinically significant personality traits or disorders given that half of them may have personality pathology.
- A personality disorder diagnosis is made using either ICD-11 or DSM-5 classificatory systems.
- Coexisting medical and psychiatric disorders are also diagnosed.
- In order to better formulate personality disorders it is vital to obtain adequate family and childhood developmental history including history of any trauma.
- Careful consideration and understanding of suicide, self-harm and aggression risk assessment is important.
- Chronic patterns of crisis and risk behaviours are noted; factors that are likely to change risk from a chronic to an acute state are elicited.
- The existing support systems, family and carers involvement, dependent children (if any) are noted.
- Accessibly, affordability and availability of proposed treatments are understood and the treatment preferences of patients are taken into account.
- Stigma, discrimination and the dynamics within health care systems are taken into consideration.

These assessment parameters will assist the clinician to collaboratively develop a crisis plan and treatment plan for consumers with personality disorders.

Personality disorders that are commonly seen in clinical practice include borderline pattern, anankastia, dissociality and narcissistic personality disorders.

ANANKASTIA OR OBSESSIVE-COMPULSIVE PERSONALITY DISORDER (OCPD)

In ICD-11 this personality pathology is classified as anankastic personality trait but DSM-5 has retained the diagnosis of obsessive-compulsive personality disorder (OCPD). Individuals with anankastia or OCPD exhibit a pattern of preoccupation with orderliness, perfectionism and control at the expense of flexibility, openness and efficiency. People with this disorder attempt to keep control through rigid attention to detail, rules, procedures and lists, to the extent that the major point of the activity is lost. They may devote themselves to work to the exclusion of social and leisure activities and friendships, and are inflexible about matters of morality, ethics and values. Individuals with this disorder can be rigid and stubborn, reluctant to delegate to others, miserly and live below the level they can afford. Individuals with OCPD may have such difficulty deciding the best way of doing some tasks that they may never get started. They are prone to become anxious, upset or angry in situations in which they are not able to maintain control of their physical or interpersonal environment, although the anger is typically not expressed directly. Individuals with this disorder usually express affection in a highly controlled or stilted fashion, with everyday relationships having a formal and serious quality with difficulty expressing tender feelings or paying compliments. They may be preoccupied with logic and intellect, and intolerant of affective behaviour in others. Individuals with this disorder may experience occupational difficulties and distress, particularly when confronted with new situations that demand flexibility and compromise. Cultural emphasis on work and productivity in some societies needs to be considered prior to making this diagnosis. In systematic studies, the disorder appears to be diagnosed about twice as often among males as among females.

Various etiological theories have been postulated. Psychoanalytic theorists have linked OCPD with the fixation and early childhood parent–child interactions during the anal psychosexual developmental stage. Cognitive behaviourists have conceptualised OCPD as a product of errors in thought process. Interpersonal theorists have suggested OCPD as a transference neurosis.

Most people with OCPD do not perceive that they have a disorder and hence do not seek treatment. There are no empirically validated biological or psychological treatments for OCPD. However, clinicians commonly use treatments such as cognitive behaviour therapy and/or antidepressant medications (SSRI's). Interpersonal therapy and psychoanalytic therapies are also options.

4.9.7 BORDERLINE PATTERN OR BORDERLINE PERSONALITY DISORDER

SATHYA RAO & JILLIAN BROADBEAR

DESCRIPTION

Borderline personality disorder (BPD) is the most frequently diagnosed and severest form of personality disorder (Chanen, McCutcheon, Jovev, Jackson, & McGorry, 2007). It is highly stigmatised and misunderstood. ICD-11 now classifies BPD as 'borderline pattern' of personality disorders, whereas DSM-5 has retained the DSM-IV description of BPD. The origins of the term 'borderline' arose from psychoanalytic theory describing clients who responded differently from those diagnosed as neurotic or psychotic. It became a means of describing symptoms that bordered on psychotic and then a way of describing the intrapsychic organisation of personality. Persons with a diagnosis of BPD experience a pattern of instability in interpersonal relationships, self-image and affect, and marked impulsivity. The disorder usually manifests in adolescence. A history of invalidating experiences in childhood is frequently reported; sexual trauma is not unusual. Physical and sexual abuse, neglect, hostility, conflict, and early parental loss or separations are overrepresented in the childhood histories of people with BPD. It is notable however that not all people with this diagnosis have a background of trauma or sexual abuse.

INTERPERSONAL RELATIONSHIPS

People with BPD have intense and unstable relationship patterns, often shifting from idealising to devaluing people with whom they have close relationships, including clinicians in therapeutic relationships. They often crave romantic relationships but may lack the interpersonal skill to maintain long-term relationships. They may make frantic efforts to avoid real or imagined abandonment. More than one-third of people with BPD find themselves in challenging and at times abusive relationships, with many becoming victims of sexual assault in adulthood (Zittel Conklin & Westen, 2005).

MOOD STATES

People diagnosed with BPD often describe their emotional state as a roller coaster of moods. They intensely experience emotions such as sadness, anxiety, panic, anger and aggression. They may overreact to real or perceived interpersonal cues or rejections and have low tolerance for frustration. They may also experience sad mood states for several years. These experiences can be difficult to differentiate from emotional states associated with bipolar disorder or major depression. Longitudinal and repeated evaluations may be required to confirm diagnosis.

IDENTITY

People with BPD may have identity disturbance characterised by unstable self-image or sense of self. This may be reflected with respect to their sexual identity, body image or an intense dislike or hatred for self. Some have described this as a state of 'identitylessness' (Zanarini et al., 1998).

SELF-HARM AND SUICIDE

Self-harm is described by Gunderson and Ridolfi (2001) as the 'behavioural specialty' of persons with BPD. Recurrent self-harm acts are often characteristic of persons with BPD, and occur in about 75–90% of clients (Mack, 1975). Some acts of self-harm are of low lethality (e.g. superficial cuts) and others may be highly lethal (e.g. severe overdoses, asphyxiation and carbon monoxide poisoning). Highly lethal self-harm acts need careful examination and management to prevent unintended accidental death (Beatson, Rao, Watson, & Victoria, 2010). It is important to ask the person their reason for the self-harm and not assume that the self-harm acts are intended towards a particular purpose, such as suicide or seeking attention of others (Shearer, 1994). The self-harm acts, although pathological, are often adaptive and may help regulate painful and unstable emotional states (Connors, 1996; see Table 4.36).

Suicidal ideation is very common in persons with BPD and is usually evident over several years. Suicidal threats and suicidal gestures may be used to communicate distress. Older studies reported suicide rates of about 10%. However, later figures (4.6%) are more optimistic (Zanarini et al., 2008). About two-thirds of people with BPD attempt suicide at least once in their lifetime; this risk is elevated when accompanied by clinical depression or substance abuse. An exploratory Australasian study (Krawitz & Batcheler, 2006) demonstrated that clinicians' defensive responses to risk of acute self-harm and chronic suicide risk is influenced by medicolegal concerns and not necessarily in the best interest of the patient.

Table 4.36 Why do people with borderline personality disorder self-harm?

Function of self-harm	Frequency reported by respondents
To feel physical pain or to overcome psychic pain	59%
To punish oneself for being 'bad'	49%
To control feelings	39%
To exert control	22%
To express anger	22%
To have sensation or overcome numbness	20%

Source: Adapted from Shearer, 1994

OTHER FEATURES

Clinical experience and client reports suggest that shame is central to the subjective experience of BPD. Intense reactions to interpersonal stressors are often followed by shame and guilt and contribute to the person feeling bad or evil. People with BPD may also act impulsively through gambling, substance abuse, eating disturbances, engaging in unsafe sexual practices or in self-harm acts. Many experience a deep sense of emptiness, a symptom most resistant to change (Price, Mahler, & Hopwood, 2019).

Zanarini and colleagues (Zanarini, Gunderson, & Frankenburg, 1990) reported partial psychotic features in about 40% of persons with BPD. These included transient episodes of psychosis with partial or true hallucinations, paranoid experiences, body image distortions, magical thinking, regressed behaviour and disturbed reality testing (Beatson et al., 2010). Transient psychosis and dissociative episodes are more likely to occur during periods of crisis.

BPD is also characterised by emotional instability, existential dilemmas, uncertainty, anxiety-provoking choices, and competing social pressures to decide on careers. BPD is diagnosed predominantly (about 70%) in females (American Psychiatric Association, 2000), however prevalence in community studies is similar for men and women (Tomko, Trull, Wood, & Sher, 2014).

Physical handicaps may result from self-inflicted injury or failed suicide attempts. Recurrent job losses, interrupted education and broken marriages are common. People with BPD are prone to metabolic syndromes because of the high prevalence of treatment with psychotropic medications. Chronic pain disorders, arthritis and urinary incontinence are also common. In the absence of appropriate care, people with BPD may live painful and miserable lives with long-term disability and functional impairment, entailing significant costs to the community.

LIVED EXPERIENCE: A CONSUMER

DANIELLE JAEGER

When I was first diagnosed with borderline personality disorder I remember feeling shattered and broken. Wondering if I would ever lead a meaningful life and get out of the darkness that consumed me. My symptoms of borderline personality disorder developed more intensely after I experienced the loss of my father and grandfather.

When I was first diagnosed, I was seeing a psychologist and psychiatrist and I think I was in denial, therefore my self-harm and suicidal ideation sky-rocketed and I was barely able to live life from day to day. Everything felt hard, overwhelming and distressing.

At the time of my diagnosis I felt my psychiatrist and psychologist were not helpful. I needed openness, honesty and transparency and I felt like I wasn't receiving this from these professionals. It wasn't until I accessed services through a specialist personality disorders service that I felt understood and treated like a human being.

My life is an evolving journey and I have definitely experienced ups and downs. The down times were consuming, distressing, overwhelming and I felt so isolated and felt like I was fighting an endless battle. However after working with the right professionals I began to see that I was in charge of my life and that in fact I could lead a meaningful life. Borderline personality disorder changed my life and I'm actually grateful for the difficult times because they make me appreciate the good times even more.

EPIDEMIOLOGY

BPD affects between 1 and 4% of Australians. It is commonly encountered in clinical practice, affecting up to 5% of primary care patients, 11% of community mental health patients and up to 20% of psychiatric inpatients, despite under-diagnosis due to poor recognition and under-reporting (reviewed in Carrotte & Blanchard, 2018).

COEXISTING DISORDERS

Common co-occurring disorders include mood disorders, substance-use disorders, eating disorders (notably bulimia), post-traumatic stress disorder, other anxiety disorders and attention deficit or hyperactivity disorder. BPD also frequently co-occurs with other personality disorders. The presence of BPD has significant implications for the prognosis of co-occurring mental illnesses, particularly depression.

BPD is associated with an increased prevalence of obesity (Frankenburg & Zanarini, 2006). Headache and nicotine dependence are also common. Management of diabetes mellitus (type I) is challenging when BPD coexists. 30% of women with BPD had polycystic ovarian syndrome (PCOS) compared to 6.9% in healthy controls (Roepke et al., 2010). It has been hypothesised that oestrogen and progesterone exert significant effects on BPD symptoms, especially feelings of social rejection, negative and positive urgency, anger rumination and lack of premeditation (Eisenlohr-Moul, DeWall, Girdler, & Segerstrom, 2015). 30% of chronic pain patients met criteria for BPD (Sansone & Sansone, 2012). The association between pain conditions and BPD is significant compared to other psychiatric disorders (McWilliams & Higgins, 2013).

AETIOLOGY

> Having BPD is not the person's own fault—it is a condition of the brain and mind.
>
> *National Health and Medical Research Council, 2012*

Genetic predisposition in combination with adverse psychosocial environmental factors may contribute to causation of BPD. An increased prevalence of mood disorders, alcohol use disorders and substance-use disorders is found in first-degree relatives (Widiger & Trull, 1992). Genetic models report a heritability effect of 0.69 (Torgersen et al., 2000), with some suggesting a genetic predisposition to a dysregulation of impulses, moods and behaviour. Many theorists (e.g. Zanarini & Frankenburg, 1997) have hypothesised that adverse childhood factors may lead to disturbed attachment which fosters the development of the disorder. Although trauma, specifically childhood sexual trauma, is common in BPD, trauma is not a prerequisite for the development of BPD. A complex gene-environment interaction seems to be implicated in the causation of BPD.

Course

> BPD improves symptomatically more often, more quickly, and more dramatically than expected and, once better, maintains improvements more enduring than for many other major psychiatric disorders.
>
> *Professor J Gunderson, 2011*

Despite the previously held belief was that the prognosis for BPD was poor and it was not amenable to treatment, evidence to the contrary is plentiful with recent studies reporting a more optimistic course and outcome for BPD.

The course of BPD is variable, generally emerging during adolescence, although a diagnosis during this time is controversial (Paris, 2003). Chanen and colleagues (Chanen et al., 2007) question whether the delay in diagnosis is counterproductive, advocating early intervention and prevention programs. Impairment from the disorder and the risk of suicide are greatest during the young adult years and gradually wane with advancing age (Beatson et al., 2016). As consumers mature into their thirties and forties, up to 60% attain some stability in relationships and vocational functioning.

The McLean Study of Adult Development (MSAD; Zanarini et al., 2014), has been prospectively following up people diagnosed with Borderline personality disorders and has entered its 24th year. The 10-, 14- and 16-year follow-up data have been published. The study included 290 severely affected and extensively treated hospitalised BPD participants and 79 controls. It defined remission as no longer meeting criteria for borderline personality disorder or another personality disorder for two years or longer and recovery as concurrent symptomatic remission with good social and full-time vocational functioning. The steady rate of remission of and recovery from BPD symptoms is shown in Table 4.37. By 16 years, 99% of BPD patients had achieved remission and 60% achieved recovery. Recurrence of BPD was rare. These results support a hopeful prognosis for remission from BPD. However there is work yet to do, as despite symptomatic remission, patients may continue to experience severe and persistent impairment in social functioning.

Table 4.37 Cumulative rates of remission and recovery from BPD

Years of follow-up data collection	Remission rates	Recovery rates
2 years	35%	14%
4 years	55%	27%
6 years	76%	36%
8 years	88%	43%
10 years	91%	47%
12 years	95%	50%
14 years	97%	56%
16 years	99%	60%

Source: Adapted from Zanarini et al., 2012

TREATMENT

PRACTICE ILLUSTRATION: PRESENTATION AND FAMILY HISTORY

Rebecca, aged 28, lives with her partner of two years, Leanne. She works at McDonald's. Rebecca has a well-established diagnosis of BPD. She has self-injured since the age of 11. Her preferred method is superficial cutting (at times requiring suturing). She cuts in order to cope with mood swings and to punish herself as she believes she is a bad or an evil person.

Rebecca describes her mood as unstable: 'Like going on a roller coaster, up and down'; 'my emotions are all over the place'. She reports that she 'snaps very easily' and that her emotional reactions and anger outbursts are often out of proportion to the triggers. However she is unable to control it in the moment. She has a very poor sense of self and chronic low self-esteem; she describes feeling sad 'always'—since her primary school years.

Rebecca has thought about suicide since she was 11 years old. She reports feeling empty most of the time: 'I feel I am nothing ...if someone cut me open they will find nothing inside of me, it will just be black'. She has always felt lonely and unloved.

Family history

Jeff, Rebecca's 58-year-old father, is alcohol dependent and lives alone. Rebecca has had no contact with him since her parents' divorce when she was aged 13, after severe domestic violence. Her mother Mary died in a car accident aged 41, when Rebecca was 16. Mary had 'chronic depression' and also self-injured by cutting. Rebecca suspects it was suicide. Rebecca had an ambivalent relationship with her mother and found her invalidating and critical.

Rebecca was sexually abused by her paternal grandfather when aged 11–13. She has a 22-year-old sister who has chronic depression.

BPD is a complex disorder and treating it can be challenging for an inexperienced clinician. However, BPD is an eminently treatable disorder (Gabbard, 2007), with several evidence-based psychotherapies emerging during recent decades. Use of these therapies (with the possible exception of supportive psychotherapy) requires clinicians to access formal training. Clinicians engaging in long-term management of BPD patients are advised to access clinical supervision in order to process the complex emotions that are encountered in therapeutic interactions. It has been argued (Weinberg, Ronningstam, Goldblatt, Schechter, & Maltsberger, 2011) that the various psychotherapies share common strategies. These include: a clear treatment framework; attention to emotions; a focus on the therapeutic relationship; an active therapist; and explanatory, change-orientated interventions. Medications, although extensively used, may provide symptomatic relief but do not appear to change the course of the disorder when used in isolation (Lieb, Vollm, Rucker, Timmer, & Stoffers, 2010).

People with BPD access treatment across a range of clinical settings. They often present to public hospital emergency departments seeking admission to inpatient psychiatric units when in crisis. Unfortunately, most Australian public mental health systems only provide crisis interventions and lack effective and evidence-based long-term psychotherapies; this creates a revolving door phenomenon. To address this, a list of essential principles in the treatment of BPD has been developed (Beatson et al., 2010; Gunderson, 2001; Paris, 2004; Trett, Dick, & Cooke, 2011; Weinberg et al., 2011; see also Table 4.35). It is important to remember that the person with BPD is doing the best they can, even when their behaviour is maladaptive and/or out of control. Crises are inevitable in the lives of persons with BPD and do not represent a failure of treatment.

PRACTICE ILLUSTRATION: TREATMENT HISTORY

Rebecca attempted suicide by hanging shortly after her mother's death and was admitted to a psychiatric hospital for three weeks and was briefly prescribed sertraline. She left school after Year 11 and worked in the sex industry for six years while abusing a range of illicit drugs. Rebecca met Mark, aged 50, and for two years stopped her drug use, took up employment and engaged minimally in self-harm behaviours. The relationship ended after Mark was unfaithful, triggering a serious self-poisoning and Rebecca, then 26, was hospitalised again. She received six ECT treatments and venlafaxine was briefly prescribed.

She met Leanne, aged 19, in hospital; Leanne also had a diagnosis of BPD. A two-year period of stability ensued, during which Rebecca was employed and continued to see her psychiatrist who prescribed escitalopram. She was also receiving psychotherapy. Her suicidal thoughts increased but she did not act on them.

Then Rebecca discovered Leanne was sleeping with another woman. Feeling rejected and angry, sad and agitated, her suicidal thoughts increased; she was sleeping poorly and lost 4 kg. She began drinking alcohol heavily and using cannabis. She reported hearing voices in her head telling her to kill herself, that she was worthless and stupid. She continued to take escitalopram.

Dialectical behaviour therapy

Dialectical behaviour therapy (DBT) was the first treatment to challenge the therapeutic nihilism that defined BPD until the 1990s and remains the most evidence-based of all BPD-specific psychotherapies. It is particularly effective at mitigating suicidal behaviours and reduces the need for frequent hospitalisations. DBT is based on mindfulness and behavioural approaches. DBT comprises weekly individual therapy, weekly group psychoeducation and skills training sessions, telephone coaching during crises and regular staff supervision groups. Dialectics is defined as a process of change that results from the interplay of two opposites. The dichotomous and extreme thinking behaviour and emotions of BPD patients are viewed as dialectical failures. Patients are stuck in polarities (good-bad, right-wrong, black-and-white thinking, idealisation-devaluation, and avoidance of conflict versus intense confrontation) and are unable to move towards synthesis. DBT encourages patients to negotiate the dialectic between the need to change and the need to accept themselves as they are. DBT programs teach mindfulness skills, emotion regulation skills, interpersonal effectiveness skills, distress tolerance skills and behavioural self-management.

DBT is likely the most commonly practised BPD-specific psychotherapy in Australia, although Australian research has yielded variable results. Brassington and Krawitz (2006) found DBT to be effective in retaining patients, decreasing the length of hospitalisations and generally improving functioning. However, Carter and colleagues (2010), using DBT in comparison to treatment as usual and a waiting list control, failed to find a reduction in deliberate self-harm or in hospital treatment time, although both treatment groups improved over time.

BOX 4.5: A MENTAL ILLNESS EXPERT REVEALS HER OWN FIGHT

In an interview with reporter Benedict Carey published in the New York Times (23 June 2011), Marsha Linehan, a psychologist and founder of DBT, revealed that she had a very troubled past, and as an adolescent and young woman she was at times suicidal and engaged in self-harming behaviour. In order to cope with feelings of being out of control, totally empty and having no way to communicate, she displayed her desperation by cutting and burning herself and banging her head against a wall and wanting to die. At that time she was admitted to an inpatient unit and treated with medication, ECT and psychoanalysis. She drew on her experiences of that time to inform and then incorporate into DBT some of the issues she was struggling with, such as the paradox of acceptance of life as it is, not as it is supposed to be, and the need to change. She also realised the importance of learning day-to-day skills. She went on to complete a PhD after deciding to work and treat people suffering in the same way she had.

Mentalisation-based therapy

Mentalisation-based therapy (MBT) is an evidence-based BPD-specific psychotherapy proposed by Bateman and Fonagy (1999). The efficacy of MBT for BPD has been demonstrated in randomised clinical trials (Bales et al., 2012; Jørgensen et al., 2013). Mentalisation describes the capacity to understand and interpret human behaviour in terms of underlying mental states. The ability to mentalise is thought to develop from having experienced oneself in the mind of another within an attachment context. Mentalisation matures best within the context of secure attachment. The central focus of the MBT approach is to assist consumers to understand mental states that underpin behaviour–their own and that of others–while helping to recognise meaning in their own actions, where meaning relates to emotional states that can be thought about and understood. Table 4.38 summarises the techniques. This therapy is available in a few centres in Australia.

Table 4.38 MBT techniques

- Focusing on mental states in the here-and-now
- Employing an active, collaborative style of interaction
- Maintaining motivation via support, reassurance and empathy
- Reflecting on what is going on in the patient's mind and encouraging the patient to consider what is in the therapist's mind
- Adopting a stance of not knowing, but seeking to understand
- Endeavouring to promote the person's interest and curiosity in their own mind
- Checking understanding that what is reached is correct
- Using simple, brief interventions
- Accepting transference as an example of a different perspective on the current situation

Source: Adapted from Beatson et al., 2010

Schema focused therapy

Schema focused therapy (SFT) proposes that clients develop maladaptive cognitive schemas in the context of adverse childhood events (Giesen-Bloo et al., 2006; Young, Klosko, & Weishaar, 2003). The therapy attempts to modify these schemas through a range of cognitive and behavioural techniques. SFT is an evidence-based BPD-specific psychotherapy. SFT is not readily available for clients in the Australian context.

Transference-focused psychotherapy

Transference-focused psychotherapy (TFP) is a psychodynamic therapy that uses the patient–therapist relationship as the primary source of information and the context for intervention (Clarkin et al., 2001). The therapy focuses on improving the client's ability to accurately perceive and respond to interpersonal relationships using the transferential relationship between patient and therapist. The therapy attempts to address the 'split' perceptions of clients into 'all good or all bad' in the context of therapeutic relationship. Although TFP is an evidence-based BPD-specific psychotherapy, it is not widely available in Australia.

Cognitive analytic therapy

A group at Orygen, Victoria, has demonstrated the effectiveness of cognitive analytic therapy (CAT) for adolescents with BPD (Chanen et al., 2008). This treatment warrants trialling in adult populations in the Australian context. CAT is a therapy that is informed by psychoanalytic and cognitive behavioural schools of psychology. It is based on a developmental model, is goal oriented and uses the relationship between the client and therapist to reflect on helpful and unhelpful ways of being.

General psychiatric management (GPM)

General psychiatric management (GPM) is a psychodynamic approach developed by the Gunderson group (Gunderson, 2001). This therapy emphasises relational aspects and early attachment relationships. GPM considers the interrelatedness of disturbed attachment relationships and emotion dysregulation as a primary deficit in BPD. Unlike DBT, this therapy is not focused on self-harm and suicidal behaviours. The primary strategies of GPM include psychoeducation about BPD, supporting relationship management, taking a here-and-now focus, emphasising validation and empathy, emotion focus and active attention to signs of negative transference. Patients are encouraged to use medications concurrently. Therapists are mandated to access supervision.

Supportive psychotherapy

This approach focuses on the patient's strengths in order to assist in developing attainable and realistic changes and containment of destructive behaviours. It depends on developing a collaborative therapeutic alliance with the client and in providing firm, clear boundaries.

Acceptance and commitment therapy

Acceptance and commitment therapy (ACT) is a recently developed mindfulness-based behaviour therapy. ACT rests on the assumption that fighting against thoughts and feelings is likely to increase symptoms. Rather than focusing on psychological events directly, ACT seeks to change the individual's relationship to them. Core principles of acceptance and commitment therapy include cognitive defusion, acceptance, contact with the present moment, the observing self, values and committed action. An RCT by the Spectrum service in Melbourne compared treatment as usual (TAU) with TAU plus twelve two-hour group ACT sessions (Morton, Snowdon, Gopold, & Guymer, 2012). The study demonstrated symptomatic improvements across a wide range of outcome measures. Further research on ACT for BPD is required. This therapy is only available in a few centres in Australia.

Conversational model

The conversational model of therapy developed by Meares evolved from the psychodynamic treatment model, placing considerable emphasis in developing an empathic understanding of the client's experience. Therapy helps clients discover and elaborate their inner world and, in so doing, mature. Attention to both empathic listening and the inevitable failures in empathy on behalf of the clinician are central aspects in the process of therapy. This therapy has been shown to be effective in uncontrolled trials (Korner, Gerull, Meares, & Stevenson, 2006).

COMMONALITIES

Although these psychotherapeutic approaches differ in their assumptions, explanations and theoretical underpinnings, they do have some features in common (see Table 4.39). All place an emphasis on therapeutic alliance and the long-term nature of therapy. All aim to enhance accuracy of cognitions and focus on emotions rather than on behaviours and regulation of emotions. Therapists need to have considerable understanding, be well versed in theory and practice, and be able to utilise consultation and supervision effectively in order to clarify and assist the process of treatment. The development of an integrative model of practice which draws on common aspects of effective treatment modalities is emerging as a model for meeting the complex needs of people diagnosed with BPD.

Table 4.39 Common factors in empirically supported treatments for BPD

- Clear, structured treatment framework
- Focus on the relationship with the therapist
- Active therapist
- Collaborative, cooperative relationship with the therapist
- Focus on affect
- Exploratory interventions
- Change-oriented interventions
- Support/supervision for the therapist
- Individual sessions are usually conducted once weekly for minimum of 12 months

Source: Adapted from Beatson & Rao, 2014

PRACTICAL ASPECTS OF DEVELOPING A JOINT CRISIS PLAN

Joint crisis planning is one of the most important aspects of treatment of BPD. Table 4.40 outlines practical aspects that should be considered when developing a joint crisis plan. This needs to be completed with the active collaboration of the person experiencing BPD, their family/carers and all other treatment providers.

Table 4.40 Factors to be considered when developing a Joint Crisis Plan

- Early warning signs:
  - Was there a particular feeling?
  - Was there a behavioural change?
  - Were thought patterns different?
  - What makes you vulnerable?
- Rate Crisis
  - 0-Control
  - 1
  - 2
  - 3-Out of control/Crisis point
- What can the patient do or not do?
  - Strategies that have been helpful in the past
  - Leaving the triggering situation
  - Calling a friend
  - Distraction
  - Distress tolerance
- What can others people do or not do?
  - How can others identify emerging crisis?
  - What might they do to help?
  - Examine last three crises situations

Source: Adapted from Bateman & Krawitz, 2013; Moran et al., 2010

BIOLOGICAL TREATMENT

Medications are often used to treat people with personality disorders, despite minimal evidence, especially in clinical settings where access to psychosocial treatments is limited. Most psychotropic medications studied in double-blind, placebo-controlled trials are at best only modestly effective (Angstman & Rasmussen, 2011; Lieb et al., 2010) and are used as adjuncts to psychosocial interventions in order to target symptom relief (see Table 4.41), rather than attempt to change the personality disorder itself (Woo-Ming & Siever, 1998). There are no medications that are specifically indicated for any of the PDs. The common practice of polypharmacy (using multiple medications) has no empirical support and may be unnecessary and potentially harmful for most clients with BPD and is therefore best avoided. Clinicians need to be aware that about 25% of persons with BPD consider overdose as a means to end their lives (Makela, Moeller, Fullen, & Gunel, 2006). Although often prescribed, there is no evidence to support the use of electroconvulsive therapy for BPD. Transcranial Magnetic Stimulation (TMS) is also used in the treatment of BPD patients however there is no credible evidence to support this.

Table 4.41 Medication treatment for BPD

- Topiramate and lamotrigine have been reported to have some effectiveness against anger, aggression and mood instability of BPD.
- Aripiprazole has been shown to be effective against anger, aggression, depression, paranoid thinking, anxiety and interpersonal sensitivity.
- Fluvoxamine has been reported to help in controlling rapid mood shifts.
- Selective serotonin reuptake inhibitors (SSRIs), such as fluoxetine, appear to have some beneficial effect on mood instability, anger and impulsivity.
- Low-dose atypical antipsychotics (olanzapine) have some positive effect on impulsivity, aggression, interpersonal relationships, depression and global functioning.
- Omega-3 fatty acids can reduce depression and aggression. The safety of this drug in pregnancy makes it an attractive option.
- Mood stabilisers and antipsychotics are more effective than antidepressants in the treatment of BPD.
- Generally, psychotropics are less effective in treating depression that is associated with BPD than in treating depression on its own.

PRACTICE ILLUSTRATION: CHALLENGES AND DEVELOPMENTS

Rebecca recovered from depression after 8 weeks, stopped using substances, and was no longer hearing voices in her head or having suicidal thoughts. She moved interstate and was lost to follow-up until returning a year later with a new female partner. Rebecca received no psychotherapy during that year and had resumed abusing substances. Rebecca had four hanging attempts and three significant overdoses requiring medical interventions. She has also tried to gas herself on two occasions. She is still grieving for her soul-mate Leanne. She has subsequently had brief relationships with five women. Rebecca re-engaged with treatment services after an emergency department attendance. She resumed seeing her psychiatrist and commenced a dialectical behaviour therapy group program. Over time she has reduced her substance use and self-harming behaviours while building skills to better manage interpersonal stressors which she understands are key triggers for her crisis-driven behaviours. Although she continues to feel empty and sad, Rebecca is not currently clinically depressed and reports no immediate suicidal plans.

4.9.8 NARCISSISTIC PERSONALITY DISORDER

JAYDIP SARKAR

INTRODUCTION

The term 'narcissism' arises from the legend of Narcissus in Greek mythology. After viewing an image of himself in a pool of water and not recognising his own reflection, he becomes infatuated with himself. After eventually realising that his love can never be reciprocated, he remains in despair, fixated by his image until death (Yakeley, 2018).

Psychoanalysts such as Otto Rank (1911) and Sigmund Freud (1914) proposed that narcissism psychologically defended the individual from feelings of low self-worth and conceptualised it as a dimensional state that ranged from normal to pathological. The most influential theories on narcissism are Kohut's self-psychology (1971) and Kernberg's object relations approach (1995). The former explanation attributes pathological narcissism to failure of parents to empathise with their child, causing narcissistic individuals to experience emptiness and depression. The latter holds that cold, indifferent or aggressive parental figures push the child to develop feelings of specialness as a retreat. In pathologically narcissistic individuals, primitive defence mechanisms of idealisation, denigration and splitting predominate, the capacity for sadness, guilt and mourning is lacking, and the main affects are shame, envy and aggression (Yakeley, 2018). Theodore Millon's (1981) social learning perspective proposes that beliefs about specialness and entitlement stem from early parental overindulgence. Beck and Freeman (Freeman, 1990) described dysfunctional core beliefs or schemas, stemming from early experiences of adverse parenting leading the person to be self-indulgent, demanding and aggressive, often accompanied by symptoms of depression.

Subtypes of narcissistic personality disorder

Pathological narcissism is widely agreed to present in two ways: an overt grandiose, arrogant and self-centred self that defends against an underlying vulnerability, or the covert aspect of narcissism which presents as overly sensitive, insecure and anxious to hide an underlying sense of shame and inadequacy. These two presentations of pathological narcissism are now accepted (Pincus, Cain, & Wright, 2014). These subtypes have also been described as 'thick-skinned' and 'thin-skinned' narcissism (Rosenfeld, 1986). This distinction suggests that the outward overconfident grandiose attitudes and behaviours conceal an underlying sense of shame and inadequacy and, conversely, manifest shyness and reticence may shield a secret sense of importance. Irrespective of the subtype, narcissistic individuals prioritise their own needs, exploiting others to meet them.

The status of narcissistic personality disorder as a diagnosis

The ICD-11 does not use narcissistic personality disorder (NPD) as a diagnostic label. In ICD-11, people presenting with this clinical picture would be found to have traits of dissociality and negative affectivity (Bach & First, 2018). NPD had low prominence in the categorical ICD-10 system, being listed as one of the 'other specific personality disorders'. This was because narcissistic personality is far less commonly recognised in many parts of the world outside of North America and Western Europe (WHO, 1992).

DSM-5 retained the NPD diagnosis and focuses entirely upon the grandiose/overt presentation of this personality within its diagnostic criteria, ignoring entirely the covert manifestation of the shy, shame-ridden, incompetent narcissist. It highlights overt features including persistent fantasies of success, power, attractiveness, intellectual superiority or ideal love, sense of specialness and entitlement, wish to be admired, lack of empathy and arrogant, contemptuous attitudes and behaviours. Much of the recent assessment and treatment literature adopts the DSM-5 conceptualisation of this condition.

Epidemiology

A large, nationally representative, epidemiological survey of 34 093 civilians in the United States using face-to-face interviews revealed an overall prevalence of NPD of 6.2%, with rates higher for men (7.7%) than for women (4.8%). NPD was also significantly more common in African-American men and women and Hispanic women, younger adults and people who were separated, divorced, widowed or never married (Hasin & Grant, 2015). High rates of co-occurring substance use, mood, anxiety and other personality disorders were observed (Stinson et al., 2008).

Treatment

The mainstay of treatment for NPD is psychological therapy, although no specific approach or modality has proven superior. The essential ingredients of successful therapy include building a working relationship and incorporation of key techniques derived from both psychoanalytic and cognitive behavioural theory, employing a spirit of 'integrative eclecticism' which synergistically utilises whichever approach or model that seems to work (Livesley, 2012). Individual work is preferable as consumers do not do well in group settings (Yakeley, 2018).

Individuals with NPD constitute some of the highest-functioning patients seen in psychiatry and also some of the most impaired and intractable (Caligor, Levy, & Yeomans, 2015). In fact, of all the personality disorders, NPD spans the broadest spectrum of severity (Kernberg, 1985). Hence it is useful to distinguish not only between grandiose/overt and vulnerable/covert clinical presentations, but also among different levels of severity of narcissistic personality disorder, consistent with the approach to diagnosis of ICD-11. In general, as severity of narcissistic pathology increases, aggression against self or others becomes more evident, with worsening interpersonal and moral functioning posing significant challenges to clinical management (Gunderson & Ronningstam, 2001; Kernberg, 2007).

Challenges in the treatment of NPD include premature termination and drop-outs, attempts to control therapy and therapist, sensitivity to diagnosis, features of grandiosity, entitlement, lack of empathy, and feeling blamed or treated unfairly treated. Poor affect tolerance, especially of feelings of shame, humiliation and vulnerability and a desire to impress the therapist exist alongside rapid switching into aggressive, antisocial or psychopathic features. They may evoke severe negative counter-transferential feelings leading to rejection from therapy.

The following tips may assist a therapist with the assessment and management of NPD:

- anticipate being treated as an audience to the patient's performance
- expect to be drawn into lengthy accounts of the patient's life
- in interviewing the patient, agree at the start how and why you will interrupt
- anticipate negative responses to perceived criticism—any comment that may be interpreted as disrespectful or generates a feeling of shame or humiliation
- avoid directly challenging a patient, even when they express very negative attitudes
- be empathic without colluding with what the patient says
- reflect on negative countertransference reactions rather than revealing these to the patient (Yakeley, 2018, p. 311).

CONCLUSION

Narcissistic pathology in consumers significantly impacts their management and treatment. Efforts should be made to distinguish between healthy and pathological narcissism, covert and overt presentations. Maintaining a grandiose sense of self can provide a more or less stable self-experience for the individual with narcissistic personality disorder, but comes at a cost, requiring a retreat from or denial of realities that do not support grandiosity, and leaving the individual excessively reliant on external feedback to support not only positive self-regard but also self-definition. Hence those with grandiose selves tend to engage in superficial relationships organised to support self-esteem and self-definition, while those who have vulnerable features tend to withdraw from social situations. For both types, self-regulatory needs leave little room for genuine interest in the needs or feelings of others.

4.9.9 ANTISOCIAL OR DISSOCIAL PERSONALITY DISORDER

JAYDIP SARKAR & JILLIAN BROADBEAR

INTRODUCTION

Antisocial personality disorder (ASPD) is one of 10 personality disorders in the DSM-5. The diagnosis of dissocial personality disorder in the ICD-10 received little or no empirical validation (De Brito & Hodgins, 2009). It appears to be defunct and is not a diagnosis within the ICD-11. The personality domain of 'dissociality'' now represents aspects of ASPD in ICD-11. This chapter will refer to empirical data on ASPD only, as conceptualised in DSM-5.

An ASPD diagnosis refers to a lifelong pattern of overt antisocial acts plus traits of impulsivity, irritability and remorselessness; it is considered one of the most reliable of all personality disorder diagnoses (Coid, 2003). Contrary to popular belief, it is a heterogenous condition, composed of distinct subtypes according to comorbid disorders such as substance abuse, anxiety, depression and psychopathy (Compton, Conway, Stinson, Colliver, & Grant, 2005; Sareen et al 2004; Robins, Tipp, & Przybeck, 1991; Patrick, 2006).

DIAGNOSIS

Like all personality disorders, the DSM-5 diagnosis of ASPD is made only in people over 18 years of age. Unlike all other diagnoses, ASPD requires that a similar disorder–conduct disorder, described as 'a pervasive pattern of disregard for and violation of the rights of others'–be present prior to the age of 15 years (APA, 2013). Associated behaviours include a failure to conform to social norms (including laws), repeated fights or assaults, reckless disregard for the safety of self and others, impulsivity or failure to plan ahead, irritability, irresponsibility and lack of remorse.

A younger age of onset and higher number of symptoms of conduct disorder increase the likelihood that ASPD will develop. About 50% of children with conduct disorder develop adult ASPD (Simonoff et al., 2004), suggesting that protective factors may mediate. A more severe version of ASPD is the entity of psychopathy, which, in addition to a stable pattern of early conduct problems, requires the presence of four traits:

- **a** arrogant and deceitful,
- **b** deficient affective experience and lack of empathy,
- **c** impulsive and irresponsible lifestyle and
- **d** versatile antisocial behaviour (Hare & Neumann, 2005).

Of these, deficient affective experience forms the core of the disorder. The prevalence of psychopathy in men in the community is thought to be less than 1% (De Brito & Hodgins, 2009). It is noteworthy that despite robust empirical validity, both diagnostic systems have not included psychopathy as an entity, probably to deny individuals involved with criminal justice systems from misusing this diagnosis as an excuse for violence.

Epidemiology

The rates of ASPD in men vary from around 1% in European nations to about 4.5–6.5% in North America. It is thought to be nearly 6–8 times more common in men than in women, depending on the nationalities of the sample, with rates in the United States (Robins et al., 1991) and Canada (Swanson, Bland, & Newman, 1994) being far higher than in Europe (Coid, Yang, Tyrer, Roberts, & Ullrich, 2006). Male criminal offenders with ASPD tend to die early, probably due to reckless behaviour (Repo-Tiihonen, Virkkunen, & Tiihonen, 2001). ASPD is 4–5 times more common in men than in women (Coid, 2003).

Aetiology

The prevalence of ASPD increases with social deprivation associated with low-socioeconomic class, with ASPD patients living in socially deprived inner-city areas with high rates of unemployment (Moran, 1999), a consequence of poor academic achievement by children with conduct disorder (Farrington & Coid, 2003). There is a strong genetic component to ASPD; two genetic polymorphisms (the low activity alleles of the MAO-A gene and the serotonin transporter gene 5HT-TLPR) are associated with a disproportionately greater degree of persistent violence, often in association with childhood adversity, thus highlighting the importance of environment in the expression of ASPD (Buades-Rotger, & Gallardo-Pujol, 2014; Cherepkova, Maksimov, & Aftanas, 2018).

Comorbidity

Co-occurring psychiatric disorders are present in 90% of individuals diagnosed with ASPD. These include substance misuse disorders (Compton et al., 2005), anxiety disorders (De Brito & Hodgins, 2009) and depression (Robins et al., 1991). Men with ASPD are three times more likely to abuse alcohol and five times more likely to abuse illicit drugs than men without ASPD. For ASPD women, the rates were 13 times and 12 times higher respectively than those without ASPD (Robins et al., 1991). Almost half of ASPD men meet criteria for at least one anxiety disorder (Goodwin & Hamilton, 2003) and they are also at least three times as likely as the general population to have a major depressive disorder (Lenzenweger et al., 2007).

Treatment

Psychological treatment for ASPD patients is essential, with treatment for comorbid disorders often requiring psychotropic treatment.

Schemas

Understanding the dysfunctional schema of the ASPD individual is the key to providing help. Such schemas (Young et al., 2003) describe the maladaptive manner in which patients perceive themselves, the world around them and how those perceptions drive their interpersonal behaviours. Such individuals view themselves as loners, autonomous, independent and strong people and the world as a jungle, where others are either dangerous or vulnerable and hence able to be exploited. They survive by attempting to deceive, attack or manipulate others in an impulsive or planned way in order to get what they need.

Basic engagement and management principles

It is beyond the scope of this chapter to provide a detailed outline of the treatment strategies but there are some useful strategies that are time-tested, which can be employed to engage the person experiencing ASPD. These can be summarised as:

- monitor one's own emotional reactions to being/feeling threatened or used
- don't become too punitive or submissive and limit expectations of quick improvement
- be positive, firm, persistent, transparent and respectful
- provide clear feedback consistently and don't make threats that you can't/won't carry out
- use the notion of 'enlightened self-interest' to help the person achieve goals (e.g. money for lifestyle vs staying out of prison) and use a CBT approach to make a cost-benefit analysis of antisocial behaviour
- be mindful of attempts to deceive and be on your guard, e.g. if you're too trusting they may get suspicious, too anxious and they may deceive you
- try not to feel defensive or humiliated if you are caught out and don't hesitate to say sorry if you've made an error.

Specialist offending behaviours programs

For individuals who have criminal behaviours, offending behaviours programs—which are usually run by psychologists working with criminal justice systems—generally target four main areas:

1. *Improving thinking and social problem-solving skills*. These are the most commonly completed short duration programmes, designed to enhance prosocial competencies including impulse control, perspective taking, reasoning skills and interpersonal problem solving.
2. *Tackling violence*. These programs tend to target either expressive violence (emotional control and anger management) or instrumental violence.
3. *Tackling sex offending*. A range of programs designed to provide the right intensity of intervention to match risk level and treatment need.
4. *Tackling substance misuse*. Includes a range individual and group work for alcohol and drug misuse (Craissati, Joseph, & Skett, 2015).

CONCLUSION

ASPD is a complex disorder with biopsychosocial causative factors. It is predominantly found in men and leads to significant amounts of distress to the person and those around them. It costs significant sums of money to the society—the direct costs of violence, deception and aggression, and the indirect costs of time lost due to poor employment records and early deaths. It is a disorder that can be successfully managed (NICE, 2009) with standard psychological approaches but requires trained and supported groups of professionals, usually within a shared responsibility model between criminal justice, social work and mental health services.

4.9.10 WHERE AND HOW DO PEOPLE GET HELP?

SATHYA RAO & RITA BROWN

Most people with personality disorders do not have access to evidence-based treatments. The lack of robust evidence-based treatments for personality disorders other than BPD only makes matters worse. Limited access to services for people with personality disorders may be due to lack of mental health staff trained in the treatment of personality disorders, as well as stigma and limited mental health resources.

Australian mental health services were not designed to treat personality disorders and lack well-articulated models of care for personality disorders. A recent report (Carrotte & Blanchard, 2018) identified that the Australian mental health system lacks specialised treatment services for personality disorder and uses a medical funding model that doesn't support long-term treatment. For example, under the current Australian scheme, the government rebate for psychological services in the private sector is generally only provided for 10 sessions in any calendar year.

The limited personality disorder services that are available cater mainly for the management and treatment of borderline personality disorder (BPD). Despite high community prevalence rates (1% or more), a substantial number of people with BPD may never obtain a formal diagnosis. This may be because they don't come into contact with mental health services, or because they receive numerous incorrect diagnoses before receiving a diagnosis of BPD. This is often a relief for the person—their distress now has a context. Diagnosis needs to be discussed with the patient to help then make sense of what it means to them.

Budgetary considerations and the dominance of treatment models that have efficacy for other mental health disorders are inadequate to meet the needs of people with significant and disabling psychological conditions such as BPD. A sense of abandonment when a psychologist's 10 session treatment under the Medicare scheme (see Section 1.7.2) ends can be overwhelming, contributing to increased self-harm or suicidal behaviours. Various ways to manage these shortcomings may be to provide a particular focus for the 10 sessions, developing mindfulness skills for example. This may reduce anxieties around abandonment by establishing the focus and structure of the treatment from the beginning. Some consumers 'dose' the psychologist sessions by attending on a monthly basis, creating a relational 'thread' when the patient is unsure of the ongoing commitment of other services to their treatment. Other patients establish an enduring relational thread with their family doctor. General practice settings are ideal for providing education about the factors common to effective treatments for BPD. The provision of access to expert advice at times of crisis would greatly assist in general practice management of patients with BPD. It is however important to note that progress towards recovery for patients with a condition of this severity would be slow when treatment contacts are infrequent (less than weekly).

The Australia's National Health and Medical Research Council (NHMRC) published a clinical practice guideline for the management of BPD (National Health and Medical Research Council, 2012), however there has been no concerted implementation effort. The consensus-based recommendations of the guideline noted:

- for most people with BPD, effective treatment with a structured psychological therapy can be provided within mainstream public or private community-based mental health services, via individual appointments (with or without group sessions), by therapists with access to peer consultation and clinical review
- people with complex care needs may benefit from treatment within a specialised BPD service.

The NHMRC Guideline recognises the significant trauma that many people with BPD have experienced and the need for trauma-informed health care. It recommends the Practice Guidelines for Treatment of Complex Trauma and Trauma-Informed Care and Service Delivery (2012) prepared by the Blue Knot Foundation (Kezelman & Stavropoulos, 2012). The Mental Health Coordinating Council of Australia published Trauma-informed Care and Practice: A National Strategic Direction in 2013, identifying the steps needed to embed trauma-informed principles and evidence into policy and practice across the health sector (Bateman, Henderson, & Kezelman, 2013). The high prevalence of complex trauma in people diagnosed with BPD makes it imperative for services to adopt a trauma-informed framework.

The NHMRC Guideline suggests the following roles for specialised BPD services:

- treatment of people with complex care needs or those at high risk for suicide or significant self-harm
- provision of consultation to primary care services and mental health services
- education, training, supervision and support for health professionals, including support for rural and remote services; education for local general mental health services; and consultation and advice for GPs managing BPD

- health promotion and advocacy (e.g. raising awareness of BPD and reducing stigma)
- provision of community education and support for families and carers
- the undertaking of research to develop better treatment models.

Although state-based initiatives exist in Victoria, South Australia and New South Wales, a unified national approach to understanding and addressing personality disorder is required. At present there are three state-based initiatives—the Project Air Strategy, a personality disorder strategy in New South Wales, Spectrum Personality Disorders Service in Victoria and Borderline Personality Disorder Collaborative in South Australia.

4.9.11 THE IMPLICATIONS OF THE DIVERSITY IN AUSTRALIA

JILLIAN BROADBEAR

There is paucity of literature about the prevalence of personality disorders and access to treatments among refugees, rural, Indigenous, LGBTIQ and Culturally and Linguistically Diverse populations (CALD). The burden of mental health disorders in Australia's Indigenous communities is three times greater than for other Australians, reflecting the significant impact of intergenerational trauma, substance misuse, and social disadvantage. With respect to the prevalence of personality disorder in Indigenous Australians, the accuracy of estimates is deemed poor, particularly in remote communities (Vos, Barker, Begg, Stanley, & Lopez, 2009). Community prevalence surveys estimate personality disorder is present in 4–16% of Aboriginal and Torres Strait Islander populations (Parker & Milroy, 2010). Guidelines and various reports recommend culturally appropriate interventions, however social and cultural impediments as well as the lack of resources and service capacity continue to hamper mental health initiatives (Hinton, Kavanagh, Barclay, Chenhall, & Nagel, 2015). The difficulty of diagnosing personality disorder in a cross-cultural context (Balaratnasingam & Janca, 2017; Morice, 1979) adds to the current inability to effectively match services with community needs. The remoteness of many communities compounds the problem.

Cultural differences may affect the expression of personality disorders, although the prevalence of personality disorder across countries doesn't appear to vary (Neacsiu et al., 2017; Paris & Lis, 2013). The authors speculate that a loss of social cohesion may increase the prevalence of personality disorder. This may interact with dominant cultural factors, which in Australia and New Zealand have been described as 'individualistic', where members of society seek 'achievement, success, and equality' (Neacsiu et al., 2017, p. 192) while following traditional and established paths and looking after their own needs. The impact of culture on the expression of personality disorder may cloud diagnosis, given the DSM-5 states 'a personality disorder is an enduring pattern of inner experience and behaviour that deviates markedly from the expectations of the individual's culture' (APA, 2013, p. 645). In terms of its cultural origins, the concept of personality disorder has been described as a checklist of behaviours that deviate from Western capitalist society norms (Fábrega, 1994). People from culturally diverse backgrounds who experience difficulties related to acculturation may have these difficulties confused with diagnoses of personality disorder. Screening instruments, normative samples and the language used to describe symptoms may not be culturally appropriate. While some instruments have been adapted and translated into other languages, their utilisation within the Australian mental health system is likely limited (Neacsiu et al., 2017).

Since the inclusion of BPD in the DSM-III (Spitzer, & Williams, 1980), gender and/or sexual identity have been listed within the definition of 'identity disturbance', with the DSM-5 stating 'there may be sudden changes in ...sexual identity' (APA, 2013). Changes in DSM definitions over time include the removal of 'unstable gender identity' from the 3rd edition and the addition of 'changes in sexual identity' in the 5th edition. Sexual diversity among clinical populations of people diagnosed with BPD varies, with reported rates of homosexuality or bisexuality among men with BPD ranging from 16.7-57% (Dulit, Fyer, Miller, Sacks, & Frances, 1993; Reich & Zanarini, 2008; Zubenko, George, Soloff, & Schulz, 1987) and from 14-31.1% of women diagnosed with BPD (Dulit et al., 1993; Hurlbert, Apt, & White, 1992; Reich & Zanarini, 2008; Schulte-Herbrüggen et al.; Singh, McMain, & Zucker, 2011; Zubenko et al., 1987). This is noticeably higher than levels reported in the general population; approximately 3.5% of adults in the United States identify as lesbian, gay or bisexual, 8.2% of adults reported having had at least one same-sex sexual experience, and 11% reported some attraction to individuals of the same-sex (Gates, 2011). Although there is no evidence for a common aetiology for sexual diversity and personality disorder, the presence of each complicates and compounds the challenges of the other, particularly given their associated stigma.

The prevalence of personality disorder in older Australians has been estimated to range from 22-60% (Quirk et al., 2016; Stevenson et al., 2011). Changes in symptom expression over a lifespan can make it difficult to diagnose personality disorder in the elderly (e.g., Beatson et al., 2016). This has become particularly problematic in residential aged care settings due to the lack of staff training around detection and management of personality disorder. This problem is particularly acute given Australia's ageing population (see Section 3.3.1).

4.9.12 COMMENTARY AND REFLECTION

SATHYA RAO

Personality disorders have received limited recognition as a public health priority in Australia: a unified national approach to understanding and servicing personality disorder is required. A perspectives paper (Grenyer et al., 2017) identifies key issues pertaining to early intervention, treatment needs, consumer and carer experiences, and the need for accurate and representative data collection in personality disorder, as starting points in mental health care reform.

Emerging evidence from the inter-related fields of neuroscience and complex trauma offers new paradigms for understanding and responding to people with a wide range of issues and symptoms that fit within the diagnosis of personality disorder. In addition, contemporary mental health policy supports a shift of focus away from the question of 'What's wrong with you?' to 'What's happened to you?' and aims to strengthen partnerships with the people who use these services, supporting each individual journey towards a self-defined experience of recovery.

Personality disorders have gained much deserved attention during the past three decades. Although important progress has been made, further research is clearly required to clarify many areas that continue to be problematic. These include classification, neurobiology, genetics, psychosocial determinants, assessment and evidence-based therapy and clinical outcomes relevant to the pathological dimensions that comprise personality disorder. The nosology of personality disorders is clearly set to undergo further refinement.

There is reason for hope as we look to the future for more effective and meaningful psychosocial interventions and treatment principles for personality disorder. An integrated, modular, stepped care treatment approach based on common psychotherapeutic factors may become a reality. As our understanding of the neurobiology of personality disorder develops, there may be scope for new and effective biological interventions that will complement evidence-based psychotherapeutic approaches.

BIBLIOGRAPHY

@indigenousx. (2020). *Indigenous X*. Retrieved from https://indigenousx.com.au.

1800Respect. (2020). *National Sexual Assault, Domestic Family Violence Counselling Service*. Retrieved from www.1800respect.org.au.

3CR 855am community radio. (2016). *Echoes Support Group for Dissociation*. Retrieved from www.3cr.org.au/brainwaves/episode-201605111700/echoes-support-group-dissociation.

Aadam, B., & Petrakis, M. (2020). Ethics, values, and recovery in mental health social work practice. In R. & A. W. C. Poon (eds.), *Mental Health and Social Work* (pp. 400). Singapore: Springer.

Aadil, J., Shah, O., Wadoo, J., & Latoo. (2010). Psychological distress in carers of people with mental disorders. *British Journal of Medical Practitioners, 33*.

Aaltonen, J., Seikkula, J., & Lehtinen, K. (2011). The comprehensive open-dialogue approach in Western Lapland: I. The incidence of non-affective psychosis and prodromal states. *Psychosis-Psychological Social and Integrative Approaches, 3*(3), 179-191.

Abbass, A., Kisely, S., & Kroenke, K. (2009). Short-term psychodynamic psychotherapy for somatic disorders systematic review and meta-analysis of clinical trials. *Psychother Psychosom, 78*(5), 265-274.

Abbass, A., Town, J., & Driessen, E. (2011). The efficacy of short-term psychodynamic psychotherapy for depressive disorders with comorbid personality disorder. *Psychiatry-Interpersonal and Biological Processes, 74*(1), 58-71.

ABC News. (2018). *ACT Mental Health Faces Staff Departure and 'Chronic Skills Shortage', Review Finds*. Retrieved from https://mobile.abc.net.au/news/2018-07-12/act-mental-health-review-highlights-staff-shortage-risks/9983814.

Aboriginal and Torres Strait Islander Suicide Prevention Evaluation Project Report (ATSISPEP). (2016). *Solutions That Work—What the Evidence and Our People Tell Us, the Aboriginal and Torres Strait Islander Suicide Prevention Evaluation Project*. Retrieved from www.atsispep.sis.uwa.edu.au

Abraha, I., Rimland, J. M., Trotta, F. M., Dell'Aquila, G., Cruz-Jentoft, A., Petrovic, M., . . . Cherubini, A. (2017). Systematic review of systematic reviews of non-pharmacological interventions to treat behavioural disturbances in older patients with dementia: The SENATOR-OnTop series. *BMJ Open, 7*(3).

Abramowitz, J. S., Deacon, B. J., Olatunji, B. O., Wheaton, M. G., Berman, N. C., Losardo, D., . . . Hale, L. R. (2010). Assessment of obsessive-compulsive symptom dimensions: Development and evaluation of the Dimensional Obsessive-Compulsive Scale. *Psychol Assess, 22*(1), 180-198.

Academy of Cognitive and Behavioral Therapies (ACT). (2020). *The Academy of Cognitive Therapy*. Retrieved from www.academyofct.org.

Access Economics. (2009). *The Economic Impact of Youth Mental Illness and the Cost Effectiveness of Early Intervention*. Melbourne: Access Economics.

Achenbach, T. M. (1997). *Empirically Based Assessment of Child and Adolescent Psychopathology*. Thousand Oaks: Sage.

Ackerman, D. L., & Greenland, S. (2002). Multivariate meta-analysis of controlled drug studies for obsessive-compulsive disorder. *J Clin Psychopharmacol, 22*(3), 309-317.

ACT Government. (2015). *ACT Mental Health Act 2015*. Retrieved from https://health.act.gov.au/about-our-health-system/consumer-involvement/community-consultation/acts-mental-health-act-2015.

Active Minds. (2020). *Let's Change the Conversation About Mental Health*. Retrieved from www.activeminds.org.

Adams, C. E., Awad, G., Rathbone, J., & Thornley, B. (1998). Chlorpromazine versus placebo for schizophrenia. *Cochrane Review*, (3).

Adams, R., Dominelli, L., & Payne, M. (2009). *Developing Integrative Practice*. In R. Adams, L. Dominelli, & M. Payne (eds.), *Practising Social Work in a Complex World*. London: Palgrave Macmillan.

Adams, Y., Drew, N., & Walker, R. (2014). *Principles of Practice in Mental Health Assessment with Aboriginal Australians*. In P. Dudgeon, H. Milroy, & R. Walker (eds.), *Working Together: Aboriginal and Torres Strait Islander Mental Health and Wellbeing Principles and Practice* (pp. 271-288). Barton: Commonwealth of Australia.

Addington, J., Coldham, E. L., Jones, B., Ko, T., & Addington, D. (2003). The first episode of psychosis: The experience of relatives. *Acta Psychiatr Scand, 108*(4), 285-289.

Agency for Healthcare Research and Quality (AHRQ). (2012). *Clinical Practice Guideline for the Management of Borderline Personality Disorder*. Melbourne: Agency for Healthcare Research and Quality.

Ainsworth, M. D. S., & Bowlby, J. (1991). An ethological approach to personality-development. *American Psychologist, 46*(4), 333-341.

Akister, J. (2011). Protecting Children: The Central Role of Knowledge. *British Association of Social Workers, 23*(5).

Alameda, L., Ferrari, C., Baumann, P. S., Gholam-Rezaee, M., Do, K. Q., & Conus, P. (2015). Childhood sexual and physical abuse: Age at exposure modulates impact on functional outcome in early psychosis patients. *Psychol Med, 45*(13), 2727-2736.

Alarcon Manchego, P., Knott, J., Graudins, A., Bartley, B., & Mitra, B. (2015). Management of mental health patients in Victorian emergency departments: A 10 year follow-up study. *Emergency Medicine Australasia, 27*(6), 529-536.

Alberts, N. M., Hadjistavropoulos, H. D., Jones, S. L., & Sharpe, D. (2013). The Short Health Anxiety Inventory: A systematic review and meta-analysis. *J Anxiety Disord, 27*(1), 68-78.

Alesi, R. (2005). Infertility and its treatment-an emotional roller coaster. *Australian Journal of General Practice, 34*(3), 135.

Alexander, J. (1999). Beyond identity: Queer values and community. *Formerly: Journal of Gay, Lesbian, and Bisexual Identity, 4*(4), 293-314.

Alexander, R. T., Green, F. N., O'Mahony, B., Gunaratna, I. J., Gangadharan, S. K., & Hoare, S. (2010). Personality disorders in offenders with intellectual disability: A comparison of clinical, forensic and outcome variables and implications for service provision. *Journal of Intellectual Disability Research, 54*(7), 650-658.

Ali, K., Farrer, L., Fassnacht, D. B., Gulliver, A., Bauer, S., & Griffiths, K. M. (2017). Perceived barriers and facilitators towards help-seeking for eating disorders: A systematic review. *International Journal of Eating Disorders, 50*(1), 9-21.

Al-Issa, I. (1982). *Gender and Psychopathology*. New York: Academic Press.

Aliyev, N. A., & Aliyev, Z. N. (2011). Lamotrigine in the immediate treatment of outpatients with depersonalization disorder without psychiatric comorbidity randomized, double-blind, placebo-controlled study. *Journal of Clinical Psychopharmacology, 31*(1), 61-65.

Allen, C. K., Austin, S. L., David, S. K., Earhart, C. A., McCraith, D. B., & Riska-Williams, L. (2007). *Manual for the Allen Cognitive Level Screen-5 (ACLS-5) and Large Allen Cognitive Level Screen-5 (LACLS-5)*. Camarillo: ACLS and LACLS Committee.

Allen, J., Balfour, R., Bell, R., & Marmot, M. (2014). Social determinants of mental health. *Int Rev Psychiatry, 26*(4), 392-407.

Allen, K. L., Byrne, S. M., Oddy, W. H., & Crosby, R. D. (2013). DSM-IV-TR and DSM-5 eating disorders in adolescents: Prevalence, stability, and psychosocial correlates in a population-based sample of male and female adolescents. *Journal of Abnormal Psychology, 122*(3), 720.

Allen, M. C. (2008). Neurodevelopmental outcomes of preterm infants. *Current Opinion in Neurology, 21*(2), 123-128.

Allison, S. E., von Wahlde, L., Shockley, T., & Gabbard, G. O. (2006). The development of the self in the era of the internet and role-playing fantasy games. *American Journal of Psychiatry, 163*(3), 381-385.

Altman, D. G., Schulz, K. F., Moher, D., Egger, M., Davidoff, F., Elbourne, D., . . . Lang, T. (2001). The revised CONSORT statement for reporting randomized trials: Explanation and elaboration. *Ann Intern Med, 134*(8), 663-694.

Altunoz, U., Kokurcan, A., Kirici, S., Bastug, G., & Ozel-Kizil, E. T. (2018). Clinical characteristics of generalized anxiety disorder: Older vs. young adults. *Nord J Psychiatry, 72*(2), 97-102.

Álvarez-Jiménez, M., Alcazar-Corcoles, M. A., González-Blanch, C., Bendall, S., McGorry, P. D., & Gleeson, J. F. (2014). Online, social media and mobile technologies for psychosis treatment: A systematic review on novel user-led interventions. *Schizophrenia Research, 156*, 96-106.

Álvarez-Jiménez, M., Bendall, S., Lederman, R., Wadley, G., Chinnery, G., Vargas, S., . . . Gleeson, J. (2013). On the HORYZON: Moderated online social therapy for long-term recovery in first episode psychosis. *Schizophrenia Research, 143*(1), 143-149.

Álvarez-Jiménez, M., Gleeson, J. F., Bendall, S., Lederman, R., Wadley, G., Killackey, E., & McGorry, P. D. (2012). Internet-based interventions for psychosis: A sneak-peek into the future. *Psychiatric Clinics, 35*(3), 735-747.

Álvarez-Jiménez, M., Gleeson, J. F., Bendall, S., Penn, D. L., Yung, A. R., Ryan, R. M., . . . Nelson, B. (2018). Enhancing social functioning in young people at Ultra High Risk (UHR) for psychosis: A pilot study of a novel strengths and mindfulness-based online social therapy. *Schizophrenia Research*.

Ambresin, A.-E., Bennett, K., Patton, G. C., Sanci, L. A., & Sawyer, S. M. (2013). Assessment of youth-friendly health care: A systematic review of indicators drawn from young people's perspectives. *Journal of Adolescent Health, 52*(6), 670-681.

American Psychiatric Association (APA). (1980). *Diagnostic and Statistical Manual of Mental Disorders,* (3rd ed.). Washington DC: American Psychiatric Association.

American Psychiatric Association (APA). (1987). *Diagnostic and Statistical Manual of Mental Disorders,* (3rd revised ed.). Washington DC: American Psychiatric Association.

American Psychiatric Association (APA). (1994). *Diagnostic and Statistical Manual of Mental Disorders (DSM-IV),* (4th ed.). Washington DC: American Psychiatric Association.

American Psychiatric Association (APA). (2000). *Diagnostic and Statistical Manual of Mental Disorders (4th ed., text rev.)*. Washington, DC: Author.

American Psychiatric Association (APA). (2013). *Diagnostic and Statistical Manual of Mental Disorders (DSM-5) 5th edition*. Arlington, VA: APA.

American Psychiatric Association (APA). (2018). *The Structured Clinical Interview for DSM-5®*. Retrieved from www.appi.org/products/structured-clinical-interview-for-dsm-5-scid-5.

American Psychiatric Association (APA). (2020). *The Structured Clinical Interview for DSM-5*. Retrieved from www.apa.org.

American Psychological Association (APA). (2020). *Cognitive Behavioral Therapy Techniques and Strategies*. Retrieved from www.apa.org/education/ce/1360500.

Amering, M., & Schmolke, M. (2009). *Recovery in Mental Health: Reshaping Scientific and Clinical Responsibilities*. Oxford: Wiley-Blackwell.

Amering, M. L., Stastny, P., & Hopper, K. (2005). Psychiatric advance directives: Qualitative study of informed deliberations by mental, health service' users. *British Journal of Psychiatry, 186*, 247-252.

Ames, D., Chiu, E., Lindesay, J., & Shulman, K. I. (2010). Assessing the elderly psychiatric patient. In *Guide to the Psychiatry of Old Age*. Cambridge, Cambridge University Press.

Ammerman, A., Smith, T. W., & Calancie, L. (2014). Practice-based evidence in public health: Improving reach, relevance, and results. *Annu Rev Public Health, 35*, 47-63.

Amminger, G. P. (2017). *The Cannabidiol Youth Anxiety Pilot Study (CAPS): A 12-Week Open-Label Pilot Study of Cannabidiol for Anxiety Disorders (ACTRN12617000825358)*. Retrieved from www.anzctr.org.au/Trial/Registration/TrialReview.aspx?id=372924.

Anderson, C., Cowlishaw, S., Dowling, N. A., Jackson, A. C., Lorains, F., Merkouris, S. S., . . . Thomas, S. (2011). Pharmacological interventions for the treatment of pathological and problem gambling. *Cochrane Database of Systematic Reviews,* (1).

Andrade, G. (2019). Medical ethics and the trolley problem. *Journal of Medical Ethics and History of Medicine, 12*, 3-3.

Andreescu, C., & Reynolds, C. F., 3rd. (2011). Late-life depression: Evidence-based treatment and promising new directions for research and clinical practice. *Psychiatr Clin North Am, 34*(2), 335-355, vii-iii.

Andresen, R., Oades, L. G., & Caputi, P. (2011). *Psychological Recovery: Beyond Mental Illness*. Oxford: Wiley.

Andrews, G., Anstey, K., Brodaty, H., Issakidis, C., & Luscombe, G. (1999). Recall of depressive episode 25 years previously. *Psychol Med, 29*(4), 787-791.

Andrews, G., Basu, A., Cuijpers, P., Craske, M. G., McEvoy, P., English, C. L., & Newby, J. M. (2018). Computer therapy for the anxiety and depression disorders is effective, acceptable and practical health care: An updated meta-analysis. *J Anxiety Disord, 55*, 70-78.

Andrews, G., Bell, C., Boyce, P., Gale, C., Lampe, L., Marwat, O., . . . Wilkins, G. (2018). Royal Australian and New Zealand College of Psychiatrists clinical practice guidelines for the treatment of panic disorder, social anxiety disorder and generalised anxiety disorder. *Australian & New Zealand Journal of Psychiatry, 52*(12), 1109-1172.

Andrews, G., Dean, K., & Genderson, M. (2014). *Management of Mental Disorders* (5th ed.). US: Createspace.

Andrews, G., Hall, W., Teesson, M., & Henderson, S. (1999). *The Mental Health of Australians*. Canberra: Commonwealth Department of Health and Aged Care.

Angell, B., & Mahoney, C. (2007). Reconceptualizing the case management relationship in intensive treatment: A study of staff perceptions and experiences. *Administration and Policy in Mental Health, 34*(2), 172-188.

Anglicare. (2018). *Rental Affordability Snapshot 2018*. Retrieved from www.anglicare.asn.au/research-advocacy/the-rental-affordability-snapshot'.

Angstman, K. B., & Rasmussen, N. H. (2011). Personality disorders: Review and clinical application in daily practice. *American Family Physician, 84*(11), 1253-1260.

Ansara, G. (2016). *Making the Count: Addressing Data Integrity Gaps in Australian Standards for Collecting Sex and Gender Information [White Paper]*. Retrieved from https://lgbtihealth.org.au/white-paper-addressing-data-integrity-gaps-in-the-abs-2016-standard-for-sex-and-gender-variables.

Anthony, W. A. (1993). Recovery from mental illness: The guiding vision of the mental health service system in the 1990s. *Psychosocial Rehabilitation Journal*, vol. 16 (no. 4), 11-23.

Antony, M. M., Orsillo, S. M., & Roemer, L. (eds.). (2001). *Practitioner's Guide to Empirically Based Measures of Anxiety*. New York: Kluwer Academic/Plenum Publishers.

Antony, M. M., & Stein, M. B. (2008). *Oxford Handbook of Anxiety and Related Disorders*. USA: Oxford University Press.

Anxiety Disorders Association of Victoria (ADAVIC). (2014). *Anxiety Disorders Association of Victoria, Inc*. Retrieved from www.adavic.org.au/PG-social-support-support-groups.aspx.

Anxiety Recovery Centre Victoria (ARCVIC). (2020). *Anxiety Recovery Centre Victoria*. Retrieved from www.arcvic.com.au.

Apte, A., Kielhofner, G., Paul-Ward, A., & Braveman, B. (2005). Therapists' and clients' perceptions of the occupational performance history interview. *Occupational Therapy in Health Care, 19*(1-2), 173-192.

Arango, C., Díaz-Caneja, C. M., McGorry, P. D., Rapoport, J., Sommer, I. E., Vorstman, J. A., . . . Carpenter, W. (2018). Preventive strategies for mental health. *The Lancet Psychiatry, 5*(7), 591-604.

Argentzell, E., Hultqvist, J., Neil, S., & Eklund, M. (2017). Measuring personal recovery—psychometric properties of the Swedish Questionnaire about the process of recovery (QPR-Swe). *Nord J Psychiatry, 71*(7), 529-535.

Argyris, C. (1993). *On Organizational Learning*. US: Blackwell.

Armitage, N., & Trethewie, S. (2014). Paediatric palliative care-the role of the GP. *Australian Journal of General Practice, 43*(4), 176.

Arnett, J. J., Žukauskienė, R., & Sugimura, K. (2014). The new life stage of emerging adulthood at ages 18-29 years: Implications for mental health. *Lancet Psychiatry, 1*(7), 569-576.

Arnstein, S. R. (1969). A ladder of citizen participation. *Journal of the American Institute of Planners, 35*(4), 216-224.

Arseneault, L., Bowes, L., & Shakoor, S. (2010). Bullying victimization in youths and mental health problems: 'Much ado about nothing'? *Psychol Med, 40*(5), 717-729.

Arunogiri, S., Keks, N. A., & Hope, J. (2016). Should ketamine be used for the clinical treatment of depression? *Australasian Psychiatry, 24*(4), 381-384.

Asad, S., & Chreim, S. (2016). Peer support providers' role experiences on interprofessional mental health care teams: A qualitative study. *Community Mental Health Journal, 52*(7), 767-774.

Ash, D., Bland, R., Brown, P., Oakley Browne, M. A., Burvill, P., Davies, J., . . . Weir, W. (2012). Mental Health Services in the Australian States and Territories. In G. Meadows, B. Singh, & M. Grigg (eds.), *Mental Health in Australia 3e; Collaborative Community Practice* (3rd ed., pp. 118-154). Melbourne: Oxford University Press.

Association for Behavioral and Cognitive Therapies (ABCT). (2020). *Association for Behavioral and Cognitive Therapies*. Retrieved from www.abct.org/Home.

Association for Contextual Behavioural Science (ACBS). (2020). *The Association for Contextual Behavioural Science*. Retrieved from https://contextualscience.org.

Astbury, J. (1996). *Crazy for You: The Making of Women's Madness*. Melbourne: Oxford University Press.

Atkins, J., Naismith, S., Luscombe, G., & Hickie, I. (2013). Psychological distress and quality of life in older persons: Relative contributions of fixed and modifiable risk factors. *BMC Psychiatry, 13*(1), 249-249.

Atkinson, J.-A., Page, A., Heffernan, M., McDonnell, G., Prodan, A., Campos, B., . . . Hickie, I. B. (2019). The impact of strengthening mental health services to prevent suicidal behaviour. *Australian & New Zealand Journal of Psychiatry, 53*(7), 642-650.

Atkinson, J. M., Garner, H. C., Gilmour, W. H., & Dyer, J. A. T. (2002). Changes to leave of absence in Scotland: The views of patients. *Journal of Forensic Psychiatry, 13*(2), 315-328.

Attwood, B., & Markus, A. (2007). *The 1967 Referendum: Race, Power and the Australian Constitution* (2nd ed.). Canberra: Aboriginal Studies Press.

Atwoli, L., Stein, D. J., Koenen, K. C., & McLaughlin, K. A. (2015). Epidemiology of posttraumatic stress disorder: Prevalence, correlates and consequences. *Curr Opin Psychiatry, 28*(4), 307-311.

Aubry, T., Goering, P., Veldhuizen, S., Adair, C. E., Bourque, J., Distasio, J., . . . Tsemberis, S. (2016). A multiple-city RCT of housing first with assertive community treatment for homeless Canadians with serious mental illness. *Psychiatric Services (Washington, DC), 67*(3), 275.

Australasian College of Emergency Medicine. (2018). *The Long Wait. An Analysis of Mental Health Presentations to Australian Emergency Departments*. Retrieved from https://acem.org.au/getmedia/60763b10-1bf5-4fbc-a7e2-9fd58620d2cf/ACEM_report_41018.

Australasian College of Emergency Medicine (ACEM). (2019). *Mental Health in the Emergency Department Consensus Statement*. Retrieved from https://acem.org.au.

Australian Association for Cognitive and Behaviour Therapy (AACBT). (2020). *Australian Association for Cognitive and Behaviour Therapy*. Retrieved from www.aacbt.org.au.

Australian Association of Social Workers. (2010). *Code of Ethics*. Retrieved from www.aasw.asn.au/document/item/1201.

Australian Bureau of Statistics (ABS). (1998a). *Census of Population and Housing: Aboriginal and Torres Strait Islander People, Northern Territory* (cat. no. 2034.7). Canberra, Australia: Author.

Australian Bureau of Statistics (ABS). (1998b). *Mental Health and Well-being: Profile of Adults, Australia, 1997* (cat. no. 4326.0). Canberra, Australia: Author. Retrieved from www.abs.gov.au/ausstats.

Australian Bureau of Statistics (ABS). (1998c). *The National Survey of Mental Health and Well-being: Confidential Unit Record File: User's Guide*. Canberra, Australia: Author.

Australian Bureau of Statistics (ABS). (2007). *National Survey of Mental Health and Wellbeing: Summary of Results, 2007* (cat. no. 4326.0.). Retrieved from www.abs.gov.au.

Australian Bureau of Statistics (ABS). (2008a). *National Survey of Mental Health and Wellbeing 2007* (cat. no. 4326.0). Canberra, Australia: Author.

Australian Bureau of Statistics (ABS). (2008b). *National Survey of Mental Health and Wellbeing: Summary of Results* (cat. no. 4326.0). Canberra, Australia: Author.

Australian Bureau of Statistics (ABS). (2009). *National Health Survey: Summary of Results, 2007-2008 (Reissue)*. Retrieved from www.abs.gov.au.

Australian Bureau of Statistics (ABS). (2010). *Australia's Health*. Retrieved from www.aihw.gov.au

Australian Bureau of Statistics (ABS). (2013). *Australian Aboriginal and Torres Strait Islander Health Survey: First Results*. Canberra, Australia: Author.

Australian Bureau of Statistics (ABS). (2014a). *Mental Health and Experiences of Homelessness*. Canberra: Australian Bureau of Statistics. Retrieved from www.abs.gov.au.

Australian Bureau of Statistics (ABS). (2014b). *Causes of Death, Australia, 2012*. Canberra: Australian Bureau of Statistics. Retrieved from www.abs.gov.au/ausstats.

Australian Bureau of Statistics (ABS). (2015a). *Mental Health Statistics, 2015*. Canberra: Australian Bureau of Statistics. Retrieved from www.abs.gov.au/ausstats.

Australian Bureau of Statistics (ABS). (2015b). *Disability, Ageing and Carers, Australia: Summary of Findings* (cat. no. 4430.0). Canberra: Australian Bureau of Statistics. Retrieved from www.abs.gov.au/ausstats.

Australian Bureau of Statistics (ABS). (2016a). *2016 Census QuickStats*. Canberra: Australian Bureau of Statistics. Retrieved from https://quickstats.censusdata.abs.gov.au.

Australian Bureau of Statistics (ABS). (2016b). *Patterns of Use of Mental Health Services and Prescription Medication*. Canberra: Australian Bureau of Statistics. Retrieved from www.abs.gov.au/ausstats.

Australian Bureau of Statistics (ABS). (2016c). *Census of Population and Housing: Reflecting Australia—Stories from the Census, 2016*. Canberra: Australian Bureau of Statistics. Retrieved from www.abs.gov.au/ausstats.

Australian Bureau of Statistics (ABS). (2017). *Australian Demographic Statistics, Dec 2017* (cat. no. 3101.0). Canberra: Australian Bureau of Statistics. Retrieved from www.abs.gov.au/AUSSTATS/abs@.nsf/Lookup/3101.0Main+Features1Dec%202017?OpenDocument.

Australian Bureau of Statistics (ABS). (2018a). *Census of Population and Housing: Characteristics of Aboriginal and Torres Strait Islander Australians, 2016* (cat. no. 2076.0). Canberra: Australian Bureau of Statistics. Retrieved from www.abs.gov.au/ausstats.

Australian Bureau of Statistics (ABS). (2018b). *Life Tables, States, Territories and Australia, 2015–2017* . Canberra: Australian Bureau of Statistics. Retreived from www.abs.gov.au/ausstats.

Australian Bureau of Statistics (ABS). (2018c). *National Health Survey; First Results, Australia 2017–18*. Canberra: Australian Bureau of Statistics. Retreived Retrieved from www.abs.gov.au.

Australian Bureau of Statistics (ABS). (2018d). *Northern Territory Population Australia*. Canberra: Australian Bureau of Statistics. Retrieved from https://itt.abs. gov.au.

Australian Bureau of Statistics (ABS). (2018e). *Causes of Death, Australia 2017*. Canberra: Australian Bureau of Statistics. Retrieved from www.abs.gov.au/ausstats.

Australian Bureau of Statistics (ABS). (2018f). *Growing Up in Australia, Australian Institute of Family Studies*. Canberra: Australian Bureau of Statistics. Retrieved from https://growingupinaustralia.gov.au/about-study#main-content.

Australian Bureau of Statistics (ABS). (2019a). *Australian Demographic Statistics, June 2019* 9 (cat. no. 3101.0). Canberra: Australian Bureau of Statistics. Retrieved from www.abs.gov.au/ausstats.

Australian Bureau of Statistics (ABS). (2019b). *Prisoners in Australia* (cat. no. 4517.0). Canberra: Australian Bureau of Statistics. Retrieved from www.abs.gov.au/ausstats.

Australian Bureau of Statistics (ABS). (2020). *Household Impacts of COVID-19 Survey, 14–17 Apr 2020*. Canberra: Australian Bureau of Statistics Retrieved from www.abs.gov.au/AUSSTATS.

Australian Charities and Not-for-profits Commission (ACNC). (2011). *Australian Infant Child Adolescent and Family Mental Health Association*. Retrieved from www.acnc.gov.au/charity

Australian Child Rights Taskforce. (2011). *Listen to Children Report*. Retrieved from www.childrights.org.au/child-rights/the-reporting-process/listen-to-children-report.

Australian College of Mental Health Nurses. (2010). *Standards of Practice for Australian Mental Health Nurses 2010*. Retrieved from www.acmhn.org/publications/standards-of-practice.

Australian College of Mental Health Nurses. (2013). *Scope of Practice of Mental Health Nurses in Australia 2013*. Retrieved from www.acmhn.org/career-resources/scope-of-practice.

Australian Commission on Safety and Quality in Health Care. (2016). *Delirium Clinical Care Standard*. Retrieved from www.safetyandquality.gov.au/sites/default/files/migrated/Delirium-Clinical-Care-Standard-Web-PDF.pdf.

Australian Government. (1994). *First National Mental Health Report 1993: Monitoring Progress Towards National Mental Health Policy*. Canberra: Australian Government.

Australian Government. (2009). *National Framework for Protecting Australia's Children 2009–2020*. Canberra: Australian Government. Retrieved from www.dss.gov.au/our-responsibilities/families-and-children/publications-articles/protecting-children-is-everyones-business.

Australian Government. (2010a). *Carer Recognition Act 2010: An Act to Provide for the Recognition of Carers and Related Purposes. Carer Recognition Act 2010*. Canberra: Australian Government. Retrieved from www.legislation.gov.au/Series/C2010A00123.

Australian Government. (2010b). *National Standards for Mental Health Service 2010s*. Canberra: Australian Government. Retrieved from www.health.gov.au/internet/main/publishing.nsf/Content.

Australian Government. (2010c). *Carer Recognition Act 2010 Guidelines*. Canberra: Australian Government. Retrieved from www.dss.gov.au/our-responsibilities/disability-and-carers/publications-articles/carer-recognition-act-2010-guidelines.

Australian Government. (2011). *Social Security (Tables for the Assessment of Work-related Impairment for Disability Support Pension) Determination 2011*. Canberra: Australian Government. Retrieved from www.legislation.gov.au.

Australian Government. (2014). *Aboriginal and Torres Strait Islander Health Curriculum Framework*. Retrieved from www1.health.gov.au/internet/main/publishing.nsf/Content/aboriginal-torres-strait-islander-health-curriculum-framework.

Australian Government. (2015a). *National Aboriginal and Torres Strait Islander Health Plan 2013–2023*. Retrieved from www1.health.gov.au/internet/main/publishing.nsf.

Australian Government. (2015b). *GP Workforce Statistics*. Canberra: Department of Health.

Australian Government. (2015c). *PHN Profiles. Primary Health Networks*. Retrieved from www1.health.gov.au/internet/main/publishing.nsf/Content/PHN-Profiles.

Australian Government. (2018). *Regional and Remote Communities*. Retrieved from www.aihw.gov.au/reports/older-people/older-australia-at-a-glance/contents/diverse-groups-of-older-australians/regional-remote-communities.

Australian Government. (2019a). *Apology to Australia's Indigenous Peoples*. Canberra: Australian Government Retrieved from www.australia.gov.au/about-australia/our-country/our-people/apology-to-australias-indigenous-peoples.

Australian Government. (2019b). *Better Access Telehealth Services for People in Rural and Remote Areas*. Canberra: Australian Government. Retrieved from www1.health.gov.au/internet/main/publishing.nsf/Content/mental-ba-telehealth.

Australian Government. (2019c). *Fourth National Mental Health Plan: Productivity Commission Mental Health draft report. Mental Health.* Canberra: Australian Government. Retrieved from www.pc.gov.au/inquiries/current/mental-health/draft.

Australian Government. (2019d). *PHN Primary Mental Health Care Flexible Funding Pool Implementation Guidance*. Canberra: Australian Government. Retrieved from www.health.gov.au/internet/main/publishing.nsf.

Australian Government. (2019e). *Programs and Initiatives*. Canberra: Australian Government. Retrieved from www.health.gov.au/about-us/what-we-do/initiatives-and-programs.

Australian Government (2019f). *Productivity Commission Report on Government Services: Mental Health Management*. Canberra: Australian Government. Retrieved from www.pc.gov.au/research/ongoing/report-on-government-services/2019/health/mental-health-management.

Australian Government Department of Health. (2009). *National Mental Health Policy 2008*. Canberra: Australian Government. Retrieved from www1.health.gov.au/internet/main/publishing.nsf/Content.

Australian Government Department of Health. (2013). *National Practice Standards for the Mental Health Workforce 2013*. Canberra: Australian Government. Retrieved from www.health.gov.au/internet/main/publishing.nsf/Content.

Australian Government Department of Health. (2015). *Australian Government Response to Contributing Lives, Thriving Communities—Review of Mental Health Programmes and Services*. Canberra: Australian Government. Retrieved from www1.health.gov.au.

Australian Government Department of Health. (2017). *Roadmap for National Mental Health Reform*. Canberra: Australian Government. Retrieved from www1.health.gov.au/internet/main/publishing.nsf/Content/mental-roadmap.

Australian Government Department of Health. (2018). Better *Access to Psychiatrists, Psychologists and General Practitioners through the MBS (Better Access) Initiative*. Canberra: Australian Government. Retrieved from www.health.gov.au/mentalhealth-betteraccess.

Australian Government Department of Health and Ageing. (2012). *Operational Guidelines for the Access to Allied Psychological Services Initiative*. Canberra: Australian Government.

Australian Government Department of Health and Ageing. (2020). *Social and Emotional Wellbeing and Mental Health Services in Aboriginal Australia*. Canberra: Australian Government. Retrieved from www.sewbmh.org.au.

Australian Government Productivity Commission. (2020). Canberra: Australian Government. Productivity Commisson *Mental Healt Report*. Retrieved from www.pc.gov.au/inquiries/current/mental-health#report.

Australian Government Department of Health. (2012). *E-mental Health Strategy for Australia*. Retrieved from www1.health.gov.au/internet/main/publishing.nsf/Content/mental-pubs-e-emstrat.

Australian Government Department of Health. (2018). Achieving Integrated Regional Planning and Service Delivery.

Australian Health Ministers. (1992a). *National Mental Health Plan*. Canberra: Australian Government.

Australian Health Ministers. (1992b). National Mental Health Policy. Retrieved from www1.health.gov.au/internet/main/publishing.nsf/Content/mental-strat.

Australian Health Ministers. (2003). *National Mental Health Plan 2003–2008*. Canberra: Australian Government.

Australian Health Ministers. (2009). *Fourth National Mental Health Plan: An Agenda for Collaborative Government Action in Mental Health 2009–2014*. Canberra: Commonwealth of Australia.

Australian Health Minister's Advisory Council (AHMAC). (2003). *Evaluation of the Second National Mental Health Plan*. Canberra: Commonwealth of Australia

Australian Health Minister's Advisory Council (AHMAC). (2013). *A National Framework for Recovery-Oriented Mental Health Services: Guide for Practitioners and Providers*. Retrieved from www1.health.gov.au/internet/main/publishing.nsf/Content/67D17065514CF8E8CA257C1D00017A90/$File/recovgde.pdf.

Australian Health Minister's Advisory Council (AHMAC). (2015). *Aboriginal and Torres Strait Islander Health Performance Framework 2014 Report*. Retrieved from www.pmc.gov.au.

Australian Health Practitioner Regulation Agency (AHPRA). (2018). *Annual Report 2017/2018*. Retrieved from www.ahpra.gov.au/annualreport/2018.

Australian Housing and Urban Research Institute (AHURI). (2017). *Census Data Shows Falling Proportion of Households in Social Housing*. Retrieved from www.ahuri.edu.au/policy.

Australian Human Rights Commission (AHRC). (1997). *Bringing Them Home: Report of the National Inquiry into the Separation of Aboriginal and Torres Strait Islander Children from Their Families*. Retrieved from www.humanrights.gov.au/our-work/bringing-them-home-report-1997.

Australian Human Rights Commission (AHRC). (2013). *Sexual Orientation, Gender Identity and Intersex Status Discrimination*. Sydney: Australian Human Rights Commission.

Australian Institute of Health and Welfare (AIHW). (2008). *The Health and Welfare of Australia's Aboriginal and Torres Strait Islander Peoples 2008* (1441–2004). Retrieved from www.aihw.gov.au/reports/indigenous-health-welfare/health-welfare-australias-indigenous-peoples-2008/contents/table-of-contents.

Australian Institute of Health and Welfare (AIHW). (2010). *A Snapshot of Men's Health in Rural and Remote Australia*. Canberra: AIHW. Retrieved from www.aihw.gov.au/reports/rural-health/a-snapshot-of-men-s-health-in-regional-and-remote-australia/contents/table-of-contents.

Australian Institute of Health and Welfare (AIHW). (2011a). *Australian Burden of Disease Study*. Canberra: AIHW.

Australian Institute of Health and Welfare (2011b). *Headline Indicators for Children's Health, Development and Wellbeing 2011*. Cat. no. PHE 144. Canberra: AIHW.

Australian Institute of Health and Welfare (AIHW). (2011c). *Young Australians: Their Health and Wellbeing 2011* (cat. no. PHE 140). Canberra: AIHW.

Australian Institute of Health and Welfare (AIHW). (2012). *Dementia in Australia*. Canberra: AIHW. Retrieved from www.aihw.gov.au/reports/dementia/dementia-in-australia/related-material.

Australian Institute of Health and Welfare (AIHW). (2014a). *Mental Health Services in Australia*. Canberra: AIHW.

Australian Institute of Health and Welfare (AIHW). (2014b). *National Drug Household Report Detailed Findings 2013*. Canberra: AIHW.

Australian Institute of Health and Welfare (AIHW). (2015). *The Health and Welfare of Australia's Aboriginal and Torres Strait Islander Peoples 2015* (cat. no. IHW 147). Canberra: AIHW.

Australian Institute of Health and Welfare (AIHW). (2015a). *Mental Health of Older Australians. Australia's Welfare 2015. Australia's Welfare Series No. 12* (cat. no. AUS 189). Canberra: AIHW. Retrieved from www.aihw.gov.au.

Australian Institute of Health and Welfare (AIHW). (2015b). *National Mental Health Performance Framework*. Canberra: AIHW. Retrieved from http://meteor.aihw.gov.au.

Australian Institute of Health and Welfare (AIHW). (2016c). *Alcohol and Other Drug Treatment Services in Australia 2014-15*. Canberra: AIHW.

Australian Institute of Health and Welfare (AIHW). (2016a). *Australian Burden of Disease Study: Impact and Causes of Illness and Death in Australia 2011. Australian Burden of Disease Study Series No. 3. BOD 4*. Canberra: AIHW.

Australian Institute of Health and Welfare (AIHW). (2016-17a). *Mental Health Establishments NMDS 2016-17*. Canberra: AIHW. Retrieved from https://meteor.aihw.gov.au.

Australian Institute of Health and Welfare (AIHW). (2016-17b). *Specialised Mental Health Care Facilities*. Canberra: AIHW. Retrieved from www.aihw.gov.au/reports.

Australian Institute of Health and Welfare (AIHW). (2017a). *Australia's Welfare 2017. Australia's Welfare Series No. 13*. Canberra: AIHW. Retrieved from www.aihw.gov.au.

Australian Institute of Health and Welfare (AIHW). (2017b). *Mental Health Workforce*. Canberra: AIHW. Retrieved from www.aihw.gov.au/reports/mental-health-services/mental-health-services-in-australia/report-contents/mental-health-workforce.

Australian Institute of Health and Welfare (AIHW). (2017, 29 May 2017). *Rural & Remote Health*. Canberra: AIHW. Retrieved from www.aihw.gov.au/reports/rural-health/rural-remote-health/notes.

Australian Institute of Health and Welfare (AIHW). (2017-18a). *Mental Health Services in Australia*. Canberra: AIHW. Retrieved from www.aihw.gov.au.

Australian Institute of Health and Welfare (AIHW). (2017-2018b). *Medicare-subsidised Mental Health-Specific Services*. Canberra: AIHW. Retrieved from www.aihw.gov.au.

Australian Institute of Health and Welfare (AIHW). (2018a). *Key Performance Indicators for Australian Public Mental Health Services*. Canberra: AIHW. Retrieved from www.aihw.gov.au.

Australian Institute of Health and Welfare (AIHW). (2018b). *Mental Health Services in Australia: In Brief 2018*. Canberra: AIHW. Retrieved from www.aihw.gov.au/reports.

Australian Institute of Health and Welfare (AIHW). (2018c). *National Hospitals Data Collection*. Canberra: AIHW. Retrieved from www.aihw.gov.au/about-our-data/our-data-collections/national-hospitals-data-collection.

Australian Institute of Health and Welfare (AIHW). (2018d). *Housing Assistance in Australia, 2018*. Canberra: AIHW. Retrieved from www.aihw.gov.au/reports.

Australian Institute of Health and Welfare (AIHW). (2018e). *Australia's Health 2018. Australia's Health Series No. 16. AUS 221*. Canberra: AIHW.

Australian Institute of Health and Welfare (AIHW). (2018f). *National Drug Household Report Detailed Findings 2016*. Canberra: AIHW.

Australian Institute of Health and Welfare. (AIHW). (2019). Australian Burden of Disease Study: Impact and causes of illness and death in Australia 2015. *Australian Burden of Disease series*, no. 19. Cat. no. BOD 22. Canberra: AIHW.

Australian Institute of Health and Welfare (AIHW). (2019a). Australia's health 2018: 6.9 Supply of the health workforce for the Indigenous population. *Australia's Health Series No 16*. AUS 221. Canberra: AIHW.

Australian Institute of Health and Welfare (AIHW). (2019b). *Classifications and Technical Notes*. Canberra: AIHW. Retrieved from www.aihw.gov.au/reports/mental-health-services/mental-health-services-in-australia/classifications-and-technical-notes.

Australian Institute of Health and Welfare (AIHW). (2019c). *Mental Health Services: In Brief 2019*. Canberra: AIHW. Retrieved from www.aihw.gov.au.

Australian Institute of Health and Welfare (AIHW). (2019d). *Mental Health Services in Australia*. Canberra: AIHW. Retrieved from www.aihw.gov.au/reports/mental-health-services/mental-health-services-in-australia/report-contents/summary-of-mental-health-services-in-australia.

Australian Institute of Health and Welfare (AIHW). (2020). *Specialised Mental Health Care Facilities*. Canberra: AIHW. Retrieved from www.aihw.gov.au/reports/mental-health-services/mental-health-services-in-australia/report-contents/specialised-mental-health-care-facilities.

Australian Mental Health Care Classification (AMHCC). *Mental Health Care*. Retrieved from www.ihpa.gov.au/what-we-do/mental-health-care.

Australian Mental Health Outcomes and Classification Network (AMHOCN). (2020). *Australian Mental Health Outcomes and Classification Network*. Retrieved from www.amhocn.org.

Australian National University. (2020). *ACACIA: The ACT Consumer and Carer Mental Health Research Unit*. Retrieved from https://rsph.anu.edu.au/study/student-projects/acacia-act-consumer-and-carer-mental-health-research-unit.

Australian New Zealand Clinical Trails Registry (ANZCTR). (2020). *Australian New Zealand Clinical Trails Registry*. Retrieved from www.anzctr.org.au.

Australian Psychological Society (APS). (2007). *Code of Ethics*. Melbourne: APA.

Australian Psychological Society (APS). (2010). *Ethical Guidelines for Psychological Practice with Lesbian, Gay and Bisexual Clients*. Retrieved from www.psychology.org.au/for-members/resource-finder/resources/ethics/Ethical-guideline-psychological-practice-LGBTI.

Australian Psychological Society (APS). (2013). *Ethical Guidelines on Working with Sex And/Or Gender Diverse Clients*. Retrieved from www.psychology.org.au/for-members/resource-finder/resources/ethics/Ethical-guidelines-working-with-sex-gender-diverse.

Australian Psychological Society (APS). (2015). *APS Ethical Guidelines*. Retrieved from www.psychology.org.au/About-Us/What-we-do/ethics-and-practice-standards/APS-Ethical-Guidelines.

Australian Psychological Society (APS). (2015). Position Statement on Psychological Practices that attempt to change Sexual Orientation. Retrieved from https://www.psychology.org.au/About-Us/What-we-do/advocacy/Position-Statements/use-of-psychological-practice-sexual-orientationAustralian Psychological Society (APS). (2018). *Ethical Guidelines for Psychological Assessment and the Use of Psychological Tests*. Melbourne: APA.

Australian Psychological Society (APS). (2020a). *Lesbian, Gay, Bisexual, Transgender and Intersex Issues*. Retrieved from www.psychology.org.au/About-Us/What-we-do/advocacy/Advocacy-social-issues/lesbian-gay-bisexual-transgender-intersex.

Australian Psychological Society (APS). (2020b). *Sexual Identity and Gender Diversity*. Retrieved from www.psychology.org.au/About-Us/What-we-do/advocacy/Advocacy-social-issues/lesbian-gay-bisexual-transgender-intersex/Information-sexual-identity-and-gender-diversity.

Australian Psychological Society (APS). (2020d). *Australian Psychological Society: Believe in Change*. Retrieved from www.psychology.org.au.

Australian Psychological Society (APS). (2020c). *Tips for Psychologists and Others Working with LGBTQI+ People*. Retrieved from www.psychology.org.au/About-Us/What-we-do/advocacy/Advocacy-social-issues/lesbian-gay-bisexual-transgender-intersex/Tips-for-psychologists-working-with-LGBTQI-peopleAustralian Psychological Society (APS). (2020e). *Royal Commission Into Aged Care Quality and Safety*. Retrieved from www.psychology.org.au.

Awad, A. G., & Voruganti, L. N. P. (2008). The burden of schizophrenia on caregivers: A review. *Pharmacoeconomics, 26*(2), 149-162.

Azzopardi, P. S., Sawyer, S. M., Carlin, J. B., Degenhardt, L., Brown, N., Brown, A. D., & Patton, G. C. (2018). Health and wellbeing of Indigenous adolescents in Australia: A systematic synthesis of population data. *Lancet, 391*(10122), 766-782.

Bach, B., & First, M. B. (2018). Application of the ICD-11 classification of personality disorders. *BMC Psychiatry, 18*(1), 351.

Bach, M., & Kerzner, L. (2010). *A New Paradigm for Protecting Autonomy and the Right to Legal Capacity*. Toronto: Law Commission.

Bacopoulos-Viau, A., & Fauvel, A. (2015). The patient's turn: Roy Porter and psychiatry's tales, thirty years on. *Medical History, 60*(1), 1-18.

Baer, L., & Blais, M. A. (eds.). (2010). *Handbook of Clinical Rating Scales and Assessment in Psychiatry and Mental Health*. New York: Humana Press.

Baer, R. (2003). Mindfulness training as a clinical intervention: A conceptual and empirical review. *Clinical Psychology: Science and Practice, 10*, 125-143.

Baggio, S., Dupuis, M., Studer, J., Spilka, S., Daeppen, J. B., Simon, O., . . . Gmel, G. (2016). Reframing video gaming and internet use addiction: Empirical cross-national comparison of heavy use over time and addiction scales among young users. *Addiction, 111*(3), 513-522.

Baier, V., Favrod, J., Ferrari, P., Koch, N., & Holzer, L. (2013). Early tailored assertive community case management for hard-to-engage adolescents suffering from psychiatric disorders: An exploratory pilot study. *Early Intervention in Psychiatry, 7*(1), 94-99.

Bailey, D., & Campling, J. (2012). *Interdisciplinary Working in Mental Health*. UK: Palgrave Macmillan.

Bailey, R., Torrie, R., & Osborne, R. (2013). *Measuring Youth Outcomes at Kapiti Youth Support. Impact Evaluation: Summary Report 2013*. New Zealand: Evaluation Works.

Baker, A. L., Heather, N., Stalwart, A., O'Neill, K., & Wodak, A. (1996). *A Manual of Cognitive Behavioural Techniques Aimed at Reducing HIV Risk-Taking Behaviour in Injecting Drug Users*. Kensington, National Drug and Alcohol Research Centre.

Baker, M., & Jeffers, H. (2016). *Continuity of Care in Modern Day General Practice*. Retrieved from www.rcgp.org.uk/-/media/Files/Policy/A-Z-policy/2016/Continuity-of-care-in-modern-day-general-practice1.ashx?la=en.

Bakker, D., Kazantzis, N., Rickwood, D., & Rickard, N. (2016). Mental health smartphone apps: Review and evidence-based recommendations for future developments. *JMIR mental health, 3*(1), e7.

Balaratnasingam, S., & Janca, A. (2017). Culture and personality disorder: A focus on Indigenous Australians. *Curr Opin Psychiatry, 30*(1), 31-35.

Balaratnasingam, S., & Janca, A. (2019). Depression in Indigenous Australians: Getting it right. *Medical Journal of Australia, 211*(1), 16-16.

Bales, D., van Beek, N., Smits, M., Willemsen, S., Busschbach, J. J., Verheul, R., & Andrea, H. (2012). Treatment outcome of 18-month, day hospital mentalization-based treatment (MBT) in patients with severe borderline personality disorder in The Netherlands. *Journal of Personality Disorders, 26*(4), 568-582.

Bambra, C., Egan, M., Thomas, S., Petticrew, M., & Whitehead, M. (2007). The psychosocial and health effects of workplace reorganisation. 2. A systematic review of task restructuring interventions. *J Epidemiol Community Health, 61*(12), 1028-1037.

Bandelow, B., & Michaelis, S. (2015). Epidemiology of anxiety disorders in the 21st century. *Dialogues in Clinical Neuroscience, 17*(3), 327-335.

Bandelow, B., Zohar, J., Hollander, E., Kasper, S., Möller, H. J., Zohar, J., . . . Vega, J. (2008). World Federation of Societies of Biological Psychiatry (WFSBP) guidelines for the pharmacological treatment of anxiety, obsessive-compulsive and post-traumatic stress disorders—first revision. *World J Biol Psychiatry*, 9(4), 248-312.

Banerjee, D., & Rai, M. (2020). Social isolation in Covid-19: The impact of loneliness. *International Journal of Social Psychiatry*. doi:10.1177/0020764020922269, on-line ahead of print.

Banfield, M., & Forbes, O. (2018). Health and social care coordination for severe and persistent mental illness in Australia: A mixed methods evaluation of experiences with the Partners in Recovery Program. *Int J Ment Health Syst*(12), 13.

Barbato, A., & D'avanzo, B. (2000). Family interventions in schizophrenia and related disorders: A critical review of clinical trials. *Acta Psychiatr Scand, 102*(2), 81-97.

Barbato, N., & Hafner, R. J. (1998). Comorbidity of bipolar and personality disorder. *Australian and New Zealand Journal of Psychiatry, 32*(2), 276-280.

Barkham, M., & Mellor-Clark, J. (2003). Bridging evidence-based practice and practice-based evidence: Developing a rigorous and relevant knowledge for the psychological therapies. *Clinical Psychology & Psychotherapy, 10*(6), 319-327.

Barlow, D. H. (1988). *Anxiety and Its Disorders: The Nature and Treatment of Anxiety and Panic*. New York: Guilford Press.

Barlow, D. H. (2002). *Anxiety and Its Disorders: The Nature and Treatment of Anxiety and Panic* (2nd ed.). New York: Guilford Press.

Barlow, D. H. (2000). Unraveling the mysteries of anxiety and its disorders from the perspective of emotion theory. *American Psychologist, 55*(11), 1247.

Barlow, D. H. (2010). Negative effects from psychological treatments: A perspective. *Am Psychol, 65*(1), 13-20.

Barlow, D. H. (2014). *Clinical Handbook of Psychological Disorders: A Step-By-Step Treatment Manual* (5th ed.). New York: Guilford Press.

Barlow, D. H., & Craske, M. G. (2014). Panic disorder and agoraphobia. In D. H. Barlow (ed.), *Clinical Handbook of Psychological Disorders: A Step-By-Step Treatment Manual* (pp. 1-61). New York: The Guilford Press.

Barlow, D. H., & Durand, V. M. (2012). *Abnormal Psychology: An Integrative Approach* (6th ed.). Belmont: Wadsworth.

Barnes, M., Davis, A., & Tew, J. (2000). Valuing Experience: Users' experiences of compulsion under the *Mental Health Act 1983*. *Mental Health Review Journal, 5*(3), 11-14.

Barnett, P., Matthews, H., Lloyd-Evans, B., Mackay, E., Pilling, S., & Johnson, S. (2018). Compulsory community treatment to reduce readmission to hospital and increase engagement with community care in people with mental illness: A systematic review and meta-analysis. *The Lancet Psychiatry, 5*(12), 1013-1022.

Baron, K., Kielhofner, G., Iyenger, A., Gladhammer, V., & Wolenski, J. (2006). *Occupational Self Assessment (OSA) Version 2.2*. Chicago: Model of Human Occupation Clearinghouse.

Barr, B., Taylor-Robinson, D., Scott-Samuel, A., McKee, M., & Stuckler, D. (2012). Suicides associated with the 2008-10 economic recession in England: Time trend analysis. *BMJ, 345*, e5142.

Barratt, M. J., & Livingston, M. (2015). *Problem Gambling in Victoria: Identifying Local Area Community and Gaming Industry Risk and Protective Factors*, Fitzroy: Victorian Government Department of Justice.

Barsky, A. J., & Ahern, D. K. (2004). Cognitive behavior therapy for hypochondriasis–A randomized controlled trial. *Jama-Journal of the American Medical Association, 291*(12), 1464-1470.

Barsky, A. J., Goodson, J. D., Lane, R. S., & Cleary, P. D. (1988). The amplification of somatic symptoms. *Psychosomatic Medicine, 50*, 510-519.

Bartnik, E. (2013). *Leading mental health reform in the Australian context*. Paper presented at the Keynote address to the International Initiative for Mental Health Leadership, Auckland New Zealand.

Bartnik, E. (2015). *Self directed support: Forging a new direction for mental health*. Paper presented at the TheMHS National Conference, Perth, WA.

Bartnik, E., & Chalmers, R. (2007). It's about more than the money: Local Area Coordination supporting people with disabilities. In S. Hunter & P. Ritchie (eds.), *Co-Production and Personalisation in Social Care: Changing Relationships in the Provision of Social Care* (pp. 19-38). London: Jessica Kingsley Publishers.

Barton, J., Hine, R., & Pretty, J. (2009). The health benefits of walking in greenspaces of high natural and heritage value. *Journal of Integrative Environmental Sciences., 6*(4), 261-278.

Bartsch, D. (2007). Prevalence of body dysmorphic disorder symptoms and associated clinical features among Australian university students. *Clinical Psychologist, 11*(1), 16-23.

Baskerville, J. R. (2010). Observer and subject bias: Lessons From Procrustes. *Academic Emergency Medicine, 17*(9), 1032-1032.

Bass, C., & Halligan, P. (2014). Factitious disorders and malingering: Challenges for clinical assessment and management. *The Lancet, 383*, 1422-1432.

Bassilios, B., Harris, M. G., Middleton, A., Gunn, J., & Pirkis, J. (2015). Characteristics of people who use telephone counseling: Findings from secondary analysis of a population-based study. *Administration and Policy in Mental Health and Mental Health Services Research, 42*(5), 633-633.

Bassilios, B., Nicholas, A., King, K., Reifels, L., Fletcher, J., & Pirkis, J. (2017). *Evaluating the Access to Allied Psychological Services (ATAPS) and Mental Health Services in Rural and Remote Areas (MHSRRA) Programs: Final ATAPS and MHSRRA Evaluation Report*. Retrieved from https://minerva-access.unimelb.edu.au/handle/11343/127221.

Bassilios, B., Nicholas, A., Reifels, L., King, K., Fletcher, J., Machlin, A., . . . Pirkis, J. (2016). Achievements of the Australian Access to Allied Psychological Services (ATAPS) program: Summarising (almost) a decade of key evaluation data. *International Journal of Mental Health Systems, 10*(1).

Bassilios, B., Telford, N., Rickwood, D., Spittal, M. J., & Pirkis, J. (2017). Complementary primary mental health programs for young people in Australia: Access to Allied Psychological Services (ATAPS) and headspace. *International Journal of Mental Health Systems, 11*, 19-19.

Bastien, M. F., & Corbiere, M. (2019). Return-to-work following depression: What work accommodations do employers and human resources directors put in place? *Journal of Occupational Rehabilitation, 29*(2), 423-432.

Bateman, A., & Fonagy, P. (1999). Effectiveness of partial hospitalization in the treatment of borderline personality disorder: A randomized controlled trial. *American Journal of Psychiatry, 156*(10), 1563-1569.

Bateman, A., & Tyrer, P. (2002). *Effective management of personality disorder*. London: Department of Health.

Bateman, A. W., & Krawitz, R. (2013). *Borderline Personality Disorder: An Evidence-Based Guide for Generalist Mental Health Professionals*. Oxford. Oxford University Press.

Bateman, J., Henderson, C., & Kezelman, C. (2013). Trauma-informed care and practice: Towards a cultural shift in policy reform across mental health and human services in Australia. *Position Paper*. Lilyfield, Mental Health Coordinating Council.

Batyr. (2020). *Giving a Voice to the Elephant in the Room*. Retrieved from www.batyr.com.au.

Bauml, J., Pitschel-Walz, G., Volz, A., Luscher, S., Rentrop, M., Kissling, W., & Jahn, T. (2016). Psychoeducation improves compliance and outcome in schizophrenia without an increase of adverse side effects: A 7-year follow-up of the Munich PIP-Study. *Schizophrenia Bulletin, 42*, S62-S70.

Baxter, A. J., Scott, K. M., Vos, T., & Whiteford, H. A. (2013). Global prevalence of anxiety disorders: A systematic review and meta-regression. *Psychol Med, 43*, 897-910.

Bayne, T., & Levy, N. (2005). Amputees By Choice: Body integrity identity disorder and the ethics of amputation. *Journal of Applied Philosophy, 22*(1), 75-86.

Baysak, E., Yertutanol, F. D. K., Dalgar, I., & Candansayar, S. (2018). How game addiction rates and related psychosocial risk factors change within 2-years: A follow-up study. *Psychiatry Investigation, 15*(10), 984.

Beange, H., McElduff, A., & Baker, W. (1995). Medical disorders of adults with mental retardation: A population study. *American Journal on Mental Retardation, 99*(6), 595-604.

Beardslee, W. R., Chien, P. L., & Bell, C. C. (2011). Prevention of mental disorders, substance abuse, and problem behaviors: A developmental perspective. *Psychiatric Services, 62*(3), 247-254.

Beardslee, W. R., Gladstone, T. R. G., Wright, E. J., & Cooper, A. B. (2003). A family-based approach to the prevention of depressive symptoms in children at risk: Evidence of parental and child change. *Pediatrics, 112*(2), e119-e131.

Beatson, J., Broadbear, J. H., Sivakumaran, H., George, K., Kotler, E., Moss, F., & Rao, S. (2016). Missed diagnosis: The emerging crisis of borderline personality disorder in older people. *Australian and New Zealand Journal of Psychiatry, 50*(12), 1139-1145.

Beatson, J., & Rao, S. (2014). Psychotherapy for borderline personality disorder. *Australasian Psychiatry, 22*(6), 529-532.

Beatson, J., Rao, S., Watson, C., & Victoria, S. P. D. S. f. (2010). *Borderline Personality Disorder: Towards Effective Treatment*. Fitzroy: Australian Postgraduate Medicine.

Beauchamp, T. L., & Childress, J. F. (2019). *Principles of Biomedical Ethics* (8th ed.). USA: Oxford University Press.

Beck, A., & Freeman, A. (1990). *Cognitive Therapy of Personality Disorders, 1990*. New York: Guilford.

Beck, A. T. (1967). *Depression: Clinical, Experimental, and Theoretical Aspects*. Michigan: Hoeber Medical Division, Harper & Row.

Beck, A. T. (1979). *Cognitive Therapy of Depression*. New York: Guilford Publications.

Beck, A. T. (1993). *Beck Anxiety Inventory Manual*. San Antonio: Psychological Corporation.

Beck, A. T., Epstein, N., Brown, G., & Steer, R. A. (1988). An inventory for measuring clinical anxiety: Psychometric properties. *J Consult Clin Psychol, 56*(6), 893-897.

BECK Cognitive Behavior Therapy. (2020). *The Home of Cognitive Behavior Therapy*. Retrieved from https://beckinstitute.org.

Beck, J. S. (2011). *Cognitive Behavior Therapy, Second Edition: Basics and Beyond*. New York: Guilford Publications.

Beckett, L., Yu, Q., & Ngoc Long, A. (2005, 2005). The *Impact of Fragile X: Prevalence, Numbers Affected, and Economic Impact*. [A White Paper Prepared for the National Fragile X Foundation].

Beckett, R., & Steer, R. A. (1993). *Beck Anxiety Inventory Manual*. San Antonio: The Psychological Corporation.

Bee, P., Brooks, H., Fraser, C., & Lovell, K. (2015). Professional perspectives on service user and carer involvement in mental health care planning: A qualitative study. *International Journal of Nursing Studies, 52*(12), 1834-1845.

Beer, A., & Faulkner, D. (2008). *The Housing Careers of People with a Disability and Carers of People with a Disability*. Melbourne: Australian Housing and Urban Research Institute Limited.

Behrendt, T. R. H. L., & Fraser, T. R. H. M. (2012). *Indigenous Australia for Dummies*. Milton: John Wiley & Sons.

Beiser, M., & Hou, F. (2001). Language acquisition, unemployment and depressive disorder among Southeast Asian refugees: A 10-year study. *Soc Sci Med, 53*(10), 1321-1334.

Bejerholm, U., Hansson, L., & Eklund, M. (2006). Profiles of occupational engagement in people with schizophrenia (POES): The development of a new instrument based on time-use diaries. *British Journal of Occupational Therapy, 69*(2), 58-68.

Bell, R., Donkin, A., & Marmot, M. (2013). *Tackling Structural and Social Issues to Reduce Inequities in Children's Outcomes in Low to Middle-Income Countries, Office of Research Discussion Paper No.2013-02*. Florence: Unicef.

Belsky, J., & de Haan, M. (2010). Annual research review: Parenting and children's brain development: The end of the beginning. *Journal of Child Psychology and Psychiatry, 52*(4), 409-428.

Bendall, S., Phelps, A., Browne, V., Metcalf, O., Cooper, J., Rose, B., . . . Fava, N. (2018). *Trauma and Young People. Moving Toward Trauma-Informed Services and Systems*. Melbourne: Orygen.

Benjamin, R., Haliburn, J., & King, S. (2019). *Humanising Mental Health Care in Australia: A Guide to Trauma-informed Approaches*. Abingdon: Taylor & Francis.

Bennetts, W. (2009). *Real Lives, Real Jobs—Final Report*. Retrieved from www.healthissuescentre.org.au/documents/items/2009/08/289454-upload-00001.pdf.

Bennetts, W., Cross, W., & Bloomer, M. (2011). Understanding consumer participation in mental health: Issues of power and change. *International Journal of Mental Health Nursing, 20*(3), 155-164.

Bennetts, W., Pinches, A., Paluch, T., & Fossey, E. (2013). Real lives, real jobs: Sustaining consumer perspective work in the mental health sector. *Advances in Mental Health, 11*(3), 313-325.

Bentall, R. P., Wickham, S., Shevlin, M., & Varese, F. (2012). Do specific early-life adversities lead to specific symptoms of psychosis? A study from the 2007 the Adult Psychiatric Morbidity Survey. *Schizophrenia Bulletin, 38*(4), 734-740.

Ben-Zeev, D., Drake, R. E., Corrigan, P. W., Rotondi, A. J., Nilsen, W., & Depp, C. (2012). Using contemporary technologies in the assessment and treatment of serious mental illness. *American Journal of Psychiatric Rehabilitation, 15*, 357-376.

Berg, S., Rortveit, K., & Aase, K. (2017). Suicidal patients' experiences regarding their safety during psychiatric in-patient care: A systematic review of qualitative studies. *BMC Health Serv. Res., 17*(1).

Berney, T. P. (2000). Autism—an evolving concept. *The British Journal of Psychiatry, 176*(1), 20-25.

Berntsen, D., & Rubin, D. C. (2007). When a trauma becomes a key to identity: Enhanced integration of trauma memories predicts posttraumatic stress disorder symptoms. *Applied Cognitive Psychology, 21*, 417-431.

Berrouiguet, S. et al. (2018) Toward mHealth Brief Contact Interventions in Suicide Prevention: Case series From the Suicide Intervention Assisted by Messages (SIAM) Randomised Controlled Trial. *JMIR*, vol 6 (1).

Berry, H. L., Bowen, K., & Kjellstrom, T. (2010). Climate change and mental health: A causal pathways framework. *International Journal of Public Health, 55*(2), 123-132.

Berry, H. L., Hogan, A., Owen, J., Rickwood, D., & Fragar, L. (2011). Climate change and farmers' mental health: Risks and responses. *Asia Pacific Journal of Public Health, 23*(2_suppl), 119S-132S.

Berry, L. M., & Laskey, B. (2012). A review of obsessive intrusive thoughts in the general population. *Journal of Obsessive-Compulsive and Related Disorders, 1*(2), 125-132.

Berry, N., Lobban, F., Emsley, R., & Bucci, S. (2016). Acceptability of interventions delivered online and through mobile phones for people who experience severe mental health problems: A systematic review. *Journal of Medical Internet Research, 18*(5), e121.

Best, L., Still, M., & Cameron, G. (2008). Supported education: Enabling course completion for people experiencing mental illness. *Australian Occupational Therapy Journal, 55*(1), 65-68.

Beveridge, A. (1997). On the origins of posttraumatic stress disorder. In D. Black, M. Newman, J. Harris-Hendriks, & G. Mezey (eds.), *Psychological Trauma: A Developmental Approach*. London: Gaskell.

Beyondblue. (2011). *Clinical Practice Guidelines: Depression in Adolescents and Young Adults*. Melbourne: Beyondblue.

Beyondblue. (2013). *National Mental Health Survey of Doctors and Medical Students*. Retrieved from www.beyondblue. org.au/docs/default-source/research-project-files/bl1132-report—nmhdmss-full-report_web.

Beyondblue. (2018). The way back support service. *Support after a suicide attempt*. Retrieved from www.beyondblue.org.au/the-facts/suicide-prevention/after-a-suicide-attempt/support-after-a-suicide-attempt.

Bhar, S. S., & Kyrios, M. (2007). An investigation of self-ambivalence in obsessive-compulsive disorder. *Behav Res Ther, 45*(8), 1845-1857.

Bickman, L., Douglas, S., Andrade, A., Tomlinson, M., Gleacher, A., Olin, S., & Hoagwood, K. (2016). Implementing a measurement feedback system: A tale of two sites. *Administration and Policy in Mental Health and Mental Health Services Research, 43*(3), 410-425.

Bigner, J. J. (1994). *Individual and Family Development: A Life-Span Interdisciplinary Approach*. New Jersey: Prentice Hall.

Binkert, F., Mutter, M., & Schinzel, A. (2002). Impact of prenatal diagnosis on the prevalence of live births with Down syndrome in the eastern half of Switzerland 1980-1996. *Swiss Medical Weekly, 132*, 478-484.

Binswanger, L. (1958). The Case of Ellen West. An Anthropological-Clinical Study. In R. May, E. Angel, & H. F. Ellenberger (eds.), *Existence: A New Dimension in Psychiatry and Psychology*. Simon and Schuster.

Birchwood, M., Michail, M., Meaden, A., Tarrier, N., Lewis, S., Wykes, T., . . . Peters, E. (2014). Cognitive behaviour therapy to prevent harmful compliance with command hallucinations (COMMAND): A randomised controlled trial. *Lancet Psychiatry, 1*(1), 23–33.

Birchwood, M., Spencer, E., & McGovern, D. (2000). Schizophrenia: Early warning signs. *Advances in Psychiatric Treatment, 6(2)*, 93–101.

Bird, M., & Henderson, C. (2005). Recognising and enhancing the role of Aboriginal and Torres Strait Islander health workers in general practice. *Aboriginal and Islander Health Worker Journal, 29*(3), 3.

Bird, V., Leamy, M., Le Boutillier, C., Williams, J., & Slade, M. (2014). *REFOCUS: Promoting Recovery in Mental Health Services* (2nd edn.). London: Rethink Mental Illness.

Bishop, L., Ransom, A., & Laverty, M. (2017). *Health Care Access, Mental Health and Preventative Health: Health Priority Survey Findings for People in the Bush*. Retrieved from www.cwaa.org.au/images/PDF/RN032-Healths-Needs-Survey-Result.pdf.

Björkman, T., Hansson, L., & Sandlund, M. (2002). Outcomes of case management based on the strengths model compared to standard care. *Social Psychiatry & Psychiatric Epidemiology, 37*(4), 147–152.

Bjornsson, A. S., Didie, E. R., Grant, J. E., Menard, W., Stalker, E., & Phillips, K. A. (2013). Age at onset and clinical correlates in body dysmorphic disorder. *Compr Psychiatry, 54*(7), 893–903.

Black, E., Ranmuthugala, G., Kondalsamy-Chennakesavan, S., Toombs, M., Nicholson, G., & Kisely, S. (2015). A systematic review: Identifying the prevalence rates of psychiatric disorder in Australia's Indigenous populations. *Australian & New Zealand Journal of Psychiatry, 49*(5), 412–429.

Black, E. B., Toombs, M. R., & Kisely, S. (2018). The cultural validity of diagnostic psychiatric measures for Indigenous Australians. *Australian Psychologist, 53*(5), 383–393.

Blackmore, S. (2003). *Consciousness: An Introduction*. London: Hodder and Stoughton.

Blackmore, S., & Troscianko, E. T. (2018). *Consciousness: An Introduction* (3rd ed.). Abingdon: Taylor & Francis.

Blackwell, T. L., & McDermott, A. N. (2014). Test review: Patient Health Questionnaire-9 (PHQ-9). *Rehabilitation Counseling Bulletin, 57*(4), 246–248.

Blanch, A., Filson, B., & Penney, D. (2012). *Engaging Women in Trauma-Informed Peer Support: A Guidebook*. US: Centre for Mental Health Services National Center for Trauma-Informed Care.

Bland, R., Farhall, J., Fernbacher, S., Fossey, E., Happell, B., Kazantzis, N., . . . Willshire, D. (2012). Assessment: Specialised assessment skills. In G. Meadows, B. Singh, & M. Grigg (eds.), *Mental Health in Australia: Collaborative Community Practice* (3rd ed., pp. 394–427). Melbourne: Oxford University Press.

Bland, R., Renouf, N., & Tullgren, A. (2015). *Social Work Practice in Mental Health: An Introduction*. Crows Nest: Allen & Unwin.

Blandon, A. Y., Calkins, S. D., & Keane, S. P. (2010). Predicting emotional and social competence during early childhood from toddler risk and maternal behavior. *Development and Psychopathology, 22*(1), 119–132.

Blaszczynski, A., & Nower, L. (2002). A pathways model of problem and pathological gambling. *Addiction, 97*(5), 487–499.

Bleiberg, K. L., & Markowitz, J. C. (2014). Interpersonal psychotherapy for depression. In D. H. Barlow (ed.), *Clinical Handbook of Psychological Disorders: A Step-By-Step Treatment Manual* (5th ed., pp. 332–352). New York: Guilford Press.

Bleichhardt, G., & Hiller, W. (2007). Hypochondriasis and health anxiety in the German population. *Br J Health Psychol, 12*(Pt 4), 511–523.

Bloch, M. H., Landeros-Weisenberger, A., Rosario, M. C., Pittenger, C., & Leckman, J. F. (2008). Meta-analysis of the symptom structure of obsessive-compulsive disorder. *American Journal of Psychiatry, 165*(12), 1532–1542.

Bloch, S., & Green, S. A. (2009). *Psychiatric Ethics*. USA. Oxford University Press.

Bloch, S., Green, S. A., Janca, A. J., Mitchell, P. B., & Robertson, M. (2017). *Foundations of Clinical Psychiatry* (4th ed.) Melbourne: Melbourne University Press.

Blom, R. M., Hennekam, R. C., & Denys, D. (2012). Body integrity identity disorder. *PLoS One, 7*(4).

Bloom, S. L. (ed.) (2000). *The Sanctuary Model*. Philadelphia: Community Works.

Blow, F. C., & Barry, K. L. (2014). Substance misuse and abuse in older adults: What do we need to know to help? *Generations: Journal of the American Society on Aging, 38*(3), 53–67.

Bluden, R., & Allen, D. (eds.). (1987). *Facing the Challenge: An Ordinary Life for People with Learning Disabilities and Challenging Behaviour*. London: King's Fund.

blue knot foundation. (2020). *National Centre of Excellence for Complex Trauma*. Retrieved from www.blueknot.org.au.

Bodenmann, G., Cina, A., Ledermann, T., & Sanders, M. R. (2008). The efficacy of the Triple P-Positive Parenting Program in improving parenting and child behavior: A comparison with two other treatment conditions. *Behav Res Ther, 46*(4), 411–427.

Bogg, D. (2010). *Values and Ethics in Mental Health Practice; Post-Qualifying Social Work Practice Series*. Exeter: Learning Matters Ltd.

Bond, K., & Anderson, I. M. (2015). Psychoeducation for relapse prevention in bipolar disorder: A systematic review of efficacy in randomized controlled trials. *Bipolar Disorders, 17*(4), 349–362.

Bonell-Pascual, E., Huline-Dickens, S., Hollins, S., Esterhuyzen, A., Sedgwick, P., Abdelnoor, A., & Hubert, J. (1999). Bereavement and grief in adults with learning disabilities: A follow-up study. *British Journal of Psychiatry, 175*, 348–350.

Bonham, C. A., & Uhlenhuth, E. (2014). Disability and comorbidity: Diagnoses and symptoms associated with disability in a clinical population with panic disorder. *Psychiatry Journal, 2014*, 619727–619727.

Book, H. E. (1998). *How to Practice Brief Psychodynamic Psychotherapy: The Core Conflictual Relationship Theme Method* (2nd ed.). Washington: DC American Psychological Association.

Boot, G. R., & Lowell, A. (2019). Acknowledging and promoting Indigenous knowledges, paradigms, and practices within health literacy-related policy and practice documents across Australia, Canada, and New Zealand. *International Indigenous Policy Journal, 10*(3).

Bordin, E. S. (1979). The generalisability of the psychoanalytic concept of the working alliance. *Psychotherapy Psychosomedic Medicine Psychology, 16*(3), 252–260.

Borg, M., & Kristiansen, K. (2004). Recovery-oriented professionals: Helping relationships in mental health services. *Journal of Mental Health, 13*(5), 493–505.

Borkovec, T. D. (1994). The nature, functions, and origins of worry. In G. Davey & F. Tallis (eds.), *Worrying: Perspectives on Theory Assessment and Treatment* (pp. 5–33). Sussex: Wiley & Sons.

Borkovec, T. D., Alcaine, O., & Behar, E. (2004). Avoidance theory of worry and generalized anxiety disorder. In R. G. Heimberg, C. L. Turk, & D. S. Mennin (eds.), *Generalized Anxiety Disorder: Advances in Research and Practice* (Vol. 2004, pp. 77–108). New York: Guilford Press.

Borson, S., Brush, M., Gil, E., Scanlan, J., Vitaliano, P., Chen, J., . . . Roques, J. (1999). The clock drawing test: Utility for dementia detection in multiethnic elders. *Journals of Gerontology Series a-Biological Sciences and Medical Sciences, 54*(11), M534-M540.

Boskind-Lodahl, M. (1976). Cinderella's stepsisters: A feminist perspective on anorexia nervosa and bulimia. *Signs: Journal of Women in Culture and Society, 2*(2), 342-356.

Bottche, M., Kuwert, P., & Knaevelsrud, C. (2012). Posttraumatic stress disorder in older adults: An overview of characteristics and treatment approaches. *International Journal of Geriatric Psychiatry, 27*(3), 230-239.

Bouman, T. K., & Buwalda, F. A. (2008). A psychoeducational approach to hypochondriasis: Background, content, and practice guidelines. *Cognitive and Behavioral Practice, 15*(3), 231-243.

Bouras, N., Martin, G., Leese, M., Vanstraelen, M., Holt, G., Thomas, C., . . . Boardman, J. (2004). Schizophrenia-spectrum psychoses in people with and without intellectual disability. *J Intellect Disabil Res, 48*(6), 548-555.

Bouton, M. E., Mineka, S., & Barlow, D. H. (2001). A modern learning theory perspective on the etiology of panic disorder. *Psychological review, 108*(1), 4.

Bower, C., Leonard, H., & Petterson, B. (2000). Intellectual disability in Western Australia. *Journal of Paediatrics and Child Health, 36*(3), 213-215.

Bower, E. S., Wetherell, J. L., Mon, T., & Lenze, E. J. (2015). Treating anxiety disorders in older adults: Current treatments and future directions. *Harvard Review of Psychiatry, 23*(5), 329-342.

Bowlby, J. (1969). Disruption of affectionate bonds and its effect on behaviour. *Canada's Mental Health, Supplement, no. 59*, p. 12.

Bowman, S., Álvarez-Jiménez, M., Wade, D., Howie, L., & McGorry, P. (2017). The positive and negative experiences of caregiving for siblings of young people with first episode psychosis. *Frontiers in Psychology, 8*, 730.

Bowman, S., Álvarez-Jiménez, M., Wade, D., McGorry, P., & Howie, L. (2015). Forgotten family members: The importance of siblings in early psychosis. *Early Intervention in Psychiatry, 8*(3), 269-273.

Bowman, S., McKinstry, C., & McGorry, P. (2017). Youth mental ill health and secondary school completion in Australia: Time to act. *Early Intervention in Psychiatry, 11*(4), 277-289.

Boyle, D., Harris, M., New Economics Foundation, & National Endowment for Science: Technology the Arts. (2009). *The Challenge of Co-Production: How Equal Partnerships Between Professionals and the Public Are Crucial to Improving Public Services*. UK: NESTA.

Braam, A. W., Visser, S., Cath, D. C., & Hoogendijk, W. J. (2006). Investigation of the syndrome of apotemnophilia and course of a cognitive-behavioural therapy. *Psychopathology, 39*(1),32-37.

Bracken, P. (2003). *Citizenship and Psychiatry.* Paper presented at the inaugural seminar of the Centre for Citizenship and Community Mental Health. University of Bradford. Retrieved from http://62.24.236.202/estep/Prison%20Officer%20Training%20programme/9.%20Mental%20Health/PO-MENTHE-BR-04.pdf.

Brackertz, N., Wilkinson, A., & Davison, J. (2018). Housing, homelessness and mental health: Towards systems change. In *AHURI Research Paper*. Melbourne: Australian Housing and Urban Research Institute (AHURI).

Bradford, D. E., Shapiro, B. L., & Curtin, J. J. (2013). How bad could it be? Alcohol dampens stress responses to threat of uncertain intensity. *Psychological Science, 24*(12), 2541-2549.

Brakoulias, V., Eslick, G. D., & Starcevic, V. (2015). A meta-analysis of the response of pathological hoarding to pharmacotherapy. *Psychiatry Res, 229*(1-2), 272-276.

Brakoulias, V., Seymour, J., Lee, J., Sammut, P., & Starcevic, V. (2013). Predictors of the length of stay in a psychiatric emergency care centre. *Australasian Psychiatry, 21*(6), 563-566.

Brakoulias, V., Starcevic, V., Belloch, A., Brown, C., Ferrao, Y. A., Fontenelle, L. F., . . . Viswasam, K. (2017). Comorbidity, age of onset and suicidality in obsessive-compulsive disorder (OCD): An international collaboration. *Compr Psychiatry, 76*, 79-86.

Brand, M., Wegmann, E., Stark, R., Muller, A., Wolfling, K., Robbins, T. W., & Potenza, M. N. (2019). The interaction of Person-Affect-Cognition-Execution (I-PACE) model for addictive behaviors: Update, generalization to addictive behaviors beyond internet-use disorders, and specification of the process character of addictive behaviors. *Neuroscience and Biobehavioral Reviews, 104*, 1-10.

Braslow, J. T. (2013). The manufacture of recovery. *Annual Review of Clinical Psychology, 9*(1), 781-809.

Brassington, J., & Krawitz, R. (2006). Australasian dialectical behaviour therapy pilot outcome study: Effectiveness, utility and feasibility. *Australasian Psychiatry, 14*(3), 313-318.

Braveman, B., Robson, M., Velozo, C., Kielhofner, G., Fisher, G., Forsyth, K., & Kerschbaum, J. (2005). *Worker Role Interview (WRI) Version 10.0*. Chicago: Model of Human Occupation Clearinghouse, Department of Occupational Therapy, College of Applied Health Sciences, University of Illinois at Chicago.

Breen, H., Hing, N., Gordon, A., & Holdsworth, L. (2013). Indigenous Australian gamblers and their help-seeking behavior. *Psychology of Gaming*. Hauppauge: Nova Science Publishers, 93-120.

Breen, L. J. (2011). Professionals' experiences of grief counseling: Implications for bridging the gap between research and practice. *Omega-Journal of Death and Dying, 62*(3), 285-303.

Brekke, E., Lien, L., & Biong, S. (2018). Experiences of professional helping relations by persons with co-occurring mental health and substance use disorders. (Report). *International Journal of Mental Health and Addiction, 16*(1), 53.

Brennan, S., Davis, M., Edgeworth, B., & Terrill, L. (2015). *Native Title From Mabo to Akiba: A Vehicle for Change and Empowerment?* Annandale: The Federation Press.

Brennand, K. J., Simone, A., Jou, J., Gelboin-Burkhart, C., Tran, N., Sangar, S., . . . Gage, F. H. (2011). Modelling schizophrenia using human induced pluripotent stem cells. *Nature, 473*(7346), 221-+.

Breslin, F. C., Sobell, L. C., Sobell, M. B., & Agrawal, S. (2000). A comparison of a brief and long version of the Situational Confidence Questionnaire. *Behav Res Ther, 38*(12), 1211-1220.

Brett, M., Norton, R., & James, R. (2012). *National Summit on the Mental Health of Tertiary Students*. Retrieved from www.cshe.unimelb.edu.au/nationalsummit/Student_Mental_Health_Checklist_and_Resources.pdf.

Breuer, J., & Freud, S. (1893-1895/1955). Studies on hysteria. In S. Freud, J. Breuer, J. Strachey, & A. Freud (eds.), *The Standard Edition of the Complete Psychological Works of Sigmund Freud* (Vol. 3). Vintage.

Brewin, C. R. (2003). *Post-traumatic Stress Disorder: Malady or Myth?* New Haven: Yale University Press.

Brewin, C. R., Andrews, B., & Valentine, J. D. (2000). Meta-analysis of risk factors for posttraumatic stress disorder in trauma-exposed adults. *J Consult Clin Psychol, 68*(5), 748-766.

Brewin, C. R., & Holmes, E. A. (2003). Psychological theories of posttraumatic stress disorder. *Clinical Psychology Review, 23*, 339-376.

Briere, J., & Lanktree, C. (2013). *Integrative Treatment of Complex Trauma for Adolescents (ITCT-A) Treatment Guide. 2nd Edition.* Los Angeles: University of Southern California.

Briere, J., & Scott, C. (2006). *Principles of Trauma Therapy: A Guide to Symptoms, Evaluation and Treatment*. Thousand Oaks. SAGE Publications.

Britt, H., Miller, G. C., Charles, J., Henderson, J., Bayram, C., Pan, Y., . . . Fahridin, S. (2010). General practice activity in Australia 2009-10. *General Practice Series, 27*.

Britt, H., Miller, G. C., Henderson, J., Bayram, C., Harrison, C., Valenti, L., . . . Gordon, J. (2016). *General Practice Activity in Australia 2015-16*. Sydney: Sydney University Press.

Brockman, R., & Dudgeon, P. (2019). Indigenous clinical psychology in Australia: A decolonising social-emotional wellbeing approach. In P. Rhodes (ed.), *Beyond the Psychology Industry: How Else Might We Heal?* (pp. 83-94). Sydney: Springer International Publishing.

Brodaty, H., Thomson, C., Thompson, C., & Fine, M. (2005). Why caregivers of people with dementia and memory loss don't use services. *International Journal of Geriatric Psychiatry, 20*(6), 537-546.

Broman, N., & Hakansson, A. (2018). Problematic gaming and internet use but not gambling may be overrepresented in sexual minorities: A pilot population web survey study. *Frontiers in Psychology, 9*.

Brook RED. (2019). *Recovery Empowerment Development Peer Support.* Retrieved from www.brookred.org.au.

Brooker, C., Saul, C., Robinson, J., King, J., & Dudley, M. (2003). Is training in psychosocial interventions worthwhile? Report of a psychosocial intervention trainee follow-up study. *International Journal of Nursing Studies, 40*(7), 731-747.

Brophy, L., Bruxner, A., Wilson, E., Cocks, N., & Stylianou, M. (2015). How social work can contribute in the shift to personalised, recovery-oriented psycho-social disability support services. *British Journal of Social Work, 45*(suppl1), i98-i116.

Brophy, L., Campbell, J., & Healy, B. (2003). Dilemmas in the case manager's role: Implementing involuntary treatment in the community. *Psychiatry, Psychology and Law, 10*(1), 154-163.

Brophy, L., Healy, B., & Maylea, C. (2018). Mental health law and its implications for social work practice. In S. Rice, A. Day, & L. Briskman (eds.), *Social Work in the Shadow of the Law* (5th ed., pp. 546). Annandale: The Federation Press.

Brophy, L., Hodges, C., Halloran, K., Grigg, M., & Swift, M. (2014). Impact of care coordination on Australia's mental health service delivery system. *Australian Health Review, 38*(4), 396-400.

Brophy, L., Kokanović, R., Flore, J., McSherry, B., & Herrman, H. (2019). Community treatment orders and supported decision-making. *Frontiers in Psychiatry, 10*.

Brophy, L., & McDermott, F. (2013). Using social work theory and values to investigate the implementation of community treatment orders. *Australian Social Work, 66*(1), 72-85.

Brophy, L., & Ring, D. (2004). The efficacy of involuntary treatment in the community: Consumer and service provider perspectives. *Social Work in Mental Health, 2*(2-3), 157-174.

Brophy, L., Ryan, C. J., & Weller, P. (2018). Community treatment orders: The evidence and the ethical implications. In C. Spivakovsky, K. Seear, & A. Carter (eds.), *Critical Perspectives on Coercive Interventions: Law, Medicine and Society* (pp. 42-55). New York Routledge.

Brosnan, L. (2018). Who's talking about us without us? A survivor research interjection into an academic psychiatry debate on compulsory community treatment orders in Ireland. *Laws, 7*(4), 33.

Brown, A., Rice, S. M., Rickwood, D. J., & Parker, A. G. (2016). Systematic review of barriers and facilitators to accessing and engaging with mental health care among at-risk young people. *Asia-Pacific Psychiatry, 8*(1), 3-22.

Brown, A. S. (2011). The environment and susceptibility to schizophrenia. *Progress in Neurobiology, 93*(1), 23-58.

Brown, C., & Dunn, W. (2002). *Adolescent-adult sensory profile: User's manual.* San Antonio: Therapy Skill Builders.

Brown, C., Moore, W. P., Hemman, D., & Yunek, A. (1996). Influence of instrumental activities of daily living assessment method on judgments of independence. *American Journal of Occupational Therapy, 50*(3), 202-206.

Brown, G. W., Birley, J. L., & Wing, J. K. (1972). Influence of family life on the course of schizophrenic disorders: A replication. *The British Journal of Psychiatry, 121*(562), 241-258.

Brown, T., Tseng, M. H., Casey, J., McDonald, R., & Lyons, C. (2010). Predictors of research utilization among pediatric occupational therapists. *OTJR Occupation, Participation and Health, 30*(4), 172-183.

Browne, A., & Finkelhor, D. (1986). Impact of child sexual abuse: A review of the research. *Psychological Bulletin, 99*(1), 66.

Browne, M., Goodwin, B. C., & Rockloff, M. J. (2018). Validation of the Short Gambling Harm Screen (SGHS): A tool for assessment of harms from gambling. *Journal of Gambling Studies, 34*(2), 499-512.

Browne, M., Greer, N., Rawat, V., & Rockloff, M. (2017). A population-level metric for gambling-related harm. *International Gambling Studies, 17*(2), 163-175.

Browne, M., Langham, E., Rawat, V., Greer, N., Li, E., Rose, J., . . . Best, T. (2016). *Assessing gambling-related harm in Victoria: A public health perspective*. Melbourne: Victorian Responsible Gambling Foundation.

Bruch, H. (1962). Perceptual and conceptual disturbances in anorexia nervosa. *Psychosom Med, 24*, 187-194.

Bruch, H. (1973). *Eating disorders: Obesity, Anorexia Nervosa, and the Person Within*. London: Routledge & Kegan Paul.

Bruno, R. (1997). Devotees, Pretenders and wannabes: Two cases of factitious disability disorder. *A Journal Devoted to the Psychological and Medical Aspects of Sexuality in Rehabilitation and Community Settings, 15*(4), 243-260.

Brunton, G., Thomas, J., O'Mara-Eves, A., Jamal, F., Oliver, S., & Kavanagh, J. (2017). Narratives of community engagement: A systematic review-derived conceptual framework for public health interventions. *BMC Public Health, 17*(1), 944.

Brylewski, J., & Duggan, L. (2004). Antipsychotic medication for challenging behaviour in people with learning disability. *Cochrane Database of Systematic Reviews*, 3 (CD000377).

Bryson, S. A., Gauvin, E., Jamieson, A., Rathgeber, M., Faulkner-Gibson, L., Bell, S., . . . Burke, S. (2017). What are effective strategies for implementing trauma-informed care in youth inpatient psychiatric and residential treatment settings? A realist systematic review. *International Journal of Mental Health Systems, 11*, 36-36.

Buades-Rotger, M., & Gallardo-Pujol, D. (2014). The role of the monoamine oxidase A gene in moderating the response to adversity and associated antisocial behavior: A review. *Psychology Research and Behavior Management, 7*, 185.

Buckmaster, L., & Clark, S. (2018). The National Disability Insurance Scheme: A chronology. *NDIS.* Retrieved from www.aph.gov.au/About_Parliament/Parliamentary_Departments/Parliamentary_Library/pubs/rp/rp1819/Chronologies/NDIS.

Buhlmann, U., Etcoff, N. L., & Wilhelm, S. (2006). Emotion recognition bias for contempt and anger in body dysmorphic disorder. *J Psychiatr Res, 40*(2), 105-111.

Bullen, C., Howe, C., Laugesen, M., McRobbie, H., Parag, V., Williman, J., & Walker, N. (2013). Electronic cigarettes for smoking cessation: A randomised controlled trial. *The Lancet, 382*(9905), 1629-1637.

Bullock, S. A., & Potenza, M. N. (2013). Update on the Pharmacological Treatment of Pathological Gambling. *Current Psychopharmacology, 2*(3), 204.

Burdekin, B., Guilfoyle, M., & Hall, D. (1993). *Human Rights and Mental Illness, Report of the National Inquiry into the Human Rights of People with Mental Illness*. Retrieved from www.humanrights.gov.au/sites/default/files/document/publication/1993_HR_Mental_Illness_Volume_%201.pdf.

Burdon, D. (2017, 23 July, 2017). ACT mental health system in grip of 'crippling' shortage of psychiatrists. *The Canberra Times*. Retrieved from www.canberratimes.com.au/story/6030252/act-mental-health-system-in-grip-of-crippling-shortage-of-psychiatrists.

Burgess, C. P., Johnston, F. H., Berry, H. L., McDonnell, J., Yibarbuk, D., Gunabarra, C., . . . Bailie, R. S. (2009). Healthy country, healthy people: The relationship between Indigenous health status and 'caring for country'. *Med J Aust, 190*(10), 567-572.

Burgess, N., Christensen, H., Leach, L. S., Farrer, L., & Griffiths, K. M. (2008). Mental health profile of callers to a telephone counselling service. *Journal of Telemedicine and Telecare, 14*(1), 42-47.

Burgess, P., Coombs, T., Clarke, A., Dickson, R., & Pirkis, J. (2012). Achievements in mental health outcome measurement in Australia: Reflections on progress made by the Australian Mental Health Outcomes and Classification Network (AMHOCN). *International Journal of Mental Health Systems, 6*(1), 4.

Burgess, P., Pirkis, J., & Coombs, T. (2006). Do adults in contact with Australia's public sector mental health services get better? *Australia and New Zealand Health Policy, 3*, 9.

Burgess, P., Pirkis, J., Coombs, T., & Rosen, A. (2010). *Australian Mental Health Outcomes and Classification Network 'Sharing Information to Improve Outcomes' Review of Recovery Measures (Version 1.01)*. Retrieved from www.mentalhealth.va.gov/communityproviders/docs/review_recovery_measures.pdf.

Burgess, P. M., Pirkis, J. E., Slade, T. N., Johnston, A. K., Meadows, G., & Gunn, J. M. (2009). Service use for mental health problems: Findings from the 2007 National Survey of Mental Health and Wellbeing. *Australian and New Zealand Journal of Psychiatry, 43*(7), 615-623.

Burns, D. (2007). *Systemic Action Research: A Strategy for Whole System Change*. Bristol: Policy Press.

Burns, J., & Birrell, E. (2014). Enhancing early engagement with mental health services by young people. *Psychology Research and Behavior Management, 7*, 303-312.

Burns, J. K. (2009). Mental health and inequity: A human rights approach to inequality, discrimination, and mental disability. *Health and Human Rights, 11*(2), 19-31.

Burns, J. M., Davenport, T. A., Durkin, L. A., Luscombe, G. M., & Hickie, I. B. (2010). The internet as a setting for mental health service utilisation by young people. *Medical Journal of Australia, 192*(11), S22-S26.

Burns, T., Catty, J., Dash, M., Roberts, C., Lockwood, A., & Marshall, M. (2007). Use of intensive case management to reduce time in hospital in people with severe mental illness: Systematic review and meta-regression. *British Medical Journal, 335*(7615), 336-342.

Burns, T., & Molodynski, A. (2014). Community treatment orders: Background and implications of the OCTET trial. *Psychiatrist, 38*(1), 3-5.

Busfield, J. (1996). *Men, Women and Madness*. London: Macmillan.

Bustillo, J. R., Lauriello, J., Horan, W. P., & Keith, S. J. (2001). The psychosocial treatment of schizophrenia: An update. *American Journal of Psychiatry, 158*(2), 163-175.

Butcher, J. N., Graham, J. R., Ben-Porath, Y. S., Tellegen, A., Dahlstrom, G., & Kaemmer, B. (2001). *Minnesota Multiphasic Personality Inventory®-2 (MMPI®-2)*. Retrieved from www.pearsonclinical.com.au/products/view/241.

Butler, T. L., Anderson, K., Garvey, G., Cunningham, J., Ratcliffe, J., Tong, A., . . . Howard, K. (2019). Aboriginal and Torres Strait Islander people's domains of wellbeing: A comprehensive literature review. *Social Science & Medicine, 233*, 138-157.

Butterworth, P., Leach, L. S., Strazdins, L., Olesen, S. C., Rodgers, B., & Broom, D. H. (2011). The psychosocial quality of work determines whether employment has benefits for mental health: Results from a longitudinal national household panel survey. *Occup Environ Med, 68*(11), 806-812.

Butterworth, P., Pymont, C., Rodgers, B., Windsor, T. D., & Anstey, K. J. (2010). Factors that explain the poorer mental health of caregivers: Results from a community survey of older Australians. *Australian and New Zealand Journal of Psychiatry, 44*(7), 616-624.

Byles, J. E., Robinson, I., Banks, E., Gibson, R., Leigh, L., Rodgers, B., . . . Jorm, L. (2014). Psychological distress and comorbid physical conditions: Disease or disability? *Depression and Anxiety, 31*(6), 524-532.

Byrne, L., Happell, B., & Reid-Searl, K. (2015). Recovery as a Lived Experience Discipline: A grounded theory study. *Issues in Mental Health Nursing, 36*(12), 935-943.

Byrne, L., Happell, B., & Reid-Searl, K. (2016). Lived experience practitioners and the medical model: World's colliding? *Journal of Mental Health, 25*(3), 217-223.

Byrne, L., Roennfeldt, H., O'Shea, P., & Macdonald, F. (2018). Taking a gamble for high rewards? Management perspectives on the value of mental health peer workers. *International Journal of Environmental Research and Public Health, 15*(4), 746.

Byrne, L., Roper, C., Happell, B., & Reid-Searl, K. (2019). The stigma of identifying as having a lived experience runs before me: Challenges for lived experience roles. *Journal of Mental Health, 28*(3), 260-266.

Byrne, L., Schoeppe, S., & Bradshaw, J. (2018). Recovery without autonomy: Progress forward or more of the same for mental health service users? *International Journal of Mental Health Nursing*, 27, 1459-1469.

Byrne, L., Stratford, A., & Davison, L. (2018). The global need for lived experience leadership. *Psychiatric Rehabilitation Journal, 41*(1), 76-79.

Byrne, S., Cooper, Z., & Fairburn, C. (2003). Weight maintenance and relapse in obesity: A qualitative study. *Int J Obes Relat Metab Disord, 27*(8), 955-962.

Cade, J. F. (1949). Lithium salts in the treatment of psychotic excitement. *Medical Journal of Australia, 2*, 349-352.

Cadence. (2015). *Improving Outcomes for People with Psychosis*. Retrieved from https://cadencetrials.com.

Cahalan, S. (2020). Insane places. *New Scientist, 245*(3268), 38-40.

Cahill, K., Stead, L., & Lancaster, T. (2009). A preliminary benefit-risk assessment of varenicline in smoking cessation. *Drug Safety, 32*(2), 119-135.

Cahn, E. S. (2000). *No More Throw-away People: The Co-production Imperative*. USA: Essential.

Cairns, A., Hill, C., Dark, F., McPhail, S., & Gray, M. (2013). The Large Allen Cognitive Level Screen as an indicator for medication adherence among adults accessing community mental health services. *British Journal of Occupational Therapy, 76*(3), 137–143.

Calado, F., & Griffiths, M. D. (2016). Problem gambling worldwide: An update and systematic review of empirical research (2000–2015). *Journal of Behavioral Addictions, 5*(4), 592–613.

Caligor, E., Levy, K. N., & Yeomans, F. E. (2015). Narcissistic personality disorder: Diagnostic and clinical challenges. *American Journal of Psychiatry, 172*(5), 415–422.

Calma, T., Dudgeon, P., & Bray, A. (2017). Aboriginal and Torres Strait Islander social and emotional wellbeing and mental health. *Australian Psychologist, 52*(4), 255–260.

Cameron, J., Sadlo, G., Hart, A., & Walker, C. (2016). Return-to-work support for employees with mental health problems: Identifying and responding to key challenges of sick leave. *British Journal of Occupational Therapy, 79*(5), 275–283.

Campbell, L. E., Hanlon, M.-C., Galletly, C. A., Harvey, C., Stain, H., Cohen, M., . . . Brown, S. (2018). Severity of illness and adaptive functioning predict quality of care of children among parents with psychosis: A confirmatory factor analysis. *Australian & New Zealand Journal of Psychiatry, 52*(5), 435–445.

Campbell, L. E., Hanlon, M.-C., Poon, A. W. C., Paolini, S., Stone, M., Galletly, C., . . . Cohen, M. (2012). The experiences of Australian parents with psychosis: The Second Australian National Survey of psychosis. *Australian & New Zealand Journal of Psychiatry, 46*(9), 890–900.

Campbell, M. K., Piaggio, G., Elbourne, D. R., & Altman, D. G. (2012). Consort 2010 statement: Extension to cluster randomised trials. *BMJ: British Medical Journal, 345*, e5661.

Campbell, N., McAllister, L., & Eley, D. (2012). The influence of motivation in recruitment and retention of rural and remote allied health professionals: A literature review. *Rural and Remote Health, 12*(3).

Campise, R. L., Geller, S. K., & Campise, M. E. (2006). Combat stress. In C. H. Kennedy & E. A. Zillmer (eds.), *Military Psychology: Clinical and Operational Applications* (pp. 215–240). New York: The Guilford Press.

Canadian Association of Occupational Therapists. (2002). *Enabling Occupation: An Occupational Therapy Perspective*. Ottowa: Canadian Association of Occupational Therapists.

Canale, N., Vieno, A., Pastore, M., Ghisi, M., & Griffiths, M. D. (2016). Validation of the 8-item Attitudes Towards Gambling Scale (ATGS-8) in a British population survey. *Addictive Behaviors, 54*, 70–74.

Caplan, G., & Felix, R. H. (1964). *Principles of Preventive Psychiatry*. New York, Basic Books.

Caqueo-Urízar, A., Rus-Calafell, M., Craig, T. K. J., Irarrazaval, M., Urzúa, A., Boyer, L., & Williams, D. R. (2017). Schizophrenia: Impact on family dynamics. *Current Psychiatry Reports, 19*(2), 1–8.

Cara, E. (2013). Groups. In E. Cara & A. MacRae (eds.), *Psychosocial Occupational Therapy: An Evolving Practice* (3rd ed., pp. 671–711). Clifton Park: Delmar.

Carers Australia Vic. (2012). *Victorian Carers Recognition Act*. Retrieved from https://www.carersvictoria.org.au/be-informed/victorian-carers-recognition-act.

Carers Trust. (2013). *The Triangle of Care Carers Included: A Guide to Best Practice in Mental Health Care in England* (2nd ed.). London: Carers Trust.

Carey, M., Jones, K., Meadows, G., Sanson-Fisher, R., D'Este, C., Inder, K., . . . Russell, G. (2014). Accuracy of general practitioner unassisted detection of depression. *Australian & New Zealand Journal of Psychiatry, 48*(6), 571–578.

Carlson, B. (2016). *The Politics of Identity: Who Counts as Aboriginal Today?* Canberra: Aboriginal Studies Press.

Carney, T., Beaupert, F., Perry, J., & Tait, D. (2008). Advocacy and participation in mental health cases: Realisable rights or pipe dreams? *Law in Context, 26*(2), 125–147.

Carnie, T. L., Berry, H. L., Blinkhorn, S. A., & Hart, C. R. (2011). In their own words: Young people's mental health in drought-affected rural and remote NSW. *Australian Journal of Rural Health, 19*(5), 244–248.

Carpenter, J. (2002). Mental health recovery paradigm: Implications for social work. *Health & Social Work, 27*(2), 86–94.

Carpenter, M. (2018). The 'normalization' of intersex bodies and 'othering' of intersex identities in Australia. *Journal of Bioethical Inquiry, 15*(4), 487–495.

Carr, A. (2018). The effectiveness of family therapy and systemic interventions for adult-focused problems. *Journal of Family Therapy, 31*(1), 46–74.

Carr, A. (2019). Family therapy and systemic interventions for child-focused problems: The current evidence base. *Journal of Family Therapy*, 41(2), 153–213.

Carroll, A., & McSherry, B. (2015). Making defensible decisions in the era of recovery and rights. *Australasian Psychiatry, 26*(5), 474–477.

Carroll, K. M., Ball, S. A., Nich, C., O'Connor, P. G., Eagan, D. A., Frankforter, T. L., . . . Rounsaville, B. J. (2001). Targeting behavioral therapies to enhance naltrexone treatment of opioid dependence: Efficacy of contingency management and significant other involvement. *Archives of General Psychiatry, 58*(8), 755–761.

Carrotte, E., & Blanchard, M. (2018). *Understanding How Best to Respond to the Needs of Australians Living with Personality Disorder*. Retrieved from www.sane.org/images/NMHC_SANE_PD_Report.pdf.

Carson, E., King, S., & Papatraianou, L. H. (2011). Resilience among social workers: The role of informal learning in the workplace. *Practice, 23*(5), 267–278.

Carter, G., Milner, A., McGill, K., Pirkis, J., Kapur, N., & Spittal, M. J. (2017). Predicting suicidal behaviours using clinical instruments: Systematic review and meta-analysis of positive predictive values for risk scales. *Br J Psychiatry, 210*(6), 387-+.

Carter, G., Page, A., Large, M., Hetrick, S., Milner, A. J., Bendit, N., . . . Christensen, H. (2016). Royal Australian and New Zealand College of Psychiatrists clinical practice guideline for the management of deliberate self-harm. *Australian & New Zealand Journal of Psychiatry, 50*(10), 939–1000.

Carter, G. L., Willcox, C. H., Lewin, T. J., Conrad, A. M., & Bendit, N. (2010). Hunter DBT project: Randomized controlled trial of dialectical behaviour therapy in women with borderline personality disorder. *Australian and New Zealand Journal of Psychiatry, 44*(2), 162–173.

Carter, J. C., McFarlane, T. L., Bewell, C., Olmsted, M. P., Woodside, D. B., Kaplan, A. S., & Crosby, R. D. (2009). Maintenance treatment for anorexia nervosa: A comparison of cognitive behavior therapy and treatment as usual. *International Journal of Eating Disorders, 42*(3), 202–207.

Casasnovas, C., Fernández-Aranda, F., Granero, R., Krug, I., Jiménez-Murcia, S., Bulik, C. M., & Vallejo-Ruiloba, J. (2007). Motivation to change in eating disorders: Clinical and therapeutic implications. *Eur Eat Disord Rev, 15*(6), 449–456.

Caselli, I., Poloni, N., Ceccon, F., Ielmini, M., Merlo, B., & Callegari, C. (2018). A systematic review on factitious disorders: Psychopathology and diagnostic classification. *Neuropsychology, 8*(1), 281-292.

Casey, L. M., Oei, T. P. S., Raylu, N., Horrigan, K., Day, J., Ireland, M., & Clough, B. A. (2017). Internet-based delivery of cognitive behaviour therapy compared to monitoring, feedback and support for problem gambling: A randomised controlled trial. *Journal of Gambling Studies*, 1-18.

Casey, R. J. (1996). Emotional competence in children with externalizing and internalizing disorders. In *Emotional development in atypical children* (pp. 161-183). Hillsdale: Lawrence Erlbaum Associates.

Caspi, A., & Moffitt, T. E. (2018). All for one and one for all: Mental disorders in one dimension. *American Journal of Psychiatry, 175*(9), 831-844.

Castle, D., Bassett, D., King, J., & Gleason, A. (2013). *A Primer of Clinical Psychiatry*. Australia, Elsevier Health Sciences.

Castle, D., Jablensky, A., McGrath, J., Carr, V., Morgan, V. A., Waterreus, A., . . . Farmer, A. (2006). The Diagnostic Interview for Psychoses (DIP): Development, reliability and applications. *Psychol Med, 36*, 69-80.

Catalano, R., Goldman-Mellor, S., Saxton, K., Margerison-Zilko, C., Subbaraman, M., LeWinn, K., & Anderson, E. (2011). The health effects of economic decline. *Annu Rev Public Health, 32*, 431-450.

Catty, J., Burns, T., Knapp, M., Watt, H., Wright, C., Henderson, J., & Healey, A. (2002). Home treatment for mental health problems: A systematic review. *Psychol Med, 32*, 383-401.

Caulley, D. W. (1994). Evaluation: Does it make a difference? *Evaluation Journal of Australasia, vol. 5*(no. 2), pp. 3-15.

Cayoun, B. A. (2011). *Mindfulness-integrated Cognitive Behaviour Therapy: Principles and Practice*. West Sussex: Wiley-Blackwell.

Cayoun, B. A. (2015). *Mindfulness-integrated CBT for Well-Being and Personal Growth*. West Sussex: Wiley-Blackwell.

Cayoun, B. A. (2017). The purpose, mechanisms, and benefits of cultivating ethics in mindfulness-integrated cognitive behavior therapy. In L. M. Monteiro, J. F. Compson, & F. Musten (eds.), *Practitioner's Guide to Ethics and Mindfulness-Based Interventions* (pp. 163-192). Cham: Springer.

Cayoun, B. A., Francis, S. E., & Shires, A. G. (2019). *The Clinical Handbook of Mindfulness-integrated Cognitive Behavior Therapy: A Step-by-Step Guide for Therapists*. West Sussex: John Wiley & Sons.

Cayoun, B. A., Simmons, A., & Shires, A. (2020). Immediate and Lasting Chronic Pain Reduction Following a Brief Self-Implemented Mindfulness-Based Interoceptive Exposure Task: a Pilot Study. *Mindfulness*, 11, 112-114.

Center for Research on Environmental Decisions (CRED). (2009). *The Psychology of Climate Change Communication: A Guide for Scientists, Journalists, Educators, Political Aides, and the Interested Public*. Retrieved from cred.columbia.edu/guide.

Centers for Disease Control and Prevention. (2014). *Step by Step: Evaluating Violence and Injury Prevention Policies*. Atlanta: CDC.

Centre for Evidence-Based Medicine. (2018). *Evidence Oxford*. Retrieved from www.cebm.net/evidence-oxford-2.

Centre of Best Practice in Aboriginal and Torres Strait Islander Suicide Prevention (CBPATISP). (2019). *Building a Stronger Tomorrow: Connecting Our Communities Through Culture. Report on the 2nd National Aboriginal and Torres Strait Islander Suicide Prevention Conference and the 2nd World Indigenous Suicide Prevention Conference*. Scarborough. WA: CBPATISP.

Centre of Excellence in Peer Support. (2011). *Charter of Peer Support*. Retrieved from www.peersupportvic.org/index.php/2014-12-15-22-41-32/2014-12-15-22-46-46.

Chaffey, L., & Fossey, E. (2004). Caring and daily life: Occupational experiences of women living with sons diagnosed with schizophrenia. *Australian Occupational Therapy Journal, 51*(4), 199-207.

Chalmers, A. (2013). *What Is This Thing Called Science?* Brisbane: University of Queensland Press.

Chamberlin, J. (1978). *On Our Own: Patient Controlled Alternatives to the Mental Health System*. Haworth Press.

Chanen, A. M., Jackson, H. J., McCutcheon, L. K., Jovev, M., Dudgeon, P., Yuen, H. P., . . . Weinstein, C. (2008). Early intervention for adolescents with borderline personality disorder using cognitive analytic therapy: Randomised controlled trial. *British Journal of Psychiatry, 193*(6), 477-484.

Chanen, A. M., McCutcheon, L. K., Jovev, M., Jackson, H. J., & McGorry, P. D. (2007). Prevention and early intervention for borderline personality disorder. *Medical Journal of Australia, 187*(S7), S18-S21.

Chang, S.-S., Stuckler, D., Yip, P., & Gunnell, D. (2013). Impact of 2008 global economic crisis on suicide: Time trend study in 54 countries. *British Medical Journal, 347*, f5239.

Chapman, C., Slade, T., Hunt, C., & Teesson, M. (2015). Delay to first treatment contact for alcohol use disorder. *Drug and Alcohol Dependence, 147*, 116-121.

Chapparo, C., & Ranka, J. (1997). The Perceive: Recall: Plan: Perform (PRPP) System of task analysis. In C. Chapparo & J. Ranka (eds.), *Occupational Performance Model (Australia): Monograph 1* (pp. 189-198). Lidcombe: University of Sydney.

Chapparo, C., Ranka, J. L., & Nott, M. T. (2017). Occupational Performance Model (Australia): A description of constructs, structure and propositions. In M. Curtin, M. Egan, & J. Adams (eds.), *Occupational Therapy for People Experiencing Illness, Injury or Impairment: Promoting Occupation and Participation* (7th ed., pp. 134-147). Edinburgh: Elsevier.

Chartres, D., & Brayley, J. (2010). *Submission to the Productivity Commission Inquiry into Disability Care and Support*. South Australia.

CHCCAG Warm Line. (2017). *Cairns and Hinterland Warm Line*. Retrieved from www.primaryhealth.com.au/wp-content/uploads/2017/04/Warm-Line-Newsletter-March.pdf.

Chen, F., & Greenberg, J. S. (2004). A positive aspect of caregiving: The influence of social support on caregiving gains for family members of relatives with schizophrenia. *Community Mental Health Journal, 40*(5), 423-435.

Cherepkova, E. V., Maksimov, V. V., & Aftanas, L. I. (2018). Polymorphism of serotonin transporter gene in male subjects with antisocial behavior and MMA fighters. *Translational Psychiatry, 8*(1), 248.

Chertkow, H., Massoud, F., Nasreddine, Z., Belleville, S., Joanette, Y., Bocti, C., . . . Bergman, H. (2008). Diagnosis and treatment of dementia: 3. Mild cognitive impairment and cognitive impairment without dementia. *Canadian Medical Association Journal, 178*(10), 1273-1285.

Cheshire, A., Ridge, D., Hughes, J., Peters, D., Panagioti, M., Simon, C., & Lewith, G. (2017). Influences on GP coping and resilience: A qualitative study in primary care. *Br J Gen Pract, 67*(659), e428-e436.

Chesler, P. (1972). *Women and Madness*. New York: Avon.

Chesler, P. (1989). *Women and Madness* (1st Harvest/HBJ ed.). San Diego: Harcourt Brace Jovanovich.

Chien, W.-T., & Norman, I. (2009). The effectiveness and active ingredients of mutual support groups for family caregivers of people with psychotic disorders: A literature review. *International Journal of Nursing Studies, 46*(12), 1604–1623.

Chiesa, A., & Malinowski, P. (2011). Mindfulness-based approaches: Are they all the same? *Journal of Clinical Psychology, 67*(4), 404–424.

Chikritzhs, T., Catalano, P., Pascal, R., & Henrickson, N. (2007). *Predicting Alcohol-Related Harms From Licensed Outlet Density: A Feasibility Study*. Retrieved from www.nabca.org/assets/Docs/predicting-alcoholrelated-harms.pdf.

Chinman, M., Allende, M., Bailey, P., Maust, J., & Davidson, L. (1999). Therapeutic agents of assertive community treatment. *Psychiatric Quarterly, 70*(2), 137–162.

Chisholm, K., Patterson, P., Greenfield, S., Turner, E., & Birchwood, M. (2016). Adolescent construction of mental illness: Implication for engagement and treatment. *Early Intervention in Psychiatry, 12*(4), 626–636.

Chisholm, L., Holttum, S., & Springham, N. (2018). Processes in an experience-based co-design project with family carers in community mental health. *SAGE Open, 8*(4).

Choi, B., & Pak, A. (2006). Multidisciplinarity, interdisciplinarity and transdisciplinarity in health research, services, education and policy: 1. Definitions, objectives, and evidence of effectiveness. *Clinical and Investigative Medicine, 29*(6), 351–364.

Chopra, P., Hamilton, B., Castle, D., Smith, J., Mileshkin, C., Deans, M., . . . Wilson, M. (2009). Implementation of the Strengths Model at an area mental health service. *Australasian Psychiatry, 17*(3), 202–206.

Chou, A. Y. M. (2010). Optimizing the use of video-tapes of clinical sessions: The data-mining approach for scale construction and theory building for bereaved persons in Hong Kong. *Social Work in Health Care, 49*, 832–855.

Christensen, D., Fahey, M. T., Giallo, R., & Hancock, K. J. (2017). Longitudinal trajectories of mental health in Australian children aged 4–5 to 14–15 years. *PLoS One, 12*(11), e0187974.

Christensen, H., Batterham, P. J., Griffiths, K. M., Gosling, J., & Hehir, K. K. (2013). Research priorities in mental health. *Australian and New Zealand Journal of Psychiatry, 47*(4), 355–362.

Christian Counsellors Association of Australia (CCAA). (2017). *Code of Ethics*. Retrieved from https://ccaa.net.au.

Christiansen, C. H., Baum, C. M., & Bass, J. D. (2015). *Occupational Therapy: Performance, Participation, and Well-Being* (4th ed.). Thorofare: SLACK Incorporated.

Christiansen, C. H., & Townsend, E. A. (2010). An introduction to occupation. In C. H. Christiansen & E. A. Townsend (eds.), *Introduction to Occupation: The Art and Science* (2nd ed., pp. 1–34). Upper Saddle River: Prentice Hall.

Churchill, R., Owen, G., Singh, S., & Hotopf, M. (2007). *International Experiences of Using Community Treatment Orders*. London: Institute Of Psychiatry.

Cicchetti, D., & Toth, S. L. (2009). The past achievements and future promises of developmental psychopathology: The coming of age of a discipline. *Journal of Child Psychology and Psychiatry, 50*(1–2), 16–25.

Cipriani, A., Furukawa, T. A., Salanti, G., Chaimani, A., Atkinson, L. Z., Ogawa, Y., . . . Geddes, J. R. (2018). Treatment of adults with major depressive disorder: A systematic review and network meta-analysis. *The Lancet, 391*(10128), 1357–1366.

Clark, L. A., Cuthbert, B., Lewis-Fernández, R., Narrow, W. E., & Reed, G. M. (2017). Three approaches to understanding and classifying mental disorder: ICD-11, DSM-5, and the National Institute of Mental Health's Research Domain Criteria (RDoC). *Psychological Science in the Public Interest, 18*(2), 72–145.

Clarke, D. M., Cook, K., Smith, G. C., & Piterman, L. (2008). What do general practitioners think depression is? A taxonomy of distress and depression for general practice. *Medical Journal of Australia, 188*, S110–S113.

Clarke, D. M., & Currie, K. C. (2009). Depression, anxiety and their relationship with chronic diseases: A review of the epidemiology, risk and treatment evidence. *Medical Journal of Australia, 190*(7), S54–S60.

Clarke, D. M., Piterman, L., Byrne, C. J., & Austin, D. W. (2008). Somatic symptoms, hypochondriasis and psychological distress: A study of somatisation in Australian general practice. *Medical Journal of Australia, 189*(10), 560–564.

Clarke, D (2007). Schizophrenia spectrum disorders in people with intellectual disabilities. In N Bouras and G Holt (eds) *Psychiatric and Behavioural Disorders in Intellectual and Developmental Disabilities*. (2nd edn.) Cambridge: Cambridge University Press.

Clarkin, J. F., Foelsch, P. A., Levy, K. N., Hull, J. W., Delaney, J. C., & Kernberg, O. F. (2001). The development of a psychodynamic treatment for patients with borderline personality disorder: A preliminary study of behavioral change. *Journal of Personality Disorders, 15*(6), 487–495.

Clayton, J., & Tse, S. (2003). An educational journey towards recovery for individuals with persistent mental illness: A New Zealand perspective. *Psychiatric Rehabilitation Journal, 27*, 72–78.

Clayton, S., Manning, C. M., Krygsman, K., & Speiser, M. (2017). *Mental Health and Our Changing Climate: Impacts, Implications, and Guidance*. Retrieved from www.apa.org/news/press/releases/2017/03/mental-health-climate.pdf.

Cleary, M., Walter, G., & Escott, P. (2006). Consumer consultant: Expanding the role of consumers in modern mental health services. *International Journal of Mental Health Nursing, 15*, 29–34.

Clinical Society. (1874). *Transactions of the Clinical Society of London*. London: Spottiswood.

Cloitre, M., Garvert, D. W., Weiss, B., Carlson, E. B., & Bryant, R. A. (2014). Distinguishing PTSD, Complex PTSD, and Borderline Personality Disorder: A latent class analysis. *European Journal of Psychotraumatology, 5*.

Cloninger, R. C., & Svrakic, D. M. (2009). Personality Disorders. In B. J. Sadock, V. A. Sadock, P. Ruiz, & H. I. Kaplan (eds.), *Kaplan & Sadock's Comprehensive Textbook of Psychiatry* (9 ed., vol. 2, pp. 4520). Philadelphia: Wolters Kluwer Health/Lippincott Williams & Wilkins.

Coid, J. (2003). Epidemiology, public health and the problem of personality disorder. *British Journal of Psychiatry, 182*(S44), s3–s10.

Coid, J., Yang, M., Tyrer, P., Roberts, A., & Ullrich, S. (2006). Prevalence and correlates of personality disorder in Great Britain. *British Journal of Psychiatry, 188*(5), 423–431.

Coker, F., Williams, A., Hayes, L., Hamann, J., & Harvey, C. (2016). Exploring the needs of diverse consumers experiencing mental illness and their families through family psychoeducation. *Journal of Mental Health*, 1–7.

Cole, M. G. (2010). Persistent delirium in older hospital patients. *Curr Opin Psychiatry, 23*(3), 250–254.

Coleman, R. (2011). *Recovery: An Alien Concept.* P & P Press.

Collacott, R. A., Cooper, S.-A., & McGrother, C. (1992). Differential rates of psychiatric disorders in adults with Down's syndrome compared with other mentally handicapped adults. *British Journal of Psychiatry, 161*, 671–674.

College of Emergency Nursing Australasia (CENA). (2019). *Treat Us Equally: South Australians with Mental Illness Getting a Raw Deal*. Retrieved from www.cena.org.au/752.

Collins, V. R., Muggli, E. E., Riley, M., Palma, S., & Halliday, J. L. (2008). Is Down syndrome a disappearing birth defect? *Journal of Pediatrics, 152*(1), 20–24.e21.

Colom, F., & Vieta, E. (2006). *Psychoeducation Manual for Bipolar Disorder.* Cambridge University Press.

Commission on Social Determinants of Health (CSDH). (2008). *Closing the Gap in a Generation: Health Equity Through Action on the Social Determinants of Health. Final Report of the Commission on Social Determinants of Health*. Retrieved from https://apps.who.int/iris/bitstream/handle/10665/43943/9789241563703_eng.pdf;jsessionid=2FBEEEB9F637FD3A4E70715B03DF350D?sequence=1.

Commonwealth of Australia. (2013). *A National Framework for Recovery Oriented Health Services*. Retrieved from www1.health.gov.au/internet/main/publishing.nsf/content/67D17065514CF8E8CA257C1D00017A90/$File/recovgde.pdf.

Commonwealth of Australia. (2018). *Mental Health National Outcomes and Casemix Collection: Technical Specification of State and Territory Reporting Requirements, Version 2.01*. Retrieved from https://docs.validator.com.au/nocc/02.01.

Commonwealth of Australia Constitution Act. (2013). *The Constitution*. Retrieved from http://classic.austlii.edu.au/au/legis/cth/consol_act/coaca430/s51.html.

Commonwealth of Australia: National Expert Advisory Committee on Alcohol. (2002). *Fetal Alcohol Syndrome: Diagnosis, Epidemiology, Prevention and Treatment*. Canberra: Commonwealth Department of Health and Ageing.

Commonwealth Ombudsman. (2016). *Accessibility of Indigenous Language Interpreters: Talking in Language Follow Up Investigation*. Retrieved from www.ombudsman.gov.au/__data/assets/pdf_file/0028/42598/December-2016-Investigation-into-Indigenous-Language-Interpreters.pdf.

Compassionate Mind Australia. (2020). *Compassionate Mind Australia*. Retrieved from www.compassionatemind.org.au.

Compton, W. M., Conway, K. P., Stinson, F. S., Colliver, J. D., & Grant, B. F. (2005). Prevalence, correlates, and comorbidity of DSM-IV antisocial personality syndromes and alcohol and specific drug use disorders in the United States: Results from the National Epidemiologic Survey on Alcohol and Related Conditions. *Journal of Clinical Psychiatry, 66*(6), 677–685.

Conigrave, K., Freeman, B., Caroll, T., Simpson, L., Lee, K. K., Wade, V., . . . Freeburn, B. (2012). The Alcohol Awareness project: Community education and brief intervention in an urban Aboriginal setting. *Health Promotion Journal of Australia, 23*(3), 219–225.

Connell, H. M. (1985). *Essentials of Psychiatry*. Melbourne: Blackwell.

Connors, R. (1996). Self-injury in trauma survivors: 1. Functions and meanings. *American Journal of Orthopsychiatry, 66*(2), 197–206.

Considine, R., Tynan, R., James, C., Wiggers, J., Lewin, T., Inder, K., . . . Kelly, B. (2017). The contribution of individual, social and work characteristics to employee mental health in a coal mining industry population. *PLoS One, 12*(1), e0168445.

Consolidated Standards of Reporting Trials. (2020). *CONSORT Transparent Reporting of Trails*. Retrieved from www.consort-statement.org.

Consumer Led Research Forum. (2015). *Enabling Consumer Led Research in a World That's Not Used to It*. Retrieved from www.youtube.com/watch?reload=9&v=PWBRJMy1gUg&t=572s.

Consumer Participation Program Orientation and Job Manual—Mental Health Staff-Consumer Consultants. (1996). *Understanding and Involvement, Consumer Evaluation of Acute Psychiatric Hospital Practice Project.* Melbourne: Victorian Mental Illness Awareness Council.

Conus, P., Lambert, M., Cotton, S., Bonsack, C., McGorry, P. D., & Schimmelmann, B. G. (2010). Rate and predictors of service disengagement in an epidemiological first-episode psychosis cohort. *Schizophrenia Research, 118*(1-3), 256–263.

Cook, J. M., Biyanova, T., Elhai, J., Schnurr, P. P., & Coyne, J. C. (2010). What do psychotherapists really do in practice? An internet study of over 2000 practitioners. *Psychotherapy, 47*(2), 260–267.

Cooper, M., Evans, Y., & Pybis, J. (2016). Interagency collaboration in children and young people's mental health: A systematic review of outcomes, facilitating factors and inhibiting factors. *Child Care Health Dev*, 42(3): 325–42.

Cooper, S., Enticott, J. C., Shawyer, F., & Meadows, G. (2019). Determinants of mental illness among humanitarian migrants: Longitudinal analysis of findings from the first three waves of a large cohort study. *Frontiers in Psychiatry, 10*(545).

Cooper, S. A. (1997). High prevalence of dementia among people with learning disabilities not attributable to Down's syndrome. *Psychol Med, 27*(3), 609–616.

Cooper, S. A. (2003). Diagnostic criteria for psychiatric disorders for use with adults with Learning Disabilities/Mental Retardation (DC-LD). *Journal of Intellectual Disability Research, 47*, 1–2.

Copeland Centre for Wellness and Recovery. (2014). *The Way WRAP Works! Strengthening Core Values & Practices*. Retrieved from https://copelandcenter.com/resources/way-wrap-works.

Copeland, W. E., Wolke, D., Angold, A., & Costello, E. J. (2013). Adult psychiatric outcomes of bullying and being bullied by peers in childhood and adolescence. *JAMA Psychiatry, 70*(4), 419–426.

Corbiere, M., Mazaniello-Chezol, M., Bastien, M. F., Wathieu, E., Bouchard, R., Panaccio, A., . . . Lecomte, T. (2019). Stakeholders' role and actions in the return-to-work process of workers on sick-leave due to common mental disorders: A scoping review. *Journal of Occupational Rehabilitation*.

Corey, G. (2001). *The Art of Integrative Counseling*. Brooks-Cole/Wadsworth.

Correll, C. U., Galling, B., Pawar, A., Krivko, A., Bonetto, C., Ruggeri, M., . . . Kane, J. M. (2018). Comparison of early intervention services vs treatment as usual for early-phase psychosis: A systematic review, meta-analysis, and meta-regression. *JAMA Psychiatry, 75*(6), 555–565.

Corrigan, P., Barr, L., Driscoll, H., & Boyle, M. (2008). The educational goals of people with psychiatric disabilities. *Psychiatric Rehabilitation Journal, 32*(1), 67–70.

Corring, D., Apos, Reilly, R., & Sommerdyk, C. (2017). A systematic review of the views and experiences of subjects of community treatment orders. *International Journal of Law and Psychiatry, 52*, 74–80.

Corryn, C. L. S., Noakes, L. A., Westine, C. D., & Schroter, D. C. (2011). Systematic review of theory-driven evaluation practice from 1990–2009. *American Journal of Evaluation, 32*(2), 199–226.

Cosgrove, E. M., Yung, A. R., Killackey, E. J., Buckby, J. A., Godfrey, K. A., Stanford, C. A., & McGorry, P. D. (2008). Met and unmet need in youth mental health. *Journal of Mental Health, 17*(6), 618–628.

Costello, A., Abbas, M., Allen, A., Ball, S., Bell, S., Bellamy, R., . . . Patterson, C. (2009). Managing the health effects of climate change. *Lancet, 373*(9676), 1693–1733.

Council of Australian Governments (COAG). (2008). *National Action Plan for Mental Health 2006-2011* Retrieved from www.mhpn.org.au/Uploads/Documents/AHMC_COAG_mental_health.pdf.

Council of Australian Governments (COAG). (2012). *The Roadmap for National Mental Health Reform 2012-2022*. Retrieved from www.coag.gov.au/sites/default/files/communique/The%20Roadmap%20for%20National%20Mental%20Health%20Reform%202012-2022.pdf.

Council of Australian Governments (COAG). (2017). *Fifth National Mental Health and Suicide Prevention Plan (2017-22)* Retrieved from www.coaghealthcouncil.gov.au/Publications/Reports.

Cowling, V. (1999). *Children of Parents with Mental Illness*. Camberwell: ACER Press.

Cowling, V. (2004). *Children of Parents with Mental Illness 2: Personal and Clinical Perspectives*. Camberwell: ACER Press.

Cowlishaw, S., Merkouris, S. S., Dowling, N. A., Anderson, C., Jackson, A., & Thomas, S. (2012). Psychological therapies for pathological and problem gambling. *Cochrane Database of Systematic Reviews, 11*, CD008937.

Cox, A. D. (1994). *Diagnostic Appraisal* (3rd ed.). Melbourne: Blackwell.

Craddock, N., & Mynors-Wallis, L. (2014). Psychiatric diagnosis: Impersonal, imperfect and important. *British Journal of Psychiatry, 204*(2), 93–95.

Craissati, J., Joseph, N., & Skett, S. (2015). *working with offenders with personality disorder: A practitioners guide*. London: Crown.

Cramer, V., Torgersen, S., & Kringlen, E. (2006). Personality disorders and quality of life. A population study. *Comprehensive Psychiatry, 47*(3), 178–184.

Crane, R. S., Brewer, J., Feldman, C., Kabat-Zinn, J., Santorelli, S., Williams, J. M., & Kuyken, W. (2017). What defines mindfulness-based programs? The warp and the weft. *Psychol Med, 47*(6), 990–999.

Cranwell, K., Polacsek, M., & McCann, T. V. (2017). Improving care planning and coordination for service users with medical co-morbidity transitioning between tertiary medical and primary care services. *Journal of Psychiatric and Mental Health Nursing, 24*(6), 337–347.

Craven, M. A., & Bland, R. (2006). Better practices in collaborative mental health care: An analysis of the evidence base. *Canadian Journal Psychiatry*, 51(6 (Suppl 1)). 7S-72S.

Cree, L., Brooks, H. L., Berzins, K., Fraser, C., Lovell, K., & Bee, P. (2015). Carers' experiences of involvement in care planning: A qualitative exploration of the facilitators and barriers to engagement with mental health services. *BMC Psychiatry, 15*.

Creed, F., & Barsky, A. (2004). A systematic review of the epidemiology of somatisation disorder and hypochondriasis. *J Psychosom Res, 56*(4), 391–408.

Creed, F. H., Tomenson, B., Chew-Graham, C., Macfarlane, G. J., Davies, I., Jackson, J., . . . McBeth, J. (2013). Multiple somatic symptoms predict impaired health status in functional somatic syndromes. *International Journal of Behavioral Medicine, 20*(2), 194–205.

Creed, T. A., Reisweber, J., & Beck, A. T. (2011). *Cognitive Therapy for Adolescents in School Settings*. Guilford Publications.

Crews, F. C. (1997). *The Memory Wars: Freud's Legacy in Dispute*. New York: Granta Books.

Crisp, K., Creek, R., Fraser, S., Stavely, H., & Woodhead, G. (2014). *In This Together: Family Work and Early Psychosis*. Melbourne: Orygen Youth Health Research Centre.

Cristea, I. A., Gentili, C., Cotet, C. D., Palomba, D., Barbui, C., & Cuijpers, P. (2017). Efficacy of psychotherapies for borderline personality disorder: A systematic review and meta-analysis. *JAMA Psychiatry, 74*(4), 319–328.

Croft, B., Battis, K., Isvan, N., & Mahoney, K. (2020). Service utilization before and after self-direction: A quasi-experimental difference-in-differences analysis of Utah's Mental Health Access to Recovery Program. *Administration and Policy in Mental Health and Mental Health Services Research, 47*(1), 36–46.

Crome, E., & Baillie, A. J. (2016). Better Access and equitable access to clinical psychology services: What do we need to know? *Med J Aust, 204*(9), 341–343.

Crome, E., Grove, R., Baillie, A. J., Sunderland, M., Teesson, M., & Slade, T. (2015). DSM-IV and DSM-5 social anxiety disorder in the Australian community. *Australian & New Zealand Journal of Psychiatry, 49*(3), 227–235.

Crone, C. C., Lackamp, J. M., & Alkis, A. R. (2018). Gastrointestinal Disorders. In J. L. Levenson (ed.), *The American Psychiatric Association Publishing Textbook of Psychosomatic Medicine and Consultation-Liaison Psychiatry*, (3rd ed., pp. 527–570). USA: American Psychiatric Association Publishing.

Crosby, R. P. (1992). *Walking the Empowerment Tightrope*. King of Prussia PA: Organisational Design and Development.

CSIRO. (2018). *State of the climate. Report at a Glance*. Retrieved from www.csiro.au/en/Research/OandA/Areas/Assessing-our-climate/State-of-the-Climate-2018/Report-at-a-glance.

Cuijpers, P. (1999). The effects of family interventions on relatives' burden: A meta-analysis. *Journal of Mental Health*.

Cuijpers, P., Driessen, E., Hollon, S. D., van Oppen, P., Barth, J., & Andersson, G. (2012). The efficacy of non-directive supportive therapy for adult depression: A meta-analysis. *Clinical Psychology Review, 32*(4), 280–291.

Cuijpers, P., Reijnders, M., & Huibers, M. J. H. (2019). The Role of Common Factors in Psychotherapy Outcomes. *Annu Rev Clin Psychol. 15*(1), 207–231.

Cuijpers, P., van Straten, A., Andersson, G., & van Oppen, P. (2008). Psychotherapy for depression in adults: A meta-analysis of comparative outcome studies. *J Consult Clin Psychol, 76*(6), 909–922.

Cummings, J., Lee, G., Ritter, A., Sabbagh, M., & Zhong, K. (2019). Alzheimer's disease drug development pipeline: 2019. *Alzheimer's & Dementia: Translational Research & Clinical Interventions, 5*(C), 272–293.

Curie, C., & Thornicroft, G. (2020). *Summative Evaluation of the National Mental Health Plan 2003–2008*.

Curry, S. J., Mermelstein, R. J., & Sporer, A. K. (2009). Therapy for specific problems: Youth tobacco cessation. *Annual Review of Psychology, 60*, 229–255.

Cyril, S., Smith, B. J., Possamai-Inesedy, A., & Renzaho, A. M. N. (2015). Exploring the role of community engagement in improving the health of disadvantaged populations: A systematic review. *Global Health Action, 8*(1), 29842.

d'Abbs, P., & MacLean, S. (2008). *Volatile Substance Misuse: A Review of Interventions*. Canberra: Australian Government Department of Health and Ageing.

da Luz, F. Q., Sainsbury, A., Mannan, H., Touyz, S., Mitchison, D., & Hay, P. (2017). Prevalence of obesity and comorbid eating disorder behaviors in South Australia from 1995 to 2015. *Int J Obes (Lond), 41*(7), 1148–1153.

Dalgleish, T. (1999). Cognitive theories of post-traumatic stress disorder. In W. Yule (ed.), *Post-traumatic Stress Disorders: Concepts and Therapy* (pp. 192–220). New York: John Wiley & Sons.

Dam, K., & Hall, E. O. C. (2016). Navigating in an unpredictable daily life: A metasynthesis on children's experiences living with a parent with severe mental illness. *Scandinavian Journal of Caring Sciences, 30*(3), 442-457.

Damasio, A. R. (2000). *The Feeling of What Happens Body, Emotion and the Making of Consciousness*. Vintage: Mariner Books.

Damasio, A. R. (2003). *Looking for Spinoza: Joy, Sorrow, and the Feeling Brain* (1st ed.). New York: Mariner Books.

Damschroder, L. J., Aron, D., Keith, R., Kirsh, S., Alexander, J., & Lowery, J. (2009). Fostering implementation of health services research findings into practice: A consolidated framework for advancing implementation science. *Implementation Science, 4*(1), 50.

Dannon, P. N., Iancu, I., & Grunhaus, L. (2002). Psychoeducation in panic disorder patients: Effect of a self-information booklet in a randomized, masked-rater study. *Depression and Anxiety, 16*(2), 71-76.

Darke, S., Hall, W., Wodaki, A., Heather, N., & Ward, J. (1992). Development and validation of a multidimensional instrument for assessing outcome of treatment among opiate users: The Opiate Treatment Index. *British Journal of Addiction, 87*(5), 733-742.

Darlington, Y., & Feeney, J. A. (2008). Collaboration between mental health and child protection services: Professionals' perceptions of best practice. *Children and Youth Services Review, 30*(2), 187-198.

Darlington, Y., Feeney, J. A., & Rixon, K. (2004). Complexity, conflict and uncertainty: Issues in collaboration between child protection and mental health services. *Children and Youth Services Review, 26*(12), 1175-1192.

Darlington, Y., Feeney, J. A., & Rixon, K. (2005a). Interagency collaboration between child protection and mental health services: Practices, attitudes and barriers. *Child Abuse & Neglect, 29*, 1085-1098.

Darlington, Y., Feeney, J. A., & Rixon, K. (2005b). Practice challenges at the intersection of child protection and mental health. *Child and Family Social Work, 10*(3), 239-247.

Darwin, C. (1877). A Biographical Sketch of an Infant. *Mind. A Quarterly Review of Psychology and Philosophy, 2*, 285-294.

Dasgupta, P., & Barber, J. (2004). Admission patterns of patients with personality disorder. *Psychiatric Bulletin, 28*(9), 321-323.

Davey, C. G., & Chanen, A. M. (2016). The unfulfilled promise of the antidepressant medications. *Medical Journal of Australia, 204*(9), 348-350.

Davey, C. G., Hetrick, S., Chanen, A., Cotton, S. M., Ratheesh, A., Amminger, G. P., . . . Berk, M. (2019). The addition of fluoxetine to cognitive behavioural therapy for youth depression: The YoDA-C randomised clinical trial. *Bipolar Disord., 21*(s1), 13-14.

Davidson, G., Brophy, L., & Campbell, J. (2016). Risk, Recovery and Capacity: Competing or Complementary Approaches to Mental Health Social Work. *Australian Social Work, 69*(2), 158-168.

Davidson, G., Brophy, L., Campbell, J., Farrell, S. J., Gooding, P., Amp, . . . Brien, A.-M. (2016). An international comparison of legal frameworks for supported and substitute decision-making in mental health services. *International Journal of Law and Psychiatry, 44*, 30-40.

Davidson, G., & Campbell, J. (2007). An examination of the use of coercion by assertive outreach and community mental health teams in Northern Ireland. *British Journal of Social Work, 37*(3), 537-555.

Davidson, L. (2003). *Living Outside Mental Illness: Qualitative Studies of Recovery in Schizophrenia*. New York: NYU Press.

Davidson, L., Hoge, M. A., Merrill, M. E., Rakfeldt, J., & Griffith, E. E. H. (1995). The experiences of long-stay inpatients returning to the community. *Psychiatry-Interpersonal and Biological Processes, 58*(2), 122-132.

Davidson, L., O'Connell, M. J., Tondora, J., Staeheli, M., & Evans, A. C. (2005). Recovery in serious mental illness: Paradigm shift or shibboleth? In L. Davidson, C. Harding, & L. Spaniol (eds.), *Recovery in Severe Mental Illness: Research Evidence and Implications for Practice* (Pp. 5-26). Boston: Center for Psychiatric Rehabilitation, Boston University.

Davidson, L., Rakfeldt, J., & Strauss, J. (2010). *The Roots of the Recovery Movement in Psychiatry: Lessons Learned*. UK: Wiley.

Davidson, L., Ridgway, P., Kidd, S. A., Topor, A., & Borg, M. (2008). Using qualitative research to inform mental health policy. *Canadian Journal of Psychiatry-Revue Canadienne De Psychiatrie, 53*(3), 137-144.

Davidson, L., Tondora, J., Lawless, M. S., O'Connell, M. J., & Rowe, M. (2009). *A Practical Guide to Recovery-Oriented Practice: Tools for Transforming Mental Health Care*. New York. Oxford University Press.

Davidson, L., Tondora, J., Staeheli, M., O'Connell, M., Frey, J., & Chinman, M. J. (2005). Recovery guides: An emerging model of community-based care for adults with psychiatric disabilities. In A. Lightburn & P. Sessions (eds.), *Handbook of Community-Based Clinical Practice*. London. Oxford University Press.

Davies, K., Gray, M., & Butcher, L. (2014). Lean on me: The potential for peer support in a non-government Australian mental health service. *Asia Pacific Journal of Social Work and Development, 24*(1-2), 109-121.

Davis, J. K. (2015). Supervision of peer specialists in community mental health centers: Practices that predict role clarity. *Social Work in Mental Health, 13*(2), 145-158.

Dawes, M., Summerskill, W., Glasziou, P., Cartabellotta, A., Martin, J., Hopayian, K., . . . Osborne, J. (2005). Sicily statement on evidence-based practice. *BMC Medical Education, 5*(1), 1.

Day, K., & Petrakis, M. (2018). Early intervention in mental health: Opportunities and challenges. In M. Petrakis (ed.), *Social Work Practice in Health: An Introduction to Contexts, Theories and Skills* (pp. 100-115). Crows Nest: Allen & Unwin.

Daya, I. (2020). *Compounding the Impact of Trauma*. Retrieved from www.indigodaya.com/trauma_context.

de Anstiss, H., Ziaian, T., Procter, N., Warland, J., & Baghurst, P. (2009). Help-seeking for mental health problems in young refugees: A review of the literature with implications for policy, practice, and research. *Transcultural Psychiatry, 46*(4), 584-607.

De Brito, S. A., & Hodgins, S. (2009). Antisocial personality disorder. *Personality, Personality Disorder and Violence, 42*, 133-153.

de Diego-Adeliño, J., Portella, M. J., Puigdemont, D., Pérez-Egea, R., Álvarez, E., & Pérez, V. (2010). A short duration of untreated illness (DUI) improves response outcomes in first-depressive episodes. *J Affect Disord, 120*(1-3), 221-225.

De Fazio, P., Gaetano, R., Caroleo, M., Pavia, M., De Sarro, G., Fagiolini, A., & Segura-Garcia, C. (2017). Lithium in late-life mania: A systematic review. *Neuropsychiatric Disease and Treatment, 13*, 755-766.

de Groot, M., Anderson, R., Freedland, K. E., Clouse, R. E., & Lustman, P. J. (2001). Association of depression and diabetes complications: A meta-analysis. *Psychosomatic Medicine, 63*(4), 619-630.

De Hert, M., Correll, C. U., Bobes, J., Cetkovich-Bakmas, M., Cohen, D. A. N., Asai, I., . . . Leucht, S. (2011). Physical illness in patients with severe mental disorders. I. Prevalence, impact of medications and disparities in health care. *World Psychiatry, 10*(1), 52-77.

de Jong, M. H., Kamperman, A. M., Oorschot, M., Priebe, S., Bramer, W., van de Sande, R., . . . Mulder, C. L. (2016). Interventions to reduce compulsory psychiatric admissions: A systematic review and meta-analysis. *JAMA Psychiatry, 73*(7), 657-664.

de Leeuw, E. (2011). Do healthy cities work? A logic of method for assessing impact and outcome of healthy cities. *J Urban Health, 89*(2), 217-231.

de Leeuw, E., & Simos, J. (eds.). (2017). *Healthy Cities. The Theory, Policy, and Practice of Value-Based Urban Planning*. New York: Springer.

de Lijster, J. M., Dierckx, B., Utens, E. M. W. J., Verhulst, F. C., Zieldorff, C., Dieleman, G. C., & Legerstee, J. S. (2017). The age of onset of anxiety disorders: A meta-analysis. *The Canadian Journal of Psychiatry, 62*(4), 237-246.

De Maio, J., Silbert, M., Jenkinson, R., & Smart, D. (2014). Building a new life in Australia. Introducing the longitudinal study of humanitarian migrants. *Family Matters, 94*, 5-14.

De Vries, T., Henning, R. H., Hogerzeil, H. V., Fresle, D., Policy, M., & Organization, W. H. (1994). *Guide to Good Prescribing: A Practical Manual*. Geneva, World Health Organization.

de Waal, M. W., Arnold, I. A., Eekhof, J. A., & van Hemert, A. M. (2004). Somatoform disorders in general practice: Prevalence, functional impairment and comorbidity with anxiety and depressive disorders. *Br J Psychiatry, 184*, 470-476.

Deacon, B., Lickel, J., & Abramowitz, J. S. (2008). Medical utilization across the anxiety disorders. *Journal of Anxiety Disorders, 22*(2), 344-350.

Dean, K., Laursen, T. M., Pedersen, C. B., Webb, R. T., Mortensen, P. B., & Agerbo, E. (2018). Risk of being subjected to crime, including violent crime, after onset of mental illness: A Danish National Registry study using police data. *JAMA Psychiatry, 75*(7), 689-696.

Dean, K., Stevens, H., Mortensen, P. B., Murray, R. M., Walsh, E., & Pedersen, C. B. (2010). Full spectrum of psychiatric outcomes among offspring with parental history of mental disorder. *Archives of General Psychiatry, 67*(8), 822-829.

Deans, E. G., Thomas, S. L., Derevensky, J., & Daube, M. (2017). The influence of marketing on the sports betting attitudes and consumption behaviours of young men: Implications for harm reduction and prevention strategies. *Harm Reduction Journal, 14*.

Dechant, K. (2014). Show Me the Money: Incorporating Financial Motives into the Gambling Motives Questionnaire. *Journal of Gambling Studies, 30*(4), 949-965.

Deegan, P. E. (2010). A web application to support recovery and shared decision making in psychiatric medication clinics. *Psychiatr Rehabil J*, 34(1), 23-28.

Deegan, P. E. (1988). Recovery: The lived experience of rehabilitation. *Psychosocial Rehabilitation Journal, 11*(4), 11.

Delfabbro, P., & King, D. (2017). Prevention paradox logic and problem gambling: Does low-risk gambling impose a greater burden of harm than high-risk gambling? *J Behav Addict, 6*(2), 163-167.

Deloitte Access Economics. (2011). *Dementia Across Australia: 2011-2050*. Retrieved from www.fightdementia.org.au/research-publications/access-economics-reports.aspx.

DeLongis, A., Folkman, S., & Lazarus, R. S. (1988). The impact of daily stress on health and mood: Psychological and social resources as mediators. *Journal of Personality and Social Psychology, 54*(3), 486-495.

Delvecchio, G., Rossetti, M. G., Caletti, E., Arighi, A., Galimberti, D., Basilico, P., . . . Brambilla, P. (2019). The Neuroanatomy of Somatoform Disorders: A Magnetic Resonance Imaging Study. *Psychosomatics, 60*(3), 278-288.

Dementia Australia. (2020). *Planning Tools*. Retrieved from www.dementia.org.au.

Denham, S. A., Wyatt, T. M., Bassett, H. H., Echeverria, D., & Knox, S. S. (2009). Assessing social-emotional development in children from a longitudinal perspective. *J Epidemiol Community Health, 63*, 137-152.

Dennett, D. C. (1991). *Consciousness Explained*. London: Penguin Books.

Department of Education and Training. (2018). *Doctors in Secondary Schools*. Retrieved from www.education.vic.gov.au/about/programs/Pages/doctors.aspx.

Department of Health. (2011). *Framework for Recovery-oriented Practice*. Melbourne: Government of Victoria.

Department of Health. (2014). *The April 2014 Medicare Benefits Schedule*. Retrieved from www.mbsonline.gov.au.

Department of Health. (2016). *Primary Health Network Mental Health Reform Lead Site Project Evaluation Framework*. Canberra: Australian Government.

Department of Health. (2018a). *Policy Frameworks*. Retrieved from https://ww2.health.wa.gov.au/About-us/Policy-Frameworks.

Department of Health. (2018b). *Sustainable Health Review: Interim Report to the Western Australian Government*. Retrieved from https://ww2.health.wa.gov.au/Improving-WA-Health/Sustainable-health-review/Interim-report.

Department of Health. (2019). *Head to Health*. Retrieved from https://headtohealth.gov.au.

Department of Health Aged Care & Deakin Human Services Australia. (1999). *Learning Together: Education and Training Partnerships in Mental Health*. Canberra: Dept of Health and Aged Care.

Department of Health and Ageing. (2005). *National Mental Health Information Priorities 2nd Edition*. Retrieved from www1.health.gov.au/internet/main/publishing.nsf/Content/AA5F407938FC9D2FCA257BF000209AA9/$File/infopri2.pdf.

Department of Health and Ageing. (2013). *National Mental Health Report 2013: Tracking Progress of Mental Health Reform in Australia 1993-2011*. Retrieved from www.health.gov.au/internet/main/publishing.nsf/Content/B090F03865A7FAB9CA257C1B0079E198/$File/rep13.pdf.

Department of Health and Human Service Victoria. (2018a). Mental health and drug and alcohol Crisis Hubs. *Delivering for all Victorians*. Retrieved from www.premier.vic.gov.au/new-mental-health-hubs-to-treat-more-victorians-sooner.

Department of Health and Human Service Victoria. (2018b). *The Hospital Outreach Post-Suicidal Engagement (HOPE) Initiative*. Retrieved from https://dhhs.vic.gov.au/news/more-support-people-who-have-attempted-suicide#.

Department of Health and Human Services. (2004). *Bridging the Gap: Review of Mental Health Services, Tasmania*. Retrieved from www.dhhs.tas.gov.au/mentalhealth/publications/strategic_documents.

Department of Health and Human Services. (2006). *Mental Health Services Strategic Plan 2006-2011*. Hobart: Department of Health and Human Services, State of Tasmania.

Department of Health and Human Services. (2015). *Victoria's 10-Year Mental Health Plan*. Retrieved from www2.health.vic.gov.au/mental-health/priorities-and-transformation/mental-health-plan.

Department of Health and Human Services. (2016). *Healthy Tasmania Five Year Strategic Plan*. Retrieved from www dhhs.tas.gov.au/about_the_department/our_plans_and_strategies/a_healthy_tasmania.

Department of Health and Human Services. (2018). *Victoria's Mental Health Services Annual Report 2017-18*. Retrieved from www2.health.vic.gov.au/Api/downloadmedia/%7B43432A35-7B8F-4E89-A87C-6AFC6E156015%7D.

Department of Health Family Services. (1998). *Second National Mental Health Plan*. Canberra: Commonwealth Department of Health and Family Services.

Department of Human Services. (2008). *Review of Mental Health Act 1986*. Melbourne: Government of Victoria.

Department of Human Services. (2009). *Because Mental Health Matters: Victorian Mental Health Reform Strategy 2009-2019*. Retrieved from www.health.vic.gov.au/mentalhealth/reformstrategy.

Department of the Prime Minister and Cabinet. (2017). *Religious Freedom Review*. Retrieved from www.pmc.gov.au/domestic-policy/religious-freedom-review.

Depue, R. M.-S., J. (2005). A neurobehavioral model of affiliative bonding. *Behavioural and Brain Sciences, 28*(28), 313-395.

Derald Wing, S., Capodilupo, C. M., Torino, G. C., Bucceri, J. M., Holder, A. M. B., Nadal, K. L., & Esquilin, M. (2007). Racial microaggressions in everyday life: Implications for clinical practice. *American Psychologist, 62*(4), 271-286.

Derubeis, R. J., Brotman, M. A., & Gibbons, C. J. (2005). A Conceptual and Methodological Analysis of the Nonspecifics Argument. *Clinical Psychology: Science and Practice, 12*(2), 174-183.

deVaus, D. (2004). Diversity and Change in Australian Families, Australian Institute of Family Studies, Melbourne. In *Families Australia*. Melbourne: Families Australia.

Devilly, G. J., Gist, R., & Cotton, P. (2006). Ready! Fire! Aim! The status of psychological debriefing and therapeutic interventions: In the work place and after disasters. *Review of General Psychology, 10*(4), 318-345.

Dewa, C. S., Corbiere, M., Durand, M.-J., & Hensel, J. (2012). Challenges related to mental health in the workplace. In R. J. Gatchel & I. Z. Schultz (eds.), *Handbook of Occupational Health and Wellness* (pp. 105-130). New York: Springer.

Dewa, C. S., Loong, D., Trojanowski, L., & Bonato, S. (2018). The effectiveness of augmented versus standard individual placement and support programs in terms of employment: A systematic literature review. *Journal of Mental Health, 27*(2), 174-183.

Dewa, C. S., & McDaid, D. (2011). Investing in the mental health of the labor force: Epidemiological and economic impact of mental health disabilities in the workplace. In I. Z. Schultz & E. S. Rogers (eds.), *Work Accommodation and Retention in Mental Health* (pp. 33-52). New York: Springer.

Diamond, A. (2013). Executive Functions. *Annual Review of Psychology, 64*(1), 135-168.

Diamond, J. (2011). *Collapse: How Societies Choose to Fail or Succeed*. Penguin Books.

Dick, D. M., Pagan, J. L., Viken, R., Purcell, S., Kaprio, J., Pulkkinen, L., & Rose, R. J. (2007). Changing environmental influences on substance use across development. *Twin Research and Human Genetics, 10*(2), 315-326.

Dickins, M., & Thomas, A. (2016). *Gambling in Culturally and Linguistically Diverse Communities in Australia (AGRC Discussion Paper No. 7)*. Retrieved from https://aifs.gov.au/agrc/publications/gambling-culturally-and-linguistically-diverse-communities-australia.

Dickinson, H. (2019). *Explainer: How Much Does the NDIS Cost and Where Does This Money Come From?* Retrieved from https://theconversation.com/explainer-how-much-does-the-ndis-cost-and-where-does-this-money-come-from-95924.

Diemer, E. W., White Hughto, J. M., Gordon, A. R., Guss, C., Austin, S. B., & Reisner, S. L. (2018). Beyond the binary: Differences in eating disorder prevalence by gender identity in a transgender sample. *Transgend Health, 3*(1), 17-23.

Dieterich, M., Irving, C., Bergman, H., Khokhar, M. A., Park, B., & Marshall, M. (2017). Intensive case management for severe mental illness. *Cochrane Database Syst Rev., 1*(1).

DiMasi, J. A., Hansen, R. W., & Grabowski, H. G. (2003). The price of innovation: New estimates of drug development costs. *Journal of Health Economics, 22*, 151-185.

DiMatteo, M. R., Lepper, H. S., & Croghan, T. W. (2000). Depression is a risk factor for noncompliance with medical treatment: Meta-analysis of the effects of anxiety and depression on patient adherence. *Archives of Internal Medicine, 160*(14), 2101-2107.

Dimidjian, S., Hollon, S. D., Dobson, K. S., Schmaling, K. B., Kohlenberg, R. J., Addis, M. E., . . . Jacobson, N. S. (2006). Randomized trial of behavioral activation, cognitive therapy, and antidepressant medication in the acute treatment of adults with major depression. *J Consult Clin Psychol, 74*, 658-670.

Dimidjian, S., & Segal, Z. V. (2015). Prospects for a clinical science of mindfulness-based intervention. *Am Psychol, 70*(7), 593-620.

Diminic, S., Hielscher, E., Harris, M. G., Lee, Y. Y., Kealton, J., & Whiteford, H. (2018). A profile of Australian mental health carers, their caring role and service needs: Results from the 2012 Survey of Disability, Ageing and Carers. *Epidemiology and psychiatric sciences*, 1-12.

Diminic, S., Hielscher, E., Lee, Y. Y., Harris, M., Schess, J., Kealton, J., & Whiteford, H. (2016). *The Economic Value of Informal Mental Health Caring in Australia*. Retrieved from www.mindaustralia.org.au/sites/default/files/Mind_value_of_informal_caring_full_report.pdf.

Dixon, L. B., Lucksted, A., Medoff, D. R., Burland, J., Stewart, B., Lehman, A. F., . . . Murray-Swank, A. (2011). Outcomes of a randomized study of a peer-taught family-to-family education program for mental illness. *Psychiatric Services, 62*(6), 591-597.

Dixon-Gordon, K. L., Turner, B. J., & Chapman, A. L. (2011). Psychotherapy for personality disorders. *International Review of Psychiatry, 23*(3), 282-302.

Dodgen, D., Donato, D., Kelly, N., La Greca, A., & Morganstein, J. (2016). *Mental Health and Well-Being. The Impacts of Climate Change on Human Health in the United States: A Scientific Assessment*. Retrieved from http://dx.doi.org/10.7930/J0TX3C9H.

Doherty, T. J., & Clayton, S. (2011). The psychological impacts of global climate change. *American Psychologist, 66*(4), 265-276.

Dolgoff, R., Harrington, D., & Loewenberg, F. M. (2012). *Brooks/Cole Empowerment Series: Ethical Decisions for Social Work Practice*. Cengage Learning.

Dols, A., Kupka, R. W., van Lammeren, A., Beekman, A. T., Sajatovic, M., & Stek, M. L. (2014). The prevalence of late-life mania: A review. *Bipolar Disorders, 16*(2), 113-118.

Don Dunstan Foundation. (2020). *Adelaide Zero Project*. Retrieved from https://dunstan.org.au/?s=Adelaide+Zero+Project+.

Donaldson, S. I., & Lipsey, M. W. (2006). *Roles for Theory in Contemporary Evaluation Practice: Developing Practical Knowledge*. London: Sage.

Dong, G. H., Liu, X. Y., Zheng, H., Du, X. X., & Potenza, M. N. (2019). Brain response features during forced break could predict subsequent recovery in internet gaming disorder: A longitudinal study. *Journal of Psychiatric Research, 113*, 17-26.

Dong, J. Y., Zhang, Y. H., Tong, J., & Qin, L. Q. (2012). Depression and risk of stroke a meta-analysis of prospective studies. *Stroke, 43*(1), 32-U108.

Donker, T., Griffiths, K. M., Cuijpers, P., & Christensen, H. (2009). Psychoeducation for depression, anxiety and psychological distress: A meta-analysis. *BMC Medicine, 7*.

Doron, G., Moulding, R., Kyrios, M., Nedeljkovic, M., & Mikulincer, M. (2009). Adult attachment insecurities are related to obsessive compulsive phenomena. *Journal of Social and Clinical Psychology, 28*(8), 1022-1049.

Doroud, N., Fossey, E., & Fortune, T. (2015). Recovery as an occupational journey: A scoping review exploring the links between occupational engagement and recovery for people with enduring mental health issues. *Australian Occupational Therapy Journal, 62*(6), 378-392.

Dowling, N. A., Brown, M., Aarsman, S., & Merkouris, S. S. (2019). Brief report: Problem gambling in international and domestic university students. *American Journal on Addictions*.

Dowling, N. A., Merkouris, S. S., Dias, S., Rodda, S. N., Manning, V., Youssef, G. J., . . . Volberg, R. A. (2019). The diagnostic accuracy of brief screening instruments for problem gambling: A systematic review and meta-analysis. *Clinical Psychology Review, 74*.

Dowling, N. A., Merkouris, S. S., Greenwood, C. J., Oldenhof, E., Toumbourou, J. W., & Youssef, G. J. (2017). Early risk and protective factors for problem gambling: A systematic review and meta-analysis of longitudinal studies. *Clinical Psychology Review, 51*, 109-124.

Dowling, N. A., Merkouris, S. S., Rodda, S., Smith, D., Lavis, T., Lubman, D., . . . Battersby, M. (2018). *Development and Evaluation of an Online Gambling Self-Directed Program: Effective Integration into Existing Services*. Retrieved from file:///E:/Brayden/Downloads/Development_and_evaluation_of_an_online_gambling_self-direct_help_program.pdf.

Dowling, N. A., Oldenhof, E., Cockman, S., Suomi, A., Merkouris, S. S., & Jackson, A. C. (2019). Problem gambling and family violence: Factors associated with family violence victimization and perpetration in treatment-seeking gamblers. *Journal of Interpersonal Violence*, 886260519835877.

Dowling, N. A., Youssef, G. J., Jackson, A. C., Pennay, D. W., Francis, K. L., Pennay, A., & Lubman, D. I. (2016). National estimates of Australian gambling prevalence: Findings from a dual-frame omnibus survey. *Addiction, 111*(3), 420-435.

Drake, R. E., Bond, G. R., & Becker, D. R. (2012). *Individual Placement and Support: An Evidence-Based Approach to Supported Employment*. USA. Oxford University Press.

Draper, B., & Low, L. F. (2009). Patterns of hospitalisation for depressive and anxiety disorders across the lifespan in Australia. *J Affect Disord, 113*(1-2), 195-200.

Driessen, E., Hegelmaier, L. M., Abbass, A. A., Barber, J. P., Dekker, J. J. M., Van, H. L., . . . Cuijpers, P. (2015). The efficacy of short-term psychodynamic psychotherapy for depression: A meta-analysis update. *Clinical Psychology Review, 42*, 1-15.

Driskell, T., Salas, E., & Driskell, J. E. (2018). Teams in extreme environments: Alterations in team development and teamwork. *Human Resource Management Review, 28*(4), 434-449.

Drug and Alcohol Multicultural Education Centre. (2014). *Respect: Best Practice Approaches Working with Culturally Diverse Clients in AOD Treatment Settings*. Sydney: Drug and Alcohol Multicultural Education Centre.

Drukker, M., van Os, J., Sytema, S., Driessen, G., Visser, E., & Delespaul, P. (2011). Function assertive community treatment (FACT) and psychiatric service use in patients diagnosed with severe mental illness. *Epidemiology and psychiatric sciences, 20*(3), 273.

Drummond, M. F., Sculpher, M. J., Claxton, K., Stoddart, G. L., & Torrance, G. W. (2015). *Methods for the Economic Evaluation of Health Care Programmes*. Oxford University Press.

D'Souza, R., & George, K. (2006). Spirituality, religion and psychiatry: Its application to clinical practice. *Australas Psychiatry, 14*(4), 408-412.

Dubois, B., Slachevsky, A., Litvan, I., & Pillon, B. (2000). The FAB: A frontal assessment battery at bedside. *Neurology, 55*(11), 1621-1626.

Duckett, S., & Swerissen, H. (2017). *Building Better Foundations for Primary Care*. Retrieved from https://grattan.edu.au/wp-content/uploads/2017/04/Building-better-foundations-for-primary-care.pdf.

Duckett, S., & Willcox, S. (2015). *The Australian Health Care System* (5th ed.). Oxford University Press.

Dudgeon, P., & Bray, A. (2018). Indigenous healing practices in Australia. *Women & Therapy, 41*(1-2), 97-113.

Dudgeon, P., Bray, A., D'Costa, B., & Walker, R. (2017). Decolonising psychology: Validating social and emotional wellbeing. *Australian Psychologist, 52*(4), 316-325.

Dudgeon, P., Calma, T., Brideson, T., & Holland, C. (2016). The Gayaa Dhuwi (Proud Spirit) Declaration: A call to action for Aboriginal and Torres Strait Islander leadership in the Australian mental health system. *Advances in Mental Health, 14*(2), 126-139.

Dudgeon, P., Calma, T., & Holland, C. (2017). Context and causes of Indigenous suicide in Australia. *Indigenous Wellbeing, 2*(2).

Dudgeon, P., Darwin, L., Hirvonen, T., Boe, M., Johnson, R., Cox, R., . . . Garrett, L. (2018). *We are Not the Problem, We Are Part of the Solution: Indigenous Lived Experience Project Report*. Retrieved from www.blackdoginstitute.org.au/docs/default-source/lifespan/lived-experience-report–final-nov-2018.pdf?sfvrsn=2.

Dudgeon, P., Darwin, L., McPhee, R., Holland, C., Von Helle, S., & Halliday, L. (2018). *Implementing Integrated Suicide Prevention in Aboriginal and Torres Strait Islander Communities, a Guide for Primary Health Networks*. Retrieved from www.cbpatsisp.com.au/wp-content/uploads/2019/03/Implementation-Guide.pdf.

Dudgeon, P., & Holland, C. (2018). Recent developments in suicide prevention among the Indigenous peoples of Australia. *Australasian Psychiatry, 26*(2), 166-169.

Dudgeon, P., Milroy, H., & Walker, R. (2014). *Working Together: Aboriginal and Torres Strait Islander Mental Health and Wellbeing Principles and Practice* (2nd ed.). Barton: Commonwealth of Australia.

Dudgeon, P., & Ugle, K. (2014). Communicating and Engaging with Diverse Communities. In P. Dudgeon, H. Milroy, & R. Walker (eds.), *Working Together: Aboriginal and Torres Strait Islander Mental Health and Wellbeing Principles and Practice* (pp. 257-268). Barton: Commonwealth of Australia.

Duffy, M. E., Henkel, K. E., & Earnshaw, V. A. (2016). Transgender clients' experiences of eating disorder treatment. *Journal of LGBT Issues in Counseling, 10*(3), 136-149.

Duggan, M. (2016). *Investing in Women's Mental Health: Strengthening the Foundations for Women, Families and the Australian Economy* Retrieved from www.vu.edu.au/sites/default/files/AHPC/pdfs/investing-in-womens-mental-health.pdf.

Dulit, R. A., Fyer, M. R., Miller, F. T., Sacks, M. H., & Frances, A. J. (1993). Gender differences in sexual preference and substance abuse of inpatients with borderline personality disorder. *Journal of Personality Disorders, 7*(2), 182–185.

Dunai, J., Labuschagne, I., Castle, D. J., Kyrios, M., & Rossell, S. L. (2010). Executive function in body dysmorphic disorder. *Psychol Med, 40*(9), 1541–1548.

Duncan, B. L. (2012). The Partners for Change Outcome Management System (PCOMS): The heart and soul of change project. *Canadian Psychology, 53*(2), 93–104.

Dunne, T., Bishop, L., Avery, S., & Darcy, S. (2017). A review of effective youth engagement strategies for mental health and substance use interventions. *Journal of Adolescent Health, 60*(5), 487–512.

Dunt, D. R., Benoy, A. W., Phillipou, A., Collister, L. L., Crowther, E. M., Freidin, J., & Castle, D. J. (2017). Evaluation of an integrated housing and recovery model for people with severe and persistent mental illnesses: The Doorway program. *Australian Health Review, 41*(5), 573–581.

Durose, C., & Richardson, L. (2016). *Designing Public Policy for Co-production: Theory, Practice and Change*. Policy Press.

Dweck, C. (2008). *Mindset: The New Psychology of Success*. New York: Ballantine Books.

Dyer, A. H., Nabeel, S., Briggs, R., O'Neill, D., & Kennelly, S. P. (2016). Cognitive assessment of older adults at the acute care interface: The informant history. *Postgraduate Medical Journal, 92*(1087), 255–259.

Dyer, S. M., Harrison, S. L., Laver, K., Whitehead, C., & Crotty, M. (2018). An overview of systematic reviews of pharmacological and non-pharmacological interventions for the treatment of behavioral and psychological symptoms of dementia. *International Psychogeriatrics, 30*(3), 295–309.

Early, J., & GlenMaye, L. F. (2000). Valuing families: Social work practice with families from a strengths perspective. *Social Work, 45*(2), 118–130.

Early Psychosis Guidelines Writing Group and EPPIC National Support Program. (2016). *Australian Clinical Guidelines for Early Psychosis, 2nd Edition Update*. Retrieved from www.orygen.org.au/Campus/Expert-Network/Resources/Free/Clinical-Practice/Australian-Clinical-Guidelines-for-Early-Psychosis/Australian-Clinical-Guidelines-for-Early-Psychosis.aspx?ext=.

Eassom, E., Giacco, D., Dirik, A., & Priebe, S. (2014). Implementing family involvement in the treatment of patients with psychosis: A systematic review of facilitating and hindering factors. *BMJ Open, 4*(10).

eCentreClinic. (2019). *Develop and Evaluate State-of-the-Art Free Online Treatment Courses for People with Common Mental Health and Chronic Physical Health Conditions*. Retrieved from www.ecentreclinic.org.

Ecker, S., & Bennett, E. (2017). *Preliminary Results of the Coping with Marriage Equality Debate Survey: Investigating the Stress Impacts Associated with the Australian Marriage Equality Debate During the Lead Up to the Postal Survey Results Announcement*. Retrieved from www.tai.org.au/sites/default/files/P447%20Briefing%20note_LGBTIQ%2B%20coping%20survey%20prelimary%20results.pdf.

Edwards, B., Gray, M., & Hunter, B. (2015). The impact of drought on mental health in rural and regional Australia. *Social Indicators Research, 121*(1), 177–194.

Egan, G. (2007). *The Skilled Helper: A Problem-Management and Opportunity-Development Approach to Helping* (8th ed.). Thomson Brooks/Cole.

Egan, G., & Reese, R. J. (2018). *The Skilled Helper: A Problem-Management and Opportunity-Development Approach to Helping* (11th ed.). Cengage Learning.

Egan, M., Bambra, C., Thomas, S., Petticrew, M., Whitehead, M., & Thomson, H. (2007). The psychosocial and health effects of workplace reorganisation. 1. A systematic review of organisational-level interventions that aim to increase employee control. *J Epidemiol Community Health, 61*(11), 945–954.

Eghigian, G. (2017). *The Routledge History of Madness and Mental Health*. Taylor & Francis.

Ehlers, A., & Clark, D. M. (2000). A cognitive model of posttraumatic stress disorder. *Behav Res Ther, 38*(4), 319–345.

Eisenberg, D., Hunt, J., & Speer, N. (2013). Mental health in American colleges and universities: Variation across student subgroups and across campuses. *Journal of Nervous and Mental Disease, 201*(1), 60–67.

Eisendrath, S. J., & Feldman, M. D. (1996). *The spectrum of factitious disorders*. Washington: American Psychiatric Pub.

Eisenlohr-Moul, T. A., DeWall, C. N., Girdler, S. S., & Segerstrom, S. C. (2015). Ovarian hormones and borderline personality disorder features: Preliminary evidence for interactive effects of estradiol and progesterone. *Biological psychology, 109*, 37–52.

Eklund, M., Leufstadius, C., & Bejerholm, U. (2009). Time use among people with psychiatric disabilities: Implications for practice. *Psychiatric Rehabilitation Journal, 32*(3), 177–191.

Elbogen, E. B., Swanson, J. W., Swartz, M. S., Van Dorn, R., Ferron, J., Wagner, H. R., & Wilder, C. (2007). Effectively implementing psychiatric advance directives to promote self-determination of treatment among people with mental illness. *Psychology Public Policy and Law, 13*(4), 273–288.

Ellis, A. (1962). *Reason and emotion in psychotherapy*. L. Stuart.

Ellis, B. H., Miller, A. B., Baldwin, H., & Abdi, S. (2011). New Directions in Refugee Youth Mental Health Services: Overcoming Barriers to Engagement. *Journal of Child & Adolescent Trauma, 4*(1), 69–85.

Ellis, I. K., & Philip, T. (2010). Improving the skills of rural and remote generalists to manage mental health emergencies. *Rural and Remote Health, 10*(3), 1503.

Emerging Minds. (2019). *Trauma Informed*. Retrieved from https://emergingminds.com.au.

Emerging Minds. (2020). *Better Mental Health Support and Approaches for Infants, Children and Families*. Retrieved from https://emergingminds.com.au.

Ende, P. C., Busschbach, J. T., Nicholson, J., Korevaar, E. L., & Weeghel, J. (2016). Strategies for parenting by mothers and fathers with a mental illness. *Journal of Psychiatric and Mental Health Nursing, 23*(2), 86–97.

Endrawes, G., O'Brien, L., & Wilkes, L. (2007). Egyptian families caring for a relative with mental illness: A hermeneutic study. *International Journal of Mental Health Nursing, 16*(6), 431–440.

Engel, G. L. (1977). The need for a new medical model: A challenge for biomedicine. *Science, 196*(4286), 129–136.

Engel, G. L. (1980). The clinical application of the biopsychosocial model. *American Journal of Psychiatry, 137*(5), 535–544.

Ennals, P., & Fossey, E. (2009). Using the OPHI-II to support people with mental illness in their recovery. *Occupational Therapy in Mental Health, 25*(2), 138–150.

Ennals, P., Fossey, E., Harvey, C., & Killackey, E. (2014). Postsecondary education: Kindling opportunities for people with mental illness *Asia-Pacific Psychiatry, 6*(2), 115–119.

Ennals, P., Fossey, E., & Howie, L. (2015). Postsecondary study and mental ill-health: A meta-synthesis of qualitative research exploring students' lived experiences. *Journal of Mental Health, 24*(2), 111–119.

Enticott, J. C., Lin, E., Shawyer, F., Russell, G., Inder, B., Patten, S., & Meadows, G. (2018). Prevalence of psychological distress: How do Australia and Canada compare? *Australian and New Zealand Journal of Psychiatry, 52*(3), 227–238.

Enticott, J. C., Meadows, G. N., Shawyer, F., Inder, B., & Patten, S. (2016). Mental disorders and distress: Associations with demographics, remoteness and socioeconomic deprivation of area of residence across Australia. *Australian and New Zealand Journal of Psychiatry, 50*(12), 1169–1179.

Enticott, J. C., Shawyer, F., Brophy, L., Russell, G., Fossey, E., Inder, B., . . . Meadows, G. (2016). The PULSAR primary care protocol: A stepped-wedge cluster randomized controlled trial to test a training intervention for general practitioners in recovery-oriented practice to optimize personal recovery in adult patients. *BMC Psychiatry, 16*(1), 451-451.

Enticott, J. C., Shawyer, F., Brophy, L., Russell, G., Mazza, D., Wilson-Evered, E., . . . Meadows, G. (Under review). Exploratory findings from the REFOCUS-PULSAR primary care intervention for general practitioners in recovery-oriented practice to optimize personal recovery in adult patients.

Enticott, J. C., Shawyer, F., Vasi, S., Buck, K., Cheng, I. H., Russell, G., . . . Meadows, G. (2017). A systematic review of studies with a representative sample of refugees and asylum seekers living in the community for participation in mental health research. *BMC Med Res Methodol, 17*(1), 37.

Epp, A. M., & Dobson, K. S. (2010). The evidence base of cognitive-behavioural therapy. In K. S. Dobson (ed.), *Handbook of Cognitive-Behavioral Therapies* (3rd ed., pp. 39). Guilford Publications.

EPPIC National Support Program Writing Group. (2014). *Medical Interventions in Early Psychosis: A Practical Guide for Early Psychosis Clinicians*. Melbourne: Orygen.

Epstein, I. (1996). In quest of a research-based model for clinical practice: Or, why can't a social worker be more like a researcher? *Social Work Research, 20*(2), 97-100.

Epstein, I. (2011). Reconciling evidence-based practice, evidence-informed practice, and practice-based research: The role of clinical data-mining. *Social Work, 56*(3), 284–288.

Epstein, M. (1997). *Developing Effective Consumer Participation in Mental Health Services: The Report of the Lemon Tree Learning Project*. Retrieved from www.ourcommunity.com.au/files/OCP/LemonTree.pdf.

Epstein, M. (2019a). Consumer Perspective. *Resource Centre for Mental Health Consumers*. Retrieved from www.ourconsumerplace.com.au/consumer/article?id=5688.

Epstein, M. (2019b). *Two Hats: Consumers Who Are Also Clinicians. Resource Centre for Mental Health Consumers*. Retrieved from www.ourconsumerplace.com.au/consumer/article?id=5646.

Epstein, M., & Wadsworth, Y. (1994). *Understanding and Involvement (U&I): Consumer Evaluation of Acute Psychiatric Hospital Practice: A Project's Beginnings* (vol. 1). Melbourne: Victorian Mental Illness Awareness Council.

Estroff, S. E., Crazy, M. I., & Lamb, H. R. (1981). *Making It Crazy: An Ethnography of Psychiatric Clients in an American Community*. University of California Press.

Etter, J.-F., & Bullen, C. (2014). A longitudinal study of electronic cigarette users. *Addictive behaviors, 39*(2), 491–494.

European Association for Behavioural and Cognitive Therapies (EABCT). (2020). *European Association for Behavioural and Cognitive Therapies*. Retrieved from https://eabct.eu.

Evans-Lacko, S., Knapp, M., McCrone, P., Thornicroft, G., & Mojtabai, R. (2013). The mental health consequences of the recession: Economic hardship and employment of people with mental health problems in 27 European countries. *PLoS One, 8*(7), e69792.

Everitt, B. S., & Wessely, S. (2004). *Clinical Trials in Psychiatry*. New York: Oxford University Press.

Ewart, S. B., Bocking, J., Happell, B., Platania-Phung, C., & Stanton, R. (2016). Mental Health Consumer Experiences and Strategies When Seeking Physical Health Care: A Focus Group Study. Global Qualitative Nursing Research, 3. 1-10.

Fábrega, H. (1994). International systems of diagnosis in psychiatry. *Journal of Nervous and Mental Disease*.

Fadden, G., James, C., & Pinfold, V. (2012). *Caring for Yourself–Self Help for Families and Friends Supporting People with Mental Health Problems*. Birmingham: White Halo Design.

Fairburn, C. G. (2008). *Cognitive Behavior Therapy and Eating Disorders*. Guilford Publications.

Fairburn, C. G. (2010). *Transdiagnostic Cognitive Behavior Therapy for Eating Disorders*. New York: Guilford Press.

Fairburn, C. G., Cooper, Z., Doll, H. A., Norman, P., & O'Connor, M. (2000). The natural course of bulimia nervosa and binge eating disorder in young women. *Arch Gen Psychiatry, 57*(7), 659–665.

Falkov, A. (2012). *The Family Model Handbook: An Integrated Approach to Supporting Mentally Ill Parents and Their Children*. Pavilion.

Falloon, I. R. H., & Fadden, G. (1993). *Integrated Mental Health Care: A Comprehensive Community-Based Approach*. Cambridge: Cambridge University Press.

Fallot, R. D., & Harris, M. (2008). trauma-informed approaches to systems of care. *Trauma Psychology: Newsletter.* Winter, vol 3, no. 1. Retrieved from http://traumapsychnews.com/wp-content/uploads/2016/01/newsletter_2008_winter.pdf#page=6.

Families Australia. (2011). *About*. Retrieved from https://familiesaustralia.org.au/about.

Families Housing Community Services and Indigenous Affairs (FaHCSIA). (2012). *Department of Families, Housing, Community Services and Indigenous Affairs (FaHCSIA)*. Retrieved from www.indigenousjustice.gov.au/publisher/department-of-families-housing-community-services-and-indigenous-affairs-fahcsia.

Farhall, J., Cugnetto, M. L., Mathews, S., Ratcliff, K., Farnan, S., Higgins, K., & Constantine, E. (2019). Outcomes and change processes of an established family education program for carers of adults diagnosed with a serious mental health condition. *Psychol Med*, 1-11.

Farhall, J., Greenwood, K. M., & Jackson, H. J. (2007). Coping with hallucinated voices in schizophrenia: A review of self-initiated strategies and therapeutic interventions. *Clinical Psychology Review, 27*(4), 476–493.

Faris, R. E. L., & Dunham, H. W. (1939). *Mental Disorders in Urban Areas*. Chicago: University of Chicago Press.

Farley, R., Askew, D., & Kay, M. (2014). Caring for refugees in general practice: Perspectives from the coalface. *Australian Journal of Primary Health, 20*(1), 85–91.

Farnworth, L. (2003). Time use, tempo and temporality: Occupational therapy's core business or someone else's business. *Australian Occupational Therapy Journal, 50*(3), 116–126.

Farrington, D. P., & Coid, J. W. (2003). *Early Prevention of Adult Antisocial Behaviour*. Cambridge University Press.

Fava, G. A., Grandi, S., Rafanelli, C., Fabbri, S., & Cazzaro, M. (2000). Explanatory therapy in hypochondriasis. *Journal of Clinical Psychiatry, 61*(4), 317-322.

Fava, M. (2003). Diagnosis and definition of treatment-resistant depression. *Biological Psychiatry, 53*(8), 649–659.

Fazel, S., Hayes, A. J., Bartellas, K., Clerici, M., & Trestman, R. (2016). Mental health of prisoners: Prevalence, adverse outcomes, and interventions. *Lancet Psychiatry, 3*(9), 871-881.

Feinstein, A. (2011). Conversion disorder: Advances in our understanding. *Canadian Medical Association Journal, 183*(8), 915-920.

Feldman, G. C., Joormann, J., & Johnson, S. L. (2008). Responses to positive affect: A self-report measure of rumination and dampening. *Cognitive Therapy and Research, 32*(4), 507-525.

Feldman, M. B., & Meyer, I. (2007). Eating disorders in diverse lesbian, gay, and bisexual populations. *International Journal of Eating Disorders, 40*(3), 218-226.

Ferris, J., & Wynne, H. (2001). *The Canadian Problem Gambling Index: Final report*. Retrieved from www.greo.ca/Modules/EvidenceCentre/files/Ferris%20et%20al(2001)The_Canadian_Problem_Gambling_Index.pdf.

Feusner, J. D., Neziroglu, F., Wilhelm, S., Mancusi, L., & Bohon, C. (2010). What causes BDD: Research findings and a proposed model. *Psychiatric Annals, 40*(7), 349-355.

Filges, T., Montgomery, E., Kastrup, M., & Jørgensen, A.M. (2015). The impact of detention on the health of asylum seekers: A systematic review. *Campbell Systematic Reviews, 13*.

Fink, P., Ewald, H., Jensen, J., Sorensen, L., Engberg, M., Holm, M., & Munk-Jørgensen, P. (1999). Screening for somatization and hypochondriasis in primary care and neurological in-patients: A seven-item scale for hypochondriasis and somatization. *J Psychosom Res, 46*(3), 261-273.

Fink, P., Hansen, M. S., & Oxhoj, M. L. (2004). The prevalence of somatoform disorders among internal medical inpatients. *Journal of Psychosomatic Research, 56*(4), 413-418.

Firn, M., Alonso-Vicente, M., Hubbeling, D., Holley, J., White, S. J., & Jones, B. (2018). The replacement of assertive outreach services by reinforcing local community teams: A replication study reporting comparative outcomes and patient reported experience. *Journal of Mental Health, 27*(2), 157-163.

Firn, M., White, S. J., Hubbeling, D., & Jones, B. (2018). The replacement of assertive outreach services by reinforcing local community teams: A four-year observational study. *Journal of Mental Health, 27*(1), 4-9.

First, M. B. (2005). Desire for amputation of a limb: Paraphilia, psychosis, or a new type of identity disorder. *Psychol Med, 35*(6), 919-928.

Firth, J., Cotter, J., Torous, J., Bucci, S., Firth, J. A., & Yung, A. R. (2015). Mobile phone ownership and endorsement of 'mHealth' among people with psychosis: A meta-analysis of cross-sectional studies. *Schizophrenia Bulletin, 42*(2), 448-455.

Fisher, A. G., & Bray Jones, K. (2012). *Assessment of Motor and Process Skills. Vol. 1: Development, standardization, and administration manual* (7th rev. ed.). Fort Collins: Three Star Press.

Fisher, A. G., & Bray Jones, K. (2014). *Assessment of Motor and Process Skills. Vol. 2: User manual* (8th ed.). Fort Collins: Three Star Press.

Fisher, D. (2017). *Heartbeats of Hope: The Empowerment Way to Recover Your Life*. Wisconsin: Daniel B. Fisher.

Fisher, J., Cabral, d. M. M., Patel, V., Rahman, A., Tran, T., Holton, S., & Holmes, W. (2012). Prevalence and determinants of common perinatal mental disorders in women in low- and lower-middle-income countries: A systematic review. *Bulletin of the World Health Organization, 90*(2), 139G-149G.

Fisher, J. R. W., Wynter, K. H., & Rowe, H. J. (2010). Innovative psycho-educational program to prevent common postpartum mental disorders in primiparous women: A before and after controlled study. *BMC Psychiatry, 10*.

Fisher, M., & Baum, F. (2010). The social determinants of mental health: Implications for research and health promotion. *Aust N Z J Psychiatry, 44*(12), 1057-1063.

Fisher, S. (1994). Identifying video game addiction in children and adolescents. *Addictive Behaviors, 19*(5), 545-553.

Flaherty, J. H. (2011). The evaluation and management of delirium among older persons. *Medical Clinics of North America, 95*(3), 555-+.

Flatau, P., Seivwright, A., Callis, Z., Thielking, M., Mackelprang, J., Taylor, K., & La Sala, L. (2018). *Chronic Homelessness in Melbourne: First-Year Outcomes of the Journey to Social Inclusion Phase 2 Study Participants*. St Kilda: Sacred Heart Missions.

Fletcher, J., Brophy, L., Killaspy, H., Ennals, P., Hamilton, B., Collister, L., & Hall, T. (2019). Prevention and recovery care services in Australia: Describing the role and function of sub-acute recovery-based residential mental health services in Victoria.(Report). *Frontiers in Psychiatry, 10*.

Fletcher, J., Spittal, M., Brophy, L., Tibble, H., Kinner, S., Elsom, S., & Hamilton, B. (2017). Outcomes of the Victorian Safewards trial in 13 wards: Impact on seclusion rates and fidelity measurement. *International Journal of Mental Health Nursing, 26*(5), 461-471.

Fletcher, K., Foley, F., Thomas, N., Michalak, E., Berk, L., Berk, M., . . . Murray, G. (2018). Web-based intervention to improve quality of life in late stage bipolar disorder (ORBIT): Randomised controlled trial protocol. *BMC Psychiatry, 18*(1), 221.

Fleury, M.-J., Grenier, G., Bamvita, J.-M., & Chiocchio, F. (2018). Associated and mediating variables related to job satisfaction among professionals from mental health teams. *Psychiatric Quarterly, 89*(2), 399-413.

Fleury, M.-J., Grenier, G., Caron, J., & Lesage, A. (2008). Patients' report of help provided by relatives and to meet their needs. *Community Mental Health Journal, 44*, 271-281.

Flewett, T. (2011). *Clinical Risk Management: An Introductory Text for Mental Health Professionals*. Elsevier Health Sciences.

Fliege, H., Grimm, A., Eckhardt-Henn, A., Gieler, U., Martin, K., & Klapp, B. F. (2007). Frequency of ICD-10 factitious disorder: Survey of senior hospital consultants and physicians in private practice. *Psychosomatics, 48*(1), 60-64.

Flood, M., & Buckwater, K. C. (2009). Recommendations for mental health care of older adults, part 2: An overview of dementia, delirium, and substance abuse. *Journal of Gerontological Nursing, 35*(2), 35-47.

Flores, A. R., Brown, T. N. T., & Herman, J. L. (2016). *Race and ethnicity of adults who identify as transgender in the United States*. The Williams Institute.

Flynn, C., & McDermott, F. (2016). *Doing Research in Social Work and Social Care: The Journey from Student to Practitioner Researcher*. SAGE Publications.

Foa, E. B., Liebowitz, M. R., Kozak, M. J., Davies, S., Campeas, R., Franklin, M. E., . . . Tu, X. (2005). Randomized, placebo-controlled trial of exposure and ritual prevention, clomipramine, and their combination in the treatment of obsessive-compulsive disorder. *American Journal of Psychiatry, 162*(1), 151-161.

Foa, E. B., & Rothbaum, B. O. (1998). *Treating the Trauma of Rape: Cognitive Behavioral Therapy for PTSD*. New York: Guilford Press.

Foley, G., Schaap, A., & Howell, E. (2014). *The Aboriginal Tent Embassy: Sovereignty, Black Power, Land Rights and the State*. Oxfordshire: Taylor & Francis.

Folkman, S., & Lazarus, R. S. (1980). An analysis of coping in a middle-aged community sample. *J Health Soc Behav, 21*(3), 219-239.

Folstein, M. F., Folstein, S. E., & McHugh, P. R. (1975). 'Mini-mental state'. A practical method for grading the cognitive state of patients for the clinician. *Journal of Psychiatric Research, 12*(3), 189–198.

Folstein, S. E. (1999). Autism. *International Review of Psychiatry, 11*(4), 269–277.

Fombonne, E. (2005). The Changing Epidemiology of Autism. *Journal of Applied Research in Intellectual Disabilities, 18*(4), 281–294.

Ford, A. H., & Almeida, O. P. (2015). Pharmacological interventions for preventing delirium in the elderly. *Maturitas, 81*(2), 287–292.

Ford, T., Parker, C., Salim, J., Goodman, R., Logan, S., & Henley, W. (2018). The relationship between exclusion from school and mental health: A secondary analysis of the British Child and Adolescent Mental Health Surveys 2004 and 2007. *Psychol Med, 48*(4), 629–641.

Ford, T., & Ramchandani, P. (2009). Common mental health problems in childhood and adolescence: The broad and varied landscape. *Child: Care, Health and Development, 35*(6), 751–753.

Forester, B. P., Patrick, R. E., & Harper, D. G. (2019). Setbacks and Opportunities in disease-modifying therapies in Alzheimer disease. *JAMA Psychiatry, 77*(1), 7–8.

Forman, E. M., Herbert, J. D., Moitra, E., Yeomans, P. D., & Geller, P. A. (2007). A randomized controlled effectiveness trial of acceptance and commitment therapy and cognitive therapy for anxiety and depression. *Behavior modification, 31*(6), 772–799.

Fossey, E., Brophy, L., Grigg, M., Hamann, J., Hamilton, B., Harvey, C., . . . Watson, S. (2012). Case Management. In G. Meadows, B. Singh, & M. Grigg (eds.), *Mental Health in Australia 3e; Collaborative Community Practice* (3rd ed., Vol. 3, pp. 428–450). Melbourne: Oxford University Press.

Fossey, E., & Harvey, C. (2010). Finding and sustaining mainstream employment: A qualitative meta-synthesis of mental health consumer views. *Canadian Journal of Occupational Therapy, 77*(5), 303–314.

Fossey, E., Harvey, C., McDermott, F., & Davidson, L. (2002). Understanding and evaluating qualitative research. *Australian and New Zealand Journal of Psychiatry, 36*(6), 717–732.

Fossey, E., Harvey, C., Plant, G., & Pantelis, C. (2006). Occupational Performance of People Diagnosed with Schizophrenia in Supported Housing and Outreach Programmes in Australia. *British Journal of Occupational Therapy, 69*(9), 409–419.

Fossey, E., & Harvey, C. A. (2001). A conceptual review of functioning: Implications for the development of consumer outcome measures. *Australian and New Zealand Journal of Psychiatry, 35*(1), 91–98.

Fossey, E., & Krupa, T. (2016). Patterns of participation: Time use and Occupational Balance. In T. Krupa, B. Kirsh, D. B. Pitts, & E. Fossey (eds.), *Bruce and Borgs' Psychosocial Frames of Reference: Theories, Models and Approaches for Occupation-Based Practice* (4th ed., pp. 151–171).

Fossey, E. M., & Harvey, C. A. (2010). Finding and sustaining employment: A qualitative meta-synthesis of mental health consumer views. *Canadian Journal of Occupational Therapy-Revue Canadienne D Ergotherapie, 77*(5), 303–314.

Foucault, M. (1967). *Madness and Civilization: A History of Insanity in the Age of Reason*. Taylor and Francis.

Foucault, M. (1973). *The Birth of the Clinic: An Archaeology of Medical Perception*. New York: Pantheon Books.

Foucault, M. (1979). *Discipline and Punish: The Birth of the Prison*. Vintage Books.

Foucault, M., & Howard, R. (1988). *Madness and Civilization: A History of Insanity in the Age of Reason*. Vintage Books.

Fournier, J. C., Derubeis, R. J., Hollon, S. D., Dimidjian, S., Amsterdam, J. D., Shelton, R. C., & Fawcett, J. (2010). Antidepressant drug effects and depression severity: A patient-level meta-analysis. *JAMA, 303*(1), 47–53.

Fox, A. (1997). *Project Eve: Internal Evaluation Methodology and Partnership Evaluation Development in Selected Health Service Sectors* (Suppl 3), Melbourne, University of Melbourne.

Fox, J., Ramon, S., & Morant, N. (2015). Exploring the meaning of recovery for carers: Implications for social work practice. *British Journal of Social Work, 45* (suppl 1), i117–i134.

Fox, M., Martin, P., & Green, G. (2007). *Doing Practitioner Research*. London: Sage.

Fox, N. A., & Pine, D. S. (2012). Temperament and the emergence of anxiety disorders. *J Am Acad Child Adolesc Psychiatry, 51*(2), 125–128.

Foxcroft, D. R., Coombes, L., Wood, S., Allen, D., & Almeida Santimano, N. M. (2014). Motivational interviewing for alcohol misuse in young adults. *The Cochrane Library*.

Framo, J. (1980). *Marriage and Marital Therapy: Issues and Initial Interview Techniques*. New York: Springer.

Francis, A. (2014). Strengths-based assessments and recovery in mental health: Reflections from practice. *International Journal of Social Work and Human Services Practice, 2*(6), 264–271.

Frank, R., Fawcett, L., & Emmerson, B. (2005). Development of Australia's first psychiatric emergency centre. *Australasian Psychiatry, 13*(3), 266–272.

Frank, R. G., & Glied, S. A. (2006). *Better but Not Well: Mental Health Policy in the United States Since 1950*. Baltimore: Johns Hopkins University Press.

Frank, R. G., & Glied, S. A. (2006). The Evolving Technology of Mental Health Care. In *Better but Not Well: Mental Health Policy in the United States since 1950* (pp. 26–47). Baltimore: Johns Hopkins University Press.

Frankenburg, F. R., & Zanarini, M. C. (2006). Personality disorders and medical comorbidity. *Curr Opin Psychiatry, 19*(4), 428–431.

Freebairn, L., Atkinson, J. A., Osgood, N. D., Kelly, P. M., McDonnell, G., & Rychetnik, L. (2019). Turning conceptual systems maps into dynamic simulation models: An Australian case study for diabetes in pregnancy. *PLoS One, 14*(6).

Freeman, D., Reeve, S., Robinson, A., Ehlers, A., Clark, D., Spanlang, B., & Slater, M. (2017). Virtual reality in the assessment, understanding, and treatment of mental health disorders. *Psychol Med, 47*(14), 2393–2400.

Freeman, J. (2005). Towards a definition of holism. *The British Journal of General Practice, 55*(511), 154–155.

Freeston, M. H., Rheaume, J., & Ladouceur, R. (1996). Correcting faulty appraisals of obsessional thoughts. *Behav Res Ther, 34*(5-6), 433–446.

Freud, S. (1896/1962). The aetiology of hysteria. In S. Freud, J. Strachey, A. Freud, C. L. Rothgeb, & S. L. Corporation (eds.), *The Standard Edition of the Complete Psychological Works of Sigmund Freud* (Vol. 3). London: Hogarth Press.

Freud, S. (1914). *On Narcissism: The Standard Edition of the Complete Psychological Works of Sigmund Freud.* Trans. and ed. James Strachey, *14*, 67–102.

Freud, S. (1985). Group Psychology and the Analysis of the Ego, Future of an Illusion and Civilization and Its Discontents. In A. Dickson (ed.), *Civilization, Society and Religion* (pp. 91–178). Penguin.

Freud, S. (2008). *Three Case Histories*. New York: Touchstone.

Friedman, E. H. (1985). *Generation to Generation: Family Process in Church and Synagogue*. New York: Guilford Press.

Froggatt, D., Fadden, G., Johnson, D., Leggatt, M., & Shankar, R. (2007). *Families as Partners in Mental Health Care: A Guidebook for Implementing Family Work*. Toronto: World Fellowship for Schizophrenia and Allied Disorders.

Frogner, B. K., Hussey, P. S., & Anderson, G. F. (2011). Health systems in industrialized countries. In S. Glied & P. C. Smith (eds.), *The Oxford Handbook of Health Economics* (pp. 8-29). New York: Oxford University Press.

Fronek, P. I. (2012, August 2). On human rights and social work: In conversation with Sharlene Nipperess [Episode 17]. In *Podsocs*.

Frost, R. O., & Hartl, T. L. (1996). A cognitive-behavioral model of compulsive hoarding. *Behav Res Ther, 34*(4), 341-350.

Frost, R. O., Ruby, D., & Shuer, L. J. (2012). The Buried in Treasures Workshop: Waitlist control trial of facilitated support groups for hoarding. *Behav Res Ther, 50*(11), 661-667.

Frost, R. O., & Steketee, G. (2002). *Cognitive Approaches to Obsessions and Compulsions: Theory, Assessment, and Treatment*. USA: Elsevier Science.

Frost, R. O., Steketee, G., & Grisham, J. (2004). Measurement of compulsive hoarding: Saving inventory-revised. *Behav Res Ther, 42*(10), 1163-1182.

Frost, R. O., Steketee, G., & Williams, L. (2000). Hoarding: A community health problem. *Health & Social Care in the Community, 8*(4), 229-234.

Fryers, T., & Brugha, T. (2013). Childhood determinants of adult psychiatric disorder. *Clinical Practice & Epidemiology in Mental Health, 9*, 1-50.

Fukui, S., Goscha, R., Rapp, C. A., Mabry, A., Liddy, P., & Marty, D. (2012). Strengths model case management fidelity scores and client outcomes. *Psychiatric Services, 63*(7), 708-710.

Fulford, K. W. M. (1989). *Moral Theory and Medical Practice*. Cambridge University Press.

Fuller, J. D., Perkins, D., Parker, S., Holdsworth, L., Kelly, B., Roberts, R., . . . Fragar, L. (2011). Building effective service linkages in primary mental health care: A narrative review part 2. *BMC Health Services Research, 11*(1), 66.

Gabbard, G. O. (2007). Do All Roads Lead to Rome? New Findings on Borderline Personality Disorder. American Journal of Psychiatry, 164(6), 853-855. https://doi.org/10.1176/ajp.2007.164.6.853.

Gaebel, W., Großimlinghaus, I., Kerst, A., Cohen, Y., Hinsche-Böckenholt, A., Johnson, B., . . . Zielasek, J. (2016). European Psychiatric Association (EPA) guidance on the quality of eMental health interventions in the treatment of psychotic disorders. *European Archives of Psychiatry and Clinical Neuroscience, 266*(2), 125-137.

Gainsbury, S. M., Russell, A., Hing, N., Wood, R., & Lubman, D. I. (2014). The prevalence and determinants of problem gambling in Australia: Assessing the impact of interactive gambling and new technologies. *Psychology of Addictive Behaviors, 28*(3), 769-779.

Galletly, C., Castle, D., Dark, F., Humberstone, V., Jablensky, A., Killackey, E., . . . Tran, N. (2016). Royal Australian and New Zealand College of Psychiatrists clinical practice guidelines for the management of schizophrenia and related disorders. *Australian & New Zealand Journal of Psychiatry, 50*(5), 410-472.

Galvin, S. W., & McCarthy, S. (1994). Multi-disciplinary community teams: Clinging to the wreckage. *Journal of Mental Health, 3*, 157-166.

Gambrill, E. (2008). Evidence-based (informed) macro practice: Process and philosophy. *J Evid Based Soc Work, 5*(3-4), 423-452.

Gammarano, R. (2019). *Work and Employment Are Not Synonyms*. Retrieved from https://ilostat.ilo.org/2019/10/29/work-and-employment-are-not-synonyms.

Gammon, D., Strand, M., Eng, L. S., Børøsund, E., Varsi, C., & Ruland, C. (2017). Shifting practices toward recovery-oriented care through an e-recovery portal in community mental health care: A mixed-methods exploratory study. *Journal of Medical Internet Research, 19*(5), e145.

Gannon, E., Delfabbro, P., & Sutherland, C. (2020). Gambling in rural and remote South Australia. *International Journal of Mental Health and Addiction*, 1-18.

Garber, J., Frankel, S. A., & Herrington, C. G. (2016). Developmental demands of cognitive behavioral therapy for depression in children and adolescents: Cognitive, social, and emotional processes. *Annual Review of Clinical Psychology, 12*(1), 181-216.

Garcia-Campayo, J., Alda, M., Sobradiel, N., Olivan, B., & Pascual, A. (2007). Personality disorders in somatization disorder patients: A controlled study in Spain. *Journal of Psychosomatic Research, 62*(6), 675-680.

Garcia-Velazquez, R., Jokela, M., & Rosenstrom, T. H. (2017). Symptom severity and disability in psychiatric disorders: The US Collaborative Psychiatric Epidemiology Survey. *J Affect Disord, 222*, 204-210.

Gardener, J., Parsons, R., & Paxton, G. (2010). *Adaptation Benchmarking Survey: Initial Report*. Retrieved from https://research.csiro.au/climate/wp-content/uploads/sites/54/2016/03/4_WorkingPaper04_CAF_pdf-Standard.pdf.

Gardiner-Garden, J. (2003). Defining Aboriginality in Australia. *Current Issues Brief*, no. 10 2002-03. Canberra: Parliament of Australia.

Gardner, B. K., & O'Connor, D. W. (2008). A review of the cognitive effects of electroconvulsive therapy in older adults. *Journal of ECT, 24*(1), 68-80.

Garner, D. M., Vitousek, K. M., & Garfinkel, P. E. (1997). Cognitive-behavioral therapy for anorexia nervosa. In D. M. Garner & P. E. Garfinkel (eds.), *Handbook of Treatments for Eating Disorders* (2 ed., pp. 94-144). New York: The Guildford Press.

Garralda, M. E. (1996). Somatisation in children. *Journal of Child Psychology and Psychiatry, vol. 37*(1), pp. 13-33.

Gask, L. (1995). *Management in Primary Care*. Oxford: Oxford University Press.

Gates, G. J. (2011). *How Many People Are Lesbian, Gay, Bisexual and Transgender?* The Williams Institute: Los Angeles.

Gee, G., Dudgeon, P., Schultz, C., Hart, A., & Kelly, K. (2014). Aboriginal and Torres Strait Islander Social and Emotional Wellbeing and Mental Health. In P. Dudgeon, H. Milroy, & R. Walker (eds.), *Working Together: Aboriginal and Torres Strait Islander Mental Health and Wellbeing Principles and Practice* (pp. 55-68). Barton: Commonwealth of Australia.

Gelder, M. G., Andreasen, N. C., Lopez-Ibor, J. J., & Geddes, J. R. (2012). *New Oxford Textbook of Psychiatry*. Oxford University Press.

General Practice New South Wales. (2014). *Primary Care Mental Health Strategy*. Retrieved from https://nswmentalhealthcommission.com.au.

Gentile, D. A., Choo, H., Liau, A., Sim, T., Li, D. D., Fung, D., & Khoo, A. (2011). Pathological video game use among youths: A two-year longitudinal study. *Pediatrics, 127*(2), E319-E329.

Gentry, S., & Badrinath, P. (2017). Defining health in the era of value-based care: Lessons from England of relevance to other health systems. *Cureus, 9*(3), e1079-e1079.

Gerstein, D., Murphy, S., Toce, M., Volberg, R., Harwood, H., Tucker, A., . . . Sinclair, S. (1999). *Gambling Impact and Behavior Study: Report to the National Gambling Impact Study Commission*. Retrieved from www.researchgate.net/publication/246284410_Gambling_impact_and_behavior_study_report_to_the_National_Gambling_Impact_Study_Commission/citation/download.

Gerull, F. C., & Rapee, R. M. (2002). Mother knows best: Effects of maternal modelling on the acquisition of fear and avoidance behaviour in toddlers. *Behav Res Ther, 40*(3), 279–287.

Gesell, A. (1926). The mental growth of the pre-school child. *Journal of Nervous and Mental Disease, 64*(2), 201.

Gewurtz, R. E., Moll, S. E., Letts, L. J., Larivière, N., Levasseur, M., & Krupa, T. M. (2016). What you do every day matters: A new direction for health promotion. *Canadian Journal of Public Health, 107*(2), e205–e208.

Gibb, S. J., Fergusson, D. M., & Horwood, L. J. (2010). Burden of psychiatric disorder in young adulthood and life outcomes at age 30. *British Journal of Psychiatry, 197*, 122–127.

Gibson, B. (2003). Beyond 'Two Communities'. In V. Lin & B. Gibson (eds.), *Evidence-based Health Policy: Problems and Possibilities* (pp. 18–31). Melbourne: Oxford University Press.

Gibson, R. W., D'Amico, M., Jaffe, L., & Arbesman, M. (2011). Occupational therapy interventions for recovery in the areas of community integration and normative life roles for adults with serious mental illness: A systematic review. *American Journal of Occupational Therapy, 65*(3), 247–256.

Giddens, A. (1991). *Modernity and Self Identity*. Cambridge: Polity Press.

Gieler, U., & Eckhardt-Henn, A. (2004). Factitious disorders. *Dermatol Psychosom, 5*, 93–98.

Giesbrecht, T., Lynn, S. J., Lilienfeld, S. O., & Merckelbach, H. (2008). Cognitive processes in dissociation: An analysis of core theoretical assumptions. *Psychological Bulletin, 134*(5), 617–647.

Giesen-Bloo, J., Van Dyck, R., Spinhoven, P., Van Tilburg, W., Dirksen, C., Van Asselt, T., . . . Arntz, A. (2006). Outpatient psychotherapy for borderline personality disorder: Randomized trial of schema-focused therapy vs transference-focused psychotherapy. *Archives of General Psychiatry, 63*(6), 649–658.

Gilat, I. and Shahar, G. (2007). Emotional first aid for a suicide crisis: Comparison between telephonic hotline and internet. *Psychiatry*, vol. 70(1).

Gilbert, E., Marwaha, S., Milton, A., Johnson, S., Morant, N., Parsons, N., . . . Cunliffe, D. (2013). Social firms as a means of vocational recovery for people with mental illness: A UK survey. *BMC Health Services Research, 13*.

Gilbert, P. (2009). Introducing compassion-focused therapy. *Advances in Psychiatric Treatment, 15*(3), 199–208.

Gilbert, P. (2010). *Compassion Focused Therapy*. East Sussex: Routledge.

Gilbert, P. (2014). Compassion-focused therapy: Preface and introduction for special section. *British Journal of Clinical Psychology, 53*(1), 1–5.

Gilbert, P. (2014). The origins and nature of compassion focused therapy. *British Journal of Clinical Psychology, 53*(1), 6–41.

Gill, K. H. (2017). Creating an environment that cultivates meaningful consumer-led or co-produced research. Are we there yet? *The Australian Journal on Psychosocial Rehabilitation, Summer 2017/18*, 49–52.

Gillard, S., Foster, R., Gibson, S., Goldsmith, L., Marks, J., & White, S. (2017). Describing a principles-based approach to developing and evaluating peer worker roles as peer support moves into mainstream mental health services. *Mental Health and Social Inclusion, 21*(3), 133–143.

Gillard, S., & Holley, J. (2014). Peer workers in mental health services: Literature overview. *Advances in Psychiatric Treatment, 20*(4), 286–292.

Gillespie, M. A. M., Derevensky, J., & Gupta, R. (2007). Adolescent problem gambling: Developing a gambling expectancy instrument. *Journal of Gambling Issues* (19), 51–68.

Gillespie, N. (2007). *Reflections: 40 Years on from the 1967 Referendum*. Adelaide: Aboriginal Legal Rights Movement Incorporated.

Gillespie, N. A., Zhu, G., Heath, A. C., Hickie, I. B., & Martin, N. G. (2000). The genetic aetiology of somatic distress. *Psychol Med, 30*(5), 1051–1061.

Gillon, R. (1986). *Philosophical Medical Ethics*. Chichester: Wiley Medical Publications.

Gillon, R. (1994). Medical ethics: Four principles plus attention to scope. *British Medical Journal, 309*, 184.

Gillon, R. (2003). Ethics needs principles—four can encompass the rest—and respect for autonomy should be 'first among equals'. *Journal of Medical Ethics, 29*(5), 307.

Ginsburg, G. S., Becker, E. M., Keeton, C. P., Sakolsky, D., Piacentini, J., Albano, A. M., . . . Kendall, P. C. (2014). Naturalistic follow-up of youths treated for pediatric anxiety disorders. *JAMA Psychiatry, 71*(3), 310–318.

Girard, N. J. (2008). Practice-based evidence. *AORN Journal, 87*(1), 15–16.

Gire, N., Farooq, S., Naeem, F., Duxbury, J., McKeown, M., Kundi, P. S., . . . Husain, N. (2017). mHealth based interventions for the assessment and treatment of psychotic disorders: A systematic review. *mHealth, 3*.

Giummarra, M. J., Bradshaw, J. L., Nicholls, M. E. R., Hilti, L. M., & Brugger, P. (2011). Body integrity identity disorder: Deranged body processing, right fronto-parietal dysfunction, and phenomenological experience of body incongruity. *Neuropsychology Review, 21*(4), 320–333.

Gleaves, D. H. (1996). The sociocognitive model of dissociative identity disorder: A reexamination of the evidence. *Psychological Bulletin, 120*(1), 42–59.

Gleaves, D. H., Smith, S. M., Butler, L. D., & Spiegel, D. (2004). False and recovered memories in the laboratory and clinic: A review of experimental and clinical evidence. *Clinical Psychology Science and Practice, 11*(1), 3–28.

Glied, S., & Smith, P., C. (2011). *The Oxford Handbook of Health Economics*. Oxford: Oxford University Press.

Glied, S., & Smith, P. C. (2013). *The Oxford Handbook of Health Economics*. Oxford: Oxford University Press.

Glover, H. (2009). Foreward. In M. Amering & M. Schmolke (eds.), *Recovery in Mental Health* (pp. xi–xiii). Oxford: Wiley-Blackwell.

Glover, H., Kalyanasundaram, V., & Tooth, B. (2008). *Unpacking Practices that Support 'Recovery': Level 1 Workbook 1*. Unpublished manuscript. Brisbane.

Gmitroski, T., Bradley, C., Heinemann, L., Liu, G., Blanchard, P., Beck, C., . . . Barbic, S. P. (2018). Barriers and facilitators to employment for young adults with mental illness: A scoping review. *BMJ Open, 8*(12).

Goenka, S. N. (1987). *The Discourse Summaries: Talks from a Ten-day Course in Vipassana Meditation Condensed by William Hart*. Maharashtra: Vipassana Research Institute.

Goffman, E. (1961). *Asylums: Essays on the Social Situation of Mental Patients and Other Inmates*. Doubleday.

Goldberg, D. (2000). Impressions of psychiatry in Australia. *Australasian Psychiatry, 8*, 307-317.

Goldberg, D., & Huxley, P. (1980). *Mental Illness in the Community: The Pathway to Psychiatric Care*. Tavistock: London.

Goldberg, D., & Williams, P. (1988). *A User's Guide to the General Health Questionnaire*. Windsor: NFER-Nelson.

Goldberg Edelson, M. (2006). Are the majority of children with autism mentally retarded?: A systematic evaluation of the data. *Focus on Autism and Other Developmental Disabilities, 21*(2), 66-83.

Goldhammer, H. B., Maston, E. D., & Keuroghlian, A. S. (2019). Addressing eating disorders and body dissatisfaction in sexual and gender minority youth. *American Journal of Preventive Medicine, 56*(2), 318-322.

Goldstein, M. J. (1987). Psychosocial issues. *Schizophrenia Bulletin, 13*(1), 157-171.

Goldstone, E., Farhall, J., & Ong, B. (2012). Modelling the emergence of hallucinations: Early acquired vulnerabilities, proximal life stressors and maladaptive psychological processes. *Social Psychiatry and Psychiatric Epidemiology, 47*(9), 1367-1380.

Goodare, H., & Lockwood, S. (1999). Involving patients in clinical research improves the quality of research. *British Medical Journal, 319*(7212), 724-725.

Goodfellow, J., & Laverty, J. (2003). Grandparents supporting working families. *Family Matters, 66*, 14-19.

Gooding, P. (2013). Supported decision-making: A rights-based disability concept and its implications for mental health law. *Psychiatry, Psychology and Law, 20*(3), 431-451.

Goodman, L. A., Salyers, M. P., Mueser, K. T., Rosenberg, S. D., Swartz, M., Essock, S. M., . . . Comm, S. H. R. S. R. (2001). Recent victimization in women and men with severe mental illness: Prevalence and correlates. *Journal of Traumatic Stress, 14*(4), 615-632.

Goodman, W. K., Price, L. H., Rasmussen, S. A., Mazure, C., Delgado, P., Heninger, G. R., & Charney, D. S. (1989). The Yale-Brown Obsessive Compulsive Scale. II. Validity. *Arch Gen Psychiatry, 46*(11), 1012-1016.

Goodman, W. K., Price, L. H., Rasmussen, S. A., Mazure, C., Fleischmann, R. L., Hill, C. L., . . . Charney, D. S. (1989). The Yale-Brown Obsessive Compulsive Scale. I. Development, use, and reliability. *Arch Gen Psychiatry, 46*(11), 1006-1011.

Goodwin, B. C., Browne, M., Rockloff, M., & Rose, J. (2017). A typical problem gambler affects six others. *International Gambling Studies, 17*(2), 276-289.

Goodwin, R. D., & Hamilton, S. P. (2003). Lifetime comorbidity of antisocial personality disorder and anxiety disorders among adults in the community. *Psychiatry Research, 117*(2), 159-166.

Goodyear, M., Cuff, R., Maybery, D., & Reupert, A. (2009). CHAMPS: A peer support program for children of parents with a mental illness. *Australian e-Journal for the Advancement of Mental Health, 8*(3), 296-304.

Goodyear, M., Hill, T. L., Allchin, B., McCormick, F., Hine, R., Cuff, R., & O'Hanlon, B. (2015). Standards of practice for the adult mental health workforce: Meeting the needs of families where a parent has a mental illness. *International Journal of Mental Health Nursing, 24*(2), 169-180.

Goodyer, I. M., Reynolds, S., Barrett, B., Byford, S., Dubicka, B., Hill, J., . . . Roberts, C. (2017). Cognitive behavioural therapy and short-term psychoanalytical psychotherapy versus a brief psychosocial intervention in adolescents with unipolar major depressive disorder (IMPACT): A multicentre, pragmatic, observer-blind, randomised controlled superiority trial. *Lancet Psychiatry, 4*(2), 109-119.

Gopalkrishnan, N. (2018). Cultural Diversity and Mental Health: Considerations for Policy and Practice. *Frontiers in public health, 6*, 179-179.

Gore, F. M., Bloem, P. J. N., Patton, G. C., Ferguson, J., Joseph, V., Coffey, C., . . . Mathers, C. D. (2011). Global burden of disease in young people aged 10-24 years: A systematic analysis. *Lancet, 377*(9783), 2093-2102.

Goslar, M., Leibetseder, M., Muench, H. M., Hofmann, S. G., & Laireiter, A. R. (2017). Efficacy of face-to-face versus self-guided treatments for disordered gambling: A meta-analysis. *J Behav Addict, 6*(2), 142-162.

Gossop, M., Darke, S., Griffiths, P., Hando, J., Powis, B., Hall, W., & Strang, J. (1995). The Severity of Dependence Scale (SDS): Psychometric properties of the SDS in English and Australian samples of heroin, cocaine and amphetamine users. *Addiction, 90*(5), 607-614.

Government of South Australia. (2009). *South Australian Mental Health Act 2009*.

Government of Western Australia. (2004). *Carers Recognition Act 2004*. Retrieved from https://dlgc.communities.wa.gov.au/Publications/Pages/Carers-Recognition-Act-2004.aspx.

Government of Western Australia. (2012-13). *Mental Health Commission Annual Report 2012/13*. Retrieved from www.mhc.wa.gov.au/media/1527/mhc-annual-report-2012-13.pdf.

Government of Western Australia. (2014). *Western Australian Mental Health Act 2014*. Retrieved from www.mhc.wa.gov.au/about-us/legislation.

Government of Western Australia. (2014-15). *Mental Health Commission Annual Report 2014/15*. Retrieved from https://issuu.com/marshadale/docs/annual_report_2015-16Government of Western Australia. (2015-16). Mental Health Commission Annual Report 2015/16. Retrieved from https://issuu.com/marshadale/docs/2016_mhc_annual_report_final.

Government of Western Australia. (2018). *Policy Frameworks*. Retrieved from https://ww2.health.wa.gov.au/About-us/Policy-Frameworks.

Government of Western Australia. (2018). *Sustainable Health Review: Interim Report to the Western Australian Government*. Retrieved from https://ww2.health.wa.gov.au/Improving-WA-Health/Sustainable-health-review/Interim-report.

Gowlland, R. W. (1981). *Troubled Asylum: The History of the ... Royal Derwent Hospital*. New Norfolk: Gowlland.

GP Psychiatry Support Line. (2020). *Helping GPs Manage the Care of Mental Health Consumers*. Retrieved from www.gpsupport.org.au.

Grace, F. C., Meurk, C. S., Head, B. W., Hall, W. D., Harris, M. G., & Whiteford, H. A. (2017). An analysis of policy success and failure in formal evaluations of Australia's national mental health strategy (1992-2012). *BMC Health Services Research, 17*(1), 374.

Grana, R. A., Popova, L., & Ling, P. M. (2014). A longitudinal analysis of electronic cigarette use and smoking cessation. *JAMA Internal Medicine, 174*(5), 812-813.

Grant, B. F., Chou, S. P., Goldstein, R. B., Huang, B., Stinson, F. S., Saha, T. D., . . . Pickering, R. P. (2008). Prevalence, correlates, disability, and comorbidity of DSM-IV borderline personality disorder: Results from the Wave 2 National Epidemiologic Survey on Alcohol and Related Conditions. *J Clin Psychiatry, 69*(4), 533.

Grant, J. E., Potenza, M. N., Weinstein, A., & Gorelick, D. A. (2010). Introduction to behavioral addictions. *American Journal of Drug and Alcohol Abuse, 36*(5), 233-241.

Gray, B., Robinson, C., & Seddon, D. (2008). Invisible children: Young carers of parents with mental health problems– the perspectives of professionals. *Child and Adolescent Mental Health, 13*(4), 169-172.

Gray, B., Robinson, C., Seddon, D., & Roberts, A. (2008). 'Confidentiality smokescreens' and carers for people with mental health problems: The perspectives of professionals. *Health & Social Care in the Community, 16*(4), 378-387.

Gray, R., Bressington, D., Ivanecka, A., Hardy, S., Jones, M., Schulz, M., . . . Chien, W. T. (2016). Is adherence therapy an effective adjunct treatment for patients with schizophrenia spectrum disorders? A systematic review and meta-analysis. *BMC Psychiatry, 16*.

Greatbatch, D., Luff, P., Heath, C., & Campion, P. (1993). Interpersonal-Communication and Human-Computer Interaction: An Examination of the Use of Computers in Medical Consultations. *Interacting with Computers, 5*(2), 193-216.

Green, A. C., Hunt, C., & Stain, H. J. (2012). The delay between symptom onset and seeking professional treatment for anxiety and depressive disorders in a rural Australian sample. *Social Psychiatry and Psychiatric Epidemiology, 47*(9), 1475-1487.

Greenhalgh, T. (2007). *Primary Health Care: Theory and Practice*. Blackwell Publishing.

Greenspan, S. (1999). What is meant by mental retardation? *International Review of Psychiatry, 11*(1), 6-18.

Greer, J., Halgin, R., & Harvey, E. (2004). Global versus specific symptom attributions: Predicting the recognition and treatment of psychological distress in primary care. *J Psychosom Res, 57*(6), 521-527.

Grenyer, B. F., Ng, F. Y., Townsend, M. L., & Rao, S. (2017). Personality disorder: A mental health priority area. *Australian & New Zealand Journal of Psychiatry, 51*(9), 872-875.

Grey, F., & O'Hagan, M. (2015). *The Effectiveness of Services Led or Run by Consumers in Mental Health: Rapid Review of Evidence for Recovery-Oriented Outcomes: An Evidence Check Rapid Review Brokered by the Sax Institute*. Retrieved from www.saxinstitute.org.au.

Griffith University NCCARF. (2020). *National Climate Change Adaptation Research Facility*. Retrieved from www.nccarf.edu.au/publications/public-risk-perceptions-final.

Griffiths, M. (2000). Does internet and computer 'addiction' exist? Some case study evidence. *CyberPsychology & Behavior, 3*, 211-218.

Griffiths, M., Kuss, D., & Pontes, H. (2016). A brief overview of internet gaming disorder and its treatment. *Australian Clinical Psychologist, 2*, 1-12.

Grimm, V., Berger, U., Deangelis, D. L., Polhill, J. G., Giske, J., & Railsback, S. F. (2010). The ODD protocol: A review and first update. *Ecological Modelling, 221*(23), 2760-2768.

Grimmer-Somers, K., Lekkas, P., Nyland, L., Young, A., & Kumar, S. (2007). Perspectives on research evidence and clinical practice: A survey of Australian physiotherapists. *Physiotherapy Research, 12*(3), 147-161.

Grisham, J. R., Frost, R. O., Steketee, G., Kim, H. J., & Hood, S. (2006). Age of onset of compulsive hoarding. *J Anxiety Disord, 20*(5), 675-686.

Guba, E. G., & Lincoln, Y. S. (1989). *Fourth Generation Evaluation*. Newbury Park: Sage.

Guba, E. G., & Lincoln, Y. S. (1994). Competing paradigms in qualitative research. In N. K. Denzin & Y. S. Lincoln (eds.), *Handbook of Qualitative Research*. SAGE Publications.

Guidano, V. F., & Liotti, G. (1986). *Cognitive Processes and Emotional Disorders: A Structural Approach to Psychotherapy*: Guilford Publications.

Gulbinat, W., Manderscheid, R., Baingana, F., Jenkins, R., Khandelwal, S., Levav, I., . . . Whiteford, H. (2004). The International Consortium on Mental Health Policy and Services: Objectives, design and project implementation. *International Review of Psychiatry, 16*(1-2), 5-17.

Gull, W.W.1874 Anorexia Nervosa (apesia hysterica, anorexia hysteria). Transactions of the Clinical Society of London 7, 22-28.

Gumley, A., Bradstreet, S., Ainsworth, J., Allan, S., Álvarez-Jimenez, M., Aucott, L., ... Gleeson, G. (2020). Early Signs Monitoring to Prevent Relapse in Psychosis and Promote Well-Being, Engagement, and Recovery: Protocol for a Feasibility Cluster Randomized Controlled Trial Harnessing Mobile Phone Technology Blended With Peer Support. *JMIR Research Protocols*, 9(1) e15058.

Gumley, A., Braehler, C., Laithwaite, H., MacBeth, A., & Gilbert, P. (2010). A compassion focused model of recovery after psychosis. *International Journal of Cognitive Therapy, 3*, 186-201.

Gumley, A., O'Grady, M., McNay, L., Reily, J., Power, K., & Norrie, J. (2003). Early intervention for relapse in schizophrenia: Results of a 12-month randomized controlled trial of cognitive behavioural therapy. *Psychol Med, 33*, 419-431.

Gunderson, J. G. (2001). *Borderline Personality Disorder: A Clinical Guide*. Arlington: American Psychiatric Association.

Gunderson, J. G., & Ridolfi, M. E. (2001). Borderline personality disorder: Suicidality and self-mutilation. *Annals of the New York Academy of Sciences, 932*(1), 61-77.

Gunderson, J. G., & Ronningstam, E. (2001). Differentiating antisocial and narcissistic personality disorders. *Journal of Personality Disorders, 15*(2), 103-109.

Gunderson, J. G., Stout, R. L., McGlashan, T. H., Shea, M. T., Morey, L. C., Grilo, C. M., . . . Sanislow, C. (2011). Ten-year course of borderline personality disorder: Psychopathology and function from the Collaborative Longitudinal Personality Disorders study. *Archives of General Psychiatry, 68*(8), 827-837.

Gunn, J., Palmer, V., Naccarella, L., Kokanović, R., Pope, C., Lathlean, J., & Stange, K. (2008). The promise and pitfalls of generalism in achieving the Alma-Ata vision of health for all. *Med J Aust, 189*, 110-112.

Gunn, J. M., Ayton, D. R., Densley, K., Pallant, J. F., Chondros, P., Herrman, H. E., & Dowrick, C. F. (2012). The association between chronic illness, multimorbidity and depressive symptoms in an Australian primary care cohort. *Social Psychiatry and Psychiatric Epidemiology, 47*(2), 175-184.

Guo, D., Kleinstauber, M., Johnson, M. H., & Sundram, F. (2019). Evaluating commonalities across medically unexplained symptoms. *International Journal of Environmental Research and Public Health, 16*(5).

Guthrie, E., Creed, F., Dawson, D., & Tomenson, B. (1991). A controlled trial of psychological treatment for the irritable bowel syndrome. *Gastroenterology, 100*(2), 450-457.

Guyatt, G. H., Meade, M. O., Jaeschke, R. Z., Cook, D. J., & Haynes, R. B. (2000). Practitioners of evidence based care. Not all clinicians need to appraise evidence from scratch but all need some skills. *BMJ, 320*(7240), 954-955.

Gynther, B., Charlson, F., Obrecht, K., Waller, M., Santomauro, D., Whiteford, H., & Hunter, E. (2019). The epidemiology of psychosis in Indigenous populations in Cape York and the Torres Strait. *EClinicalMedicine, 10*, 68.

Gyollai, A., Griffiths, M. D., Barta, C., Vereczkei, A., Urban, R., Kun, B., . . . Demetrovics, Z. (2014). The genetics of problem and pathological gambling: A systematic review. *Current Pharmaceutical Design, 20*(25), 3993-3999.

Haagsma, M. C., Pieterse, M. E., & Peters, O. (2012). The prevalence of problematic video gamers in The Netherlands. *Cyberpsychology Behavior and Social Networking, 15*(3), 162-168.

Haber, P., Lintzeris, N., Proude, E., & Lopatko, O. (2009). Guidelines for the treatment of alcohol problems. Retrieved from www.drugsandalcohol.ie/20201/1/Gudelines_for_treatment_of_alcohol_problems.pdf.

Habermas, T. (1989). The psychiatric history of anorexia nervosa and bulimia nervosa: Weight concerns and bulimic symptoms in early case reports. *International Journal of Eating Disorders, 8*(3), 259-273.

Hackett, M. L., Anderson, C. S., House, A., & Xia, J. (2008). Interventions for treating depression after stroke. *Cochrane Database of Systematic Reviews*, (4), CD003437-CD003437, https://doi.org/10.1002/14651858.CD003437.pub3.

Hackett, M. L., Anderson, C. S., & House, A. O. (2005). Management of depression after stroke: A systematic review of pharmacological therapies. *Stroke, 36*(5), 1092-1097.

Hagberg, B., & Kyllerman, M. (1983). Epidemiology of mental retardation: A Swedish survey. *Brain Dev, 5*, 441 449.

Hagman, J., Gralla, J., Sigel, E., Ellert, S., Dodge, M., Gardner, R., . . . Wamboldt, M. Z. (2011). A double-blind, placebo-controlled study of risperidone for the treatment of adolescents and young adults with anorexia nervosa: A pilot study. *J Am Acad Child Adolesc Psychiatry, 50*(9), 915-924.

Hales, R. E., Yudofsky, S. C., & Gabbard, G. O. (2010). *American Psychiatric Publishing Textbook of Psychiatry* (3rd ed.). Arlington, VA: American Psychiatric Pub.

Hall, A. (2013). Enabling Risk to Aid Recovery. In A. Hall, M. Wren, & S. Kirby (eds.), *Care Planning in Mental Health: Promoting Recovery* (pp. 248). Wiley.

Hall, W. D., & Mattick, R. P. (2007). Clinical update: Codeine maintenance in opioid dependence. *The Lancet, 370*(9587), 550-552.

Halldorsson, B., & Salkovskis, P. M. (2017). Why do people with OCD and health anxiety seek reassurance excessively? An investigation of differences and similarities in function. *Cognitive Therapy and Research, 41*(4), 619-631.

Haller, H., Cramer, H., Lauche, R., & Dobos, G. (2015). Somatoform disorders and medically unexplained symptoms in primary care: A systematic review and meta-analysis of prevalence. *Deutsches Arzteblatt International, 112*(16), 279-287.

Hambridge, J. A., & Rosen, A. (1994). Assertive community treatment for the seriously mentally ill in suburban Sydney: A programme description and evaluation. *Australian and New Zealand Journal of Psychiatry, 28*, 438-445.

Hamera, E., & Brown, C. E. (2000). Developing a context-based performance measure for persons with schizophrenia: The test of grocery shopping skills. *American Journal of Occupational Therapy, 54*(1), 20-25.

Hamilton, B., Bichara, E., Roper, C., & Easton, C. (2012). *Gaining Strength: Consumers' Experiences of Case Management with the Strengths Model*. Melbourne, St Vincent's Mental Health.

Hamilton, M. P., Hetrick, S. E., Mihalopoulos, C., Baker, D., Browne, V., Chanen, A. M., . . . McGorry, P. D. (2017a). Identifying attributes of care that may improve cost-effectiveness in the youth mental health service system. *Medical Journal of Australia, 207*(10), S27-s37.

Hamilton, M. P., Hetrick, S. E., Mihalopoulos, C., Baker, D., Browne, V., Chanen, A. M., . . . McGorry, P. D. (2017b). Targeting mental health care attributes by diagnosis and clinical stage: The views of youth mental health clinicians. *Medical Journal of Australia, 207*(10), S19-S26.

Hammen, C. (1992). Cognitive, life stress, and interpersonal approaches to a developmental psychopathology model of depression. *Dev Psychopathol, 4*(1), 189-206.

Hampton, R., & Toombs, M. (2013). *Indigenous Australians and Health*. Melbourne: Oxford University Press.

Hamrin, V., Gray Deering, C., & Scahill, L. (2008). Mental Health Assessment of children and adolescents. In M. A. Boyd (ed.), *Psychiatric Nursing: Contemporary Practice* (pp. 596-816). Wolters Kluwer Health/Lippincott Williams & Wilkins.

Han, J. H., Wilson, A., & Ely, E. W. (2010). Delirium in the older emergency department patient: A quiet epidemic. *Emergency Medicine Clinics of North America, 28*(3), 611-+.

Hancock, N., Honey, A., & Bundy, A. C. (2015). Sources of meaning derived from occupational engagement for people recovering from mental illness. *British Journal of Occupational Therapy, 78*(8), 508-515.

Hanlon, P., Carlisle, S., Hannah, M., Lyon, A., & Reilly, D. (2012). A perspective on the future public health: An integrative and ecological framework. *Perspectives in Public Health, 132*(6), 313-319.

Hannigan, B., Simpson, A., Coffey, M., Barlow, S., & Jones, A. (2018). Care coordination as imagined, care coordination as done: Findings from a cross-national mental health systems study. *International Journal of Integrated Care, 18*(3).

Hansen, M., Andersen, T. E., Armour, C., Elklit, A., Palic, S., & Mackrill, T. (2010). PTSD-8: A short PTSD inventory. *Clinical Practice & Epidemiology in Mental Health, 6*, 101-108.

Happell, B., Bennetts, W., Harris, S., Platania-Phung, C., Tohotoa, J., Byrne, L., & Wynaden, D. (2015). Lived experience in teaching mental health nursing: Issues of fear and power. *International Journal of Mental Health Nursing, 24*(1), 19-27.

Happell, B., Curtis, J., Banfield, M., Goss, J., Niyonsenga, T., Watkins, A., . . . Stanton, R. (2018). Improving the cardiometabolic health of people with psychosis: A protocol for a randomised controlled trial of the Physical Health Nurse Consultant service. *Contemporary Clinical Trials, 73*, 75-80.

Happell, B., Ewart, S. B., Bocking, J., Platania-Phung, C., & Stanton, R. (2016). 'That red flag on your file': Misinterpreting physical symptoms as mental illness. *Journal of Clinical Nursing, 25*(19-20), 2933-2944.

Happell, B., Ewart, S. B., Platania-Phung, C., Bocking, J., Griffiths, K., Scholz, B., & Stanton, R. (2016). Embedding a physical health nurse consultant within mental health services: Consumers' perspectives. *International Journal of Mental Health Nursing, 25*(4), 377-384.

Happell, B., Gordon, S., Bocking, J., Ellis, P., Roper, C., Liggins, J., . . . Platania-Phung, C. (2018a). 'Chipping away': Non-consumer researcher perspectives on barriers to collaborating with consumers in mental health research. *Journal of Mental Health*, 1-7.

Happell, B., Gordon, S., Bocking, J., Ellis, P., Roper, C., Liggins, J., . . . Platania-Phung, C. (2018b). Turning the tables: Power relations between consumer researchers and other mental health researchers. *Issues in Mental Health Nursing, 39*(8).

Happell, B., Platania-Phung, C., Gaskin, C., & Stanton, R. (2016). Use of an electronic metabolic monitoring form in a mental health service: A retrospective file audit. *BMC Psychiatry, 16*(1), 109.

Happell, B., Platania-Phung, C., Watkins, A., Scholz, B., Curtis, J., Goss, J., . . . Stanton, R. (2019). Developing an evidence-based specialist nursing role to improve the physical health care of people with mental illness. *Issues in Mental Health Nursing, 40*(10), 832-838.

Happell, B., Platania-Phung, C., Webster, S., McKenna, B., Millar, F., Stanton, R., . . . Scott, D. (2015). Applying the World Health Organization Mental Health Action Plan to evaluate policy on addressing co-occurrence of physical and mental illnesses in Australia. *Australian Health Review, 39*(4), 370–378.

Happell, B., & Roper, C. (2006). The myth of representation: The case for consumer leadership. *Australian e-Journal for the Advancement of Mental Health (AeJAMH), 5*(3), 177-184.

Happell, B., & Roper, C. (2009). Promoting genuine consumer participation in mental health education: A consumer academic role. *Nurse Education Today, 29*(6), 575–579.

Happell, B., & Scholz, B. (2018). Doing what we can, but knowing our place: Being an ally to promote consumer leadership in mental health. *International Journal of Mental Health Nursing, 27*(1), 440–447.

Happell, B., Stanton, R., Hoey, W., & Scott, D. (2015). Reduced ambivalence to the role of the cardiometabolic health nurse following a 6-month trial. *Perspectives in Psychiatric Care, 51*(2), 80–85.

Happell, B., Stanton, R., Platania-Phung, C., McKenna, B., & Scott, D. (2014). The cardiometabolic health nurse: Physical health behaviour outcomes from a randomised controlled trial. *Issues in Mental Health Nursing, 35*(10), 768–775.

Happell, B., Wilson, K., Platania-Phung, C., & Stanton, R. (2016). Physical health nurse consultant role to improve physical health in mental health services: A carer's perspective. *International Journal of Mental Health Nursing, 25*(3), 243–250.

Happell, B., Wilson, K., Platania-Phung, C., & Stanton, R. (2017). Filling the gaps and finding our way: Family carers navigating the healthcare system to access physical health services for the people they care for. *Journal of Clinical Nursing, 26*(13/14), 1917-1926.

Hardaker, L., Halcomb, E., Griffiths, R., Bolzan, N., & Arblaster, K. (2011). A survey of 63 Australian occupational therapists working in youth mental health. *Occupational Therapy in Mental Health, 27*(2), 140–154.

Hare, R. D., & Neumann, C. S. (2005). Structural models of psychopathy. *Current Psychiatry Reports, 7*(1), 57–64.

Harper, D., & Speed, E. (2012). Uncovering recovery: The resistible rise of recovery and resilience. *Studies in Social Justice, 6*(1), 8–25.

Harris, A., Chen, W., Jones, S., Hulme, M., Burgess, P., & Sara, G. (2019). Community treatment orders increase community care and delay readmission while in force: Results from a large population-based study. *Australian & New Zealand Journal of Psychiatry, 53*(3), 228–235.

Harris, M., & Fallot, R. D. (2001). Ensivioning a trauma-informed service system: a vital paradigm shift. New directions for mental health services, 89(Spring 2001), 3-22.Harrison, P. J. (1997). Schizophrenia: A disorder of neurodevelopment? *Current Opinion in Neurobiology, 7*(2), 285–289.

Harrison, P. L., & Oakland, T. (2015). *Adaptive Behavior Assessment System: Third Edition (ABAS-3)*. WPS.

Hart, C. R., Berry, H. L., & Tonna, A. M. (2011). Improving the mental health of rural New South Wales communities facing drought and other adversities. *Australian Journal of Rural Health, 19*(5), 231–238.

Hart, G., Panayi, M. C., Harris, J. A., & Westbrook, R. F. (2014). Benzodiazepine treatment can impair or spare extinction, depending on when it is given. *Behav Res Ther, 56*, 22-29.

Hart, W., & Goenka, S. N. (1987). *The Art of Living.* Onalaska: Pariyatti Publishing.

Hartmann, J. A., Nelson, B., Ratheesh, A., Treen, D., & McGorry, P. D. (2019). At-risk studies and clinical antecedents of psychosis, bipolar disorder and depression: A scoping review in the context of clinical staging. *Psychol Med, 49*(2), 177-189.

Hartmann, P., & Bräunling, S. (2007). Finding strength together: The Berlin Runaway House. In P. Stastny, P. Lehmann, & V. Aderhold (eds.), *Alternatives Beyond Psychiatry* (pp. 431). Peter Lehmann Publishing.

Harvey, C. (2018). Family psychoeducation for people living with schizophrenia and their families. *BJPsych Advances, 24*(1), 9-19.

Harvey, C., Brophy, L., Tibble, H., Killaspy, H., Spittal, M. J., Hamilton, B., . . . Fletcher, J. (2019). Prevention and recovery care services in Australia: Developing a state-wide typology of a subacute residential mental health service model. *Frontiers in Psychiatry, 10*, 383–383.

Harvey, C., Killaspy, H., Martino, S., & Johnson, S. (2012). Implementation of assertive community treatment in Australia: Model fidelity, patient characteristics and staff experiences. *Community Mental Health Journal, 48*(5), 652–661.

Harvey, C., Killaspy, H., Martino, S., White, S., Priebe, S., Wright, C., & Johnson, S. (2011). A comparison of the implementation of assertive community treatment in Melbourne, Australia and London, England. *Epidemiol Psychiatr Sci, 20*(2), 151-161.

Harvey, C., & O'Hanlon, B. (2013). Family psycho-education for people with schizophrenia and other psychotic disorders and their families. *Aust N Z J Psychiatry, 47*(6), 516–520.

Harvey, S. B., Deady, M., Wang, M.-J., Mykletun, A., Butterworth, P., Christensen, H., & Mitchell, P. B. (2017). Is the prevalence of mental illness increasing in Australia? Evidence from national health surveys and administrative data, 2001-2014. *Medical Journal of Australia, 206*(11), 490–493.

Harvey, S. B., Joyce, S., Tan, L., Johnson, A., Nguyen, H., Modini, M., & Groth, M. (2014). *Developing A Mentally Healthy Workplace: A Review of the Literature. A Report for the National Mental Health Commission and the Mentally Healthy Workplace Alliance*. Retrieved from www.headsup.org.au/docs/default-source/resources/developing-a-mentally-healthy-workplace_final-november-2014.pdf?sfvrsn=8.

Hasin, D. S., & Grant, B. F. (2015). The National Epidemiologic Survey on Alcohol and Related Conditions (NESARC) Waves 1 and 2: Review and summary of findings. *Soc Psychiatry Psychiatr Epidemiol, 50*(11), 1609-1640.

Hauser, M., Lautenschlager, M., Gudlowski, Y., Ozgurdal, S., Witthaus, H., Bechdolf, A., . . . Juckel, G. (2009). Psychoeducation with patients at-risk for schizophrenia: An exploratory pilot study. *Patient Education and Counseling, 76*(1), 138-142.

Hawe, P. (2009). *Community Recovery After the February 2009 Victorian Bushfires: An Evidence Check Rapid Review Brokered by the Sax Institute*. Retrieved from www.saxinstitute.org.au.

Hay, P., Chinn, D., Forbes, D., Madden, S., Newton, R., Sugenor, L., . . . Ward, W. (2014). Royal Australian and New Zealand College of Psychiatrists clinical practice guidelines for the treatment of eating disorders. *Aust N Z J Psychiatry, 48*(11), 977-1008.

Hay, P., Mitchison, D., Collado, A. E. L., González-Chica, D. A., Stocks, N., & Touyz, S. (2017). Burden and health-related quality of life of eating disorders, including Avoidant/Restrictive Food Intake Disorder (ARFID), in the Australian population. *Journal of Eating Disorders, 5*, 21-21.

Hay, P., & Sachdev, P. (2011). Brain dysfunction in anorexia nervosa: Cause or consequence of under-nutrition? *Curr Opin Psychiatry, 24*(3), 251-256.

Hay, P., Touyz, S., Arcelus, J., Pike, K., Attia, E., Crosby, R. D., . . . Meyer, C. (2018). A randomized controlled trial of the compuLsive Exercise Activity TheraPy (LEAP): A new approach to compulsive exercise in anorexia nervosa. *International Journal of Eating Disorders, 51*(8), 999–1004.

Hay, P. J., & Claudino, A. d. M. (2010). Evidence-based treatment for the eating disorders. In A. W. Stewart (ed.), *The Oxford Handbook of Eating Disorders* (pp. 452–479). New York: Oxford University Press.

Hay, P. J., Loukas, A., & Philpott, H. (2005). Prevalence and characteristics of men with eating disorders in primary care: How do they compare to women and what features may aid in identification? *Primary Care & Community Psychiatry, 10*(1), 1–6.

Hayes, K., Blashki, G., Wiseman, J., Burke, S., & Reifels, L. (2018). Climate change and mental health: Risks, impacts and priority actions. *International Journal of Mental Health Systems, 12*.

Hayes, L., Hawthorne, G., Farhall, J., O'Hanlon, B., & Harvey, C. (2015). Quality of life and social isolation among caregivers of adults with schizophrenia: Policy and outcomes. *Community Mental Health Journal, 51*(5), 591–597.

Hayes, S. C. (2002). Buddhism and acceptance and commitment therapy. *Cognitive and Behavioral Practice, 9*, 58–66.

Hayes, S. C. (2016). Acceptance and commitment therapy, relational frame theory, and the third wave of behavioral and cognitive therapies: Republished article. *Behavior Therapy, 47*(6), 869–885.

Hayes, S. C., Barnes-Holmes, D., & Roche, B. (eds.). (2001). *Relational Frame Theory: A Post-Skinnerian Account of Human Language and Cognition*. New York: Kluwer Academic/Plenum.

Hayes, S. C., Luoma, J. B., Bond, F. W., Masuda, A., & Lillis, J. (2006). Acceptance and commitment therapy: Model, processes and outcomes. *Psychology Faculty Publications, 44*, 1–25.

Hayes, S. C., Strosahl, K. D., & Wilson, K. G. (2012). *Acceptance and Commitment Therapy: The Process and Practice of Mindful Change*. (2nd ed.). New York: Guilford Press.

Hayley, J. (1987). *Problem Solving Therapy* (2nd ed.). San Francisco: Jossey-Bass.

Haynes, R. B., Devereaux, P. J., & Guyatt, G. H. (2002). Clinical expertise in the era of evidence-based medicine and patient choice. *Evidence-Based Medicine, 7*(2), 36–38.

Hayward, M., Strauss, C., & Kingdon, D. (2018). *Overcoming Distressing Voices: A Self-Help Guide Using Cognitive Behavioural Techniques* (2nd ed.). London: Robinson.

Hazell, C. M., Hayward, M., Cavanagh, K., & Strauss, C. (2016). A systematic review and meta-analysis of low intensity CBT for psychosis. *Clinical Psychology Review, 45*, 183–192.

headspace. (2013). *headspace Psychosocial Assessment for Young People*. headspace National Youth Mental Health Foundation.

headspace. (2017). *Annual Report 2016–17*. headspace National Youth Mental Health Foundation.

headspace. (2019). *Increasing Demand in Youth Mental Health: A Rising Tide of Need*. headspace National Youth Mental Health Foundation.

Healing Foundation. (2019). *A Theory of Change for Healing*. Retrieved from https://healingfoundation.org.au/app/uploads/2019/04/HF_Theory_of_Change_A4_Mar2019_WEB.pdf.

Health Workforce Australia. (2014). *Mental health peer workforce literature scan*. Adelaide: Health Workforce Australia.

Heard, H. L., & Linehan, M. M. (1994). Dialectical behavior therapy: An integrative approach to the treatment of borderline personality disorder. *Journal of Psychotherapy Integration, 4*(1), 55–82.

Hegarty, K., Forsdike-Young, K., Tarzia, L., Schweitzer, R., & Vlais, R. (2016). Identifying and responding to men who use violence in their intimate relationships. *Australian Family Physician, 45*(4), 176.

Hegarty, K., & O'Doherty, L. (2011). Intimate partner violence: Identification and response in general practice. *Australian Family Physician, 40*(11), 852.

Heimberg, R. G., & Magee, L. (2014). Social anxiety disorder. In D. H. Barlow (ed.), *Clinical Handbook of Psychological Disorders* (5th ed., pp. 114–154). New York: The Guilford Press.

Hemming, K., Taljaard, M., McKenzie, J. E., Hooper, R., Copas, A., Thompson, J. A., . . . Grimshaw, J. M. (2018). Reporting of stepped wedge cluster randomised trials: Extension of the CONSORT 2010 statement with explanation and elaboration. *BMJ, 363*, k1614.

Henderson, C., Swanson, J. W., Szmukler, G., Thornicroft, G., & Zinkler, M. (2008). A Typology of Advance Statements in Mental Health Care. *Psychiatric Services, 59*(1), 63–71.

Hennessy, S., & Cocoman, A. M. (2018). What is the impact of targeted health education for mental health nurses in the provision of physical health care? An integrated literature review. *Issues in Mental Health Nursing, 39*(8), 700–706.

Henningsen, P., Zipfel, S., & Herzog, W. (2007). Management of functional somatic syndromes. *Lancet, 369*(9565), 946–955.

Henningsen, P., Zipfel, S., Sattel, H., & Creed, F. (2018). Management of functional somatic syndromes and bodily distress. *Psychother Psychosom, 87*(1), 12–31.

Henry, K. A., & Cohen, C. I. (1983). The role of labeling processes in diagnosing borderline personality disorder. *The American Journal of Psychiatry*, 140(11), 1527–1529.

Herrman, H., Trauer, T., & Warnock, J. (2002). The roles and relationships of psychiatrists and other service providers in mental health services. *Australian and New Zealand Journal of Psychiatry*, 36(1), 75–80.

Herman, J. L. (2015). *Trauma and Recovery: The Aftermath of Violence: From Domestic Abuse to Political Terror*. Basic Books.

Hernandez-Martinez, C., Canals Sans, J., & Fernandez-Ballart, J. (2011). Parents perceptions of their neonates and their relation to infant development. *Child: Care, health and development, 37*(4), 484–492.

Herrman, H., Humphreys, C., Halperin, S., Monson, K., Harvey, C., Mihalopoulos, C., . . . Moeller-Saxone, K. (2016). A controlled trial of implementing a complex mental health intervention for carers of vulnerable young people living in out-of-home care: The ripple project. *BMC Psychiatry, 16*(1), 436–436.

Herrman, H., Trauer, T., & Warnock, J. (2002). The roles and relationships of psychiatrists and other service providers in mental health services. *Australian and New Zealand Journal of Psychiatry, 36*(1), 75–80.

Hershberger, S. L., & Bogaert, A. F. (2005). Male and female sexual orientation differences in gambling. *Personality and Individual Differences, 38*(6), 1401–1411.

Herston Imaging Research Facility (HIRF). (2020). *Providing Researchers Unprecedented Access to High Quality Imaging Equipment*. Retrieved from www.hirf.com.au/main.

Hetrick, S. E., Bailey, A. P., Smith, K. E., Malla, A., Mathias, S., Singh, S. P., . . . McGorry, P. D. (2017). Integrated (one-stop shop) youth health care: Best available evidence and future directions. *Medical Journal of Australia, 207*(10), S5–18.

Hetrick, S. E., Cox, G. R., Fisher, C. A., Bhar, S. S., Rice, S. M., Davey, C. G., & Parker, A. G. (2015). Back to basics: Could behavioural therapy be a good treatment option for youth depression? A critical review. *Early Intervention in Psychiatry, 9*(2), 93–99.

Hetrick, S. E., Simmons, M., Thompson, A., & Parker, A. G. (2011). What are specialist mental health clinician attitudes to guideline recommendations for the treatment of depression in young people? *Australian & New Zealand Journal of Psychiatry, 45*(11), 993–1001.

Hick, S. F., Bien, T., & Segal, Z. V. (2008). *Mindfulness and the Therapeutic Relationship*. Guilford Publications.

Hickie, I., & Groom, G. (2004). Surveying Perceptions of the Progress of National Mental Health Reform. *Australasian Psychiatry, 12*(2), 123–125.

Hickie, I. B., Fogarty, A. S., Davenport, T. A., Luscombe, G. M., & Burns, J. (2007). Responding to experiences of young people with common mental health problems attending Australian general practice. *Medical Journal of Australia, 187*(7), S47.

Hiday, V. A. (2006). Putting community risk in perspective: A look at correlations, causes and controls. *International Journal of Law and Psychiatry, 29*(4), 316–331.

Higgs, J., Jensen, G., Loftus, S., & Christensen, N. (2018). Clinical reasoning in medicine. In J. Higgs, G. Jensen, S. Loftus, & N. Christensen (eds.), *Clinical Reasoning in the Health Professions* (pp. 532). Elsevier.

Higgs, J., Jensen, G., Loftus, S., & Christensen, N. (2018). *Clinical Reasoning in the Health Professions*. Elsevier.

Highet, N. J., Gemmill, A. W., & Milgrom, J. (2011). Depression in the prenatal period: Awareness, attitudes and knowledge in the Australian population. *Aust N Z J Psychiatry, 45*(3), 223–231.

Highet, N. J., Hickie, I. B., & Davenport, T. A. (2002). Monitoring awareness of and attitudes to depression in Australia. *Medical Journal of Australia, 176*, S63–68.

Hilferty, F., Cassells, R., Muir, K., Duncan, A., Christensen, D., Mitrou, F., . . . Katz, I. (2015). *Is headspace Making a Difference to Young People's Lives? Final Report of the Independent Evaluation of the headspace Program*. Sydney: Social Policy Research Centre.

Hing, N., & Breen, H. (2014). *Indigenous Australians and Gambling (AGRC Discussion Paper No. 2)*. Melbourne: Australian Gambling Research Centre.

Hinton, R., Kavanagh, D. J., Barclay, L., Chenhall, R., & Nagel, T. (2015). Developing a best practice pathway to support improvements in Indigenous Australians' mental health and well-being: A qualitative study. *BMJ Open, 5*(8), e007938.

Hitch, D. (2012). Better access to mental health: Mapping the evidence supporting participation in meaningful occupations. *Advances in Mental Health, 10*(2), 181–189.

Hjelmgren, J., Berggren, F., & Andersson, F. (2001). Health economic guidelines: Similarities, differences and some implications. *Value Health, 4*(3), 225–250.

Hochstenbach, R., Buizer-Voskamp, J. E., Vorstman, J. A. S., & Ophoff, R. A. (2011). Genome arrays for the detection of copy number variations in idiopathic mental retardation, idiopathic generalized epilepsy and neuropsychiatric disorders: Lessons for diagnostic workflow and research. *Cytogenetic and genome research, 135*(3–4), 174–202.

Hodge, A., Almeida, O., English, D., Giles, G., & Flicker, L. (2013). Patterns of dietary intake and psychological distress in older Australians: Benefits not just from a Mediterranean diet. *International Psychogeriatrics, 25*(3), 456–466.

Hodgins, D. C., & Makarchuk, K. (2003). Trusting problem gamblers: Reliability and validity of self-reported gambling behavior. *Psychology of Addictive Behaviors, 17*(3), 244–248.

Hodson, S., & McFarlane, A. (2016). Australian veterans: Identification of mental health issues. *Australian Family Physician, 45*(3), 98.

Hoenig, J., & Hamilton, M. W. (1966). The schizophrenic patient in the community and his effect on the household. *International Journal of Social Psychiatry, 12*(3), 165–176.

Hofer, A., & McDonald, M. (2019). Continuity of care: why it matters and what we can do. *Australian Journal of Primary Health*, 25(3), 214–218.

Hoffman, R. E. (2007). A social deafferentation hypothesis for induction of active schizophrenia. *Schizophrenia Bulletin, 33*(5), 1066–1070.

Hoffmann, T. C., Légaré, F., Simmons, M. B., McNamara, K., McCaffery, K., Trevena, L. J., . . . Del Mar, C. B. (2014). Shared decision making: What do clinicians need to know and why should they bother? *Medical Journal of Australia, 201*(1), 35–39.

Hoffnung, M., Hoffnung, R. J., Seifert, K. L., Burton Smith, R., Hine, A., Ward, L., & Quinn, A. (2010). The role of temperament in the contributions of individuals to their development. In A. Thomas & S. Chess (eds.), *Lifespan Development* (1st ed., pp. 839). Australia: John Wiley & Sons.

Hofmann, S. G., Sawyer, A. T., Witt, A. A., & Oh, D. (2010). The effect of mindfulness-based therapy on anxiety and depression: A meta-analytic review. *J Consult Clin Psychol, 78*(2), 169–183.

Holland, C. (2018). *Close the Gap—A Ten-Year Review: The Closing the Gap Strategy and Recommendations for Reset*. Retrieved from www.humanrights.gov.au/our-work/aboriginal-and-torres-strait-islander-social-justice/publications/close-gap-10-year-review.

Hollander, E., DeCaria, C. M., Mari, E., Wong, C. M., Mosovich, S., Grossman, R., & Begaz, T. (1998). Short-term single-blind fluvoxamine treatment of pathological gambling. *American Journal of Psychiatry, 155*(12), 1781–1783.

Hollins, S., & Sinason, V. (2000). Psychotherapy, learning disabilities and trauma: New perspectives. *British Journal of Psychiatry, 176*, 22–36.

Hollon, S. D., & DeRubeis, R. J. (2009). Mediating the effects of cognitive therapy for depression. *Cognitive Behaviour Therapy, 38*(1), 43–47.

Holloway, F., & Carson, J. (2001). Review article case management: An update. *International Journal of Social Psychiatry, 47*(3), 21–31.

Holmbeck, G. N., Devine, K. A., Wasserman, R., Schellinger, K., & Tuminello, E. (2012). *Guides From Developmental Psychology for Therapy with Adolescents* (P. C. Kendall Ed.). New York: Guilford Press.

Holmes, A. (2013). Is risk assessment the new clinical model in public mental health? *Australasian Psychiatry, 21*(6), 541–544.

Holtman, M. C., Frost, J. S., Hammer, D. P., McGuinn, K., & Nunez, L. M. (2011). Interprofessional professionalism: Linking professionalism and interprofessional care. *Journal of Interprofessional Care, 25*(5), 383–385.

Honey, A., Nugent, A., Hancock, N., & Scanlan, J. (2017). 'It's hard work, believe me!': Active efforts to optimise housing by people who live with mental illness and access housing assistance. *Australian Journal of Social Issues, 52*(4), 347–366.

Hood, R. (2012). A critical realist model of complexity for interprofessional working. *Journal of Interprofessional Care, 26*, 6–12.

Horn, S. D., & Gassaway, J. (2007). Practice-based evidence study design for comparative effectiveness research. *Medical Care, 45*(10), S50–S57.

Hornung, W. P., Feldman, R., Klingberg, S., Buchkremer, G., & Reker, T. (1999). Long-term effects of a psychoeducational psychotherapeutic intervention for schizophrenic outpatients and their key-persons: Results of a five-year follow-up. *European Archives of Psychiatry and Clinical Neurosciences, 249*, 162–167.

Horvath, T., Friedman, J., & Meares, R. (1980). Attention in hysteria: A study of Janet's hypothesis by means of habituation and arousal measures. *American Journal of Psychiatry, 137*(2), 217–220.

Horwitz, A. V., & Wakefield, J. C. (2007). *The Loss of Sadness: How Psychiatry Transformed Normal Sorrow into Depressive Disorder*. Oxford University Press.

Hosie, A., Vogl, G., Carden, J., Hoddinott, J., & Lim, S. (2015). *A Way Forward: Equipping Australia's Mental Health System for the Next Generation*. Australia: EY and ReachOut.

Hotopf, M., Churchill, R., & Lewis, G. (1999). Pragmatic randomised controlled trials in psychiatry. *Br J Psychiatry, 175*, 217–223.

Hoult, J. (1986). Community care of the acutely mentally ill. *British Journal of Psychiatry, 149*(2), 137–144.

Hoult, J., Rosen, A., & Reynolds, I. (1984). Community orientated treatment compared to psychiatric hospital orientated treatment. *Social Science & Medicine, 18*(11), 1005–1010.

Howard, R., & Jeste, D. (2011). Late-onset schizophrenia. In D. R. Weinberger & P. Harrison (eds.), *Schizophrenia* (3rd ed., pp. 47–61). Oxford: Wiley-Blackwell.

Howgego, I. M., Yellowlees, P., Owen, C., Meldrum, L., & Dark, F. (2003). The therapeutic alliance: The key to effective patient outcome? A descriptive review of the evidence in community mental health case management. *Australian & New Zealand Journal of Psychiatry, 37*(2), 169–183.

Howlin, P., Goode, S., Hutton, J., & Rutter, M. (2004). Adult outcome for children with autism. *J Child Psychol & Psychiat, 45*(2), 212–229.

HSBC. (2018). *Fragile Planet: Scoring Climate Risks Around the World*. Retrieved from www.sustainablefinance.hsbc.com/reports/fragile-planet.

Huang, Y., Kotov, R., De Girolamo, G., Preti, A., Angermeyer, M., Benjet, C., . . . Karam, A. N. (2009). DSM-IV personality disorders in the WHO World Mental Health Surveys. *The British Journal of Psychiatry, 195*(1), 46–53.

Hudson, J. I., Coit, C. E., Lalonde, J. K., & Pope, H. G. (2012). By how much will the proposed new DSM-5 criteria increase the prevalence of binge eating disorder? *International Journal of Eating Disorders, 45*(1), 139–141.

Hudson, J. I., Hiripi, E., Pope, H. G., & Kessler, R. C. (2007). The Prevalence and Correlates of Eating Disorders in the National Comorbidity Survey Replication. *Biological Psychiatry, 61*(3), 348–358.

Hughes, J. R., Stead, L. F., Hartmann-Boyce, J., Cahill, K., & Lancaster, T. (2014). Antidepressants for smoking cessation. *Cochrane Database of Systematic Reviews*(1).

Hughes, K., Corcoran, T., & Slee, R. (2016). Health-inclusive higher education: Listening to students with disabilities or chronic illnesses. *Higher Education Research & Development, 35*(3), 488–501.

Huguelet, P., & Mohr, S. (2009). Religion / Spirituality and Psychosis. In H. Philippe & K. Harold G (eds.), *Religion and Spirituality in Psychiatry* (pp. 65–80). New York: Cambridge University Press.

Huhn, M., Nikolakopoulou, A., & Schneider-Thoma, J. (2019). Comparative efficacy and tolerability of 32 oral antipsychotics for the acute treatment of adults with multi-episode schizophrenia: A systematic review and network meta-analysis. *Lancet, 394*(10202), 918–918.

Human Services Victoria Mental Health Branch. (1994). *Victoria's Mental Health Services: The Framework for Service Delivery*. Melbourne: Human Services Victoria Mental Health Branch.

Humphrey, N., Kalambouka, A., Wigelsworth, M., Lendrum, A., Lennie, C., & Farrell, P. (2010). Cited in Headline Indicators for children's health, development and wellbeing, 2011 (pp. 151). Australian Institute of Health and Welfare.

Hunter, E. (2016). Commentary on Galletly et al. (2016), The Royal Australian and New Zealand College of Psychiatrists clinical practice guidelines for the management of schizophrenia and related disorders. *Australian and New Zealand Journal of Psychiatry, 50*(11), 1105–1106.

Hunter, E., Milroy, H., Brown, N., & Calma, T. (2012). Human rights, health, and Indigenous Australians. In M. Dudley, D. Silove, & F. Gale (eds.), *Mental Health and Human Rights: Vision, Praxis, and Courage* (pp. 448–464). Oxford: Oxford University Press.

Hunter, E. C. M., Baker, D., Phillips, M. L., Sierra, M., & David, A. S. (2005). Cognitive-behaviour therapy for depersonalisation disorder: An open study. *Behav Res Ther, 43*(9), 1121–1130.

Hunter, E. C. M., Phillips, M. L., Chalder, T., Sierra, M. J., & David, A. S. (2003). Depersonalisation disorder: A cognitive-behavioural conceptualisation. *Behav Res Ther, 41*(12), 1451–1467.

Hunter, E. C. M., Sierra, M., & David, A. S. (2004). The epidemiology of depersonalisation and derealisation: A systematic review. *Social Psychiatry and Psychiatric Epidemiology, 39*(1), 9–18.

Huppert, D., & Griffiths, M. (2015). Police Mental Health Partnership project: Police Ambulance Crisis Emergency Response (PACER) model development. *Australasian Psychiatry, 23*(5), 520–523.

Huppert, J. D., Simpson, H. B., Nissenson, K. J., Liebowitz, M. R., & Foa, E. B. (2009). Quality of life and functional impairment in obsessive-compulsive disorder: A comparison of patients with and without comorbidity, patients in remission, and healthy controls. *Depress Anxiety, 26*(1), 39–45.

Hurlbert, D. F., Apt, C., & White, L. C. (1992). An empirical examination into the sexuality of women with borderline personality disorder. *Journal of Sex & Marital Therapy, 18*(3), 231–242.

Hyde, B., Bowles, W., & Pawar, M. (2014). Challenges of recovery-oriented practice in inpatient mental health settings: The potential for social work leadership. *Asia Pacific Journal of Social Work and Development, 24*(1–2), 5–16.

Hyde, Z., Doherty, M., Tilley, M., McCaul, K., Rooney, R., & Jancey, J. (2013). *The First Australian National Trans Mental Health Study: Summary of Results*. Retrieved from https://espace.curtin.edu.au/handle/20.500.11937/55239.

Ibrahim, A. K., Kelly, S. J., Adams, C. E., & Glazebrook, C. (2013). A systematic review of studies of depression prevalence in university students. *Journal of Psychiatric Research, 47*(3), 391–400.

Ibrahim, N., Michail, M., & Callaghan, P. (2014). The strengths based approach as a service delivery model for severe mental illness: A meta-analysis of clinical trials. *BMC Psychiatry, 14*(1).

Idstad, M., Ask, H., & Tambs, K. (2010). Mental disorder and caregiver burden in spouses: The Nord-Trøndelag health study. *BMC Public Health, 10*, 516.

Iervolino, A. C., Perroud, N., Fullana, M. A., Guipponi, M., Cherkas, L., Collier, D. A., & Mataix-Cols, D. (2009). Prevalence and heritability of compulsive hoarding: A twin study. *American Journal of Psychiatry, 166*(10), 1156–1161.

Iglewicz, A., Meeks, T. W., & Jeste, D. V. (2011). New wine in old bottle: Late-life psychosis. *Psychiatric Clinics of North America, 34*(2), 295–+.

IHRA. (2017). *Darlington Statement*. Retrieved from https://ihra.org.au/darlington-statement.

IHRA. (2020). *Intersex Human Rights Australia*. Retrieved from https://ihra.org.au/16601/intersex-numbers.

Illich, I. (1976). *Limits to Medicine: Medical Nemesis: The Expropriation of Health*. London: Marion Boyars.

Independent Hospital Pricing Authority (IHPA). (2017). *Mental Health Care*. Retrieved from www.ihpa.gov.au/what-we-do/mental-health-care.

Independent Hospital Pricing Authority (IHPA). (2020). *Independent Hospital Pricing Authority*. Retrieved from www.ihpa.gov.au.

Independent Mental Health Advocacy. (2020). *New Self-Help Tool for Treatment and Recovery*. Retrieved from www.imha.vic.gov.au/about-us/news/new-self-help-tool-for-treatment-and-recovery.

Indigenous Allied Health Australia (IAHA). (2015; 2019). *Cultural Responsiveness in Action: An IAHA Framework*. Retrieved from https://iaha.com.au.

Ingenhoven, T. J. M. (2015). The place of trauma in the treatment of personality disorders. *European Journal of Psychotraumatology, 6*, 10.3402/ejpt.v3406.27629.

Ingram, R. E., & Luxton, D. D. (2005). Vulnerability-stress models. In B. L. Hankin & J. R. Z. Abela (eds.), *Development of Psychopathology: A Vulnerability-stress Perspective* (pp. 32–46). Thousand Oaks: Sage.

Ingram, R. E., & Price, J. M. (2001). The role of vulnerability in understanding psychopathology. In R. E. Ingram & J. M. Price (eds.), *Vulnerability to Psychopathology: Risk Across the Lifespan*. New York: The Guildford Press.

Inouye, S. K., Westendorp, R. G. J., & Saczynski, J. S. (2014). Delirium in elderly people. *Lancet, 383*(9920), 911–922.

Insel, T. R., & Fenton, W. S. (2005). Psychiatric epidemiology: It's not just about counting anymore. *Archives of General Psychiatry, 62*(6), 590–592.

Insight. (2020). *Mental Health: Developing Aboriginal and Torres Strait Islander Expertise*. Retrieved from https://insight.study.csu.edu.au/mental-health-developing-aboriginal-and-torres-strait-islander-expertise.

Integrated Regional Planning Working Group. (2018). *Joint Regional Planning for Integrated Mental Health and Suicide Prevention Services: A Guide for Local Health Networks (LHNs) and Primary Health Networks (PHNs)*. Retrieved from www.health.gov.au/internet/main/publishing.nsf/Content/68EF6317847840E3CA25832E007FD5E2/$File/Regional%20Planning%20Guide%20-%20master%20at%2023%20October.pdf.

inter voice. (2020). *The International Hearing Voices Network*. Retrieved from www.intervoiceonline.org.

International Panel on Climate Change. (2018). *Global Warming of 1.5°C. An IPCC Special Report on the Impacts of Global Warming of 1.5°C Above Pre-Industrial Levels and Related Global Greenhouse Gas Emission Pathways, in the Context of Strengthening the Global Response to the Threat of Climate Change, Sustainable Development, and Efforts to Eradicate Poverty*. Retrieved from www.ipcc.ch/sr15/faq/faq-chapter-1.

International Society for the Study of Trauma Dissociation. (2011). Guidelines for treating dissociative identity disorder in adults, third revision. *Journal of Trauma & Dissociation, 12*(2), 115–187.

IPCC. (2014). *Climate Change 2014: Synthesis Report. Contribution of Working Groups I, II and III to the Fifth Assessment Report of the Intergovernmental Panel on Climate Change*. Retrieved from www.ipcc.ch/site/assets/uploads/2018/05/SYR_AR5_FINAL_full_wcover.pdf.

Isaacs, A. N., Enticott, J. C., Meadows, G. N., & Inder, B. (2018). Lower income levels in Australia are strongly associated with elevated psychological distress: Implications for healthcare and other policy areas. *Frontiers in Psychiatry, 9*, 536.

Isaacs, A. N., & Sutton, K. (2016). An Aboriginal youth suicide prevention project in rural Victoria. *Advances in Mental Health, 14*(2), 118–125.

Isaacs, A. N., Sutton, K., Dalziel, K., & Maybery, D. (2017). Outcomes of a care coordinated service model for persons with severe and persistent mental illness: A qualitative study. *International Journal of Social Psychiatry, 63*(1), 40–47.

Isenwater, W., Lanham, W., & Thornhill, H. (2002). The College Link Program: Evaluation of a supported education initiative in Great Britain. *Psychiatric Rehabilitation Journal, 26*(1), 43–50.

Ising, H. K., Smit, F., Veling, W., Rietdijk, J., Dragt, S., Klaassen, R. M. C., . . . van der Gaag, M. (2015). Cost-effectiveness of preventing first-episode psychosis in ultra-high-risk subjects: Multi-centre randomized controlled trial. *Psychol Med, 45*(7), 1435–1446.

Issakidis, C., Sanderson, K., Teeson, M., Johnson, S., & Buhrich, N. (1999). Intensive case management in Australia: A randomized controlled trial. *Acta Psychiatr Scand, 99*, 360–367.

Ivbijaro, G., Goldberg, D., Kolkiewicz, L., Edwards, T. M., McReynolds, C., & Svab, I. (2019). Bodily Distress Syndrome (BDS), Bodily Stress Syndrome (BSS) and Health Anxiety in Older Adults. In C. A. de Mendonça Lima & G. Ivbijaro (eds.), *Primary Care Mental Health in Older People: A Global Perspective* (pp. 177–188). Springer International Publishing.

Jablensky, A., McGrath, J., Herrman, H., Castle, D., Gureje, O., Morgan, V. A., . . . on behalf of the Low Prevalence Disorders Study Group. (1999). *People Living with Psychotic Illness: An Australian Study 1997–98. National Survey of Mental Health and Wellbeing: Report 4. National Mental Health Strategy* Retrieved from www.mentalhealth.gov.au/internet/mentalhealth/publishing.nsf/Content/doha-living-psychotic-illness-1.

Jablensky, A., McGrath, J., Herrman, H., Castle, D., Gureje, O., Morgan, V. A., . . . on behalf of the Low Prevalence Disorders Study Group. (2000). Psychotic disorders in urban areas: An overview of the methods and findings of the Study on Low Prevalence Disorders, National Survey of Mental Health and Wellbeing 1996–1998. *Australian and New Zealand Journal of Psychiatry, 34*, 221–236.

Jacob, S., Munro, I., Taylor, B. J., & Griffiths, D. (2017). Mental health recovery: A review of the peer-reviewed published literature. *Collegian, 24*(1), 53–61.

Jami, C. (2016). *Healology*. CreateSpace.

Jamoulle, M. (2015). Quaternary prevention, an answer of family doctors to overmedicalization.(Perspective Report). *International Journal of Health Policy and Management, 4*(2), 61.

Janet, P. (1889). *L'automatisme psychologique*. Paris: Felix Alcan.

Jansen, J. E., Gleeson, J., & Cotton, S. (2015). Towards a better understanding of caregiver distress in early psychosis: A systematic review of the psychological factors involved. *Clinical Psychology Review, 35*, 56–66.

Jansen, J. E., Haahr, U. H., Harder, S., Trauelsen, A. M., Lyse, H.-G., Pedersen, M. B., & Simonsen, E. (2015). Caregiver distress in first-episode psychosis: The role of subjective appraisal, over-involvement and symptomatology. *Social Psychiatry and Psychiatric Epidemiology, 50*(3), 371–378.

Jansen, J. E., Pedersen, M. B., Hastrup, L. H., Haahr, U. H., & Simonsen, E. (2018). Important first encounter: Service user experience of pathways to care and early detection in first-episode psychosis. *Early Intervention in Psychiatry, 12*(2), 169–176.

Janssen, I., Krabbendam, L., Bak, M., Hanssen, M., Vollebergh, W., de Graaf, R., & van Os, J. (2004). Childhood abuse as a risk factor for psychotic experiences. *Acta Psychiatr Scand, 109*(1), 38–45.

Jarrett, R. B., Vittengl, J. R., & Clark, L. A. (2008). Preventing recurrent depression. In M. A. Whisman (ed.), *Adapting Cognitive Therapy for Depression: Managing Complexity and Comorbidity* (pp. 132-156). New York: Guilford Publications.

Jarvis, T., Tebbut, J., & Mattick, R. P. (1995). *Treatment Approaches for Alcohol and Drug Dependence: An Introductory Guide.* Sydney: Wiley & Sons.

Jaspers, K. (1963). *General psychopathology* (J. Hoeing & M. W. Hamilton, Trans.). Manchester: Manchester University Press.

Jeffers, H., & Baker, M. (2016). Continuity of care: Still important in modern-day general practice. *British Journal of General Practice, 66*(649), 396-397.

Jenkins, R., & Minoletti, A. (2013). Promoting mental health: A crucial component of all public policy. In K. Leppo, E. Ollila, S. Peña, M. Wismar, & S. Cook (eds.), *Health in All Policies: Seizing Opportunities, Implementing Policies.* (pp. 163-182). Helsinki: Ministry of Social Affairs and Health.

Jespersen, S., Chong, T., Gray, K., Carrin, D., Morton, L., Robinson, T., & Inglis, S. (2009). Clinical characteristics and patterns of referral to a primary mental health team. *Asia-Pacific Psychiatry, 1*(2), 81-87.

Jesuit Social Services. (2009). *Strong Bonds Building Family Connections.* Retrieved from www.strongbonds.jss.org.au/workers/working/family.html.

Jewell, T., Blessitt, E., Stewart, C., Simic, M., & Eisler, I. (2016). Family therapy for child and adolescent eating disorders: A critical review. *Family Process, 55*(3), 577-594.

Jewell, T., Smith, A., Hoh, B., Ladd, S., Evinger, J., Lamberti, J. S., . . . Salerno, A. J. (2012). Consumer centered family consultation: New York State's recent efforts to include families and consumers as partners in recovery. *American Journal of Psychiatric Rehabilitation, 15*(1), 44–60.

Jimenez, D. E., Bartels, S. J., Cardenas, V., Dhaliwal, S. S., & Alegría, M. (2012). Cultural beliefs and mental health treatment preferences of ethnically diverse older adult consumers in primary care. *The American Journal of Geriatric Psychiatry, 20*(6), 533–542.

Jimenez, M. A. (1997). Gender and psychiatry: Psychiatric conceptions of mental disorders in women, 1960-1994. *Affilia, vol. 12* (no. 2, Summer), pp. 154–175.

Johansson, B. A., Berglund, M., & Lindgren, A. (2006). Efficacy of maintenance treatment with naltrexone for opioid dependence: A meta-analytical review. *Addiction, 101*(4), 491-503.

Johns, L., Jolley, S., Garety, P., Khondoker, M., Fornells-Ambrojo, M., Onwumere, J., . . . Byrne, M. (2019). Improving access to psychological therapies for people with severe mental illness (IAPT-SMI): Lessons from the South London and Maudsley psychosis demonstration site. *Behav Res Ther, 116*, 104-110.

Johnson, B. A., Rosenthal, N., Capece, J. A., Wiegand, F., Mao, L., Beyers, K., . . . Anton, R. F. (2008). Improvement of physical health and quality of life of alcohol-dependent individuals with topiramate treatment: US multisite randomized controlled trial. *Archives of Internal Medicine, 168*(11), 1188-1199.

Johnson, B. A., Rosenthal, N., Capece, J. A., Wiegand, F., Mao, L., Beyers, K., . . . Ciraulo, D. A. (2007). Topiramate for treating alcohol dependence: A randomized controlled trial. *Jama, 298*(14), 1641-1651.

Johnson, C. (2007). Managing mental health issues in general practice. *Australian Family Physician, 36*(4), 202–205.

Johnson, J. G., Cohen, P., Kasen, S., & Brook, J. S. (2006). Dissociative disorders among adults in the community, impaired functioning, and axis I and II comorbidity. *Journal of Psychiatric Research, 40*(2), 131-140.

Johnson, R. L., Floyd, M., Pilling, D., Boyce, M. J., Grove, B., Secker, J., . . . Slade, J. (2009). Service users' perceptions of the effective ingredients in supported employment. *Journal of Mental Health, 18*(2), 121-128.

Johnston, L. D., O'Malley, P. M., Bachman, J. G., Schulenberg, J. E., & Miech, R. A. (2014). *Monitoring the Future National Survey Results on Drug Use, 1975-2013. Volume 2, College Students & Adults Ages 19–55.* Institute for Social Research.

Johnstone, E. C., Owens, D. C., Lawrie, S. M., McIntosh, A. M., & Sharpe, M. D. (2010). *Companion to Psychiatric Studies.* Elsevier Health Sciences.

Johnstone, L., Boyle, M. w., Cromby, J., Dillon, J., Harper, D., Kinderman, P., . . . Read, J. (2018). *The Power Threat Meaning Framework: Towards the Identification of Patterns in Emotional Distress, Unusual Experiences and Troubled or Troubling Behaviour, as an Alternative to Functional Psychiatric Diagnosis.* Retrieved from www.bps.org.uk/PTM-Main.

Jones, B. A., Haycraft, E., Murjan, S., & Arcelus, J. (2016). Body dissatisfaction and disordered eating in trans people: A systematic review of the literature. *Int Rev Psychiatry, 28*(1), 81-94.

Jones, L. (1996). *George III and Changing Views of Madness.* London: Macmillan Press.

Jones, T., Hart, B., & Carpenter, M. (2016). *Intersex: Stories and Statistics from Australia.* Open Book Publishers.

Jorenby, D. E., Leischow, S. J., Nides, M. A., Rennard, S. I., Johnston, J. A., Hughes, A. R., . . . Doan, K. (1999). A controlled trial of sustained-release bupropion, a nicotine patch, or both for smoking cessation. *New England Journal of Medicine, 340*(9), 685-691.

Jørgensen, C. R., Freund, C., Bøye, R., Jordet, H., Andersen, D., & Kjølbye, M. (2013). Outcome of mentalization-based and supportive psychotherapy in patients with borderline personality disorder: A randomized trial. *Acta Psychiatr Scand, 127*(4), 305-317.

Jorm, A. F. (2012). Mental health literacy: Empowering the community to take action for better mental health. *American Psychologist, 67*(3), 231.

Jorm, A. F. (2014). Why hasn't the mental health of Australians improved? The need for a national prevention strategy. *Australian & New Zealand Journal of Psychiatry, 48*(9), 795–801.

Jorm, A. F. (2018). Australia's 'Better Access' scheme: Has it had an impact on population mental health? *Australian & New Zealand Journal of Psychiatry, 52*(11), 1057-1062.

Jorm, A. F. (2019). Impact of Australia's 'Better Access' scheme on population mental health: Response to commentaries. *Australian and New Zealand Journal of Psychiatry, 53*(3), 184-186.

Jorm, A. F., Griffiths, K. M., Christensen, H., Parslow, R. A., & Rogers, B. (2004). Actions taken to cope with depression at different levels of severity: A community survey. *Psychol. Med., 34*(2), 293-299.

Jorm, A. F., Patten, S. B., Brugha, T. S., & Mojtabai, R. (2017). Has increased provision of treatment reduced the prevalence of common mental disorders? Review of the evidence from four countries. *World Psychiatry, 16*(1), 90-99.

Josephson, A., Larson, D., & Juthani, N. (2000). What's happening in psychiatry regarding spirituality. *Psychiatric Annals.* vol. 30, 533-41.

Jovev, M., & Jackson, H. J. (2006). The relationship of borderline personality disorder, life events and functioning in an

Australian psychiatric sample. *Journal of Personality Disorders, 20*(3), 205–217.

Joyce, S., Modini, M., Christensen, H., Mykletun, A., Bryant, R., Mitchell, P. B., & Harvey, S. B. (2016). Workplace interventions for common mental disorders: A systematic meta-review. *Psychol Med, 46*(4), 683–697.

Judd, F., Armstrong, S., & Kulkarni, J. (2009). Gender-sensitive mental health care. *Australasian Psychiatry, 17*(2).

Jungbluth, N. J., & Shirk, S. R. (2009). Therapist strategies for building involvement in cognitive-behavioral therapy for adolescent depression. *J Consult Clin Psychol, 77*(6), 1179–1184.

Jurd, S., de Beer, W., Aimer, M., Fletcher, S., Halley, E., Schapper, C., & Orkin, M. (2015). Introducing a competency based fellowship programme for psychiatry in Australia and New Zealand. *Australas Psychiatry, 23*(6), 699–705.

Kabat-Zinn, J. (1982). An outpatient program in behavioral medicine for chronic pain patients based on the practice of mindfulness meditation: Theoretical considerations and preliminary results. *General Hospital Psychiatry, 4*(1), 33–47.

Kabat-Zinn, J. (1990). *Full Catastrophe Living: Using the Wisdom of Your Body and Mind to Face Stress, Pain and Illness*. New York: Delacorte.

Kabat-Zinn, J. (1996). Mindfulness meditation: What it is, what it isn't, and it's role in health care and medicine. In Y. Haruki, Y. Ishii, & M. Suzuki (eds.), *Comparative and Psychological Study on Meditation* (pp. 161–169). Netherlands: Eburon Publishers.

Kabat-Zinn, J. (1999). Indra's net at work: The mainstreaming of Dharma practice in society. In G. Watson, S. Batchelor, & G. Claxton (eds.), *The Psychology of Awaking: Buddhism, Science and Our Day-to-Day Lives* (pp. 226–249). London: Rider.

Kabat-Zinn, J. (2003). Mindfulness-based interventions in context: Past, present, and future. *Clinical Psychology: Science and Practice, 10*(2), 144–156.

Kafantaris, V., Leigh, E., Hertz, S., Berest, A., Schebendach, J., Sterling, W. M., . . . Malhotra, A. K. (2011). A placebo-controlled pilot study of adjunctive olanzapine for adolescents with anorexia nervosa. *J Child Adolesc Psychopharmacol, 21*(3), 207–212.

Kaiser, M. (2017). Mechanisms of Connectome Development. *Trends in Cognitive Sciences, 21*(9), 703–717.

Kaite, C. P., Karanikola, M., Merkouris, A., & Papathanassoglou, E. D. E. (2015). 'An ongoing struggle with the self and illness': A meta-synthesis of the studies of the lived experience of severe mental illness. *Archives of Psychiatric Nursing, 29*(6), 458–473.

Kandel, E., Schwartz, J., & Jessell, T. (2013). Overall Perspective. In S. Mack, E. R. Kandel, T. M. Jessell, J. H. Schwartz, S. A. Siegelbaum, & A. J. Hudspeth (eds.), *Principles of Neural Science* (5th ed.). New York: McGraw-Hill Education.

Kanner, A., Coyne, J., Schaefer, C., & Lazarus, R. (1981). Comparison of two modes of stress measurement: Daily hassles and uplifts versus major life events. *Journal of Behavioral Medicine, 4*(1), 1–39.

Kanter, J. (1989). Clinical case management: Definition, principles, components. *Hospital and Community Psychiatry, 40*, 361- 368.

Kaplan, I. (1998). *Rebuilding Shattered Lives*. Victorian Foundation for Survivors of Torture Inc. Parkville: Australia.

Kaptsis, D., King, D. L., Delfabbro, P. H., & Gradisar, M. (2016). Withdrawal symptoms in internet gaming disorder: A systematic review. *Clinical Psychology Review, 43*, 58–66.

Karatzias, T., Howard, R., Power, K., Socherel, F., Heath, C., & Livingstone, A. (2017). Organic vs. functional neurological disorders: The role of childhood psychological trauma. *Child Abuse & Neglect, 63*, 1–6.

Karp, D. A. (2017). *Speaking of Sadness: Depression, Disconnection, and the Meanings of Illness*. Oxford University Press.

Kates, N., Arroll, B., Currie, E., Hanlon, C., Gask, L., Klasen, H., . . . Williams, M. (2018). Improving collaboration between primary care and mental health services. *The World Journal of Biological Psychiatry*, 1–18.

Katz, L. Y., Fotti, S. A., & Postl, L. (2009). Cognitive-behavioral therapy and dialectical behavior therapy: Adaptations required to treat adolescents. *Psychiatric Clinics of North America, 32*, 95–109.

Kausman, R. (2004). *If Not Dieting, Then What?* Allen & Unwin.

Kays, J. L., Hurley, R. A., & Taber, K. H. (2012). The dynamic brain: Neuroplasticity and mental health. *Journal of Neuropsychiatry and Clinical Neurosciences, 24*(2), 118–124.

Kazantzis, N., Dattilio, F. M., & Dobson, K. (2017). *The Therapeutic Relationship in Cognitive-Behavioral Therapy: A Clinician's Guide*. New York: Guilford Publications.

Kazantzis, N., Deane, F. P., Ronan, K. R., & L'Abate, L. (2005). *Using Homework Assignments in Cognitive Bevior Therapy*. Taylor & Francis.

Kazantzis, N., Luong, H., Usatoff, A., Impala, T., Yew, R., & Hofmann, S. (2018). The processes of cognitive behavioral therapy: A review of meta-analyses. *Cognitive Therapy and Research, 42*(4), 349–357.

Kazantzis, N., & Stuckey, M. E. (2018). Inception of a discovery: Re-defining the Use of Socratic dialogue in cognitive behavioral therapy. *International Journal of Cognitive Therapy, 11*(2), 117–123.

Kazantzis, N., Whittington, C., & Dattilio, F. M. (2010). Meta-analysis of homework effects in cognitive and behavioral therapy: A replication and extension. *Clinical Psychology Science and Practice, 17*(2), 144–156.

Kazantzis, N., Whittington, C., Zelencich, L., Kyrios, M., Norton, P. J., & Hofmann, S. G. (2016). Quantity and quality of homework compliance: A meta-analysis of relations with outcome in cognitive behavior therapy. *Behavior Therapy, 47*(5), 755–772.

Kebe, N., Chiocchio, F., Bamvita, J.-M. W., & Fleury, M.-J. (2018). Variables associated with interprofessional collaboration: The case of professionals working in Quebec local mental health service networks. *Journal of Interprofessional Care, 33*, 1–9.

Keel, P. K., Brown, T. A., Holm-Denoma, J., & Bodell, L. P. (2011). Comparison of DSM-IV versus proposed DSM-5 diagnostic criteria for eating disorders: Reduction of eating disorder not otherwise specified and validity. *International Journal of Eating Disorders, 44*(6), 553–560.

Keks, N. A., Altson, K., Hope, J., Krapivensky, N., Culhane, C., Tanaghow, A., . . . Bootle, A. (1999). Use of antipsychosis and adjunctive medications by an inner urban community psychiatric service. *Australian and New Zealand Journal of Psychiatry, 33*, 896–901.

Kelly, B. J., Lewin, T. J., Stain, H. J., Coleman, C., Fitzgerald, M., Perkins, D., . . . Beard, J. R. (2011). Determinants of mental health and well-being within rural and remote communities. *Soc Psychiatry Psychiatr Epidemiol, 46*(12), 1331–1342.

Kelly, E., Fulginiti, A., Pahwa, R., Tallen, L., Duan, L., & Brekke, J. (2014). A pilot test of a peer navigator intervention for improving the health of individuals with serious mental illness. *Community Mental Health Journal, 50*(4), 435–446.

Kelly, Y., Sacker, A., Del, B. E., M., F., & Marmot, M. (2011). What role for the home learning environment and parenting in reducing the socioeconomic gradient in child development? Findings from the Millennium Cohort Study. *Archives of Disease in Childhood, 96*(9), 832–837.

Kendler, K. S. (2016). The phenomenology of major depression and the representativeness and nature of DSM criteria. *American Journal of Psychiatry, 173*(8), 771–780.

Kendler, K. S., Myers, J., & Prescott, C. A. (2007). Specificity of genetic and environmental risk factors for symptoms of cannabis, cocaine, alcohol, caffeine, and nicotine dependence. *Archives of General Psychiatry, 64*(11), 1313–1320.

Kernberg, O. F. (1985). *Borderline Conditions and Pathological Narcissism*. Rowman & Littlefield.

Kernberg, O. F. (1995). *Object Relations Theory and Clinical Psychoanalysis*. Jason Aronson.

Kernberg, O. F. (2007). The almost untreatable narcissistic patient. *Journal of the American Psychoanalytic Association, 55*(2), 503–539.

Keski-Rahkonen, A., Hoek, H. W., Susser, E. S., Linna, M. S., Sihvola, E., Raevuori, A., . . . Rissanen, A. (2007). Epidemiology and course of anorexia nervosa in the community. *American Journal of Psychiatry, 164*(8), 1259–1265.

Kessler, R. C., Abelson, J., Demler, O., Escobar, J. I., Gibbon, M., Guyer, M. E., . . . Zheng, H. (2004). Clinical calibration of DSM-IV diagnoses in the World Mental Health (WMH) version of the World Health Organization (WHO) Composite International Diagnostic Interview (WMHCIDI). *Int J Methods Psychiatr Res, 13*(2), 122–139.

Kessler, R. C., Andrews, G., Colpe, L. J., Hiripi, E., Mroczek, D. K., Normand, S. L., . . . Zaslavsky, A. M. (2002). Short screening scales to monitor population prevalences and trends in non-specific psychological distress. *Psychol Med, 32*(6), 959–976.

Kessler, R. C., Berglund, P., Demler, O., Jin, R., Merikangas, K. R., & Walters, E. E. (2005). Lifetime prevalence and age-of-onset distributions of DSM-IV disorders in the National Comorbidity Survey Replication. *Archives of General Psychiatry, 62*(6), 593–602.

Kessler, R. C., Rose, S., Koenen, K. C., Karam, E. G., Stang, P. E., Stein, D. J., . . . Carmen Viana, M. (2014). How well can post-traumatic stress disorder be predicted from pre-trauma risk factors? An exploratory study in the WHO World Mental Health Surveys. *World Psychiatry, 13*(3), 265–274.

Kessler, R. C., & Ustun, T. B. (2004). The World Mental Health (WMH) Survey Initiative Version of the World Health Organization (WHO) Composite International Diagnostic Interview (CIDI). *Int J Methods Psychiatr Res, 13*(2), 93–121.

Kester, M. I., & Scheltens, P. (2009). Dementia: The bare essentials. *Pract Neurol, 9*(4), 241–251.

Keys, A. (1950). *The Biology of Human Starvation*. Oxford University Press.

Kezelman, C., Hossack, N., Stavropoulos, P., & Burley, P. (2015). *The Cost of Unresolved Childhood Trauma and Abuse in Adults in Australia*. Retrieved from www.blueknot.org.au/Portals/2/Economic%20Report/The%20cost%20of%20unresolved%20trauma_budget%20report%20fnl.pdf.

Kezelman, C., & Stavropoulos, P. (2012). *Practice Guidelines for Treatment of Complex Trauma and Trauma Informed Care and Service Delivery*. Kirribilli: Adults Surviving Child Abuse.

Kezelman, C., & Stavropoulos, P. (2017). *Talking About Trauma: Guide to Everyday Conversations for the General Public*. Retrieved from www.blueknot.org.au/Resources/Publications/Talking-about-trauma/Talking_About_Trauma_Public.

Kielhofner, G. (2009). *Conceptual Foundations of Occupational Therapy* (4th ed.). Philadelphia: F. A. Davis.

Kielhofner, G., Braveman, B., Fogg, L., & Levin, M. (2008). A controlled study of services to enhance productive participation among people with HIV/AIDS. *American Journal of Occupational Therapy, 62*(1), 36–45.

Kielhofner, G., Mallinson, T., Crawford, C., Nowak, M., Rigby, M., Henry, A., & Walens, D. (2004). *The Occupational Performance History Interview-II (OPHI-II), Version 2.1*. Chicago: Model of Human Occupation Clearinghouse.

Kiely, K. M., & Butterworth, P. (2013). Social disadvantage and individual vulnerability: A longitudinal investigation of welfare receipt and mental health in Australia. *Aust N Z J Psychiatry, 47*(7), 654–666.

Kilcullen, M., & Day, A. (2018). Culturally informed case conceptualisation: Developing a clinical psychology approach to treatment planning for non-Indigenous psychologists working with Aboriginal and Torres Strait Islander clients. *Clinical Psychologist, 22*(3), 280–289.

Killackey, E., Allott, K., Jackson, H. J., Scutella, R., Tseng, Y.-P., Borland, J., . . . Cotton, S. M. (2019). Individual placement and support for vocational recovery in first-episode psychosis: Randomised controlled trial. *British Journal of Psychiatry, 214*(2), 76–82.

Killackey, E., Allott, K., Woodhead, G., Connor, S., Dragon, S., & Ring, J. (2017). Individual placement and support, supported education in young people with mental illness: An exploratory feasibility study. *Early Intervention in Psychiatry, 11*(6), 526–531.

Killackey, E., & Cotton, S. (2017). Employment and education outcomes from a RCT of individual placement and support for young people with first-episode psychosis. *Schizophrenia Bulletin, 43*(Suppl 1), S50.

Killaspy, H. (2007). Assertive community treatment in psychiatry. *British Medical Journal, 335*(7615), 311–312.

Killaspy, H., Bebbington, P., Blizard, R., Johnson, S., Nolan, F., Pilling, S., & King, M. (2006). The REACT study: Randomised evaluation of assertive community treatment in north London. *British Medical Journal, 332*(7545), 815–820.

Killaspy, H., Johnson, S., Pierce, B., Bebbington, P., Pilling, S., Nolan, F., & King, M. (2009). Successful engagement: A mixed methods study of the approaches of assertive community treatment and community mental health teams in the REACT trial. *Social Psychiatry and Psychiatric Epidemiology, 44*(7), 532–540.

Killen, M., & Smetana, J. (2007). The biology of morality: Human development and moral neuroscience. *Human Development, 50*(5), 241–243.

Killerman, S. (2015). *Breaking Through the Binary: Gender Explained Using Continuums*. Retrieved from https://itspronouncedmetrosexual.com/genderbread-person.

Kim, E. J., Pellman, B., & Kim, J. J. (2015). Stress effects on the hippocampus: A critical review. *Learning & Memory, 22*(9), 411–416.

Kim, M. M., van Dorn, R. A., Scheyett, A. M., Elbogen, E. E., Swanson, J. W., Swartz, M. S., & McDaniel, L. A. (2007). Understanding the personal and clinical utility of psychiatric advance directives: A qualitative perspective. *Psychiatry-Interpersonal and Biological Processes, 70*(1), 19–29.

Kim, S. W., Grant, J. E., Potenza, M. N., Blanco, C., & Hollander, E. (2009). The Gambling Symptom Assessment Scale (G-SAS): A reliability and validity study. *Psychiatry Research, 166*(1), 76–84.

Kim-Cohen, J., Caspi, A., Moffitt, T. E., Harrington, H., Milne, B. J., & Poulton, R. (2003). Prior juvenile diagnoses in adults with mental disorder: Developmental follow-back of a prospective-longitudinal cohort. *Archives of General Psychiatry, 60*(7), 709–717.

King, D., Koster, E., & Billieux, J. (2019). Study what makes games addictive. *Nature, 573*(7774), 346.

King, D. L., Chamberlain, S. R., Carragher, N., Billieux, J., Stein, D., Mueller, K., . . . Delfabbro, P. H. (2020). Screening and assessment tools for gaming disorder: A comprehensive systematic review. *Clinical Psychology Review, 77*, 101831.

King, D. L., Delfabbro, P. H., Gainsbury, S. M., Dreier, M., Greer, N., & Billieux, J. (2019). Unfair play? Video games as exploitative monetized services: An examination of game patents from a consumer protection perspective. *Computers in Human Behavior, 101*, 131-143.

King, D. L., Delfabbro, P. H., & Griffiths, M. D. (2011). The role of structural characteristics in problematic video game play: An empirical study. *International Journal of Mental Health and Addiction, 9*(3), 320-333.

King, D. L., Delfabbro, P. H., & Griffiths, M. D. (2012). Clinical interventions for technology-based problems: Excessive internet and video game use. *Journal of Cognitive Psychotherapy, 26*(1), 43-56.

King, D. L., Delfabbro, P. H., Wu, A. M. S., Doh, Y. Y., Kuss, D. J., Pallesen, S., . . . Sakuma, H. (2017). Treatment of internet gaming disorder: An international systematic review and CONSORT evaluation. *Clinical Psychology Review, 54*, 123-133.

King, R. (2009). Caseload management, work-related stress and case manager self-efficacy among Victorian mental health case managers. *Australian & New Zealand Journal of Psychiatry, 43*(5), 453-459.

King, R., Lloyd, C., & Holewa, V. (2008). Can identified stressors be used to predict profession for mental health professionals? *Australian e-Journal for the Advancement of Mental Health, 7*(2), 97-103.

King, R., Meadows, G., & Le Bas, J. (2004). Compiling a caseload index for mental health case management. *Australian & New Zealand Journal of Psychiatry, 38*(6), 455-462.

Kinn, L. G., Holgersen, H., Aas, R. W., & Davidson, L. (2014). 'Balancing on skates on the icy surface of work': A metasynthesis of work participation for persons with psychiatric disabilities. *Journal of Occupational Rehabilitation, 24*(1), 125-138.

Kinn, L. G., Tanaka, K., Bellamy, C., & Davidson, L. (2018). 'Pushing the boat out': A meta-synthesis of how members, staff and family experience the clubhouse model. *Community Mental Health Journal, 54*(8), 1199-1211.

Kinsey, A. C., Pomeroy, W. R., & Martin, C. E. (2003). Sexual behavior in the human male. 1948. *American Journal of Public Health, 93*(6), 894-898.

Kiraly, O., Sleczka, P., Pontes, H. M., Urban, R., Griffiths, M. D., & Demetrovics, Z. (2017). Validation of the ten-item internet Gaming Disorder Test (IGDT-10) and evaluation of the nine DSM-5 internet gaming disorder criteria. *Addictive Behaviors, 64*, 253-260.

Kirkhart, K. E. (2010). Eyes on the prize: Multicultural validity and evaluation theory. *American Journal of Evaluation, 31*(3), 400-413.

Kirmayer, L. J., & Robbins, J. M. (1996). Patients who somatise in primary care: A longitudinal study of cognitive and social characteristics. *Psychol Med, 26*, 937-951.

Kirsh, B., & Cockburn, L. (2009). The Canadian Occupational Performance Measure: A tool for recovery-based practice. *Psychiatric Rehabilitation Journal, 32*(3), 171-176.

Kirsh, B., & Gewurtz, R. E. (2012). Promoting mental health within workplaces. In R. J. Gatchel & I. Z. Schultz (eds.), *Handbook of Occupational Health and Wellness* (pp. 243-265). United States: Springer.

Kirsh, B., & Tate, E. (2006). Developing a comprehensive understanding of the working alliance in community mental health. *Qualitative Health Research, 16*(8), 1054-1074.

Kisely, S. R., Campbell, L. A., & O'Reilly, R. (2017). Compulsory community and involuntary outpatient treatment for people with severe mental disorders. *Cochrane Database Syst Rev., 3*(3).

Kissane, D. (2009). Beyond the psychotherapy and survival debate: The challenge of social disparity, depression and treatment adherence in psychosocial cancer care. *Psycho-Oncology, 18*(1), 1-5.

Kitto, S. (2011). Sociology of interprofessional health care practice : critical reflections and concrete solutions. New York: Nova Science Publishers.

Kitzman, H. J., Olds, D. L., Cole, R. E., Hanks, C. A., Anson, E. A., Arcoleo, K. J., . . . Holmberg, J. R. (2010). Enduring effects of prenatal and infancy home visiting by nurses on children: Follow-up of a randomized trial among children at age 12 years. *Arch Pediatr Adolesc Med, 164*(5), 412-418.

Klerman, G. L. (1990). Paradigm shifts in USA psychiatric epidemiology since World War II. *Journal of Social Psychiatry & Psychiatric Epidemiology*, vol. 25, pp. 27-32.

Klinic Community Health Centre. (2008). *Trauma-Informed Toolkit. A Resource for Service Organizations and Providers to Deliver Services That Are Trauma-Informed.* Retrieved from www.Trauma-informed.ca.

Klinkman, M. S., & Gask, L. (2009). Mental and general health comorbidities in persons presenting in primary care. In I. M. Salloum & J. E. Mezzich (eds.), *Psychiatric Diagnosis Challenges and Prospects* (pp. 197-212). Chichester: Wiley-Blackwell.

Kluft, R. P. (1994). Multiple personality disorder: Observations on the etiology, natural history, recognition, and resolution of a long-neglected condition. In R. M. Klein & B. K. Doane (eds.), *Psychological Concepts and Dissociative Disorders* (pp. 9-50). L. Erlbaum.

Knol, M. J., Twisk, J. W. R., Beekman, A. T. F., Heine, R. J., Snoek, F. J., & Pouwer, F. (2006). Depression as a risk factor for the onset of type 2 diabetes mellitus. A meta-analysis. *Diabetologia, 49*(5), 837-845.

Koelen, J. A., Houtveen, J. H., Abbass, A., Luyten, P., Eurelings-Bontekoe, E. H., Van Broeckhuysen-Kloth, S. A., . . . Geenen, R. (2014). Effectiveness of psychotherapy for severe somatoform disorder: Meta-analysis. *Br J Psychiatry, 204*(1), 12-19.

Koenen, K. C., Ratanatharathorn, A., Ng, L., McLaughlin, K. A., Bromet, E. J., Stein, D. J., . . . Survey, W. W. M. H. (2017). Posttraumatic stress disorder in the World Mental Health Surveys. *Psychol Med, 47*(13), 2260-2274.

Kohut, H. (1971). *The analysis of the self: A systematic approach to the psychoanalytic treatment of narcissistic personality disorders.* Chicago: University of Chicago Press.

Kokanović, R., Brophy, L., McSherry, B., Flore, J., Moeller-Saxone, K., & Herrman, H. (2018). Supported decision-making from the perspectives of mental health service users, family members supporting them and mental health practitioners. *Australian & New Zealand Journal of Psychiatry, 52*(9), 826-833.

Kokanović, R., Butler, E., Halilovich, H., Palmer, V., Griffiths, F., Dowrick, C., & Gunn, J. (2013). Maps, models, and narratives: The ways people talk about depression. *Qualitative Health Research, 23*(1), 114-125.

Kokanović, R., Petersen, A., & Klimidis, S. (2006). 'Nobody can help me. . .I am living through it alone': Experiences of caring for people diagnosed with mental illness in ethno-cultural and linguistic minority communities. *Journal of Immigrant and Minority Health, 8*(2), 125-135.

Komiti, A., Judd, F., & Jackson, H. (2006). The influence of stigma and attitudes on seeking help from a GP for mental health problems. *Social Psychiatry and Psychiatric Epidemiology, 41*(9), 738-745.

Konstantareas, M. M., & Hewitt, T. (2001). Autistic disorder and schizophrenia: Diagnostic overlaps. *Journal of Autism & Developmental Disorders, 31*(1).

Koob, G. F., & Le Moal, M. (2008). Addiction and the brain antireward system. *Annu. Rev. Psychol., 59*, 29-53.

Koran, L. M., Abujaoude, E., Large, M. D., & Serpe, R. T. (2008). The prevalence of body dysmorphic disorder in the United States adult population. *CNS Spectr, 13*(4), 316-322.

Korn, D., Gibbins, R., & Azmier, J. (2003). Framing public policy towards a public health paradigm for gambling. *Journal of Gambling Studies, 19*(2), 235-256.

Korn, D., & Shaffer, H. (1999). Gambling and the health of the public: Adopting a public health perspective. *Journal of Gambling Studies, 15*(4), 289-365.

Korner, A., Gerull, F., Meares, R., & Stevenson, J. (2006). Borderline personality disorder treated with the conversational model: A replication study. *Comprehensive Psychiatry, 47*(5), 406-411.

Kozlowska, K. (2005). Healing the disembodied mind: Contemporary models of conversion disorder. *Harvard Review of Psychiatry, 13*(1), 1-13.

Kranzler, H. R., & Van Kirk, J. (2001). Efficacy of naltrexone and acamprosate for alcoholism treatment: A meta-analysis. *Alcoholism: Clinical and Experimental Research, 25*(9), 1335-1341.

Krawitz, R., & Batcheler, M. (2006). Borderline personality disorder: A pilot survey about clinician views on defensive practice. *Australasian Psychiatry, 14*(3), 320-322.

Kristeller, J. L., & Wolever, R. Q. (2011). Mindfulness-based eating awareness training for treating binge eating disorder: The conceptual foundation. *Eating Disorders, 19*(1), 49-61.

Kroenke, K. (2007). Efficacy of treatment for somatoform disorders: A review of randomized controlled trials. *Psychosomatic Medicine, 69*(9), 881-888.

Kroenke, K., Spitzer, R. L., & Williams, J. B. (2003). The Patient Health Questionnaire-2: Validity of a two-item depression screener. *Medical Care, 41*(11), 1284-1292.

Kroenke, K., Spitzer, R. L., Williams, J. B., Linzer, M., Hahn, S. R., Degruy, F. V., & Brody, D. (1994). Physical symptoms in primary care. Predictors of psychiatric disorders and functional impairment. *Archives of Family Medicine, 3*(9), 774.

Kroenke, K., Spitzer, R. L., & Williams, J. B. W. (2001). The PHQ-9. Validity of a brief depression severity measure. *Journal of General Internal Medicine, 16*, 606-613.

Krotofil, J., McPherson, P., & Killaspy, H. (2018). Service user experiences of specialist mental health supported accommodation: A systematic review of qualitative studies and narrative synthesis. *Health & Social Care in the Community, 26*(6), 787-800.

Krupa, T. (2016). Defining psychosocial practice in occupational therapy. In T. Krupa, B. Kirsh, D. B. Pitts, & E. Fossey (eds.), *Bruce and Borgs' Psychosocial Frames of Reference: Theories, Models and Approaches for Occupation-Based Practice* (4th ed., pp. 3-16). Thorofare: Slack Inc.

Krupa, T., Eastabrook, S., Hern, L., Lee, D., North, R., Percy, K., . . . Wing, G. (2005). How do people who receive assertive community treatment experience this service? *Psychiatric Rehabilitation Journal, 29*(1), 18-24.

Krupa, T., Fossey, E., Anthony, W. A., Brown, C., & Pitts, D. B. (2009). Doing daily life: How occupational therapy can inform psychiatric rehabilitation practice. *Psychiatric Rehabilitation Journal, 32*(3), 155-161.

Krupa, T., McLean, H., Eastabrook, S., Bonham, A., & Baksh, L. (2003). Daily time use as a measure of community adjustment for persons served by assertive community treatment teams. *American Journal of Occupational Therapy, 57*(5), 558-565.

Krupa, T. M. (2011). Approaches to improving employment outcomes for people with serious mental illness. In I. Z. Schultz & E. S. Rogers (eds.), *Work Accommodation and Retention in Mental Health*. New York: Springer.

Krupa, T. M., Edgelow, M., Chen, S., Mieras, C., Almas, A., Perry, A., . . . Bransfield, M. (2010). *Action Over Inertia: Addressing the Activity-Health Needs of Individuals with Serious Mental Illness.* Ottawa: CAOT Publications.

Krupa, T. M., Fossey, E., Anthony, W. A., Brown, C., & Pitts, D. (2009). Doing daily life as a means to health, personal growth and empowerment: Occupational therapy, psychiatric rehabilitation and recovery. *Psychiatric Rehabilitation Journal, 32*(3), 155-161.

Krystal, J. H., Cramer, J. A., Krol, W. F., Kirk, G. F., & Rosenheck, R. A. (2001). Naltrexone in the treatment of alcohol dependence. *New England Journal of Medicine, 345*(24), 1734-1739.

Kuerbis, A., Sacco, P., Blazer, D. G., & Moore, A. A. (2014). Substance abuse among older adults. *Clinics in Geriatric Medicine, 30*(3), 629-+.

Kuhn, T. S. (1970). *The Structure of Scientific Revolutions* (2nd ed.). Chicago: University of Chicago Press.

Kuipers, E. (2006). Family interventions in schizophrenia: Evidence for efficacy and proposed mechanisms of change. *Journal of Family Therapy, 28*(1), 73-80.

Kujala, V., Jokinen, J., Ebeling, H., & Pohjola, A. (2017). Let's Talk about Children Evaluation (LTCE) study in northern Finland: A multiple group ecological study of children's health promotion activities with a municipal and time-trend design. *BMJ Open, 7*(7), e015985-e015985.

Kunoe, N., Lobmaier, P., Vederhus, J. K., Hegstad, S., Gossop, M., Kristensen, Ø., & Waal, H. (2009). Naltrexone implants after in-patient treatment for opioid dependence: Randomised controlled trial. *British Journal of Psychiatry, 194*(6), 541-546.

Kurlansik, S. L., & Maffei, M. S. (2016). Somatic symptom disorder. *Am Fam Physician, 93*(1), 49-54.

Kuss, D. J., & Griffiths, M. D. (2012). Online gaming addiction in children and adolescents: A review of empirical research. *Journal of Behavioral Addictions, 1*(1), 3-22.

Kyrios, M. (2003). Exposure and response prevention for OCD. In R. G. Menzies & P. de Silva (eds.), *Obsessive-Compulsive Disorder: Theory, Research and Treatment* (pp. 259-274). West Sussex: John Wiley & Sons.

Kyrios, M., Ahern, C., Fassnacht, D. B., Nedeljkovic, M., Moulding, R., & Meyer, D. (2018). Therapist-assisted internet-based cognitive behavioral therapy versus progressive relaxation in obsessive-compulsive disorder: Randomized controlled trial. *Journal of Medical Internet Research, 20*(8), e242.

Kyrios, M., Mogan, C., Moulding, R., Frost, R. O., Yap, K., & Fassnacht, D. B. (2018). The cognitive-behavioural model of hoarding disorder: Evidence from clinical and non-clinical cohorts. *Clinical Psychology & Psychotherapy, 25*(2), 311-321.

Kyrios, M., Mouding, R., & Nedeljkovic, M. (2011). Anxiety disorders: Assessment and management in general practice. *Australian Family Physician, 40*(6), 370.

Kyrios, M., Moulding, R., & Bhar, S. (2014). A clinician's quick guide of evidence-based approaches: Obsessive-compulsive disorder. *Clinical Psychologist, 18*(2), 96-97.

Kyrios, M., Moulding, R., Doron, G., Bhar, S. S., Nedeljkovic, M., & Mikulincer, M. (2016). *The Self in Understanding and Treating Psychological Disorders*. Cambridge: Cambridge University Press.

Kyrios, M., Sanavio, E., Bhar, S., & Liguori, L. (2001). Associations between obsessive-compulsive phenomena, affect and beliefs: Cross-cultural comparisons of Australian and Italian data. *Behavioural and Cognitive Psychotherapy, 29*(4), 409-422.

Labbate, L. A., Fava, M., Rosenbaum, J. F., & Arana, G. W. (2010). *Handbook of Psychiatric Drug Therapy* (6th ed.). Philadelphia, PA: Lippincott Williams & Wilkins.

Labuschagne, I., Castle, D. J., Dunai, J., Kyrios, M., & Rossell, S. L. (2010). An examination of delusional thinking and cognitive styles in body dysmorphic disorder. *Aust N Z J Psychiatry, 44*(8), 706-712.

Ladwig, K.-H., Marten-Mittag, B., Erazo, N., & Gündel, H. (2001). Identifying somatization disorder in a population-based health examination survey: Psychosocial burden and gender differences. *Psychosomatics, 42*(6), 511-518.

Lagger, G., Pataky, Z., & Golay, A. (2010). Efficacy of therapeutic patient education in chronic diseases and obesity. *Patient Education and Counseling, 79*(3), 283-286.

Lakhan, S. E., & Schofield, K. L. (2013). Mindfulness-based therapies in the treatment of somatization disorders: A systematic review and meta-analysis. *PLoS One, 8*(8), e71834.

Lambert, T. J., Singh, B. S., & Patel, M. X. (2009). Community treatment orders and antipsychotic long-acting injections. *British Journal of Psychiatry, 195*(52), s57-s62.

Lampe, L., Shadbolt, N., Starcevic, V., Boyce, P., Brakoulias, V., Hitching, R., . . . Malhi, G. (2012). Diagnostic processes in mental health: GPs and psychiatrists reading from the same book but on a different page. *Australasian Psychiatry, 20*(5), 374-378.

Lander, B. (2019). *Troubling Ambiguity: Governance in SA Health*. Retrieved from https://icac.sa.gov.au/system/files/Troubling_Ambiguity_Governance_in_SA_Health.pdf.

Lang, P. (1968). *Fear Reduction and Fear Behavior: Problems in Treating a Construct*. Washington: American Psychological Association.

Langarizadeh, M., Tabatabaei, M. S., Tavakol, K., Naghipour, M., Rostami, A., & Moghbeli, F. (2017). Telemental health care, an effective alternative to conventional mental care: A systematic review. *Acta Informatica Medica, 25*(4), 240.

Langham, E., Thorne, H., Browne, M., Donaldson, P., Rose, J., & Rockloff, M. (2016). Understanding gambling related harm: A proposed definition, conceptual framework, and taxonomy of harms. *BMC Public Health, 16*.

Langton, M. (2018). *Welcome to Country: A Travel Guide to Indigenous Australia*. Hardie Grant Travel.

LaPlante, D. A., Nelson, S. E., LaBrie, R. A., & Shaffer, H. J. (2008). Stability and progression of disordered gambling: Lessons from longitudinal studies. *Canadian Journal of Psychiatry-Revue Canadienne De Psychiatrie, 53*(1), 52-60.

Larcombe, W., Finch, S., Sore, R., Murray, C. M., Kentish, S., Mulder, R. A., . . . Williams, D. A. (2014). Prevalence and socio-demographic correlates of psychological distress among students at an Australian university. *Studies in Higher Education, 41*(6), 1074-1091.

Large, M., Kaneson, M., Myles, N., Myles, H., Gunaratne, P., & Ryan, C. (2016). Meta-analysis of longitudinal cohort studies of suicide risk assessment among psychiatric patients: Heterogeneity in results and lack of improvement over time. *PLoS One, 11*(6), e0156322.

Large, M., Sharma, S., Cannon, E., Ryan, C., & Nielssen, O. (2011). Review of Risk Factors for Suicide Within a Year of Discharge from Psychiatric Hospital: A Systematic Meta-Analysis. *Australian and New Zealand Journal of Psychiatry*, 45(8), 619-628.

Large, M. M., & Ryan, C. J. (2014). Violence risk assessment has not been shown to reduce violence. *Australian & New Zealand Journal of Psychiatry, 49*(1), 91-91.

Larson, D., Thielman, S., & Greenwold, M. (1993). Religious content in the DSM-III-R glossary of technical terms. *American Journal of Psychiatry, vol. 150*, pp. 1884-1885.

Larsson, H., Dilshad, R., Lichtenstein, P., & Barker, E. D. (2011). Developmental trajectories of DSM-IV symptoms of attention-deficit/hyperactivity disorder: Genetic effects, family risk and associated psychopathology. *Journal of Child Psychology and Psychiatry, 52*(9), 954-963.

Lasègue, C. (1873). Hysterical anorexia [De l'anorexie hystérique]. *Archives Generates de. Medecine, 32*(1), 385-403.

Laska, K. M., Gurman, A. S., & Wampold, B. E. (2014). Expanding the lens of evidence-based practice in psychotherapy: A common factors perspective. *Psychotherapy, 51*(4), 467-481.

Laugharne, J., Waterreus, A. J., Castle, D. J., & Dragovic, M. (2016). Screening for the metabolic syndrome in Australia: A national survey of psychiatrists' attitudes and reported practice in patients prescribed antipsychotic drugs. *Australasian Psychiatry*, 24(1), 62-66.

Laumann, E. O., Gagnon, J. H., Michael, R. T., & Michaels, S. (1994). *The Social Organization of Sexuality: Sexual Practices in the United States*. University of Chicago Press.

Laverty, M., McDermott, D. R., & Calma, T. (2017). Embedding cultural safety in Australia's main health care standards. *Medical Journal of Australia, 207*(1), 15-+.

Lavis, A., Lester, H., Everard, L., Freemantle, N., Amos, T., Fowler, D., . . . Sharma, V. (2015). Layers of listening: Qualitative analysis of the impact of early intervention services for first-episode psychosis on carers' experiences. *The British Journal of Psychiatry, 207*(2), 135-142.

Law Council of Australia. (2020). *The Justice Project*. Retrieved from www.lawcouncil.asn.au/justice-project/final-report.

Law, M., Baptiste, S., Carswell, A., McColl, M., Polatajko, H., & Pollock, N. (2005). *Canadian Occupational Performance Measure* (4th ed.). Ottowa: Canadian Association of Occupational Therapists.

Lawn, S., & Mcmahon, J. (2014). The importance of relationship in understanding the experiences of spouse mental health carers. *Qualitative Health Research, 24*(2), 254-266.

Lawn, Zabeen, Rowlands, & Picot. (2018). Hidden care: Revelations of a case-note audit of physical health care in a community mental health service. *International Journal of Mental Health Nursing*, 27(6), 1742-1755.

Lawrence, D., Hancock, K. J., & Kisely, S. (2013). The gap in life expectancy from preventable physical illness in psychiatric patients in Western Australia: Retrospective analysis of population based registers. *BMJ, 346*, f2539.

Lawrence, D., Johnson, S., Hafekost, J., Boterhoven de Haan, K., Sawyer, M., Ainley, J., & Zubrick, S. R. (2015). *The Mental Health of Children and Adolescents. Report on the Second Australian Child and Adolescent Survey of Mental Health and Wellbeing*. Canberra Department of Health Retrieved from www1.health.gov.au/internet/main/publishing.nsf/Content/9DA8CA21306FE6EDCA257E2700016945/$File/child2.pdf.

Lawton, G. (2019). Simulating the world. *New Scientist, 244*(3250), 38-41.

Lazarus, R. S. (1990). Theory-based stress measurement. *Psychological Inquiry, 1*(1), 3-13.

Lazarus, R. S. (1999). *Stress and Emotion: A New Synthesis*. New York: Springer.

Lazarus, R. S., & Folkman, S. (1984). *Stress, Appraisal, and Coping*. New York: Springer.

Le Boutillier, C., Slade, M., Lawrence, V., Bird, V. J., Chandler, R., Farkas, M., . . . Leamy, M. (2015). Competing priorities: Staff perspectives on supporting recovery. *Administration and Policy in Mental Health and Mental Health Services Research, 42*(4), 429-438.

Le Grande, M., Ski, C. F., Thompson, D. R., Scuffham, P., Kularatna, S., Jackson, A. C., & Brown, A. (2017). Social and emotional wellbeing assessment instruments for use with Indigenous Australians: A critical review. *Social Science & Medicine, 187*, 164-173.

Lea, T., de Wit, J., & Reynolds, R. (2014). Minority stress in lesbian, gay, and bisexual young adults in Australia: Associations with psychological distress, suicidality, and substance use. *Archives of Sexual Behavior, 43*(8), 1571-1578.

Leamy, M., Bird, V., Le Boutillier, C., Williams, J., & Slade, M. (2011). Conceptual framework for personal recovery in mental health: Systematic review and narrative synthesis. *British Journal of Psychiatry, 199*(6), 445-452.

Leamy, M., Clarke, E., Le Boutillier, C., Bird, V., Choudhury, R., Macpherson, R., . . . Slade, M. (2016). Recovery practice in community mental health teams: National survey. *British Journal of Psychiatry, 209*(4), 340.

Leaviss, J., & Uttley, L. (2015). Psychotherapeutic benefits of compassion-focused therapy: An early systematic review. *Psychol Med, 45*(5), 927-945.

LeBeau, R. T., Glenn, D., Liao, B., Wittchen, H. U., Beesdo-Baum, K., Ollendick, T., & Craske, M. G. (2010). Specific phobia: A review of DSM-IV specific phobia and preliminary recommendations for DSM-V. *Depression and Anxiety, 27*(2), 148-167.

Lebel, C., & Beaulieu, C. (2011). Longitudinal development of human brain wiring continues from childhood into adulthood. *Journal of Neuroscience, 31*(30), 10937-10947.

Lebourgeois, H.W., III. (2007). Malingering: Key Points in Assessment.(Medical condition overview*). Psychiatric Times*, 24(5), 21.

Ledgerwood, D. M., & Petry, N. M. (2006). Psychological experience of gambling and subtypes of pathological gamblers. *Psychiatry Research, 144*(1), 17-27.

Lee, C. C., Liem, S. K., Leung, J., Young, V., Wu, K., Wong Kenny, K. K., . . . Lo, W. (2015). From deinstitutionalization to recovery-oriented assertive community treatment in Hong Kong: What we have achieved. *Psychiatry Research, 228*(3), 243-250.

Lee, K. K., Harrison, K., Mills, K., & Conigrave, K. M. (2014). Needs of Aboriginal Australian women with comorbid mental and alcohol and other drug use disorders. *Drug and Alcohol Review, 33*(5), 473-481.

Lee, S., Keating, C., de Castella, A., & Kulkarni, J. (2010). *Fitting Together the Pieces: Collaborative Care Models for Adults with Severe and Persistent Mental Illness*. Retrieved from www.health.gov.au/internet/main/publishing.nsf/content/C23F4021F98C0540CA25792C00790B5D/$File/colsev.pdf.

Lee, S. M., & LoGiudice, D. (2012). Phenomenology of squalor, hoarding and self-neglect: An Australian aged care perspective. *Internal Medicine Journal, 42*(1), 98-101.

Lee, Y. C., Chatterton, M. L., Magnus, A., Mohebbi, M., Le, L. K., & Mihalopoulos, C. (2017). Cost of high prevalence mental disorders: Findings from the 2007 Australian National Survey of Mental Health and Wellbeing. *Australian & New Zealand Journal of Psychiatry, 51*(12), 1198-1211.

LeFrançois, B. A., Menzies, R., & Reaume, G. (2013). *Mad Matters: A Critical Reader in Canadian Mad Studies*. Canadian Scholars' Press Incorporated.

Leggatt, M. (2005). The role of family organizations in mental health care. In N. Sartorius, J. Leff, J. J. Lopez-Ibor, M. Maj, & A. Okasha (eds.), *Families and mental disorders* (pp. 196-215). Great Britain: John Wiley & Sons.

Leggatt, M. (2011). Families as partners in mental health care. *New Paradigm: The Australian Journal of Psychosocial Rehabilittation*, Summer 2011, 15-18.

Leichsenring, F., & Rabung, S. (2011). Long-term psychodynamic psychotherapy in complex mental disorders: Update of a meta-analysis. *Br. J. Psychiatry, 199*(1), 15-22.

Leijdesdorff, S., van Doesum, K., Popma, A., Klaassen, R., & van Amelsvoort, T. (2017). Prevalence of psychopathology in children of parents with mental illness and/or addiction: An up to date narrative review. *Curr Opin Psychiatry, 30*(4), 312-317.

Lemaire, J. B., & Wallace, J. E. (2017). Burnout among doctors. *BMJ*, 358, j3360.

Lemenager, T., Gwodz, A., Richter, A., Reinhard, I., Kammerer, N., Sell, M., & Mann, K. (2013). Self-concept deficits in massively multiplayer online role-playing games addiction. *European Addiction Research, 19*(5), 227-234.

Lenzenweger, M. F., Lane, M. C., Loranger, A. W., & Kessler, R. C. (2007). DSM-IV personality disorders in the National Comorbidity Survey Replication. *Biol Psychiatry, 62*(6), 553-564.

Leonard, W., Lyons, A., & Bariola, E. (2015). *A Closer Look at Private Lives 2: Addressing the Mental Health and Wellbeing of Lesbian, Gay, Bisexual, and Transgender (LGBT) Australians*. Retrieved from https://apo.org.au/node/53996.

Lereya, S. T., Copeland, W. E., Costello, E. J., & Wolke, D. (2015). Adult mental health consequences of peer bullying and maltreatment in childhood: Two cohorts in two countries. *Lancet Psychiatry, 2*(6), 524-531.

Lerner, A., Sigal, M., Bacalu, A., Shiff, R., Burganski, I., & Gelkopf, M. (1992). A naltrexone double blind placebo controlled study in Israel. *Israel Journal of Psychiatry and Related Sciences*, 29(1), 36-43.

Lesieur, H. R., & Blume, S. B. (1987). The South Oaks Gambling Screen (Sogs): A new instrument for the identification of pathological gamblers. *American Journal of Psychiatry, 144*(9), 1184-1188.

Leucht, S., Arbter, D., Engel, R. R., Kissling, W., & Davis, J. M. (2009). How effective are second-generation antipsychotic drugs? A meta-analysis of placebo-controlled trials. *Mol Psychiatry, 14*(4), 429-447.

Leucht, S., Corves, C., Arbter, D., Engel, R. R., Li, C., & Davis, J. M. (2009). Second-generation versus first-generation antipsychotic drugs for schizophrenia: A meta-analysis. *Lancet, 373*(9657), 31-41.

Levitas, A. S., & Silka V R. (2001). Mental health clinical assessment of persons with mental retardation and developmental disabilities. *Mental Health Aspects of Developmental Disabilities, 4*(1), 31-42.

Levula, A., Harr, M., & Wilson, A. (2018). The association between social network factors with depression and anxiety at different life stages. *Community Ment Health J, 54*(6), 842-854.

Levy, K. N., & Johnson, B. N. (2016). Personality disorders. In J. C. Norcross, G. R. VandenBos, D. K. Freedheim, & N. Pole (eds.), *APA Handbook of Clinical Psychology: Psychopathology and Health,* (Vol. 4, pp. 173-207). Washington: American Psychological Association.

Levy, R. L., Whitehead, W. E., Walker, L. S., Von Korff, M., Feld, A. D., Garner, M., & Christie, D. (2004). Increased somatic complaints and health-care utilization in children: Effects of parent IBS status and parent response to gastrointestinal symptoms. *Am J Gastroenterol, 99*(12), 2442-2451.

Lewis, L. (2009). *Mental Health and Human Rights: A Common Agenda for Service User/Survivor Groups*. Retrieved from http://wrap.warwick.ac.uk/163/2/WRAP_Lewis_mental_health_and_human_rights_-_revised_article_submitted_to_Policy_and_Politics1.pdf.

Lewis, M., & Volkmar, F. (1990). *Clinical Aspects of Child and Adolescent Development* (3rd ed.). Philadelphia, Lea & Febiger.

Lexén, A., & Svensson, B. (2016). Mental health professional experiences of the flexible assertive community treatment model: A grounded theory study. *Journal of Mental Health, 25*(4), 379-384.

Leyhe, T., Reynolds, C. F., Melcher, T., Linnemann, C., Kloppel, S., Blennow, K., . . . Hampel, H. (2017). A common challenge in older adults: Classification, overlap, and therapy of depression and dementia. *Alzheimers & Dementia, 13*(1), 59-71.

Liamputtong, P. (2013). *Qualitative research methods* (4th ed.). South Melbourne: Oxford University Press.

Lichtenstein, P., Yip, B. H., Björk, C., Pawitan, Y., Cannon, T. D., Sullivan, P. F., & Hultman, C. M. (2009). Common genetic determinants of schizophrenia and bipolar disorder in Swedish families: A population-based study. *Lancet, 373*(9659), 234-239.

Lieb, K., Vollm, B., Rucker, G., Timmer, A., & Stoffers, J. M. (2010). Pharmacotherapy for borderline personality disorder: Cochrane systematic review of randomised trials. *Br J Psychiatry, 196*(1), 4-12.

Lieberman, J. A., Stroup, T. S., McEvoy, J. P., Swartz, M. S., Rosenheck, R. A., Perkins, D. O., . . . Hsiao, J. K. (2005). Effectiveness of antipsychotic drugs in patients with chronic schizophrenia. *New England Journal of Medicine, 353*(12), 1209-1223.

Liegghio, M. (2017). 'Not a good person': Family stigma of mental illness from the perspectives of young siblings. *Child & Family Social Work, 22*(3), 1237-1245.

Light, E. (2019). Rates of use of community treatment orders in Australia. *International Journal of Law and Psychiatry, 64*, 83-87.

Light, E., Kerridge, I., Ryan, C., & Robertson, M. (2012). Community treatment orders in Australia: Rates and patterns of use. *Australasian Psychiatry, 20*(6), 478-482.

Light, E. M., Robertson, M. D., Boyce, P., Carney, T., Rosen, A., Cleary, M., . . . Kerridge, I. H. (2016). How shortcomings in the mental health system affect the use of involuntary community treatment orders. *Australian Health Review, 41*(3), 351-356.

Lightburn, A., & Sessions, P. (2006). Recovery guides: An emerging model of community-based care for adults with psychiatric disabilities. In L. Davidson, J. Tondora, M. Staeheli, M. O'Connell, J. Frey, & M. J. Chinman (eds.), *Handbook of Community-Based Clinical Practice* (pp. 476-501). USA: Oxford University Press.

Like Mind. (2020). *Connecting Mental Health Care*. Retrieved from https://likemind.org.au.

Lin, E., Durbin, J., Guerriere, D., Volpe, T., Selick, A., Kennedy, J., . . . Lero, D. S. (2018). Assessing care-giving demands, resources and costs of family/friend caregivers for persons with mental health disorders: A scoping review. *Health and Social Care in the Community.*

Lincoln, T. M., Wilhelm, K., & Nestoriuc, Y. (2007). Effectiveness of psychoeducation for relapse, symptoms, knowledge, adherence and functioning in psychotic disorders: A meta-analysis. *Schizophrenia Research, 96*(1-3), 232-245.

Lincoln, Y. (1994). Tracks toward a postmodern politics of evaluation. *Evaluation Practice, vol. 15*(3), pp. 299-309.

Linehan, M. M. (1993). *Cognitive-Behavioral Treatment of Borderline Personality Disorder.* New York: The Guilford Press.

Linehan, M. M. (2015). *DBT Skills Training Manual* (2nd ed.). New York: Guilford Press.

Lipowski, Z. J. (1988). Somatization: The concept and its clinical application. *American Journal of Psychiatry, 145*(11), 1358-1368.

Lippmann, L. (1982). *Melville Evaluated: An Experiment in Community Mental Health Care, Special Publication no. 11*. Melbourne: Mental Health Research Institute, Health Commission of Victoria.

Little, A. (2011). Political action, error and failure: The epistemological limits of complexity. *Political Studies, 60*(1), 3-19.

Li, W., Yang, Y., Liu, Z.-H., Zhao, Y.-J., Zhang, Q., Zhang, L., . . . Xiang, Y.-T. (2020). Progression of mental health services during the COVID-19 outbreak in China. *Int J Biol Sci, 16*(10), 1732-1738.

Liu, J., Gill, N. S., Teodorczuk, A., Li, Z. J., & Sun, J. (2019). The efficacy of cognitive behavioural therapy in somatoform disorders and medically unexplained physical symptoms: A meta-analysis of randomized controlled trials. *J Affect Disord, 245*, 98-112.

Lived Experience Workforce Strategies Stewardship Group. (2019). *Strategy for the Consumer Mental Health Workforce in Victoria.* Retrieved from https://cmhl.org.au/sites/default/files/resources-pdfs/Consumer-Workforce-Strategy-web.pdf.

Livesley, W. J. (2007). A framework for integrating dimensional and categorical classifications of personality disorder. *Journal of Personality Disorders, 21*(2), 199-224.

Livesley, W. J. (2012). Integrated treatment: A conceptual framework for an evidence-based approach to the treatment of personality disorder. *Journal of Personality Disorders, 26*(1), 17-42.

Livesley, W. J., & Larstone, R. (2018). *Handbook of Personality Disorders: Theory, Research, and Treatment*. Guilford Publications.

Ljungberg, A., Denhov, A., & Topor, A. (2015). The art of helpful relationships with professionals: A meta-ethnography of the perspective of persons with severe mental illness. *Psychiatric Quarterly, 86*(4), 471-495.

Llewellyn-Beardsley, J., Rennick-Egglestone, S., Callard, F., Crawford, P., Farkas, M., Hui, A., . . . Slade, M. (2019). Characteristics of mental health recovery narratives: Systematic review and narrative synthesis. *PLoS One, 14*(3).

Lloyd, C., & Williams, P. L. (2010). Occupational therapy in the modern adult acute mental health setting: A review of current practice. *International Journal of Therapy and Rehabilitation, 17*(9), 483-493.

Lobban, F., Postlethwaite, A., Glentworth, D., Pinfold, V., Wainwright, L., Dunn, G., . . . Haddock, G. (2013). A systematic review of randomised controlled trials of interventions reporting outcomes for relatives of people with psychosis. *Clinical Psychology Review, 33*(3), 372-382.

Lock, J., Le Grange, D., Agras, W. S., & Dare, C. D. (2001). *Treatment Manual for Anorexia Nervosa: A Family-Based Approach* (1st ed.). New York: Guilford Publications.

Lock, J. D., & Fitzpatrick, K. K. (2009). Anorexia nervosa. *BMJ Clinical Evidence, 2009: 1011*.

Lockett, H., Waghorn, G., & Kydd, R. (2018). A framework for improving the effectiveness of evidence-based practices in vocational rehabilitation. *Journal of Vocational Rehabilitation, 49*(1), 15-31.

Long, K. M., McDermott, F., & Meadows, G. N. (2018). Being pragmatic about health care complexity: Our experiences applying complexity theory and pragmatism to health services research. *BMC Medicine, 16*(94), 1-9.

Long, K. M., & Meadows, G. N. (2017). Simulation modelling in mental health: A systematic review. *Journal of Simulation, 12*(1), 76-85.

Longhofer, J., Kubek, P. M., & Floersch, J. (2010). *On Being and Having a Case Manager: A Relational Approach to Recovery in Mental Health*. New York: Columbia University Press.

Loomes, R., Hull, L., & Mandy, W. P. L. (2017). What is the male-to-female ratio in autism spectrum disorder? A systematic review and meta-analysis. *J Am Acad Child Adolesc Psychiatry, 56*(6), 466-474.

López-Solà, C., Fontenelle, L. F., Alonso, P., Cuadras, D., Foley, D. L., Pantelis, C., . . . Harrison, B. J. (2014). Prevalence and heritability of obsessive-compulsive spectrum and anxiety disorder symptoms: A survey of the Australian Twin Registry. *American Journal of Medical Genetics Part B: Neuropsychiatric Genetics, 165*(4), 314-325.

Lorenzo-Luaces, L., & DeRubeis, R. (2018). Miles to go before we sleep: Advancing the understanding of psychotherapy by modeling complex processes. *Cognitive Therapy and Research, 42*(2), 212-217.

Loureiro, D., Pio-Abreu, J. L., Machado, A., Gonçalves, R., & Cerejeira, J. (2015). Instruments for the assessment of autism spectrum disorders in adults without intellectual disabilities: A systematic review. *European Psychiatry, 30*(S1), 1857-1857.

Love, S. M., Sanders, M. R., Turner, K. M. T., Maurange, M., Knott, T., Prinz, R., . . . Ainsworth, A. T. (2016). Social media gamification: Engaging vulnerable parents in an online evidence-based parenting program. *Child Abuse & Neglect, 53*, 95-107.

Lovibond, P. F., & Lovibond, S. H. (1995). The structure of negative emotional states: Comparison of the Depression Anxiety Stress Scales (DASS) with the Beck Depression and Anxiety Inventories. *Behav Res Ther, 33*(3), 335-343.

Lowe, B., Grafe, K., Zipfel, S., Witte, S., Loerch, B., & Herzog, W. (2004). Diagnosing ICD-10 depressive episodes: Superior criterion validity of the Patient Health Questionnaire. *Psychother Psychosom, 73*(6), 386-390.

Lowe, B., Spitzer, R. L., Grafe, K., Kroenke, K., Quenter, A., Zipfel, S., . . . Herzog, W. (2004). Comparative validity of three screening questionnaires for DSM-IV depressive disorders and physicians' diagnoses. *J Affect Disord, 78*(2), 131-140.

Luborsky, L. (1984). *Principles of Psychoanalytic Psychotherapy: A Manual for Supportive-expressive Treatment*. Basic Books.

Luby, J. (1994). New developments in infant psychiatry. *Curr Opin Psychiatry, vol. 7*(4), pp. 311-314.

Lucassen, M., Samra, R., Iacovides, I., Fleming, T., Shepherd, M., Stasiak, K., & Wallace, L. (2018). How LGBT+ young people use the internet in relation to their mental health and envisage the use of e-Therapy: Exploratory study. *JMIR serious games, 6*(4), e11249.

Luck, A. J., Morgan, J. F., Reid, F., O'Brien, A., Brunton, J., Price, C., . . . Lacey, J. (2002). The SCOFF questionnaire and clinical interview for eating disorders in general practice: Comparative study. *BMJ: British Medical Journal, 325*(7367), 755-756.

Lucksted, A., McFarlane, W., Downing, D., & Dixon, L. (2012). Recent developments in family psychoeducation as an evidence-based practice. *Journal of Marital and Family Therapy, 38*(1), 101-121.

Lum, T. Y., & Lightfoot, E. (2005). The effect of volunteering on the physical and mental health of older people. *Research on Aging, 27*, 31-35.

Lunt, M. F., & Shaw, I. (2009). *Practitioner Research in Social Services: A Literature Review (Summary)*. Retrieved from www.york.ac.uk/media/spsw/documents/research-and-publications/NeilLuntPractitionerResearchLitReview.pdf.

Luntz, J. J. (1999). What is mental health consultation? *Children Australia, 24*(3), 28-33.

Luntz, J. J. (2000). Mental health consultation: Stages in the consultation process. *Children Australia, 25*(1), 21-26.

Lydon, J. (2018). *Remembering the Myall Creek Massacre*. Lyndall Ryan: UNSW Press.

Lynch, J. M., Askew, D. A., Mitchell, G. K., & Hegarty, K. L. (2012). Beyond symptoms: Defining primary care mental health clinical assessment priorities, content and process. *Social Science & Medicine, 74*(2), 143-149.

Lyons, C., Casey, J., Brown, T., Tseng, M., & McDonald, R. (2010). Research knowledge, attitudes, practices and barriers among paediatric occupational therapists in the United Kingdom. *British Journal of Occupational Therapy, 73*(5), 200-209.

Lyons, C., Hopley, P., Burton, C. R., & Horrocks, J. (2009). Mental health crisis and respite services: Service user and carer aspirations. *Journal of Psychiatric and Mental Health Nursing, 16*(5), 424-433.

Ma, S. H., & Teasdale, J. D. (2004). Mindfulness-based cognitive therapy for depression: Replication and exploration of differential relapse prevention effects. *J Consult Clin Psychol, 72*(1), 31-40.

Mack, J. E. (1975). *Borderline States in Psychiatry*. Grune & Stratton.

MacKellar, D. (2016). *My Country*. Retrieved from www.dorotheamackellar.com.au/archive/mycountry.htm.

MacKenzie, D., Flatau, P., Steen, A., & Thielking, M. (2016). *The Cost of Youth Homelessness in Australia: Research Briefing*. Melbourne: Swinburne University.

Macneil, C., Creek, R., Fraser, S., Coulson, L., Dodd, S., Nicoll, M., . . . Stavely, H. (2014). *Get on Board: Engaging Young People and their Families in Early Psychosis*. Melbourne: Orygen Youth Health Research Centre.

Macpherson, R., Varah, M., Summerfield, L., Foy, C., & Slade, M. (2003). Staff and patient assessments of need in an epidemiologically representative sample of patients with psychosis. *Social Psychiatry and Psychiatric Epidemiology, 38*(11), 662-667.

Madden, S., Morris, A., Zurynski, Y. A., Kohn, M., & Elliot, E. J. (2009). Burden of eating disorders in 5-13-year-old children in Australia. *Medical Journal of Australia, 190*(8), 410-414.

Maddock, A. (2015). Consensus or contention: An exploration of multidisciplinary team functioning in an Irish mental health context. *European Journal of Social Work, 18*(2), 1-16.

Maercker, A., Forstmeier, S., Pielmaier, L., Spangenberg, L., Brahler, E., & Glaesmer, H. (2012). Adjustment disorders: Prevalence in a representative nationwide survey in Germany. *Soc Psychiatry Psychiatr Epidemiol, 47*(11), 1745-1752.

Maercker, A., Hecker, T., Augsburger, M., & Kliem, S. (2018). ICD-11 prevalence rates of posttraumatic stress disorder and complex posttraumatic stress disorder in a German nationwide sample. *J Nerv Ment Dis, 206*(4), 270-276.

Magliano, L., Fiorillo, A., Fadden, G., Gair, F., Economou, M., Kallert, T., . . . Maj, M. (2005). Effectiveness of a psychoeducational intervention for families of patients with schizophrenia: Preliminary results of a study funded by the European Commission. *World Psychiatry, 4*(1), 45-49.

Mahlke, I. C., Krämer, M. U., Becker, M. T., & Bock, M. T. (2014). Peer support in mental health services. *Curr Opin Psychiatry, 27*(4), 276-281.

Main, M., & Solomon, J. (1993). Procedures for Identifying Infants as disorganized disoriented during the Ainsworth Strange Situation. In M. T. Greenberg, D. Cicchetti, & E. M. Cummings (eds.), *Attachment in the Preschool Years: Theory, Research, and Intervention* (pp. 122-161). Chicago: University of Chicago Press.

Makela, E. H., Moeller, K. E., Fullen, J. E., & Gunel, E. (2006). Medication utilization patterns and methods of suicidality in borderline personality disorder. *Annals of Pharmacotherapy, 40*(1), 49-52.

Malhi, G., Adams, D., Bernardi, E., Miller, M., Mulder, R., Walter, G., & Smith, B. (2010). Time to 'get real': Preliminary insights into the long-term management of schizophrenia. *Australasian Psychiatry, 18*(2), 115-119.

Malhi, G. S., Bassett, D., Boyce, P., Bryant, R., Fitzgerald, P. B., Fritz, K., . . . Murray, G. (2015). Royal Australian and New Zealand College of Psychiatrists clinical practice guidelines for mood disorders. *Australian & New Zealand Journal of Psychiatry, 49*(12), 1087-1206.

Mancini, M. A. (2007). The role of self-efficacy in recovery from serious psychiatric disabilities: A qualitative study with fifteen psychiatric survivors. *Qualitative Social Work, 6*(1), 49-74.

Mandiberg, J. M. (2012). The failure of social inclusion: An alternative approach through community development. *Psychiatric Services, 63*(5), 458-460.

Manning, M., & Hudgins, L. (2010). Array-based technology and recommendations for utilization in medical genetics practice for detection of chromosomal abnormalities. *Genet Med, 12*(11), 742-745.

Mansfield, C., Hopfer, S., & Marteau, T. M. (1999). Termination rates after prenatal diagnosis of Down syndrome, spina bifida, anencephaly, and Turner and Klinefelter syndromes: A systematic literature review. *Prenatal Diagnosis, 19*(9), 808-812.

Marel, C., Mills, K., Deady, M., & Teesson, M. (2009). *Guidelines on the Management of Co-Occurring Alcohol and Other Drug and Mental Health Conditions in Alcohol and Other Drug Treatment Settings* (2nd ed.). Sydney: National Drug and Alcohol Research Centre.

Marinker, M. (1970). Balint seminars and vocational training in general practice. *J R Coll Gen Pract, 19*(91), 79-91.

Mark, M. M., Henry, G. T., & Jules, G. (2000). *Evaluation: An Integrative Framework for Understanding and Guiding and Improving Policies and Programs*. San Francisco: Jossey-Bass.

Marmot Review Team. (2010). *Fair Society, Healthy Lives. The Marmot Review. Strategic Review of Health Inequalities in England Post-2010*. Retrieved from www.instituteofhealthequity.org/resources-reports/fair-society-healthy-lives-the-marmot-review/fair-society-healthy-lives-full-report-pdf.pdf.

Marsh, A., O'Toole, S., Dale, A., Willis, L., & Helfgott, S. (2013). *Counselling Guidelines: Alcohol and Other Drug Issues*. Drug and Alcohol Office.

Marsh, P., & Kelly, L. (2018). Review of Dignity of risk in the community: a review of and reflections on the literature. Health, Risk & Society, 20(5-6), 297-311.

Marshall, M., & Lockwood, A. (1998). Assertive community treatment for people with severe mental disorders. *Cochrane Database Systematic Review 2011; (4): CD001089.*

Martell, C. R., Dimidjian, S., & Herman-Dunn, R. (2010). *Behavioral Activation for Depression: A Clinician's Guide*. Guilford Publications.

Martin, L. A., Neighbors, H. W., & Griffith, D. M. (2013). The experience of symptoms of depression in men vs women: Analysis of the National Comorbidity Survey Replication. *JAMA Psychiatry, 70*(10), 1100-1106.

Martin, P. R., & Birnbrauer, J. S. (1996). *Clinical Psychology: Profession and Practice in Australia*. South Melbourne: Macmillan Education Australia.

Martin-Latry, K., Goumy, M. P., Latry, P., Gabinski, C., Begaud, B., Faure, I., & Verdoux, H. (2007). Psychotropic drugs use and risk of heat-related hospitalisation. *European Psychiatry, 22*(6), 335-338.

Mason, B. J. (2001). Treatment of alcohol-dependent outpatients with acamprosate: A clinical review. *J Clin Psychiatry, 62*, 42-48.

Masten, A. S., Burt, K. B., Roisman, G. I., Obradovic, J., Long, J. D., & Tellegen, A. (2004). Resources and resilience in the transition to adulthood: Continuity and change. *Development and Psychopathology, 16*(4), 1071-1094.

Mataix-Cols, D., Boman, M., Monzani, B., & et al. (2013). Population-based, multigenerational family clustering study of obsessive-compulsive disorder. *JAMA Psychiatry, 70*(7), 709-717.

Matilainen, R., Airaksinen, E., Mononen, T., Launiala, K., & Kääriäinen, R. (1995). A population-based study on the causes of mild and severe mental retardation. *Acta Pœdiatrica, 84*(3), 261-266.

Matosin, N., Halldorsdottir, T., & Binder, E. B. (2018). Understanding the molecular mechanisms underpinning gene by environment interactions in psychiatric disorders: The FKBP5 Model. *Biological Psychiatry, 83*(10), 821-830.

Mattick, R. P., Breen, C., Kimber, J., & Davoli, M. (2009). Methadone maintenance therapy versus no opioid replacement therapy for opioid dependence. *Cochrane Database of Systematic Reviews*(3).

Mattick RP, Kimber J, Breen C, Davoli M. (2003) Buprenorphine maintenance versus placebo or methadone maintenance for opioid dependence. *Cochrane Database of Systematic Reviews*, issue 2. art. no.: CD002207. doi: 10.1002/14651858.CD002207.pub2.

Mattick, R. P., Jarvis, Tracey J, & National Drug Strategy. (1993). *An Outline for the Management of Alcohol Problems*. Canberra: Australian Govt. Pub. Service.

Mattingly, C., & Fleming, M. H. (1994). *Clinical Reasoning: Forms of Inquiry in a Therapeutic Practice*. Philadelphia: F. A. Davis.

Maybery, D., Goodyear, M., Reupert, A., Sheen, J., Cann, W., Dalziel, K., . . . von Doussa, H. (2017). Developing an Australian-first recovery model for parents in Victorian mental health and family services: A study protocol for a randomised controlled trial. *BMC Psychiatry, 17*(1), 198.

Maybery, D., & Reupert, A. (2006). Workforce capacity to respond to children whose parents have a mental illness. *Australian and New Zealand Journal of Psychiatry, 40*(8), 657-664.

Maybery, D., & Reupert, A. (2018). The number of parents who are patients attending adult psychiatric services. *Curr Opin Psychiatry, 31*(4), 358-362.

Maybery, D., Reupert, A., Patrick, K., Goodyear, M., & Crase, L. (2009). Prevalence of parental mental illness in Australian families. *Psychiatric Bulletin, 33*(1), 22-26.

Mayfield, D., McLeod, G., & Hall, P. (1974). The Cage Questionnaire: Validation of a new alcoholism screening test. *American Journal of Psychiatry, vol. 131*, pp. 1121-1123.

Maylea, C. (2017). Minimising coerciveness in coercion: A case study of social work powers under the Victorian Mental Health Act. *Australian Social Work, 70*(4), 465–476.

Maylea, C., Jørgensen, A., Matta, S., Ogilvie, K., & Wallin, P. (2018). Consumers' experiences of mental health advance statements. *Laws, 7*(22).

Maylea, C. H. (2016). An end to involuntary treatment in Australian mental health social work. In N. Paul & P. Jones (eds.), *Social Work and Health: Inclusive Practice Research and Education* (pp. 94–119). Kerala: Depaul Centre for Research and Development.

Maylea, C. H. (2017). Minimising coerciveness in coercion: A case study of social work powers under the Victorian Mental Health Act. *Australian Social Work, 70*(4), 465–476.

Maylea, C. H. (2017). A rejection of involuntary treatment in mental health social work. *Ethics and Social Welfare, 11*(4), 336–352.

Maynard, B. R., Wilson, A. N., Labuzienski, E., & Whiting, S. W. (2015). Mindfulness-based approaches in the treatment of disordered gambling. *Research on Social Work Practice, 28*(3), 348–362.

Mayou, R. (2014). Is the DSM-5 chapter on somatic symptom disorder any better than DSM-IV somatoform disorder? *Br J Psychiatry, 204*(6), 418.

McAllister, M., & Walsh, K. (2004). Different voices: Reviewing and revising the politics of working with consumers in mental health. *International Journal of Mental Health Nursing, 13*, 22–32.

McBeth, R. (2018). Digital mental health tool trialled at three DHBs. *eHealthNews*. Retrieved from www.hinz.org.nz/news/425517/Digital-mental-health-tool-trialled-at-three-DHBs.htm.

McCann, T. V., & Baker, H. (2002). Community mental health nurses and authority to prescribe medications: The way forward? *Journal of Psychiatric and Mental Health Nursing, 9*(2), 175–182.

McClain, Z., & Peebles, R. (2016). Body image and eating disorders among lesbian, gay, bisexual, and transgender youth. *Pediatr Clin North Am, 63*(6), 1079–1090.

McCloughen, A., Gillies, D., & O'Brien, L. (2011). Collaboration between mental health consumers and nurses. *International Journal of Mental Health Nursing, 20*, 47–55.

McCrone, J. (1997). Wild minds. *New Scientist, 156*(2112), 26–30.

McCrone, J. (1999). *Going Inside: A Tour Round a Single Moment of Consciousness*. London: Faber and Faber.

McCullumsmith, C. B., & Ford, C. V. (2011). Simulated illness: The factitious disorders and malingering. *Psychiatric Clinics of North America, 34*(3), 621–+.

McDermott, E., Hughes, E., & Rawlings, V. (2016). *Queer Futures: Understanding Lesbian, Gay, Bisexual and Trans (LGBT) Adolescents' Suicide, Self-Harm and Help-Seeking Behaviour.* United Kingdom: Department of Health Policy Research Programme Project.

McFarlane, W. R., Dixon, L., Lukens, E., & Lucksted, A. (2003). Family psychoeducation and schizophrenia: A review of the literature. *Journal of Marital and Family Therapy, 29*(2), 223–245.

McGahey, E., Waghorn, G., Lloyd, C., Morrissey, S., & Williams, P. L. (2016). Formal plan for self-disclosure enhances supported employment outcomes among young people with severe mental illness. *Early Intervention in Psychiatry, 10*(2), 178–185.

McGorry, P., & Purcell, R. (2009). Youth mental health reform and early intervention: Encouraging early signs. *Early Intervention in Psychiatry, 3*, 161–162.

McGorry, P. D. (2007). The specialist youth mental health model: Strengthening the weakest link in the public mental health system. *Medical Journal of Australia, 187*(7 Suppl), S53–56.

McGorry, P. D. (2012). Mental ill-health in young people: Assessment and early treatment. *Medicine Today, 13*(5), 46–52.

McGorry, P. D. (2015). Early intervention in psychosis: Obvious, effective, overdue. *Journal of Nervous and Mental Disease, 203*(5), 310–318.

McGorry, P. D., Chanen, A. M., & Robinson, J. (2018). Upstream of EDs, downstream of headspace: Helping the 'missing middle'. *MJA InSight, Issue 17*.

McGorry, P. D., Edwards, J., Mihalopoulos, C., Harrigan, S. M., & Jackson, H. J. (1996). The Early Psychosis Prevention and Intervention Centre (EPPIC): An evolving system of early detection and optimal management. *Schizophrenia Bulletin, vol. 22*(2), pp. 305–326.

McGorry, P. D., & Goldstone, S. (2011). Is this normal? Assessing mental health in young people. *Australian Family Physician, 40*(3), 94–97.

McGorry, P. D., Goldstone, S. D., Parker, A. G., Rickwood, D. J., & Hickie, I. B. (2014). Cultures for mental health care of young people: An Australian blueprint for reform. *Lancet Psychiatry, 1*(7), 559–568.

McGorry, P. D., & Hamilton, M. P. (2017). Broken promises and missing steps in mental health reform. *Medical Journal of Australia, 206*(11), 487–489.

McGorry, P. D., Hickie, I. B., Yung, A. R., Pantelis, C., & Jackson, H. J. (2006). Clinical staging of psychiatric disorders: A heuristic framework for choosing earlier, safer and more effective interventions. *Australian and New Zealand Journal of Psychiatry, 40*(8), 616–622.

McGorry, P. D., Nelson, B., Markulev, C., Yuen, H. P., Schäfer, M. R., Mossaheb, N., . . . Amminger, G. P. (2017). Effect of ω-3 polyunsaturated fatty acids in young people at ultrahigh risk for psychotic disorders: The NEURAPRO randomized clinical trial. *JAMA Psychiatry, 74*(1), 19–27.

McGorry, P. D., Purcell, R., Goldstone, S., & Amminger, G. P. (2011). Age of onset and timing of treatment for mental and substance use disorders: Implications for preventive intervention strategies and models of care. *Curr Opin Psychiatry, 24*(4), 301–306.

McGrath, A., Crome, P., & Crome, I. B. (2005). Substance misuse in the older population. *Postgraduate Medical Journal, 81*(954), 228–231.

McGuffin, P. C., Farmer, A., & Harvey, I. (1991). A polydiagnostic application of operational criteria in studies of psychotic illness. Development and reliability of the OPCRIT system. *Archives of General Psychiatry, 48*, 764–770.

McGuiness, M., & Wadsworth, Y. (1992). *Understanding Anytime: A Consumer Evaluation of an Acute Psychiatric Hospital* (1st ed.). Melbourne: Victorian Mental Illness Awareness Council.

McHugh, R. K., Hearon, B. A., & Otto, M. W. (2010). Cognitive behavioral therapy for substance use disorders. *Psychiatric Clinics, 33*(3), 511–525.

McIntosh, V. V., Jordan, J., Carter, F. A., Luty, S. E., McKenzie, J. M., Bulik, C. M., . . . Joyce, P. R. (2005). Three psychotherapies for anorexia nervosa: A randomized, controlled trial. *The American Journal of Psychiatry, 162*(4), 741–747.

McKendrick, J., Brooks, R., Hudson, J., Thorpe, M., & Bennett, P. (2014). *Aboriginal and Torres Strait Islander Healing Programs: A Literature Review*. Retrieved from https://healingfoundation.org.au.

McKenna, B., Furness, T., Wallace, E., Happell, B., Stanton, R., Platania-Phung, C., . . . Castle, D. (2014). The effectiveness of specialist roles in mental health metabolic monitoring: A retrospective cross-sectional comparison study. *BMC Psychiatry, 14*, 234.

McKenna, M. C., Zevon, M. A., Corn, B., & Rounds, J. (1999). Psychosocial factors and the development of breast cancer: A meta-analysis. *Health Psychology, 18*(5), 520-531.

McKenzie, S., Jenkin, G., & Collings, S. (2016). Men's perspectives of common mental health problems: A metasynthesis of qualitative research. *International Journal of Men's Health, 15*(1), 80-104.

McKown, C., & Strambler, M. J. (2009). Developmental antecedents and social and academic consequences of stereotype-consciousness in middle childhood. *Child Development, 80*(6), 1643-1659.

McMichael, A. J., Neira, M., Bertollini, R., Campbell-Lendrum, D., & Hales, S. (2009). Climate change: A time of need and opportunity for the health sector. *Lancet, 374*(9707), 2123-2125.

McMillen, J., & Donnelly, K. (2008). Gambling in Australian Indigenous communities: The state of play. *Australian Journal of Social Issues, 43*(3), 397-426.

McNab, C., & Meadows, G. (2005). The General-Practice Users' Perceived-Need Inventory ('GUPI'): A brief general practice tool to assist in bringing mental healthcare needs to professional attention. *Primary Care Mental Health, 3*(2), 93-101.

McQueen, D. V., Wismar, M., Lin, V., Jones, C. M., & Davies, M. (eds.). (2012). *Intersectoral Governance for Health in All Policies. Structures, Actions and Experiences. Observatory Studies Series 26*. Copenhagen: World Health Organization.

McSherry, B., & Wilson, K. (2015). The concept of capacity in Australian mental health law reform: Going in the wrong direction? *International Journal of Law and Psychiatry, 40*, 60-69.

McWade, B. (2016). Recovery-as-policy as a form of neoliberal state making. *Intersectionalities: A Global Journal of Social Work Analysis, Research, Polity, and Practice, 5*(3), 62-81.

McWilliams, L. A., & Higgins, K. S. (2013). Associations between pain conditions and borderline personality disorder symptoms: Findings from the National Comorbidity Survey Replication. *Clinical Journal of Pain, 29*(6), 527-532.

Mead, N., Lester, H., Chew-Graham, C., Gask, L., & Bower, P. (2010). Effects of befriending on depressive symptoms and distress: Systematic review and meta-analysis. *Br J Psychiatry, 196*(2), 96-101.

Mead, S. (n.d). *Peer Support as a Socio-Political Response to Trauma and Abuse*. Retrieved from www. intentionalpeersupport org.

Mead, S., Hilton, D., & Curtis, L. (2001). Peer support: A theoretical perspective. *Psychiatric Rehabilitation Journal, 25*(2), 134-141.

Mead, S., & Macneil, C. (2006). Peer support: What makes it unique? *Int J Psychosoc Rehab, 10*(2), 29-37.

Meadows, G. (2016). *PULSAR Manual Recovery Promoting Relationships and Working Practices for Specialist and Community Mental Health Services (Or Secondary Care Staff)*. Retrieved from www.monash.edu/__data/assets/pdf_file/0017/1452410/PULSAR-Secondary_Care_Manual-FINAL.pdf.

Meadows, G., Brophy, L., Shawyer, F., Enticott, J. C., Fossey, E., Thornton, C. D., . . . Slade, M. (2019). REFOCUS-PULSAR recovery-oriented practice training in specialist mental health care: A stepped-wedge cluster randomised controlled trial. *The Lancet Psychiatry, 6*(2), 103-114.

Meadows, G., & Burgess, P. M. (2009). Perceived need for mental health care: Findings from the 2007 Australian Survey of Mental Health and Wellbeing. *Australian and New Zealand Journal of Psychiatry, 43*(7), 624-634.

Meadows, G., Burgess, P. M., Fossey, E., & Harvey, C. (2000). Perceived need for mental health care, findings from the Australian National Survey of Mental Health and Well-being. *Psychol Med, 30*(3), 645-656.

Meadows, G., Enticott, J., & Rosenberg, S. (2018). Three charts on: Why rates of mental illness aren't going down despite higher spending. *The Conversation*. Retrieved from https://theconversation.com/three-charts-on-why-rates-of-mental-illness-arent-going-down-despite-higher-spending-97534.

Meadows, G., Gielewski, H., Falconer, B., Kelly, H., Joubert, L., & Clarke, M. (1997). The pattern of care model: A tool for planning community mental health services. *Psychiatric Services, 48*(2), 218-223.

Meadows, G. N., Prodan, A., Patten, S., Shawyer, F., Francis, S., Enticott, J., . . . Kakuma, R. (2019). Resolving the paradox of increased mental health expenditure and stable prevalence. *Australian & New Zealand Journal of Psychiatry*, 53(9), 844-850.

Meadows, G., & Singh, B. (2003). 'Victoria on the move': Mental health services in a decade of transition 1992-2002. *Australasian Psychiatry, 11*(1), 62-67.

Meadows, G., Turner, T., Campbell, L., Lewis, S. W., & et al. (1991). Assessing schizophrenia in adults with mental retardation: A comparative study. *British Journal of Psychiatry, 158*, 103-105.

Meadows, G. N. (1998). Establishing a collaborative model for primary mental health care. *Medical Journal of Australia, 168*, 162-165.

Meadows, G. N. (2003). Overcoming barriers to reintegration of patients with schizophrenia: Developing a best-practice model for discharge from specialist care. *Medical Journal of Australia, 178*(9), Suppl 5:S53-S56.

Meadows, G. N., & Bobevski, I. (2011). Changes in met perceived need for mental healthcare in Australia from 1997 to 2007. *British Journal of Psychiatry, 199*(6), 479-484.

Meadows, G. N., Enitcott, J. C., Inder, B., Russell, G. M., & Gurr, R. (2015). Better access to mental health care and the failure of the Medicare principle of universality. *Med J Aust, 4*(202), 190-194.

Meadows, G. N., Harvey, C. A., Joubert, L., Barton, D., & Bedi, G. (2007). The Consultation-Liaison in Primary-Care Psychiatry (CLIPP) Program: A structured approach to long-term collaboration in mental health care. *Psychiatric Services, 58*(8), 1036-1038.

Meadows, G. N., Liaw, T., Burgess, P., Bobevski, I., & Fossey, E. (2001). Australian general practice and the meeting of needs for mental health care. *Social Psychiatry and Psychiatric Epidemiology, 36*(12), 595-603.

Meadows, G. N., Monash, D., & Cichello, A. (2007). Collaborative care for common mental disorders. In G. Blashki, F. Judd, & L. Piterman (eds.), *General Practice Psychiatry* (pp. 373-383). Melbourne: McGraw-Hill.

Meadows, G. N., Prodan, A., Patten, S., Shawyer, F., Francis, S., Enticott, J., . . . Kakuma, R. (2019). Resolving the paradox of increased mental health expenditure and stable prevalence. *Australian & New Zealand Journal of Psychiatry, 53*(9), 844-850.

Meares, R., Hampshire, R., Gordon, E., & Kraiuhin, C. (1985). Whose hysteria: Briquet's, Janet's or Freud's? *Australian and New Zealand Journal of Psychiatry, 19*(3), 256-263.

Mechanic, D. (1968). *Medical Sociology*. New York: Free Press.

Medicare program. (2019). *Education Guide: Better Access to Mental Health Care for Eligible Practitioners and Allied Health Professionals*. Retrieved from www.humanservices.gov.au/organisations/health-professionals/topics/education-guide-better-access-mental-health-care-eligible-practitioners-and-allied-health/35591.

Megivern, D., Pellerito, S., & Mowbray, C. (2003). Barriers to higher education for individuals with psychiatric disabilities. *Psychiatric Rehabilitation Journal, 26*(3), 217-231.

Meichenbaum, D. H. (1973). Cognitive factors in behaviour modification: Modifying what clients say to themselves. In C. M. Franks & G. T. Wilson (eds.), *Annual Review of Behavior Therapy: Theory & Practice* (Vol. 1). Brunner/Mazel.

Melle, I., Larsen, T. K., Haahr, U., Friis, S., Johannessen, J. O., Opjordsmoen, S., . . . McGlashan, T. (2004). Reducing the duration of untreated first-episode psychosis: Effects on clinical presentation. *Archives of General Psychiatry, 61*(2), 143-150.

Meltzer, H., Vostanis, P., Dogra, N., Doos, L., Ford, T., & Goodman, R. (2009). Children's specific fears. *Child Care, Health & Development, 35*(6), 781-789.

Melzer, D., Fryers, T., Jenkins, R., Brugha, T., & McWilliams, B. (2003). Social position and the common mental disorders with disability: Estimates from the National Psychiatric Survey of Great Britain. *Social Psychiatry and Psychiatric Epidemiology, 38*(5), 238-243.

Menchon, J., Mestre-Bach, G., Steward, T., & Fernández-Aranda, F. (2018). An overview of gambling disorder: from treatment approaches to risk factors. F1000Research, 7, 434. https://doi.org/10.12688/f1000research.12784.1.

Mendelson, T., & Eaton, W. W. (2018). Recent advances in the prevention of mental disorders. *Social Psychiatry and Psychiatric Epidemiology, 53*(4), 325-339.

Mendoza, J., Bresnan, A., Rosenberg, S., Elson, A., Gilbert, Y., & Long, P. (2013). *Obsessive hope disorder: Reflections on 30 years of mental health reform and visions for the future. Summary Report*. ConNetica, Caloundra, QLD.

Mental Health Alcohol and Drug Directorate. (2015). Better mental health and wellbeing—a long-term plan for mental health in Tasmania 2015-25. *Rethink Mental Health*. Retrieved from www.dhhs.tas.gov.au/mentalhealth/rethink_mental_health_project.

Mental Health Carers Australia. (2019). *Supporting and Promoting the Well-Being of Mental Health Carers and Their Families*. Retrieved from www.mentalhealthcarersaustralia.org.au/about-us/our-members.

Mental Health Commission of NSW. (2018). *Lived Experience Framework for NSW*. Retrieved from https://nswmentalhealthcommission.com.au/sites/default/files/documents/final_lef_a4_layout_for_web.pdf.

Mental Health Commission of NSW. (2020). *Living Well Mid-term Review: Gold Card Clinics—Emotional Health Clinic and Research Unit*. Retrieved from https://nswmentalhealthcommission.com.au/living-well-ag.

Mental Health Commission. (2013). *Mental Health Commission 2012/13 Annual Report*. Retrieved from www.mhc.wa.gov.au/media/1527/mhc-annual-report-2012-13.pdf.

Mental Health Commission. (2015). *Mental Health Commission 2014/15 Annual Report*. Retrieved from www.mhc.wa.gov.au/media/1215/annual-report-2015-16-final-interactive-mhc.pdf.

Mental Health Commission. (2016). *Mental Health Commission 2015/16 Annual Report*. Retrieved from www.mhc.wa.gov.au/media/1283/2016-mhc-annual-report_final.pdf.

Mental Health Commission. (2017). *Mental Health Commission 2016/17 Annual Report*. Retrieved from www.mhc.wa.gov.au/media/2152/mhc17-54276-final-approved-interactive-pdf-12-sept-2017.pdf.

Mental Health Commission. (2018). *Mental Health Commission 2017/18 Annual Report*. Retrieved from www.mhc.wa.gov.au/media/2512/mhcar2018.pdf.

Mental Health Commission. (2019). *Western Australian Mental Health, Alcohol and Other Drug Services Plan 2015-2025 (Plan) Update 2018*. Retrieved from www.mhc.wa.gov.au/media/2830/plan-update-2018.pdf.

Mental Health Coordinating Council (MHCC). (2018). *Recovery Oriented Language Guide: Second Edition Revised*. Retrieved from www.mhcc.org.au.

Mental Health Coordinating Council (MHCC). (2020). *Empowering Community Managed Mental Health in NSW*. Retrieved from www.mhcc.org.au.

Mental Health Coordinating Council (MHCC). (2020). *Trauma-Informed Care and Practice (TICP)*. Retrieved from www.mhcc.org.au/project/trauma-informed-care-and-practice-ticp.

Mental Health First Aid Australia. (2018). *Mental Health First Aid Training*. Retrieved from https://mhfa.com.au.

Mental Health in Multicultural Australia. (2014). *Framework for Mental Health in Multicultural Australia: Towards Culturally Inclusive Service Delivery*. Upper Mt Gravatt: Mental Health in Multicultural Australia.

Mental Health Services Commission. (1988). *The Mental Health Services Commission: Report for Year 1986-87*. Hobart, Government of Tasmania.

Mentzoni, R. A., Brunborg, G. S., Molde, H., Myrseth, H., Skouveroe, K. J. M., Hetland, J., & Pallesen, S. (2011). Problematic video game use: Estimated prevalence and associations with mental and physical health. *Cyberpsychology Behavior and Social Networking, 14*(10), 591-596.

Menzies, I. E. P. (1970). *The Functioning of Social Systems as a Defence Against Anxiety: A Report on a Study of the Nursing Service of a General Hospital*. London: Tavistock Institute of Human Relations.

Menzies School of Health Research. (2019). *Mental Health & Wellbeing*. Retrieved from www.menzies.edu.au/page/Research/Indigenous_Health/Mental_health_and_prevention/Mental_Health_and_wellbeing.

Merikangas, K. R., He, J.-p., Burstein, M., Swanson, S. A., Avenevoli, S., Cui, L., . . . Swendsen, J. (2010). Lifetime prevalence of mental disorders in US adolescents: Results from the National Comorbidity Survey Replication–Adolescent Supplement (NCS-A). *Journal of the American Academy of Child & Adolescent Psychiatry, 49*(10), 980-989.

Merkouris, S., Greenwood, C., Manning, V., Oakes, J., Rodda, S., Lubman, D., & Dowling, N. (2020). Enhancing the utility of the problem gambling severity index in clinical settings: Identifying refined categories within the problem gambling category. *Addictive Behaviors*, 103, 106257. doi: https://doi.org/10.1016/j.addbeh.2019.106257.

Merskey, H. (1992). The manufacture of personalities: The production of multiple personality-disorder. *British Journal of Psychiatry, 160*, 327-340.

Metropolitan Police Service. (2018). *Fixated Threat Assessment Centre (FTAC). Preventing Harm and Facilitating Care*. Retrieved from www.fixatedthreat.com/ftac-welcome.php.

Meurk, C., Leung, J., Hall, W., Head, B. W., & Whiteford, H. (2016). Establishing and governing e-mental health care in Australia: A systematic review of challenges and a call for policy-focussed research. *Journal of Medical Internet Research, 18*(1), e10.

Mewton, L., Teesson, M., Slade, T., & Grove, R. (2011). The epidemiology of DSM-IV alcohol use disorders amongst young adults in the Australian population. *Alcohol and alcoholism, 46*(2), 185-191.

Meyer, A. (1922/1977). The philosophy of occupational therapy. *American Journal of Occupational Therapy, 31*(10), 639-642.

Meyer, T. J., Miller, M. L., Metzger, R. L., & Borkovec, T. D. (1990). Development and validation of the Penn State Worry Questionnaire. *Behav Res Ther, 28*(6), 487-495.

Micali, N., Martini, M. G., Thomas, J. J., Eddy, K. T., Kothari, R., Russell, E., . . . Treasure, J. (2017). Lifetime and 12-month prevalence of eating disorders amongst women in mid-life: A population-based study of diagnoses and risk factors. *BMC Med, 15*(1), 12.

Michelson, D. J., Shevell, M. I., Sherr, E. H., Moeschler, J. B., Gropman, A. L., & Ashwal, S. (2011). Evidence report: Genetic and metabolic testing on children with global developmental delay: Report of the Quality Standards Subcommittee of the American Academy of Neurology and the Practice Committee of the Child Neurology Society. *Neurology, 77*(17), 1629-1635.

Miklowitz, D. J. (2004). The role of family systems in severe and recurrent psychiatric disorders: A developmental psychopathology view. *Dev Psychopathol, 16*(3), 667-688.

Miklowitz, D. J., & Chung, B. (2016). Family-focused therapy for bipolar disorder: Reflections on 30 years of research. *Family Process, 55*(3), 483-499.

Milanovic, B. (2016). *Global Inequality: A New Approach for the Age of Globalization*. Harvard University Press.

Miletic, T., & Victorian Transcultural Psychiatry Unit. (2006). Guidelines for working effectively with interpreters in mental health settings. Fitzroy: Victorian Transcultural Psychiatry Unit.

Miller, C., Freeman, M., & Ross, N. (2001). *Interprofessional practice in health and social care: Challenging the shared learning agenda*. London: Arnold.

Miller, D. T., Adam, M. P., Aradhya, S., Biesecker, L. G., Brothman, A. R., Carter, N. P., . . . Ledbetter, D. H. (2010). Consensus statement: Chromosomal microarray is a first-tier clinical diagnostic test for individuals with developmental disabilities or congenital anomalies. *Am J Hum Genet, 86*(5), 749-764.

Miller, W. R., & Rollnick, S. (2012). *Motivational Interviewing: Helping People Change* (3rd ed.). New York: Guilford Publications.

Millon, T. (1981). *Disorders of Personality: DSM-III, Axis II*. New York: Wiley.

Millon, T., Grossman, S., & Millon, C. (2015). *Millon Clinical Multiaxial Inventory-IV (MCMI-IV)*. Sydney: Pearson.

Mills, K. L., McFarlane, A. C., Slade, T., Creamer, M., Silove, D., Teesson, M., & Bryant, R. (2011). Assessing the prevalence of trauma exposure in epidemiological surveys. *Australian & New Zealand Journal of Psychiatry, 45*(5), 407-415.

Mills-Koonce, W. R., Appleyard, K., Barnett, M., Deng, M., Putallaz, M., & Cox, M. (2011). Adult attachment style and stress as risk factors for maternal sensitivity and negativity. *Infant Mental Health Journal, 32*(3), 277-285.

Milner, A., King, T. L., LaMontagne, A. D., Aitken, Z., Petrie, D., & Kavanagh, A. M. (2017). Underemployment and its impacts on mental health among those with disabilities: Evidence from the HILDA cohort. *J Epidemiol Community Health, 71*(12), 1198-1202.

Milroy, H. (2003). The dance of life: The bio-psycho-social-spiritual-cultural model of health. *Australian and New Zealand Journal of Psychiatry, 37*, A42-A43.

Minas, H. (2005). Leadership for change in complex systems. *Australas Psychiatry, 13*(1), 33-39.

Minas, H., Kakuma, R., Too, L. S., Vayani, H., Orapeleng, S., Prasad-Ildes, R., . . . Oehm, D. (2013). Mental health research and evaluation in multicultural Australia: Developing a culture of inclusion. *Int J Ment Health Syst, 7*(1), 23.

Minas, H., Klimidis, S., & Tuncer, C. (2007). Illness causal beliefs in Turkish immigrants. *BMC Psychiatry*, 7(1), 34.

Mind and Helping Minds. (2016). *A Practical Guide for Working with Carers of People with Mental Illness*. Retrieved from www.carerguide.com.au.

mind Australia. (2020). *Carers*. Retrieved from www.mindaustralia.org.au/resources/carers.

MindSpot. (2020). *Online Assessment and Treatment for Anxiety and Depression*. Retrieved from https://mindspot.org.au.

Minozzi, S., Amato, L., Vecchi, S., Davoli, M., Kirchmayer, U., & Verster, A. (2011). Oral naltrexone maintenance treatment for opioid dependence. *Cochrane Database of Systematic Reviews*, (4), CD001333.

Minuchin, S. (1974). *Family and Family Therapy*. Cambridge: Harvard University.

Mioshi, E., Dawson, K., Mitchell, J., Arnold, R., & Hodges, J. R. (2006). The Addenbrooke's Cognitive Examination Revised (ACE-R): A brief cognitive test battery for dementia screening. *International Journal of Geriatric Psychiatry, 21*(11), 1078-1085.

Mitchell, F., Lunt, N., & Shaw, I. (2010). Practitioner research in social work: A knowledge review. *Evidence & Policy, 6*(1), 7-31.

Mitchell, G. (2014). End-of-life care for patients with cancer. *Australian Family Physician, 43*(8), 514.

Mitchell, G. K., Burridge, L., Zhang, J., Donald, M., Scott, I. A., Dart, J., & Jackson, C. L. (2015). Systematic review of integrated models of health care delivered at the primary-secondary interface: How effective is it and what determines effectiveness? *Australian Journal of Primary Health, 21*(4), 391-408.

Mitchell, R. J., Parker, V., & Giles, M. (2011). When do interprofessional teams succeed? Investigating the moderating roles of team and professional identity in interprofessional effectiveness. *Human Relations, 64*(10), 1321-1343.

Mitchison, D., & Hay, P. J. (2014). The epidemiology of eating disorders: Genetic, environmental, and societal factors. *Clin Epidemiol, 6*, 89-97.

Mittal, D., Drummond, K. L., Blevins, D., Curran, G., Corrigan, P., & Sullivan, G. (2013). Stigma Associated With PTSD: Perceptions of Treatment Seeking Combat Veterans. *Psychiatric Rehabilitation Journal, 36*(2), 86-92.

Mittal, V., Muralee, S., Williamson, D., McEnerney, N., Thomas, J., Cash, M., & Tampi, R. R. (2011). Delirium in the elderly: A comprehensive review. *American Journal of Alzheimers Disease and Other Dementias, 26*(2), 97-109.

Modini, M., Tan, L., Brinchmann, B., Wang, M. J., Killackey, E., Glozier, N., . . . Harvey, S. B. (2016). Supported employment for people with severe mental illness: Systematic review and meta-analysis of the international evidence. *British Journal of Psychiatry, 209*(1), 14-+.

Mogan, C., Kyrios, M., Schweitzer, I., Yap, K., & Moulding, R. (2012). Phenomenology of hoarding: What is hoarded by individuals with hoarding disorder? *Journal of Obsessive-Compulsive and Related Disorders, 1*(4), 306-311.

Mok, P. L. H., Pedersen, C. B., Springate, D., Astrup, A., Kapur, N., Antonsen, S., . . . Webb, R. T. (2016). Parental psychiatric disease and risks of attempted suicide and violent criminal offending in offspring: A population-based cohort study. *JAMA Psychiatry, 73*(10), 1015-1022.

Moll, S. E., Gewurtz, R. E., Krupa, T. M., Law, M. C., Larivière, N., & Levasseur, M. (2015). 'Do-Live-Well': A Canadian framework for promoting occupation, health, and well-being: « Vivez-Bien-Votre Vie »: Un cadre de référence canadien pour promouvoir l'occupation, la santé et le bien-être. *Canadian Journal of Occupational Therapy, 82*(1), 9-23.

Money, J., Jobaris, R., & Furth, G. (1977). Apotemnophilia: Two cases of self-demand amputation as a paraphilia. *Journal of Sex Research, 13*(2), 115-125.

Monroe, S. M., & Simons, A. D. (1991). Diathesis-stress theories in the context of life stress research: Implications for the depressive disorders. *Psychological Bulletin, 110*(3), 406-425.

Monshat, K., Carty, B., Olver, J., Castle, D., & Bosanac, P. (2010). Trends in antipsychotic prescribing practices in an urban community mental health clinic. *Australas Psychiatry, 18*(3), 238-241.

Montazer, S., & Wheaton, B. (2011). The impact of generational and country of origin on the mental health of children of immigrants. *Journal of Health and Social Behaviour, 52*(1), 23-42.

Monzani, B., Rijsdijk, F., Harris, J., & Mataix-Cols, D. (2014). The structure of genetic and environmental risk factors for dimensional representations of DSM-5 obsessive-compulsive spectrum disorders. *JAMA Psychiatry, 71*(2), 182-189.

moodgym. (2020). *Online Self-Help Program*. Retrieved from https://moodgym.com.au.

Moore, L., & Seu, I. (2011). Giving children a voice: Children's positioning in family therapy. *Journal of Family Therapy, 33*(3), 279-301.

Moore-Corner, R. A., Kielhofner, G., & Olson, L. (1998). *Work Environment Impact Scale (WEIS) Version 2.0*. Chicago: Model of Human Occupational Clearinghouse.

Moran, P. (1999). The epidemiology of antisocial personality disorder. *Social Psychiatry and Psychiatric Epidemiology, 34*(5), 231-242.

Moran, P., Borschmann, R., Flach, C., Barrett, B., Byford, S., Hogg, J., . . . Rose, D. (2010). The effectiveness of joint crisis plans for people with borderline personality disorder: Protocol for an exploratory randomised controlled trial. *Trials, 11*(1), 18.

Morey, L. C. (2010). *Personality Assessment Inventory (PAI)*. Retrieved from https://shop.acer.edu.au/personality-assessment-inventory-pai.

Morgan, J. F. (2007). Giving up the culture of blame. Risk assessment and management in psychiatric practice. *Briefing Document for the Royal College of Psychiatrists*.

Morgan, V. A., McGrath, J. J., Jablensky, A., Badcock, J. C., Waterreus, A., Bush, R., . . . Mackinnon, A. (2013). Psychosis prevalence and physical, metabolic and cognitive co-morbidity: Data from the Second Australian National Survey of Psychosis. *Psychol Med, 44*(10), 2163-2176.

Morgan, V. A., Waterreus, A., Carr, V., Castle, D., Cohen, M., Harvey, C., . . . Jablensky, A. (2017). Responding to challenges for people with psychotic illness: Updated evidence from the Survey of High Impact Psychosis. *Australian and New Zealand Journal of Psychiatry, 51*(2), 124-140.

Morgan, V. A., Waterreus, A., Jablensky, A., Mackinnon, A., McGrath, J. J., Carr, V., . . . Saw, S. (2011). *People Living with Psychotic Illness 2010. Report on the Second Australian National Survey*. Retrieved from www1.health.gov.au/internet/main/publishing.nsf/Content/717137A2F9B9FCC2CA257BF0001C118F/$File/psych10.pdf.

Morgan, V. A., Waterreus, A., Jablensky, A., Mackinnon, A., McGrath, J. J., Carr, V., . . . Saw, S. (2011). *People Living with Psychotic Illness in 2010*. (D0556). Canberra: Australian Government.

Morgan, V. A., Waterreus, A., Jablensky, A., Mackinnon, A., McGrath, J. J., Carr, V., . . . Saw, S. (2012). People living with psychotic illness in 2010: The Second Australian National Survey of Psychosis. *Australian and New Zealand Journal of Psychiatry, 46*(8), 735-752.

Morice, R. (1979). Personality disorder in transcultural perspective. *Australian and New Zealand Journal of Psychiatry, 13*(4), 293-300.

Morris, G. P. (2010). Ecological public health and climate change policy. *Perspectives in Public Health, 130*(1), 34-40.

Morrison, A. P. (2017). A manualised treatment protocol to guide delivery of evidence-based cognitive therapy for people with distressing psychosis: Learning from clinical trials. *Psychosis, 9*(3), 271-281.

Morrison, J. (1989). Childhood sexual histories of women with somatization disorder. *American Journal of Psychiatry, 146*(2), 239-241.

Morse, B. D., Scott, D. F., Lackie, J. B., & Homchenko, M. E. (2014). *An Analysis of Hoarding and Squalor Related Incidents and Responses by the Metropolitan Fire and Emergency Services Board*. Retrieved from https://digitalcommons.wpi.edu/iqp-all/2690.

Morgan, S. (2004). Risk taking. In P. Ryan & S. Morgan. *Assertive Outreach: A Strengths Approach to Policy and Practice* (pp. 223-246). Edinburgh: Churchill Livingstone.

Morton, J., Snowdon, S., Gopold, M., & Guymer, E. (2012). Acceptance and commitment therapy group treatment for symptoms of borderline personality disorder: A public sector pilot study. *Cognitive and Behavioral Practice, 19*(4), 527-544.

Moser, S. C. (2013). Navigating the political and emotional terrain of adaptation: Community engagement when climate change comes home. In S. C. Moser & M. T. Boykoff (eds.), *Successful Adaptation to Climate Change: Linking Science and Policy in a Rapidly Changing World*. Taylor & Francis.

Mosher, L. R., & Burti, L. (1989). *Community Mental Health: Principles and Practice*. New York: Norton.

Mottaghipour, Y., & Bickerton, A. (2005). The pyramid of family care: A framework for family involvement with adult mental health services *Australian e-Journal for the Advancement of Mental Health, 4*(3).

Mowbray, C., Collins, M., Bellamy, C., Megivern, D., Bybee, D., & Szilvagyi, S. (2005). Supported education for adults with psychiatric disabilities: An innovation for social work and psychosocial rehabilitation practice. *Social Work, 50*(1), 14.

Mowrer, O. H. (1960). *Learning theory and behaviour*. New York: Wiley.

Mrazek, P. J., & Haggerty, P. J. (1994). *Reducing the risks for mental disorder: Frontiers for preventive intervention research*. Washington: National Academy Press.

Mueser, K., Bond, G., Drake, R., & Resnick, S. (1998). Models of community care for severe mental illness: A review of research on case management. *Schizophrenia Bulletin, 24*(1), 37-74.

Mulder, R., Rucklidge, J., & Wilkinson, S. (2017). Why has increased provision of psychiatric treatment not reduced the prevalence of mental disorder? *Aust NZ J Psych, 51*(12), 1176-1177.

Mulders-Jones, B., Mitchison, D., Girosi, F., & Hay, P. (2017). Socioeconomic correlates of eating disorder symptoms in an Australian population-based sample. *PLoS One, 12*(1), e0170603.

Muller, K. W., Janikian, M., Dreier, M., Wolfling, K., Beutel, M. E., Tzavara, C., . . . Tsitsika, A. (2015). Regular gaming behavior and internet gaming disorder in European adolescents: Results from a cross-national representative survey of prevalence, predictors, and psychopathological correlates. *European Child & Adolescent Psychiatry, 24*(5), 565-574.

Müller, S. (2009). Body integrity identity disorder (BIID)—Is the amputation of healthy limbs ethically justified? *The American Journal of Bioethics, 9*(1), 36-43.

Munetz, M. R., & Frese, F. J. (2001). Getting ready for recovery: Reconciling mandatory treatment with the recovery vision. *Psychiatric Rehabilitation Journal, 25*(1), 35-42.

Munn-Giddings, C., & McVicar, A. (2007). Self-help groups as mutual support: What do carers value? *Health & Social Care in the Community, 15*(1), 26-34.

Munoz, R. F., Beardslee, W. R., & Leykin, Y. (2012). Major depression can be prevented. *American Psychologist, 67*(4), 285-295.

Munoz-Murillo, A., Esteban, E., Avila, C. C., Fheodoroff, K., Haro, J. M., Leonardi, M., & Olaya, B. (2018). Furthering the evidence of the effectiveness of employment strategies for people with mental disorders in Europe: A systematic review. *International Journal of Environmental Research and Public Health, 15*(5).

Murphy, K. C., Jones, L. A., & Owen, M. J. (1999). High rates of schizophrenia in adults with velo-cardio-facial syndrome. *Archives of General Psychiatry, 56*(10), 940–945.

Murray, A. M., Toussaint, A., Althaus, A., & Lowe, B. (2016). The challenge of diagnosing non-specific, functional, and somatoform disorders: A systematic review of barriers to diagnosis in primary care. *J Psychosom Res, 80*, 1-10.

Murray, C. J., & Lopez, A. D. (1996). *The Global Burden of Disease.* Geneva: World Health Organization.

NACCHO. (2019). Why ACCS are needed. Retrieved from www.naccho.org.au/member-services/why-acchs-are-needed.

Nagel, T. (2006). The need for relapse prevention strategies in Top End remote indigenous mental health. *Australian e-Journal for the Advancement of Mental Health, 5*(1), 48–52.

Nagel, T. (2007). Mental health in the states and territories. In G. Meadows, B. Singh, & M. Grigg (eds.), *Mental Health in Australia: Collaborative Community Practice* (2nd ed.). South Melbourne: Oxford University Press.

Nagel, T., Kavanagh, D., Barclay, L., Trauer, T., Chenhall, R., Frendin, J., & Griffin, C. (2011). Integrating treatment for mental and physical disorders and substance misuse in Indigenous primary care settings. *Australasian Psychiatry, 19*(1_suppl), S17–S19.

Nair, N., Newton, N., Barrett, E., Slade, T., Conrod, P., Baillie, A., & Teesson, M. (2016). Personality and early adolescent alcohol use: Assessing the four factor model of vulnerability. *Journal of Addiction & Prevention, 4*(2), 1–6.

Nancarrow, S. A., Booth, A., Ariss, S., Smith, T., Enderby, P., & Roots, A. (2013). Ten principles of good interdisciplinary team work. (Report). *Human Resources for Health, 11*(1).

Nanni, V., Uher, R., & Danese, A. (2012). Childhood maltreatment predicts unfavorable course of illness and treatment outcome in depression: A meta-analysis. *American Journal of Psychiatry, 169*(2), 141-151.

Nasir, B. F., Toombs, M. R., Kondalsamy-Chennakesavan, S., Kisely, S., Gill, N. S., Black, E., . . . Nicholson, G. C. (2018). Common mental disorders among Indigenous people living in regional, remote and metropolitan Australia: A cross-sectional study. *BMJ Open, 8*(6).

Naslund, J. A., Marsch, L. A., Mchugo, G. J., & Bartels, S. J. (2015). Review of Emerging mHealth and eHealth interventions for serious mental illness: a review of the literature. *Journal of Mental Health*, 24(5), 321-332.

Nasreddine, Z. S., Phillips, N. A., Bedirian, V., Charbonneau, S., Whitehead, V., Collin, I., . . . Chertkow, H. (2005). The Montreal Cognitive Assessment, MoCA: A brief screening tool for mild cognitive impairment. *Journal of the American Geriatrics Society, 53*(4), 695–699.

National Aboriginal and Torres Strait Islander Health Workers Association (NATSIHWA). (2018). *National Framework for Determining Scope of Practice for the Aboriginal and/or Torres Strait Islander Health Workforce and Health Practitioner Workforce.* Retrieved from www.natsihwa.org.au/sites/default/files/natsihwa_scope_of_practice_2018.pdf.

National Aboriginal and Torres Strait Islander Leadership in Mental Health Ltd. (NATSILMH). (2016). *Gayaa Dhuwi (Proud Spirit) Declaration.* Retrieved from https://natsilmh.org.au/sites/default/files/gayaa_dhuwi_declaration_A4.pdf.

National Academy of Sciences. (2009). *Preventing Mental, Emotional and Behavioral Disorders Among Young People—Progress and Possibilities.* Retrieved from www.nap.edu/resource/12480/Preventing-Mental-Emotional-and-Behavioral-Disorders-2009–Report-Brief-for-Researchers.pdf.

National Accreditation Authority for Translators and Interpreters (NAATI). (2020). *Enabling a Linguistically Connected Community.* Retrieved from www.naati.com.au.

National Center for Advancing Translational Sciences. (2015). *Translational Science Spectrum.* Retrieved from https://ncats.nih.gov/translation/spectrum.

National Institute for Health & Care Excellence (2014*). Psychosis and Schizophrenia in Adults: Prevention and Management. NICE Clinical Guideline CG178.* London: National Institute for Health & Care Excellence.

National Disability Insurance Agency (NDIS). (2019). *Intergovernmental Agreements.* Retrieved from www.ndis.gov.au/about-us/governance/intergovernmental-agreements.

National Health and Medical Research Council (NHMRC). (2003). *Dietary Guidelines for Australian Adults.* Retrieved from www.nhmrc.gov.au/about-us/publications/australian-dietary-guidelines.

National Health and Medical Research Council (NHMRC). (2009). *A Guide to the Development, Implementation and Evaluation of Clinical Practice Guidelines.* Retrieved from www.nhmrc.gov.au/about-us/publications/guide-development-evaluation-and-implementation-clinical-practice-guidelines.

National Health and Medical Research Council (NHMRC). (2012). *Clinical Practice Guideline for the Management of Borderline Personality Disorder.* Melbourne: National Health and Medical Research Council.

National Health and Medical Research Council (NHMRC). (2018). *Ethical Conduct in Research with Aboriginal and Torres Strait Islander Peoples and Communities: Guidelines for Researchers and Stakeholders.* Retrieved from www.nhmrc.gov.au/about-us/resources/ethical-conduct-research-aboriginal-and-torres-strait-islander-peoples-and-communities.

National Health and Medical Research Council; Australian Research Council; Universities Australia. (2007, Updated 2018). *National Health and Medical Research Council 2007 (Updated 2018)*. Canberra: Commonwealth of Australia.

National Indigenous Times. (2017). *NT Aboriginal Men Fall Behind in Life Expectancy.* Retrieved from https://nit.com.au/nt-aboriginal-men-fall-behind-life-expectancy.

National Indigenous Australians Agency (NIAA). (2017). *National Strategic Framework for Aboriginal and Torres Strait Islander Peoples' Mental Health and Social and Emotional Wellbeing 2017-2023.* Retrieved from www.niaa.gov.au/sites/default/files/publications/mhsewb-framework_0.pdf.

National Institute for Health and Care Excellence (NICE). (2004, May 2017). Eating disorders: Core interventions in the treatment and management of anorexia nervosa, bulimia nervosa and related disorders. *Clinical Guideline Number 9.* Retrieved from www.nice.org.uk/guidance/ng69.

National Institute for Health and Care Excellence (NICE). (2005a). *Depression in Children and Young People: Identification and Management. Clinical guideline (CG28) [updated 2017].* UK: National Institute for Health and Care Excellence.

National Institute for Health and Care Excellence (NICE). (2005b). *Obsessive-Compulsive Disorder and Body Dysmorphic Disorder: Treatment.* UK: National Institute for Health and Care Excellence.

National Institute for Health and Care Excellence (NICE). (2009a). *Depression in Adults: Recognition and Management. Clinical*

Guideline (CG90) [Updated 2018]. UK: National Institute for Health and Care Excellence.

National Institute for Health and Care Excellence (NICE). (2009b). *Depression: The Treatment and Management of Depression in Adults*. Retrieved from www.nice.org.uk/guidance.

National Institute for Health and Care Excellence (NICE). (2009c). *Antisocial Personality Disorder: Prevention and Management*. Retrieved from www.nice.org.uk/guidance/

National Institute for Health and Care Excellence (NICE). (2011a). *Generalised Anxiety Disorder and Panic Disorder in Adults: Management. Clinical Guideline (CG113)*. UK: National Institute for Health and Care Excellence (NICE). Retrieved from www.nice.org.uk/guidance/cg113.

National Institute for Health and Care Excellence (NICE). (2011b). *Self-harm in Over 8s: Long-Term Management. Clinical Guideline [CG133]*. UK: National Institute for Health and Care Excellence.

National Institute for Health and Care Excellence (NICE). (2013). *Social Anxiety Disorder: Recognition, Assessment and Treatment. Clinical Guideline (CG159)*. UK: National Institute for Health and Care Excellence.

National Institute for Health and Care Excellence (NICE). (2014). *Anxiety Disorders: Quality Standard*. UK: National Institute for Health and Care Excellence.

National Institute of Health and Clinical Excellence (NICE). (2016). *Depression: The Treatment and Management of Depression in Adults (Update). Clinical Guideline [CG90]*. Retrieved from http://guidance.nice.org.uk/CG90.

National Mental Health Commission. (2013). *A Contributing Life: The 2013 National Report Card on Mental Health and Suicide Prevention*. Retreived from www.mentalhealthcommission.gov.au/monitoring-and-reporting/national-reports/2013-national-report.

National Mental Health Commission. (2014). *The National Review of Mental Health Programmes and Services*. Sydney: National Mental Health Commission.

National Mental Health Commission (2016). *Equally Well: Consensus Statement to Improve the Physical Health and Wellbeing of People Living with Mental Illness in Australia*. Sydney, National Mental Health Commission

National Mental Health Commission. (2018). *Monitoring Mental Health and Suicide Prevention Reform: National Report 2018*. Retrieved from www.mentalhealthcommission.gov.au/media-centre/news/monitoring-mental-health-and-suicide-prevention-reform-national-report-2018.aspx.

National Mental Health Commission (NMHC). (2019a). *Monitoring Mental Health and Suicide Prevention Reform: National Report 2019*. Retrieved from www.mentalhealthcommission.gov.au/getmedia.

National Mental Health Commission (NMHC). (2019b). *2030 Vision for Mental Health and Suicide Prevention—National Mental Health Commission to Connect with Communities*. Retrieved from www.mentalhealthcommission.gov.au/news/2019/july/2030-vision-for-mental-health-and-suicide-preventi.

National Mental Health Consumer & Carer Forum. (2011). *Privacy, Confidentiality and Information Sharing—Consumers, Carers and Clinicians*. Retrieved from https://nmhccf.org.au.

National Mental Health Consumer & Carer Forum. (2017). *Advocacy Brief: Co-design and Co-production*. Retrieved from https://nmhccf.org.au.

National Mental Health Service Planning Framework (NMHSPF). (2017). *National Mental Health Service Planning Framework*. Retrieved from https://nmhspf.org.au.

National Mental Health Strategy. (2008). *National Mental Health Policy*. Retrieved from www1.health.gov.au/internet/main/publishing.nsf/Content/B4A903FB48158BAECA257BF0001D3AEA/$File/finpol08.pdf.

National Mental Health Strategy Evaluation Steering Committee. (1997). *For the Australian Health Ministers Advisory Council, Evaluation of the National Mental Health Strategy: Final Report*. Retrieved from www1.health.gov.au/internet/main/publishing.nsf/content/73F924C1ADDB5FA1CA257BF000209C61/$File/strateval.pdf.

National Oceanic and Atmospheric Administration (NOAA). (2016). *Global Climate Report—Annual 2016*. Retrieved from www.ncdc.noaa.gov/sotc/global/201613.

National Rural Health Alliance Inc. (2008). *Improving the Rural and Remote Health Workforce* Retrieved from www.ruralhealth.org.au/sites/default/files/submissions/sub-08-02-08.pdf.

Neacsiu, A. D., Eberle, J. W., Keng, S.-L., Fang, C. M., & Rosenthal, M. Z. (2017). Understanding borderline personality disorder across sociocultural groups: Findings, issues, and future directions. *Current Psychiatry Reviews, 13*(3), 188-223.

Neal, P., Delfabbro, P. H., & O'Neil, M. G. (2005). *Problem M*. Melbourne: Office of Gaming and Racing, Victorian Government Department of Justice.

Nedeljkovic, M., Kyrios, M., Moulding, R., & Doron, G. (2011). Neuropsychological changes following cognitive-behavioral treatment of obsessive-compulsive disorder (OCD). *International Journal of Cognitive Therapy, 4*(1), 8-20.

Nedeljkovic, M., Kyrios, M., Moulding, R., Doron, G., Wainwright, K., Pantelis, C., . . . Maruff, P. (2009). Differences in neuropsychological performance between subtypes of obsessive-compulsive disorder. *Aust N Z J Psychiatry, 43*(3), 216-226.

Nedeljkovic, M., Moulding, R., Foroughi, E., Kyrios, M., & Doron, G. (2011). Cultural issues in understanding and treating obsessive-compulsive and spectrum disorders. In G. Steketee (ed.), *Oxford Handbook of Obsessive Compulsive and Spectrum Disorders* (pp. 496-520). New York: Oxford University Press.

Neff, K. D., & Germer, C. K. (2013). A pilot study and randomized controlled trial of the mindful self-compassion program. *Journal of Clinical Psychology, 69*(1), 28-44.

Neil, S. T., Kilbride, M., Pitt, L., Nothard, S., Welford, M., Sellwood, W., & Morrison, A. P. (2009). The questionnaire about the process of recovery (QPR): A measurement tool developed in collaboration with service users. *Psychosis, 1*(2), 145-155.

Net Balance. (2013). *Social Return on Investment Study of Lifeline Online Crisis Chat Service*. Retrieved from www.lifeline.org.au/static/uploads/files/lifeline-online-crisis-support-chat-sroi-report-final-wfsijexrtqgq.pdf.

Nettelbeck, A., & Ryan, L. (2018). Salutary lessons: Native police and the 'civilising' role of legalised violence in colonial Australia. *Journal of Imperial and Commonwealth History, 46*(1), 47-68.

Neuman, W. L. (1994). *Social Research Methods: Qualitative and Quantitative Approaches* (2nd ed.). Boston: Allyn and Bacon.

Neuman, W. L. (2003). *Social Research Methods: Qualitative and Quantitative Approaches* (5th ed.). Boston: Allyn & Bacon.

Nevo, I., & Slonim-Nevo, V. (2011). The myth of evidence-based practice: Towards evidence-informed practice. *British Journal of Social Work, 41*(6), 1176-1197.

New South Wales Government. (2007). *Mental Health Act 2007, No 8*. Retrieved from www.legislation.nsw.gov.au/#/view/act/2007/8.

Newton, D., Day, A., Gillies, C., & Fernandez, E. (2015). A review of evidence-based evaluation of measures for assessing social and emotional well-being in Indigenous Australians: The assessment of social and emotional well-being in Indigenous patients. *Australian Psychologist, 50*(1), 40-50.

Newton, L., Rosen, A., Tennant, C., Hobbs, C., Lapsley, H. M., & Tribe, K. (2000). Deinstitutionalisation for long-term mental illness: An ethnographic study. *Australian and New Zealand Journal of Psychiatry, 34*(3), 484–490.

Newton, N. C., Barrett, E. L., Castellanos-Ryan, N., Kelly, E., Champion, K. E., Stapinski, L., . . . Teesson, M. (2016). The validity of the Substance Use Risk Profile Scale (SURPS) among Australian adolescents. *Addictive behaviors, 53*, 23–30.

Newton, N. C., Conrod, P. J., Slade, T., Carragher, N., Champion, K. E., Barrett, E. L., ... Teesson, M. (2016). The long-term effectiveness of a selective, personality-targeted prevention program in reducing alcohol use and related harms: A cluster randomized controlled trial. *Journal of Child Psychology and Psychiatry*, 57(9), 1056–1065.

Newton-Howes, G., Clark, L. A., & Chanen, A. (2015). Personality disorder across the life course. *Lancet, 385*(9969), 727–734.

Neziroglu, F., Roberts, M. A., & Yaryura-Tobias, J. A. (2004). A behavioral model for body dysmorphic disorder. *Psychiatric Annals, 34*(12), 915–920.

Nezu, A. M., Ronan, G. F., Meadows, E. A., & McClure, K. S. (eds.). (2000). *Practitioner's Guide to Empirically Based Measures of Depression*. New York: Kluwer Academic/Plenum Publishers.

Ngaanyatjarra Pitjantjatjar Yankunytjatjara (NPY), & Women's Council Aboriginal Corporation. (2013). *Traditional Healers of Central Australia: Ngangkari*. Broome: Magabala Press.

Nguyen, B., Ding, D., & Mihrshahi, S. (2017). Fruit and vegetable consumption and psychological distress: Cross-sectional and longitudinal analyses based on a large Australian sample. *BMJ Open, 7*(3).

NHMRC & Universities Australia (2018). *National Statement on Ethical Conduct in Human Research (2007)—Updated 2018*. Retrieved from: https://www.nhmrc.gov.au.

NHMRC Centre of Research Excellence in Suicide Prevention (C.R.E.S.P.) (2014). *Care After a Suicide Attempt: A report prepared for the National Mental Health Commission*. Barton: in partnership with Black Dog Institute, the University of New South Wales, in partnership with The University of Melbourne, Lifeline, and the Australian National University.

Nicholson, J., Carpenter-Song, E. A., MacPherson, L. H., Tauscher, J. S., Burns, T. C., & Lord, S. E. (2017). Developing the WorkingWell mobile app to promote job tenure for individuals with serious mental illnesses. *Psychiatric Rehabilitation Journal, 40*(3), 276–282.

Nielssen, O. (2013). Scientific and ethical problems with risk assessment in clinical practice. *Australian & New Zealand Journal of Psychiatry, 47*(12), 1198–1199.

Nigatu, Y. T., Liu, Y., Uppal, M., McKinney, S., Gillis, K., Rao, S., & Wang, J. L. (2017). Prognostic factors for return to work of employees with common mental disorders: A meta-analysis of cohort studies. *Social Psychiatry and Psychiatric Epidemiology, 52*(10), 1205–1215.

Nijenhuis, E. R. S. (2001). Somatoform dissociation: Major symptoms of dissociative disorders. *Journal of Trauma & Dissociation, 1*(4), 7–32.

Noordsy, D., Torrey, W., Mueser, K., Mead, S., O'Keefe, C., & Fox, L. (2002). Recovery from severe mental illness: An intrapersonal and functional outcome definition. *International Review of Psychiatry, 14*(4), 318–326.

Norcross, J. C. (2001). Purposes, processes and products of the Task Force on Empirically Supported Therapy Relationships. *Psychotherapy: Theory, Research, Practice, Training, 38*(4), 345–356.

Norcross, J. C. (2011). *Psychotherapy Relationships That Work: Evidence-Based Responsiveness* (2nd ed.). New York: Oxford University Press.

Norcross, J. C., & Goldfried, M. R. (2019). *Handbook of Psychotherapy Integration*. Oxford University Press.

Norcross, J. C., & Lambert, M. J. (2011). Psychotherapy relationships that work II. *Psychotherapy, 48*(1), 4–8.

Norcross, J. C., & Wampold, B. E. (2011). Evidence-based therapy relationships: Research conclusions and clinical practices. *Psychotherapy, 48*(1), 98–102.

Nordentoft, M., Melau, M., Iversen, T., Petersen, L., Jeppesen, P., Thorup, A., . . . Jørgensen, P. (2015). From research to practice: How OPUS treatment was accepted and implemented throughout Denmark. *Early Intervention in Psychiatry, 9*(2), 156–162.

Nordsletten, A. E., Reichenberg, A., Hatch, S. L., de la Cruz, L. F., Pertusa, A., Hotopf, M., & Mataix-Cols, D. (2018). Epidemiology of hoarding disorder. *British Journal of Psychiatry, 203*(6), 445–452.

Norman, I. J., & Peck, E. (1999). Working together in adult community mental health services: An inter-professional dialogue. *Journal of Mental Health, 8*(3), 217–230.

Norris, F. H., Friedman, M. J., Watson, P. J., Byrne, C. M., Diaz, E., & Kaniasty, K. (2002). 60 000 disaster victims speak: Part I. An empirical review of the empirical literature, 1981–2001. *Psychiatry—Interpersonal and Biological Processes, 65*(3), 207–239.

Northern Territory Government. (2002). *Northern Territory Mental Health and Related Services Act 2002*. Retrieved from https://health.nt.gov.au/professionals/mental-health-information-for-health-professional.

Northern Territory Government. (2020). *Northern Territory Government Information and Services*. Retrieved from https://nt.gov.au.

Northern Territory Health. (2018). *NT Health Strategic Plan 2018–2022*. Retrieved from https://digitallibrary.health.nt.gov.au/prodjspui/bitstream/10137/2729/3/Northern%20Territory%20Health%20Strategic%20Plan.pdf.

Northern Territory Mental Health Coalition & Queensland Alliance for Mental Health. (2018). *Joint Submission to Senate Standing Committee on Community Affairs Accessibility and Quality of Mental Health Services in Rural and Remote Australia*. Retrieved from www.ntmhc.org.au/wp-content/uploads/2018/05/Final-Senate-inquiry-into-rural-and-remote-mental-health.pdf.

Northern Territory Primary Health Network. (2018). *Northern Territory PHN*. Retrieved from www.ntphn.org.au.

Nøttestad, J. A., & Linaker, O. M. (2003). Psychotropic drug use among people with intellectual disability before and after deinstitutionalization. *Journal of Intellectual Disability Research, 47*(6), 464–471.

Nouwen, A., Adriaanse, M. C., van Dam, K., Iversen, M. M., Viechtbauer, W., Peyrot, M., . . . EDID, E. D. D. (2019). Longitudinal associations between depression and diabetes complications: A systematic review and meta-analysis. *Diabetic Medicine, 36*(12), 1562–1572.

NSW Government and Agency for Clinical Innovation. (2019). *A Guide to Build Co-Design Capability: Consumers and Staff Coming Together to Improve Healthcare*. Retrieved from www.aci.health.nsw.gov.au/__data/assets/pdf_file/0013/502240/Guide-Build-Codesign-Capability.pdf.

NSW Government. (2007). *NSW Mental Health Act 2007*. Retrieved from www.legislation.nsw.gov.au/#/view/act/2007/8.

NSW Government. (2010). *NSW Carers (Recognition) Act 2010*. Retrieved from www.health.nsw.gov.au/mentalhealth/services/carers/Pages/family-mh-NSWcarersact.aspx.

NSW Government. (2018–2022). *NSW Strategic Framework and Workforce Plan for Mental Health 2018–2022: A Framework and Workforce Plan for NSW Health Services*. Retrieved from www.health.nsw.gov.au/mentalhealth/resources/Pages/mh-strategic-framework.aspx.

NSW Government. (2020). *The NSW Budget 2019-2020 Half-Yearly Review*. Retrieved from www.budget.nsw.gov.au.

NSW Mental Health Commission. (2014). *Living Well: A Strategic Plan for Mental Health in NSW*. Retrieved from https://nswmentalhealthcommission.com.au/sites/default/files/Living%20Well%20-%20A%20Strategic%20Plan%20full%20version.pdf.

NSW Police Force. (2008). *Mental Health Intervention Team (MHIT)*. Retrieved from www.police.nsw.gov.au/safety_and_prevention/your_community/mental_health.

Nuechterlein, K., Dawson, M. E., Ventura, J., Gitlin, M., Subotnik, K., Snyder, K. S., . . . Bartzokis, G. (1994). The vulnerability/stress model of schizophrenic relapse: A longitudinal study. *Acta Psychiatr Scand, 89*, 58-64.

Nyttingnes, O., Ruud, T., & Rugkåsa, J. (2016). 'It's unbelievably humiliating'—Patients' expressions of negative effects of coercion in mental health care. *International Journal of Law and Psychiatry, 49*(Pt A), 147-153.

O'Brien, G. (2006). Behavioural phenotypes: Causes and clinical implications. *Advances in Psychiatric Treatment, 12*(5), 338-348.

O'Hagan, M. (2009). Foreword. In A. Sweeney, P. Beresford, A. Faulkner, M. Nettle, & D. Rose (eds.), *This is Survivor Research*. UK: PCCS Books.

O'Hagan, M. (2009). We don't start off with the agenda tied up. In *This is Survivor Research* (pp. 168-169). UK: PCCS Books.

O'Hagan, M. (2011). 'Rethinking Risk.' August 8 [workshop] 2020. Retrieved from https://insideoutconversations.com.au/#.

O'Mara-Eves, A., Brunton, G., McDaid, D., Oliver, S., Kavanagh, J., Jamal, F., . . . Thomas, J. (2013). Community engagement to reduce inequalities in health: A systematic review, meta-analysis and economic analysis. *Public Health Res, 1*(4).

O'Mara-Eves, A., Brunton, G., Oliver, S., Kavanagh, J., Jamal, F., & Thomas, J. (2015). The effectiveness of community engagement in public health interventions for disadvantaged groups: A meta-analysis. *BMC Public Health, 15*(1), 129.

Oades, L. G., Crowe, T. P., & Nguyen, M. (2009). Leadership coaching transforming mental health systems from the inside out: The Collaborative Recovery Model as person-centred strengths based coaching psychology. *International Coaching Psychology Review, 4*(1), 25-36.

Oades, L. G., Deane, F. P., & Crowe, T. P. (2017). Collaborative Recovery Model: From mental health recovery to wellbeing. In M. Slade, L. Oades, & A. Jarden (eds.), *Wellbeing, Recovery and Mental Health* (pp. 99-110). Cambridge: Cambridge University Press.

Oakes, J., Gardiner, P., McLaughlin, K., & Battersby, M. (2012). A pilot group cognitive behavioural therapy program for problem gamblers in a rural Australian setting. *International Journal of Mental Health and Addiction, 10*(4), 490-500.

O'Brien, C. P., Greenstein, R. A., Mintz, J., & Woody, G. E. (1975). Clinical experience with naltrexone. *American Journal of Drug and Alcohol Abuse, 2*(3-4), 365-377.

O'Brien, G., & Trudgett, M. (2020). School House to Big House. *The Australian Journal of Indigenous Education*, 49(1), 98-106. doi:10.1017/jie.2018.13.

O'Connor, D. W., Gardner, B., Eppingstall, B., & Tofler, D. (2010). Cognition in elderly patients receiving unilateral and bilateral electroconvulsive therapy: A prospective, naturalistic comparison. *J Affect Disord, 124*(3), 235-240.

O'Donnell, M., Maclean, M. J., Sims, S., Morgan, V. A., Leonard, H., & Stanley, F. J. (2015). Maternal mental health and risk of child protection involvement: Mental health diagnoses associated with increased risk. *J Epidemiol Community Health, 69*(12), 1175-1183.

OECD. (2012). *Sick on the Job? Myths and Realities about Mental Health and Work*. OECD Publishing.

OECD. (2019). *Alcohol Consumption (Indicator)*. Retrieved from https://data.oecd.org/healthrisk/alcohol-consumption.htm.

Office of Parliamentary Counsel. (2018). *Health Insurance (Allied Health Services) Determination 2014, Compilation No. 8*. Retrieved from www.legislation.gov.au/Details/F2018C00854.

Office of the Auditor General. (2019). *Western Australian Auditor General's Report: Access to State-Managed Adult Mental Health Services*. Retrieved from https://audit.wa.gov.au/reports-and-publications/reports/access-to-state-managed-adult-mental-health-services/finding-1.

Office of the High Commissioner for Human Rights. (1991). *Principles for the Protection of Persons with Mental Illness and the Improvement of Mental Health Care*. Retrieved from www.who.int/mental_health/policy/en/UN_Resolution_on_protection_of_persons_with_mental_illness.pdf.

Office of the High Commissioner for Human Rights. (2009). *Office of the United Nations High Commissioner for Human Rights*. Retrieved from www.ohchr.org.

O'Hagan, M. (2004). Recovery in New Zealand: Lessons for Australia? *Australian e-Journal for the Advancement of Mental Health, 3*(1), 5-7.

O'Hanlon, S. (2018). *City life: The new urban Australia*. NewSouth Publishing.

O'Keeffe, L., O'Reilly, A., O'Brien, G., Buckley, R., & Illback, R. (2015). Description and outcome evaluation of Jigsaw: An emergent Irish mental health early intervention programme for young people. *Irish Journal of Psychological Medicine, 32*(1), 71-77.

O'Keeffe, N., & Ranjith, G. (2007). Depression, demoralisation or adjustment disorder? Understanding emotional distress in the severely medically ill. *Clinical Medicine, 7*(5), 478-481.

Olatunji, B. O., Kauffman, B. Y., Meltzer, S., Davis, M. L., Smits, J. A., & Powers, M. B. (2014). Cognitive-behavioral therapy for hypochondriasis/health anxiety: A meta-analysis of treatment outcome and moderators. *Behav Res Ther, 58*, 65-74.

Olde Hartman, T. C., Borghuis, M. S., Lucassen, P. L., van de Laar, F. A., Speckens, A. E., & van Weel, C. (2009). Medically unexplained symptoms, somatisation disorder and hypochondriasis: Course and prognosis. A systematic review. *Journal of Psychosomatic Research, 66*(5), 363-377.

Oldershaw, A., Richards, C., Simic, M., & Schmidt, U. (2008). Parents' perspectives on adolescent self-harm: Qualitative study. *British Journal of Psychiatry, 193*(2), 140-144.

Olesen, S. C., Macdonald, E., Raphael, B., & Butterworth, P. (2010). Children's exposure to parental and familial adversities. *Family Matters, 43, 84*, 43-52.

Olfson, M., Gerhard, T., Huang, C., Crystal, S., & Stroup, T. S. (2015). Premature mortality among adults with schizophrenia in the United States. *JAMA Psychiatry, 72*(12), 1172-1181.

Oliver, N., & Kuipers, E. (1996). Stress and its relationship to expressed emotion in community mental health workers. *International Journal of Social Psychiatry, 42*(2), 150-159.

Oliver, S. J. (2013). The role of traditional medicine practice in primary health care within Aboriginal Australia: A review of the literature. *Journal of Ethnobiology and Ethnomedicine, 9*.

Olson, M., Seikkula, J., & Ziedonis, D. (2014). *The Key Elements of Dialogic Practice in Open Dialogue, Version 1.1*.

Retrieved from www.do-ge.ch/uploads/1/3/9/9/13993272/keyelementsv1.109022014.pdf.

Olthuis, J. V., Watt, M. C., Bailey, K., Hayden, J. A., & Stewart, S. H. (2015). Therapist-supported Internet cognitive behavioural therapy for anxiety disorders in adults. *Cochrane Database of Systematic Reviews*, (3), CD011565.

O'Malley, P. G., Jackson, J. L., Santoro, J., Tomkins, G., Balden, E., & Kroenke, K. (1999). Antidepressant therapy for unexplained symptoms and symptom syndromes. *Journal of Family Practice, 48*(12), 980–990.

Oman, D. (ed.) (2018). *Why Religion and Spirituality Matter for Public Health: Evidence, Implications, and Resources.* (Vol. 2). Switzerland: Springer International Publishing.

O'Mara-Eves, A., Brunton, G., McDaid, D., Oliver, S., Kavanagh, J., Jamal, F., . . . Thomas, J. (2013). Public health research. In *Community Engagement to Reduce Inequalities in Health: A Systematic Review, Meta-Analysis and Economic Analysis.* Southampton: NIHR Journals Library.

O'Neill, T. A., & Salas, E. (2018). Creating high performance teamwork in organizations. *Human Resource Management Review, 28*(4), 325–331.

Onken, L. S., Carroll, K. M., Shoham, V., Cuthbert, B. N., & Riddle, M. (2014). Reenvisioning clinical science: Unifying the discipline to improve the public health. *Clinical Psychological Science, 2*(1), 22–34.

Onnis, L. A. L., & Pryce, J. (2016). Health professionals working in remote Australia: A review of the literature. *Asia Pacific Journal of Human Resources, 54*(1), 32–56.

Onyett, S. (1995). Responsibility and accountability in community mental health teams. *Psychiatric Bulletin*, 19, 281-285.

Onyett, S. (1999). Community Mental Health Team Working as a Socially Valued Enterprise. *Journal of Mental Health, 8*(3), 245–251.

Onyett, S., & Campling, J. (2002). *Teamworking in Mental Health.* Palgrave Macmillan.

Open Arms. (2020). *Veterans & Families Counselling*. Retrieved from www.openarms.gov.au.

OQ Measures. (2020). *The Measure of Mental Health Vital Signs.* Retrieved from www.oqmeasures.com.

Organisation for Economic Co-operation and Development. *Psychiatric Bed Numbers*. Retrieved from https://stats.oecd.org.

Organisation for Economic Co-operation and Development. (2014). *Australia at the Forefront of Mental Health Care Innovation but Should Remain Attentive to Population Needs, Says OECD.* Retrieved from www.oecd.org/els/health-systems/MMHC-Country-Press-Note-Australia.pdf.

Orr, S. P., Metzger, L. J., Lasko, N. B., Macklin, M. L., Peri, T., & Pitman, R. K. (2000). De novo conditioning in trauma-exposed individuals with and without posttraumatic stress disorder. *Journal of Abnormal Psychology, 109*(2), 290–298.

Orygen. (2015a). *Clinical Practice in Youth Mental Health. Assessing and Managing Risk of Violence in Early Psychosis.* Melbourne: Orygen.

Orygen. (2015a). *Psychological Interventions: Why, How and When to Use in Early Psychosis.* Melbourne: Orygen.

Orygen. (2016). *Clinical Practice in Early Psychosis. Working with Cultural Diversity in Early Psychosis*. Melbourne: Orygen.

Orygen. (2017a). *Clinical Practice in Depression and Suicide. Managing Ongoing Suicidality in Young People Diagnosed with Major Depressive Disorder (MDD)*. Melbourne: Orygen.

Orygen. (2017b). *Clinical Practice in Youth Mental Health. Addressing Barriers to Engagement: Working with Challenging Behaviour*. Melbourne: Orygen.

Orygen. (2018). *What Is Trauma-Informed Care and How Can I Help Implement It in My Organisation*? Retrieved from www.orygen.org.au/Training/Resources/Trauma/Toolkits/What-is-trauma-informed-care-and-how-can-I-help-i/Trauma-informed-care-toolkit?ext=.

Orygen. (2019). *Clinical Practice in Youth Mental Health. Working Safely and Inclusively with Sexuality Diverse Young People.* Melbourne: Orygen.

Osborn, R. L., Demoncada, A. C., & Feuerstein, M. (2006). Psychosocial interventions for depression, anxiety, and quality of life in cancer survivors: Meta-analyses. *International Journal of Psychiatry in Medicine, 36*(1), 13–34.

Osborne, R. B., & Hatcher, J. W. (1989). The role of social modeling in unexplained paediatric pain. *Journal of Paediatric Psychology, 14*, 43–61.

Öst, L. G., Havnen, A., Hansen, B., & Kvale, G. (2015). Cognitive behavioral treatments of obsessive-compulsive disorder. A systematic review and meta-analysis of studies published 1993–2014. *Clin Psychol Rev, 40*, 156–169.

Ostler, T. (2010). Assessing parenting risk within the context of severe and persistent mental illness: Validating an observational measure for families with child protective service involvement. *Infant Mental Health Journal, 31*(5), 467–485.

Ostrove, J. M., & Brown, K. T. (2018). Are allies who we think they are?: A comparative analysis. *Journal of Applied Social Psychology, 48*(4), 195–204.

Ostrow, L., Smith, C., Penney, D., & Shumway, M. (2019). 'It suits my needs': Self-employed individuals with psychiatric disabilities and small businesses. *Psychiatric Rehabilitation Journal, 42*(2), 121-131.

Ovretveit, J. (1998). *Evaluating Health Interventions.* Buckingham: Open University Press.

Oxenham, D. (1999). *A Dialogue on Indigenous Identity: Warts 'n' All.* Gunada Press.

Oxfam Australia. (2018). *Growing Gulf Between Work and Wealth Australian Fact Sheet, January 2018*. Retrieved from www.oxfam.org.au/wp-content/uploads/2018/01/2018-Davos-fact-sheets.pdf.

Paalanen, T., & Hopia, H. (2017). Introduction to professional ethics. *Study Materials for the Master Students.* Retrieved from https://oppimateriaalit.jamk.fi/ethics.

Padesky, C. A. (1993). *Socratic Questioning: Changing Minds or Guiding Discovery? A Keynote Address.* Paper presented at the European Congress of Behavioural and Cognitive Therapies, London.

Padgett, D., Henwood, B. F., & Tsemberis, S. J. (2016). *Housing First: Ending Homelessness, Transforming Systems, and Changing Lives.* New York: Oxford University Press.

Page, A., Atkinson, J. A., Heffernan, M., McDonnell, G., Prodan, A., Osgood, N., & Hickie, I. (2018). Static metrics of impact for a dynamic problem: The need for smarter tools to guide suicide prevention planning and investment. *Australian and New Zealand Journal of Psychiatry, 52*(7), 660–667.

Pagnini, Deanna. & NSW Health. & Carers NSW. (2005). Carer life course framework: An evidence-based approach to effective carer support and education. Sydney: Carers NSW.

Pahl, K. M., & Barrett, P. M. (2007). *Headline Indicators for Children's Health, Development and Wellbeing, 2011*, pp. 50. Australian Institute of Health and Welfare.

Paley, G., Cahill, J., Barkham, M., Shapiro, D., Jones, J., Patrick, S., & Reid, E. (2008). The effectiveness of psychodynamic-interpersonal therapy (PIT) in routine clinical practice: A benchmarking comparison. *Psychology and Psychotherapy-Theory Research and Practice, 81*, 157–175.

Palmer, J., Chondros, P., Piper, D., Callander, R., Weavell, W., Godbee, K., Potiriadis, M., Richard, L., Densley, K., Herman, H., Furler, J., Pierce, D., Schuster, T., Iedema, R., Gunn, J. (2015). The CORE study protocol: A stepped wedge cluster randomised controlled trial to test a co-design technique to optimise psychosocial recovery outcomes for people affected by mental illness in the community mental health setting. *BMJ Open*, 5:e006688.

Palmer, V. J., Johnson, C. L., Furler, J. S., Densley, K., Potiriadis, M., & Gunn, J. M. (n.d.). Written plans: an overlooked mechanism to develop recovery-oriented primary care for depression? Australian Journal of Primary Health, 20(3), 241-249.Palmer, V. J., Weavell, W., Callander, R., Piper, D., Richard, L., Maher, L., . . . Robert, G. (2019). The Participatory Zeitgeist: An explanatory theoretical model of change in an era of coproduction and codesign in healthcare improvement. *Medical Humanities, 45*(3), 247.

Paradies, Y., Ben, J., Denson, N., Elias, A., Priest, N., Pieterse, A., . . . Gee, G. (2015). Racism as a determinant of health: A systematic review and meta-analysis. *PLoS One, 10*(9).

Paris, J. (2003). Personality disorders over time: Precursors, course and outcome. *Journal of Personality Disorders, 17*(6), 479–488.

Paris, J. (2004). Is hospitalization useful for suicidal patients with borderline personality disorder? *Journal of Personality Disorders, 18*(3), 240–247.

Paris, J. (2008). *Treatment of Borderline Personality Disorder: A Guide to Evidence-Based Practice*. Guilford Press.

Paris, J., & Lis, E. (2013). Can sociocultural and historical mechanisms influence the development of borderline personality disorder? *Transcultural Psychiatry, 50*(1), 140-151.

Park, J., Jeong, E., & Seomun, G. (2018). The clock drawing test: A systematic review and meta-analysis of diagnostic accuracy. *Journal of Advanced Nursing, 74*(12), 2742-2754.

Park, M., & Unutzer, J. (2011). Geriatric depression in primary care. *Psychiatric Clinics of North America, 34*(2), 469–+.

Parker, A., Hetrick, S., & Purcell, R. (2010). Psychosocial assessment of young people: Refining and evaluating a youth friendly assessment interview. *Australian Family Physician, 39*(8), 585.

Parker, A., Scantlebury, A., Booth, A., Macbryde, J. C., Scott, W. J., Wright, K., & McDaid, C. (2018). Interagency collaboration models for people with mental ill health in contact with the police: A systematic scoping review. *BMJ Open, 8*(3).

Parker, A. G., Hetrick, S. E., Jorm, A. F., Mackinnon, A. J., McGorry, P. D., Yung, A. R., . . . Purcell, R. (2016). The effectiveness of simple psychological and physical activity interventions for high prevalence mental health problems in young people: A factorial randomised controlled trial. *J Affect Disord, 196*, 200-209.

Parker, G., Cheah, Y.-C., & Roy, K. (2001). Do the Chinese somatize depression? A cross-cultural study. [Lifeline]. *Social Psychiatry and Psychiatric Epidemiology, 36*, 287-293.

Parker, R., & Milroy, H. (2010). Mental illness in Aboriginal and Torres Strait Islander people. In N. Purdie, P. Dudgeon, R. Walker, & Department of Health and Ageing (eds.), *Working Together: Aboriginal and Torres Strait Islander Mental Health and Wellbeing Principles and Practice* (1st ed., pp. 113-124). Australian Institute of Health and Welfare.

Parker, R., & Milroy, H. (2014). Mental illness in Aboriginal and Torres Strait Islander peoples. In P. Dudgeon, H. Milroy, & R. Walker (eds.), *Working Together: Aboriginal and Torres Strait Islander Mental Health and Wellbeing Principles and Practice* (pp. 113-124). Barton: Commonwealth of Australia.

Parliament of Australia. (2006). *A National Approach to Mental Health—From Crisis to Community. Final Report*. Retrieved from www.aph.gov.au/Parliamentary_Business/Committees/Senate/Former_Committees/mentalhealth/report02/index.

Parliament of Australia. (2017a). *Uluru Statement: A Quick Guide*. Retrieved from www.aph.gov.au/About_Parliament/Parliamentary_Departments/Parliamentary_Library/pubs/rp/rp1617/Quick_Guides/UluruStatement.

Parliament of Australia. (2017b). *The Constant Battle: Suicide by Veterans*. Retrieved from www.aph.gov.au/Parliamentary_Business/Committees/Senate/Foreign_Affairs_Defence_and_Trade/VeteranSuicide/Report.

Parliament of Australia. (2018). *Top 10 Countries of Birth for the Overseas-Born Population Since 1901*. Australia: Commonwealth of Australia.

Pascoe, B. (2018). *Dark Emu: Aboriginal Australia and the Birth of Agriculture, New Edition*. Broome, Magabala Books.

Patel, V., Saxena, S., Lund, C., Thornicroft, G., Baingana, F., Bolton, P., . . . Prince, M. (2018). The Lancet Commission on global mental health and sustainable development. *The Lancet, 392*(10157), 1553-1598.

Paterson, C. F. (1997). Rationales for the use of occupation in 19th century asylums. *British Journal of Occupational Therapy, vol. 60*(4), pp. 179-183.

Pathare, S., & Shields, L. S. (2012). Supported decision-making for persons with mental illness: A review. *Public Health Reviews, 34*(2), 1-40.

Patient Health Questionnaire (PHQ) Screeners. (2020). *Screener Overview*. Retrieved from www.phqscreeners.com/select-screener.

Paton, N., & Sanders, F. (2011). *Best Models for Carer Workforce Development: Carer Peer Support Workers, Carer Consultants, Carer Advocates and Carer Advisors*. Retrieved from https://helpingminds.org.au/wp-content/uploads/2018/07/Best-Models-for-Carer-Peer-Workforce-Nov-2011.pdf.

Patrick, C. J. (2019). *Handbook of Psychopathy, Second Edition*. New York: Guilford Publications.

Patten, S. B. (2003). Recall bias and major depression lifetime prevalence. *Social Psychiatry and Psychiatric Epidemiology, 38*(6), 290–296.

Patten, S. B., Gordon-Brown, L., & Meadows, G. (2010). Simulation studies of age-specific lifetime major depression prevalence. *BMC Psychiatry, 10*(85).

Patterson, T. L., Goldman, S., McKibbin, C. L., Hughs, T., & Jeste, D. V. (2001). UCSD Performance-based skills assessment: Development of a new measure of everyday functioning for severely mentally ill adults. *Schizophrenia Bulletin, 27*(2), 235–245.

Patton, G. C., Sawyer, S. M., Santelli, J. S., Ross, D. A., Afifi, R., Allen, N. B., . . . Viner, R. M. (2016). Our future: A Lancet Commission on adolescent health and wellbeing. *Lancet, 387*(10036), 2423-2478.

Patton, M. Q. (1990). *Qualitative Evaluation and Research Methods* (2nd ed.). Newbury Park: Sage.

Patton, M. Q. (1997). *Utilisation-Focused Evaluation: The New Century Text* (3rd ed.). Thousand Oaks: Sage.

Patton, M. Q. (2010). *Developmental Evaluation: Applying Complexity Concepts to Enhance Innovation and Use*. New York: Guilford Press.

Paus, T., Keshavan, M., & Giedd, J. N. (2008). Why do many psychiatric disorders emerge during adolescence? *Nature Reviews: Neuroscience, 9*(12), 947-957.

Pawson, H., Parsell, C., Saunders, P., Hill, T., & Liu, E. (2018). *Australian Homelessness Monitor 2018*. Collingwood, Victoria: Launch Housing.

Paxton, S. J., Hay, P., Touyz, S. W., Forbes, D., Madden, S., Girosi, F., & Morgan, C. (2012). *Paying the Price: The Economic and Social Impact of Eating Disorders in Australia*. Retrieved from https://thebutterflyfoundation.org.au/about-us/information-and-resources/paying-the-price.

Payne, M. (2000). *Teamwork in Multiprofessional Care*. Basingstoke: Lyceum Books.

Pearce, C., Trumble, S., Arnold, M., Dwan, K., & Phillips, C. (2008). Computers in the new consultation: Within the first minute. *Family Practice, 25*(3), 202-208.

Percudani, M., Corradin, Moreno, Indelicato, & Vita. (2020). Mental Health Services in Lombardy during COVID-19 outbreak. *Psychiatry Research*, 288, 112980. Retrieved from: https://doi.org/10.1016/j.psychres.2020.112980

PeerZone. (2019). *PeerZone Toolkit*. Retrieved from www.peerzonetoolkit.com.

Pence, B. W., O'Donnell, J. K., & Gaynes, B. N. (2012). The depression treatment cascade in primary care: A public health perspective. *Current Psychiatry Reports, 14*(4), 328-335.

Penfold, P. S., & Walker, G. A. (1983). *Women and the Psychiatric Paradox*. Montreal: Eden Press.

Peplau, H. E. (1952). *Interpersonal Relations in Nursing*. New York: Putnam.

Perkins, R., Meddings, S., Williams, S., & Repper, J. (2018). *Recovery Colleges 10 Years On*. Nottingham: ImROC, Nottinghamshire Healthcare.

Perkins, S. J., Murphy, R., Schmidt, U., & Williams, C. (2006). Self-help and guided self-help for eating disorders. *Cochrane Database of Systematic Reviews*, (3), CD004191.

Perlman, L. (2000). Adults with Asperger disorder misdiagnosed as schizophrenic. Professional Psychology—Research & Practice, 31(2) Apr 2000Perry, B., Pollard, R. A., Blakley, T. L., & Vigilante, D. (1995). Childhood trauma, the neurobiology of adaptation, and 'use-dependent' development of the brain: How 'states' become 'traits'. *Infant Mental Health Journal, 1*(16(4)).

Persons, J. (1995). Are all psychotherapies cognitive? *Journal of Cognitive Psychotherapy, 9*(3), 185-194.

Pertusa, A., Frost, R. O., Fullana, M. A., Samuels, J., Steketee, G., Tolin, D., . . . Mataix-Cols, D. (2010). Refining the diagnostic boundaries of compulsive hoarding: A critical review. *Clin Psychol Rev, 30*(4), 371-386.

Perugi, G., Akiskal, H. S., Giannotti, D., Frare, F., Di Vaio, S., & Cassano, G. B. (1997). Gender-related differences in body dysmorphic disorder (dysmorphophobia). *J Nerv Ment Dis, 185*(9), 578-582.

Peters, S. (2010). Qualitative research methods in mental health. *Evidence-Based Mental Health, 13*(2), 35-40.

Petersen, M. W., Schroder, A., Jørgensen, T., Ornbol, E., Dantoft, T. M., Eliasen, M., . . . Fink, P. (2019). Prevalence of functional somatic syndromes and bodily distress syndrome in the Danish population: The DanFunD study. *Scandinavian Journal of Public Health*.

Petersen, R. C. (2011). Mild cognitive impairment. *New England Journal of Medicine, 364*(23), 2227-2234.

Petersen, R. C., Lopez, O., Armstrong, M. J., Getchius, T. S. D., Ganguli, M., Gloss, D., . . . Rae-Grant, A. (2018). Author response: Practice guideline update summary: Mild cognitive impairment: Report of the Guideline Development, Dissemination, and Implementation Subcommittee of the American Academy of Neurology. *Neurology, 91*(8), 373-374.

Peterson, J. K., Skeem, J., Kennealy, P., Bray, B., & Zvonkovic, A. (2014). How often and how consistently do symptoms directly precede criminal behavior among offenders with mental illness? *Law and Human Behavior, 38*(5), 439-449.

Petrakis, M. (2015). Implementing the strengths model in a clinical mental health service. In A. P. Francis, V. Pulla, M. Clark, I. Ponnuswami, & E. S. Mariscal (eds.), *Advancing Social Work in Mental Health Through Strengths Based Practice* (pp. 304-321). Primrose Hall Publishing Group.

Petrakis, M. (2018). *Social Work Practice in Health: An Introduction to Contexts, Theories and Skills*. Crows Nest: Allen & Unwin.

Petrakis, M., & Lethborg, C. (2018). An introduction to health and health services practice, and the social determinants of health. In M. Petrakis (ed.), *Social Work Practice in Health: An Introduction to Contexts, Theories and Skills*. Crows Nest: Allen & Unwin.

Petrakis, M., Robinson, R., Myers, K., Kroes, S., & O'Connor, S. (2018). Dual diagnosis competencies: A systematic review of staff training literature. *Addictive Behaviors Reports, 7*, 53-57.

Petrakis, M., Wilson, M., & Hamilton, B. (2013). Implementing the strengths model of case management: Group supervision fidelity outcomes. *Community Mental Health Journal, 49*(3), 331-337.

Petrik, A. M., Kazantzis, N., & Hofmann, S. G. (2013). Distinguishing integrative from eclectic practice in cognitive behavioral therapies. *Psychotherapy, 50*(3), 392-397.

Pharoah F, Mari JJ, Rathbone J, Wong W. (2010). Family intervention for schizophrenia. *Cochrane Database of Systematic Reviews*, issue 12. art. no.: CD000088.

Phelan, M., M. Slade, et al. (1995). The Camberwell Assessment of Need: The validity and reliability of an instrument to assess the needs of people with severe mental illness. *British Journal of Psychiatry, 167*, 589-595.

Phillipou, A., Rossell, S. L., Wilding, H. E., & Castle, D. J. (2016). Randomised controlled trials of psychological & pharmacological treatments for body dysmorphic disorder: A systematic review. *Psychiatry Res, 245*, 179-185.

Phillips, K. A. (2007). Suicidality in body dysmorphic disorder. *Primary Psychiatry, 14*(12), 58-66.

Phillips, K. A. (2009). *Understanding Body Dysmorphic Disorder: An Essential Guide*. New York: Oxford University Press.

Phillips, K. A., Didie, E. R., Menard, W., Pagano, M. E., Fay, C., & Weisberg, R. B. (2006). Clinical features of body dysmorphic disorder in adolescents and adults. *Psychiatry Res, 141*(3), 305-314.

Phillips, K. A., Hollander, E., Rasmussen, S. A., Aronowitz, B. R., DeCaria, C., & Goodman, W. K. (1997). A severity rating scale for body dysmorphic disorder: Development, reliability, and validity of a modified version of the Yale-Brown Obsessive Compulsive Scale. *Psychopharmacology Bulletin, 33*(1), 17-22.

Phillips, K. A., Menard, W., & Fay, C. (2006). Gender similarities and differences in 200 individuals with body dysmorphic disorder. *Comprehensive Psychiatry, 47*(2), 77-87.

Phillips, K. A., Menard, W., Fay, C., & Weisberg, R. (2005). Demographic characteristics, phenomenology, comorbidity, and family history in 200 individuals with body dysmorphic disorder. *Psychosomatics, 46*(4), 317-325.

Phillips, L. J., Francey, S. M., Edwards, J., & McMurray, N. (2007). Stress and psychosis: Towards the development of new models of investigation. *Clinical Psychology Review, 27*(3), 307-317.

PHN Mental Health Tools and Resources. (2019). *Aboriginal and Torres Strait Islander Mental Health Services*. Retrieved from www1.health.gov.au/internet/main/publishing.nsf/content/phn-mental_tools.

Phoenix Australia. (2013). Australian Guidelines for the Treatment of Acute Stress Disorder and Posttraumatic Stress Disorder. Melbourne: Centre for Posttraumatic Mental Health.

Phoenix Australia. (2019). *Centre for Posttraumatic Mental Health*. Melbourne: Centre for Posttraumatic Mental Health Retrieved from www.phoenixaustralia.org.

Phongsavan, P., Chey, T., Bauman, A., Brooks, R., & Silove, D. (2006). Social capital, socio-economic status and psychological distress among Australian adults. *Social Science & Medicine, 63*(10), 2546–2561.

Pickersgill, M. D. (2014). Debating DSM-5: Diagnosis and the sociology of critique. *Journal of Medical Ethics, 40*(8), 521–525.

Pickles, A., Dunn, G., & Vázquez-Barquero, J. L. (1995). Screening for stratification in two-phase ('two-stage') epidemiological surveys. *Statistical Methods in Medical Research, 4*, 73–89.

Pieper, M. J. C., van Dalen-Kok, A. H., Francke, A. L., van der Steen, J. T., Scherder, E. J. A., Husebo, B. S., & Achterberg, W. P. (2013). Interventions targeting pain or behaviour in dementia: A systematic review. *Ageing Research Reviews, 12*(4), 1042–1055.

Pierce, J., Petry, N., Stitzer, M., Blaine, J., Kellogg, S., Satterfield, F., . . . Silva-Vazquez, L. (2006). Effects of lower-cost incentives on stimulant abstinence in methadone maintenance treatment. *Archives of General Psychiatry, 63*, 201–208.

Pigott, T. A., & Seay, S. M. (1999). A review of the efficacy of selective serotonin reuptake inhibitors in obsessive-compulsive disorder. *J Clin Psychiatry, 60*(2), 101–106.

Pike, K. M., Walsh, B. T., Vitousek, K., Wilson, G. T., & Bauer, J. (2003). Cognitive behavior therapy in the posthospitalization treatment of anorexia nervosa. *American Journal of Psychiatry, 160*(11), 2046–2049.

Piketty, T., & Goldhammer, A. (2017). *Capital in the Twenty-First Century*. Harvard University Press.

Pilcher, H. (2009). The science of voodoo: When mind attacks body. New Scientist, 2708, 5. *New Scientist, 202*(2708), 30–33.

Pilgrim, D. (2008). 'Recovery' and current mental health policy. *Chronic Illness, 4*(4), 309–310.

Pilgrim, D. (2014). *Key Concepts in Mental Health*. London: SAGE Publications.

Pilgrim, D., & McCranie, A. (2013). *Recovery and Mental Health: A Critical Sociological Account*. Palgrave Macmillan.

Pilling, S., Bebbington, P., Kuipers, E., Garety, P., Geddes, J., Orbach, G., & Morgan, C. (2002). Psychological treatments in schizophrenia: I. Meta-analysis of family intervention and cognitive behaviour therapy. *Psychol Med, 32*(5), 763–782.

Pilowsky, I. (1997). *Abnormal Illness Behaviour*. Chichester: John Wiley.

Pinches, A. (2004). *Pathfinders: Consumer participation in Mental Health & Other Services—Evidence based strategies for the ways ahead*. Kingsbury: Communityscope Research & Development.

Pinches, A. (2011). Northern CCU Peer Support Research and Development Project: Putting the Community in Community Care Unit. Final Report 2011. eEtreived from www.ourcommunity.com.au/files/OCP/NCCU_Peer_Support.doc.

Pincus, A. L., Cain, N. M., & Wright, A. G. (2014). Narcissistic grandiosity and narcissistic vulnerability in psychotherapy. *Personality Disorders: Theory, Research, and Treatment, 5*(4), 439.

Piri Pono. (2019). *Ember Korowai Takitini*. Auckland, Ember. Retrieved from https://ember.org.nz.

Pirkis, J., Burgess, P., Hardy, J., Harris, M., Slade, T., & Johnston, A. (2010). Who cares? A profile of people who care for relatives with a mental disorder. *Australian and New Zealand Journal of Psychiatry, 44*(10), 929–937.

Pirkis, J., Ftanou, M., Williamson, M., Machlin, A., Spittal, M. J., Bassilios, B., & Harris, M. (2011). Australia's Better Access initiative: An evaluation. *Australian and New Zealand Journal of Psychiatry, 45*(9), 726–739.

Pirkis, J., Kohn, F., Morley, B., Burgess, P., & Blashki, G. (2004). Better outcomes in mental healthcare. *Primary Care Mental Health, 2*(3–4), 141–149.

Pleace, N. (2018). *Using Housing First in Integrated Homelessness Strategies: A Review of the Evidence*. Retrieved from http://eprints.whiterose.ac.uk/127547.

Plos Medicine Editors. (2013). The paradox of mental health: Over-treatment and under-recognition. *PLoS Medicine, 10*(5), e1001456-e1001456.

Ploubidis, G. B., & Grundy, E. (2009). Later-life mental health in Europe: A country-level comparison. *J Gerontol B Psychol Sci Soc Sci, 64*(5), 666–676.

Point of Care Foundation. (2018). *Experience Based Co-design Tool Kit*. Retrieved from www.pointofcarefoundation.org.uk/resource/experience-based-co-design-ebcd-toolkit.

Polderman, T. J. C., Benyamin, B., de Leeuw, C. A., Sullivan, P. F., van Bochoven, A., Visscher, P. M., & Posthuma, D. (2015). Meta-analysis of the heritability of human traits based on fifty years of twin studies. *Nature Genetics, 47*, 702.

Political Psychology Research Group. (2020). *American Public Opinion on Global Warming*. Retrieved from https://climatepublicopinion.stanford.edu.

Pontin, E., Peters, S., Lobban, F., Rogers, A., & Morriss, R. K. (2009). Enhanced relapse prevention for bipolar disorder: A qualitative investigation of value perceived for service users and care coordinators. *Implementation Science, 4*.

Poon, A. W. C., Curtis, J., Ward, P., Loneragan, C., & Lappin, J. (2018). Physical and psychological health of carers of young people with first episode psychosis. *Australasian Psychiatry, 26*(2), 184–188.

Poon, A. W. C., Harvey, C., Fuzzard, S., & O'Hanlon, B. (2017). Implementing a family-inclusive practice model in youth mental health services in Australia. *Early Intervention in Psychiatry*, 1–8.

Poon, A. W. C., Harvey, C., Mackinnon, A., & Joubert, L. (2017). A longitudinal population-based study of carers of people with psychosis. *Epidemiology and Psychiatric Sciences, 26*(3), 265–275.

Poon, A. W. C., Hayes, L., & Harvey, C. (2019). Care-giving by people with psychotic disorders in the second Australian prevalence study of psychosis. *Health & Social Care in the Community*, 27(4), 1042–1052.

Poon, A. W. C., Joubert, L., & Harvey, C. (2015). A longitudinal study of the health and wellbeing of culturally and linguistically diverse caregivers of people with psychosis in Australia. *International Journal of Social Psychiatry, 61*(8), 743–753.

Poon, A. W. C., Joubert, L., & Harvey, C. (2018). Perceived needs of carers of people with psychosis: An Australian longitudinal population-based study of caregivers of people with psychotic disorders. *Health and Social Care in the Community, 26*(3), 412–422.

Poon, A. W. C., Joubert, L., Mackinnon, A., & Harvey, C. (2017). Recovery for carers of people with psychosis: A longitudinal population-based study with implications for social work. *British Journal of Social Work, 48*(6), 1754–1773.

Popay, J., Rogers, A., & Williams, G. (1998). Rationale and standards for the systematic review of qualitative literature in health services research. *Qualitative Health Research, 8*(3), 341–351.

Porta, M., Greenland, S., Hernán, M., dos Santos Silva, I., & Last, J. M. (2014). *A Dictionary of Epidemiology* (6th ed.). Oxford University Press.

Porter, M. E., Lee, T. H., Sattenspiel, J. E., & Couillard, F. (2013). The Strategy That Will Fix Health Care: Interaction. *Harvard Business Review*, 91(12), 23.

Porter, R. (1985). The patient's view: Doing medical history from below. *Theory Soc, 14*, 175–198.

Potenza, M. (2013). How central is dopamine to pathological gambling or gambling disorder? *Frontiers in Behavioral Neuroscience*, 7, 206. https://doi.org/10.3389/fnbeh.2013.00206.

Potenza, M. N. (2018). Do gaming disorder and hazardous gaming belong in the ICD-11? Considerations regarding the death of a hospitalized patient that was reported to have occurred while a care provider was gaming. (Letter to the editor). *Journal of Behavioral Addictions, 7*(2), 206.

Power, P., & McGorry, P. D. (1999). Initial assessment of first-episode psychosis. *The Recognition and Management of Early Psychosis. A Preventive Approach* (p. 155-183). Cambridge: Cambridge University Press.

Predmore, Z. et al. (2017). Expanding suicide crisis services to text and chat. *Crisis*, vol 38(4).

Pretty, J., Peacock, J., Hine, R., Sellens, M., South, N., & Griffin, M. (2007). Green exercise in the UK countryside: Effects on health and psychological well-being, and implications for policy and planning. *Journal of Environmental Planning and Management., 50*(2), 211–231.

Price-Robertson, R., Obradovic, A., & Morgan, B. (2017). Relational recovery: Beyond individualism in the recovery approach. *Advances in Mental Health, 15*(2), 108-120.

Price-Robertson, R., Smart, D., & Bromfield, L. (2010). Family is for life: Connections between childhood family experiences and wellbeing in early adulthood. *Family Matters* (85), 7-17.

Prince, M., Stewaart, R., Ford, T., & Hotopf, M. (2002). Practical psychiatric epidemiology. In M. T. Tsuang & M. Tohen (eds.), *Textbook in Psychiatric Epidemiology*. Oxford University Press.

Prince, M., Stewart, R., Ford, T., & Das-Munshi, J. (2020). *Practical Psychiatric Epidemiology*. Oxford University Press.

Problem Gambling Research and Treatment Centre. (2011). *Guideline for Screening, Assessment and Treatment of Problem Gambling*. Retrieved from https://www.greo.ca/Modules/EvidenceCentre/Details/guideline-screening-assessment-and-treatment-problem-gambling.

Probst, B. (2012). Not quite colleagues: Issues of power and purview between social work and psychiatry. *Social Work in Mental Health, 10*(5), 367-383.

Prochaska, J., Diclemente, C., & Norcross, J. (1992). In search of how people change: Applications to addictive behaviors. *American Psychologist, 47*(9), 1102.

Prochaska, J., & DiClemente, C. C. (1982). Transtheoretical therapy: Toward a more integrative model of change. *Psychotherapy: Theory, Research & Practice, 19*(3), 276.

Productivity Commission. (2010). Gambling 2010. Retrieved from https://www.pc.gov.au.

Productivity Commission. (2014). Report on Government Services 2014. Retrieved from Canberra: https://www.pc.gov.au.

Project Air Strategy. (2020). *Project Air: A Personality Disorders Strategy*. Retrieved from www.projectairstrategy.org/content/groups/public/@web/@ihmri/documents/doc/uow225679.pdf.

Psychology Board of Australia. (2019). *Psychology Board of Australia Registrant Data*. Retrieved from www.psychologyboard.gov.au/About/Statistics.aspx.

Pulla, V. R. (2017). Strengths-based approach in social work: A distinct ethical advantage. *International Journal of Innovation, Creativity and Change, 3*(2), 97–114.

Puras, D. (2018). *Report of the Special Rapporteur on the Right of Everyone to the Enjoyment of the Highest Attainable Standard of Physical and Mental Health*. Retrieved from https://digitallibrary.un.org.

Purcell, R., Maruff, P., Kyrios, M., & Pantelis, C. (1998). Neuropsychological deficits in obsessive-compulsive disorder: A comparison with unipolar depression, panic disorder, and normal controls. *Arch Gen Psychiatry, 55*(5), 415-423.

Purdie, N., Dudgeon, P., & Walker, R. (2010). *Working Together: Aboriginal and Torres Strait Islander Mental Health and Wellbeing Principles and Practice*. Retrieved from www.ichr.uwa.edu.au/files/user5/Working_Together_book_web_0.pdf.

Queensland Centre For Mental Health Research. (2020). *Queensland's Premier Mental Health Research Facility*. Retrieved from https://qcmhr.uq.edu.au.

Queensland Government. (2016). *Queensland Mental Health Act 2016*. Retrieved from www.health.qld.gov.au/clinical-practice/guidelines-procedures/clinical-staff/mental-health/act.

Quilty, S., Bachmayer, L., & Congdon, A. (2015). Telehealth in remote NT: Bridging the gap. *Medical Journal of Australia, 203*(1), 18-18.

Quinlan, F. (2014). *Getting the NDIS Right for People with Psychosocial Disability*. Retrieved from https://mhaustralia.org/general/getting-ndis-right-people-psychosocial-disability.

Quirk, S. E., Berk, M., Chanen, A. M., Koivumaa-Honkanen, H., Brennan-Olsen, S. L., Pasco, J. A., & Williams, L. J. (2016). Population prevalence of personality disorder and associations with physical health comorbidities and health care service utilization: A review. *Personality Disorders: Theory, Research, and Treatment, 7*(2), 136.

RACGP 'Red Book' Taskforce, Harris M, Bailey L, Bridges-Webb C, Furler J, Joyner B, . . . Y., Z. (2005). *Guidelines for Preventive Activities in General Practice (The Red Book)* (6th ed., vol. 2006). South Melbourne: The Royal Australian College of General Practitioners.

Rachman, S. (1998). A cognitive theory of obsessions: Elaborations. *Behav Res Ther, 36*(4), 385-401.

Rahman, A., Fisher, J., Bower, P., Luchters, S., Tran, T., Yasamy, M. T., . . . Waheed, W. (2013). Interventions for common perinatal mental disorders in women in low- and middle-income countries: A systematic review and meta-analysis. *Bull World Health Organ, 91*(8), 593-601i.

Ramon, S. (2009). Adult mental health in a changing international context: The relevance to social work. *British Journal of Social Work, 39*(8), 1615-1622.

Ramos, K., & Stanley, M. A. (2018). Anxiety disorders in late life. *Psychiatric Clinics of North America, 41*(1), 55-+.

Rank, O. (1911). Ein beitrag zum narzissismus. *Jahrbuch Für Psychoanalytische Und Psychopathologische Forschung, 3*(1), 401-426.

Rapee, R. M. (2012). Anxiety disorders in children and adolescents: Nature, development, treatment and prevention. In J. M. Rey (ed.), *IACAPAP e-Textbook of Child and Adolescent Mental Health*. Geneva: International Association for Child and Adolescent Psychiatry and Allied Professions.

Rapp, C. A. (1993). Chronic mental illness. In M. Harris & H. C. Bergman (eds.), *Case management for Mentally Ill Patients: Theory and Practice* (vol. 1, pp. 143-164). Langhorne: Harwood Academic Publishers.

Rapp, C. A., & Goscha, R. J. (2004). The principles of effective case management of mental health services. *Psychiatric Rehabilitation Journal, 27*(4), 319-333.

Rapp, C. A., & Goscha, R. J. (2006). *The Strengths Model: Case Management with People with Psychiatric Disabilities* (2nd ed.). New York: Oxford University Press.

Rapp, C. A., & Goscha, R. J. (2012). *The Strengths Model: A Recovery-Oriented Approach to Mental Health Services*. Oxford University Press.

Rapp, C. A., & Goscha, R. J. (2015). Three decades of strengths: Reflections of the past and challenges of the future. In A. P. Francis, V. Pulla, M. Clark, E. S. Mariscal, & I. Ponnuswami (eds.), *Advancing Social Work in Mental Health Through Strengths Based Practice* (pp. 31-38). Primrose Hall Publishing Group.

Rask, M. T., Ornbol, E., Rosendal, M., & Fink, P. (2017). Long-Term outcome of bodily distress syndrome in primary care: A follow-up study on health care costs, work disability, and self-rated health. *Psychosomatic Medicine, 79*(3), 345-357.

Ratcliffe, S., Stewart, A., Melville, M., Jacobs, P., & Keay, A. J. (1970). Chromosome studies on 3500 newborn male infants. *The Lancet, 295*(7638), 121-122.

Ravindran, L. N., & Stein, M. B. (2010). The pharmacologic treatment of anxiety disorders: A review of progress. *J Clin Psychiatry, 71*(7), 839-854.

Rawls, J. (1999). *A Theory of Justice*. Oxford University Press.

Rawson, R. A., & Tennant, F. S. (1984). Five-year follow-up of opiate addicts with naltrexone and behavior therapy. *NIDA Res Monogr Ser, 49*, 289-295.

Raylu, N., & Oei, T. P. S. (2004a). The gambling related cognitions scale (GRCS): Development, confirmatory factor validation and psychometric properties. *Addiction, 99*(6), 757-769.

Raylu, N., & Oei, T. P. S. (2004b). The gambling urge scale: Development, confirmatory factor validation, and psychometric properties. *Psychology of Addictive Behaviors, 18*(2), 100-105.

Razzaque, R., & Wood, L. (2015). Open dialogue and its relevance to the NHS: Opinions of NHS staff and service users. *Community Mental Health Journal, 51*(8), 931-938.

Read, J., Fink, P., Rudegeair, T., Felitti, V., & Whitfield, C. (2008). Child maltreatment and psychosis: A return to a genuinely integrated bio-psycho-social model. *Clinical Schizophrenia & Related Psychoses, 2*(3), 235-254.

Reas, D. L. (2017). Public and healthcare professionals' knowledge and attitudes toward binge eating disorder: A narrative review. *Nutrients, 9*(11).

Reavley, N. J., Cvetkovski, S., Jorm, A. F., & Lubman, D. I. (2010). Help-seeking for substance use, anxiety and affective disorders among young people: Results from the 2007 Australian National Survey of Mental Health and Wellbeing. *Australian and New Zealand Journal of Psychiatry, 44*(8), 729-735.

Reavley, N. J., & Jorm, A. F. (2011). Recognition of mental disorders and beliefs about treatment and outcome: Findings from an Australian National Survey of Mental Health Literacy and Stigma. *Australian and New Zealand Journal of Psychiatry, 45*(11), 947-956.

Reavley, N. J., Jorm, A. F., Cvetkovski, S., & Mackinnon, A. J. (2011). National depression and anxiety indices for Australia. *Australian and New Zealand Journal of Psychiatry, 45*(9), 780-787.

Reavley, N. J., McCann, T. V., & Jorm, A. F. (2012). Actions taken to deal with mental health problems in Australian higher education students. *Early Intervention in Psychiatry, 6*(2), 159-165.

Reavley, N. J., Ross, A., Martin, A., Lamontagne, A. D., & Jorm, A. F. (2014). Development of guidelines for workplace prevention of mental health problems: A Delphi consensus study with Australian professionals and employees. *Mental Health & Prevention, 2*(1-2), 26-34.

Recovery in the Bin: A critical theorist and activist collective. (2020). *The Unrecovery Star*. Retrieved from https://recoveryinthebin.org/unrecovery-star-2.

Recovery Rocks Community Inc. (2019). *Peers Standing Stronger*. Retrieved from https://recoveryrockscommunity.org.

Refugee Council of Australia. (2019). *How Generous is Australia's Refugee Program Compared to Other Countries?* Retrieved from www.refugeecouncil.org.au/2018-global-trends.

Reger, M. A., Stanley, I. H., & Joiner, T. E. (2020). Suicide mortality and coronavirus disease 2019—A perfect storm? *JAMA Psychiatry*. doi:10.1001/jamapsychiatry.2020.1060 on-line ahead of print.

Regier, D. A., Narrow, W. E., Kuhl, E. A., & Kupfer, D. J. (2011). *Introduction: The Conceptual Evolution of DSM-5*. Arlington: American Psychiatric Publishing.

Rehbein, F., Kliem, S., Baier, D., Mossle, T., & Petry, N. M. (2015). Prevalence of internet gaming disorder in German adolescents: Diagnostic contribution of the nine DSM-5 criteria in a state-wide representative sample. *Addiction, 110*(5), 842-851.

Reich, D. B., & Zanarini, M. C. (2008). Sexual orientation and relationship choice in borderline personality disorder over ten years of prospective follow-up. *Journal of Personality Disorders, 22*(6), 564-572.

Reid, S. C., Teesson, M., Sannibale, C., Matsuda, M., & Haber, P. S. (2005). The efficacy of compliance therapy in pharmacotherapy for alcohol dependence: A randomized controlled trial. *Journal of Studies on Alcohol, 66*(6), 833-841.

Reifels, L., Bassilios, B., King, K. E., Fletcher, J. R., Blashki, G., & Pirkis, J. E. (2013). Innovations in primary mental healthcare. *Australian Health Review, 37*(3), 312-317.

Reifels, L., Ftanou, M., Krysinska, K., Machlin, A., Robinson, J., & Pirkis, J. (2018). Research priorities in suicide prevention: Review in Australian research from 2010-2017 highlights continued need for intervention research. *International Journal of Environmental Research and Public Health, 15*(4), pii: E807.

Reilly, J., & Atkinson, J. M. (2010). The content of mental health advance directives: Advance statements in Scotland. *International Journal of Law and Psychiatry, 33*(2), 116-121.

Reilly, R. L., Keegan, D. L., Corring, D., Shrikhande, S., & Natarajan, D. (2006). A qualitative analysis of the use of community treatment orders in Saskatchewan. *International Journal of Law and Psychiatry, 29*(6), 516-524.

Reiss, S., & Aman, M. G. (1997). The international consensus process on psychopharmacology and intellectual disability. *Journal of Intellectual Disability Research, 41*(6), 448-455.

Repo-Tiihonen, E., Virkkunen, M., & Tiihonen, J. (2001). Mortality of antisocial male criminals. *Journal of Forensic Psychiatry, 12*(3), 677-683.

Repper, J., & Perkins, R. (2009). Recovery and social inclusion: The changing mental health agenda. In C. Booker & J. Repper (eds.), *Mental Health from Policy to Practice* (pp. 1-13). New York: Churchill Livingstone Elsevier.

Reser, J. P., Bradley, G. L., & Ellul, M. C. (2012). Coping with climate change: Bringing psychological adaptation in from the cold. In B. Molinelli & V. Grimaldo (eds.), *Handbook of the Psychology of Coping: New Research* (pp. 1-34). Nova Science Publishers.

Resick, P. A., & Calhoun, K. S. (2001). Posttraumatic stress disorder. In D. H. Barlow (ed.), *Clinical Handbook of Psychological Disorders: A Step-by-Step Treatment Manual* (3rd ed., pp. 60-113). New York: Guilford Press.

Resick, P. A., Monson, C. M., & Chard, K. M. (2017). *Cognitive Processing Therapy for PTSD: A Comprehensive Manual*. New York: The Guilford Press.

Resources for University Educators. (2020). *Enhancing Student Wellbeing*. Retrieved from http://unistudentwellbeing.edu.au.

Rethink Mental Illness. (2020). *Bristol Siblings Group*. Retrieved from www.rethink.org/help-in-your-area/support-groups/bristol-siblings-group.

Rethink Mental Illness. (2020). *Carer's Hub*. Retrieved from www.rethink.org/advice-and-information/carers-hub.

Reupert, A., & Maybery, D. (2016). What do we know about families where parents have a mental illness? *Child & Youth Services, 37*(2), 98-111.

Reynolds, J., Griffiths, K. M., Cunningham, J. A., Bennett, K., & Bennett, A. (2015). Clinical practice models for the use of e-mental health resources in primary health care by health professionals and peer workers: A conceptual framework. *JMIR Mental Health, 2*(1), e6.

Rice, S. M., Simmons, M. B., Bailey, A. P., Parker, A. G., Hetrick, S. E., Davey, C. G., . . . Edwards, J. (2014). Development of practice principles for the management of ongoing suicidal ideation in young people diagnosed with major depressive disorder. *SAGE Open Medicine*, 2. doi:10.1177/2050312114559574.

Richard, J., Martin-Storey, A., Wilkie, E., Derevensky, J. L., Paskus, T., & Temcheff, C. E. (2019). Variations in gambling disorder symptomatology across sexual identity among college student-athletes. *Journal of Gambling Studies, 35*(4), 1303-1316.

Richards, R. E., Oliver, J. E. C., Morris, E., Iervolino, A. C., Wingrove, J., & Aherne, K. (2011). Acceptance and Commitment Therapy training for clinicians: An evaluation. *Cognitive Behaviour Therapist*, 4(3), 114-121.

Richardson, L. K., & Simpson, S. (2015). The future of telemental health and psychology in Australia: Restoring the psychologically 'clever country'? *Australian Psychologist, 50*, 301-310.

Richardson, T., Elliott, P., Roberts, R., & Jansen, M. (2017). A longitudinal study of financial difficulties and mental health in a national sample of British undergraduate students. *Community Mental Health Journal, 53*(3), 344-352.

Rickwood, D. (2005). *Pathways of Recovery: Preventing Further Episodes of Mental Illness (Monograph): Prepared for the National Mental Health Promotion and Prevention Working Party.* Retrieved from www1.health.gov.au/internet/main/publishing.nsf/Content/85A27F4558113287CA257BF00021207D/$File/mono.pdf.

Rickwood, D., Paraskakis, M., Quin, D., Hobbs, N., Ryall, V., Trethowan, J., & McGorry, P. (2019). Australia's innovation in youth mental health care: The headspace centre model. *Early Intervention in Psychiatry, 13*, 159-166.

Rickwood, D. J., Deane, F. P., & Wilson, C. J. (2007). When and how do young people seek professional help for mental health problems? *Medical Journal of Australia, 187*(7 Suppl), S35-39.

Rickwood, D. J., Mazzer, K. R., & Telford, N. R. (2015). Social influences on seeking help from mental health services, in-person and online, during adolescence and young adulthood. *BMC Psychiatry, 15*(1), 40.

Rickwood, D. J., Telford, N., Mazzer, K., Anile, G., Thomas, K., Parker, A. G., . . . Soong, P. (2015). *Service Innovation Project Component 2: Social Inclusion Model Project.* Retrieved from https://headspace.org.au/assets/Uploads/Corporate/Publications-and-research/HSP201-Service-Innovation-Part-2-FA-LR.pdf.

Rickwood, D. J., Telford, N. R., Parker, A. G., Tanti, C. J., & McGorry, P. D. (2014). Headspace—Australia's innovation in youth mental health: Who are the clients and why are they presenting? *Medical Journal of Australia, 200*(2), 108-111.

Rider, G. N., McMorris, B. J., Gower, A. L., Coleman, E., & Eisenberg, M. E. (2019). Gambling behaviors and problem gambling: A population-based comparison of transgender/gender diverse and cisgender adolescents. *Journal of Gambling Studies, 35*(1), 79-92.

Rigby, C. W., Rosen, A., Berry, H. L., & Hart, C. R. (2011). If the land's sick, we're sick: The impact of prolonged drought on the social and emotional well-being of Aboriginal communities in rural New South Wales. *Australian Journal of Rural Health, 19*(5), 249-254.

Riley, R. D., Lambert, P. C., & Abo-Zaid, G. (2010). Meta-analysis of individual participant data: Rationale, conduct, and reporting. *BMJ, 340*, c221.

Rind, B., & Tromovitch, P. (1997). A meta-analytic review of findings from national samples on psychological correlates of child sexual abuse. *Journal of Sex Research, 34*(3), 237-255.

Ringeisen, H., Langer Ellison, M., Ryder-Burge, A., Biebel, K., Alikhan, S., & Jones, E. (2017). Supported education for individuals with psychiatric disabilities: State of the practice and policy implications. *Psychiatric Rehabilitation Journal, 40*(2), 197.

Ritter, A. (2015). New Australian lesbian, gay, bisexual and transgender research—and the need for more. *Drug and Alcohol Review, 34*(4), 347-348.

Roaldset, J. O. (2014). Risk assessment and clinical decision-making. *Australian & New Zealand Journal of Psychiatry, 49*(1), 90-90.

Robbins, L. N. (1990). Psychiatric epidemiology: A historic review. *Journal of Social Psychiatry & Psychiatric Epidemiology*, vol. 25, pp. 16-24.

Rober, P. (2005). The therapist's self in dialogical family therapy: Some ideas about not-knowing and the therapist's inner conversation. *Family Process, 44*(4), 477-495.

Roberts, N. P., Kitchiner, N. J., Kenardy, J., Robertson, L., Lewis, C., & Bisson, J. I. (2019). Multiple session early psychological interventions for the prevention of post-traumatic stress disorder. *Cochrane Database of Systematic Reviews* (8).

Robins LN, Tipp J, Przybeck T. (1991). Antisocial personality. In: LN Robins, Regier D (eds). *Psychiatric Disorders In America*. New York: Free Press, pp. 258-290.

Robinson, D. G., Woerner, M. G., Alvir, J. M. J., Bilder, R. M., Hinrichsen, G. A., & Lieberman, J. A. (2002). Predictors of medication discontinuation by patients with first-episode schizophrenia and schizoaffective disorder. *Schizophrenia Research, 57*(2-3), 209-219.

Robinson, J., Hill, N., Thorn, P., Teh, Z., Battersby, R., & Reavley, N. (2018). *#chatsafe: A Young Person's Guide for Communicating Safely Online About Suicide*. Melbourne: Orygen.

Robinson, J., McCutcheon, L., Browne, V., & Witt, K. (2016). *Looking the Other Way: Young People and Self-harm.* Melbourne: Orygen.

Robson, E., Waghorn, G., Sherring, J., & Morris, A. (2010). Preliminary outcomes from an individualised supported education service delivered by a community mental health service. *British Journal of Occupational Therapy, 73*(10), 481-486.

Rock, P., Roiser, J. P., Riedel, W., & Blackwell, A. D. (2014). Cognitive impairment in depression: A systematic review and meta-analysis. *Psychol Med, 44*(10), 2029-2040.

Rodda, S., & Lubman, D. I. (2014). Characteristics of gamblers using a national online counselling service for problem gambling. *Journal of Gambling Studies, 30*(2), 277-289.

Rodda, S. N., Lubman, D. I., Iyer, R., Gao, C. X., & Dowling, N. A. (2015). Subtyping based on readiness and confidence: The identification of help-seeking profiles for gamblers accessing web-based counselling. *Addiction, 110*(3), 494-501.

Roemer, L., & Orsillo, S. M. (2014). An acceptance-based behavioral therapy for generalized anxiety disorder. In D. H. Barlow (ed.),

Clinical Handbook of Psychological Disorders, Fifth Edition: A Step-By-Step Treatment Manual (pp. 206-236). Guilford Publications.

Roepke, S., Ziegenhorn, A., Kronsbein, J., Merkl, A., Bahri, S., Lange, J., . . . Lammers, C.-H. (2010). Incidence of polycystic ovaries and androgen serum levels in women with borderline personality disorder. *Journal of Psychiatric Research, 44*(13), 847-852.

Rogers, C. R. (1957). The necessary and sufficient conditions of therapeutic personality change. *Journal of Consulting Psychology, 21*(2), 95-103.

Rogers, J. C., & Holm, M. B. (2016). Functional assessment in mental health: Lessons from occupational therapy. *Dialogues in Clinical Neuroscience, 18*, 145-154.

Rogers, E. S., Kash-MacDonald, M., Bruker, D., & Maru, M. (2010). *Systematic Review of Supported Education Literature, 1989-2009*. Boston: Boston University, Sargent College, Center for Psychiatric Rehabilitation.

Rolfe, T., Sheehan, B., & Davidson, R. (2008). Are consumers on community treatment orders informed of their legal and human rights? A West Australian study. *International Journal of Mental Health Nursing, 17*(1), 36-43.

Rolland, J. S. (2017). Neurocognitive impairment: Addressing couple and family challenges. *Family Process, 56*(4), 799-818.

Rood, B. A., Reisner, S. L., Surace, F. I., Puckett, J. A., Maroney, M. R., & Pantalone, D. W. (2016). Expecting rejection: Understanding the minority stress experiences of transgender and gender-nonconforming individuals. *Transgender Health, 1*(1), 151.

Roper, C. (2009). We don't start off with the agenda tied up. In A. Sweeney, P. Beresford, A. Faulkner, M. Nettle, & D. Rose (eds.), *This is Survivor Research* (pp. 168-169). UK: PCCS Books.

Roper, C. (2016a). *Coproduction as a Methodology*. Retrieved from www.mhvic.org.au/images/PDF/newparadigm_/2016WinterNewParadigm.pdf.

Roper, C. (2016b). Is partnership a dirty word? In J. Russo & A. Sweeney (eds.), *Searching for a Rose Garden Challenging Psychiatry, Fostering Mad Studies* (pp. 201-209). Wyastone Leys: PCCS Books.

Roper, C. (2018). Capacity does not reside in me. In C. Spivakovsky, K. Seear, & A. Carter (eds.), *Critical Perspectives on Coercive Interventions: Law, Medicine and Society*. New York: Routledge.

Roper, C., Grey, F., & Cadogan, E. (2018). *Co-production—Putting Principles into Practice in Mental Health Contexts*. Retrieved from https://recoverylibrary.unimelb.edu.au/__data/assets/pdf_file/0010/2659969/Coproduction_putting-principles-into-practice.pdf.

Rose, J. E., & Behm, F. M. (2014). Combination treatment with varenicline and bupropion in an adaptive smoking cessation paradigm. *American Journal of Psychiatry, 171*(11), 1199-1205.

Rosen, A., Killaspy, H., & Harvey, C. (2013). Specialisation and marginalisation: How the assertive community treatment debate affects individuals with complex mental health needs. *Psychiatrist, 37*(11), 345-348.

Rosen, A., McGorry, P., Groom, G., Hickie, I., Gurr, R., Hocking, B., . . . Stanley, F. (2004). Australia needs a Mental Health Commission. *Australasian Psychiatry, 12*(3), 213-219.

Rosen, A., Mueser, K. T., & Teesson, M. (2007). Assertive community treatment: Issues from scientific and clinical literature with implications for practice. *Journal of rehabilitation research and development, 44*(6), 813.

Rosen, D. C., Nakash, O., & Alegría, M. (2016). The impact of computer use on therapeutic alliance and continuance in care during the mental health intake. *Psychotherapy, 53*(1), 117-123.

Rosenbaum, J. F., Biederman, J., Bolduc-Murphy, E. A., Faraone, S. V., Chaloff, J., Hirshfeld, D. R., & Kagan, J. (1993). Behavioral inhibition in childhood: A risk factor for anxiety disorders. *Harvard Review of Psychiatry, 1*(1), 2-16.

Rosenbaum, S., Nijjar, S., Watkins, A., Garwood, N., Sherrington, C., & Tiedemann, A. (2014). Nurse-assessed metabolic monitoring: A file audit of risk factor prevalence and impact of an intervention to enhance measurement of waist circumference. *International Journal of Mental Health Nursing*, 23(3), 252-256.

Rosenberg S., Hickie I. B., McGorry P. D., Salvador-Carulla, L., Burns, J., Christensen, H., ... Sinclair S. (2015). Using accountability for mental health to drive reform. *Med J Aust*, 203 (8), 328-330.

Rosenberg, S., & Hickie, I. (2019). The runaway giant: Ten years of the Better Access program. *Medical Journal of Australia, 210*(7), 299-+.

Rosenberg, S., & Rosen, A. (2012). Can mental health commissions really drive reform? Towards better resourcing, services, accountability and stakeholder engagement. *Australasian Psychiatry, 20*(3), 193-198.

Rosenberg, S., & Salvador-Carulla, L. (2017). PERSPECTIVES: Accountability for mental health: The Australian experience. *J Ment Health Policy Econ, 20*(1), 37-54.

Rosenberg, S., Redmond, C., Boyer, P., Gleeson, P., & Russell, P. (2019). Culture clash? Recovery in mental health under Australia's National Disability Insurance Scheme—A case study. *Public Health Research & Practice.*

Rosenfeld, H. (1986). Destructive narcissism and the death instinct. In impasse and interpretation. London: Tavistock Publications.

Rosengren, D. B. (2017). *Building Motivational Interviewing Skills: A Practitioner Workbook* (2nd ed.). Guilford Publications.

Rosenhan, D. L. (1973). On being sane in insane places. *Science*, vol. 179, pp. 250-258.

Rosenstreich, G. (2013). *LGBTI People Mental Health and Suicide* (revised 2 ed.). Sydney: National LGBTI Health Alliance.

Rosling, H., Rosling, O., & Rönnlund, A. R. (2018). *Factfulness: Ten Reasons We're Wrong About the World—And Why Things Are Better Than You Think*. Hodder & Stoughton.

Rösner S, Hackl-Herrwerth A, Leucht S, Lehert P, Vecchi S, Soyka M. (2010) Acamprosate for alcohol dependence. *Cochrane Database of Systematic Review*, issue 9. art. no.: CD004332.

Ross, E., & Oliver, C. (2003). The assessment of mood in adults who have severe or profound mental retardation. *Clinical Psychology Review, 23*(2), 225-245.

Ross, S., Curry, N., & Goodwin, N. (2011). *Case Management: What It Is and How It Can Best Be Implemented.* Retrieved from www.kingsfund.org.uk/ sites/default/files/Case-Management-paper-The-Kings-Fund-Paper-November-2011_0.pdf.

Rothmann, S., & Coetzer, E. P. (2003). The big five personality dimensions and job performance. *SA Journal of Industrial Psychology, 29*(1), 68-74.

Rowe, J. (2012). Great expectations: A systematic review of the literature on the role of family carers in severe mental illness, and their relationships and engagement with professionals. *Journal of Psychiatric and Mental Health Nursing, 19*(1), 70-82.

Rowe, L., & Kidd, M. (2018). *Every Doctor: Healthier Doctors = Healthier Patients*. CRC Press.

Roy, M. J., Donaldson, C., Baker, R., & Kerr, S. (2014). The potential of social enterprise to enhance health and well-being: A model and systematic review. *Social Science & Medicine, 123*, 182-193.

Royal Australian & New Zealand College of Psychiatrists (RANZCP). (2010). *Report from the Faculty of Child and Adolescent Psychiatry*. Retrieved from www.ranzcp.org/files/

resources/reports/prevention-and-early-intervention-of-mental-illnes.aspx.

Royal Australian & New Zealand College of Psychiatrists (RANZCP). (2014). *RANZCP Workforce Report Australian Membership 2014*. Retrieved from www.ranzcp.org/news-policy/policy-and-advocacy/reports.

Royal Australian & New Zealand College of Psychiatrists (RANZCP). (2016). *The Economic Cost of Serious Mental Illness and Comorbidities in Australia and New Zealand*. Retrieved from www.ranzcp.org/files/resources/reports/ranzcp-serious-mental-illness.aspx.

Royal Australian & New Zealand College of Psychiatrists (RANZCP). (2017). *Powers and Duties of Psychiatrists in Australian and New Zealand Mental Health Acts: A Literature Review*. Retrieved from www.ranzcp.org/files/resources/college_statements/mental-health-legislation-tables/powers-and-duties-of-psychiatrists-in-australian-a.aspx.

Royal Australian & New Zealand College of Psychiatrists (RANZCP). (2017). *The Provision of Mental Health Services for Asylum Seekers and Refugees*. Retrieved from www.ranzcp.org/news-policy/policy-and-advocacy/position-statements/the-provision-of-mental-health-services-for-asylum.

Royal Australian & New Zealand College of Psychiatrists (RANZCP). (2018). *Code of Ethics*. Retrieved from www.ranzcp.org/files/about_us/code-of-ethics.aspx.

Royal Australian & New Zealand College of Psychiatrists (RANZCP). (2019). Dance of Life. *Your Health in Mind.* Retrieved from www.ranzcp.org/practice-education/indigenous-mental-health/aboriginal-torres-strait-islander-mental-health/the-dance-of-life.

Royal Australian College of General Practitioners (RACGP). (2019). *National Guide to a Preventive Health Assessment for Aboriginal and Torres Strait Islander People.* Retrieved from www.racgp.org.au/clinical-resources/clinical-guidelines/key-racgp-guidelines/view-all-racgp-guidelines/national-guide/chapter-4-the-health-of-young-people/social-emotional-wellbeing.

Royal College of Psychiatrists. (2001). *Diagnostic Criteria for Psychiatric Disorders for Use with Adults with Learning Disabilities/Mental Retardation*. London: Royal College of Psychiatrists,.

Roy-Byrne, P. P., Davidson, K. W., Kessler, R. C., Asmundson, G. J., Goodwin, R. D., Kubzansky, L., . . . Laden, S. K. (2008). Anxiety disorders and comorbid medical illness. *General Hospital Psychiatry, 30*(3), 208–225.

Ruscio, A. M., Stein, D. J., Chiu, W. T., & Kessler, R. C. (2010). The epidemiology of obsessive-compulsive disorder in the National Comorbidity Survey Replication. *Mol Psychiatry, 15*(1), 53–63.

Rush, A. J., First, M. B., & Blacker, D. (eds.). (2008). *Handbook of Psychiatric Measures* (2nd ed.). Washington: American Psychiatric Publishing.

Russell, D. (1995). *Women, Madness and Medicine.* Cambridge: Polity Press.

Russell, G. (1979). Bulimia nervosa: An ominous variant of anorexia nervosa. *Psychol Med, 9*(3), 429–448.

Russell, G. F. M. (1970). Anorexia nervosa: Its identity as an illness and its treatment. In J. H. Price (ed.), *Modern Trends in Psychological Medicine* (vol. 2). California: Appleton-Century-Crofts.

Russo, J., & Sweeney, A. (2016). *Searching for a Rose Garden: Challenging Psychiatry, Fostering Mad Studies*. PCCS Books.

Rutter, M. K.-C., Julia; Maughan, Barbara. (2006). Continuities and discontinuities in psychopathology between childhood and adult life. *Journal of Child Psychology and Psychiatry, 47*(3-4), 276–295.

Ruusuvuori, J. (2001). Looking means listening: Coordinating displays of engagement in doctor-patient interaction. *Social Science & Medicine, 52*(7), 1093–1108.

Ryan, C., Nielssen, O., Paton, M., & Large, M. (2010). Clinical decisions in psychiatry should not be based on risk assessment. *Australasian Psychiatry, 18*(5), 398–403.

Ryan, C. J. (2019). Community treatment orders are (somewhat) effective: Their future in the context of rights-based mental health law. *Australian & New Zealand Journal of Psychiatry, 53*(1), 11–12.

Ryan, P., & Morgan, S. (2004). Risk taking. In *Assertive Outreach: A Strengths Approach to Policy and Practice*. Edinburgh: Churchill Livingstone, pp. 223–246.

Ryan, R., & Sunada, K. (1997). Medical evaluation of persons with mental retardation referred for psychiatric assessment. *General Hospital Psychiatry, 19*(4), 274–280.

Saakvitne, K. W., Gamble, S., Pearlman, L. A., & Lev, B. T. (2000). *Risking Connection: A Training Curriculum for Working with Survivors of Childhood Abuse.* Retrieved from https://psycnet.apa.org/record/2000-08464-000.

Sadock, B. J., Sadock, V. A., & Ruiz, P. (2014). *Kaplan and Sadock's Synopsis of Psychiatry: Behavioral Sciences/Clinical Psychiatry*. Wolters Kluwer Health.

Sadock, B. J., Sadock, V. A., & Ruiz, P. (2017). *Kaplan and Sadock's Comprehensive Textbook of Psychiatry* (10th ed.). Wolters Kluwer Health.

Sadock, B. J., Sadock, V. A., Ruiz, P., & Kaplan, H. I. (2009). *Kaplan & Sadock's Comprehensive Textbook of Psychiatry* (9th ed.). Wolters Kluwer Health/Lippincott Williams & Wilkins.

Sælør, K. T., Ness, O., & Semb, R. (2015). Taking the plunge: Service users' experiences of hope within the mental health and substance use services. *Scandinavian Psychologist, 2*(9), 1–19.

Salbach, N. M., Jaglal, S. B., Korner-Bitensky, N., Rappolt, S., & Davis, D. (2007). Practitioner and organizational barriers to evidence-based practice of physical therapists for people with stroke. *Phys Ther, 87*(10), 1284–1303.

Salkovskis, P. M. (1985). Obsessional-compulsive problems: A cognitive-behavioural analysis. *Behav Res Ther, 23*(5), 571–583.

Salkovskis, P. M., Rimes, K. A., Warwick, H. M., & Clark, D. M. (2002). The Health Anxiety Inventory: Development and validation of scales for the measurement of health anxiety and hypochondriasis. *Psychol Med, 32*(5), 843–853.

Salmon, G., & Rapport, F. (2005). Multi-agency voices: A thematic analysis of multi-agency working practices within the setting of a child and adolescent mental health service. *Journal of Interprofessional Care, 19*(5), 429–443.

Salomon, C., & Hamilton, B. (2013). 'All roads lead to medication?': Qualitative responses from an Australian first-person survey of antipsychotic discontinuation. *Psychiatr Rehabil J*, 36(3), 160–165.

Salomon, C., Hamilton, B., & Elsom, S. (2014). Experiencing antipsychotic discontinuation: Results from a survey of Australian consumers. *Journal of Psychiatric and Mental Health Nursing*, 21.

Saltman, D. (1991). *Women and Health: An Introduction to Issues.* Marrickville: Harcourt Brace Jovanovich.

Salyers, M., Fukui, S., Rollins, A., Firmin, R., Gearhart, T., Noll, J., . . . Davis, C. (2015). Burnout and self-reported quality of care in community mental health. *Administration and Policy in Mental Health and Mental Health Services Research, 42*(1), 61–69.

San, L., Pomarol, G., Peri, J., Olle, J., & Cami, J. (1991). Follow-up after a six-month maintenance period on naltrexone versus placebo in heroin addicts. *British Journal of Addiction, 86*(8), 983–990.

Sanders, A., & Szymanski, K. (2013). Having a mentally ill sibling: Implications for attachment with parental figures. *Social Work in Mental Health, 11*(6), 516–529.

Sanders, A., Szymanski, K., & Fiori, K. (2014). The family roles of siblings of people diagnosed with a mental disorder: Heroes and lost children. *International Journal of Psychology, 49*(4), 257–262.

Sanders, M. R., Ralph, A., Sofronoff, K., Gardiner, P., Thompson, R., Dwyer, S., & Bidwell, K. (2008). Every family: A population approach to reducing behavioral and emotional problems in children making the transition to school. *J Prim Prev, 29*(3), 197–222.

Sanderson, C., Swenson, C., & Bohus, M. (2002). A critique of the American psychiatric practice guideline for the treatment of patients with borderline personality disorder. *Journal of Personality Disorders, 16*(2), 122–129.

Sansone, R. A., & Sansone, L. A. (2012). Chronic pain syndromes and borderline personality. *Innovations in Clinical Neuroscience, 9*(1), 10.

Santorelli, S. F., Meleo-Meyer, F., Koerbel, L., & Kabat-Zinn, J. (2017). *Mindfulness-Based Stress Reduction (MBSR) Authorized Curriculum Guide*. Retrieved from www.umassmed.edu.

Saquib, N., Saquib, J., Wahid, A., Ahmed, A. A., Dhuhayr, H. E., Zaghloul, M. S., . . . Al-Mazrou, A. (2017). Video game addiction and psychological distress among expatriate adolescents in Saudi Arabia. *Addictive Behaviors Reports, 6*, 112–117.

Şar, V. (2011). Epidemiology of dissociative disorders: An overview. *Epidemiology Research International, 2011*, 8.

Şar, V., Akyüz, G., & Doğan, O. (2007). Prevalence of dissociative disorders among women in the general population. *Psychiatry Research, 149*(1), 169–176.

Saraf, S. (2015). Advance statements in the new Victorian Mental Health Act. *Australasian Psychiatry, 23*(3), 230–232.

Sareen, B. J., Stein, J. M., Cox, T. B., & Hassard, T. S. (2004). Understanding comorbidity of anxiety disorders with antisocial behavior: Findings From two large community surveys. *Journal of Nervous and Mental Disease, 192*(3), 178–186.

Sargant, W., & Slater, E. (1941). Amnesic Syndromes in War. *Journal of the Royal Society of Medicine, 34*(12), 757–764.

Sarkar, J., & Duggan, C. (2010). Diagnosis and classification of personality disorder: Difficulties, their resolution and implications for practice. *Advances in Psychiatric Treatment, 16*(5), 388–396.

Sasson, R., Grinspoon, A., Lachman, M., & Ponizovsky, A. (2005). A program of supported education for adult Israeli students with schizophrenia. *Psychiatric Rehabilitation Journal, 29*, 139–141.

Saunders, J. B., Aasland, O. G., Babor, T. F., De la Fuente, J. R., & Grant, M. (1993). Development of the alcohol use disorders identification test (AUDIT): WHO collaborative project on early detection of persons with harmful alcohol consumption-II. *Addiction, 88*(6), 791–804.

Saunders, J. B., Hao, W., Long, J., King, D. L., Mann, K., Fauth-Buhler, M., . . . Poznyak, V. (2017). Gaming disorder: Its delineation as an important condition for diagnosis, management, and prevention. *Journal of Behavioral Addictions, 6*(3), 271–279.

Sauter, F. M., Heyne, D., & Westenberg, P. M. (2009). Cognitive behavior therapy for anxious adolescents: Developmental influences on treatment design and delivery. *Clinical Child and Family Psychology Review, 12*, 310–335.

Sawyer, A.-M. (2008). Risk and new exclusions in community mental health practice. *Australian Social Work, 61*(4), 327–341.

Sawyer, A.-M., & Green, D. (2013). Social inclusion and individualised service provision in high risk community care: Balancing regulation, judgment and discretion. *Social Policy and Society, 12*(2), 299–308.

Sawyer, M. G., Arney, F. M., Baghurst, P. A., Clark, J. J., Graetz, B. W., Kosky, R. J., . . . Zubrick, S. R. (2001). The mental health of young people in Australia: Key findings from the child and adolescent component of the national survey of mental health and well-being. *Australian and New Zealand Journal of Psychiatry, 35*(6), 806–814.

Sawyer, M. G., Reece, C. E., Sawyer, A. C. P., Hiscock, H., & Lawrence, D. (2019). Adequacy of treatment for child and adolescent mental disorders in Australia: A national study. *Australian & New Zealand Journal of Psychiatry, 53*(4), 326–335.

Sawyer, M. G., Reece, C. E., Sawyer, A. C. P., Johnson, S. E., & Lawrence, D. (2018). Has the prevalence of child and adolescent mental disorders in australia changed between 1998 and 2013 to 2014? *Journal of the American Academy of Child & Adolescent Psychiatry, 57*(5), 343–350.

Sawyer, S. M., Azzopardi, P. S., Wickremarathne, D., & Patton, G. C. (2018). The age of adolescence. *Lancet Child & Adolescent Health, 2*(3), 223–228.

Sayfan, L., & Lagattuta, K. H. (2009). Scaring the monster away: What children now about managing fears of real and imagined creatures. *Child Development, 80*(6), 1756–1774.

Scanlan, J. N., & Novak, T. (2015). Sensory approaches in mental health: A scoping review. *Australian Occupational Therapy Journal, 62*(5), 277–285.

Schady, N. (2011). Parents' education, mothers' vocabulary, and cognitive development in early childhood: Longitudinal evidence from Ecuador. *American Journal of Public Health, 101*(12), 2299–2307.

Schatzberg, A. F., & Nemeroff, C. B. (2017). *The American Psychiatric Association Publishing Textbook of Psychopharmacology*. American Psychiatric Publishing.

Schimmelmann, B. G., Conus, P., Schacht, M., McGorry, P., & Lambert, M. (2006). Predictors of service disengagement in first-admitted adolescents with psychosis. *Journal of the American Academy of Child & Adolescent Psychiatry, 45*(8), 990–999.

Schley, C., Pace, N., Mann, R., McKenzie, C., McRoberts, A., & Parker, A. (2019). The headspace Brief Interventions Clinic: Increasing timely access to effective treatments for young people with early signs of mental health problems. *Early Intervention in Psychiatry, 13*(5), 1073–1082.

Schmaling, K. B., & Fales, J. L. (2018). The association between borderline personality disorder and somatoform disorders: A systematic review and meta-analysis. *Clinical Psychology: Science and Practice, 25*(2), e12244.

Schmitz, N., Lesage, A., & Wang, J. (2009). should psychological distress screening in the community account for self-perceived health status? *Canadian Journal of Psychiatry, 54*(8), 526–533.

Schneider, D., & Lilienfeld, D. E. (2015). *Lilienfeld's Foundations of Epidemiology*. Oxford University Press.

Schneider, S. C., Baillie, A. J., Mond, J., Turner, C. M., & Hudson, J. L. (2018). The classification of body dysmorphic disorder symptoms in male and female adolescents. *J Affect Disord, 225*, 429–437.

Schofield, G., & Beek, M. (2014). *The Secure Base Model: Promoting Attachment and Resilience in Foster Care and Adoption*. British Association for Adoption and Fostering (BAAF).

Scholz, B., Bocking, J., & Happell, B. (2018). Improving exchange with consumers within mental health organisations: Recognising mental ill health experiences as a 'sneaky, special degree'. *International Journal of Mental Health Nursing, 27*(1), 227–235.

Schore, A. N. (2001). The effects of early relational trauma on right brain development, affect regulation, and infant mental health. *Infant Mental Health Journal, 22*(1-2), 201–269.

Schulte-Herbrüggen, O., Ahlers, C. J., Kronsbein, J. M., Rüter, A., Bahri, S., Vater, A., & Roepke, S. Impaired sexual function in patients with borderline personality disorder is determined by history of sexual abuse. *Journal of Sexual Medicine, 6*(12), 3356–3363.

Schwartz, A., & Elstein, A. S. (2008). Clinical reasoning in medicine. In J. Higgs (ed.), *Clinical Reasoning in the Health Professions* (3rd ed.). Elsevier Butterworth-Heinemann.

Schwartz, C., & Gidron, R. (2002). Parents of mentally ill adult children living at home rewards of caregiving. *Health & Social Work, 27*(2), 145–154.

Schweitzer, R. D., Brough, M., Vromans, L., & Asic-Kobe, M. (2011). Mental health of newly arrived Burmese refugees in Australia: Contributions of pre-migration and post-migration experience. *Australian and New Zealand Journal of Psychiatry, 45*(4), 299–307.

Schweizer, R., Honey, A., Hancock, N., Berry, B., Waks, S., & Scanlan, J. N. (2018). Consumer-provider relationships in a care coordination model of service: Consumer perspectives. *Advances in Mental Health, 16*(1), 88–100.

Scott, A. I. F., & Freeman, C. P. L. (1992). Edinburgh Primary Care Depression Study—Treatment outcome, patient satisfaction, and cost after 16 Weeks. *British Medical Journal, 304*(6831), 883–887.

Scott, D. (1993). Inter-agency collaboration: Why is it so difficult? Can we do it better? *Children Australia, 18*(4), 4–9.

Scott, D. (2009). 'Think Child, Think Family': How Adult Specialist Services Can Support Children at Risk of Abuse and Neglect. *Family Matters* (81), 37.

Scott, I., & Jayathissa, S. (2010). Quality of drug prescribing in older patients: Is there a problem and can we improve it? *Internal Medicine Journal, 40*(1), 7–18.

SCRGSP (Steering Committee for the Review of Government Service Provision). (2016). *Overcoming Indigenous Disadvantage Key Indicators*. Retrieved from www.pc.gov.au/research/ongoing/overcoming-indigenous-disadvantage/2016/report-documents/oid-2016-overcoming-indigenous-disadvantage-key-indicators-2016-report.pdf.

Scriven, M. (1991). *Evaluation Thesaurus* (4th ed.). Newbury Park: SAGE Publications.

Scull, A. (1989). *Social Order/Mental Disorder*. Cambridge: Cambridge University Press.

Scull, A. (2017). The asylum, hospital and clinic. In G. Eghigian (ed.), *The Routledge History of Madness and Mental Health*. Taylor & Francis.

Seedhouse, D. (2009a). *Ethics: The Heart of Health Care* (3rd ed.). Wiley-Blackwell.

Seedhouse, D. (2009b). Growing pains. In *Ethics: The Heart of Health Care* (3rd ed., pp. 1–15). Wiley-Blackwell.

Segal, S. P., Hayes, S. L., & Rimes, L. (2017a). The utility of outpatient commitment: I. A need for treatment and a least restrictive alternative to psychiatric hospitalization. *Psychiatric Services, 68*(12), 1247–1254.

Segal, S. P., Hayes, S. L., & Rimes, L. (2017b). The utility of outpatient commitment: II. Mortality risk and protecting health, safety, and quality of life. *Psychiatric Services, 68*(12), 1255–1261.

Segal, Z. V., Williams, J. M. G., & Teasdale, J. (2002). *Mindfulness-based Cognitive Therapy for Depression: A New Approach to Preventing Relapse*. New York: Guilford.

Segal, Z. V., Williams, J. M. G., & Teasdale, J. D. (2013). *Mindfulness-based Cognitive Therapy for Depression* (2nd revised ed.). New York: Guilford Publications.

Segal, Z. V., Williams, M., Teasdale, J., Crane, R. S., Dimidjian, S., Ma, S. H., . . . Kuyken, W. (2016). Mindfulness-based Cognitive Therapy: Training Pathway. Version 1.0. Retrieved from http://oxfordmindfulness.org/wp-content/Seikkula, J., Aaltonen, J., Alakare, B., Haarakangas, K., Keränen, J., & Lehtinen, K. (2006). Five-year experience of first-episode nonaffective psychosis in open-dialogue approach: Treatment principles, follow-up outcomes, and two case studies. *Psychotherapy Research, 16*(02), 214–228.

Seikkula, J., Alakare, B., & Aaltonen, J. (2011). The comprehensive Open-Dialogue approach in Western Lapland: II. Long-term stability of acute psychosis outcomes in advanced community care. *Psychosis-Psychological Social and Integrative Approaches, 3*(3), 192–204.

Seikkula, J., & Olson, M. E. (2003). The open dialogue approach to acute psychosis: Its poetics and micropolitics. *Family Process, 42*(3), 403–418.

Selener, D. (1997). *Participatory Action Research and Social Change*. Cornell Participatory Action Research Network.

Self Help Addiction Resource Centre (SHARC). (2019). *Family Drug Help, APSU and Recovery Support Service*. Retrieved from www.sharc.org.au.

Senge, P. M. (1990). *The Fifth Discipline: The Art and Practice of the Learning Organization*. Doubleday/Currency.

Seok, S., & DaCosta, B. (2012). The world's most intense online gaming culture: Addiction and high-engagement prevalence rates among South Korean adolescents and young adults. *Computers in Human Behavior, 28*(6), 2143–2151.

Shaffer, H. J., Hall, M. N., & Vander Bilt, J. (2000). 'Computer addiction': A critical consideration. (statistical data included). *American Journal of Orthopsychiatry, 70*(2), 162.

Shalin, D. N. (2014). Goffman on mental illness: Asylums and 'The insanity of place' revisited. *Symbolic Interaction, 37*(1), 122–144.

Shanafelt, T., Ripp, J., & Trockel, M. (2020). Understanding and addressing sources of anxiety among health care professionals during the COVID-19 pandemic. *JAMA*. doi:10.1001/jama.2020.5893, online ahead of print.

Shankar, J., & Muthuswamy, S. S. (2007). Support needs of family caregivers of people who experience mental illness and the role of mental health services. *Families in Society: Journal of Contemporary Social Services, 88*(2), 302–310.

Shapiro, D. A., Rees, A., Barkham, M., Hardy, G., Reynolds, S., & Startup, M. (1995). Effects of treatment duration and severity of depression on the maintenance of gains after cognitive-behavioral and psychodynamic-interpersonal psychotherapy. *J Consult Clin Psychol, 63*(3), 378–387.

Shapiro, F. (2007). EMDR, adaptive information processing, and case conceptualization. *Journal of EMDR Practice and Research, 1*(2), 68–87.

Sharpe, L. (2002). A reformulated cognitive-behavioral model of problem gambling—A biopsychosocial perspective. *Clinical Psychology Review, 22*(1), 1–25.

Sharpe, M. C., Hawton, K., Simkin, S., Surawy, C., Hackmann, A., Klimes, I., . . . Seagroatt, V. (1996). Cognitive behaviour therapy for the chronic fatigue syndrome: A randomized controlled trial. *British Medical Journal, 312*(7022), 22–26.

Sharpe, M. C., & O'Malley, P. G. (2018). Chronic fatigue and fibromyalgia syndromes. In J. L. Levenson (ed.), *The American*

Psychiatric Association Publishing Textbook of Psychosomatic Medicine and Consultation-Liaison Psychiatry (3rd ed., pp. 709-736). USA: American Psychiatric Association.

Shaw, I., & Faulkner, A. (2006). Practitioner evaluation at work. *American Journal of Evaluation, 27*(1), 44-63.

Shawyer, F., Enticott, J. C., Block, A. A., Cheng, I. H., & Meadows, G. N. (2017). The mental health status of refugees and asylum seekers attending a refugee health clinic including comparisons with a matched sample of Australian-born residents. *BMC Psychiatry, 17*(1), 76.

Shawyer, F., Enticott, J. C., Brophy, L., Bruxner, A., Fossey, E., Inder, B., . . . Meadows, G. N. (2017). The PULSAR Specialist Care protocol: A stepped-wedge cluster randomized control trial of a training intervention for community mental health teams in recovery-oriented practice. *BMC Psychiatry, 17*(1), 172.

Shawyer, F., Enticott, J. C., Ozmen, M., Inder, B., & Meadows, G. N. (2016). Mindfulness-based cognitive therapy for recurrent major depression: A 'best buy' for health care? *Australian and New Zealand Journal of Psychiatry, 50*, 1001-1013.

Shear, M. K., Brown, T. A., Barlow, D. H., Money, R., Sholomskas, D. E., Woods, S. W., . . . Papp, L. A. (1997). Multicenter collaborative panic disorder severity scale. *American Journal of Psychiatry, 154*(11), 1571-1575.

Shearer, S. L. (1994). Phenomenology of self-injury among inpatient women with borderline personality disorder. *Journal of Nervous and Mental Disease, 182*(9), 524-526.

Shedler, J. (2010). The efficacy of psychodynamic psychotherapy. *American Psychologist, 65*(2), 98-109.

Sheehan, D. V., Lecrubier, Y., Sheehan, K. H., Amorim, P., Janavs, J., Weiller, E., . . . Dunbar, G. C. (1998). The Mini-International Neuropsychiatric Interview (M.I.N.I.): The development and validation of a structured diagnostic psychiatric interview for DSM-IV and ICD-10. *J Clin Psychiatry, 59 Suppl 20*, 22-33;quiz 34-57.

Sheehan, H. L., & Summers, V. K. (1949). The syndrome of hypopituitarism. *Q J Med, 18*(72), 319-378.

Sheline, Y. I., Price, J. L., Yan, Z. Z., & Mintun, M. A. (2010). Resting-state functional MRI in depression unmasks increased connectivity between networks via the dorsal nexus. *Proceedings of the National Academy of Sciences of the United States of America, 107*(24), 11020-11025.

Shepherd, C. C. J., Li, J., Cooper, M. N., Hopkins, K. D., & Farrant, B. M. (2017). The impact of racial discrimination on the health of Australian Indigenous children aged 5-10 years: Analysis of national longitudinal data. *Int J Equity Health, 16*(1), 116.

Shiue, I. (2014). Prevalence and psychiatric correlates of neighbourhood satisfaction and its impact on adolescent behaviours: UK understanding society cohort, 2011-2012. *Environ Res, 134*, 390-395.

Shor, R. (2017). Difficulties experienced by university students with severe mental illness who participate in supported education programs. *Community Mental Health Journal, 53*(3), 281-287.

Shorter, K. R., & Miller, B. H. (2015). Epigenetic mechanisms in schizophrenia. *Progress in Biophysics and Molecular Biology, 118*(1), 1-7.

Shufman, E. N., Porat, S., Witztum, E., Gandacu, D., Bar-Hamburger, R., & Ginath, Y. (1994). The efficacy of naltrexone in preventing reabuse of heroin after detoxification. *Biological Psychiatry, 35*(12), 935-945.

Sibley, M. H., Rohde, L. A., Swanson, J. M., Hechtman, L. T., Molina, B. S. G., Mitchell, J. T., . . . Stehli, A. (2018). Late-onset ADHD reconsidered with comprehensive repeated assessments between ages 10 and 25. *American Journal of Psychiatry, 175*(2), 140-149.

Siebert, B. (2017). *Mental Health ED Wait Times Lowest in a Decade: SA Health*. Retrieved from https://indaily.com.au/news/local/2017/03/24/mental-health-ed-wait-times-lowest-in-a-decade-sa-health.

Siegenthaler, E., Munder, T., & Egger, M. (2012). Effect of preventive interventions in mentally ill parents on the mental health of the offspring: Systematic review and meta-analysis. *J Am Acad Child Adolesc Psychiatry, 51*(1), 8-17.

Silburn, K. (2015). *Recommissioning Community Mental Health Support Services and Alcohol and Other Drugs Treatment Services in Victoria: Report on Findings From Interviews with Senior Personnel From Both Sectors*. Bundoora, Australian Institute for Primary Care and Ageing.

Silverman, J., & Kinnersley, P. (2010). Doctors' non-verbal behaviour in consultations: Look at the patient before you look at the computer. *British Journal of General Practice, 60*(571), 76-78.

Simeon, D. (2004). Depersonalisation disorder–A contemporary overview. *CNS Drugs, 18*(6), 343-354.

Simeon, D., & Knutelska, M. (2005). An open trial of naltrexone in the treatment of depersonalization disorder. *Journal of Clinical Psychopharmacology, 25*(3), 267-270.

Simmons, M., Rice, S., Hetrick, S., Bailey, A., & Parker, A. (2012). *Evidence Summary: Shared Decision Making (SDM) for Mental Health—What is the Evidence?* Melbourne: Orygen.

Simmons, M. B., Batchelor, S., Dimopoulos-Bick, T., & Howe, D. (2017). The Choice Project: Peer workers promoting shared decision making at a youth mental health service. *Psychiatric Services, 68*(8), 764-770.

Simone Reinders, A. A. T., Willemsen, A. T. M., Vos, H. P. J., den Boer, J. A., & Nijenhuis, E. R. S. (2012). Fact or factitious? A psychobiological study of authentic and simulated dissociative identity states (Dissociative identity disorder: Fact or factitious?). *PLoS One, 7*(6), e39279.

Simonoff, E., Elander, J., Holmshaw, J., Pickles, A., Murray, R., & Rutter, M. (2004). Predictors of antisocial personality—Continuities from childhood to adult life. *British Journal of Psychiatry, 184*, 118-127.

Simpson, A., Miller, C., & Bowers, L. (2003). Case management models and the care programme approach: How to make the CPA effective and credible. *Journal of Psychiatric and Mental Health Nursing, 10*(4), 472-483.

Simpson, D. M., Inka, W., & E., S. S. (2011). Extreme weather-related events: Implications for mental health and well-being. In I. Weissbecker (ed.), *Climate Change and Human Well-Being: Global Challenges and Opportunities* (pp. 57-78). New York: Springer.

Sindahl, T. et al. (2019) Texting for help: Processes and impact of text counseling with children and youth with suicide ideation. *Suicide and Life Threatening Behavior*, vol. 49 (5).

Singer, P., Robertson, G., & Roy, D. (1996). Bioethics for clinicians, 6: Advance care planning. *Canadian Medical Association. Journal, 155*(12), 1689-1692.

Singh, D., McMain, S., & Zucker, K. J. (2011). Gender identity and sexual orientation in women with borderline personality disorder. *Journal of Sexual Medicine, 8*(2), 447-454.

Singh, S. P., Paul, M., Ford, T., Kramer, T., Weaver, T., McLaren, S., . . . White, S. (2010). Process, outcome and experience of transition from child to adult mental healthcare: Multiperspective study. *British Journal of Psychiatry, 197*(4), 305-312.

Slade, M. (2009a). *Personal Recovery and Mental Illness: A Guide for Mental Health Professionals*. Cambridge University Press.

Slade, M. (2009b). *100 Ways to Support Recovery: A Guide for Mental Health Professionals*. London: Rethink.

Slade, M., Amering, M., Farkas, M., Hamilton, B., O'Hagan, M., Panther, G., . . . Whitley, R. (2014). Uses and abuses of recovery: Implementing recovery-oriented practices in mental health systems. *World Psychiatry, 13*(1), 12-20.

Slade, M., Amering, M., & Oades, L. (2008). Recovery: An international perspective. *Epidemiologia E Psichiatria Sociale, 17*(2), 128-137.

Slade, M., Bird, V., Clarke, E., Le Boutillier, C., McCrone, P., Macpherson, R., . . . Leamy, M. (2015). Supporting recovery in patients with psychosis through care by community-based adult mental health teams (REFOCUS): A multisite, cluster, randomised, controlled trial. *Lancet Psychiatry, 2*(6), 503-514.

Slade, M., Bird, V., Le Boutillier, C., Farkas, M., Grey, B., Larsen, J., . . . Williams, J. (2015). Development of the REFOCUS intervention to increase mental health team support for personal recovery. *Br J Psychiatry, 207*(6), 544.

Slade, M., Bird, V., Le Boutillier, C., Williams, J., & Leamy, M. et al (2016). *REFOCUS PULSAR Project Team PULSAR Manual: Recovery-promoting relationships and working practices for specialist and community mental health services (or secondary care staff)*. (2nd ed., pp. 48). Melbourne: Monash University.

Slade, M., Leese, M., Cahill, S., Thornicroft, G., & Kuipers, E. (2005). Patient-rated mental health needs and quality of life improvement. *British Journal of Psychiatry, 187*, 256-261.

Slade, M., Oades, L., & Jarden, A. (2017). *Wellbeing, Recovery and Mental Health*. Cambridge University Press.

Slade, T., Grove, R., & Burgess, P. (2011). Kessler psychological distress scale: normative data from the 2007 Australian National Survey of Mental Health and Wellbeing. *Australian & New Zealand Journal of Psychiatry*, 45(4), 308-316.

Slade, T., Chapman, C., Swift, W., Keyes, K., Tonks, Z., & Teesson, M. (2016). Birth cohort trends in the global epidemiology of alcohol use and alcohol-related harms in men and women: Systematic review and metaregression. *BMJ Open, 6*(10), e011827.

Slade, T., Grove, R., & Burgess, P. (2011). Kessler Psychological Distress Scale: Normative data from the 2007 Australian National Survey of Mental Health and Wellbeing. *Australian & New Zealand Journal of Psychiatry, 45*(4), 308-316.

Slade, T., Johnston, A., Oakley Browne, M. A., Andrews, G., & Whiteford, H. (2009). 2007 National Survey of Mental Health and Wellbeing: Methods and key findings. *Australian and New Zealand Journal of Psychiatry, 43*(7), 594-605.

Slade, T., Johnston, A., Teeson, M., Whiteford, H., Burgess, P., Pirkis, J., & Saw, S. (2009). *The Mental Health of Australians 2. Report on the 2007 National Survey of Mental Health and Wellbeing*. Retrieved from www.health.gov.au/internet/main/publishing.nsf/content/46AB7A3FEF9664E4CA2575D2000A6D09/$File/mhaust2.pdf.

Slay, J. & Stephens, L. (2013). *Co-production in mental health: A literature review*. London: New Economics Foundation.

Smail, D. (1994). Community psychology and politics. *Journal of Community & Applied Social Psychology, 4*(1), 3-10.

Smiley, E. (2005). Epidemiology of mental health problems in adults with learning disability: An update. *Advances in Psychiatric Treatment, 11*, 214-222.

Smiley, E., & Cooper, S.-A. (2003). Intellectual disabilities, depressive episode, diagnostic criteria and Diagnostic Criteria for Psychiatric Disorders for Use with Adults with Learning Disabilities/Mental Retardation (DC-LD) papers. *Journal of Intellectual Disability Research, 47*(s1), 62-71.

Smith, C., Stewart, S. H., O'Connor, R. M., Collins, P., & Katz, J. (2011). Development and psychometric evaluation of a 10-item short form inventory of gambling situations. *Journal of Gambling Studies, 27*(1), 115-128.

Smith, G. (2012). Mental Health Services in the Australian States and Territories, Western Australia. In G. Meadows, B. Singh, & M. Grigg (eds.), *Mental Health in Australia: Collaborative Community Practice* (3rd ed., pp. 118-154). Melbourne: Oxford University Press.

Smith, L. M., Onwumere, J., Craig, T., & Kuipers, E. (2019). Role of poor sleep in determining distress in caregivers of individuals with early psychosis. Early Intervention in Psychiatry, 13(3), 613-618.Smith, L. T. (1999). *Decolonizing Methodologies: Research and Indigenous People*. London and New York: Zed Books.

Smith, R., & Rennie, D. (2014). Evidence-based medicine—An oral history. *Jama, 311*(4), 365-367.

Smith-Merry, J., Hancock, N., Gilroy, J., Llewellyn, G., Yen, I., & Bresnan, A. (2018). *Mind the Gap: The National Disability Insurance Scheme and Psychosocial Disability: Final Report: Stakeholder Identified Gaps and Solutions*. Retrieved from www.qfcc.qld.gov.au/mind-gap-national-disability-insurance-scheme-and-psychosocial-disability-final-report-stakeholder.

Smucny, J., Olincy, A., Eichman, L. C., Lyons, E., & Tregellas, J. R. (2013). Early sensory processing deficits predict sensitivity to distraction in schizophrenia. *Schizophrenia Research, 147*(1), 196-200.

Smullen, A. (2016). Not centralisation but decentralised integration through Australia's National Mental Health Policy. *Australian Journal of Public Administration, 75*(3), 280-290.

Sobell, M. B., & Sobell, L. C. (1995). Controlled drinking after 25 years. *Addiction, 90*, 1149-1153.

Sobral, D., & Figueiredo-Braga, M. (2016). Family Physician Communication, Quality Of Care And The Use Of Computer In The Consultation—The patient's perspective. *Procedia Computer Science, 100*, 594-601.

Social Ventures Australia. (2020). *Resolve SBB*. Retrieved from www.socialventures.com.au/work/resolve-sbb.

Solantaus, T., Paavonen, E. J., Toikka, S., & Punamäki, R. (2010). Preventive interventions in families with parental depression: Children's psychosocial symptoms and prosocial behaviour. *European Child & Adolescent Psychiatry, 19*(12), 883-892.

Solomi, V. L., & Casiday, R. E. (2017). In sickness and in health: The strains and gains of caring for a chronically ill or disabled spouse. *Chronic Illness, 13*(2), 75-87.

Song, F., Eastwood, A. J., Gilbody, S., Duley, L., & Sutton, A. J. (2000). Publication and related biases. *Health Technol Assess, 4*(10), 1-115.

Soomro, G. M., Altman, D., Rajagopal, S., & Oakley-Browne, M. (2008). Selective serotonin re-uptake inhibitors (SSRIs) versus placebo for obsessive compulsive disorder (OCD). *Cochrane Database of Systematic Reviews* (1), Cd001765.

Sorrell, J. M. (2016). Community-based older adults with mental illness: We can do better. *Journal of Psychosocial Nursing and Mental Health Services, 54*(11), 25-29.

Sosso, F. A. E., Kuss, D. J., Vandelanotte, C., Jasso-Medrano, J. L., Husain, M. E., Curcio, G., . . . Toth, A. J. (2020). Insomnia, sleepiness, anxiety and depression among different types of gamers in African countries. *Scientific Reports, 10*(1), 1937.

South Australian Social Inclusion Board. (2007-2012). *Stepping Up: A Social Inclusion Action Plan for Mental Health Reform*. Retrieved from www.sahealth.sa.gov.au/wps/wcm/connect/8ea68b804308c5cfb076fa2cf7cfa853/steppingupmentalhlthreform0712-socinclusion-2010.

pdf?MOD=AJPERES&CACHEID=ROOTWORKSPACE-8ea68b804308c5cfb076fa2cf7cfa853-mHVT.Vg.

Souza, A. C., Alexandre, N. M. C., & Guirardello, E. B. (2017). Psychometric properties in instruments evaluation of reliability and validity. *Epidemiol Serv Saude, 26*(3), 649–659.

Sovner, R. (1986). Limiting factors in the use of DSM-III with mentally ill/mentally retarded persons. *Psychopharmocology Bulletin*, vol. 22, pp. 1055–1059.

Spaniol, L., & Nelson, A. (2015). Family recovery. *Community Mental Health Journal, 51*(7), 761–767.

Spaniol, L., Wewiorski, N. J., Gagne, C., & Anthony, W. A. (2002). The process of recovery from schizophrenia. *International Review of Psychiatry, 14*(4), 327–336.

Sparrow, S. S., & Cicchetti, D. V. (1985). Diagnostic uses of the Vineland Adaptive Behavior Scales. *Journal of Pediatric Psychology, 10*(2), 215–225.

Spencer, M., Dineen, R., & Phillips, A. (2013). *Co-Producing Services—Co-Creating Health*. Retrieved from www.1000livesplus.wales.nhs.uk/sitesplus/documents/1011/T4I%20%288%29%20Co-production.pdf.

Spicer, B., Smith, D. I., Conroy, E., Flatau, P. R., & Burns, L. (2015). Mental illness and housing outcomes among a sample of homeless men in an Australian urban centre. *Australian & New Zealand Journal of Psychiatry, 49*(5), 471–480.

Spillane, A., Matvienko-Sikar, K., Larkin, C., Corcoran, P., & Arensman, E. (2018). What are the physical and psychological health effects of suicide bereavement on family members? An observational and interview mixed-methods study in Ireland. *BMJ Open, 8*(1), e019472.

Spitzer, R. L., Kroenke, K., Williams, J. B., & Lowe, B. (2006). A brief measure for assessing generalized anxiety disorder: The GAD-7. *Archives of Internal Medicine, 166*(10), 1092–1097.

Sroufe, L. A., & Fleeson, F. (1986). *Attachment and Construction of Relationships*. New Jersey: Lawrence Erlbaum Associates.

St Luke's Innovative Resources. (2019). *Innovative Resources*. Retrieved from https://innovativeresources.org.

St Vincents Hospital. (2014). *Strengths Model: A Recovery-Oriented Approach to Mental Health Services Core Training Manual*. Melbourne, St Vincent's Hospital.

Stacey, D., Légaré, F., Lewis, K., Barry, M. J., Bennett, C. L., Eden, K. B., . . . Thomson, R. (2017). Decision aids for people facing health treatment or screening decisions. *Cochrane Database of Systematic Reviews* (4).

Stacey, G., Felton, A., Morgan, A., Stickley, T., Willis, M., Diamond, B., . . . Dumenya, J. (2016). A critical narrative analysis of shared decision-making in acute inpatient mental health care. *Journal of Interprofessional Care, 30*(1), 35–41.

Stacy, A. W., Newcomb, M. D., & Bentler, P. M. (1991). Cognitive motivation and drug use: A 9-year longitudinal study. *Journal of Abnormal Psychology, 100*(4), 502.

Stafford, A., & Wood, L. (2017). Tackling health disparities for people who are homeless? Start with social determinants. *International Journal of Environmental Research and Public Health, 14*(12), 1535.

Stallard, P. (2002). *A Clinicians Guide to Think Good, Feel Good: Using CBT with Children and Young People*. West Sussex: Wiley.

Stallard, P. (2002). *Think Good—Feel Good: A Cognitive Behaviour Therapy Workbook for Children and Young People*. West Sussex: John Wiley & Sons.

Stanbridge, R., & Burbach, F. (2007). Involving carers in staff training and service development in Somerset UK. In D. Froggatt (ed.), *Families as Partners in Mental Health Care: A Guidebook for Implementing Family Work*. Toronto: World Fellowship for Schizophrenia and Allied Disorders.

Stanford, S., Sharland, E., Heller, N. R., & Warner, J. (2017). *Beyond the Risk Paradigm in Mental Health Policy and Practice*. UK: Macmillan Education.

Stanghellini, G., Broome, M., Fernandez, A. V., Fusar-Poli, P., Raballo, A., & Rosfort, R. (2019). *The Oxford Handbook of Phenomenological Psychopathology*. Oxford: Oxford University Press.

Stanners, M. N., Barton, C. A., Shakib, S., & Winefield, H. R. (2012). A qualitative investigation of the impact of multimorbidity on GP diagnosis and treatment of depression in Australia. *Aging & Mental Health, 16*(8), 1058–1064.

Stansfeld, S., Smuk, M., Onwumere, J., Clark, C., Pike, C., McManus, S., . . . Bebbington, P. (2014). Stressors and common mental disorder in informal carers—An analysis of the English Adult Psychiatric Morbidity Survey 2007. *Social Science & Medicine, 120*, 190–198.

Stanton, R., Happell, B., & Reaburn, P. (2015). Investigating the exercise-prescription practices of nurses working in inpatient mental health settings. *International Journal of Mental Health Nursing, 24*(2), 112–120.

Stanton, R., Platania-Phung, C., Gaskin, C. J., & Happell, B. (2016). Screening for metabolic syndrome in mental health consumers using an electronic metabolic monitoring form. *Issues in Mental Health Nursing, 37*(4), 239–244.

Stapelberg, N. J. C., Neumann, D. L., Shum, D. H. K., McConnell, H., & Hamilton-Craig, I. (2011). A topographical map of the causal network of mechanisms underlying the relationship between major depressive disorder and coronary heart disease. *Australian and New Zealand Journal of Psychiatry, 45*(5), 351–369.

Stapinski, L. A., Edwards, A. C., Hickman, M., Araya, R., Teesson, M., Newton, N. C., . . . Heron, J. (2016). Drinking to cope: A latent class analysis of coping motives for alcohol use in a large cohort of adolescents. *Prevention Science, 17*(5), 584–594.

Starcevic, V., & Berle, D. (2015). Cyberchondria: An Old Phenomenon in a New Guise? In E. Aboujaoude & V. Starcevic (eds.), *Mental Health in the Digital Age: Grave Dangers, Great Promise*. Oxford: Oxford University Press.

State Government of Victoria (Department of Human Services). (2009). *After the Bushfires: Victoria's Psychosocial Recovery Framework*. Retrieved from www.health.vic.gov.au/mentalhealth.

State Government of Victoria (Department of Premier and Cabinet). (2017). *Free from Violence: Victoria's Strategy to Prevent Family Violence and All Forms of Violence Against Women*. Retrieved from https://iepcp.org.au/wp-content/uploads/2017/05/Free-from-violence-Victorias-prevention-strategy1.pdf.

State Government of Victoria. (2018–19). *Royal Commission into Victoria's Mental Health System, Interim Report, Parl Paper No. 87* Retrieved from https://rcvmhs.vic.gov.au/interim-report.

State Government of Victoria. (2019). *Royal Commission into Victoria's Mental Health System, Interim Report*. Retrieved from https://rcvmhs.vic.gov.au.

State Government of Victoria. (2019). *Royal Commission into Victoria's Mental Health System*. Retrieved from www2.health.vic.gov.au/mental-health/priorities-and-transformation/royal-commission.

Steel, C. (ed.) (2012). *CBT for Schizophrenia: Evidence-based Interventions and Future Directions*. Chicester: Wiley-Blackwell.

Steel, Z., Silove, D., Phan, T., & Bauman, A. (2002). Long-term effect of psychological trauma on the mental health of

Vietnamese refugees resettled in Australia: A population-based study. *Lancet, 360*(9339), 1056–1062.

Stefancic, A., Tsemberis, S., Messeri, P., Drake, R., & Goering, P. (2013). The Pathways Housing First Fidelity Scale for individuals with psychiatric disabilities. *American Journal of Psychiatric Rehabilitation, 16*(4), 240–261.

Stefano, S. C., Bacaltchuk, J., Blay, S. L., & Hay, P. (2006). Self-help treatments for disorders of recurrent binge eating: A systematic review. *Acta Psychiatr Scand, 113*(6), 452–459.

Steffen, W., Rockström, J., Richardson, K., Lenton, T. M., Folke, C., Liverman, D., . . . Schellnhuber, H. J. (2018). Trajectories of the Earth System in the Anthropocene. *Proceedings of the National Academy of Sciences, 115*(33), 8252.

Stein, L., & Test, M. (1980). Alternatives to mental hospital treatment: I. Conceptual model, treatment program and clinical evaluation. *Archives of General Psychiatry,* vol. 37, pp. 392–397.

Stein, M. B., Roy-Byrne, P. P., Craske, M. G., Bystritsky, A., Sullivan, G., Pyne, J. M., . . . Sherbourne, C. D. (2005). Functional impact and health utility of anxiety disorders in primary care outpatients. *Medical Care,* 1164–1170.

Stein, M. B., & Sareen, J. (2015). Generalized anxiety disorder. *New England Journal of Medicine, 373*(21), 2059–2068.

Steinert, C., Munder, T., Rabung, S., Hoyer, J., & Leichsenring, F. (2017). Psychodynamic therapy: As efficacious as other empirically supported treatments? A meta-analysis testing equivalence of outcomes. *American Journal of Psychiatry, 174*(10), 943–953.

Steinhausen, H. C. (2002). The outcome of anorexia nervosa in the 20th century. *American Journal of Psychiatry, 159*(8), 1284–1293.

Steinhausen, H. C., & Weber, S. (2009). The outcome of bulimia nervosa: Findings from one-quarter century of research. *American Journal of Psychiatry, 166*(12), 1331–1341.

Stephens, A., Bohanna, I., & Graham, D. (2017). Expert consensus to examine the cross-cultural utility of substance use and mental health assessment instruments for use with Indigenous clients. *Evaluation Journal of Australasia, 17*(3), 14–22.

Stephens, J. R., Farhall, J., Farnan, S., & Ratcliff, K. M. (2011). An evaluation of Well Ways, a family education programme for carers of people with a mental illness. *Aust N Z J Psychiatry, 45*(1), 45–53.

Stephenson, C. P., Karanges, E., & McGregor, I. S. (2012). Trends in the utilisation of psychotropic medications in Australia from 2000 to 2011. *Australian & New Zealand Journal of Psychiatry, 47*(1), 74–87.

Stevens, M. W. R., King, D. L., Dorstyn, D., & Delfabbro, P. H. (2019). Cognitive-behavioral therapy for internet gaming disorder: A systematic review and meta-analysis. *Clinical Psychology & Psychotherapy, 26*(2), 191–203.

Stevenson, J., Datyner, A., Boyce, P., & Brodaty, H. (2011). The effect of age on prevalence, type and diagnosis of personality disorder in psychiatric inpatients. *International Journal of Geriatric Psychiatry, 26*(9), 981–987.

Stewart, C., Kerridge, I., & Parker, M. (2008). Mental Health. In *The Australian Medico-Legal Handbook* (pp. 174–204). Marickville: Churchill Livingstone Elsevier.

Stice, E. (2002). Risk and maintenance factors for eating pathology: A meta-analytic review. *Psychological Bulletin, 128*(5), 825–848.

Stice, E., Killen, J. D., Hayward, C., & Taylor, C. B. (1998). Age of onset for binge eating and purging during late adolescence: A 4-year survival analysis. *J Abnorm Psychol, 107*(4), 671–675.

Stickley, A. J., & Hall, K. J. (2017). Social enterprise: A model of recovery and social inclusion for occupational therapy practice in the UK. *Mental Health and Social Inclusion, 21*(2), 91–101.

Stickley, T., Higgins, A., Meade, O., Sitvast, J., Doyle, L., Ellilä, H., . . . Kilkku, N. (2016). From the rhetoric to the real: A critical review of how the concepts of recovery and social inclusion may inform mental health nurse advanced level curricula—The eMenthe project. *Nurse Education Today, 37*, 155–163.

Stinchfield, R. (2014). A review of problem gambling assessment instruments and brief screens. In D. C. S. Richard, A. Blaszczynski, & L. Nower (eds.), *The Wiley-Blackwell Handbook of Disordered Gambling*. John Wiley & Sons.

Stinson, F. S., Dawson, D. A., Goldstein, R. B., Chou, S., Huang, B., Smith, S. M., . . . Grant, B. F. (2008). Prevalence, correlates, disability, and comorbidity of DSM-IV narcissistic personality disorder: Results from the Wave 2 National Epidemiologic Survey on Alcohol and Related Conditions. *J Clin Psychiatry, 69*(7), 1033–1045.

Stinson, F. S., Dawson, D. A., Patricia Chou, S., Smith, S., Goldstein, R. B., June Ruan, W., & Grant, B. F. (2007). The epidemiology of DSM-IV specific phobia in the USA: Results from the National Epidemiologic Survey on Alcohol and Related Conditions. *Psychol Med, 37*(7), 1047–1059.

Stirling, Y., Higgins, K., & Petrakis, M. (2018). Challenges in implementing individual placement and support in the Australian mental health service and policy context. *Australian Health Review, 42*(1), 82–88.

Stockwell, T., Auld, M. C., Zhao, J., & Martin, G. (2012). Does minimum pricing reduce alcohol consumption? The experience of a Canadian province. *Addiction, 107*(5), 912–920.

Stockwell, T., Sitharthan, T., McGrath, D., & Lang, E. (1994). The measurement of alcohol dependence and impaired control in community samples. *Addiction, 89*(2), 167–184.

Stokes, B. (2012). *Review of the Admission or Referral to and the Discharge and Transfer Practices of Public Mental Health Facilities/Services in Western Australia*. Retrieved from https://ww2.health.wa.gov.au/Reports-and-publications/Review-of-the-admission-referral-and-discharge-transfer-practices-of-public-mental-health-facilities.

Stokes, Helen. & Turnbull, Malcolm. & Wyn, Johanna. & Australian Youth Research Centre, issuing body. (2013). *Young People with a Disability: Independence and Opportunity: A Literature Review.* Retrieved from http://web.education.unimelb.edu.au.

Stokes, J. (1994). The unconscious at work in groups and teams: Contributions from the work of Wilfred Bion. In A. Obholzer & V. Z. Roberts (eds.), *The Unconscious at Work* (pp. 19–27). London: Routledge.

Stolk, Y., Minas, H., & Klimidis, S. (2008). *Access to Mental Health Services in Victoria: A Focus on Ethnic Communities*. Melbourne: Victorian Transcultural Psychiatry Unit.

Stone, L. (2013). Being a botanist and a gardener: Using diagnostic frameworks in general practice patients with medically unexplained symptoms. *Australian Journal of Primary Health, 19*, 90–97.

Stone, L. (2014). Blame, shame and hopelessness: Medically unexplained symptoms and the 'heartsink' experience. *Australian Family Physician, 43*(4), 191.

Stone, L. (2015). Managing medically unexplained illness in general practice. *Australian Family Physician, 44*(9), 624.

Stoppard, J. M. (1999). *Understanding Depression: Feminist Social Constructionist Approaches*. UK: Routledge.

Stoppard, J. M., & McMullen, L. M. (2003). *Situating Sadness: Women and Depression in Social Context*. New York: New York University Press.

Storey, J. E., Rowland, J. T. J., Conforti, D. A., & Dickson, H. G. (2004). The Rowland Universal Dementia Assessment Scale (RUDAS): A multicultural cognitive assessment scale. *International Psychogeriatrics, 16*(1), 13-31.

Strand, M., Gammon, D., Eng, L. S., & Ruland, C. (2017). Exploring working relationships in mental health care via an e-recovery portal: Qualitative study on the experiences of service users and health providers. *JMIR Mental Health, 4*(4), e54.

Stratford, A. C., Halpin, M., Phillips, K., Skerritt, F., Beales, A., Cheng, V., . . . Davidson, L. (2017). The growth of peer support: An international charter. *Journal of Mental Health*, 1-6.

Stratford, A. C., Halpin, M., Phillips, K., Skerritt, F., Beales, A., Cheng, V., . . . Davidson, L. (2019). The growth of peer support: An international charter. *Journal of Mental Health, 28*(6), 627-632.

Streiner, D., & Geddes, J. (1998). Some useful concepts and terms used in articles about diagnosis. *Evidence Based Mental Health, 1*(1), 6-8.

Strober, M. (2010). The chronically ill patient with anorexia nervosa development: Phenomenology and therapeutic considerations. In C. M. Grilo & J. E. Mitchell (eds.), *The Treatment of Eating Disorders: A Clinical Handbook* (pp. 225-238). New York: The Guilford Press.

Stuckler, D., Basu, S., Suhrcke, M., Coutts, A., & McKee, M. (2009). The public health effect of economic crises and alternative policy responses in Europe: An empirical analysis. *Lancet, 374*(9686), 315-323.

Student Minds. (2020). *UK's Student Mental Health Charity*. Retrieved from www.studentminds.org.uk.

Stunkard, A. (1959). Eating patterns and obesity. *Psychiatric Quarterly, 33*(2), 284-295.

Sturmey, P. (1993). The use of DSM and ICD diagnostic criteria in people with mental retardation: A review of empirical studies. *Journal of Nervous and Mental Disease, 181*(1), 38-41.

Subjective Emptiness: A Clinically Significant Trans-diagnostic Psychopathology Construct. (2020, April 20). *Mental Health Weekly Digest*, 861. Retrieved from https://link.gale.com.

Substance Abuse and Mental Health Services Administration (SAMHSA). (2014a). *SAMHSA's Concept of Trauma and Guidance for a Trauma-Informed Approach*. Retrieved from https://store.samhsa.gov/system/files/sma14-4884.pdf.

Substance Abuse and Mental Health Services Administration (SAMHSA). (2014b). *Trauma-Informed Care in Behavioral Health Services* (Vol. Treatment Improvement Protocol (TIP) Series 57. HHS Publication No. (SMA) 13-4801). Rockville, MD: Substance Abuse and Mental Health Services Administration. Retreived from https://store.samhsa.gov.

Substance Abuse and Mental Health Services Administration (SAMHSA). (2018). *Substance Abuse and Mental Health Services Administration*. Retrieved from www.samhsa.gov/programs.

Substance Abuse and Mental Health Services Administration (SAMHSA). (2020). Programs. *Samhsa's Programs and Campaigns Offer Information, Training, and Technical Assistance to Improve the Quality and Delivery of Behavioral Health Services Across the Nation*. Retrieved from https://www.samhsa.gov/programs.

Sue, D. W., Capodilupo, C. M., Torino, G. C., Bucceri, J. M., Holder, A. M. B., Nadal, K. L., & Esquilin, M. (2007). Racial microaggressions in everyday life: Implications for clinical practice. *American Psychologist, 62*(4), 271-286.

Sullivan, P. F., Neale, M. C., & Kendler, K. S. (2000). Genetic epidemiology of major depression: Review and meta-analysis. *American Journal of Psychiatry, 157*(10), 1552-1562.

Summers, M., & McKenzie, P. (2006). Not for service: Experiences of injustice and despair in mental health care in Australia. (Mental Health Council of Australia, Brain and Mind Research Institute). *Australian Health Review, 30*(2), 261.

Sunderland, M., Newby, J. M., & Andrews, G. (2013). Health anxiety in Australia: Prevalence, comorbidity, disability and service use. *British Journal of Psychiatry, 202*(1), 56-61.

Surawy, C., Roberts, J., & Silver, A. (2005). The effect of mindfulness training on mood and measures of fatigue, activity, and quality of life in patients with chronic fatigue syndrome on a hospital waiting list: A series of exploratory studies. *Behavioural and Cognitive Psychotherapy, 33*, 103-109.

Surkan, P. J., Kennedy, C. E., Hurley, K. M., & Black, M. M. (2011). Maternal depression and early childhood growth in developing countries: Systematic review and meta-analysis. *Bulletin of the World Health Organization, 89*(8), 608-615.

Survivor Researcher Network. (2018). *Survivor Researcher Network*. Retrieved from www.nsun.org.uk/Handlers/Download.ashx?IDMF=941b61f7-4a71-4eba-8099-1269177a7858.

Sutherland, G., Edwards, G., Taylor, C., Phillips, G., Gossop, M., & Brady, R. (1986). The measurement of opiate dependence. *British Journal of Addiction, 81*(4), 485-494.

Suurvali, H., Cordingley, J., Hodgins, D. C., & Cunningham, J. A. (2009). Barriers to seeking help for gambling problems: A review of the empirical literature. *Journal of Gambling Studies, 25*(3), 407-424.

Suurvali, H., Hodgins, D., Toneatto, T., & Cunningham, J. (2008). Treatment seeking among Ontario problem gamblers: Results of a population survey. *Psychiatric Services, 59*(11), 1343-1346.

Swainston, K., & Summerbell, C. (2008). *The Effectiveness of Community Engagement Approaches and Methods for Health Promotion Interventions*. Teeside: National Institute for Health and Clinical Excellence.

Swan, P., & Raphael, B. (1995). *Ways Forward: National Aboriginal and Torres Strait Islander Mental Health Policy National Consultancy Report*. Retrieved from https://healthinfonet.ecu.edu.au/key-resources/publications/8608.

Swanson, M. C. J., Bland, R. C., & Newman, S. C. (1994). Antisocial personality disorders. *Acta Psychiatr Scand, 89*, 63-70.

Swisher, A. K. (2010). Practice-based evidence. *Cardiopulmonary Physical Therapy Section of the American Physical Therapy Association*, 21 (2) 4.

Sykes, M. J., Brabban, A., & Reilly, J. (2015). Balancing harms in support of recovery. *Journal of Mental Health, 24*(3), 140-144.

Sytema, S., Jörg, F., Nieboer, R., & Wunderink, L. (2014). Adding evidence-based interventions to assertive community treatment: A feasibility study. *Psychiatric Services, 65*(5), 689-692.

Sytema, S., Wunderink, L., Bloemers, W., Roorda, L., & Wiersma, D. (2007). Assertive community treatment in The Netherlands: A randomized controlled trial. *Acta Psychiatr Scand, 116*(2), 105-112.

Szasz, T. S., & Szasz, T. (1974). *The Myth of Mental Illness Revised Edition*. HarperCollins.

Szmukler, G. I., Burgess, P., Herrman, H., Bloch, S., Benson, A., & Colusa, S. (1996). Caring for relatives with serious mental illness: The development of the Experience of Caregiving Inventory. *Social Psychiatry and Psychiatric Epidemiology, 31*(3), 137-148.

Tabak, I., Zabłocka-Żytka, L., Ryan, P., Poma, S. Z., Joronen, K., Viganò, G., . . . Smith, M. (2016). Needs, expectations and consequences for children growing up in a family where the parent has a mental illness. *International Journal of Mental Health Nursing, 25*(4), 319-329.

Tackett, J. L. (2010). Toward an externalizing spectrum in DSM-V: Incorporating developmental concerns. *Child Development Perspectives, 4*(3), 161-167.

Taichman, D. B., Backus, J., Baethge, C., Bauchner, H., de Leeuw, P. W., Drazen, J. M., . . . Wu, S. (2016). Sharing clinical trial data: A proposal from the International Committee of Medical Journal Editors. *PLoS Medicine, 13*(1).

Taichman, D. B., Sahni, P., Pinborg, A., Peiperl, L., Laine, C., James, A., . . . Backus, J. (2017). Data sharing statements for clinical trials: A requirement of the International Committee of Medical Journal Editors. *Bull World Health Organ, 95*(7), 482-483.

Taipale, H., Mittendorfer-Rutz, E., Alexanderson, K., Majak, M., Mehtala, J., Hoti, F., . . . Tiihonen, J. (2018). Antipsychotics and mortality in a nationwide cohort of 29 823 patients with schizophrenia. *Schizophrenia Research, 197*, 274-280.

Talmon, M. (2012). When less is more: Lessons from 25 years of attempting to maximize the effect of each (and often only) therapeutic encounter. *Australian and New Zealand Journal of Family Therapy, 33*(1), 6-14.

Tapsell, R., Mathews, L., & Toi, L. (2018). *Waka: Digital Self-Management Tool for Service Users Who Experience Schizophrenia*. Paper presented at the RANZCP Annual Congress.

Tarzia, L., Maxwell, S., Valpied, J., Novy, K., Quake, R., & Hegarty, K. (2017). Sexual violence associated with poor mental health in women attending Australian general practices. *Australian and New Zealand Journal of Public Health, 41*(5), 518-523.

Tasman, A., Kay, J., Lieberman, J. A., First, M. B., & Riba, M. B. (2015). *Psychiatry* (4th ed., vol. 1 & 2). Chichester: John Wiley & Sons.

Tasmanian Government. (2013). *Mental Health Act*. Retrieved from www.legislation.tas.gov.au.

Taylor, B. (2019, 29 April, 2020). Record $19.7 million for suicide prevention and expanded mental health services. *Ministerial Press Release*. Retrieved from www.health.nsw.gov.au/news.

Taylor, J., & Kukutai, T. (2016). Indigenous data sovereignty: Toward an agenda. *Centre for Aboriginal Economic Policy Research (CAEPR)*. Retrieved from https://press.anu.edu.au/publications/series/caepr/indigenous-data-sovereignty.

Taylor, R. R. (2017). *Kielhofner's Model of Human Occupation: Theory and Application* (5th ed.). Philadelphia: Wolters Kluwer.

Taylor, S. C., Pugh, J., Goodwach, R., & Coles, J. (2012). Sexual trauma in women: The importance of identifying a history of sexual violence. *Australian Family Physician, 41*(7), 538.

Tchernegovski, P., Reupert, A., & Maybery, D. (2015). 'Let's talk about children': A pilot evaluation of an e-learning resource for mental health clinicians. *Clinical Psychologist, 19*(1), 49-58.

Teasdale, J. D., Segal, Z. V., Williams, J. M. G., Ridgeway, V. A., Soulsby, J. M., & Lau, M. A. (2000). Prevention of relapse/recurrence in major depression by mindfulness-based cognitive therapy. *J Consult Clin Psychol, 68*(4), 615-623.

Tee, J., & Kazantzis, N. (2011). Collaborative empiricism in cognitive therapy: A definition and theory for the relationship construct. *Clinical Psychology—Science and Practice, 18*(1), 47-61.

Teesson, M (1998) Substance use disorders. *World Health Organization Management of Mental Disorders*. Sydney: World Health Organization Collaborating Centre in Mental Health and Substance Use Disorders, St Vincent's Hospital.

Teesson, M., Hall, W., Slade, T., Mills, K., Grove, R., Mewton, L., . . . Haber, P. (2010). Prevalence and correlates of DSM-IV alcohol abuse and dependence in Australia: Findings of the 2007 National Survey of Mental Health and Wellbeing. *Addiction, 105*(12), 2085-2094.

Teesson, M., Sannibale, C., Reid, S., Proudfoot, H., Gournay, K., & Haber, P. (2003). *Manual for Compliance Therapy in Alcohol Pharmacotherapy*. Retrieved from https://ndarc.med.unsw.edu.au/resource/manual-compliance-therapy-alcohol-pharmacotherapy.

Teesson, M., Slade, T., & Mills, K. (2009). Comorbidity in Australia: Findings of the 2007 National Survey of Mental Health and Wellbeing. *Australian and New Zealand Journal of Australia, 43*(7), 606-614.

Teesson, M., Slade, T., Swift, W., Mills, K., Memedovic, S., Mewton, L., . . . Hall, W. (2012). Prevalence, correlates and comorbidity of DSM-IV cannabis use and cannabis use disorders in Australia. *Australian and New Zealand Journal of Psychiatry, 46*(12), 1182-1192.

Teicher, M. H., & Samson, J. A. (2016). Annual research review: Enduring neurobiological effects of childhood abuse and neglect. *Journal of Child Psychology and Psychiatry, 57*(3), 241-266.

Telfer, M. M., Tollit, M. A., Pace, C. C., & Pang, K. C. (2018). *Australian Standards of Care and Treatment Guidelines for Trans and Gender Diverse Children and Adolescents Version 1.1*. Retrieved from www.rch.org.au/uploadedFiles/Main/Content/adolescent-medicine/australian-standards-of-care-and-treatment-guidelines-for-trans-and-gender-diverse-children-and-adolescents.pdf.

Temes, C. M., & Zanarini, M. C. (2018). The longitudinal course of borderline personality disorder. *Psychiatric Clinics, 41*(4), 685-694.

ten Brinke, A., Sterk, P. J., Masclee, A. A. M., Spinhoven, P., Schimdt, J. T., Zwinderman, A. H., . . . Bel, E. H. (2005). Risk factors of frequent exacerbations in difficult-to-treat asthma. *European Respiratory Journal, 26*(5), 812-818.

Teyber, E., & Holmes McClure, F. (2011). *Interpersonal Process in Therapy: An Integrative Model* (6th ed.). USA: Cengage.

Thapliyal, P., Hay, P., & Conti, J. (2018). Role of gender in the treatment experiences of people with an eating disorder: A metasynthesis. *J Eat Disord, 6*, 18.

The Bouverie Centre. (2016). *From Individual to Families: A Client-Centred Framework for Involving Families*. Retrieved from www.bouverie.org.au/images/uploads/Bouverie_Centre_Framework.pdf.

The Gambia Hepatitis Study Group. (1987). The Gambia Hepatitis Intervention Study. *Cancer Research, 47*(21), 5782-5787.

The Getting it Right Collaborative Group. (2019). Getting it right: Validating a culturally specific tool for depression (aPHD-9) in Aboriginal and Torres Strait Islander Australians. *MJA, 211*(1), 24-30.

The Lancet. (2019). *The Best Science for Better Lives*. Retrieved from www.thelancet.com/about-us.

The Stanford Encyclopedia of Philosophy. (2011). *Culture and Cognitive Science*. Retrieved from https://plato.stanford.edu/entries/culture-cogsci.

The Stanford Encyclopedia of Philosophy. (2016). *Positive and Negative Liberty*. Retrieved from https://plato.stanford.edu/entries/liberty-positive-negative.

The Territory. (2020). *Grow Your Career in The Territory*. Retrieved from https://boundlesspossible.nt.gov.au/career.

The Trevor Project. (2018). *Eating Disorders Among LGBTQ Youth: A National Assessment*. Retrieved from https://www.thetrevorproject.org.

The University of Melbourne. (2020). *Centre for Psychiatric Nursing, Recovery Library*. Retrieved from https://healthsciences.unimelb.edu.au/departments/nursing/about-us/centre-for-psychiatric-nursing.

The World Bank. (2019). *GINI Index (World Bank Estimate). World Bank*. Retrieved from https://data.worldbank.org.

Thege, B. K., Woodin, E. M., Hodgins, D. C., & Williams, R. J. (2015). Natural course of behavioral addictions: A 5-year longitudinal study. *BMC Psychiatry, 15*.

Thigpen, C. H., & Cleckley, H. M. (1957). *The Three Faces of Eve*: Thigpen & Cleckley.

Thisted, C. N., Nielsen, C. V., & Bjerrum, M. (2018). Work Participation Among Employees with Common Mental Disorders: A Meta-synthesis. *Journal of Occupational Rehabilitation, 28*(3), 452–464.

Thistlethwaite, J. (2009). Breaking bad news—skills and evidence. *InnovAiT*.

Thistlethwaite, J. E. (2012). *Values-Based Interprofessional Collaborative Practice: Working Together in Health Care*. Cambridge University Press.

Thomas, A. (2013). Psychiatric assessment of older people. In T. Dening & A. Thomas (eds.), *Oxford Textbook of Old Age Psychiatry* (2nd ed., pp. 141-148). Oxford: Oxford University Press

Thomas, A. J., Kalaria, R. N., & O'Brien, J. T. (2004). Depression and vascular disease: What is the relationship? *J Affect Disord, 79*(1-3), 81–95.

Thomas, M., & Hall, A. (2016). *Housing Affordability in Australia*. Retrieved from www.aph.gov.au/About_Parliament/Parliamentary_Departments/Parliamentary_Library/pubs/BriefingBook45p/HousingAffordability.

Thomas, N., Farhall, J., Foley, F., Leitan, N. D., Villagonzalo, K., Ladd, E., . . . Kyrios, M. (2016). Promoting personal recovery in people with persisting psychotic disorders: Development and pilot study of a novel digital intervention.(Report) (Author abstract). *Frontiers in Psychiatry, 7*.

Thomas, N., Foley, F., Lindblom, K., & Lee, S. (2017). Access and use of the internet in Australian mental health service users. *Australasian Psychiatry, 25*(3), 257–261.

Thomas, N, Nedeljkovic, M, Foroughi, E, Seabrook, E. Foley, F, Shaw, R. (2020) *Mental Health Online*. Retrieved from www.mentalhealthonline.org.au.

Thomas, S. A., Merkouris, S. S., Radermacher, H. L., Dowling, N. A., Misso, M. L., Anderson, C. J., & Jackson, A. C. (2011). Australian guideline for treatment of problem gambling: An abridged outline. *Med J Aust, 195*(11), 664–665.

Thombs, B., Ziegelstein, R., Roseman, M., Kloda, L., & Ioannidis, J. (2014). There are no randomized controlled trials that support the United States Preventive Services Task Force guideline on screening for depression in primary care: A systematic review. *BMC Medicine, 12*(1), 13.

Thompson, A., Issakidis, C., & Hunt, C. (2008). Delay to seek treatment for anxiety and mood disorders in an Australian clinical sample. *Behaviour Change, 25*(2), 71–84.

Thompson, L., & McCabe, R. (2012). The effect of clinician-patient alliance and communication on treatment adherence in mental health care: A systematic review. *BMC Psychiatry, 12*(1), 87.

Thorne, S. E. (1990). Constructive noncompliance in chronic illness. *Holist Nurs Pract, 5*(1), 62–69.

Thornicroft, G., & Betts, V. (2002). *International Mid-Term Review of the Second National Mental Health Plan for Australia*. Canberra: Australian Government.

Thornicroft, G., Rose, D., Kassam, A., & Sartorius, N. (2007). Stigma: Ignorance, prejudice or discrimination? *British Journal of Psychiatry, 190*(3), 192–193.

Tiihonen, J., Lönnqvist, J., Wahlbeck, K., Klaukka, T., Niskanen, L., Tanskanen, A., & Haukka, J. (2009). Mortality in schizophrenia: An 11-Year follow-up study of the total Finnish population (FIN11 Study). *The Lancet, 374*(9690), 620–627.

Tiihonen, J., Mittendorfer-Rutz, E., Majak, M., Mehtala, J., Hoti, F., Jedenius, E., . . . Taipale, H. (2017). Real-world effectiveness of antipsychotic treatments in a nationwide cohort of 29 823 patients with schizophrenia. *JAMA Psychiatry, 74*(7), 686–693.

Timpano, K. R., Exner, C., Glaesmer, H., Rief, W., Keshaviah, A., Brahler, E., & Wilhelm, S. (2011). The epidemiology of the proposed DSM-5 hoarding disorder: Exploration of the acquisition specifier, associated features, and distress. *J Clin Psychiatry, 72*(6), 780–786; quiz 878–789.

Titov, N., Schofield, C., Staples, L., Dear, B. F., & Nielssen, O. (2019). A comparison of Indigenous and non-Indigenous users of MindSpot: An Australian digital mental health service. *Australasian Psychiatry, 27*(4), 352–357.

Tolin, D. F., Frost, R. O., & Steketee, G. (2010). A brief interview for assessing compulsive hoarding: The Hoarding Rating Scale-Interview. *Psychiatry Research, 178*(1), 147–152.

Tolin, D. F., Frost, R. O., Steketee, G., & Muroff, J. (2015). Cognitive behavioral therapy for hoarding disorder: A meta-analysis. *Depression & Anxiety, 32*(3), 158–166.

Tomizawa, R., Shigeta, M., & Reeves, S. (2017). Framework development for the assessment of interprofessional teamwork in mental health settings. *Journal of Interprofessional Care, 31*(1), 43–50.

Tomko, R. L., Trull, T. J., Wood, P. K., & Sher, K. J. (2014). Characteristics of borderline personality disorder in a community sample: Comorbidity, treatment utilization, and general functioning. *Journal of Personality Disorders, 28*(5), 734–750.

Tondora, J., Miller, R., Slade, M., & Davidson, L. (2014). *Partnering for Recovery in Mental Health: A Practical Guide to Person-Centered Planning*. Wiley.

Toombs, M., Nasir, B., Kisely, S., Ranmuthugala, G., Gill, N. S., Beccaria, G., . . . Nicholson, G. C. (2019). Cultural validation of the structured clinical interview for Diagnostic and Statistical Manual of Mental Disorders in Indigenous Australians. *Australasian Psychiatry, 27*(4), 362–365.

Torales, J., O'Higgins, M., Castaldelli-Maia, J. M., & Ventriglio, A. (2020). The outbreak of COVID-19 coronavirus and its impact on global mental health. *Int J Soc Psychiatry*, 20764020915212. doi:10.1177/0020764020915212, online ahead of print.

Torgersen, S., Lygren, S., Øien, P. A., Skre, I., Onstad, S., Edvardsen, J., . . . Kringlen, E. (2000). A twin study of personality disorders. *Comprehensive Psychiatry, 41*(6), 416–425.

Torgerson, D. J., & Roland, M. (1998). What is Zelen's design? *BMJ, 316*(7131), 606–606.

Touyz, S., Le Grange, D., Lacey, H., Hay, P., Smith, R., Maguire, S., . . . Crosby, R. D. (2013). Treating severe and enduring anorexia nervosa: A randomized controlled trial. *Psychol Med, 43*(12), 2501–2511.

Townsend, C., Whiteford, H., Baingana, F., Gulbinat, W., Jenkins, R., Baba, A., . . . Parameshvara Deva, M. (2004). The Mental Health Policy Template: Domains and elements for mental health policy formulation. *International Review of Psychiatry, 16*(1–2), 18–23.

Townsend, E. A., & Polatajko, H. J. (2007). *Enabling Occupation II: Advancing an Occupational Therapy Vision for Health, Well-Being, & Justice Through Occupation*. Ottawa: Canadian Association of Occupational Therapists.

Townsend, E. A., & Polatajko, H. J. (2013). *Enabling Occupation II: Advancing an Occupational Therapy Vision for Health,*

Well-Being, & Justice Through Occupation (2nd ed.). Ottowa: Canadian Association of Occupational Therapists.

Trachtenberg, M., Parsonage, M., Shepherd, G., & Boardman, J. (2013). *Peer Support in Mental Health Care: Is It Good Value for Money?* Retrieved from http://eprints.lse.ac.uk/60793/1/Trachtenberg_etal_Report-Peer-support-in-mental-health-care-is-it-good-value-for-money_2013.pdf.

Tramatic Stress Clinic. (2020). *Evidence-based Treatments and Research for PTSD and Prolonged Grief.* Retrieved from www.traumaticstressclinic.com.

Transcultural Mental Health Centre. (2020). *Support Positive Mental Health for People From Culturally and Linguistically Diverse Communities.* Retrieved from www.dhi.health.nsw.gov.au/transcultural-mental-health-centre.

Trauer, T., Tobias, G., & Slade, M. (2008). Development and evaluation of a patient-rated version of the Camberwell Assessment of Need short appraisal schedule (CANSAS-P). *Community Mental Health Journal, 44*, 113-124.

Travelbee, J. (1971). *Interpersonal Aspects of Nursing* (2nd ed.). Philadelphia: F. A. Davis Company.

Treasure, J., & Russell, G. (2011). The case for early intervention in anorexia nervosa: Theoretical exploration of maintaining factors. *Br J Psychiatry, 199*(1), 5-7.

Treasure, J., & Schmidt, U. (2013). The cognitive-interpersonal maintenance model of anorexia nervosa revisited: A summary of the evidence for cognitive, socio-emotional and interpersonal predisposing and perpetuating factors. *J Eat Disord, 1*, 13.

Trett, R., Dick, D., & Cooke, K. (2011). Borderline Personality Disorder. In K.-L. Edward, I. L. Munro, A. J. Welch, & A. N. Robins (eds.), *Mental Health Nursing: Dimensions of Praxis* (pp. 198-219). South Melbourne: Oxford University Press.

Trevillion, S. (1999). *Networking and Community Partnership.* Ashgate: Aldershot.

Triangle Consulting. (2010). *Recovery Star.* Retrieved from www.outcomesstar.org.uk.

Tropea, J., Slee, J. A., Brand, C. A., Gray, L., & Snell, T. (2008). Clinical practice guidelines for the management of delirium in older people in Australia. *Australasian Journal on Ageing, 27*(3), 150-156.

Tsang, W. H., Siu, A. M. H., & Lloyd, C. (2010). Evidence-based practice in mental health. In C. Brown & G. Stoffel (eds.), *Occupational Therapy in Mental Health: A Vision for Participation* (pp. 57-69). Philadelphia: FA Davis.

Tse, S., Tsoi, E. W., Hamilton, B., O'hagan, M., Shepherd, G., Slade, M., . . . Petrakis, M. (2016). Uses of strength-based interventions for people with serious mental illness: A critical review. *International Journal of Social Psychiatry, 62*(3), 281-291.

Tsemberis, S. (2010). Housing first: Ending homelessness, promoting recovery and reducing costs. *How to House the Homeless*, 37-56.

Tsoi, E. W. S., Tse, S., Yu, C.-H., Chan, S.-K., Wan, E., Wong, S., & Liu, L. (2019). A nonrandomized controlled trial of strengths model case management in Hong Kong. *Research on Social Work Practice, 29*(5), 540-554.

Tsouros, A. D. (1991). *World Health Organization Healthy Cities Project: A Project Becomes a Movement. Review of Progress 1987-1990.* Retrieved from

Tsouros, A. D. (2015). Twenty-seven years of the WHO European Healthy Cities movement: A sustainable movement for change and innovation at the local level. *Health Promot Int, 30 Suppl 1*, i3-i7.

Tsuang, M. T., Tohen, M., & Jones, P. B. (2011). *Textbook of Psychiatric Epidemiology* (3rd ed.). Wiley.

Tucker, T. K., Ritter, A. J., Maher, C., & Jackson, H. (2004). Naltrexone maintenance for heroin dependence: Uptake, attrition and retention. *Drug and Alcohol Review, 23*(3), 299-309.

Turk, J. (1992). The fragile-X syndrome. On the way to a behavioural phenotype. *British Journal of Psychiatry, 160*(1), 24-35.

Turner, B. S., & Samson, C. (1995). *Medical Power and Social Knowledge.* SAGE Publications.

Turner, N. E., Jain, U., Spence, W., & Zangeneh, M. (2008). Pathways to pathological gambling: Component analysis of variables related to pathological gambling. *International Gambling Studies, 8*(3), 281-298.

Tyrer, P. (2014). A comparison of DSM and ICD classifications of mental disorder. *Advances in Psychiatric Treatment, 20*(4), 280-285.

Tyrer, P., Coombs, N., Ibrahimi, F., Mathilakath, A., Bajaj, P., Ranger, M., . . . Din, R. (2007). Critical developments in the assessment of personality disorder. *British Journal of Psychiatry, 190*(S49), s51-s59.

Tyrer, P., Gunderson, J., Lyons, M., & Tohen, M. (1997). Special feature: Extent of comorbidity between mental state and personality disorders. *Journal of Personality Disorders, 11*(3), 242-259.

Uher, R., & Zwicker, A. (2017). Etiology in psychiatry: Embracing the reality of poly-gene-environmental causation of mental illness. *World Psychiatry, 16*(2), 121-129.

UMass Memorial Health Care. (2020). *MBSR Teacher Training.* Retrieved from www.umassmemorialhealthcare.org.

Undrill, G. (2007). The risks of risk assessment. *Advances in Psychiatric Treatment, 13*(4), 291-297.

UNICEF. (2020). *The Convention on the Rights of the Child.* Retrieved from www.unicef.org/child-rights-convention/what-is-the-convention.

United Nations Committee on the Rights of Persons with Disabilities. (2014). *General Comment No 1 on Article 12 of the Convention—Equal Recognition before the Law.* Retrieved from www.ohchr.org/documents/hrbodies/crpd/gc/dgcarticle12.doc.

United Nations Department of Public Information. (1991). Principles for protection of persons with mental illness and the improvement of mental health care. In *Human Rights: A Compilation of International Instruments, Universal Instruments* (vol. 1, pp. 517-530). New York and Geneva: United Nations.

United Nations General Assembly Human Rights Council (2017). *Special Rapporteur on the Right of Everyone to the Enjoyment of the Highest Attainable Standard of Physical and Mental Health.* Retrieved from http://www.ohchr.org.

United Nations General Assembly. (2017). *Report of the Special Rapporteur on the Right of Everyone to the Enjoyment of the Highest Attainable Standard of Physical and Mental Health.* (A/HRC/35/21). Retrieved from https://documents-dds-ny.un.org/doc/UNDOC/GEN/G17/076/04/pdf/G1707604.pdf?OpenElement.

United Nations High Commissioner for Refugees (UNHCR). (2015). *World at War. UNHCR Global Trends Forced Displacement in 2014.* Retrieved from www.unhcr.org/556725e69.pdf.

United Nations High Commissioner for Refugees (UNHCR). (2019). *Global Trends Forced Displacement in 2018.* Geneva: United Nations High Commissioner for Refugees.

United Nations. (1948). The Universal Declaration of Human Rights. Retrieved from https://www.un.org/en/universal-declaration-human-rights/

United Nations. (2003). *International Norms and Standards Relating to Disability.* Retrieved from www.un.org/esa/socdev/enable/comp00.htm.

United Nations. (2007b). *Convention on the Rights of Persons with Disabilities (CRPD).* Retrieved from www.un.org/development/desa/disabilities/resources/general-assembly/convention-on-the-rights-of-persons-with-disabilities-ares61106.html.

United Nations. (2007a). *United Nations Adopts Declaration on Rights of Indigenous Peoples*. Retrieved from https://news.un.org/en/story/2007/09/231062-united-nations-adopts-declaration-rights-indigenous-peoples.

United Nations. (2013). *Indigenous Peoples and the United Nations Human Rights System Fact Sheet No.9/Rev.2*. Retrieved from www.ohchr.org/Documents/Publications/fs9Rev.2.pdf.

United Nations. (2019). *Universal Declaration of Human Rights*. Retrieved from www.un.org/en/universal-declaration-human-rights.

United Nations. (2020). Goal 11: Make cities inclusive, safe, resilient and sustainable. *Sustainable Development Goals*. Retrieved from www.un.org/sustainabledevelopment/cities.

University of New South Wales. (2018). *Inequality in Australia*. Retrieved from www.acoss.org.au/wp-content/uploads/2018/07/Inequality-in-Australia-2018.pdf.

Ursano, R. J., Fullerton, C. S., Weisaeth, L., & Raphael, B. (2017). *Textbook of Disaster Psychiatry* (2nd ed.). Cambridge: Cambridge University Press.

Uskul, A. K. (2010). Socio-cultural aspects of health and illness. In D. French, K. Vedhara, A. A. Kaptein, & J. Weinman (eds.), *Health Psychology* (2nd ed., pp. 347-359). BPS Blackwell.

Ussher, J. (1992). *Women's Madness: Mysogyny or Mental Illness?* New York: Harvester Wheatsheaf.

Vachon, D. D., & Bagby, R. M. (2009). Pathological gambling subtypes. *Psychol Assess, 21*(4), 608-615.

Vall, E., & Wade, T. D. (2015). Predictors of treatment outcome in individuals with eating disorders: A systematic review and meta-analysis. *Int J Eat Disord, 48*(7), 946-971.

Vallesi, S., Wood, N., Wood, L., Cumming, C., Gazey, A., & Flatau, P. (2018). *50 Lives 50 Homes: A Housing First Response to Ending Homelessness in Perth. Second Evaluation Report*. Retrieved from www.uwa.edu.au/projects/evaluation-of-50-lives-50-homes.

van der Gaag, M., Smit, F., Bechdolf, A., French, P., Linszen, D. H., Yung, A. R., . . . Cuijpers, P. (2013). Preventing a first episode of psychosis: Meta-analysis of randomized controlled prevention trials of 12 month and longer-term follow-ups. *Schizophrenia Research, 149*(1-3), 56-62.

van der Kolk, B. A., Roth, S., Pelcovitz, D., Sunday, S., & Spinazzola, J. (2005). Disorders of extreme stress: The empirical foundation of a complex adaptation to trauma. *International Society for Traumatic Stress Studies, 18*(5 October), 389-399.

van der Wurff, F. B., Stek, M. L., Hoogendijk, W. J. G., & Beekman, A. T. F. (2003). The efficacy and safety of ECT in depressed older adults: A literature review. *International Journal of Geriatric Psychiatry, 18*(10), 894-904.

Van Gordon, W., Shonin, E., & Griffiths, M. D. (2015). Towards a second generation of mindfulness-based interventions. *Australian and New Zealand Journal of Psychiatry, 49*(7), 591-592.

van Melle, J. P., de Jonge, P., van den Berg, M. P., Pot, H. J., & van Veldhuisen, D. J. (2006). Treatment of depression in acute coronary syndromes with selective serotonin reuptake inhibitors. *Drugs, 66*(16), 2095-2107.

van Os, J., Guloksuz, S., Vijn, T. W., Hafkenscheid, A., & Delespaul, P. (2019). The evidence-based group-level symptom-reduction model as the organizing principle for mental health care: Time for change? *World Psychiatry, 18*(1), 88-96.

van Rooij, A. J., Schoenmakers, T. M., Vermulst, A. A., van den Eijnden, R. J. J. M., & van de Mheen, D. (2011). Online video game addiction: Identification of addicted adolescent gamers. *Addiction, 106*(1), 205-212.

van Vugt, M. D., Kroon, H., Delespaul, P. A. E. G., Dreef, F. G., Nugter, A., Roosenschoon, B. J., . . . Mulder, C. L. (2011). Assertive community treatment in The Netherlands: Outcome and model fidelity. *Canadian Journal of Psychiatry-Revue Canadienne De Psychiatrie, 56*(3), 154-160.

vanderKolk, B. A., Pelcovitz, D., Roth, S., Mandel, F. S., McFarlane, A., & Herman, J. L. (1996). Dissociation, somatization, and affect dysregulation: The complexity of adaptation to trauma. *American Journal of Psychiatry, 153*(7), 83-93.

Vandewalle, J., Debyser, B., Beeckman, D., Vandecasteele, T., Van Hecke, A., & Verhaeghe, S. (2016). Peer workers' perceptions and experiences of barriers to implementation of peer worker roles in mental health services: A literature review. *International Journal of Nursing Studies, 60*, 234-250.

Vaughn, C., & Leff, J. (1976). The measurement of expressed emotion in the families of psychiatric patients. *British Journal of Social and Clinical Psychology, 15*(2), 157-165.

Veale, D. (2004). Advances in a cognitive behavioural model of body dysmorphic disorder. *Body Image, 1*(1), 113-125.

Veale, D., Gledhill, L. J., Christodoulou, P., & Hodsoll, J. (2016). Body dysmorphic disorder in different settings: A systematic review and estimated weighted prevalence. *Body Image, 18*, 168-186.

Vecchio, N., Stevens, S., & Cybinski, P. (2008). Caring for people with a mental disability at home: Australian carers' perceptions of service provision. *Community Mental Health Journal, 44*(2), 125-134.

Velligan, D. I., Sajatovic, M., Hatch, A., Kramata, P., & Docherty, J. P. (2017). Why do psychiatric patients stop antipsychotic medication? A systematic review of reasons for nonadherence to medication in patients with serious mental illness. *Patient Preference and Adherence*, 11, 449-468.

Veness, B. (2016). *The Wicked Problem of University Student Mental Health. Report to The Winston Churchill Memorial Fund.* Sydney: Australia.

Venn Brown, A. (2018). *Gay Conversion Therapy in Australia—Report*. Retrieved from www.abbi.org.au/2018/05/gay-conversion-therapy-in-australia.

Ventriglio, A., Watson, C., & Bhugra, D. (2020). Pandemics, panic and prevention: Stages in the life of COVID-19 pandemic. *International Journal of Social Psychiatry*. doi: https://doi.org/10.1177/0020764020924449, online ahead of print.

Venville, A., Street, A., & Fossey, E. (2013). Student perspectives on disclosure of mental illness in post-compulsory education: Displacing doxa. *Disability & Society*, 1-15.

Verheul, R., & Widiger, T. A. (2004). A meta-analysis of the prevalence and usage of the personality disorder not otherwise specified (PDNOS) diagnosis. *Journal of Personality Disorders, 18*(4), 309-319.

Verwijk, E., Comijs, H. C., Kok, R. M., Spaans, H. P., Tielkes, C. E. M., Scherder, E. J. A., & Stek, M. L. (2014). Short- and long-term neurocognitive functioning after electroconvulsive therapy in depressed elderly: A prospective naturalistic study. *International Psychogeriatrics, 26*(2), 315-324.

verywell mind. (2019). *The Stages of Change Model of Overcoming Addiction*. Retrieved from www.verywellmind.com/the-stages-of-change-model-of-overcoming-addiction-21961.

VicHealth & CSIRO. (2015). *Bright Futures: Megatrends Impacting the Mental Wellbeing of Young Victorians Over the Coming 20 Years*. Melbourne: Victorian Health Promotion Foundation.

Victoria State Government. (2014). *Victoria Mental Health Act 2014*. Retrieved from www2.health.vic.gov.au/mental-health/practice-and-service-quality/mental-health-act-2014.

Victoria State Government. (2018). *Mental Health Act 2014 Handbook*. Retrieved from www2.health.vic.gov.au/mental-health/practice-and-service-quality/mental-health-act-2014-handbook.

Victoria State Government. (2019). *Labor Government to Make Conversion 'Therapy' Against the Law*. Retrieved from www.premier.vic.gov.au/labor-government-to-make-conversion-therapy-against-the-law.

Victoria State Services Authority. (2007). *Victorian Approaches to Joined Up Government: An Overview*. Melbourne: State Services Authority.

Victorian Agency for Health Information. (2019). *Value Based Healthcare*. Retrieved from www.bettersafercare.vic.gov.au/reports-and-publications/value-based-healthcare.

Victorian and Tasmanian PHN Alliance. (2018). *Place-based Suicide Prevention*. Retrieved from https://vtphna.org.au/place-based-suicide-prevention.

Victorian Auditor General Report. (2009). *Responding to Mental Health Crises in the Community*. Melbourne: Government Printer.

Victorian Department of Human Services. (1997). *Tailoring Services to Meet the Needs of Women*.

Victorian Government. (2018). *Latrobe Health Innovation Zone*. Retrieved from www2.health.vic.gov.au/about/health-strategies/latrobe-health-innovation-zone.

Victorian Government Department of Health. (2011). *National Mental Health Workforce Strategy*. Retrieved from www.aihw.gov.au.

Vidal, J. (2002). Updated review on the benefits of weight loss. *Int J Obes Relat Metab Disord, 26 Suppl 4*, S25-28.

Villotti, P., Corbiere, M., Fossey, E., Fraccaroli, F., Lecomte, T., & Harvey, C. (2017). work accommodations and natural supports for employees with severe mental illness in social businesses: An international comparison. *Community Mental Health Journal, 53*(7), 864-870.

Vine, R., & Judd, F. (2019). Contextual issues in the implementation of mental health legislation. *International Journal of Law and Psychiatry, 62*, 16-19.

Virtanen, M., Kawachi, I., Oksanen, T., Salo, P., Tuisku, K., Pulkki-Raback, L., . . . Kivimaki, M. (2011). Socio-economic differences in long-term psychiatric work disability: Prospective cohort study of onset, recovery and recurrence. *Occup Environ Med, 68*(11), 791-798.

Visa, B., & Harvey, C. (2019). Mental health carers' experiences of an Australian Carer Peer Support program: Tailoring supports to carers' needs. *Health & Social Care in the Community, 27*(3), 729-739.

Visser, J. C., Smeekens, S., Rommelse, N., Verkes, R. J., Van der Gaag, R. J., & Buitelaar, J. K. (2010). Assessment of psychopathology in 2 to 5 year olds: Applying the infant-toddler social emotional assessment. *Infant Mental Health Journal, 31*(6), 611-629.

Voices Vic. (2020). *Voices Vic—A Proud Initiative of Uniting Prahran*. Retrieved from www.unitingprahran.org.au/ourservices/voices-vic/#page_1.

von Peter, S., Aderhold, V., Cubellis, L., Bergstrom, T., Stastny, P., Seikkula, J., & Puras, D. (2019). Open Dialogue as a Human Rights-Aligned Approach. *Frontiers in Psychiatry, 10*.

von Stumm, S., Deary, I. J., Kivimaki, M., Jokela, M., Clark, H., & Batty, G. D. (2011). Childhood behavior problems and health at midlife: 35-year follow-up of a Scottish birth cohort. *Journal of Child Psychology and Psychiatry, 52*(9), 992-1001.

Vos, T., Barker, B., Begg, S., Stanley, L., & Lopez, A. D. (2009). Burden of disease and injury in Aboriginal and Torres Strait Islander Peoples: The Indigenous health gap. *International Journal of Epidemiology, 38*(2), 470-477.

Vrklevski, L. P., Eljiz, K., & Greenfield, D. (2017). The evolution and devolution of mental health services in Australia. *Inquiries Journal, 9*(10).

VTMH. (2019). *Working with Interpreters. A Resource for Service Providers Engaging with Interpreters in Mental Health Settings*. Retrieved from www.vtmh-workingwithinterpreters.online.

Waddell, G., & Burton, K. (2006). *Is Work Good for Your Health and Wellbeing?*. London: The Stationery Office.

Wade, D., Crompton, D., Howard, A., Stevens, N., Metcalf, O., Brymer, M., . . . Forbes, D. (2014). Skills for psychological recovery: Evaluation of a post-disaster mental health training program. *Disaster Health, 2*(3-4), 138-145.

Wade, D., Forbes, D., Nursey, J., & Creamer, M. (2013). A multi-level framework to guide mental health response following a natural disaster. *Drying Technology, 31*(2), 109-113.

Wade, D., Howard, A., Fletcher, S., Cooper, J., & Forbes, D. (2013). Early response to psychological trauma: What GPs can do. *Australian Family Physician, 42*(9), 610.

Wadsworth, Y. (2010). *Building in Research and Evaluation: Human Inquiry for Living Systems*. Hawthorn: Action Research Press.

Wadsworth, Y. (2011). *Do It Yourself Social Research: The Bestselling Practical Guide to Doing Social Research Projects* (3rd ed.). Sydney: Allen & Unwin.

Wadsworth, Y., & Epstein, M. (1996). *Understanding and Involvement (U&I)-Consumer Evaluation of Acute Psychiatric Hospital Practice: A Project Concludes* (vol. 3). Melbourne: Victorian Mental Illness Awareness Council.

Wadsworth, Y., & Epstein, M. (1996). *Understanding and Involvement (U&I)-Consumer Evaluation of Acute Psychiatric Hospital Practice: A Project Unfolds...* (Vol. 2). Melbourne: Victorian Mental Illness Awareness Council.

Wadsworth, Y., & Epstein, M. (1998). Building in dialogue between consumers and staff in acute mental health services. *Systemic Practice and Action Research, 11*(4), 353-379.

Wadsworth Yoland (ed.) in ongoing association with Merinda Epstein (ed.). (1998-2001). *The Essential U&I—A One-Volume Presentation of the Findings of a Lengthy Grounded Study of Whole Systems Change Towards Staff-Consumer Collaboration for Enhancing Mental Health Services*. Carlton South: VicHealth.

Wagenaar, A. C., Salois, M. J., & Komro, K. A. (2009). Effects of beverage alcohol price and tax levels on drinking: A meta-analysis of 1003 estimates from 112 studies. *Addiction, 104*(2), 179-190.

Waghorn, G., Chant, D., Lloyd, C., & Harris, M. (2011). Earning and learning among Australian community residents with psychiatric disorders. *Psychiatry Research, 186*(1), 109-116.

Waghorn, G., Killackey, E., Dickson, P., Brock, L., & Skate, C. (2020). Evidence-Based Supported Employment for People With Psychiatric Disabilities in Australia: Progress in the Past 15 Years. *Psychiatric Rehabilitation Journal*, 43(1), 32-39.

Waghorn, G., Saha, S., Harvey, C., Morgan, V. A., Waterreus, A., Bush, R., . . . McGrath, J. J. (2012). 'Earning and learning' in those with psychotic disorders: The Second Australian National Survey of Psychosis. *Australian and New Zealand Journal of Psychiatry, 46*(8), 774-785.

Waghorn, G., Still, M., Chant, D., & Whiteford, H. (2004). Specialised supported education for Australians with psychotic disorders. *Australian Journal of Social Issues, 39*(4), 443-458.

Wahlbeck, K., & McDaid, D. (2012). Actions to alleviate the mental health impact of the economic crisis. *World Psychiatry, 11*(3), 139-145.

Wakefield, M. A., Coomber, K., Durkin, S. J., Scollo, M., Bayly, M., Spittal, M. J., ... Hill, D. (2014). Time series analysis of the impact of tobacco control policies on smoking prevalence among Australian adults, 2001-2011. *Bulletin of the World Health Organization*, 92(6), 413-422.

Waks, S., Scanlan, J. N., Berry, B., Schweizer, R., Hancock, N., & Honey, A. (2017). Outcomes identified and prioritised by consumers of partners in recovery: A consumer-led study. *BMC Psychiatry, 17.*

Waldman, S. A., & Terzic, A. (2010). Clinical and translational science: From bench-bedside to global village. *Clinical and Translational Science, 3*(5), 254-257.

Walker, C., Emmens, A., & Simpson, H. (2012). Integrating the recovery approach into everyday clinical practice. *Mental Health Practice, 15*(6), 19-22.

Walker, G., & Bryant, W. (2013). Peer support in adult mental health services: A metasynthesis of qualitative findings. *Psychiatric Rehabilitation Journal, 36*(1), 28-34.

Walker, M., Toneatto, T., Potenza, M. N., Petry, N., Ladouceur, R., Hodgins, D. C., . . . Blaszczynski, A. (2006). A framework for reporting outcomes in problem gambling treatment research: The Banff, Alberta Consensus. *Addiction, 101*(4), 504-511.

Walker, R. (2014). Introduction to National Standards for the Mental Health Workforce. In P. Dudgeon, H. Milroy, & R. Walker (eds.), *Working Together: Aboriginal and Torres Strait Islander Mental Health and Wellbeing Principles and Practice* (pp. 181-194). Barton: Commonwealth of Australia.

Walker, R., & Mason, W. (2015). *Climate Change Adaptation for Health and Social Services.* CSIRO Publishing.

Wallace, G., Bird, V., Leamy, M., Bacon, F., Le Boutillier, C., Janosik, M., . . . Slade, M. (2016). Service user experiences of REFOCUS: A process evaluation of a pro-recovery complex intervention. *Social Psychiatry and Psychiatric Epidemiology, 51*(9), 1275-1284.

Waller, G., Cordery, H., Corstorphine, E., Hinrichsen, H., Lawson, R., Mountford, V., & Russell, K. (2007). *Cognitive Behavioral Therapy for Eating Disorders: A Comprehensive Treatment Guide.* Cambridge University Press.

Wallerstein, N., & Duran. (2003). The conceptual, historical and practice roots of community based participatory research and related participatory traditions. In M. Minkler & N. Wallerstein (eds.), *Community Based Participatory Research for Health* (pp. 512). Jossey-Bass.

Walter, T., Stevens, P., Verhoeven, A., & Boxall, A.-m. (2014). *Impacts of Climate Change on Public Health in Australia: Recommendations for New Policies and Practices for Adaptation Within the Public Health Sector.* Retrieved from https://ahha.asn.au/system/files/docs/publications/deeble_issues_brief_no_7_walter_t_et_al_impacts_of_climate_change_on_public_health.pdf.

Walterfang, M., Siu, R., & Velakoulis, D. (2006). The NUCOG: Validity and reliability of a brief cognitive screening tool in neuropsychiatric patients. *Australian and New Zealand Journal of Psychiatry, 40*(11-12), 995-1002.

Waluk, O. R., Youssef, G. J., & Dowling, N. A. (2016). The relationship between problem gambling and attention deficit hyperactivity disorder. *Journal of Gambling Studies, 32*(2), 591-604.

Wampold, B. E. (2001). *The Great Psychotherapy Debate: Models, Methods, and Findings* (2nd ed.).Taylor & Francis.

Wampold, B. E., Minami, T., Baskin, T. W., & Tierney, S. C. (2002). A meta-(re)analysis of the effects of cognitive therapy versus 'other therapies' for depression. *J Affect Disord, 68*(2-3), 159-165.

Wampold, B. E., Mondin, G. W., Moody, M., Stich, F., Benson, K., & Ahn, H. N. (1997). A meta-analysis of outcome studies comparing bona fide psychotherapies: Empirically, 'all must have prizes'. *Psychological Bulletin, 122*(3), 203-215.

Wand, T. (2012). Investigating the evidence for the effectiveness of risk assessment in mental health care. *Issues in Mental Health Nursing, 33*(1), 2-7.

Wand, T. (2015). Recovery is about a focus on resilience and wellness, not a fixation with risk and illness. *Australian & New Zealand Journal of Psychiatry, 49*(12), 1083-1084.

Wand, T., Amp, Apos, Abrew, N., Acret, L., & White, K. (2016). Evaluating a new model of nurse-led emergency department mental health care in Australia: Perspectives of key informants. *International Emergency Nursing, 24*(1), 16-21.

Wang, C.E.,, Chan, C., Sai-Yin, H., Wong, P., & Ho, R. (2014). Prevalence and Correlates of Video and Internet Gaming Addiction among Hong Kong Adolescents: A Pilot Study. *The Scientific World Journal*, article ID 874648.

Wang, J., & Du, W. (2019). Factors associated with high psychological distress in primary carers of people with disability. *Australian Journal of General Practice, 48*(4), 234.

Wang, Q., Ren, H., Long, J., Liu, Y., & Liu, T. (2019). Research progress and debates on gaming disorder. *General Psychiatry, 32*(3).

Ware, J. E. J., Kosinski, M., & Keller, S. D. (1996). A 12-item short form health survey: Construction of scales and preliminary tests of reliability and validity. *Medical Care, 34*, pp. 220-233.

Wareham, J. D., & Potenza, M. N. (2010). Pathological gambling and substance use disorders. *American Journal of Drug and Alcohol Abuse, 36*(5), 242-247.

Warren, S. L., Huston, L., Egeland, B., & Sroufe, L. A. (1997). Child and adolescent anxiety disorders and early attachment. *Journal of the American Academy of Child & Adolescent Psychiatry, 36*(5), 637-644.

Warshaw, C. (2007). Domestic violence, trauma & mental health—framing the issues. The need for cross-sector collaboration. Conference paper presented at 'Towards better practice: Enhancing collaboration between mental health services & women's domestic violence services', Sydney.

Waters, F. (2016). *Good Practice Guidelines for Engaging with Families and Carers in Adult Mental Health Services Government of Western Australia Department of Health.* Retrieved from www.chiefpsychiatrist.wa.gov.au/wp-content/uploads/2017/04/Good-Practice-Guidelines-for-engaging-with-families-and-carers-May-2016.pdf.

Waters, K. A., Suresh, S., & Nixon, G. M. (2013). Sleep disorders in children. *Medical Journal of Australia, 199*(8), S31-S35.

Watson, J., Fossey, E., & Harvey, C. (2019). A home but how to connect with others? A qualitative meta-synthesis of experiences of people with mental illness living in supported housing. *Health & Social Care in the Community, 27*(3), 546-564.

Watson, M., Haviland, J. S., Greer, S., Davidson, J., & Bliss, J. M. (1999). Influence of psychological response on survival in breast cancer: A population-based cohort study. *Lancet, 354*(9187), 1331-1336.

Watt, T. T. (2017). Paradigm shifts don't come easy: Confrontations between the trauma perspective and the DSM in mental health treatment for abused and neglected children. *Journal of Child & Adolescent Trauma, 10*(4), 395-403.

Way, K., Kannis-Dymand, L., Lastella, M., & Lovell, G. P. (2018). Mental health practitioners' reported barriers to prescription of exercise for mental health consumers. *Mental Health and Physical Activity, 14*, 52-60.

WayAhead. (2016). *Mental Health Association NSW.* Retrieved from https://wayahead.org.au/about.

Weathers, F. W., Blake, D.D., Schnurr, P.P., Kaloupek, D.G., Marx, B.P., & Keane, T.M. (2013). *The Life Events Checklist for DSM-5 (LEC-5)*. Retrieved from www.ptsd.va.gov.

Weathers, F. W., Blake, D. D., Schnurr, P. P., Kaloupek, D. G., Marx, B. P., & Keane, T. M. (2013). *The Clinician-Administered PTSD Scale for DSM-5 (CAPS-5)*. Retrieved from www.ptsd.va.gov asp.

Weathers, F. W., Litz, B. T., Keane, T. M., Palmieri, P. A., Marx, B. P., & Schnurr, P. P. (2013). *PTSD Checklist for DSM-5 (PCL-5)*. Retrieved from www.ptsd.va.gov.

Webber, M., McCree, C., & Angeli, P. (2013). Inter-agency joint protocols for safeguarding children in social care and adult mental-health agencies: A cross-sectional survey of practitioner experiences. *Child & Family Social Work*, 18(2), 149–158.

Webster-Stratton, C., Jamila Reid, M., & Stoolmiller, M. (2008). Preventing conduct problems and improving school readiness: Evaluation of the Incredible Years Teacher and Child Training Programs in high-risk schools. *J Child Psychol Psychiatry, 49*(5), 471–488.

Wechsler, D. (1997). *Weschsler Adult Intelligence Scale-III*. San Antonio: The Psychological Corporation .

Wechsler, D. (2008). *Wechsler Adult Intelligence Scale—Fourth Edition*. Retrieved from www.pearsonclinical.com.au/products/view/19.

Weersing, V. R., Gonzalez, A., Campo, J. V., & Lucas, A. N. (2008). Brief behavioral therapy for pediatric anxiety and depression: Piloting an integrated treatment approach. *Cognitive and Behavioral Practice, 15*(2), 126–139.

Weinberg, I., Ronningstam, E., Goldblatt, M. J., Schechter, M., & Maltsberger, J. T. (2011). Common factors in empirically supported treatments of borderline personality disorder. *Current Psychiatry Reports, 13*(1), 60–68.

Weise, M. (2016). Medical ethics made easy. *Professional Case Management, 21*(2), 88–94.

Weissbecker, I. (2011). *Climate Change and Human Well-Being: Global Challenges and Opportunities*. New York: Springer.

Welford, M. (2016). *Compassion Focused Therapy for Dummies*. United Kingdom: John Wiley & Sons.

Weller, P. (2013). *New law and Ethics in Mental Health Advance Directives: The Convention on the Rights of Persons with Disabilities and the Right to Choose*. East Sussex: Routledge.

Wells, A. (2005). The metacognitive model of GAD: Assessment of meta-worry and relationship with DSM-IV generalized anxiety disorder. *Cognitive Therapy and Research, 29*, 107–121.

Wells, A. (2013). *Cognitive Therapy of Anxiety Disorders: A Practice Manual and Conceptual Guide*. John Wiley & Sons.

Wells, J. E., Oakley Browne, M. A., Scott, K. M., McGee, M. A., Baxter, J., & Kokaua, J. (2006). Te Rau Hinengaro: The New Zealand Mental Health Survey: Overview of methods and findings. *Australian and New Zealand Journal of Psychiatry, 40*(10), 835–844.

Wells, J. E., Oakley Browne, M. A., Scott, K. M., McGee, M. A., Baxter, J., Kokaua, J., & New Zealand Mental Health Survey Research Team. (2006). Prevalence, interference with life and severity of 12-month DSM-IV disorders in Te Rau Hinengaro: The New Zealand Mental Health Survey. *Australian and New Zealand Journal of Psychiatry, 40*(10), 845–854.

wellways. (2020). *Peer Education*. Retrieved from www.wellways.org/understanding-mental-health/peer-education.

Wen X 1997. The definition and prevalence of intellectual disability in Australia. AIHW Catalogue no. DIS 2. Canberra: AIHW. Retrieved from www.aihw.gov.au.

Wenger, E. (2000). Communities of practice and social learning systems. *Organization, 7*(2), 225–246.

Wenzel, A., Brown, G. K., & Beck, A. T. (2009). *Cognitive Therapy for Suicidal Patients: Scientific and Clinical Applications*. American Psychological Association.

Wessely, S., Rose, S., & Bisson, J. (2000). Brief psychological interventions ('debriefing') for trauma-related symptoms and the prevention of post traumatic stress disorder. *Cochrane Database of Systematic Reviews* , CD000560.

West, W. (2000). *Psychotherapy and Spirituality: Crossing the Line Between Therapy and Religion*. London: Sage.

Westen, D., & Shedler, J. (2000). A prototype matching approach to diagnosing personality disorders: Toward DSM-V. *Journal of Personality Disorders, 14*(2), 109–126.

Western Australian Association for Mental Health. (2014). *Peer Work Strategic Framework for the Mental Health and Alcohol and Other Drug Sectors in WA*. Retrieved from https://waamh.org.au/assets/documents/projects/peer-work-strategic-framework-report-final-october-2014.pdf.

Western Australian Government. (2018). *Delivering Community Services in Partnership Policy: A Policy to Achieve Better Outcomes for Western Australians through the Procurement of Community Services*. Retrieved from www.wa.gov.au/government/publications.

Western, D. (2018). Women and domestic and family violence. In M. Petrakis (ed.), *Social Work Practice in Health: An Introduction to Contexts, Theories and Skills*. Allen & Unwin.

Western Mass Recovery Learning Community (WMRLC). (2013). Are we 'anti'? *Recovery Learning Community*. Retrieved from www.westernmassrlc.org/rlc-articles/213-are-we-anti.

Western Mass Recovery Learning Community (WMRLC). (2019). Healing and recovery through peer support. *Recovery Learning Community*. Retrieved from www.westernmassrlc.org.

Western Mass Recovery Learning Community (WMRLC). (2019). *Western Massachusetts Recovery Learning Community (WMRLC)*. Retrieved from www.westernmassrlc.org.

Westra, H. A., Stewart, S. H., & Conrad, B. E. (2002). Naturalistic manner of benzodiazepine use and cognitive behavioral therapy outcome in panic disorder with agoraphobia. *Journal of Anxiety Disorders, 16*(3), 233–246.

Wheeler, A. J., Roennfeldt, H., Slattery, M., Krinks, R., & Stewart, V. (2018). Codesigned recommendations for increasing engagement in structured physical activity for people with serious mental health problems in Australia. *Health & Social Care in the Community, 26*(6), 860–870.

Whelan, R., Watts, R., Orr, C. A., Althoff, R. R., Artiges, E., Banaschewski, T., . . . Carvalho, F. M. (2014). Neuropsychosocial profiles of current and future adolescent alcohol misusers. *Nature, 512*(7513), 185–189.

White, M. (1987). Family therapy and schizophrenia: Addressing the 'in-the-corner lifestyle'. *Dulwich Centre Newsletter* (Spring), 14-21.

Whiteford, H. A., & Buckingham, W. J. (2005). Ten years of mental health service reform in Australia: Are we getting it right? *Medical Journal of Australia, 182*(8), 396–400.

Whiteford, H. A., Buckingham, W. J., Harris, M. G., Burgess, P. M., Pirkis, J. E., Barendregt, J. J., & Hall, W. D. (2014). Estimating treatment rates for mental disorders in Australia. *Australian Health Review, 38*(1), 80–85.

Whittington, C. (2003). Collaboration and partnership in context. In J. Weinstein, C. Whittington, & T. Leiba (eds.), *Collaboration in Social Work Practice*. USA: Jessica Kingsley Publishers.

Whittle, S., Yücel, M., Lorenzetti, V., Byrne, M. L., Simmons, J. G., Wood, S. J., . . . Allen, N. B. (2012). Pituitary volume mediates the relationship between pubertal timing and depressive symptoms during adolescence. *Psychoneuroendocrinology, 37*(7), 881-891.

WHO. (2020). *Supported Decision Making*. Retrieved from www.who.int/mental_health/policy/quality_rights/en.

WHO Regional Office for Europe. (2018). *Mental Health Promotion and Mental Health Care in Refugees and Migrants*. Retrieved from: https://www.euro.who.int/_ pdf.

Wickrama, K. A., Conger, R. D., Lorenz, F. O., & Jung, T. (2008). Family antecedents and consequences of trajectories of depressive symptoms from adolescence to young adulthood: A life course investigation. *J Health Soc Behav, 49*(4), 468-483.

Widiger, T. A., & Trull, T. J. (1992). Personality and psychopathology: An application of the Five-Factor Model. *Journal of Personality, 60*(2), 363-393.

Wikipedia. (2019). *Pre- and Post-Test Probability*. Retrieved from https://en.wikipedia.org/wiki/Pre-_and_post-test_probability.

Wilcock, A. A. (2001). *Occupation for Health: A Journey From Self Health to Prescription*. London: British College of Occupational Therapists.

Wilhelm, S., Phillips, K. A., & Steketee, G. (2012). *Cognitive-Behavioral Therapy for Body Dysmorphic Disorder: A Treatment Manual*. Guilford Publications.

Wilkes, E., Gray, D., Casey, W., Stearne, A., & Dadd, L. (2014). Harmful substance use and mental health. In P. Dudgeon, H. Milroy, & R. Walker (eds.), *Working Together: Aboriginal and Torres Strait Islander Mental Health and Wellbeing Principles and Practice* (pp. 125-146). Barton: Commonwealth of Australia.

Wilkinson, C., & McAndrew, S. (2008). 'I'm not an outsider, I'm his mother!' A phenomenological enquiry into carer experiences of exclusion from acute psychiatric settings. *International Journal of Mental Health Nursing, 17*(6), 392-401.

Wilkinson, R., & Pickett, K. (2011). *The Spirit Level: Why Greater Equality Makes Societies Stronger*. USA: Bloomsbury.

Wilkinson, R., & Pickett, K. (2018). *The Inner Level: How More Equal Societies Reduce Stress, Restore Sanity and Improve Everyone's Well-being*. UK: Penguin Books.

Wilkinson, R. G., & Marmot, M. (2003). *Social Determinants of Health: The Solid Facts*: World Health Organization.

Williams, A., Fossey, E., Farhall, J., Foley, F., & Thomas, N. (2018). Recovery after psychosis: Qualitative study of service user experiences of lived experience videos on a recovery-oriented website. *Journal of Medical Internet Research Mental Health, 5*(2), e:37.

Williams, A., Fossey, E., & Harvey, C. (2010). Sustaining employment in a social firm: Use of the Work Environment Impact Scale v2.0 to explore views of employees with psychiatric disabilities. *The British Journal of Occupational Therapy, 73*(11), 531-539.

Williams, A. E., Fossey, E., Corbiere, M., Paluch, T., & Harvey, C. (2016). Work participation for people with severe mental illnesses: An integrative review of factors impacting job tenure. *Australian Occupational Therapy Journal, 63*(2), 65-85.

Williams, J., Leamy, M., Bird, V., Le Boutillier, C., Norton, S., Pesola, F., & Slade, M. (2015). Development and evaluation of the INSPIRE measure of staff support for personal recovery. *Soc Psychiatry Psychiatr Epidemiol, 50*(5), 777-786.

Williams, J. R. (2009). *World Medical Association Medical Ethics Manual* (2nd ed.). Geneva: World Medical Association.

Williams, L., Jacka, F., Pasco, J., Henry, M., Dodd, S., Nicholson, G., . . . Berk, M. (2010). The prevalence of mood and anxiety disorders in Australian women. *Australasian Psychiatry, 18*(3), 250-255.

Williams, R. J., Volberg, R. A., & Stevens, R. M. G. (2012). *The Population Prevalence of Problem Gambling: Methodological Influences, Standardized Rates, Jurisdictional Differences, and Worldwide Trends*. Retrieved from https://opus.uleth.ca/handle/10133/3068.

Williams, S., & Dale, J. (2006). The effectiveness of treatment for depression/depressive symptoms in adults with cancer: A systematic review. *British Journal of Cancer, 94*(3), 372-390.

Lester, D. (2002). *Crisis Intervention and Counseling By Telephone*. (2nd ed.). Springfield: Charles C Thomas Publisher.

Williams, T. M., & Smith, G. P. (2014). Can the National Disability Insurance Scheme work for mental health? *Australian & New Zealand Journal of Psychiatry, 48*(5), 391-394.

Williamson, A. B., Raphael, B., Redman, S., Daniels, J., Eades, S. J., & Mayers, N. (2010). Emerging themes in Aboriginal child and adolescent mental health: Findings from a qualitative study in Sydney, New South Wales. *Med J Aust, 192*(10), 603-605.

Willie, C. V. (1995). *Mental Health, Racism and Sexism*. Pittsburgh: University of Pittsburgh Press.

Wilson, A., & Childs, S. (2002). The relationship between consultation length, process and outcomes in general practice: A systematic review. *The British Journal of General Practice: Journal of the Royal College of General Practitioners, 52*(485), 1012-1020.

Wing, J. K., Babor, T., Brugha, T., & Burke, J. (1990). SCAN: Schedules for Clinical Assessment in Neuropsychiatry. *Archives of General Psychiatry, 47*, 589-593.

Wing, J. K., Beevor, A. S., Curtis, R. H., Park, S. B. G., Hadden, S., & Burns, A. (1998). Health of the Nation Outcome Scales (HoNOS): Research and development. *British Journal of Psychiatry, 172*, 11-18.

Wing, L. (1997). The autistic spectrum. *The Lancet, 350*(9093), 1761-1766.

Wirtz, P. H., & von Kanel, R. (2017). Psychological stress, inflammation, and coronary heart disease. *Current Cardiology Reports, 19*(11).

Wittchen, H.-U. (1994). Reliability and validity studies of the WHO Composite International Diagnosis Interview (CIDI): A critical review. *Journal of Psychiatric Research, vol. 28*, pp. 57-84.

Wittchen, H.-U., & Jacobi, F. (2005). Size and burden of mental disorders in Europe: A critical review and appraisal of 27 studies. *Eur Neuropsychopharmacol, 15*(4), 357-376.

Wittchen, H.-U., Kessler, R. C., Beesdo, K., Krause, P., Höfler, M., & Hoyer, J. (2002). Generalized anxiety and depression in primary care: Prevalence, recognition, and management. *J Clin Psychiatry, 63*(Suppl 8), 24-34.

Woicik, P. A., Stewart, S. H., Pihl, R. O., & Conrod, P. J. (2009). The substance use risk profile scale: A scale measuring traits linked to reinforcement-specific substance use profiles. *Addictive behaviors, 34*(12), 1042-1055.

Wolfensberger, W. (1972). *Principle of Normalization in Human Services*. Canadian Assoc for the Mentally Retarded.

Wolfling, K., Beutel, M. E., & Muller, K. W. (2012). Construction of a standardized clinical interview to assess internet addiction: First findings regarding the usefulness of AICA-C. *Addiction Research & Therapy, S6*.

Wolfling, K., Muller, K. W., Dreier, M., Ruckes, C., Deuster, O., Batra, A., . . . Beutel, M. E. (2019). Efficacy of short-term treatment of internet and computer game addiction: A randomized clinical trial. *JAMA Psychiatry, 76*(10), 1018-1025.

Wolstencroft, K. E., Deane, F. P., Jones, C. L., Zimmermann, A., & Cox, M. (2018). Consumer and staff perspectives of the implementation frequency and value of recovery and wellbeing oriented practices. *International Journal of Mental Health Systems, 12.*

Women's Health Victoria. (2019). *The Social and Economic Benefits of Improving Mental Health: Submission to the Productivity Commission Inquiry April 2019.* Retrieved from https://whv.org.au/resources/whv-publications/submission-inquiry-social-and-economic-benefits-improving-mental-health.

Women's Mental Health Network Victoria. (2020). *Victorian Women and Mental Health Network.* Retrieved from https://wmhnv.org.au.

Woodhouse, D., & Pengelly, P. (1991). *Anxiety and the Dynamics of Collaboration.* Aberdeen: Aberdeen University Press.

Woody, C. A., Baxter, A. J., Harris, M. G., Siskind, D. J., & Whiteford, H. A. (2018). Identifying characteristics and practices of multidisciplinary team reviews for patients with severe mental illness: A systematic review. *Australasian Psychiatry, 26*(3), 267–275.

Woody, S. R., Kellman-McFarlane, K., & Welsted, A. (2014). Review of cognitive performance in hoarding disorder. *Clin Psychol Rev, 34*(4), 324–336.

Wooff, D., Schneider, J., Carpenter, J., & Brandon, T. (2003). Correlates of stress in carers. *Journal of Mental Health, 12*(1), 29–40.

Woo-Ming, A. M., & Siever, L. J. (1998). Psychopharmacological treatment of personality disorders. In P. E. Nathan & J. M. Gorman (Eds.), A Guide To Treatments That Work (4th ed., pp. 554–567). New York, NY: Oxford University Press.Workplace Prevention of Mental Health Problems. (2020). *Prevention Guidelines.* Retrieved from www.prevention.workplace-mentalhealth.net.au.

World Health Organization (WHO). (1978). *International Classification of Diseases: Ninth Revision, Basic Tabulation List with Alphabetic Index.* Geneva: World Health Organization.

World Health Organization (WHO). (1992). *The ICD-10 Classification of Mental and Behavioural Disorders: Clinical Descriptions and Diagnostic Guidelines, 10th Edn.* Geneva: World Health Organization.

World Health Organization (WHO). (1993). *International Classification of Diseases (ICD-10)* (10th ed.). Geneva: World Health Organization.

World Health Organization (WHO). (1994). *The Composite International Diagnostic Interview (CIDI)*. Geneva, World Health Organization.

World Health Organization (WHO). (1996). *Diagnostic and Management Guidelines for Mental Disorders in Primary Care: ICD-lO Chapter V Primary Care Version.* Gottingen, Germany: WHO/Hogrefe & Huber.

World Health Organization (WHO). (2007). Monitoring and evaluation of mental health policies and plans. Retrieved from www.who.int.

World Health Organization (WHO). (2009). *Pharmacological Treatment of Mental Disorders in Primary Health Care.* Geneva: World Health Organization.

World Health Organization (WHO). (2010). *Framework for Action on Interprofessional Education and Collaborative Practice.* Retrieved from www.who.int/hrh/resources/framework_action/en.

World Health Organization (WHO). (2013a). *Family as Centre of Health Development.* Retrieved from http://apps.searo.who.int/PDS_DOCS/B4972.pdf.

World Health Organization (WHO). (2013c). *Mental Health Action Plan 2013–2020.* Retrieved from www.who.int/mental_health/action_plan_2013/en.

World Health Organization (WHO). (2014). *Review of Social Determinants and the Health Divide in the WHO European Region: Final Report.* Geneva, WHO.

World Health Organization (WHO). (2013d). *WHO Evaluation Practice Handbook.* Retrieved from https://apps.who.int.

World Health Organization (WHO). (2016). *Life Expectancy Increased by 5 Years Since 2000, but Health Inequalities Persist.* Retrieved from www.who.int/en/news-room/detail/19-05-2016-life-expectancy-increased-by-5-years-since-2000-but-health-inequalities-persist.

World Health Organization (WHO). (2017a). *Mental Health ATLAS 2017.* Retrieved from www.who.int/mental_health/evidence/atlas/mental_health_atlas_2017/en.

World Health Organization (WHO). (2017b). *The World Health Organization World Mental Health Composite International Diagnostic Interview (WHO WMH-CIDI)*. Retrieved from www.hcp.med.harvard.edu/wmhcidi.

World Health Organization (WHO). (2018a). *International Classification of Diseases: 11th Revision (ICD-11)*. Geneva: World Health Organization. Retrieved from https://icd.who.int/en.

World Health Organization (WHO). (2018b). *Mental Health ATLAS 2017.* Retrieved from www.who.int/mental_health/evidence/atlas/mental_health_atlas_2017/en.

World Health Organization (WHO). (2018c). *Mental Health in Primary Care: Illusion or Inclusion? Technical Series on Primary Health Care.* Geneva: World Health Organization.

World Health Organization (WHO). (2019a). *Suicide Data.* Retrieved from www.who.int/mental_health/prevention/suicide/suicideprevent/en.

World Health Organization (WHO). (2019b). *WHO Strategic Meeting on Social Determinants of Health.* Retrieved from www.who.int/social_determinants/strategic-meeting/en.

World Health Organization (WHO). (2019c). *ICD-11 Implementation or Transition Guide.* Retrieved from https://icd.who.int/en.

World Health Organization and Calouste Gulbenkian Foundation. (2014). *Social Determinants of Mental Health.* Retrieved from www.who.int/mental_health/publications/gulbenkian_paper_social_determinants_of_mental_health/en.

World Medical Association. (2006). *WMA International Code of Ethics.* Geneva.

World Professional Association for Transgender Health (WPATH). (2012). *Standards of Care for the Health of Transsexual, Transgender, and Gender-Nonconforming People.* Retrieved from www.wpath.org/media/cms/Documents/SOC%20v7/Standards%20of%20Care_V7%20Full%20Book_English.pdf.

World Psychiatric Association (WPA). (2011). *Madrid Declaration on Ethical Standards for Psychiatric Practice.* Retrieved from www.wpanet.org/current-madrid-declaration.

Worthington, A., & Rooney, P. (2010). *The Triangle of Care, Carers Included: A Guide to Best Practice in Acute Mental Health Care* (2nd ed.). London: Carers Trust. Retrieved from https://professionals.carers.org/sites/default/files/thetriangleofcare_guidetobestpracticeinmentalhealthcare_england.pdf.

Wray, N. R., Ripke, S., Mattheisen, M., Trzaskowski, M., Byrne, E. M., Abdellaoui, A., . . . Working, M. D. D. (2018). Genome-wide association analyses identify 44 risk variants and refine the genetic architecture of major depression. *Nature Genetics, 50*(5), 668–+.

Wulfert, E., Hartley, J., Lee, M., Wang, N., Franco, C., & Sodano, R. (2005). Gambling screens: Does shortening the time frame affect their psychometric properties? *Journal of Gambling Studies, 21*(4), 521–536.

Wulsin, L. R. (2004). Is depression a major risk factor for coronary disease? A systematic review of the epidemiologic evidence. *Harvard Review of Psychiatry, 12*(2), 79–93.

Wyatt, C., Harper, B., & Weatherhead, S. (2014). The experience of group mindfulness-based interventions for individuals with mental health difficulties: A meta-synthesis. *Psychotherapy Research, 24*(2), 214–228.

Wyatt, K. (2019). *National Press Club Address—'Walking in Partnership to Effect Change'*. Retrieved from https://ministers.pmc.gov.au/wyatt/2019/national-press-club-address-walking-partnership-effect-change.

Wyder, M., & Bland, R. (2014). The recovery framework as a way of understanding families' responses to mental illness: Balancing different needs and recovery journeys. *Australian Social Work, 67*(2), 179–196.

Wynaden, D., & Orb, A. (2005). Impact of patient confidentiality on carers of people who have a mental disorder. *International Journal of Mental Health Nursing, 14*(3), 166–171.

Wynne, L. C. (1994). The rationale for consultation with the families of schizophrenic patients. *Acta Psychiatr Scand, 90*, 125–132.

Xia J, Merinder LB, Belgamwar MR .(2011) Psychoeducation for schizophrenia. *Cochrane Database of Systematic Reviews*, issue 6. art. no.: CD002831.

Xie, H. (2013). Strengths-based approach for mental health recovery. *Iranian Journal of Psychiatry and Behavioral Sciences, 7*(2), 5.

Xie, H., Yuan, P., Cui, S. S., & Yen, M. S. S. (2015). A study to examine the uses of personal strength in relation to mental health recovery in adults with serious mental illnesses: A research protocol. *Health Psychology Research, 3*(2), 2209.

Xin, M., Xing, J., Pengfei, W., Houru, L., Mengcheng, W., & Hong, Z. (2018). Online activities, prevalence of internet addiction and risk factors related to family and school among adolescents in China. (Report) (Author abstract). *Addictive Behaviors Reports, 7*, 14.

Xuan, Y.-H., Li, S., Tao, R., Chen, J., Rao, L.-L., Wang, X. T., & Zheng, R. (2017). Genetic and environmental influences on gambling: A meta-analysis of twin studies. *Frontiers in Psychology*, 8, 2121.

Y Foundation. (2017). *A Home of Your Own: Housing First and Ending Homelessness in Finland*. Keuruu: Otava Book Printing.

Yakeley, J. (2018). Current understanding of narcissism and narcissistic personality disorder. *BJPsych Advances, 24*(5), 305–315.

Yakovenko, I., Quigley, L., Hemmelgarn, B. R., Hodgins, D. C., & Ronksley, P. (2015). The efficacy of motivational interviewing for disordered gambling: Systematic review and meta-analysis. *Addictive behaviors, 43*, 72–82.

Yale Program on Climate Change Communication. (2020). *Climate Change*. Retrieved from https://climatecommunication.yale.edu.

Yao, Y. W., Liu, L., Ma, S. S., Shi, X. H., Zhou, N., Zhang, J. T., & Potenza, M. N. (2017). Functional and structural neural alterations in internet gaming disorder: A systematic review and meta-analysis. *Neuroscience and Biobehavioral Reviews, 83*, 313–324.

Yates, G. P., & Feldman, M. D. (2016). Factitious disorder: A systematic review of 455 cases in the professional literature. *General Hospital Psychiatry, 41*, 20–28.

Yates, S., & Gatsou, L. (2017). Enhancing family communication in families where a parent has a mental illness. *Journal of Parent and Family Mental Health, 2*(3), 1.

Yatham, L. N., Kennedy, S. H., Parikh, S. V., Schaffer, A., Bond, D. J., Frey, B. N., . . . Berk, M. (2018). Canadian Network for Mood and Anxiety Treatments (CANMAT) and International Society for Bipolar Disorders (ISBD) 2018 guidelines for the management of patients with bipolar disorder. *Bipolar Disorders, 20*(2), 97–170.

Yee, N. Y., Large, M. M., Kemp, R. I., & Nielssen, O. B. (2011). Severe non-lethal violence during psychotic illness. *Australian and New Zealand Journal of Psychiatry, 45*(6), 466–472.

Yellowlees, M. H. P. (1997). An evaluation study of clinical case management using clinical case management standards. *Journal of Mental Health, 6*(6), 589–598.

Yerkes, R., & Dodson, J. (1908). The relation of strength of stimulus to rapidity of habit formation. *Journal of Comparative Neurological Psychology, 18*(3), 459–482.

Young, J. E., Klosko, J. S., & Weishaar, M. E. (2003). *Schema Therapy: A Practitioner's Guide*. New York: Guilford Press.

Ypinazar, V. A., Margolis, S. A., Haswell-Elkins, M., & Tsey, K. (2007). Indigenous Australians' understandings regarding mental health and disorders. *Australian and New Zealand Journal of Psychiatry, 41*(6), 467–478.

Yücel, M., Harrison, B. J., Wood, S. J., Fornito, A., Wellard, R. M., Pujol, J., . . . Pantelis, C. (2007). Functional and biochemical alterations of the medial frontal cortex in obsessive-compulsive disorder. *Arch Gen Psychiatry, 64*(8), 946–955.

Yull, D. G., & Wilson, M. A. F. (2018). Allies, accomplices, or troublemakers: Black families and scholar activists working for social justice in a race-conscious parent engagement program. *Critical Education, 9*(8), 1–18.

Yung, A. R., Cotter, J., Wood, S. J., McGorry, P., Thompson, A. D., Nelson, B., & Lin, A. (2015). Childhood maltreatment and transition to psychotic disorder independently predict long-term functioning in young people at ultra-high risk for psychosis. *Psychol Med, 45*(16), 3453–3465.

Zajac, K., Ginley, M. K., Chang, R., & Petry, N. M. (2017). Treatments for internet gaming disorder and internet addiction: A systematic review. *Psychology of Addictive Behaviors, 31*(8), 979–994.

Zanarini, M. C., & Frankenburg, F. R. (1997). Pathways to the development of borderline personality disorder. *Journal of Personality Disorders, 11*(1), 93–104.

Zanarini, M. C., Frankenburg, F. R., DeLuca, C. J., Hennen, J., Khera, G. S., & Gunderson, J. G. (1998). The pain of being borderline: Dysphoric states specific to borderline personality disorder. *Harvard Review of Psychiatry, 6*(4), 201–207.

Zanarini, M. C., Frankenburg, F. R., Reich, D. B., Fitzmaurice, G., Weinberg, I., & Gunderson, J. G. (2008). The 10-year course of physically self-destructive acts reported by borderline patients and axis II comparison subjects. *Acta Psychiatr Scand, 117*(3), 177–184.

Zanarini, M. C., Frankenburg, F. R., Reich, D. B., Wedig, M. M., Conkey, L. C., & Fitzmaurice, G. M. (2014). Prediction of time-to-attainment of recovery for borderline patients followed prospectively for 16 years. *Acta Psychiatr Scand, 130*(3), 205–213.

Zanarini, M. C., Gunderson, J. G., & Frankenburg, F. R. (1990). Cognitive features of borderline personality disorder. *American Journal of Psychiatry, 147*(1), 57–63.

Zanarini, M.C., Frankenburg, F.R., Reich, D.B., Fitzmaurice, G. et al. (2012). Attainment and stability of sustained symptomatic remission and recovery among patients with borderline personality disorder and axis ii comparison subjects: A 16-year prospective follow-up study. *American Journal of Psychiatry,* 69, 476–483.

Zarkowska, E., & Clements, C. (1994). *Problem Behaviour and People with Severe Learning Disabilities: The STAR Approach* (2nd ed.). London: Chapman & Hall.

Zeanah, C. H., Berlin, L. J., & Boris, N. W. (2011). Practitioner review: Clinical applications of attachment theory and research for infants and young children. *Journal of Child Psychology and Psychiatry, 52*(8), 819–833.

Zimmerman, M., Chelminski, I., & Young, D. (2008). The frequency of personality disorders in psychiatric patients. *Psychiatric Clinics of North America, 31*(3), 405–420.

Zimmerman, M., Pfohl, B., Coryell, W. H., Corenthal, C., & Stangl, D. (1991). Major depression and personality disorder. *J Affect Disord, 22*(4), 199–210.

Zisman-Ilani, Y., Shern, D., Deegan, P., Kreyenbuhl, J., Dixon, L., Drake, R., . . . Elwyn, G. (2018). Continue, adjust, or stop antipsychotic medication: Developing and user testing an encounter decision aid for people with first-episode and long-term psychosis. *BMC Psychiatry*, 18(1), 142.

Zink, M., Englisch, S., & Meyer-Lindenberg, A. (2010). Polypharmacy in schizophrenia. *Curr Opin Psychiatry, 23*(2), 103–111.

Zisook, S., Lesser, I., Stewart, J. W., Wisniewski, S. R., Balasubramani, G. K., Fava, M., . . . Rush, A. J. (2007). Effect of age at onset on the course of major depressive disorder. *American Journal of Psychiatry, 164*(10), 1539–1546.

Zittel Conklin, C., & Westen, D. (2005). Borderline personality disorder in clinical practice. *American Journal of Psychiatry, 162*(5), 867–875.

Zubenko, G. S., George, A. W., Soloff, P. H., & Schulz, P. (1987). Sexual practices among patients with borderline personality disorder. *American Journal of Psychiatry, 144*(6), 748–752.

Zubin, J., & Spring, B. (1977). Vulnerability: A new view of schizophrenia. *Journal of Abnormal Psychology, 86*(2), 103–126.

Zubrick, S., Shepherd, C. C., Dudgeon, P., Gee, G., Paradies, Y., Scrine, C., & Walker, R. (2014). Social determinants of social and emotional wellbeing. In P. Dudgeon, H. Milroy, & R. Walker (eds.), *Working Together: Aboriginal and Torres Strait Islander Mental Health and Wellbeing Principles and Practice* (pp. 93–112). Barton: Commonwealth of Australia.

INDEX